SHOULDER RECONSTRUCTION

SHOULDER RECONSTRUCTION

CHARLES S. NEER, II, M.D.

Professor Emeritus of Clinical Orthopaedic Surgery,
Columbia University; Chief of Shoulder Service,
Columbia-Presbyterian Medical Center, New York, NY;
Inaugural President, American Shoulder and Elbow Surgeons

Illustrated by
Robert J. Demarest

1990
W.B. SAUNDERS COMPANY
Harcourt Brace Jovanovich, Inc.
Philadelphia ▪ London ▪ Toronto ▪ Montreal ▪ Sydney ▪ Tokyo

W. B. SAUNDERS COMPANY
Harcourt Brace Jovanovich, Inc.

The Curtis Center
Independence Square West
Philadelphia, PA 19106

Library of Congress Cataloging-in-Publication Data

Neer, Charles S., 1917–

Shoulder reconstruction / Charles S. Neer II : illustrated by Robert J. Demarest.

p. cm.

Includes bibliographical references.

1. Shoulder—Surgery. 2. Shoulder—Surgery—Patients—Rehabilitation. I. Title. [DNLM: 1. Shoulder—injuries. 2. Shoulder—surgery. 3. Shoulder Dislocation—surgery. 4. Shoulder Fractures—surgery. WE 810 N381s]

RD557.5.N44 1990 817.5′72059—dc20 89–70286

ISBN 0–7216–2832–x

Editor: Lewis Reines
Designer: Bill Donnelly
Production Manager: Peter Faber
Manuscript Editors: Tom Stringer and Ruth Low
Illustration Coordinator: Peg Shaw
Page Layout Artists: Paul Fry and Kris Hartzell
Indexer: Nancy Newman
Cover Designer: Joanne Carroll

Shoulder Reconstruction ISBN 0–7216–2832–X

Printed in the United States of America.

Last digit is the print number: 9 8 7 6 5 4 3 2 1

To the unification and intellectual exchange of the shoulder surgeons all over the world.

CHARLES S. NEER, II, M.D.

Inaugural Speaker of Honor,
Japanese Shoulder Society, 1976

Inaugural President,
American Shoulder and Elbow Surgeons, 1982

Inaugural Speaker of Honor,
European Shoulder Society, 1987

Co-Chairman,
Fourth International Congress on Surgery of the Shoulder, 1989

Patron of Honor,
Australian Shoulder Society

Preface

Most modern shoulder surgery has been developed during the last forty years. This book is written in response to requests from surgeons all over the world, as well as from radiologists, rheumatologists, residents in orthopaedic surgery, students of rehabilitation medicine, and those in family practice for a comprehensive book on the advanced techniques of diagnosis and reconstruction of the shoulder.

The objective of this book is to describe in detail the system I have found to be most effective for recognizing the pathology and treating painful shoulders. No attempt is made to discuss all other methods. Instead, I have devoted the space to the many practical details found to be important for optimum results with this method. Result studies are included for each operation.

The points of anatomy and kinesiology discussed in the first chapters of this book are those forming the background and anatomical rationale for the operative procedures and aftercare programs to follow. The reader is spared a reiteration of the embryology and general anatomy of the shoulder. A resume of the differential diagnoses of shoulder pain is included.

Since it is now generally recognized that the vast majority of tears of the rotator cuff and biceps lesions are either primarily or secondarily related to subacromial impingement, in the second chapter these lesions are considered with impingement. Anterior acromioplasty is now said to be the most frequently performed shoulder operation. A recently devised classification of impingement is given, which provides logical indications for anterior acromioplasty as well as for the treatment of all types of impingement problems. A systematic method for repairing tears of the rotator cuff is described, which is backed by a long-term follow-up report.

The chapter on glenohumeral arthroplasty might well have been a separate, free-standing book. However, since the reconstruction and the rehabilitation of the soft tissue (the rotator cuff and ligaments) are of more importance to the success of arthoplasties in the shoulder than in those of other joints, and since 20 percent of glenohumeral arthroplasties are necessitated by fractures, it seems important that shoulder arthroplasties be considered with rotator cuff repairs, dislocation repairs, and with fractures rather than separately. The principles and fine points are shown of freeing and reconstructing the soft tissue and the orientation of the components as applies to any anatomically designed make of nonconstrained implant, existing now or in the future.

The quality of function after shoulder reconstruction depends on the aftercare, although rehabilitation following shoulder surgery is recognized to be more difficult than that after surgery on other joints. Simple exercise programs are illustrated without complex apparatus. The earlier passive motion program is described, which has been a great advance in care after rotator cuff repairs and arthroplasties. Also, the rehabilitation programs for formidable problems of shoulders with inadequate bone and soft tissue and those in patients with paraplegia are described.

CHARLES S. NEER, II, M.D.

Acknowledgments

Authors recall many important people in their professional lives. I must pay particular tribute to a few of them.

First, a tribute to my father, who was an extremely dedicated doctor and a son of a doctor. He never once thought of me being anything other than a doctor.

Second, my teacher, Professor of Anatomy at Dartmouth College, Professor George A. Lord, who ignited my interest in musculoskeletal surgery and has remained an inspiration.

I am forever grateful to Doctor Isadore Ravdin, Professor of Surgery, University of Pennsylvania, who allowed me to work in his surgical research laboratory when I was a medical student and set a lasting example in teaching, research, and patient care.

In my surgical training, a special tribute to my "Chief," Doctor William Darrach, who at one time or another had been many things to Columbia University, including Director of Surgery, Professor of Anatomy, Dean of the Medical School, and, when I knew him, Director of the Fracture Service of the Columbia-Presbyterian Medical Center. I think of him daily as I use his retractors in anatomical approaches. Also, special thanks to two of the outstanding teachers on Dr. Darrach's staff: Dr. Clay Ray Murray, whose genius introduced to the world the principles of the operative treatment of fractures, and Harrison L. McLaughlin, a pioneer in shoulder surgery, who, with Dr. Darrach, encouraged me as a resident to pursue my interest in glenohumeral fracture-dislocations and in replacement arthroplasty of the shoulder.

I owe much to the many wonderful fellows, residents, and therapists on our Shoulder Service at the Columbia-Presbyterian Medical Center, and to the many visitors from all corners of America and abroad. They never resented the long hours, and they were constantly coming up with stimulating ideas. They made it fun and exciting to work in the field of shoulder surgery.

Finally, I have been fortunate indeed that Mr. Robert Demarest has always been the illustrator for my articles and illustrated this work. He is the best at what he does. He depicts the concepts better than words. He and my office manager, Eileen, should rank as co-authors. Eileen is a constant advisor and trusted friend. She organized my records and follow-up system as well as transcribed and edited this manuscipt.

CHARLES S. NEER, II, M.D.

Contents

CHAPTER 1

CHAPTER 2

CHAPTER 3

CHAPTER 4

CHAPTER 5

CHAPTER 6

CHAPTER 7

1

ANATOMY OF SHOULDER RECONSTRUCTION

For optimal success in shoulder reconstruction, the surgeon must respect the unique functional demands on the shoulder and the special anatomical features that permit it to meet these demands. The glenohumeral joint is subjected to great mechanical stress and yet has more motion than any other joint. Consider how the shoulder differs from other joints.

SHOULDER MOVEMENT

Four Joints

Normal shoulder function depends on four joints: the glenohumeral joint, the acromioclavicular joint, the sternoclavicular joint, and the scapulothoracic "joint" (in which the bursae between the scapula and chest wall function as a fourth joint) (Fig. 1–1). Some European authors[1] refer to the subacromial space as a fifth joint and have introduced the term "degenerative arthritis of the subacromial joint" in place of "impingement le-

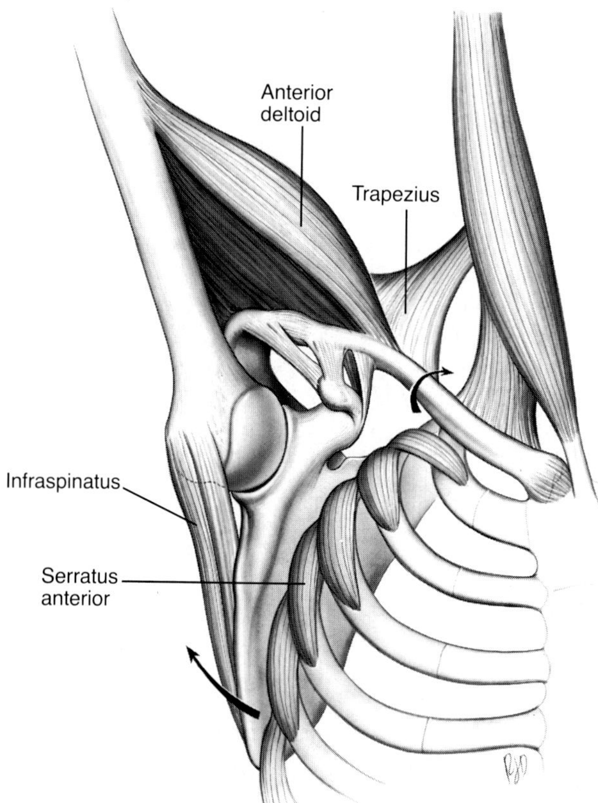

Figure 1–1. ***Normal Mechanism of Elevation.*** "Elevation" is the term used to indicate raising the arm in the scapular plane. The scapula is rotated synchronously as the humerus is raised so that the glenoid receives the thrust of the humeral head. The acromion is tilted upward out of the way of the greater tuberosity. The humerus rises approximately twice as far and twice as fast, and is simultaneously externally rotated, giving the greater tuberosity more clearance under the acromion and causing more of the articular surface of the head to become available, as explained in Figure 1–20. The coracoclavicular ligaments rotate the clavicle in its long axis as the scapula moves. Motion at the sternoclavicular joint plus that at the acromioclavicular joint equals the motion of the scapula. Motion at the sternoclavicular joint is much more than that at the acromioclavicular joint, occurs in all planes, and accommodates virtually all 40 degrees of clavicular rotation.

The key muscles in elevation are the anterior deltoid, raising the humerus; the infraspinatus, giving 90 per cent of the power for external rotation of the humerus; and the serratus anterior and trapezius, rotating the scapula forward and laterally.

sions." It seems important to clarify this difference from the concept in the United States, where wear changes beneath the acromion are termed "subacromial impingement lesions," as in Chapter 2. The pathology and treatment of impingement lesions are entirely different from those of degenerative arthritis of the glenohumeral joint (see Chapter 3). In degenerative osteoarthritis of the glenohumeral joint, the rotator cuff and long head of the biceps are almost always intact,[2] in contrast to subacromial impingement, which is now considered to be the most common cause of cuff tears and biceps lesions, and these tendons are ruptured in advanced impingement lesions.

The four joints move synchronously and simultaneously rather than separately and independently. There have been many attempts to ascribe a precise number of degrees of motion for each of these four joints; however, this is impossible because there are such individual variations in joint laxity and *variations in shoulder movement* in different age groups and between men and women. In older patients, overhead movement is restricted by two factors: first, the usual stiffening that occurs in all joints in later life; and second, the rounding of the dorsal spine that often occurs. Rounding of the dorsal spine restricts elevation of the scapula by causing it to be tilted forward (Fig. 1–2). The shoulders of women are generally more supple than those of men. An old man often has 40 degrees less upward excursion than a young woman. Because of these individual variations, it is important when examining range of motion to record the movements of the uninvolved side as an index of what is probably normal for that individual (see Figs. 1–5 and 1–6, pp. 8 and 9).

Although it is not possible to cite a standard amount of *motion at the glenohumeral joint*, if there is a total of 180 degrees of upward movement of the arm, the glenohumeral joint contributes in the neighborhood of 120 degrees. Scapulothoracic motion accounts for approximately 60 degrees. The glenohumeral joint provides virtually all rotation. To permit this large amount of motion at the glenohumeral joint, the glenoid is small and flat, unlike the acetabulum. Its articular surface is little more than one-quarter the size of the humeral head, and the radius of curve is larger than that of the head. The ligaments of the glenohumeral joint are normally loose, unlike the knee and most other joints. The capsule is normally large enough to contain two humeral heads. Rotation is greatest with the arm at the side because in this position the ligaments are at maximum relaxation. When the arm is raised, rotation diminishes because the ligaments are twisted and progressively tightened (see Fig. 1–20). With the arm at the side, it is usually possible to rotate the glenohumeral joint at least 170 degrees.

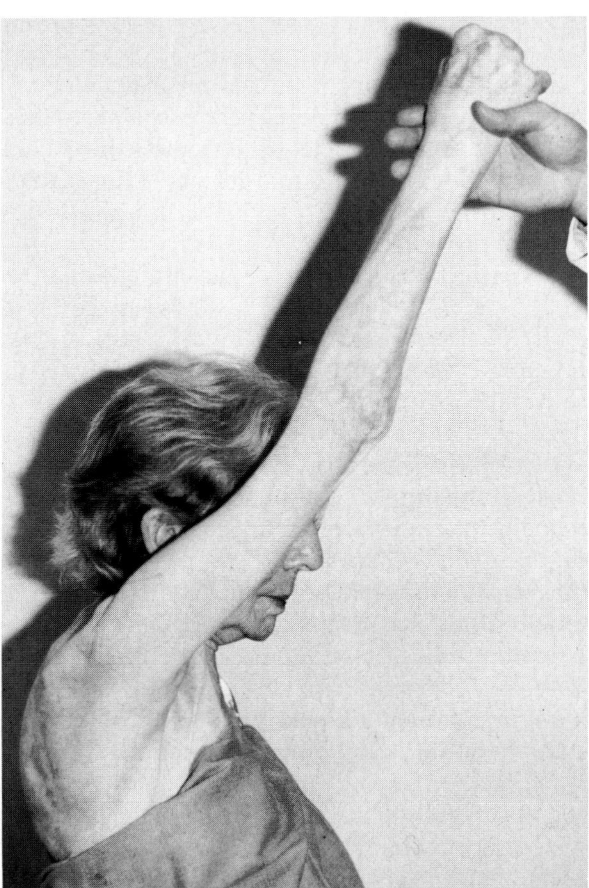

Figure 1–2. Individual variations in age, sex, ligamentous laxity, and posture of the dorsal spine cause marked differences in the range of shoulder motion. The rounding of the dorsal spine and stiffness with aging cause this elderly patient to have 45 degrees less elevation than she probably had in her youth. Some youthful patients are hypermobile. These variations make it impossible to establish a normal for all and make it necessary to record the range of both shoulders. The opposite side, if it is uninvolved, is used as the normal.

Biomechanical calculations of the *forces on the glenohumeral joint* are thwarted to some extent by the many movements taking place simultaneously and also by individual variations in the rhythm of the movements. The joint reaction force on the humeral head is greatest when erect with the arm held outstretched at 90 degrees parallel to the ground.[3–5] The maximum shear force between the humeral head and glenoid is thought to occur at 60 degrees of abduction.[5] Such biomechanical calculations become less exacting, however, when one considers that with the arm held at the horizontal the scapula has rotated approximately 30 degrees and the angle between the humerus and scapula is only approximately 60 degrees. There are individual differences in the way the simultaneous movements of the humerus and scapula occur. In addition, the simultaneous external rotation of the humerus takes place as the arm is raised (see Fig. 1–20). Rotation of the humerus causes different parts of the head to contact the glenoid and introduces changing neck-shaft angles to complicate biomechanical calculations. In glenohumeral osteoarthritis, most wear on the head is seen to occur on the superior part corresponding to this area of contact when the arm is raised 90 degrees in the position of maximum joint reaction force. Most wear on the glenoid is posterior.[2] Posterior glenoid wear corresponds to the forward position in which the arm is most often used (see Fig. 1–3). Forces on this joint are considered further on page 24 and in Chapter 3 (Fig. 3–21, p. 164).

The *scapula* is suspended by the suspensory mechanism (see Figs. 1–13 and 1–14) on the clavicle in muscles. It rests like the palm of the hand on the chest wall to provide stability for the base of the upper extremity. It is rotated in synchrony with the glenohumeral movements to receive the thrust of the humerus (see Fig. 1–15). Scapulothoracic movement is usually about 60 degrees. The sum of the motion of the clavicle plus that of its two joints, the sternoclavicular and acromioclavicular joints, is equal to the amount of movement of the scapula on the thorax. The *sternoclavicular joint* is very moveable and tilts 40 degrees in all directions and accommodates virtually all of the 40 degrees of rotation of the clavicle. *Acromioclavicular joint* movement is limited by the extensive connection of the coracoclavicular ligaments, which extends all along the distal clavicle from the coranoid tubercle to the acromioclavicular joint capsule. Because of the firm connection of these ligaments to the clavicle, which causes the clavicle to move in unison with movements of the scapula, acromioclavicular joint motion is limited to less than 20 degrees.

The movement of these four joints is depicted in Figure 1–1. The humerus moves twice as far and twice as fast as the scapula. As the scapula rotates forward, the coracoclavicular ligaments cause the clavicle to rotate backward about 40 degrees in its long axis. The rotation of the clavicle occurs on the sternoclavicular joint with only minimal tilting at the acromioclavicular joint. The scapula rotates upward and forward to receive the thrust of the humerus. The patterns and rhythm of these movements have often been described in terms of the *three phases of shoulder motion: Phase I ("setting phase")—0 to 30 degrees; Phase II—30 to 90 degrees; and Phase III—above 90 degrees.* In observing patients, however, the exact patterns of active motion vary too much from one individual to another to permit an exacting analysis of the events of each phase. For example, the "setting phase" is often almost entirely scapular motion, as Poppen and Walker[4,5] state; however, in some patients one sees humeral motion start during this phase. Normally after the first 30 degrees, scapular rotation occurs synchronously with the humerus. Those directing post-operative exercises should be made to understand this. It is a deterrent to recovery if, during the post-operative exercise program, the patient is told to keep the scapula down as the arm is raised on the false assumption that this will better develop "pure glenohumeral motion" (see Chapter 7). Keeping the scapula down during exercises retards the recovery of glenohumeral motion because without scapular rotation the acromion impedes elevation of the humerus (see Fig. 1–20).

Abnormalities of any one of the four joints may reduce the efficiency of the others. The result of a perfect glenohumeral arthroplasty in a rheumatoid patient may be spoiled by a painful acromioclavicular joint (see Chapter 3). Derangements of the glenohumeral joint can cause scapular pain because of strain and fatigue of the scapular muscles that result if the patient compensates with scapular movement (see Chapter 5). Loss of scapular rotation, as in trapezius muscle paralysis, may interfere with glenohumeral movement by causing subacromial impingement (see Chapter 2). Because each joint may affect the function of the others, all four joints must be evaluated during an examination before shoulder surgery (p. 14 and Figs. 1–10 and 1–11).

"Plane of Maximum Elevation"

The term "elevation" is used in this book to indicate upward motion in the scapular plane rather than in the coronal plane ("abduction") or sagittal plane ("flexion" and "extension") (Fig. 1–3). Glenohumeral motion is centered on the scapular plane rather than, as has been considered in the past, the coronal or sagittal plane. There are practical reasons for thinking of shoulder motion as being centered on the scapular plane. First, the highest upward excursion and the greatest ease and freedom for raising the arm are in this plane. Second, this is the plane in which the glenohumeral joint is most often used.

The scapular plane offers the greatest ease and height of upward movement because the glenohumeral joint capsule tightens, restricting movement if the arm is raised more toward either the coronal plane or the sagittal plane. The reader can self-demonstrate this as shown in Figure 1–4. Place the arm in neutral rotation by holding it in the anatomical position and bending the elbow 90 degrees. Without allowing rotation, raise the humerus as high as possible in the coronal plane. Upward motion in this plane is restricted unless the arm is externally rotated. Next, with the arm at the side in the same neutral rotation with the elbow bent 90 degrees, raise it straightforward in the sagittal plane. Upward movement without rotation in this plane is also restricted. Finally, starting with the arm at the side in the same neutral rotation with elbow bent, raise the arm as high as possible in the scapular plane (about midway between the coronal and sagittal planes). In the scapular plane, the arm can be raised higher. This is the "plane of maximum elevation."

The reader has but to consider the position of the arm in daily use to realize that the scapular plane is also important as the plane in which the glenohumeral joint is most often used. In almost all activities, the hands are in front. When the elbows are bent and the hands are in front, the humeral head is directed toward the scapula because of its retroversion, as shown in Figure 1–17. The arm is rarely raised in abduction or flexion but is raised somewhere in between—near the scapular plane. The retroversion of the proximal humerus and tracking by the scapula as the arm is raised make upward movement in this plane more

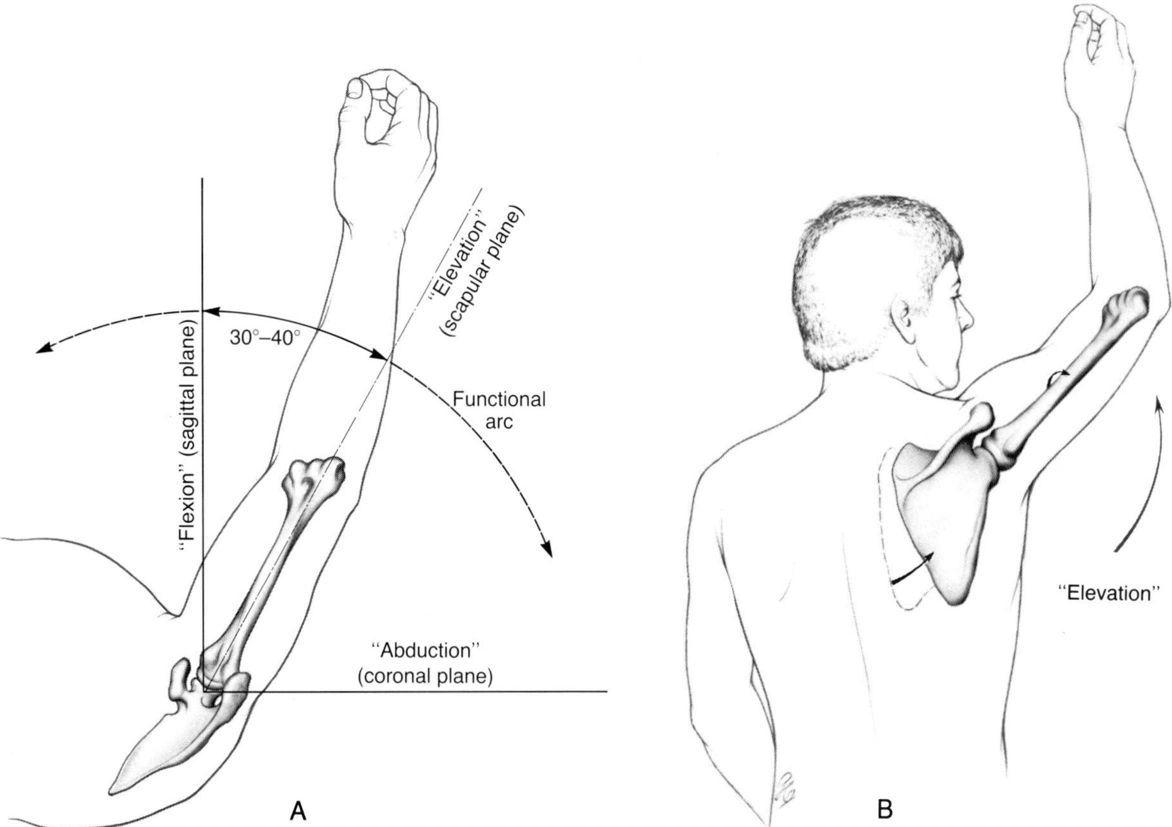

Figure 1–3. The "plane of maximum elevation" is centered on the scapular plane rather than the coronal plane ("abduction") or sagittal plane ("flexion"). Two important reasons for thinking of shoulder movements as centered on this plane are (A) the capsule of the glenohumeral joint is most relaxed in the scapular plane, allowing the highest upward excursion with the greatest ease and freedom of movement; and (B) the glenohumeral joint is most often used in this plane. Movements here are more natural and with less effort. The body may be rotated to cause the arm to be raised in the scapular plane rather than the coronal plane, as when serving a tennis ball.

This concept is stressed in the postoperative exercise programs.

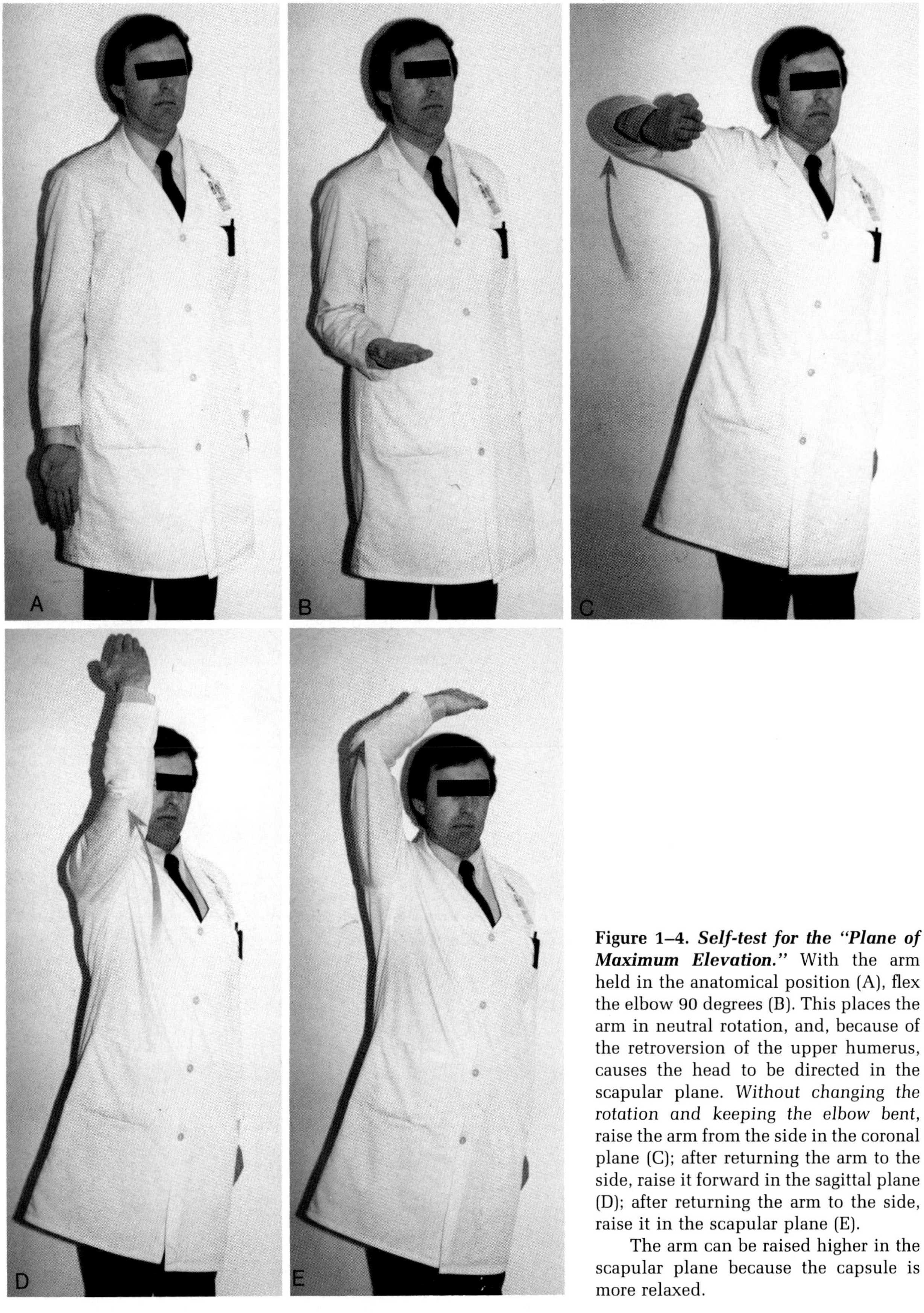

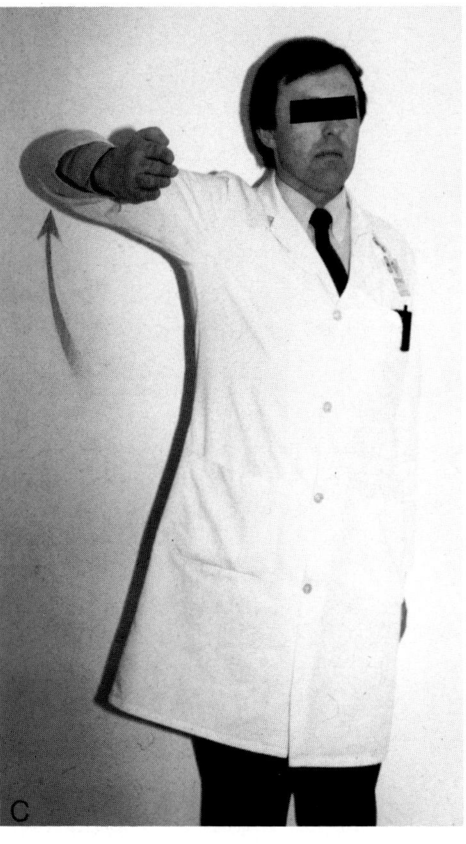

Figure 1–4. ***Self-test for the "Plane of Maximum Elevation."*** With the arm held in the anatomical position (A), flex the elbow 90 degrees (B). This places the arm in neutral rotation, and, because of the retroversion of the upper humerus, causes the head to be directed in the scapular plane. *Without changing the rotation and keeping the elbow bent,* raise the arm from the side in the coronal plane (C); after returning the arm to the side, raise it forward in the sagittal plane (D); after returning the arm to the side, raise it in the scapular plane (E).

The arm can be raised higher in the scapular plane because the capsule is more relaxed.

natural. The body may be rotated, as in serving a tennis ball, to cause the arm to be raised in the scapular plane rather than in the coronal plane.

This concept of the glenohumeral joint being centered on the scapular plane is important clinically. In this text, this concept is emphasized in the post-operative exercise program, in the system for measuring motion, and in roentgen projections of the glenohumeral joint.

Recording Shoulder Motion

The shoulder allows motion in every plane. There has been much confusion as to how this motion can best be recorded. Methods that attempt to describe both upward and rotary movement in all possible directions are too complicated to be of practical use. A simple and reproducible system should be adopted universally so that each examiner can see what was found at previous examinations. The method of recording motion and the terminology used in this book are shown in Figures 1–5 and 1–6. This system has eliminated confusion among our house staff members and in the records of our general orthopaedic service. It can be recommended for general use and has been adopted in principle by the American Shoulder and Elbow Surgeons.

Measurement of motion is primarily concerned with passive motion and is intended for following progress during treatment. Physical examination when making a diagnosis requires testing motion in other directions. Active motion and strength are recorded separately, since these measurements are less accurate because they may be altered by pain, skeletal instability, or motivation of the patient.

In this system for recording shoulder motion, rotation is measured with the arm at the side (Fig. 1–5). Almost all rotation occurs at the glenohumeral joint, and the glenohumeral ligaments and capsule are most relaxed when the arm is at the side. This position permits maximum rotation. The ligaments tighten as the arm is raised, progressively restricting rotation. When the arm is held straight up overhead, no rotation is possible because the ligaments are tight. Codman[6] referred to this as the "pivotal position." As shown in Figure 1–5, "*external rotation*" (A) is measured with the patient supine because this eliminates rotation of the body and the table serves as a point of reference. "*Internal rotation*" (B) is measured with the patient sitting. The level that the patient's thumb can be brought up the spine by the examiner is recorded. This measurement, of course, reflects shoulder extension and elbow flexion rather than pure internal rotation, but because the body is in the way and prevents direct measurement of internal rotation, this method is practical. It works well, but allowance must be made when the elbow is stiff or painful.

A measurement of *rotation in abduction* can be important in diagnosis and in following the effectiveness of treatment of some conditions. Loss of rotation or excessive rotation may occur in abduction that cannot be detected with the arm at the side. This is especially important in evaluating malunion of the greater tuberosity or a throwing arm in an athlete. Rotation in abduction can be measured either with the patient sitting, as in Figure 1–6A, or with the patient lying with the arm off the side of a table, as in Figure 1–7.

As previously discussed (p. 4), upward motion is measured with the arm in the scapular plane rather than in the coronal plane ("abduction") or sagittal plane ("flexion"). The term "*elevation*" is used to indicate that the arm is being raised in the scapular plane. In recording motion, the term "*total elevation*" indicates upward excursion of the humerus and scapula combined. In the initial examination when the examiner is making the diagnosis, it is important to consider scapular and humeral motion separately; however, it is impractical to measure these components separately in every routine re-examination when following the progress of patients under treatment. As shown in Figure 1–5, *total passive elevation* is measured with the patient supine because the table gives a point of reference and eliminates spine motion and knee motion, making the measurement more accurate.

Active motion can be altered by pain, an unstable glenohumeral fulcrum, patient motivation, strength, and passive range of motion. Its measurement is less consistent. It is recorded separately. *Total active elevation* (glenohumeral and scapular motion combined) is measured by having the patient raise the arm against gravity in the sitting position. In the sitting position, the scapular muscles are unrestricted by the table (as they are when the patient is supine) and knee and spine movements (which confuse this measurement if made in the standing position) are eliminated. This is illustrated in Figure 1–6B. *Active internal and external rotation* can also be tested with the patient in the sitting position. Brems[7] developed a strain gauge with a numerical reading for measuring strength, which greatly enhances the accuracy of this measurement (Fig. 1–8).

The progress of the patient is documented by recording these measurements at each examination on the sheet illustrated in Figure 1–9.

Text continued on page 14

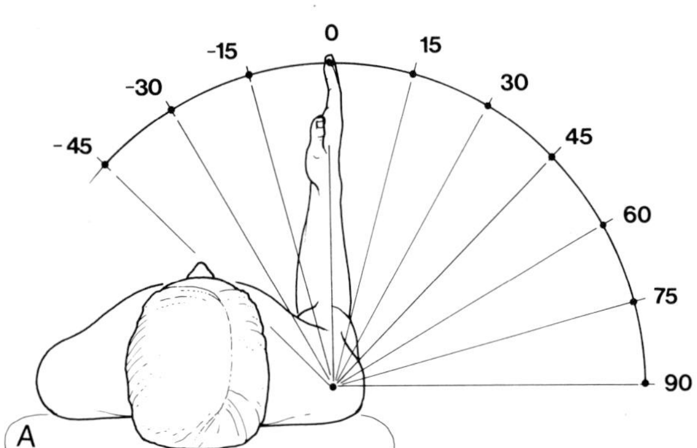

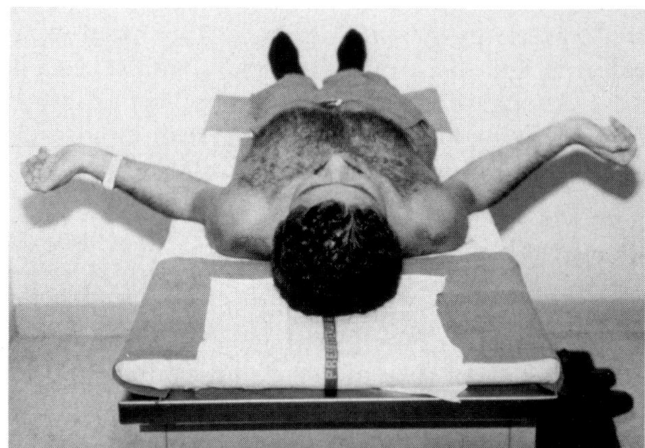

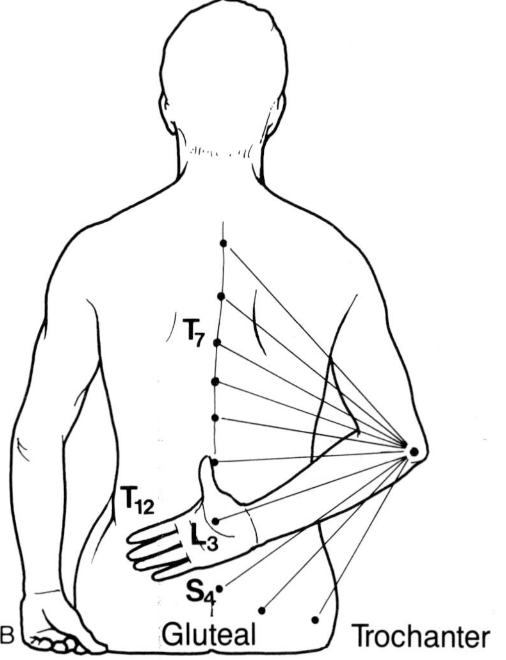

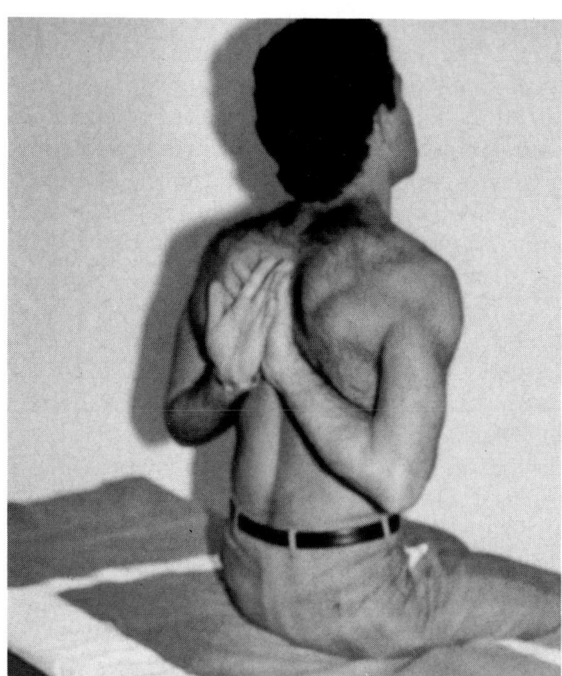

Figure 1–5. ***Recording Shoulder Motion.*** This system of recording the excursion of movement is easily reproduced by the next examiner and has proved to be an efficient method for following the progress of a patient under treatment and valuable in the analysis of results.

Passive motion is measured separately from active motion. Motion of the opposite shoulder is recorded for comparison.

Since almost all rotation occurs at the glenohumeral joint and the glenohumeral ligaments and capsule are most relaxed when the arm is at the side, passive rotation is measured with the arm at the side. As shown in Figure 1–5A, external rotation is measured with the patient supine and the elbow flexed 90 degrees and held against the side as the examiner externally rotates the arm as far as possible. An internal rotation contracture is recorded in minus degrees of external rotation. Internal rotation is measured with the patient sitting (Fig. 1–5B). The highest level that the thumb can be brought up the spine by the examiner is recorded. In the figure illustrated, the thumb is at the third lumbar spine. Allowance must be made when the elbow is stiff and painful.

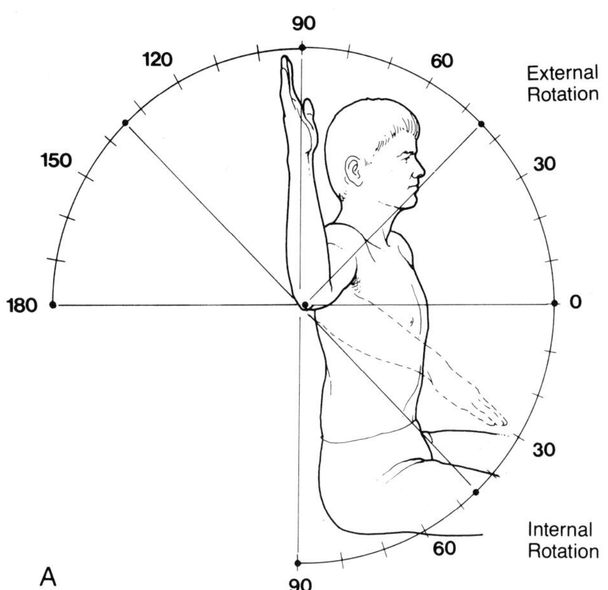

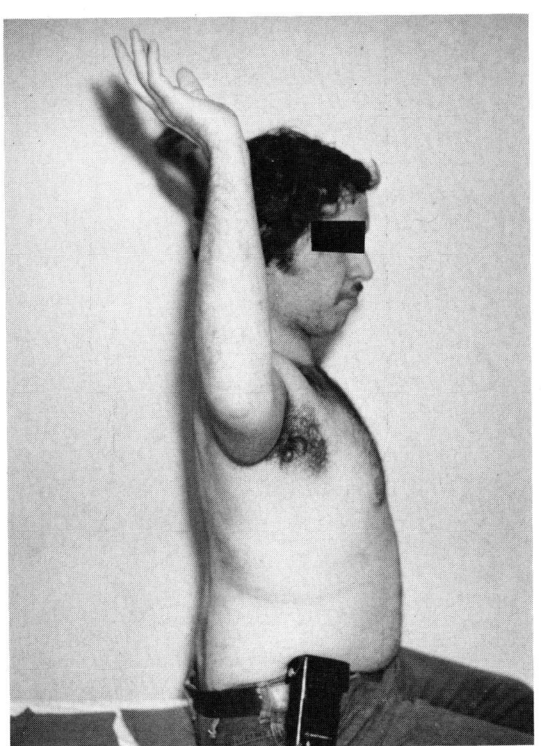

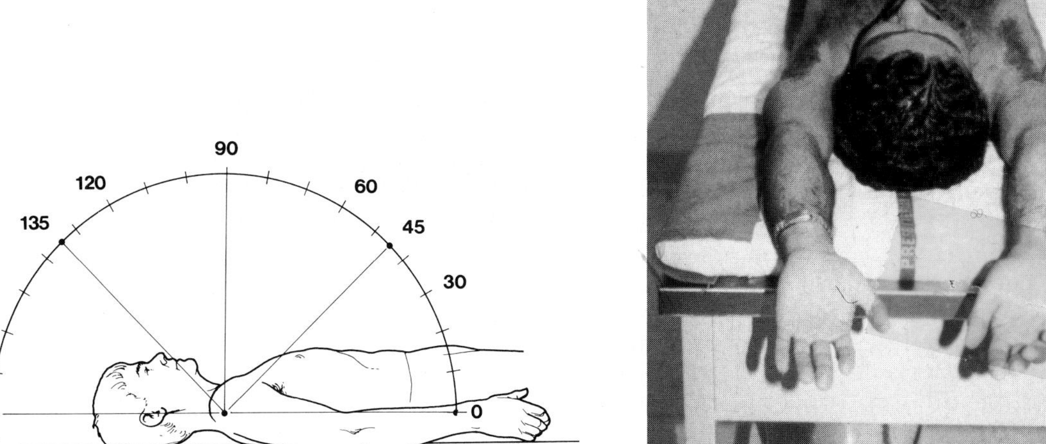

Figure 1–6. ***Recording Shoulder Motion.*** It is important in special cases, as in the throwing arm (see Chapter 6) or after surgery for malunion of the greater tuberosity (see Chapter 5), to follow the range of rotation in 90 degrees of abduction. The patient may be sitting, as in Figure 1–6A; or supine, as in Figure 1–7. The elbow is flexed 90 degrees. When the patient is sitting, the zero position is with the forearm parallel to the horizontal. When the patient is supine, the zero position is with the forearm vertical.

Total passive elevation is measured with the patient supine (to eliminate knee and spine movements) as the examiner raises the arm to the highest level possible (Fig. 1–6B). The arm is raised in the scapular plane, which is generally about 30 degrees or 40 degrees lateral to the sagittal plane. No attempt is made to eliminate scapular motion. Motion of both the glenohumeral joint and the scapula is recorded.

Illustration continued on following page

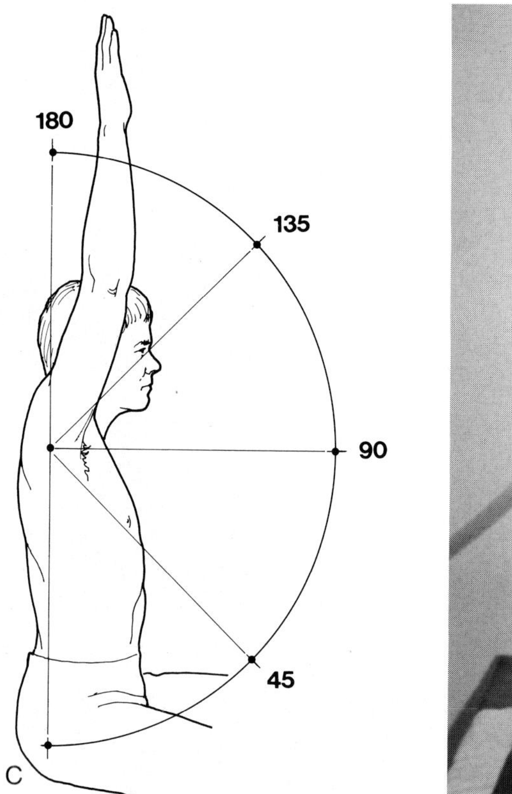

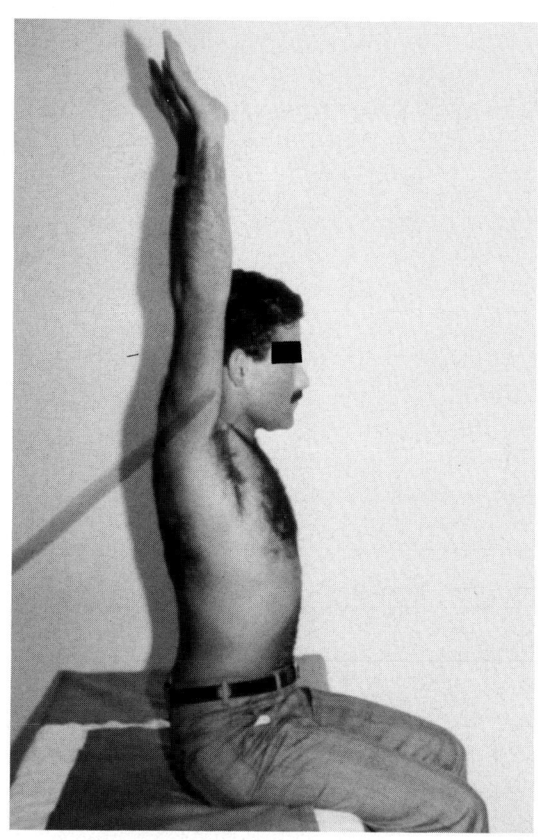

Figure 1–6 *Continued* Measurements of strength and active motion are less consistent and are recorded separately. Total active elevation is measured with the patient sitting, as in Figure 1–6C (to eliminate knee and spine motion). The arm is raised by the patient as high as possible in the scapular plane. It may be important in the initial examination and special cases to estimate the ratio of glenohumeral motion to scapular motion, but this is not recorded at every routine follow-up examination. Numerical recordings of strength may be made, as in Figure 1–8.

These measurements are recorded at each examination, as illustrated in Figure 1–9.

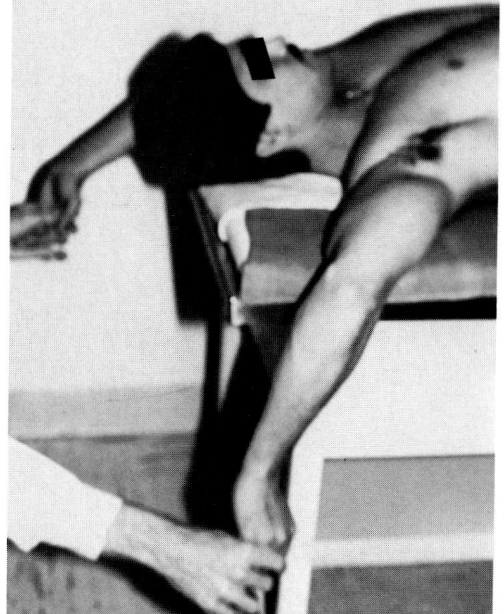

Figure 1–7. Measuring passive external rotation of the right shoulder at 90 degrees abduction with the patient supine. This was found to be more than that of the opposite side in this 25 year old right-handed professional baseball pitcher. This measurement can be made with the patient supine rather than sitting (see Fig. 1–6A). Abnormal rotation at 90 degrees abduction, either excess or less, may be discovered even though measurement at the side is normal. This is discussed further in connection with malunion of the greater tuberosity (Chapter 5) and "pitchers' shoulders" (Chapter 6).

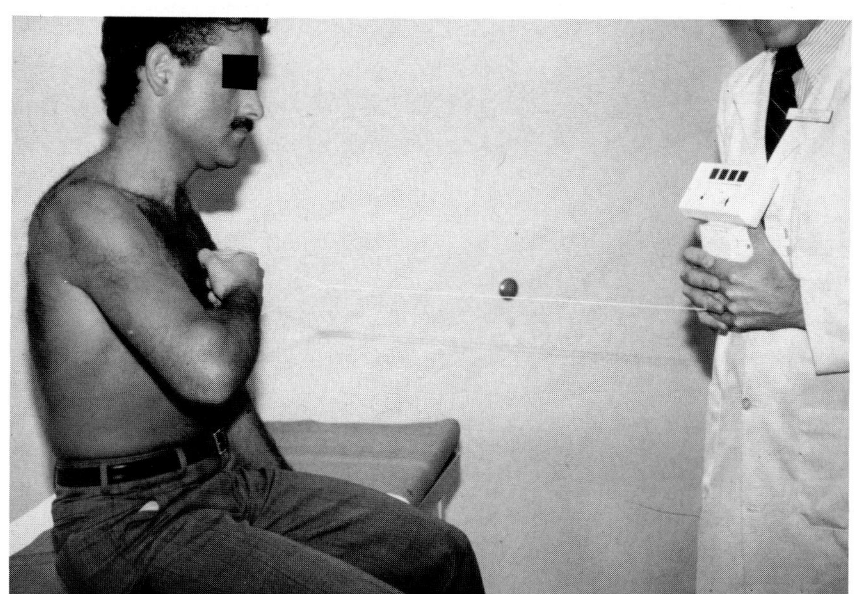

Figure 1–8. Brems developed a strain gauge with a numerical reading that is useful for measuring the strength of the internal rotators, external rotators, and deltoid.[7] It has the advantage of being more portable and less expensive than the more complex isokinetic machines. It can be mounted on a wall or, as shown, held by the examiner. The numerical readout (which can be converted to pounds or kilograms) makes it possible to compare more accurately with the last examination. Unfortunately, measurement of strength is less accurate because it is altered by pain, an unstable glenohumeral fulcrum, patient motivation, and the range of motion. Since measurement of strength is less consistent and less reproducible, it is recorded separately from passive motion.

THE PRESBYTERIAN HOSPITAL
in the City of New York

Charles S. Neer II, M.D.
Department of Orthopaedic Surgery
Columbia-Presbyterian Medical Center

PREOPERATIVE AND POSTOPERATIVE
EVALUATION FOR SHOULDER SURGERY

Unit No. ____________

Type Operation ____________

Date Operation ____________

Surgeon ____________

Right ________ Left ________

Diagnosis ____________

Dominant Side ____________

Last Name First Name Occupation Age

PAIN

1	2	3	4	5	6
Complete shoulder disability interrupts sleep.	Marked with serious limitations of shoulder activity. Occasionally requires medication & interrupts sleep.	Moderate, interfering with some activities. Makes concessions.	Only after unusual activity but disappears quickly.	Slight or occasional. No compromise in activity.	None

Type & number pain tablets/day ____________ Pain at night? Yes ____ No ____

Incision from prior surgery: Location ____________ Length ________ Shape ________

STRENGTH

	PARALYSIS	SEVERE WEAKNESS	MILD WEAKNESS	NORMAL
Deltoid				
Internal Rotators				
External Rotators				

Strength evaluation precluded because of pain? Yes ________ No ________

INITIAL EXAMINATION

DATE ________

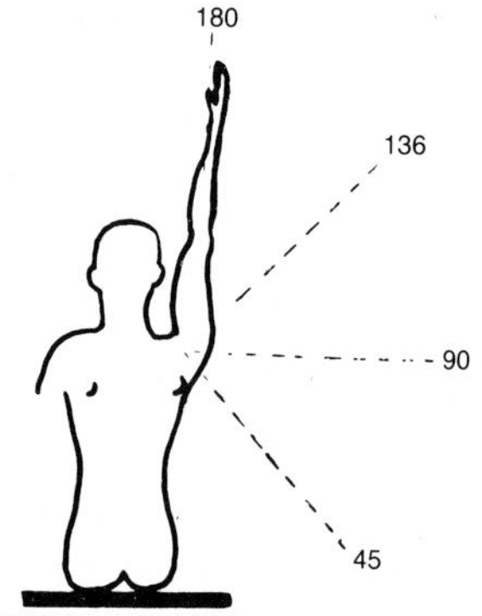

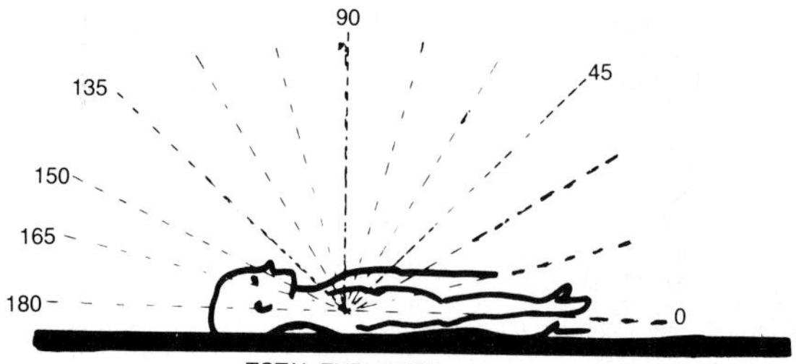

	+	−
Impingement Sign		
Anterior Apprehension		
Posterior "Fukuda"		
Inferior Apprehension		

Injection Test Relieve Pain ____ / 10

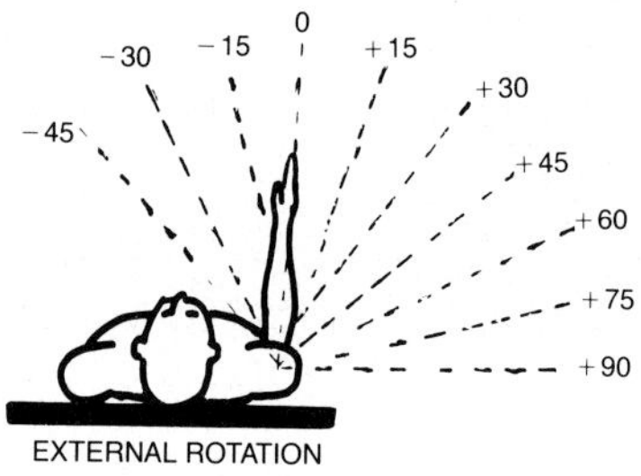

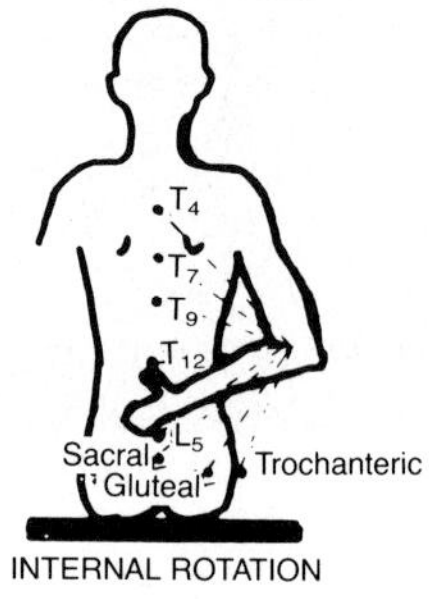

Figure 1–9. *See legend on opposite page*

GENERAL FUNCTION

DATE	Yes	No	Yes	No	Yes	No	Yes	No
Sleep on that side								
Reach overhead								
Comb hair								
Reach mouth								
Reach opposite axilla								
Reach belt buckle								
Reach back pocket								
Reach between shoulder blades								
Carry 10 pounds								
Do usual work								
Do usual sports (__________ specify type)								

Mental Attitude:

Physical condition:

Prior Surgery:
Scar:

Other remarks:

FOLLOW-UP EXAM

DATE	Elevation Passive	Elevation Active	ER	IR	DATE	Elevation Passive	Elevation Active	ER	IR

Figure 1–9 *Continued* Evaluation sheet used by the author before and following shoulder surgery. A similar sheet is being developed for adoption by the American Shoulder and Elbow Surgeons. Pain, strength, range of motion, and function are recorded, as discussed in Chapter 7.

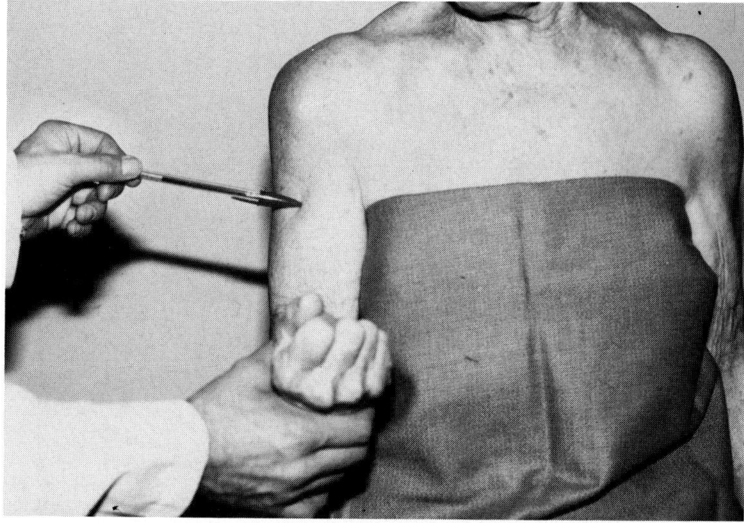

Figure 1–10. ***System for Evaluation of the Shoulder.*** Since it is impossible to interpolate local physical signs without having excluded infection, tumors, and systemic conditions causing joint pains, laboratory data (erythrocyte sedimentation rate, complete blood count, chemical profile, and serologic testing) and basic x-ray studies of the shoulder are required prior to the examination. Routine x-ray views are anterior-posterior in internal and external rotation and an axillary (including the glenoid) (see Fig. 1–12A). When there has been an injury, an anterior-posterior view and lateral view in the scapular plane with the arm in a sling and a "Velpeau axillary" view (see Fig. 1–12B) are made. Records of previous treatment are routinely requested.

A system is followed during the initial examination; otherwise, less obvious but important diagnostic signs will be missed. The patient is seated in a good light on the examination table with both shoulders and upper extremities completely exposed and the table arranged so that the examiner can stand both in front and in back of the patient.

At the start of the examination, from the front, the patient is asked to point to the site of pain and to demonstrate movements provoking pain. Next the acromioclavicular joint, sternoclavicular joint, biceps, elbows, and hands are examined, including neurological tests. The patient illustrated has a rupture of the long head of the biceps with self-reattachment and only partial retraction. This is discussed in Chapter 2, Figure 2–26, page 72. This is very suggestive of an impingement lesion with a tear of the rotator cuff.

INITIAL INVESTIGATION OF THE SHOULDER AND NECK

Interpretation of physical findings is impossible without having excluded infection, tumors, and systemic conditions causing shoulder pain. The routine (Table 1–2) includes erythrocyte sedimentation rate, blood count, chemical profile, and serologic studies, as well as the basic x-ray films made in internal and external rotation and an axillary view showing the head and glenoid (see Fig. 1–12). If there has been an injury,[8] anterior-posterior and lateral scapular plane views are made with the arm in a sling (without moving the arm), supplemented with a Velpeau axillary view to exclude any possibility of posterior dislocation. Routine and glenoid skyline and Velpeau[15] x-ray views are illustrated in Figure 1–12. Previous treatment records and operating reports are requested.

A system is followed in the examination, as discussed in Figures 1–10 and 1–11. The initial examination of the shoulder includes routine testing of the neck and scapular muscles from behind as well as biceps and hand strength in front. The C5–C6 root is critical so far as glenohumeral motion is concerned because it is a major component of both the suprascapular nerve (to the supraspinatus and infraspinatus) and the axillary nerve

Text continued on page 20

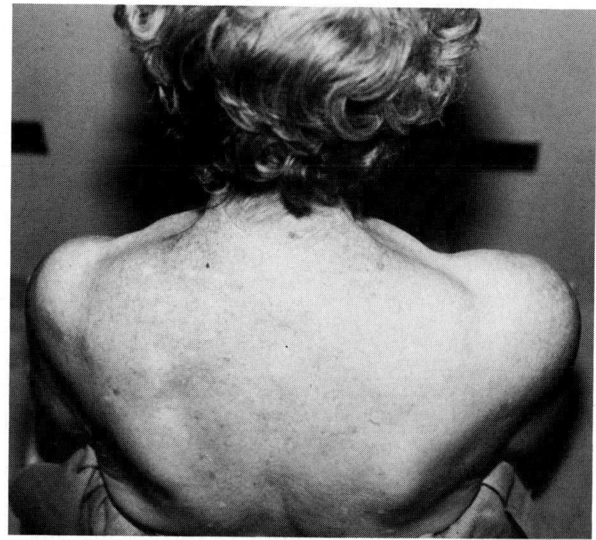

Figure 1–11. The importance of the examination from behind is stressed. An examination for shoulder pain must include a careful evaluation of the neck and cervical motion. This is best checked from behind, as are the supraclavicular and scapular regions for masses and motion, and the scapula for winging.

Only then is the examination of the glenohumeral joint begun. Here the specific signs and tests are elicited as specifically discussed in each part of the book. The patient illustrated in Figures 1–10 and 1–11 has enlargement of the subacromial bursa, discussed in Chapter 2 as the "fluid sign," which further confirms the diagnosis of a complete tear of the rotator cuff.

Table 1–1. FREQUENT CAUSES OF SHOULDER PAIN (DIFFERENTIAL DIAGNOSIS)

	TYPICAL AGE (YEARS)	HISTORY	TENDERNESS	STIFFNESS	ROENTGEN FINDINGS	IMPINGEMENT INJECTION TEST STOPS PAIN	SPECIAL TESTS
Impingement							
Stage I	Under 40	Overuse	Bursa and biceps +	Guard at extremes	None	Yes	
Stage II	30–40	Pain after activities	After activities	Guard after activities. May stiffen later	None	Yes	
Cuff tear (Stage III)	Over 40	No injury in 50%	Bursa and biceps ±	Guarding. May freeze later	Changes late in Stage III	Yes, unless large or frozen	Biceps rupture common Arthrogram (Sonogram? or MRI?) Arthroscopy
Acute traumatic subacromial bursitis	Under 30	Injury	Bursa + + +	Guarding	None	Yes	May aspirate blood
Acute calcium deposit	33–55	Pain varies (intermittent to severe)	+ + + + (cuff)	Guarding; may freeze later	Yes		Rotation and axillary views
Frozen shoulder	30–40	Insidious	None	+ + +	None Disuse later	No	Therapeutic test: trial of exercises
Recurrent dislocations	Under 30	No initial injury in 50%	Minimal	Apprehension at extremes	None to changes (see Chapter 4)	No	Loose joints, sulcus sign, apprehension tests, axillary and weight views, evaluation under anesthesia (EUA), arthroscopy
Acromio-clavicular arthritis	Any	Weight lifter, arthritis	+ + + + AC joint	Pain on horizontal adduction and extremes	Yes	No	Horizontal adduction test AC joint injection test Tomograms, CT scan
Glenohumeral arthritis	Any	Insidious	Posterior joint line + +	+ + + elevation and external rotation	Yes	No	Posterior joint line tenderness Axillary view, CT scan Tomograms
C5–C6 nerve root	Over 40	Neck problems	Tilt and extend neck + +	None (may freeze later)	Cervical spine	No	Neck x-ray, neck CT scan, electromyogram, biceps weakness
Neoplasms	Any	24 hour (night and day) pain	Over tumor ±	None	Yes	No	Tomograms, CT scans, bone scan, MRI
Infections	Any	Prior injection or surgery	+ + + +	Guarding	Late	No	Erythrocyte sedimentation rate, aspirate and cultures

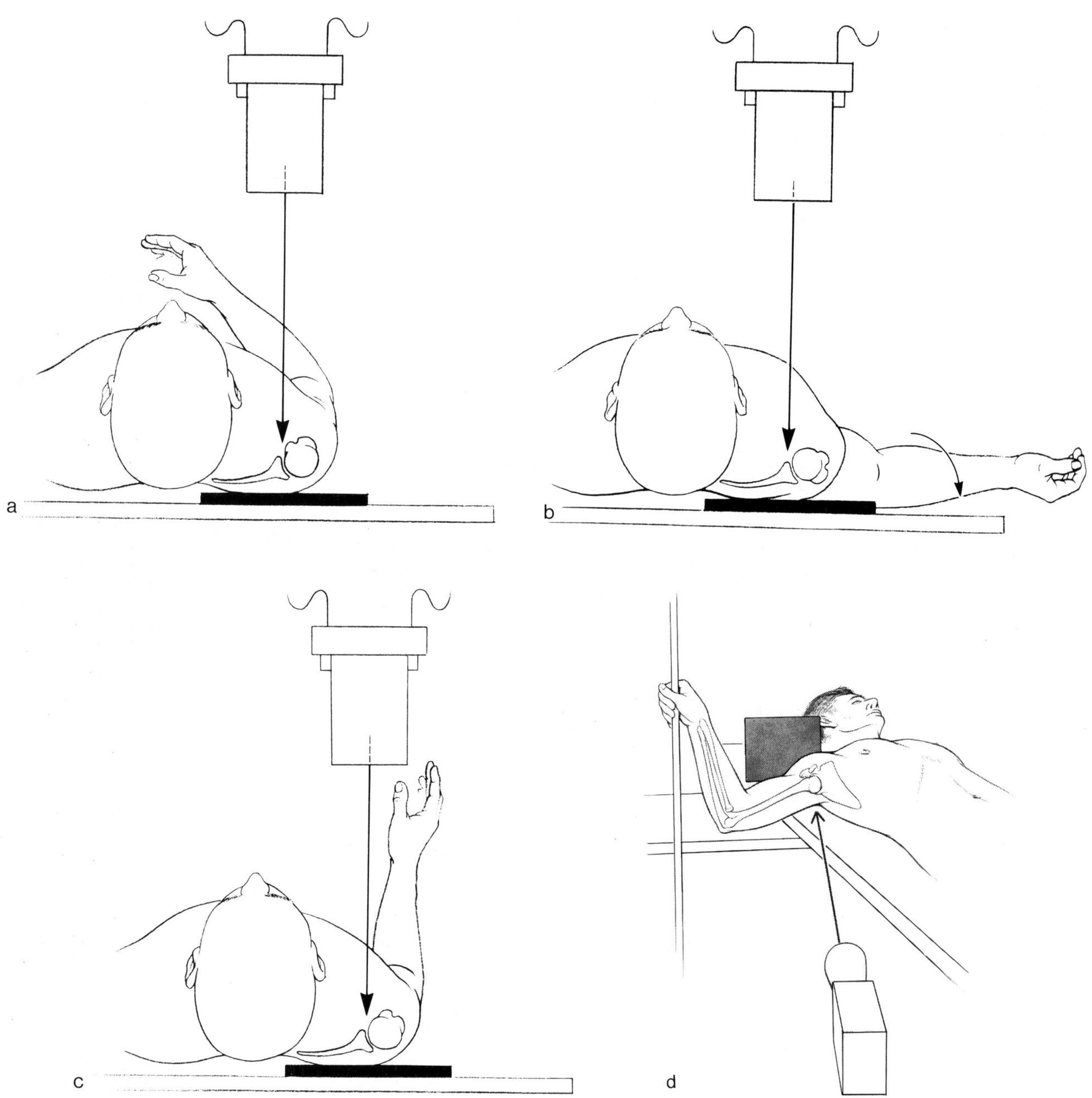

Figure 1–12A. Routine x-ray vews. "Routine" anterior-posterior view with the arm in (a) internal rotation and (b) external rotation and (c) neutral position; (d) an axillary view with the patient supine.

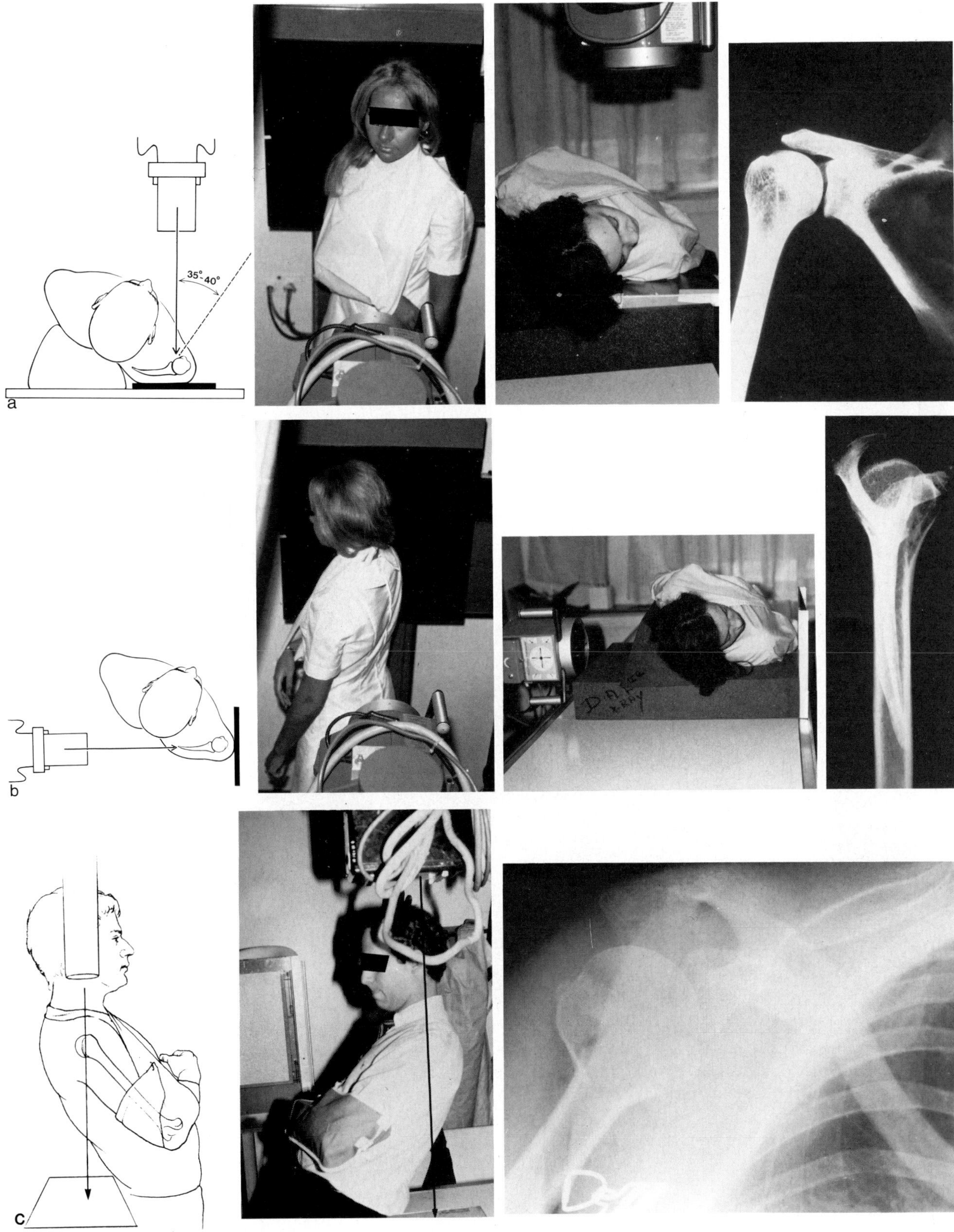

Figure 1–12B. "Trauma series." When there has been an injury and the possibility of a fracture, (a) anterior-posterior, (b) lateral in the scapular plane, and (c) "Velpeau axillary" views are made. The arm remains in a sling (without being moved). The anterior-posterior and lateral views can be made with the patient standing; sitting; or, when multiple injuries are present, lying down.

Illustration continued on following page

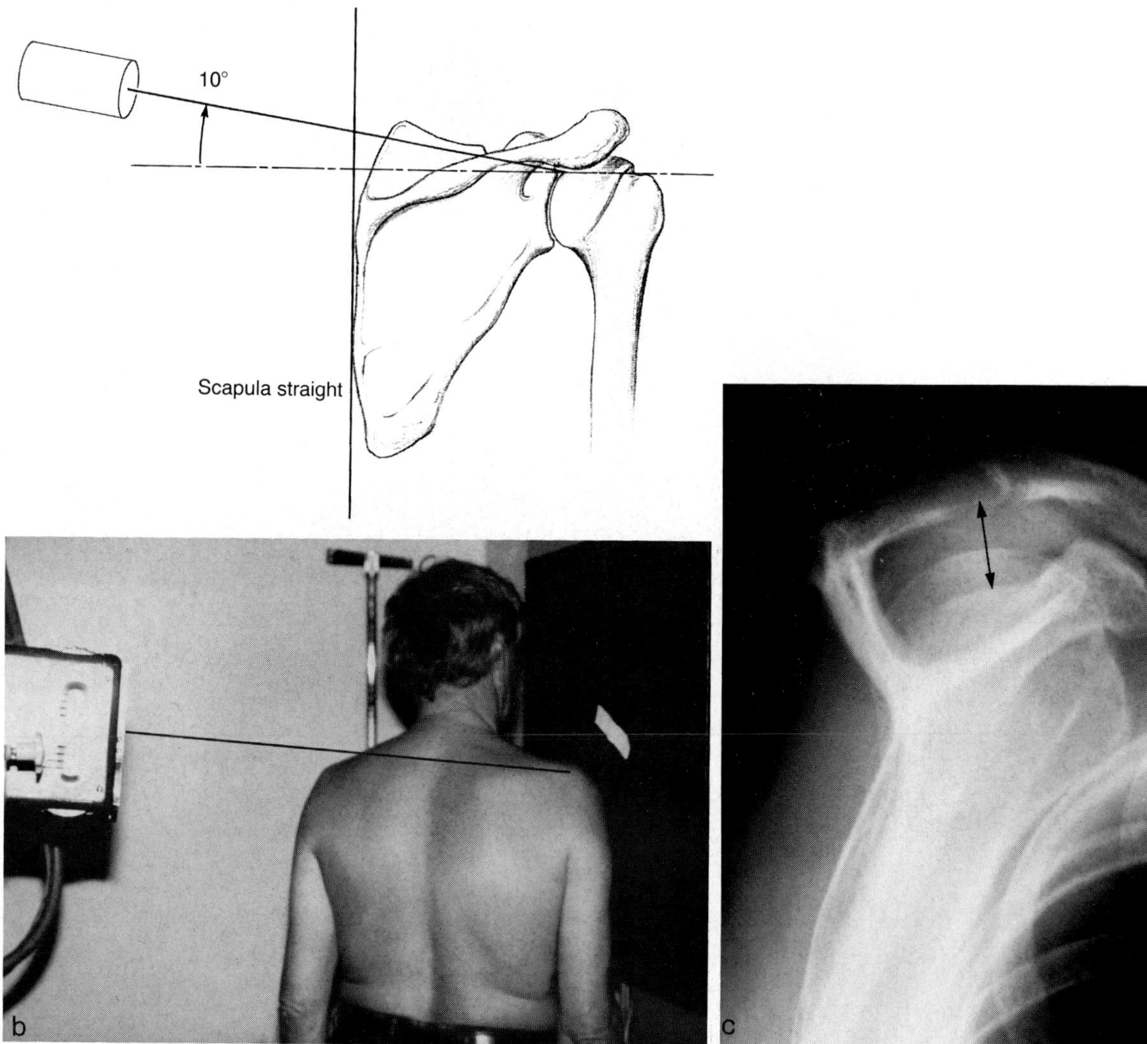

Figure 1–12C. Special views. "Supraspinatus outlet view" is a lateral of the scapula when the scapula is held upward so that the spine of the scapula is parallel to the floor and the ray is angled downward 10 degrees. This view is used for impingement lesions to show encroachment on the supraspinatus outlet and to allow a more accurate measurement of the acromiohumeral distance.

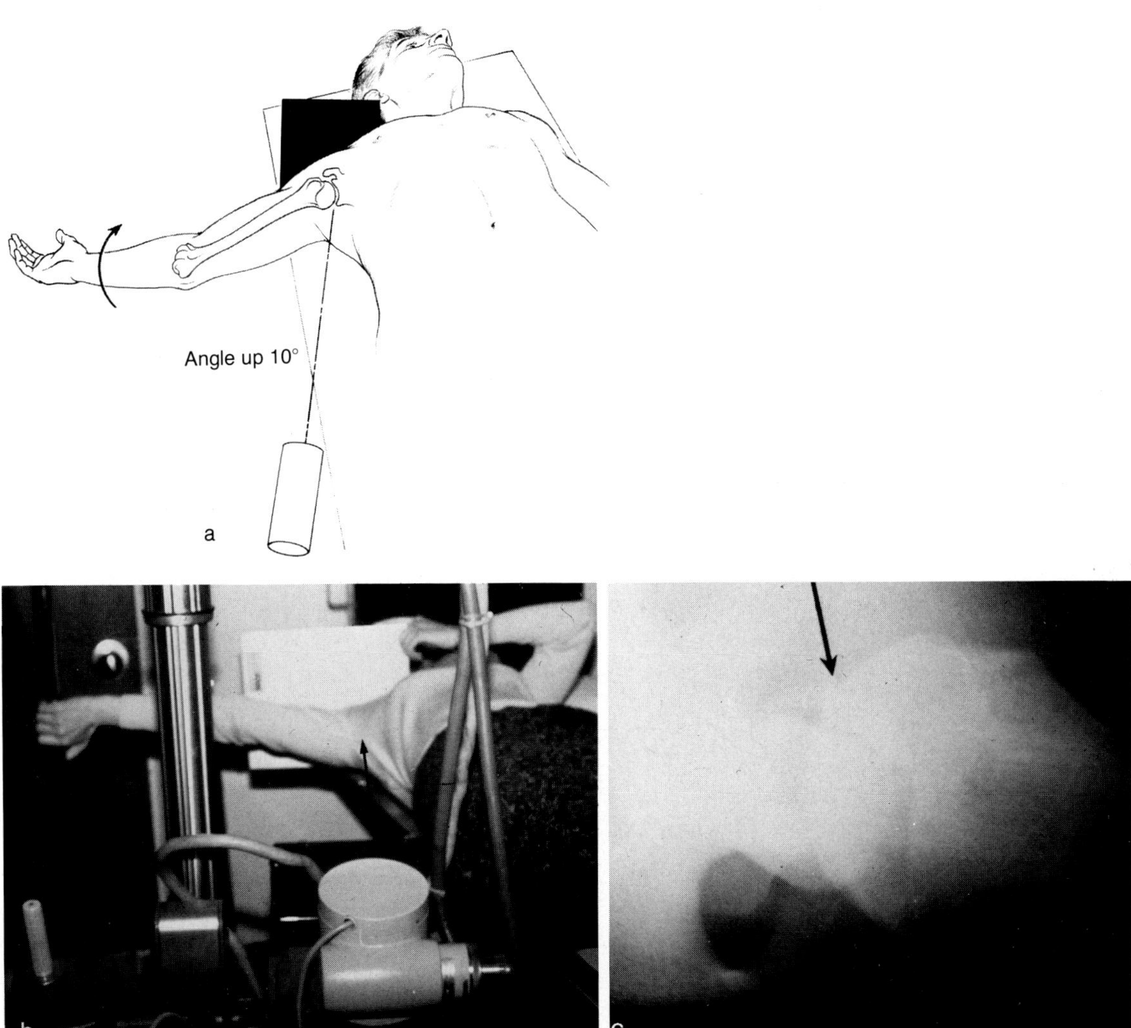

Figure 1–12D. Supine axillary view with the arm in external rotation and the tube angled upward 10 degrees (a) (glenoid skyline axillary view). Used for instability to show the skyline of the anterior glenoid rim for reactive bone or fragments (arrow in b), indicative of anterior dislocations (c). This view has replaced the "West Point" axillary view, once used for the same purpose, as discussed in Chapter 4.

Illustration continued on following page

Table 1–2. LABORATORY ROUTINES

BLOOD STUDIES	
	Complete blood count, erythrocyte sedimentation rate, rheumatoid factor, chemistry profile (SMA-20*)
X-RAY VIEWS	
No Injury	"Routine" (anterior-posterior in neutral, internal rotation, external rotation, and supine axillary)
Injury	"Trauma series" (anterior-posterior and lateral in the scapular plane [arm at side] and Velpeau axillary)
SPECIAL X-RAY STUDIES	
Impingement	Outlet view (see Fig. 1–12)
Instability	Supine axillary with 10 degree upward tilt (see Fig. 1–12) Weights (see Fig. 1–12)
Acromioclavicular	Less exposure than glenohumeral
Clavicle	45 degree angle view (see Fig. 1–12)
Sternoclavicular	45 degree angle view, tomograms, CT scan
Scapular	Lateral of scapula with arm raised

*Sequential multiple analyzer.

(to the deltoid and teres minor). Thus, it innervates the only external rotators of the shoulder as well as the prime motor itself. It also innervates the biceps. A test for biceps weakness as part of the examination of the shoulder may make the diagnosis of a C5–C6 lesion (see Fig. 2–37B). Involvement of higher roots can cause scapular pain and scapular muscle weakness.

Cervical root lesions not only lead to errors in diagnosis but also can occur unnoticed concomitantly with shoulder pathology interfering with recovery of function after shoulder surgery. Root involvement can lead to failure of a perfect shoulder reconstruction by causing both radicular pain and motor weakness.

Patients with arthritis or injuries as well as older patients should be especially scrutinized for cervical spine lesions before major surgical reconstruction is undertaken. Pre-operative roentgenograms of the cervical spine are routine, and electromyography is performed when symptoms warrant this study.

An overview of the common causes of chronic shoulder pain in those with normal laboratory data is presented in Table 1–1. Clinical tests of special value are as indicated.

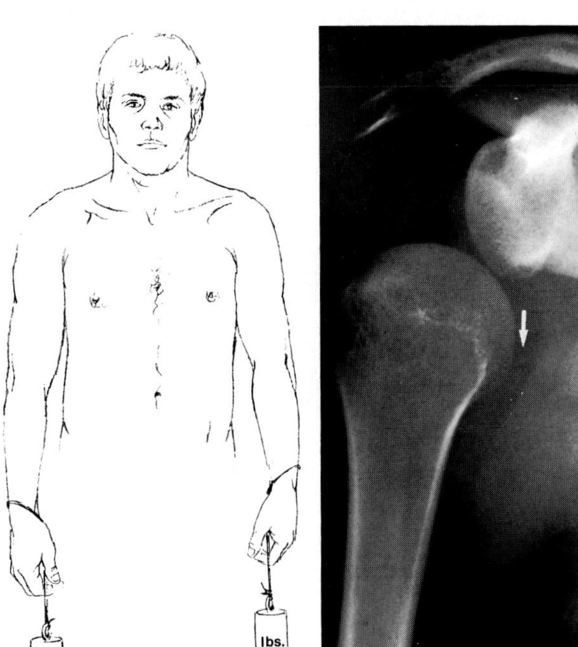

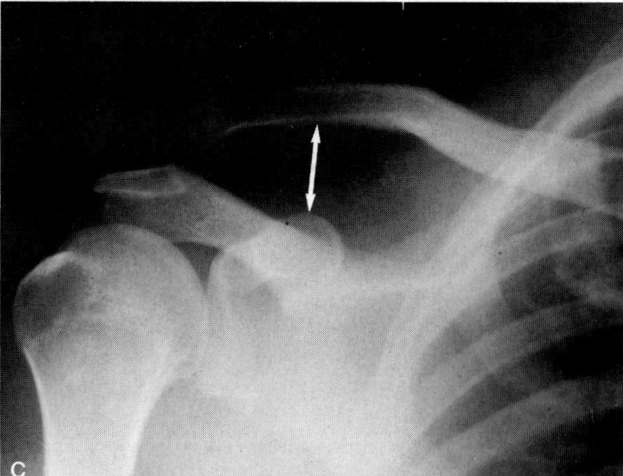

Figure 1–12E. Anterior-posterior view (a) of both shoulders on one plate, patient erect; weights are used on each wrist (b). Used with 25 lb. weights to show inferior instability (patient must relax the deltoid muscle). Used with 10 lb. weights (c) to show acromioclaviclar separation (comparing the coracoclavicular distance (arrow).

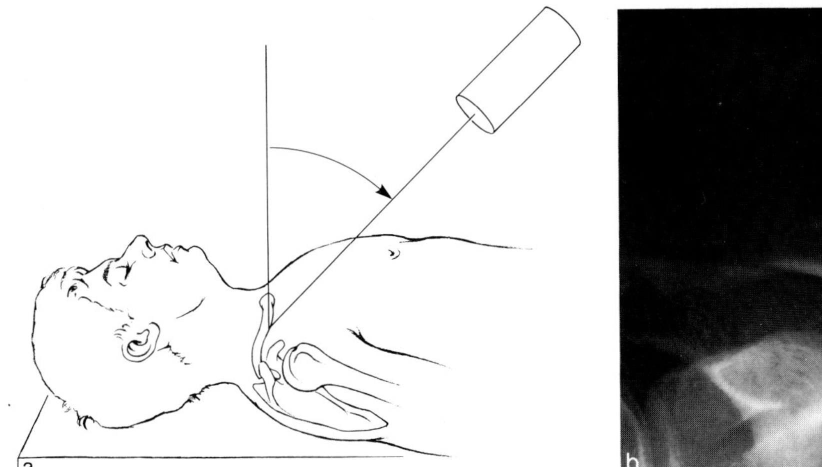

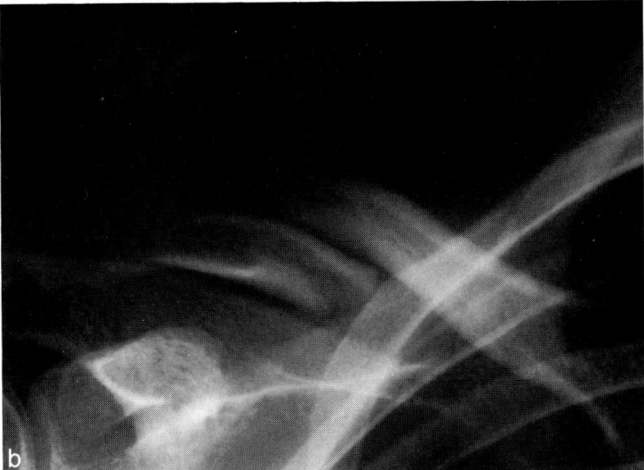

Figure 1–12F. Forty-five degree cephalic angle view of the clavicle (a). Used to show displacement fractures of the clavicle (b) and sternoclavicular dislocations (see Chapter 4).

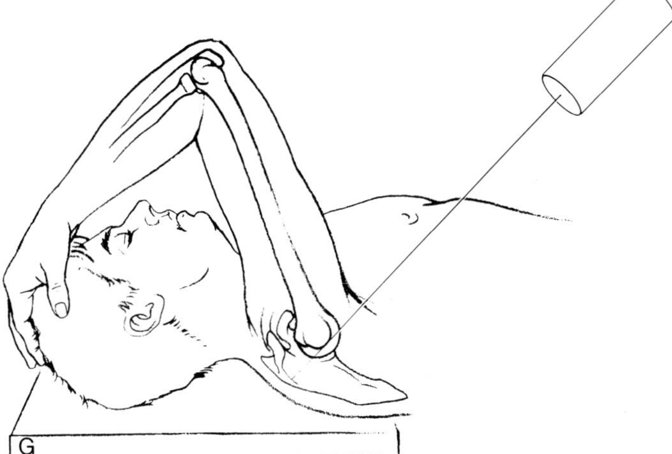

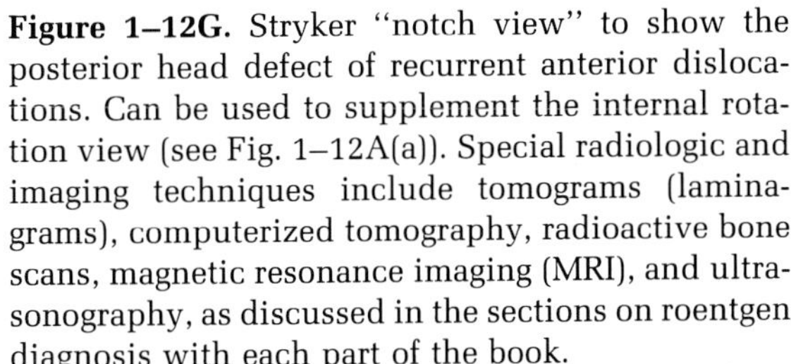

Figure 1–12G. Stryker "notch view" to show the posterior head defect of recurrent anterior dislocations. Can be used to supplement the internal rotation view (see Fig. 1–12A(a)). Special radiologic and imaging techniques include tomograms (laminagrams), computerized tomography, radioactive bone scans, magnetic resonance imaging (MRI), and ultrasonography, as discussed in the sections on roentgen diagnosis with each part of the book.

SCAPULOTHORACIC FUNCTION

There are two scapulothoracic functions: suspension and motion. In this section, they are considered separately.

Suspensory Mechanism

During most daily activities, whenever the body is erect, the *trapezius and levator scapulae* muscles must support the entire weight of the upper extremity (Fig. 1–13). These muscles are aided by the *clavicle*, which provides leverage and maintains the width of the shoulder. Loss of the clavicle makes the shoulder narrow and more subject to fatigue. The *coracoclavicular ligaments* are termed the "suspensory ligaments" because they are the main connection between the arm and the trunk.

The Coracoclavicular Ligaments

The coracoclavicular ligaments have an extensive attachment all along the undersurface of the distal clavicle from the coracoid tubercle to the acromioclavicular joint (see Fig. 1–24). They prevent the scapula from dropping and prevent posterior displacement of the clavicle. The ligaments and capsule of the acromioclavicular joint have a major role in stabilizing against anterior motion at the clavicle.[9] The glenohumeral and coracohumeral ligaments act to check against excessive external rotation, but they are normally loose when the arm is at the side and fail to maintain the humerus against the glenoid when the muscles lose tone (see Figs. 1–18 and 1–24). The supraspinatus and middle deltoid are aided by all of the long muscles crossing the glenohumeral joint in preventing downward displacement of the humerus on the scapula.

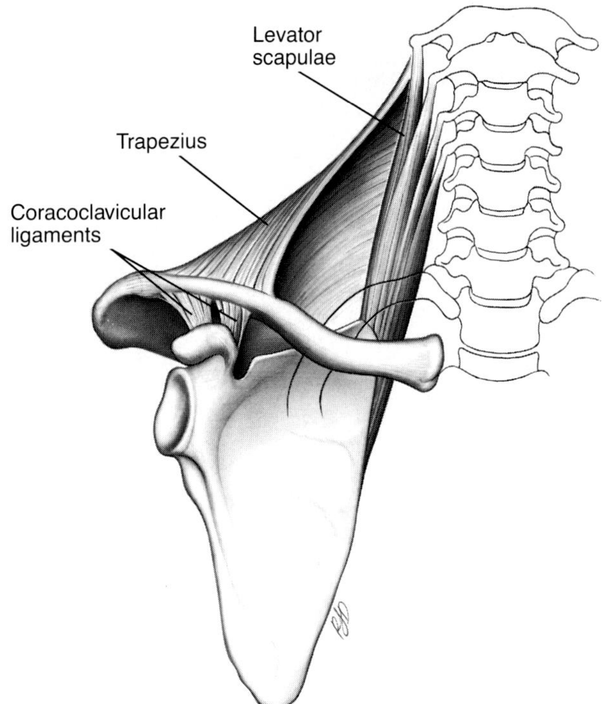

Figure 1–13. ***Suspensory Mechanism.*** The trapezius and levator scapulae muscles support the weight of the upper extremity whenever the body is erect. They are aided by the clavicle, providing leverage. Loss of the clavicle makes the shoulder subject to fatigue. The coracoclavicular ligaments are termed the "suspensory ligaments." They carry the weight of the upper extremity during most daily activities. They have an extensive attachment all along the undersurface of the distal clavicle from the coronoid tubercle to the capsule of the acromioclavicular joint. When these ligaments are disrupted, as in a complete acromioclavicular separation or when there is paralysis of the trapezius muscle, the scapula drops and its rotation becomes abnormal.

Several different types of pain may be seen after loss of the trapezius muscle or loss of the suspensory ligaments: (1) fatigue symptoms from the remaining scapular muscles, (2) infraclavicular plexus symptoms from the downward displacement of the coracoid, (3) subacromial impingement because of the faulty scapular rotation, and, in the case of acromioclavicular dislocations, (4) incongruity pain at the acromioclavicular joint.

When there is a complete disruption of the coracoclavicular ligaments, as in a Grade III acromioclavicular dislocation, the scapula drops. It is remarkable how well some patients function with old acromioclavicular dislocations; however, many have disabling symptoms.[10, 11, 199] Symptoms may be due to the scapula dropping with trapezius muscle fatigue, neurological traction symptoms, acromioclavicular incongruity, or impingement.[202] This is discussed further in Chapter 2 and Chapter 6. This potential impairment makes a strong case in favor of surgical repair of complete acromioclavicular dislocations in active patients. In resection of the distal clavicle, care is taken to preserve the acromioclavicular ligaments; otherwise, the scapula will drop, with the same threat of problems posed by a complete acromioclavicular dislocation as illustrated in Figure 1–14.

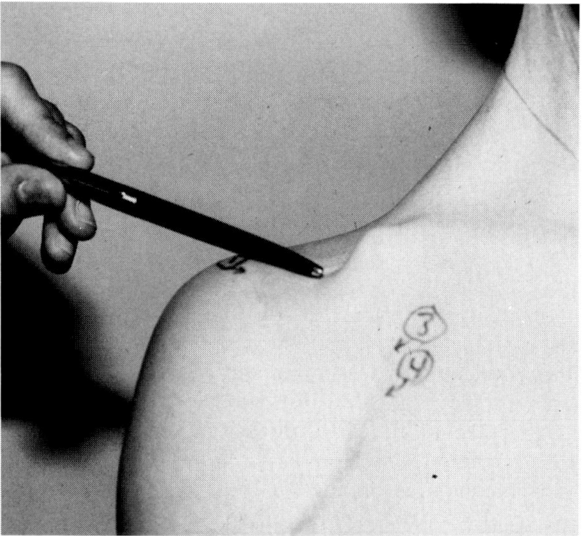

Figure 1–14. Patient seen after four failed procedures because of loss of the suspensory ligaments caused by the resection of too much distal clavicle. The incisional scars were numbered with a skin marker in order. There had been (1) attempt to relieve fatigue pain in the scapular muscles by neurolysis of the suprascapular nerve in its notch; (2) attempt to relieve incongruity pain by resecting more clavicle (which resulted only in more riding up of the clavicle); (3) attempt to compensate for the lost suspensory ligaments with Mercylene tape, which soon pulled loose, and (4) attempt to eliminate impingement symptoms by division of the coracoacromial ligament, which proved to be inadequate.

Restoration of normal anatomy by correcting the dropped scapula was thought to be the key to successful reconstruction. This was accomplished by at rebuilding the coracoacromial ligament by transfer of the coracoacromial ligament from the acromion to the clavicle (Dunne Weaver)[10] with reinforcement from part of the short head of the biceps (Vargas)[11] and with internal fixation with No. 5 nonabsorbable subcoracoid suture fixation. In addition, an anterior acromioplasty (see Chapter 2) was performed to further ensure relief of the impingement symptoms.

Sternoclavicular Joint

The sternoclavicular joint is very moveable. It allows at least 40 degrees angulation upward and downward as well as anteriorly and posteriorly; and, as shown in Figure 1–1, allows the clavicle to rotate 40 degrees in its long axis. Because of the strong connection of the coracoclavicular ligaments, clavicular rotation occurs with every scapular movement. Clavicular movements cannot be prevented by a cast. The sternoclavicular joint should never be transfixed with a pin, as is tempting in sternoclavicular dislocations, because breakage of the pin is almost certain to occur. Migration of a broken pin from this joint into the mediastinum has been known to be fatal.

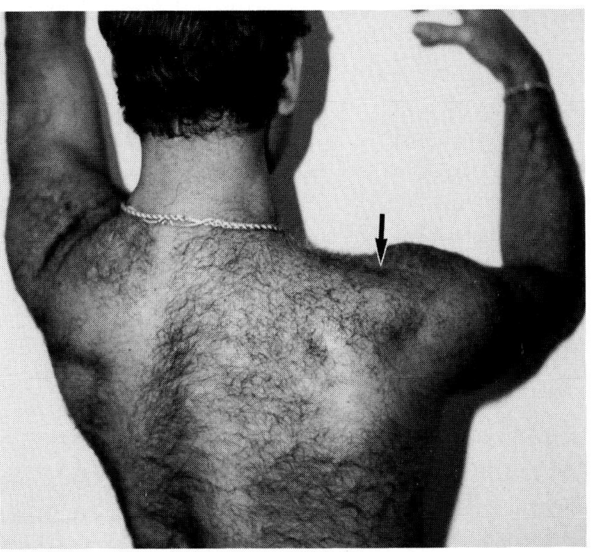

Figure 1–16. Trapezius muscle palsy. Patient with permanent trapezius muscle paralysis caused by division of the spinal accessory nerve during a lymph node biopsy. He was unable to raise the arm overhead, and in addition to some fatigue pain, had symptoms of subacromial impingement. Note how the acromion remains down (arrow), impinging against the humerus as the patient attempts to raise the arm.

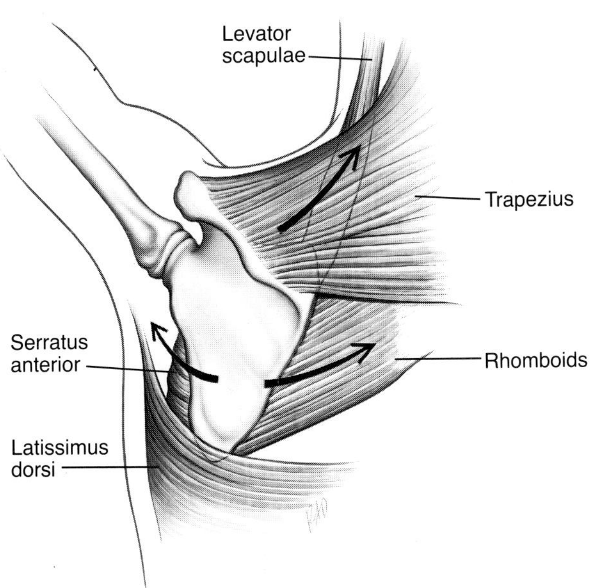

Figure 1–15. ***Scapulothoracic Movements.*** The scapula is rotated to receive the thrust of the humerus in a synergy involving the most complex muscle couplings imaginable. The upper trapezius with the levator scapulae lifts the scapula cephalad (as when lifting a suitcase), and this is done in coordination with the middle deltoid and supraspinatus. The lower trapezius acts with the rhomboids and latissimus dorsi in coordination with the posterior deltoid and teres major to pull backward. The key muscles in elevating the arm are the upper trapezius, rotating the scapula in the scapular plane into abduction; the serratus anterior, rotating the scapula forward; the anterior deltoid, raising the humerus; and the infraspinatus, externally rotating the humerus.

It is important to remember the scapular muscles become atrophied and require attention in the postoperative exercise program in patients with old injuries or long-standing arthritis of the glenohumeral joint.

Scapulothoracic Movements

Considering the movements of the scapula apart from those of its suspensory mechanism, the glenoid is rotated to receive the thrust of the humerus in synchrony with glenohumeral motion. This involves the most complex muscle couplings (Fig. 1–15). The trapezius muscle not only suspends the scapula but also is a key muscle in scapular rotation. The upper trapezius (with the levator scapula) lifts the scapula cephalad as when *lifting* a suitcase off the ground. This is done in coordination with the middle deltoid and supraspinatus. The lower trapezius acts (with the rhomboids and latissimus dorsi) in coordination with the posterior deltoid and teres major to *pull the arm backward.* The key muscles involved in *elevation* are the upper trapezius (which rotates the scapula in scapular plane abduction), the serratus anterior (which rotates the scapula forward), the anterior deltoid (which elevates the humerus), and the infraspinatus (which is the main external rotator of the humerus) (Figs. 1–15 and 1–16).

The scapula must be properly positioned and stabilized for effective glenohumeral movements. Loss of the spinal accessory nerve with paralysis of the trapezius muscle may cause subacromial impingement because of failure of lateral rotation of the scapula (see Fig. 2–7). Loss of the long thoracic nerve with paralysis of the serratus anterior limits active elevation and causes fatigue pain.

Patients with long-standing disability from arthritis or injury should be expected to have atrophy of the scapular muscles as well as of the rotator cuff and deltoid. For optimal results following reconstruction of long-standing shoulder problems, the surgeon should appreciate the need in the rehabilitation program for strengthening the scapular muscles in addition to those acting on the glenohumeral joint.

GLENOHUMERAL JOINT

There are three requirements for glenohumeral motion: a fulcrum (the humeral head and the glenoid), the rotator cuff, and the deltoid muscle. This discussion considers each separately.

Humeral Head and Glenoid

The importance of the humeral head and glenoid should be considered first. In 1951, after investigators completed a study of a group of patients in whom the humeral head had been removed for severe fractures or fracture-dislocations, the original prosthesis to replace the articular surface of the humeral head was designed.[12] The typical result of removal of the head was a weak, flail, unstable shoulder because there was no fulcrum for leverage. The shoulder was usually painful because of skeletal incongruity and muscle fatigue. In time, with fibrosis and scarring, a few patients became complacent after humeral head removal, but the majority of patients were permanently dissatisfied. The initial prosthesis was designed to restore a normal-sized, painless fulcrum for the muscles when the head had been destroyed by trauma. Replacement arthroplasty has now advanced to a point at which it supersedes "resection arthroplasty" and fusion for all types of destruction of the articular surfaces except infection, as discussed in Chapter 3.

Version at the Glenohumeral Joint

The contribution of proper version of the head and glenoid for the stability of the glenohumeral joint has received little careful consideration. Rotational osteotomy of the humerus or glenoid osteotomy aimed at eliminating recurrent glenohumeral dislocations by altering the version of the humerus alone (without concomitant capsular repair) has proved to be inadequate (Chapter 4). This is because in patients with recurrent dislocations the version of the humerus and glenoid is almost always within normal limits, and the problem is almost always in the ligaments and capsule. Altering version for the correction of instability is inappropriate except in the very rare shoulder with a true skeletal abnormality. On the other hand, in nonconstrained replacement arthroplasty the version of the components is of great importance for stability, especially because the ligaments and capsule are released without repair (Chapter 3).

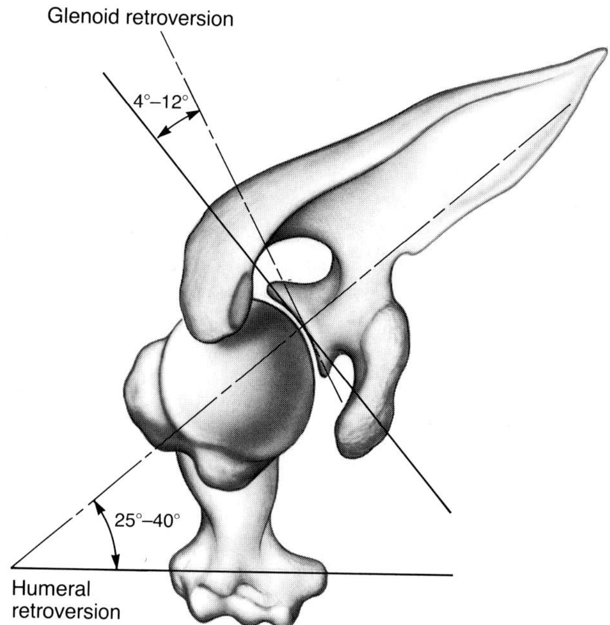

Figure 1–17. ***Humeral Head and Glenoid.*** With the arm held in the anatomical position, the humeral head is directed toward the scapula (in the scapular plane) in approximately 25 to 40 degrees retroversion. The articular surface of the glenoid normally has 4 to 12 degrees retroversion, is much smaller than the head, and its surface is flatter with a larger radius of curve. When the arm is raised, the glenoid rotates laterally and forward to receive the head.

Stability of the glenohumeral joint is dependent on four factors: (1) the glenohumeral ligaments functioning as check reins; (2) the capsule inhibiting dislocation by its volume; (3) the rotator cuff functioning as active ligaments, and; (4) the version and fulcrum action of the humeral head and glenoid.

Skeletal abnormalities are rarely of importance in treating recurrent dislocations (see Chapter 4); however, in nonconstrained glenohumeral arthroplasties the version of the head and glenoid become very important for stability. If the head is in excessive anteversion, anterior dislocation is prone to occur. If directed in excessive retroversion, posterior dislocation may occur. Uneven wear of the glenoid may, in effect, alter its version and cause instability.

The *normal version* at the glenohumeral joint is shown in Figure 1–17. With the arm held at the side in the anatomical position, the normal 25 to 40 degrees retroversion of the humeral head cause it to be directed toward the articular surface of the glenoid in the scapular plane. The normal articular surface of a glenoid has 4 to 12 degrees of retroversion. The surface area of the glenoid is much smaller, and its radius of curve is larger than that of the humeral head. The glenohumeral ligaments are normally loose. The ligaments act only as check reins. When the arm is elevated, the scapula rotates forward and upward to receive the full thrust of the head. If the head is directed in too much anteversion, anterior subluxation may occur. If the head is in too much retroversion, posterior subluxation may occur. Uneven wear of the glenoid, as in osteoarthritis and arthritis of dislocations, may also cause instability.

Forces on the Glenohumeral Joint

Although the glenohumeral joint is referred to as a "non–weight-bearing joint," surprisingly large *forces* are brought to bear upon it in everyday use. As discussed on page 2, accurate measurements are difficult to obtain because of the complex simultaneous movements of the scapula and humerus. The joint reaction force when the arm is held empty-handed out to the side in 90 degrees of abduction is estimated to be approximately 8.9 times body weight.[3–5] This force is greatly magnified if a weight is held in the hand or if a sudden movement occurs such as in lifting overhead, throwing, or pushing. The use of crutches or wheelchair transfers, as in paraplegics, causes the force to approximate that on the hip, and it can be magnified tremendously by impact loads such as falling.

There are three reasons why properly implanted, nonconstrained glenohumeral prostheses are capable of withstanding these loads. The surface of the glenoid is small and flat; the forces between it and the humeral head are largely compressive; and finally, the scapula "gives" with impact loads. Some shear force occurs, greatest when the angle between the humerus and the glenoid is between 30 and 60 degrees,[5] but clinically this is within the tolerance of a well-anchored glenoid component. Despite the large forces acting on the glenohumeral joint, the durability of a nonconstrained glenoid component has been remarkably good (see Chapter 3). However, constrained, fixed-fulcrum implants introduce abnormal shear and distraction forces beyond the tolerance of the frail scapula.

Glenohumeral Ligaments and Labrum

The glenohumeral ligaments are thickened bands in the anterior and inferior capsule. They are better seen from inside the joint than outside (Fig. 1–18).

The "Cleft"

At surgery when the capsule has been exposed from the front, there is an almost constant opening

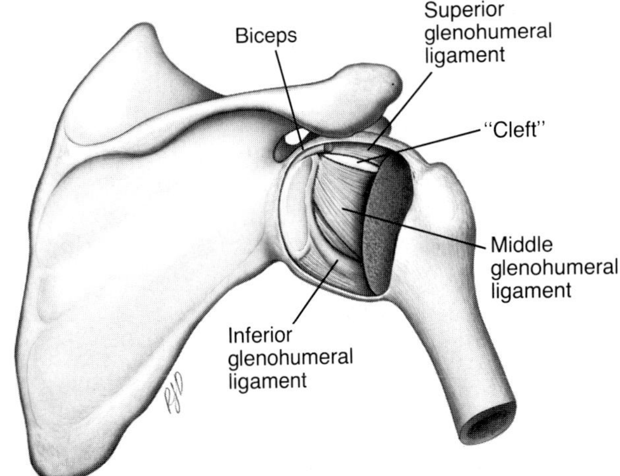

Figure 1–18. ***Glenohumeral Ligaments and "Cleft" (from behind).*** The inferior glenohumeral ligament is the largest and most important. Its medial attachment to the scapula forms the anterior glenoid labrum.[14] Therefore, it is logical when performing repairs for recurrent dislocations to re-attach the anterior labrum whenever it is found to be detached from the scapula.[15, 16]

The middle glenohumeral ligament is underdeveloped and deficient in approximately 10 percent of the population.[17, 18] Therefore, it is usually reinforced with half the thickness of the subscapularis tendon in repairs for multidirectional[13] and anterior dislocations.[14]

Between the superior and middle glenohumeral ligaments is an almost-constant opening through which dye passes to reach the subcoracoid bursa in an arthrogram. This opening we term the "cleft."[13] The cleft is often enlarged in patients with recurrent anterior and multidirectional subluxations and dislocations and is closed in the repairs for these conditions.

The superior glenohumeral ligament is a separate structure from the coracohumeral ligament. It is thin. It covers the long head of the biceps in the rotator interval (see Fig. 1–27).

The posterior labrum is formed by a continuum of the long head of the biceps, and since there are no ligaments posteriorly it is an unimportant structure in contrast to the anterior labrum. The posterior capsule is separated from it.

between the middle and superior glenohumeral ligaments, which is a useful guide. I term this the "cleft."[13] It is the normal communication between the subcoracoid bursa and the glenohumeral joint. It is the opening through which the dye in arthrograms enters the subcoracoid bursa beneath the coracoid. It may be enlarged and contribute to instability and is routinely closed in repairing recurrent anterior and multidirectional dislocations (see Chapter 4).

Inferior Glenohumeral Ligament and Anterior Labrum

The inferior glenohumeral ligament is the largest and most important of the three glenohumeral ligaments. As Professor J. C. Boileau Grant[14] of Toronto has shown, the *anterior labrum* is in fact the medial attachment of the inferior glenohumeral ligament (Fig. 1–18). Grant's observing the anterior labrum and inferior glenohumeral ligament to be one and the same clarifies the importance of reattaching the anterior labrum to the scapula, as described by Perthes[15] in 1906 and Bankart[16] in 1923, whenever it is found to be detached during a repair for recurrent anterior dislocation[15, 19] (see Chapter 4). Repair of the capsule and its ligaments is the most important consideration in surgery for recurrent dislocation.

Middle Glenohumeral Ligament

The middle glenohumeral ligament has been found to be underdeveloped or absent in about 20 percent of the specimens in anatomical studies.[17, 18] This deficiency can lead to recurrent anterior dislocations. For this reason, the middle glenohumeral ligament is routinely reinforced in the repair for anterior instability (see Chapter 4).

Superior Glenohumeral Ligament

The superior glenohumeral ligament is small and barely covers the long head of the biceps in the "rotator interval" (Figs. 1–18 and 1–27). In frozen shoulders (see Chapter 6) and arthritic shoulders (see Chapter 3), division of the coracohumeral ligament, which is a much more imposing structure than the superior glenohumeral ligament, is critical to the optimal success of releases. The anterior capsule and ligaments may also require release to restore external rotation.

Posterior Labrum

The *posterior labrum* is formed by a continuation of the attachment of the long head of the biceps and, in contrast to the anterior labrum, is of little significance in glenohumeral stability. There are no named ligaments posteriorly.

Rotator Cuff and Long Head of Biceps

The rotator cuff has three essential functions: stability, movement, and nutrition of the glenohumeral joint. In shoulder reconstruction, every effort is made to preserve or restore the cuff. No other joint has a similar second layer of muscles, and this is what makes shoulder surgery and its rehabilitation unique. The long head of the biceps assists in stabilizing the humeral head and is preserved whenever possible.

Rotator Cuff As a Stabilizer

Function of the rotator cuff as a stabilizer is summarized in Figure 1–19. The supraspinatus snubs up the humeral head to prevent its ascent when the deltoid contracts. With the arm raised, the teres minor and the inferior parts of the infraspinatus and subscapularis become "*depressors of the head*" acting to prevent its ascent.[30] This action is increased by the normal lateral rotation of the scapula. With the arm raised, the teres major and latissimus dorsi also become head depressors. The importance of the long head of the biceps as a stabilizer against upward excursion of the humeral head has too often been ignored. The *anterior stabilizers* against excessive external rotation that might lead to anterior dislocation are the subscapularis, latissimus dorsi, teres major, and pectoralis major, with the glenohumeral ligaments and capsule acting as check reins. *Posterior stabilizers* against excessive internal rotation and against posterior dislocation are few, consisting of only the infraspinatus and teres minor. *Inferior stabilizers* against inferior subluxation are primarily the supraspinatus and middle deltoid, aided in some degree by all of the other muscles crossing the joint.

Rotator Cuff in Glenohumeral Movement

Active external rotation is essential for use of the arm overhead or away from the side. There are many strong internal rotators outside the rotator cuff (the teres major, pectoralis major, and latissimus dorsi) capable of substituting for a weak subscapularis, but the only effective external rotators

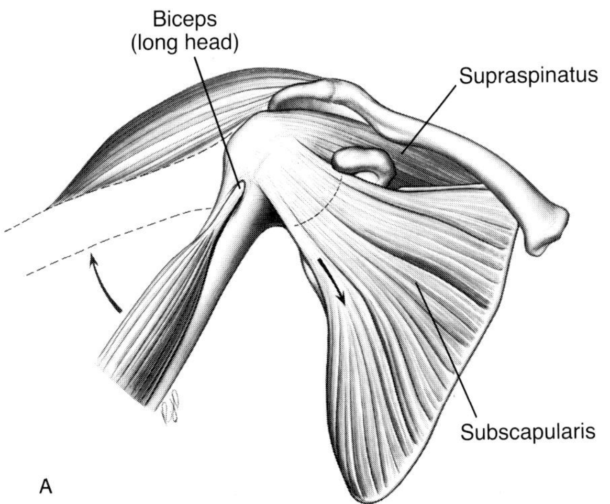

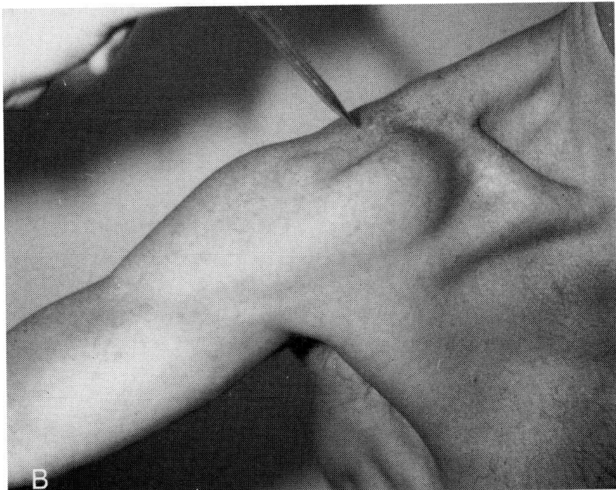

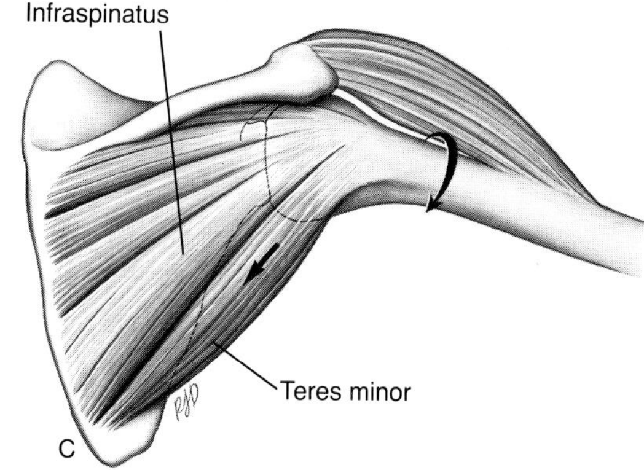

Figure 1–19. ***Rotator Cuff and Biceps in Glenohumeral Stability.*** To permit the large amount of motion normally present at the glenohumeral joint, its ligaments are loose in most positions. The rotator cuff functions as active ligaments to stabilize against subluxation or dislocation and against ascent of the head. The long head of the biceps assists in stabilizing the humerus.

When the arm is at the side, the head depressors against the ascent of the head, which would otherwise be caused by the contraction of the deltoid, are the supraspinatus and long head of the biceps. When the humerus is elevated, the lower part of the subscapularis, lower part of the infraspinatus, teres minor, and teres major act as head depressors *(A)*. This action is enhanced by scapular rotation, which improves the alignment of these muscles for preventing the head from riding up against the acromion. The latissimus dorsi and sternal head of pectoralis major also act as head depressors as the arm is raised *(B)*.

The anterior stabilizers against excessive external rotation and anterior dislocation are numerous. The subscapularis is augmented by a number of powerful muscles outside the rotator cuff, e.g., pectoralis major, teres major, and latissimus dorsi. The teres major is anatomically like the same muscle or is an extension of the subscapularis. It inserts just below it and has a similar origin and nerve supply.

The posterior stabilizers *(C)* are few, consisting of only the infraspinatus and teres minor. The infraspinatus is larger and supplies 90 per cent of the power. There are no muscles outside the rotator cuff to substitute when these muscles are nonfunctional.

Inferior stabilizers against downward displacement of the head are primarily the supraspinatus and middle deltoid augmented by the triceps, biceps, and coracobrachialis.

are rotator cuff muscles—the infraspinatus and teres minor. Of these, the infraspinatus contributes 90 per cent of external rotation power.

Consider the importance of *external rotation in overhead movement,* as seen in Figure 1–20. When the arm is raised, external rotation prevents impingement of the greater tuberosity against the acromion, provides more articular surface, and releases tension on the capsule. An injury with continuing upward movement of the arm without external rotation causes the greater tuberosity to lever against the acromion and is a common mechanism for producing an anterior dislocation.

Consider the importance of *external rotation when the arm is at the side.* Rotation of the humerus positions the hand where it can be used by bending or straightening the elbow. Rotation is the most used shoulder movement. The glenohumeral and elbow joints act as a functional unit (see p. 31). With the arm at the side, the shoulder can be rotated approximately 170 degrees, and virtually all of this is glenohumeral motion. When the infraspinatus has been detached or denervated, the hand cannot be held away from the side of the body, demonstrated by a positive "dropping sign," shown in Figure 1–21.

Figures 1–20 and 1–21. ***Rotator Cuff in Glenohumeral Movements.*** External rotation is essential for use of the hand overhead, as shown in Figure 1–20, and also for use at the side, as shown in Figure 1–21.

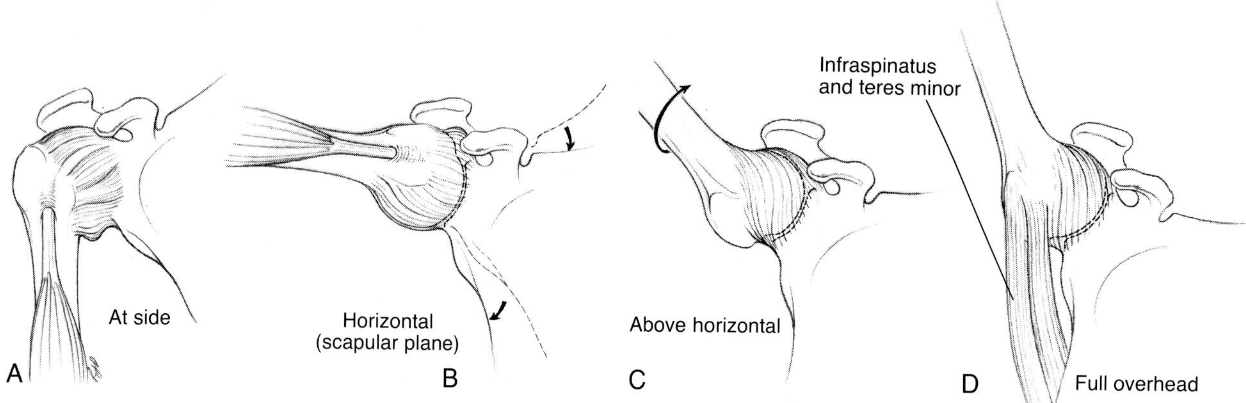

Figure 1–20. ***Role of the External Rotators in Use of the Hand Overhead.*** When the arm is at the side (A), the capsule is relaxed. At elevation to the horizontal (B), the inferior capsule becomes tight, all of the articular surface of the humeral head has been expended, and the greater tuberosity levers against the acromion. With external rotation (C), more articular surface is provided and the greater tuberosity is rotated away from the acromion so that the arm can be raised overhead (D). Raising the hand overhead is facilitated by scapular rotation, which points the acromion upward providing better clearance for the greater tuberosity and directs the glenoid to receive the force of the humeral head. These synergistic movements in raising the arm are centered on the scapular plane ("elevation") rather than on the coronal plane ("abduction"), as shown in Figures 1–1, 1–3, and 1–4.

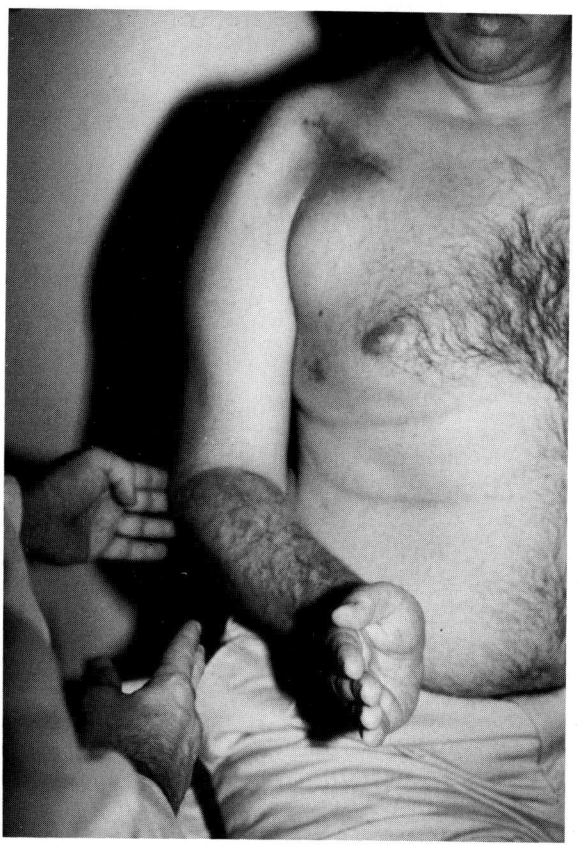

Figure 1–21. ***Role of the External Rotators in Use of the Hand Below the Horizontal.*** "Dropping sign" illustrates the role of the external rotators in use of the hand below the horizontal. With detachment or denervation of the infraspinatus, the hand cannot be moved or held away from the side of the body, as demonstrated in this patient, who has a massive cuff tear. This sign is elicited with the patient sitting. The examiner supports the foream and hand in the externally rotated position with the elbow bent 90 degrees and instructs the patient to maintain this position after he lets go at the wrist. If the infraspinatus is nonfunctioning, the arm falls against the side of the body despite efforts of the patient to the contrary. The patient shown had a nonunion of the greater tuberosity that rendered the infraspinatus and teres minor nonfunctional following a gunshot wound. This sign is useful in evaluating the size of a tear of the rotator (see Fig. 2–32C) or the severity of a paralytic problem. It demonstrates the importance of the external rotators in the use of the arm below the horizontal. Without the infraspinatus and the teres minor, the use of the hand in front (as in inserting a key) and reaching to the side (as in paying a toll) becomes impossible. The lack of stability of the arm makes such simple activities as writing difficult. The main function of the glenohumeral joint in daily activities is to provide rotation. This positions the hand.

Rotator Cuff in Nutrition of Articular Surfaces

The importance of the rotator cuff in the nutrition of the articular surfaces of the glenohumeral joint has only recently been appreciated.[20–25] Large tears with instability can lead to cuff-tear arthropathy with atrophy of the articular cartilage; fragmentation of the subchondral bone; and eventually, complete destruction of the joint surfaces, as discussed on page 124, Chapter 2. This phenomenon is seen only in the glenohumeral joint because of the unique anatomical arrangement of the rotator cuff.

Synergy Between Biceps and Rotator Cuff

The long head of the biceps assists the rotator cuff in stabilizing the humeral head against riding upward (Fig. 1–22). Clinically, as reported to the American Academy of Orthopaedic Surgeons in 1977,[26, 27] the long head of the biceps is observed to be important in its action against subacromial impingement. It should be preserved during shoulder surgery whenever possible. A thoughtless tenodesis of the long head destroys its function as a head depressor and may precipitate or escalate an impingement problem. Transfer of the long head to the coracoid is even less desirable than tenodesis to the humerus. This not only causes loss of its stabilizing effect against ascent of the humerus, but also causes the long head to pull the humerus upward, further intensifying impingement. The pathomechanics of biceps lesions is discussed further in Chapter 2, pages 50, 70, 84, 91, and 134.

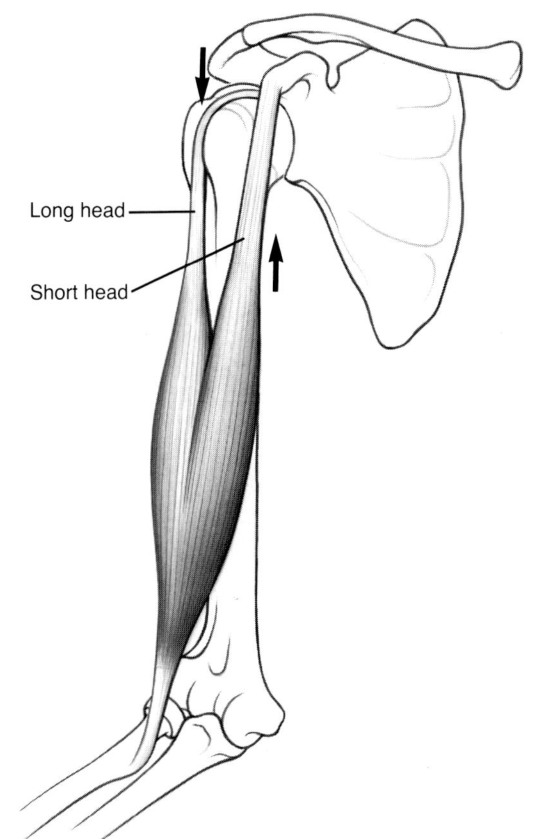

Figure 1–22. ***The Dual Action of the Long Head of the Biceps.*** The long head of the biceps stabilizes and acts against ascent of the head of the humerus. When the patient lifts a heavy object, the dual action of the long head becomes apparent. It stabilizes the humeral head against ascent and at the same time bends the elbow. Tenodesis of the long head removes this action at the shoulder and may escalate an impingement problem. Transfer of the long head to the coracoid process, as has been advocated by some surgeons, makes the long head function like the short head and, by pulling the humeral head upward, may further escalate impingement.

Deltoid Muscle

The deltoid muscle is the prime mover of the glenohumeral joint. It has three parts: anterior, middle, and posterior. The latissimus dorsi extends the shoulder and can substitute for loss of the posterior deltoid, but there are no muscles to substitute for loss of either the middle or the anterior deltoid muscle. Surgical approaches should spare the origins of the anterior and middle deltoid. Detachment, even if carefully repaired, causes a peculiar atrophy and weakness of the portion involved.

In regard to the *anterior deltoid*, because the arm is used in front of the body more than at the side, the anterior part of the deltoid is the most important part in everyday activities. As shown in Figures 1–1, 1–20, and 1–21, the external rotators (infraspinatus and teres minor) are essential for overhead elevation as well as for use of the arm at the side. Because there are no other muscles capable of substituting for either the anterior deltoid or the infraspinatus, they are the key muscles in glenohumeral reconstruction (Fig. 1–23). They must be spared in approaches,[22, 27–29] as shown in Figure 1–26. If damaged, they must be repaired whenever possible.

The *middle deltoid* acts in unison with the supraspinatus.[3] However, if the middle deltoid is nonfunctioning, the supraspinatus is inadequate to substitute for raising the arm. Radical acromionectomy, in which the attachment for the origin of the middle deltoid is removed, causes a devastating

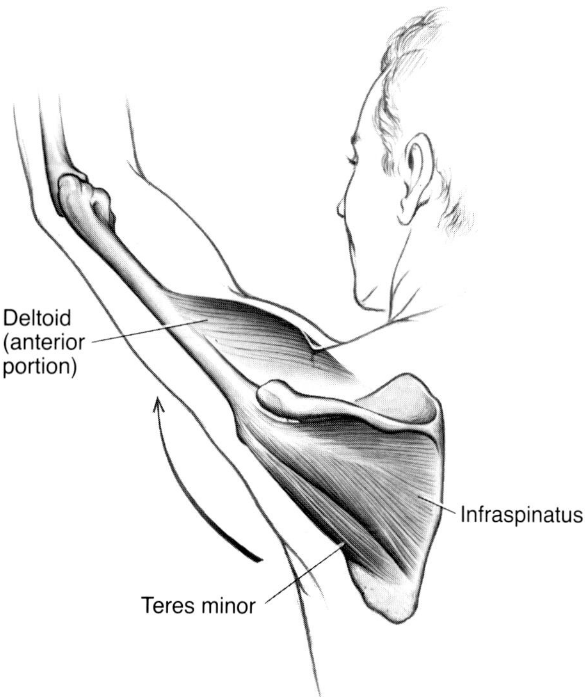

Figure 1–23. The anterior deltoid and infraspinatus are the key muscles in glenohumeral reconstruction. The arm is used in front of the body more than at the side, so these muscles are the most often used in everyday activities. There are no other muscles capable of substituting for them. They must be spared in approaches, and if damaged, they must be repaired.

In the past, the supraspinatus and middle deltoid have been accorded more importance and received the emphasis; but, as shown in Figures 1–20 and 1–21, the external rotators and anterior deltoid are more important in everyday activities.

disability and should be forever abandoned[29] (see Chapter 2, pp. 122–124, Fig. 2–46).

When the deltoid has been detached or denervated by injury or surgery, *deltoidplasty* has, to date, been inadequate. Transfer of the pectoralis, either one or both heads, has failed. The posterior deltoid origin can be shifted to a more anterior position to restore anterior deltoid function if the latissimus dorsi is intact to give power for extension. However, this has also been inadequate to raise the arm. There is current interest in transfer of the latissimus dorsi for loss of the anterior deltoid. This has not been used enough for adequate clinical assessment. In considering this procedure, however, it is important for the patient to know that transfer of the latissimus, when the posterior deltoid is nonfunctioning, would take away all power for extending the shoulder or pulling.

Subacromial Mechanism and Bursa

The subacromial space has been considered by some investigators as a fifth joint space.[1] It is nearly as large as the knee joint. It is lined by the subacromial and subdeltoid bursae. The *subacromial space may be encroached upon in many different ways.* The bursa can be thickened by chemical irritation, as from a calcium deposit (see Chapter 6); by the hemorrhage and fibrosis of trauma; or by inflammation and disease. The most common cause of subacromial impingement is some variation in the shape or slope of the acromion or acromioclavicular joint,[27, 28] which causes narrowing of the "supraspinatus outlet,"[32] discussed in Chapter 2. Less frequent ("nonoutlet") causes of subacromial impingement are listed in Table 2–1 and are discussed further in Chapter 2, p. 48; they include: loss of "head depressors" (such as in rupture of the rotator cuff or long head of the biceps), upward displacement of the greater tuberosity because of loss of the "spacer" effect of the articular surfaces of the humeral head or glenoid (as in rheumatoids) (see Chapter 3), prominence of the greater tuberosity (as in a malunion of a fracture of the proximal humerus) (Chapter 5), abnormalities of the acromion (as from old fractures (Chapter 5) or an unfused epiphysis) (Chapter 2), and loss of the suspensory mechanism (Chapter 2, Chapter 4, Chapter 5, and Chapter 6). It is important to understand each of these causes of subacromial impingement because the surgical treatment differs according to the cause. The restoration of this space is a basic step in many different types of shoulder reconstruction.

Three Coracoid Ligaments

There are three major ligaments attaching to the coracoid that are of surgical importance (Fig. 1–24). The coracoacromial ligament is important in subacromial impingement. The coracohumeral ligament has heretofore been overlooked as important in surgical releases of the glenohumeral joint or mobilization of a torn rotator cuff. The importance of the coracoclavicular ligament as the "suspensory ligament" is discussed in Chapter 4 and Chapter 6. It is responsible for supporting the weight of the upper extremity, for congruity of the acromioclavicular joint, and for the proper rotation of the scapula.

Because the *coracoacromial ligament* (Fig. 1–24) connects two prominences of the scapula and

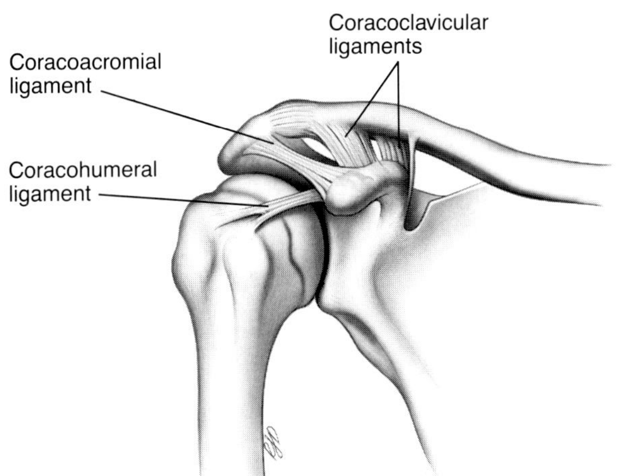

Figure 1–24. ***Three Coracoid Ligaments.*** There are three major ligaments attaching to the coracoid that are of surgical importance. The function of the coracoacromial ligament has long been disputed. Understanding anterior acromial spurs as traction spurs (see pp. 46 and 47, Chapter 2) has clarified the function of this ligament. It is resected only when there is good reason, and at times it is re-attached in acromioplasties.

does not bridge a joint, many surgeons have labeled it useless and expendable. A surgical cliché of the past has been: "Whenever you can see the coracoacromial ligament, it should be divided." It must be wrong to divide it without good reason. Anterior acromial spurs that form within this ligament in many impingement lesions are now understood to be traction spurs caused by the humerus striking against this ligament.[27, 28] This proves that the ligament functions as a buffer. When the depressor muscles (see p. 26) are weak, as in rheumatoid arthritis, a special effort is made to preserve the coracoacromial ligament (Chapter 3) to retain its buffering action. When there is chronic impingement from an overhanging acromion, this ligament is detached because the bone on the undersurface of the acromion where it attaches is excised in an anterior acromioplasty (Chapter 2). However, in the rarely indicated acromioplasty in a rheumatoid, the coracoacromial ligament is re-attached after the acromioplasty (Chapter 3).

The *coracohumeral ligament* (Fig. 1–24) is a more significant structure in shoulder reconstruction than has generally been appreciated. Its release is a key step in many procedures. It normally tightens when the shoulder is externally rotated and relaxes when the shoulder is internally rotated. If chronic pain causes the shoulder to be held against the side of the chest to splint the arm against painful movements, in internal rotation (the "protected position"), the coracohumeral ligament becomes permanently contracted. This structure usually requires division in an open release for frozen shoulder (see Chapter 6) and during glenohumeral arthroplasties (see Chapter 3) to restore external rotation. Its division for mobilizing the rotator cuff is described on page 111, Figure 2–43G, Chapter 2.

The *coracoclavicular ligaments* have an extensive attachment on the undersurface of the clavicle extending from the coronoid tuberosity to the acromioclavicular joint capsule. These ligaments are responsible for supporting the weight of the upper extremity (preventing fatigue symptoms or infraclavicular plexus traction symptoms), for preserving the congruity of the acromioclavicular joint against upward or posterior displacement of the clavicle,[9] for preventing acromioclavicular joint symptoms, and for proper rotation of the scapula during overhead use (preventing impingement symptoms), as discussed on page 52, Chapter 2; and in Chapter 4, pages 343 to 355.

THE UPPER EXTREMITY UNIT

The dual role of the biceps, as shown in Figure 1–22, illustrates how their functions are so closely related. The shoulder and elbow form a functional unit. Shoulder rotation and elbow flexion and extension act together to place the hand where it is needed in both heavy and light activities. These joints act in unison for throwing, pushing, lifting, reaching the face, and virtually every upper extremity movement. Decisions regarding the indications and priorities for shoulder arthroplasties cannot be made without knowing the condition of the elbow joint. Both joints may be involved in conditions such as rheumatoid arthritis, paralysis, and trauma. It is quite logical that a new specialty organization has been formed—The American Shoulder and Elbow Surgeons—to consider these two joints together.

Chronic shoulder pain, as in rheumatoid arthritis, may have an adverse effect on the entire "upper extremity unit."[21, 39] The patient guards against movement of a painful shoulder by holding the arm closely to the side in a position of internal rotation and adduction, with the elbow flexed. Gravity tends to pull the wrist and hand toward ulnar deviation. Actually, this "protective position" (to splint the shoulder against painful movements) influences the entire length of the extremity from the scapula to the fingertips. The flexed elbow eventually develops a flexion contracture. The hand develops contractures with attenuation for ulnar drift, stiffness, and vasomotor instability. This has been referred to as the "shoulder-hand syndrome." In addition, glenohumeral splinting often causes strain and fatigue of the scapular muscles with scapular pain and eventually disuse atrophy of these muscles (Chapter 3 and Chapter 6). Relief of glenohumeral pain, by either nonoperative or surgical means, often has a beneficial effect on the entire upper extremity, including the scapular region, elbow, and hand. For this reason, the shoulder lesion should usually have first priority when multiple joints in the upper extremity are involved equally and are being considered for arthroplasty (Chapter 3).

SHOULDER MOTION NECESSARY FOR FUNCTION

The amount of active motion and strength necessary for "adequate function" depends upon the normal activities of the patient and varies tremendously, ranging from the perfection of a high performance athlete to the simple objective of personal care and hygiene needed for independent daily self-care sought by a severe rheumatoid. The condition of the elbow influences the range of active shoulder motion needed. In this discussion, normal elbow function is assumed.

Active patients with normal elbows and good strength usually have full function if active elevation is 150 degrees, external rotation is 50 degrees, and internal rotation is to T8. This amount of motion permits such activities as high level tennis and most other sports, with the exception of baseball pitching, javelin throwing, and perhaps one or two less common sports requiring full external rotation for optimal throwing performance (see Chapter 6). In the criteria for rating the results of a shoulder arthroplasty (Chapter 3), a patient with an "excellent" rating is required to have at least 135 degrees active elevation and near-normal rotation and strength. This amount of motion implies essential function.

The cutoff between a "satisfactory" and an "unsatisfactory" rating for a shoulder arthroplasty is 90 degrees active elevation and 20 degrees active external rotation. This is the active range required for reaching the top of the head and for grooming the hair. Active external rotation beyond neutral is necessary to raise the hand above the eyebrows, as explained in Figure 1–20.

When there has been severe bone loss, inadequate rotator cuff, and/or deltoid deficiency, as in severe rheumatoid arthritis, cuff-tear arthropathy, and some old injuries, "limited goals" rehabilitation is usually employed post-operatively. This is aimed at less motion and more stability (see Chapters 3 and 7). The surgeon makes the decision as to the type of rehabilitation program based on the amount of tissue loss encountered at surgery. The activities for self-care, e.g., reaching the mouth, opposite armpit, and anal region, can be achieved with only neutral external rotation and a few degrees of active elevation. Even with the most massive rotator cuff tears, the pectoralis major, teres major, and latissimus dorsi remain to give internal rotation and extension. If surgery accomplishes only a few degrees of active elevation and external rotation and relief of pain, the patient will have gained independent self-care and comfort. These patients are extremely grateful for this improvement.

PRINCIPLES OF SHOULDER INCISIONS

A good scar is important. No scar in orthopaedic surgery is more noticed by the patient than one on the front of the shoulder. Men notice it each time they shave, and women are much more upset by an ugly scar on the shoulder than by one on the hip, knee, or trunk. Beyond appearance, patients see an unsightly scar as a reflection of the quality of the surgery beneath it. This can affect their attitude during the rehabilitation period. Continuous subcuticular pullout closure is used to avoid the crossmarks of interrupted skin. Buried subcutaneous sutures are avoided because they often cause a reaction that is apparently due to the large excursion of motion of the shoulder.

The incision should follow the *tension lines* of the skin (Langer's lines), but this is not always practical because of the location of the sensory nerves. Skin incisions are placed between *zones of sensory nerve distribution,* to avoid areas of hypesthesia and traumatic neuromas (Fig. 1–25). The three supraclavicular nerves supply a very large area of skin over the pectoralis and anterior deltoid as well as on the top of the shoulder. The axillary nerve supplies the skin over the middle deltoid. The posterior rami of the spinal nerves C3–C4 and T2 through T7 supply the skin over the trapezius muscle and scapula. The incisions described in this book are placed between these sensory zones but also follow the skin lines as closely as possible.

The blood supply to the skin in the shoulder region is especially good. Skin flaps remain viable even with extensive undermining, provided it is performed just superficial to the muscles, at the level of the deep fascia, leaving thick flaps. This makes it possible to perform extensive surgical procedures on the glenohumeral joint through a relatively small skin incision, such as the anterior axillary incision, which is undermined all the way up to the clavicle in repair of anterior dislocations (see Chapter 4).

Because the glenohumeral joint is so moveable,

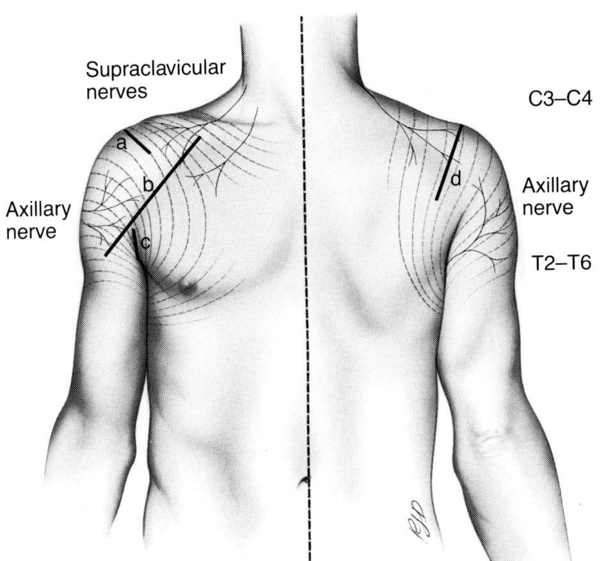

Figure 1–25. ***Skin Incisions.*** Because the glenohumeral joint is so moveable, small incisions provide a lot of exposure provided that the humerus is positioned properly (Rule 3, p. 34). The incisions follow Langer's lines for a thinner scar, are placed between the zones of the sensory nerves to avoid numbness or neuromas, and are closed with removable subcuticular sutures to avoid the cross-matching caused by interrupted sutures and staples. Shown are the incisions for (a) anterior acromioplasty and cuff repair; (b) arthroplasties and most open reductions (extended deltopectoral approach); (c) repair of recurrent anterior dislocations; and (d) the posterior approach to the glenohumeral joint in which a vertical skin incision is preferred.

the tuberosities and cuff can be reached through small openings in the deltoid, as in the anterior deltoid-split or anterior acromioplasty approach, provided that the humerus is rotated in proper position to give the exposure desired.

Special pre-operative skin preparation is used before shoulder surgery. Skin appears to be the most important source of *bacterial contamination* during surgery in this region. The level of the bacterial count of the skin at the axilla is second only to that of the groin. Acne and other skin blemishes are frequently present at the shoulder in young patients. Inflamed acne in the region of the incision must be under control before the procedure. Prior to entering the hospital for elective shoulder surgery, patients apply antiseptic soap to their shoulder and axilla during showers. In fracture patients, a bulky pad in the axilla is changed daily to avoid maceration of the skin.

Regarding *old scars* in patients who have had previous surgery, because the appearance of scars on the shoulder is important to these patients, every effort should be made to excise, undermine, or extend previous scars rather than create new scars.

Incisions in young patients almost invariably become wider, whereas those in old patients remain hairline. The wide scar in the young is more gracefully accepted when patients and parents have been warned pre-operatively to expect it.

PRINCIPLES OF APPROACHES TO THE GLENOHUMERAL JOINT

Principles of the surgical approaches to the glenohumeral joint, illustrated in Figure 1–26, should be briefly summarized.

1. ***Preserve the origin of the anterior and middle deltoid.*** Detachment of the posterior deltoid is tolerated because the latissimus dorsi is a strong extensor and can compensate for residual weakness of this part of the deltoid muscle. However, there are no muscles to compensate for weakening of the anterior and middle parts of the deltoid.

This principle differs from most existing anatomical texts on surgical approaches. The anatomists see that all of the origin of the deltoid can be detached without encountering a single significant structure, and this certainly gives extensive exposure. Unfortunately, however, the deltoid muscle has a peculiar intolerance to detachment of its origin and is weakened and permanently impaired by this approach. It shrivels and never regains full strength even if meticulously re-attached.

Detachment of the middle deltoid origin, as in the "saber approach" and lateral acromionectomy approach, has been widely used despite adverse effect. These approaches cause loss of strength, retractions of the middle deltoid, a high incidence of joint sinuses, and other wound complications. Wound complications and residual impingement following saber approaches and acromionectomies have done much to prejudice surgeons against repairing tears of the rotator cuff. These approaches have been replaced by the anterior acromioplasty approach,[27–29] which preserves nearly all of the deltoid origin, provides better decompression of the subacromial space, and has dramatically improved results, as discussed on pages 96 to 106, Chapter 2.

Detachment of the anterior deltoid origin has been an error in shoulder surgery repeated for many years in the approaches for replacement arthroplasties and open reduction of fractures. The detrimental effect on the deltoid was obvious; therefore, superior approaches (from above) and posterior approaches were tried in an effort to avoid weakening the anterior deltoid (see below and Chapter 3, p. 171). It was not until 1977 that

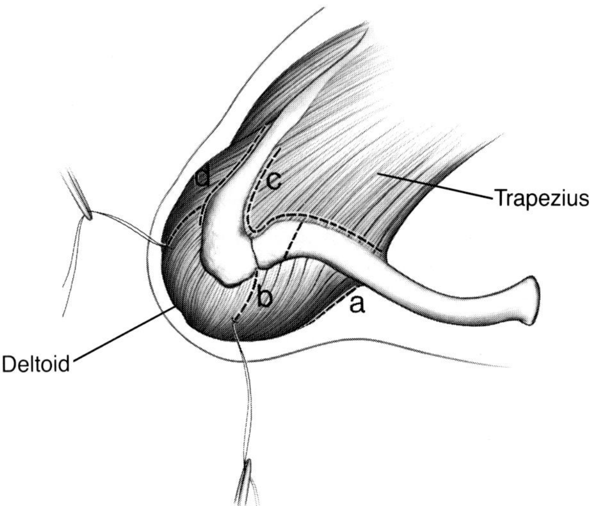

Figure 1–26. ***Approaches to the Glenohumeral Joint Spare the Origins of the Anterior and Middle Deltoid.***

(a) The "extended deltopectoral approach" used for arthroplasties and fractures. A small part of the anterior insertion of the deltoid may be elevated or detached if necessary to prevent injury to the muscle from retraction, but all of the origin of the deltoid is preserved (see p. 171, Fig. 3–25, Chapter 3).

(b) The anterior acromioplasty approach used for impingement lesions and tears of the rotator cuff. Not more than 1.0 cm. of deltoid origin is detached from the acromion as a flap of tendinous origin is elevated intact from the acromion to facilitate a strong repair of this small defect. If more exposure of the distal clavicle is needed, the capsule of the acromioclavicular joint is divided, leaving deltoid origin attached to the capsule (see p. 101, Fig. 2–41D, Chapter 2).

(c) Extension of the anterior acromioplasty approach through the acromioclavicular joint with detachment of the trapezius (and, if necessary, posterior deltoid) for mobilizing massive tears of the rotator cuff. The deltoid origin and trapezius insertion are left attached to the acromioclavicular joint capsule so that these structures can be sutured together for a strong repair (see p. 103, Fig. 2–41H, Chapter 2; and p. 435, Fig. 6–8C, Chapter 2).

(d) Detachment of the origin of the posterior deltoid is better tolerated because the latissimus dorsi compensates for residual weakness of this part of the deltoid, as for repair of posterior glenohumeral dislocation (see Chapter 4).

the long or "extended" deltopectoral approach was developed.[22] In this approach, a small part of the insertion of the deltoid may be elevated or temporarily detached if necessary to prevent injury to the muscle from excessive retraction (see p. 171), but all of the origin of the deltoid is preserved. It has made a tremendous improvement in the ease of rehabilitation and recovery of strength following shoulder arthroplasties.

In the repair of recurrent anterior dislocations (see Chapter 4), the full length of the deltopectoral interval is developed through a short skin incision placed in the anterior axillary skin creases, as described by Leslie and Ryan.[31]

2. ***Preserve the infraspinatus.*** There are many strong internal rotators to compensate for a weak subscapularis, but no muscle exists to substitute for the infraspinatus. The teres minor is too small. The infraspinatus provides 90 percent of the power for external rotation, and, as explained in Figures 1–20 and 1–21, external rotation is critical for many shoulder activities. This muscle is maintained intact or restored whenever possible.

The suprascapular nerve entering the infraspinatus from above and the axillary nerve entering the teres minor from below make the interval between these two muscles a safe and preferred route for posterior approaches to the glenohumeral joint (see Fig. 1–32). The infraspinatus is detached in only a few circumstances, such as when the capsule is attenuated and needs reinforcement in repair of multidirectional or recurrent posterior glenohumeral dislocations (see Chapter 4). If detached, it is carefully repaired and is given special attention later in the exercise program.

In the early 1970s, a posterior approach was tried for glenohumeral arthroplasty in an effort to avoid injury to the anterior deltoid (see p. 171). This approach was unsatisfactory for three reasons: exposure is obstructed by the overhanging posterior acromion; release of the soft tissue in front for the correction of an internal rotation contracture is extremely hazardous; and thirdly, it detaches the important infraspinatus tendon unnecessarily.

3. ***Rotate the humerus into the wound for exposure.*** The large amount of motion at the glenohumeral joint makes it possible to get adequate exposure for many procedures through small openings provided that the arm is positioned to bring the desired structures into the wound. For example, through the anterior acromioplasty approach, the subscapularis tendon is seen if the shoulder is held in a flexed and externally rotated position, the infraspinatus and teres minor tendons are seen if the arm is extended and internally rotated, and the supraspinatus tendon is best seen if the arm is held in neutral rotation.

4. ***Rotator interval is preferred for entering the joint.*** The "rotator interval," as described in Figure 1–27 and discussed further on page 35 is the usual route for entering the glenohumeral joint. There are no tendons in this location to be damaged, and the coracohumeral ligament is readily available for release as indicated. The long head of the biceps is a guide during surgery to the location of this interval.

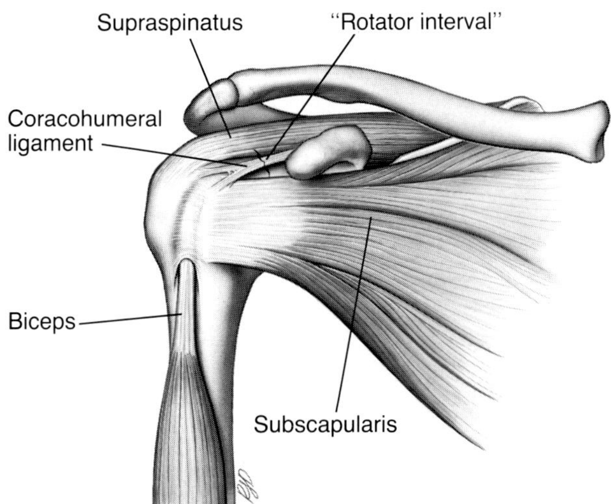

Figure 1–27. The "rotator interval" is a term introduced in 1970[8] to indicate the space between the supraspinatus and subscapularis tendons. The coracohumeral ligament lies superficially along its anterior edge, where it is readily available for release as indicated. The long head of the biceps lies deep along its posterior edge and serves as a guide to this interval during surgery.

5. ***Release coracohumeral ligament and lengthen subscapularis if tight.*** Restoring external rotation is critical for overhead function, and release of these structures will be referred to in connection with many procedures.

6. ***Anterior acromioplasty if impingement due to the contour of acromion or acromioclavicular joint is present.*** An adequate space for the supraspinatus tendon should be made by *anterior acromioplasty* whenever dictated by the shape or slope of the acromion or undersurface of the acromioclavicular joint or by evidence of subacromial impingement (see Chapter 2). This removes prominences on the undersurface of the anterior acromion and acromioclavicular joint to enlarge the "supraspinatus outlet"[32] (see p. 96). Radical acromionectomy is never performed. Resection of the undersurface of the acromioclavicular joint (leaving the superficial surface intact) preserves a significant amount of anterior deltoid origin and is preferred to complete resection of the distal clavicle except when there is painful arthritis of the acromioclavicular joint or if more exposure of the supraspinatus is needed.

7. ***Distal clavicle excision if acromioclavicular arthritis or exposure is needed.*** There are two indications for excision of the distal clavicle. The first is painful arthritis of the acromioclavicular joint. This can spoil the result of a perfect arthroplasty or cuff repair. The determination as to whether this joint is sufficiently symptomatic to require excision must be made pre-operatively by examination or by lidocaine (Xylocaine) injection. The second indication—when more exposure of the supraspinatus is needed—usually applies to massive cuff repairs. As shown in Figure 1–27, resection of the acromioclavicular joint and detachment of the trapezius insertion offer unlimited additional exposure of the supraspinatus without deltoid detachment[28, 29] (see Chapter 2).

"ROTATOR INTERVAL"

The term "rotator interval" was first introduced in 1970 in describing the pathology of displaced proximal humeral fractures.[8] The rotator interval (Fig. 1–27) is formed by the coracoid process projecting between the subscapularis and supraspinatus tendons creating an interval in the rotator cuff where there is no tendon. As stated previously in Principle 4, this is the preferred site for opening the glenohumeral joint because no rotator cuff tendon is divided and good exposure of the whole interior of the joint is obtained when it is opened its full length. In displaced fractures, the rotator interval is often torn, at least in part, as the greater and lesser tuberosities retract. The long head of the biceps is an excellent guide to this interval.

The coracohumeral ligament lies along the anterior edge of the rotator interval. In frozen or arthritic shoulders, old tears of the rotator cuff, and old fractures, this ligament becomes shortened and limits external rotation. Release of it is almost always an important step in surgery for these conditions. It is readily available for release if the rotator interval route is used in entering the joint, mobilizing frozen and arthritic shoulders, and freeing up the subscapularis and supraspinatus tendons when repairing tears of the rotator cuff.

AVOIDING NERVE INJURIES

Nerve injuries are especially threatening during shoulder reconstruction and are constantly in mind. Some practical points in positioning the patient and in the approaches are shown in Figures 1–28 through 1–33.

In *positioning the patient*, as shown in Figure 1–28, care is taken to support the head to prevent hyperextension of the neck. Those with degenerative or arthritic lesions of the shoulder usually have changes in the cervical spine as well. Compression of the cervical roots is easily produced by prolonged hyperextension or tilting of the neck. To avoid this, the head is taped on the headrest securely in the "military position" with the chin in

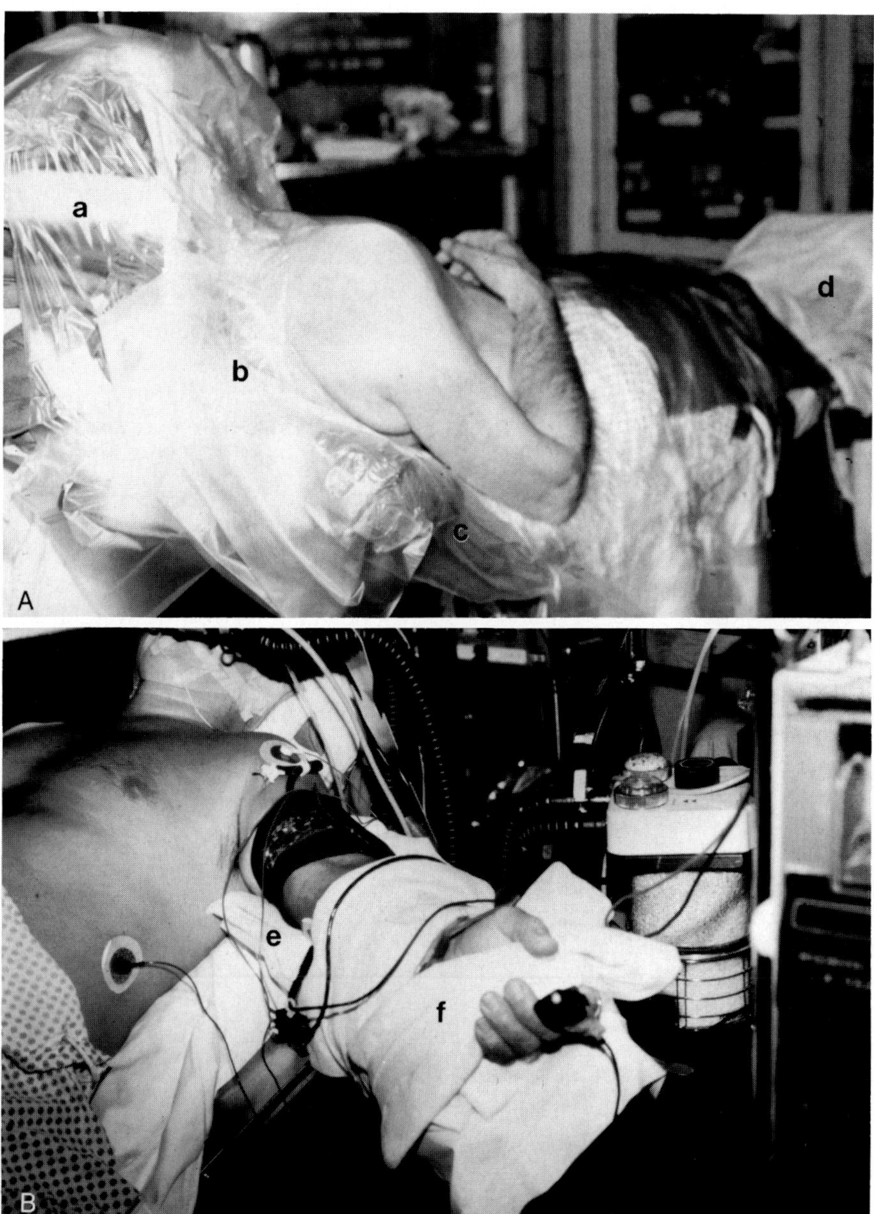

Figure 1–28. ***Avoiding Nerve Injuries.*** In positioning the patient, the head of the table is raised 35 degrees, the knees are flexed enough to prevent sliding down, and the shoulder protrudes over the corner of the table for access posteriorly as well as to the midline anteriorly. The following sites especially threaten nerve compression and are checked before beginning the skin scrub.

A, The head is secured on a padded headrest to maintain the neck in neutral rotation and slight flexion (a). Arthritic changes of the cervical spine, as are often present in patients having shoulder reconstruction, can cause cervical root compression if the neck is maintained in a hyperextended or rotated position during surgery.

The scapula is supported on a pad not only to enhance exposure of the shoulder but also to maintain the position of the neck during the procedure despite manipulations of the arm (b).

The mattress is shifted to cover the edge of the operating table to prevent contusing the ulnar nerve (c).

The knees and feet are padded and supported (d).

B, The opposite elbow is padded and, if arthritic, as in rheumatoids, is supported in the position of deformity (e).

The opposite wrist is secured to avoid a prolonged period in the flexed position, which can cause carpal tunnel symptoms (f).

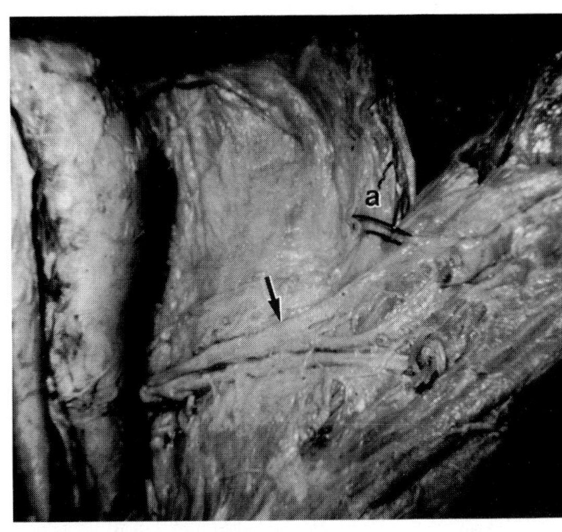

Figure 1–29. ***Avoiding Nerve Injuries.*** Photographs of the deep surface of the deltoid muscle of a cadaver after a 5.0 cm. deltoid-splitting approach made from the acromion downward between the anterior and middle parts of the deltoid with a stay suture (a), at the lower end of the split. The arrow points to the axillary nerve seen only on the deep surface. It is less than 1.0 cm. from the stay suture!

An anterior deltoid-splitting approach must not exceed 5.0 cm. in length, and a stay suture is used at the lower end to prevent further splitting by retraction.

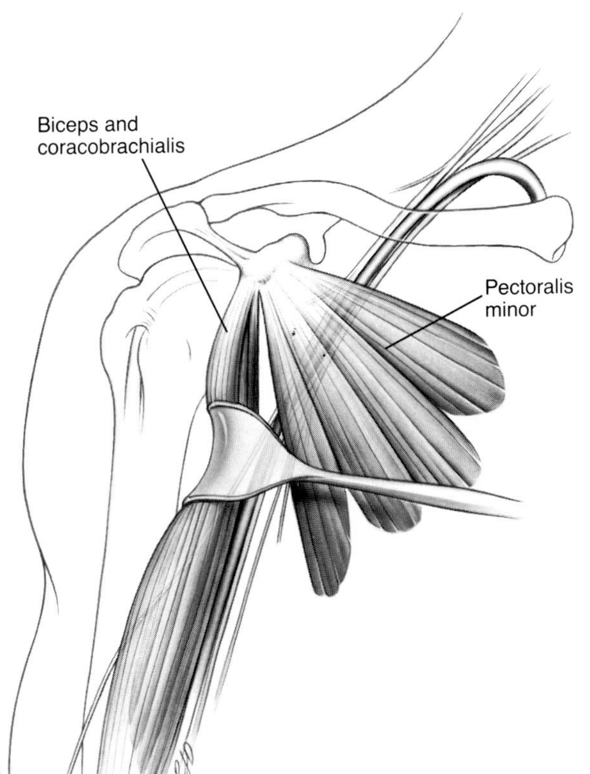

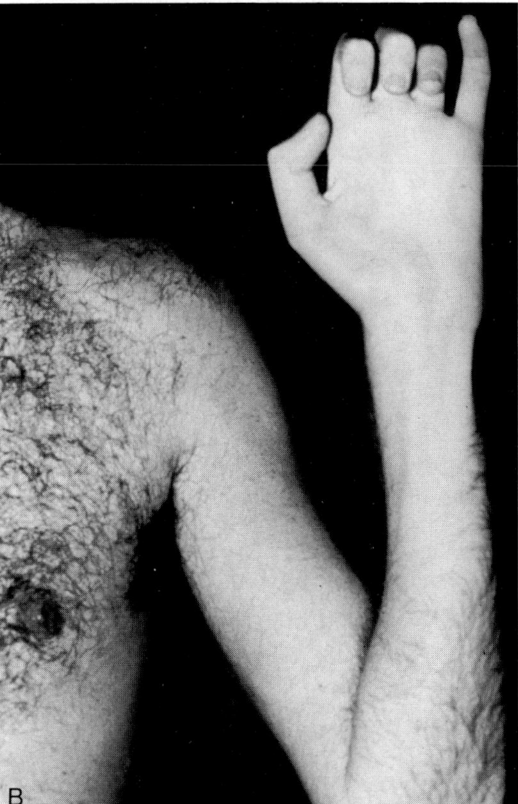

Figure 1–30. ***Avoiding Nerve Injuries.*** The coracoid muscles protect the infraclavicular plexus from retractors during an anterior approach except in unusual circumstances. The drawing (A) illustrates this, and the photograph (B) shows a patient with an extensive infraclavicular plexus paralysis from retraction during a repair for recurrent anterior dislocations in which the coracoid had been detached.

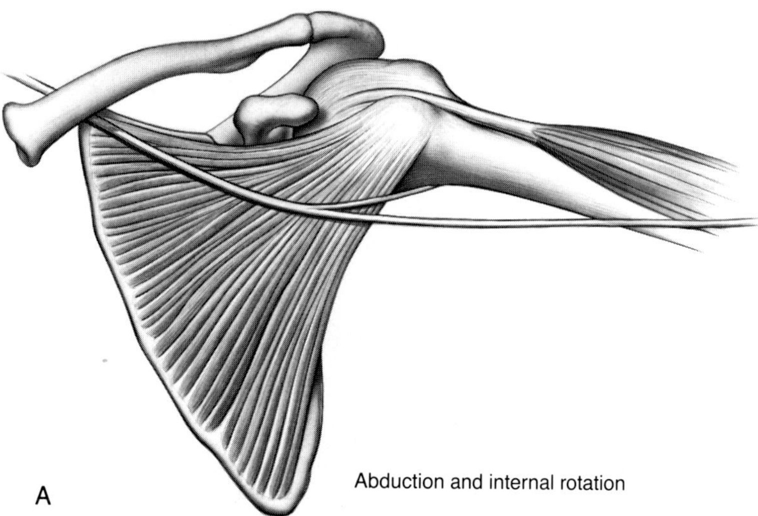

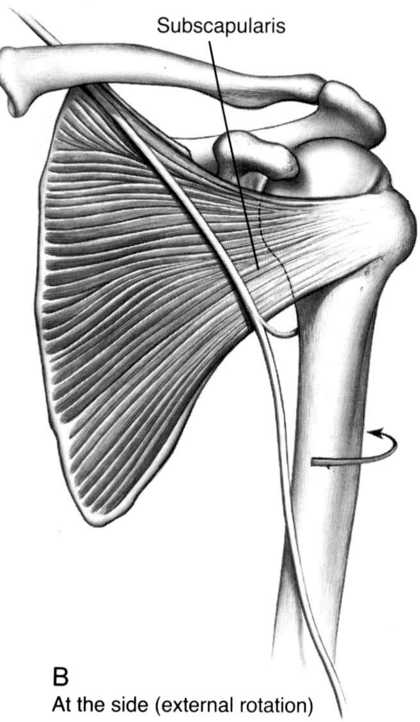

Figure 1–31. ***Avoiding Nerve Injuries.*** Drawings to show how the axillary nerve is displaced upward in peril by abduction and internal rotation (A) and is much safer during anterior approaches when the arm is at the side and in external rotation (B).

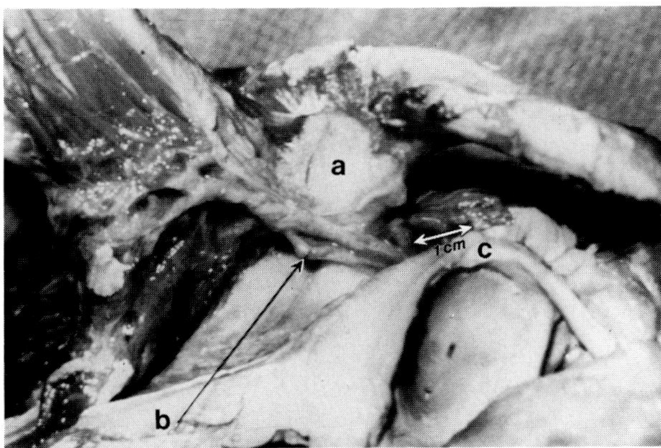

Figure 1–32. ***Avoiding Nerve Injuries.*** Posterior view of the glenohumeral joint with the infraspinatus tendon raised showing (a) the base of the acromion, (b) the suprascapular nerve entering the infraspinatus muscle, and (c) the long head of the biceps arising from the posterosuperior edge of the glenoid.

The suprascapular nerve winds around the base of the acromion, where it is in danger of being damaged during mobilization of the supraspinatus and infraspinatus tendons in rotator cuff repairs (see Chapter 2) and old fractures (Chapter 3). At this point, it is less than 1.0 cm. from the edge of the glenoid and is easily hit with an elevator.

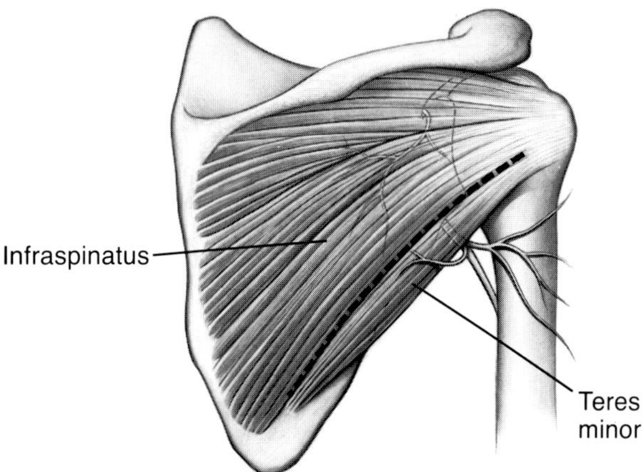

Figure 1–33. ***Avoiding Nerve Injuries.*** In the posterior approach, the suprascapular nerve going to the infraspinatus above and the axillary nerve going to the teres minor below make it safe to develop the interval between these two muscles for entering the joint. Since the infraspinatus is so important for external rotation (see p. 26 to 28 and Figs. 1–20 and 1–21), it is preserved intact except in a few special situations. If ever detached, it is carefully repaired.

and the back of the head held forward and without rotation. This opens the neural foramen. Contusion of the ulnar nerve against the side of the operating table can be avoided by shifting the edge of the mattress so that it extends over the edge of the table. Prolonged flexion of the wrist during surgery is also to be avoided because it may produce neuritis of the median nerve at the carpal tunnel. Care to pad and position the opposite elbow, wrist, and arm is important, especially in rheumatoid patients.

In a *deltoid-splitting approach*, it is important for the surgeon to know the precise location of the axillary nerve in the deltoid muscle. This is shown beautifully in Figure 1–29. The length of the split is limited to 5.0 cm. from the acromion, and a stay suture is placed at the lower end of the split to prevent splitting further down; otherwise, a heavy retractor may denervate the anterior deltoid.

The coracoid muscles are left intact during an anterior approach to protect the infraclavicular plexus from a heavy retractor (Fig. 1–30). Their detachment is often recommended as a routine in repairing recurrent anterior dislocations; however, serious brachial plexus injuries, as seen in Figure 1–30B, have occurred from retraction. It may be necessary to detach the coracoid muscles for more exposure in special situations, as in some re-operations or old fractures in which the subscapularis is retracted or buried in scar; otherwise, they are left intact.

In *inferior approaches* from the front, as in an inferior capsular shift or repair of comminuted fractures, the axillary nerve lies in close proximity to the capsule and requires fail-proof location by palpation or exposure (see Chapters 4 and 5).

In *anterior approaches* to the glenohumeral joint, the axillary nerve is placed in peril if the arm is held in abduction[111] and internal rotation, as shown in Figure 1–31. Having the arm at the side and in external rotation is safer.

In *superior approaches* to the glenohumeral joint, as in mobilization and repair of a tear of the rotator cuff (see Chapter 2), the suprascapular nerve is easily injured (Fig. 1–32). This nerve is in peril if the surgeon dissects more than 1.0 cm. medial to the rim of the glenoid against the base of the spine of the scapula, where it is only 1.0 cm. medial to the rim of the glenoid. It is also easily injured medial to the coracoid process where it is tethered in the suprascapular notch.

In *posterior approaches*, the interval between the infraspinatus muscle, supplied by the suprascapular nerve from above, and the teres minor, supplied by the axillary nerve from below, affords a safe route to the posterior capsule between two areas of motor nerve supply (Fig. 1–33). As discussed on page 314 and shown in Figure 4–34, the infraspinatus is detached only in special situations. If the infraspinatus is detached, the suprascapular nerve receives special care. The base of the spine of the scapula is first palpated to locate the nerve, and the division of the tendon is made so that the deep part is further lateral away from the nerve (see Fig. 4–34D).

2

CUFF TEARS, BICEPS LESIONS, AND IMPINGEMENT

Although subacromial impingement has long been recognized as a cause of chronic shoulder pain,[35–38, 40] only recently has the close relationship of impingement to lesions of the rotator cuff, biceps, subacromial bursa, and acromioclavicular joint become appreciated (Fig. 2–1). In 1972,[28] the most frequent type of impingement (see Table 2–1) was first described as occurring beneath the anterior third of the acromion and undersurface of the acromioclavicular joint rather than laterally, and this type of impingement was recognized as the most common cause of cuff tears and biceps lesions. Since 1985,[32] this type of impingement has been referred to as "outlet impingement." As the progressive stages in the pathology of outlet impingement have become better understood[27] (see Fig. 2–13), impingement lesions are seen to occur in patients of all ages, from the early teens to senility, and are now considered the most frequent cause of chronic shoulder disability.

Most of the confusion in the literature of the past regarding cuff tears and biceps lesions was caused by thinking of them separately without recognizing their close relationship. There was disagreement between Codman[6, 43] and Meyer,[44, 45] the most distinguished pioneers in ruptures of shoulder tendons, as to whether ruptures of the supraspinatus tendon were the major source of shoulder pain or whether lesions of the long head

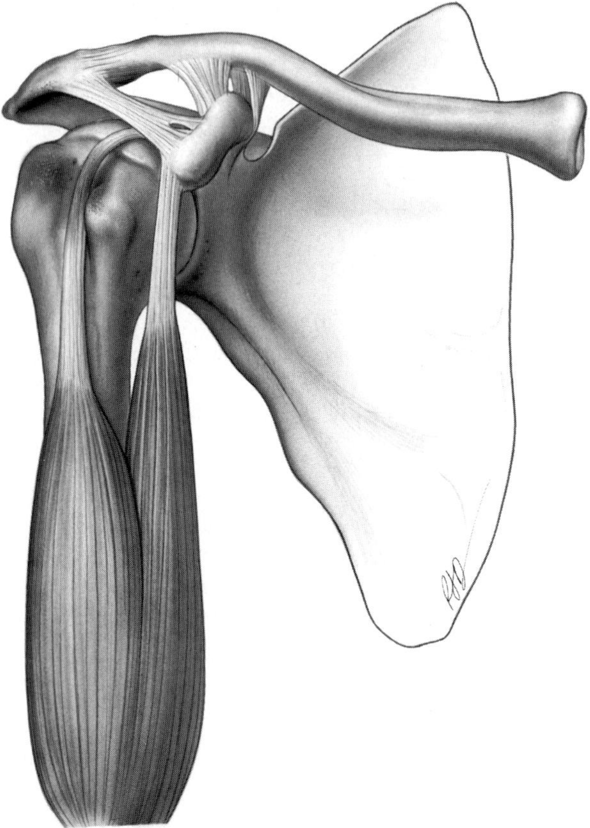

Figure 2–1. ***Impingement Lesions.*** The close anatomical relationship between the anterior acromion, rotator cuff, long head of the biceps, subacromial bursa, and acromioclavicular joint is illustrated, all of which may be involved in "outlet impingement" (explained in Figure 2–2). Tears of the rotator cuff and ruptures of the long head of the biceps are no longer thought of as isolated lesions but are interpreted as the result of impingement beneath the anterior acromion and acromioclavicular joint, which may affect all of these closely related structures simultaneously.

An understanding of this impingement mechanism is essential; for diagnosis and treatment. Only recently has "outlet impingement" come to be recognized as the most frequent cause of chronic shoulder pain.

of the biceps were more important. In 1931, Codman[43] wrote:

> Doctor Meyer's attention has been concentrated on the biceps tendon, while I believe the rupture of the supraspinatus tendon is the primary and important lesion. I cannot agree with Doctor Meyer, but his work demands respectful study as one explanation for some of the lesions discussed here.

The literature continued to consider clinical disorders of these structures separately until, in 1977,[26] the clinical importance of relating them to each other and to impingement was shown.

In this book, for the first time, details of the pathology and treatment of all of these lesions are considered together, and the observations leading to the conclusion that "outlet impingement" is the primary cause of most cuff tears and biceps lesions are described. Understanding this relationship has proved to be most helpful. The treatment of chronic outlet impingement is anterior acromioplasty, whereas the treatment of the less frequent types of impingement, as listed in Table 2–1, usually entails additional steps in reconstruction with or without anterior acromioplasty, depending on the specific lesion. They will be considered separately. In complete cuff tears, the action of the cuff to depress the head as the arm is raised is impaired, causing a second type of impingement (Table 2–1, item II-B-1). This second type of impingement is another reason for performing an anterior acromioplasty at the time of repairing tears of the rotator cuff.

CLASSIFICATION AND PATHOMECHANICS OF IMPINGEMENT

My classification of impingement lesions is outlined in Table 2–1. The usual cause of impinge-

Table 2–1. AUTHOR'S CLASSIFICATION OF IMPINGEMENT

I. *"OUTLET IMPINGEMENT"*—narrowing of the "supraspinatus outlet"
   - A. Anterior acromial spur
   - B. Shape of acromion (e.g., overhang or curve)
   - C. Slope of acromion (e.g., flat)
   - D. Prominent acromioclavicular joint (e.g., excrescences)

II. *LESS FREQUENT IMPINGEMENT MECHANISMS ("NON-OUTLET IMPINGEMENT")*
   - A. Prominent greater tuberosity
     1. Malunion or nonunion
     2. Low set humeral component
   - B. Loss of head depressors
     1. Rotator cuff tear
     2. Biceps rupture
   - C. Loss of glenohumeral fulcrum
     1. Loss of head or glenoid (e.g., rheumatoid arthritis, head resection)
     2. Ligamentous laxity (e.g., multidirectional dislocator)
   - D. Loss of suspensory mechanism
     1. Old acromioclavicular separation
     2. Trapezius palsy
   - E. Defects of the acromion
     1. Unfused acromial epiphysis
     2. Malunion or nonunion
     3. Congenital (Erb's palsy)
   - F. Thickened bursa or cuff
     1. Large, chronic calcium deposit
     2. Chronic bursitis
   - G. Loss of the lower extremities (e.g., abnormal use)
     1. Paraplegia
     2. Amputations
     3. Chronic arthritis

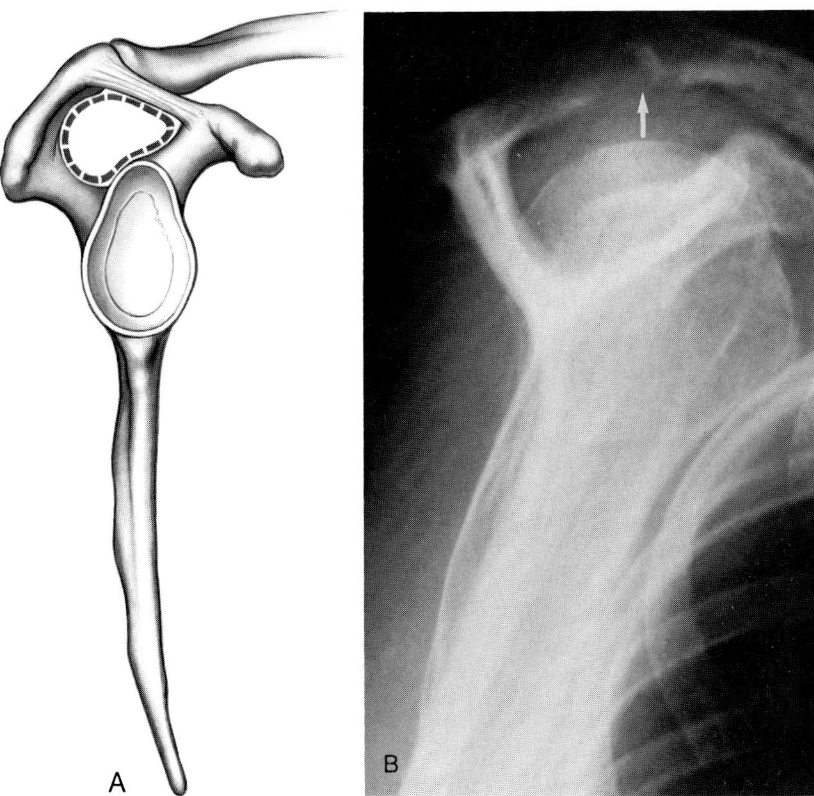

Figure 2–2. ***The "Supraspinatus Outlet."*** A, "supraspinatus outlet" is a term that was introduced to indicate the space beneath the anterior acromion, coracoacromial ligament, and acromioclavicular joint, as illustrated in this drawing. The supraspinatus muscle lies in the supraspinatus fossa, and its tendon passes beneath these structures. Narrowing of this outlet is the most frequent cause of impingement. The narrowing may be due to the shape or slope of the acromion, prominence of the undersurface of the acromioclavicular joint, or an anterior acromial spur. B, The supraspinatus outlet can be seen in a lateral view of the scapula, provided that the tube is angled downward 10 degrees (using the spine of the scapula as a guide) and the patient keeps the scapula perpendicular to the floor, as shown in Figure 1–12.

ment is narrowing of the supraspinatus outlet (Fig. 2–2). The evidence that this accounts for most cuff tears and biceps lesions can be seen in advanced lesions in the anatomy laboratory and at surgery, as discussed on pages 53 to 63. We will consider this type of impingement first, followed by the less frequent, non-outlet causes of impingement.

"Outlet Impingement"

By far the most frequent cause of impingement is narrowing of the supraspinatus outlet. Until fairly recently, impingement was thought to occur against the lateral edge of the acromion and the surgical treatment recommended was complete acromionectomy or lateral acromionectomy. The crippling effects of these procedures, because of weakening of the deltoid muscle and wound complications,[29] as shown in Figure 2–46, suggested the need for a study of the undersurface of the acromion and acromioclavicular joint. This study was started in 1962 in the anatomy laboratory and resulted in the article of 1972 describing how this type of impingement occurs anteriorly rather than laterally.[28]

Most movements of the shoulder are in the scapular plane or even more anterior rather than in the coronal plane (Fig. 2–3). "Outlet impingement" occurs against the anterior third of the acromion and the undersurface of the acromioclavicular joint (see Figs. 2–4, 2–5, 2–6, 2–14, and 2–15), but not against the lateral edge of the posterior half of the acromion. Complete acromionectomy and lateral acromionectomy remove an innocent part of the acromion and weaken the deltoid unnecessarily. These observations led to the development of anterior acromioplasty (pp. 96 to 106 and Fig. 2–39). This procedure removes prominences on the undersurface of the acromion and acromioclavicular joint with minimal detachment of the origin of the deltoid muscle. It enlarges the supraspinatus tendon beneath the acromion and acromioclavicular joint. The term "subacromial decompression" was introduced to describe the objectives of this procedure.

"Coracoid Impingement"

Theoretically, in addition to prominences of the anterior acromion and acromioclavicular joint, narrowing of the outlet might be caused by cephalic protrusion of the rim of the glenoid, the posterior

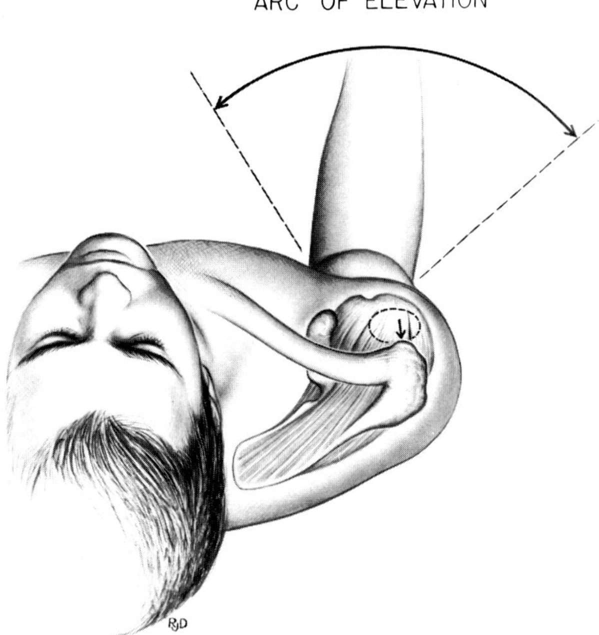

Figure 2–3. The arc of use and function is anterior to the acromion—not lateral to the acromion. Impingement is against the anterior one-third of the acromion and undersurface of the acromioclavicular joint, and not against the posterior part of the acromion. This is as should be expected because the upper extremity is usually used in front rather than out to the side. (From Neer, C. S., II: Anterior acromioplasty for the chronic impingement syndrome in the shoulder. J. Bone Joint Surg. 54-A:41, 1972.)

location or anterolateral overhang of the coracoid process, or the anterior location of the spine of the scapula. In practice, however, these structures have not needed to be altered in the surgical treatment of outlet impingement.

Recently, the rather vague term "coracoid impingement" has been introduced. It should be clear that an overhanging coracoid process, as in a longstanding Erb's palsy, as a result of a malunion or nonunion of an osteotomized coracoid, or as a result of deep wear of the glenoid in severe glenohumeral arthritis, may encroach on the subscapularis and require partial removal of the coracoid. However, this does not affect the supraspinatus tendon and does not cause outlet impingement.

Anterior Acromial Spur

As shown in Figure 2–4, traction spurs in the acromial attachment of the coracoacromial ligament may protrude into the supraspinatus outlet and cause impingement. These lesions almost never occur prior to age 40. If they are associated with chronic impingement symptoms, they are removed as a part of the anterior acromioplasty. However, the mere presence of a spur in x-ray films cannot be interpreted as invariable evidence that pain is present as a result of impingement. They may be seen in routine chest x-rays of patients who have no shoulder pain.

The decision as to whether anterior acromioplasty for removal of a spur is indicated requires clinical interpretation. The impingement injection test (see Fig. 2–30) is particularly helpful. The absence of a spur does not exclude outlet impingement caused by variations in the shape or slope of the acromion or by variations in the prominence of the acromioclavicular joint. Thus, anterior acromioplasty may be indicated even though no spur is present.

Shape of the Acromion

A curved or elongated, overhanging acromion may cause outlet impingement[28, 82–84] (Fig. 2–5A). In an acromioplasty, any of the anterior edge of the acromion protruding beyond the line of the clavicle is removed and a curved, overhanging anterior edge is also beveled so that the undersurface becomes straight.

Slope of the Acromion

Narrowing of the supraspinatus outlet may be caused by a flat angle, as shown in Figure 2–5B.[28] A higher incidence of tears of the rotator cuff and evidences of impingement have been demonstrated in cadavers when the angle of the acromion is flat.[82–84]

Variations in the shape and slope of the acromion in dried human scapula can be seen in Figure 2–5B.

Prominences of the Acromioclavicular Joint

The supraspinatus outlet may be narrowed by prominences of the undersurface of the acromioclavicular joint, as in Figure 2–6. Excision of the undersurface of this joint is an important part of anterior acromioplasty whenever such prominences are present. I now prefer beveling the undersurface of this joint for impingement rather than excising the entire distal clavicle because more of the origin of the deltoid is maintained intact. The thought has occurred that this might lead to acromioclavicular joint pain because of incongruity of the joint surfaces; however, this has not been seen as a complication. The indications to excise the distal 1.5 to 2.0 cm. of clavicle (rather than beveling the undersurface) are (1) if the acromioclavicular

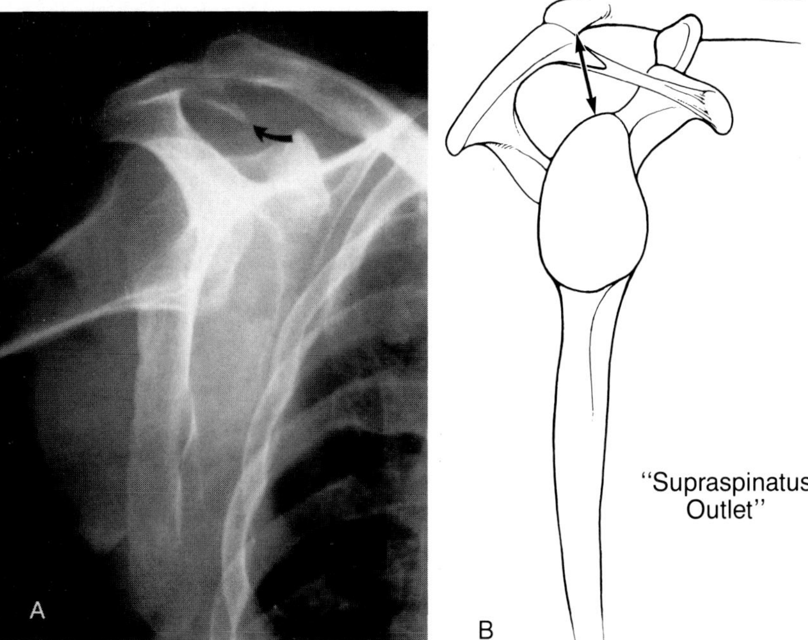

Figure 2–4. Lateral view of the scapula ("outlet view") x-ray film (A) and drawing (B) to show how an anterior acromial spur encroaches upon the supraspinatus outlet. This spur is thought to result from intermittent traction on the coracoacromial ligament caused by the impact of the humerus. Because the spur encroaches on the outlet, it may cause impingement.

joint is tender and painful pre-operatively because of arthritis, and (2) if more exposure of the supraspinatus is needed in a difficult cuff repair. The technique is shown in Figure 2–40.

X-ray Evaluation with the "Outlet View"

The shape of the supraspinatus outlet can be seen in true lateral views of the scapula (see Figs. 2–2 and 2–4). Poppen and I tried to develop a standard projection[32] for obtaining lateral views to be used for visualizing the shape and size of the outlet and also for a better measurement of the true acromiohumeral distance (see Fig. 1–12). A more accurate measurement of the acromiohumeral distance can be made in a lateral view than in an anterior-posterior view because of the normal curve of the acromion. Poppen developed a measuring device, the "scapulometer," which consists of a transparent scale of concentric circles at 1.0 mm.

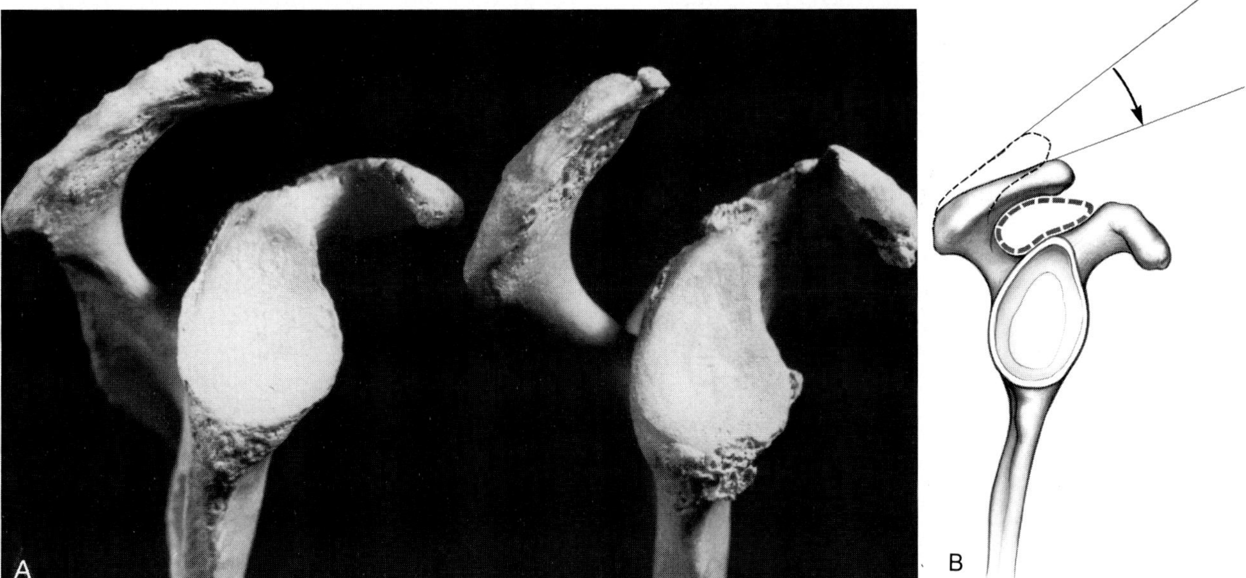

Figure 2–5. The shape or slope of the acromion may cause encroachment on the supraspinatus outlet leading to outlet impingement.[28] A, Photograph of dried bones illustrating variations in the shape, slope, or overhang of the acromion seen in the anatomy laboratory. B, Drawing illustrating how a flat angle of the acromion can cause outlet impingement in the absence of an anterior acromial spur or other gross evidence of impingement.

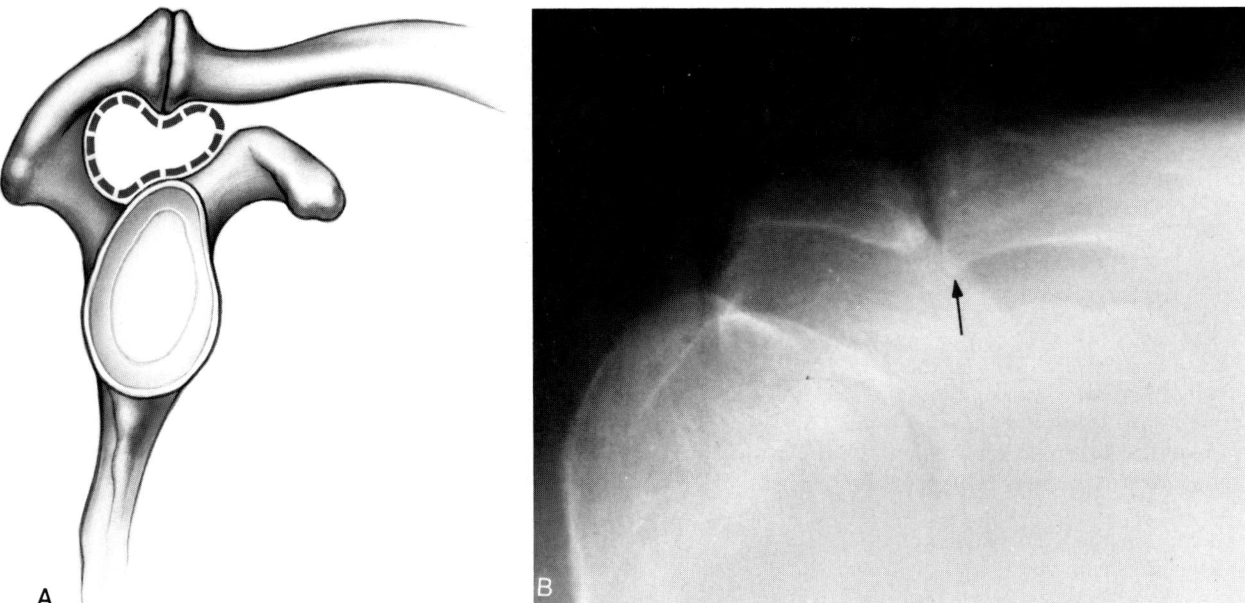

Figure 2–6. Prominence of the undersurface of the acromioclavicular joint may encroach on the supraspinatus outlet causing outlet impingement, as illustrated in the drawing (A) and the x-ray (B).

intervals combined with a protractor. This instrument is placed over the outlet view (lateral view) film. The purpose of this instrument is to more accurately demonstrate the slope of the acromion; the size of the outlet; the precise site of narrowing of the outlet, if such exists; and the true acromiohumeral distance. The difficulty has been lack of consistency in obtaining true lateral projections without tilt or rotation of the scapula. Clinical correlation and the impingement injection test (see Fig. 2–30) are necessary for the interpretation of the findings in an outlet view film, and are discussed on page 80.

Non-outlet Impingement

The less frequent causes of impingement, with the exception of items II–B-1 and II–B-2 in Table 2–1, usually occur with a normal supraspinatus outlet. The technique of treating these lesions is discussed in detail in a later section (pp. 138 to 142). However, the pathomechanics of each of these types of impingement is discussed in this section to show how they differ from outlet impingement, and to show the practical value of this classification in surgical reconstruction.

Prominence of the Greater Tuberosity

Theoretically, congenital or developmental variations in the height and orientation of the greater tuberosity could account for impingement; however, these have not been recognizable as a clinical problem. Excrescences may develop on the greater tuberosity as a result of outlet impingement (see Figs. 2–18 and 2–35), which may be prominent enough to catch against the acromion and require removal at the time of acromioplasty (see Fig. 2–41J).

Examples of the greater tuberosity being the primary cause of subacromial impingement are malunited fractures of the greater tuberosity, malunion of the surgical neck, and low placement of a humeral prosthesis. Their treatments differ.

Malunion of the Greater Tuberosity

Malunion of the greater tuberosity occurs with displacement posteriorly, superiorly, and medially, depending on the size of the fragment and the proportions of the attachments of the supraspinatus compared with the external rotators[140] (Fig. 2–7B). There is an important difference between this and the type of impingement caused by narrowing of the supraspinatus outlet. The displaced tuberosity covers a portion of the articular surface of the humeral head, and when the glenohumeral joint is externally rotated, especially in the abducted position, the displaced tuberosity strikes against the glenoid. Re-location of the tuberosity is required to solve this problem rather than acromioplasty alone (see Chapter 5).

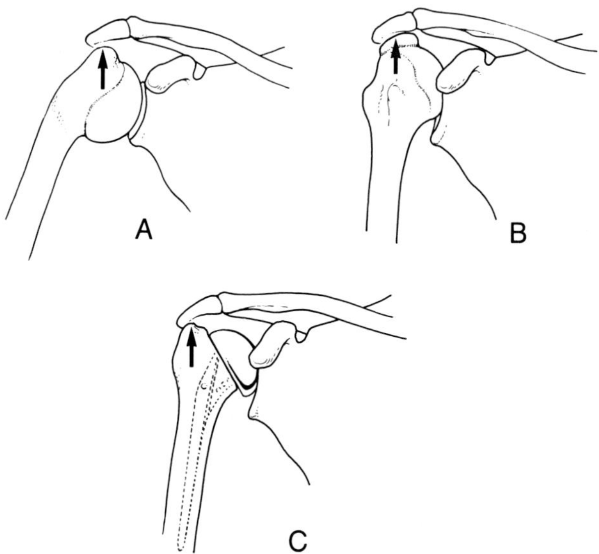

Figure 2–7. Prominence of the greater tuberosity is one of the causes of non-outlet impingement as seen in a varus malunion of the surgical neck of the proximal humerus (A), a malunion of the greater tuberosity (B), and a low placement of a humeral prosthesis (C). Surgical treatment, as discussed in the text, differs from that for outlet impingement in that more than anterior acromioplasty is usually required.

Malunion of the Surgical Neck

Varus malunion of the surgical neck differs in that the tuberosity does not cover a part of the articular surface (Fig. 2–7A). The tuberosity may impinge against the acromion, but if the articular surface of the head is in good contact with the glenoid and in good condition, it may be possible to alleviate the condition with a acromioplasty. When there is marked displacement and a tear of the rotator cuff, it is better to remove some of the greater tuberosity at the time of repairing the rotator cuff (see Chapter 5).

Low Placement of a Humeral Component

Distal displacement of the humeral component in a shoulder arthroplasty is shown in Figure 2–7C. The treatment usually required for this is revision rather than acromioplasty, with placement of the humeral component at the proper height so that its articular surface extends cephalad to the top of the greater tuberosity (see Chapter 3, Fig. 3–26).

Loss of the Humeral Head Depressors

When the deltoid muscle contracts, it displaces the humeral head upward, causing impingement and rendering its contraction less efficient in raising the arm, unless the head is stabilized by the rotator cuff and long head of the biceps.

The stabilizing action of the *rotator cuff* against the ascent of the head is impaired and subacromial impingement escalated when there is a complete tear of the rotator cuff (Fig. 2–8). Almost all tears begin in the supraspinatus tendon with impairment of this action of the supraspinatus against the head riding upward. This creates a vicious cycle. As the head displaces upward, more rapid wear of the tendon occurs, causing more rapid enlargement of the tear. With enlargement of the tear, there is more ascent of the head and further escalation of the impingement wear. Loss of the acromiohumeral distance is important roentgen evidence (see Fig. 2–36). The vicious cycle of the escalation of im-

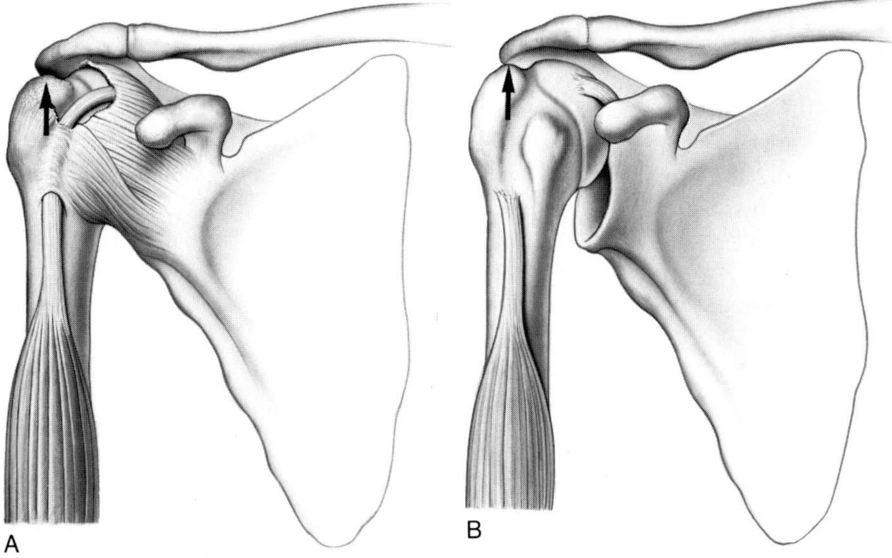

Figure 2–8. Loss of the depressors of the humeral head, such as with a cuff tear (A) or rupture of the long head of the biceps (B), may cause non-outlet impingement.

pingement wear as the tear enlarges makes early repair and decompression of impingement tears the logical course to follow in healthy patients. Even in the case of tears in which narrowing of the supraspinatus outlet is of less importance in the etiology, this second type of impingement after complete tears gives a logical basis for anterior acromioplasty at the time of repair of these lesions as well.

The *long head of the biceps* also acts to stabilize the head against ascent (Fig. 2–8). When the long head ruptures, it would be most ideal to repair the tendon end-on to preserve its motion in the groove, maintaining its stabilizing function. Unfortunately, no satisfactory way to achieve this type of repair has yet been developed. Tenodesis of the ruptured long head to the humerus does not alter the threat of impingement; therefore, acromioplasty should be considered when the biceps is tenodesed. Transfer of the long head to the coracoid process, as advised by some surgeons should be avoided because this would cause the long head to displace the humerus upward even more (see Figs. 1–22 and 2–31B).

Loss of the Glenohumeral Fulcrum

Impingement can be caused by loss of the fulcrum function of the glenohumeral joint from destruction of the articular surfaces or from ligamentous laxity.

In *rheumatoid arthritis with loss of the articular surfaces*, the humerus translocates upward (Fig. 2–9), causing the greater tuberosity to impinge against the acromion. The loss of the acromiohumeral distance gives the appearance of a massive tear of the rotator cuff; however, the rotator cuff is usually intact at the time of shoulder arthroplasty unless impingement has gone on too long. In rheumatoid patients, once the articular surfaces have been destroyed beyond medical treatment, arthroplasty should be advised before the rotator cuff becomes destroyed. Further delay may also allow more granulation erosion of the bone on both sides of the joint, causing the humerus to displace medially, a process that I have termed "centralization." Centralization escalates impingement, and the loss of bone makes arthroplasty even more difficult.

The roentgen appearance of rheumatoid shoulders with the upward displacement of the greater tuberosity from loss of the articular surfaces created a false reputation for a high incidence of rotator cuff tears in rheumatoids, necessitating constrained rather than unconstrained arthroplasty. Only 20 percent of our rheumatoid patients have a complete thickness rotator cuff tear at the time of shoulder arthroplasty, and these lesions are usually small and easily repaired. The incidence of complete thickness tears at the time of arthroplasty in Cofield's series of rheumatoids is also low.[103] Of course, if shoulder arthroplasty is delayed until the end stages, the incidence of larger cuff tears is much higher.

Although I once thought that anterior acromioplasty was indicated almost routinely at the time of shoulder arthroplasty in rheumatoids,[21] further experience has shown that it is rarely needed because an adequate subacromial space can be maintained by proper placement of the prosthetic components[39] (see Fig. 2–51). Furthermore, it is now thought important to preserve the buffering and cushioning function of the coracoacromial ligaments especially in rheumatoids, because the rotator cuff muscles, which may be weakened by the rheumatoid disease, may be acting as another cause for the humerus to ascend against the acromion. Therefore, anterior acromioplasty is avoided. In the rare instances when anterior acromioplasty is necessary, because of a bony prominence that has developed on the acromion from long-standing impingement, the coracoacromial ligament is re-attached to the acromion after completing the acromioplasty (see p. 220, Chapter 3).

Surgical removal of the head or avascular necrosis may be complicated by impingement as a result of translocation of the proximal humerus upward against the acromion (Fig. 2–9C). Obviously, this type of impingement is logically treated with a prosthetic head with care to eliminate contact between the tuberosities and the acromion. The head of the humeral component is placed cephalad to the level of the tuberosities. In old fractures with avascular necrosis, malunion of the greater tuberosity and traumatic tears of the rotator cuff might also be present to cause impingement beyond that due to the loss of the fulcrum. Therefore, at the time of arthroplasty for old trauma, it may be necessary to osteotomize and reposition the greater tuberosity and to repair the rotator cuff in addition to providing a prosthetic head for the fulcrum, as shown in Figs. 3–62 and 3–63.

In multidirectional instability, an unstable head that dislocates anteriorly, posteriorly, and inferiorly because of capsular laxity may also displace upward against the acromion (Fig. 2–9B). This has created two clinical problems. First, the theoretical coexistence of instability and impingement has been misconstrued by some surgeons as

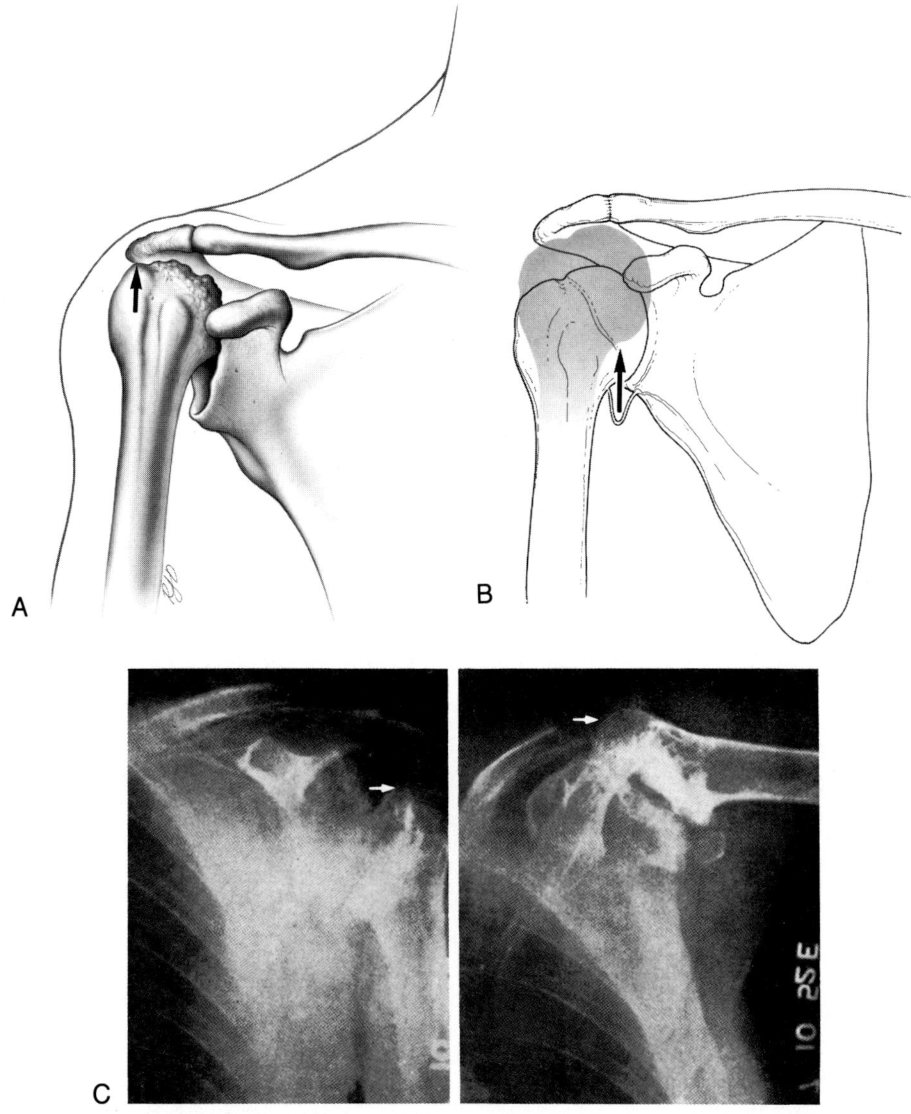

Figure 2–9. Loss of the fulcrum action of the glenohumeral joint may cause non-outlet impingement, as in rheumatoid destruction of the glenohumeral joint (see Fig. 2–9A and Chapter 3), multidirectional glenohumeral instability (see Fig. 2–9B, Fig. 2–36, and Chapter 4), and resection of the humeral head (see Fig. 2–9C and Chapter 3). The x-rays in Figure 2–9C, made with the arm at the side and with impingement occurring on attempting to raise the arm, are from the initial article in 1953 on the logic of a humeral head prosthesis to supply a fulcrum against impingement when the humeral head has been destroyed by trauma.[12]

an indication for anterior acromioplasty at the time of repairing recurrent dislocating shoulders. In my experience, a repair for the recurrent dislocations stabilizes the shoulder sufficiently, so that this type of impingement is almost always eliminated. Only two patients in my series have had persistent symptoms of impingement after surgical repair of the instability, as discussed in Chapter 4. Both of these patients had obvious deformities of the anterior acromion. The number of patients with continuing impingement pain after surgical stabilization of unstable shoulders are too few to make anterior acromioplasty at the time of repairing instability a serious consideration.

The second clinical problem has been the treatment of this type of impingement with anterior acromioplasty alone without stabilizing the dislocating shoulder. This fails, of course, because of failure to eliminate the underlying cause (see Fig. 2–31). Lidocaine (Xylocaine) injected subacromially (see Fig. 2–30) temporarily stops the pain that is due to impingement, but does not relieve that caused by instability. This test has been a very accurate guide. If the injection fails to relieve the pain, factors other than outlet impingement (e.g., glenohumeral instability, frozen shoulder, etc.) are usually present, making it unlikely that anterior acromioplasty will be successful.

Loss of the Suspensory Mechanism; Impaired Scapular Rotation

It has not generally been appreciated that loss of the suspensory mechanism can cause impingement. I am convinced that it can. In both paralysis of the trapezius muscle and complete acromioclavicular separations, the acromion drops and, more importantly, is no longer properly rotated out of the way of the greater tuberosity as the arm is raised.

Trapezius palsy (paralysis of the spinal accessory nerve) is usually caused by surgeons either intentionally at the time of head and neck surgery for neoplasms or accidentally at the time of biopsy of a cervical lymph node. Some patients with this condition have no significant pain. Others have either fatigue symptoms in the shoulder girdle muscles or impingement symptoms (Fig. 2–10). Those with persistent and disabling fatigue symptoms are considered for a modified Dewar-Harris procedure (see Fig. 6–20B). Those with relief of pain after the subacromial injection of xylocaine (see Fig. 2–30) may be relieved by anterior acromioplasty (see Fig. 2–40; Chapter 6, p. 451).

Old acromioclavicular dislocations with disruption of the coracoclavicular ligaments may likewise cause several types of pain, or the pain may be minimal. Pain may be due to fatigue of the shoulder girdle muscles, to incongruity between the end of the clavicle and the displaced scapula, or to subacromial impingement (Fig. 2–10). Injection tests into both the acromioclavicular joint and the subacromial space are helpful in analyzing the type of pain present, as outlined in Table 4–3. As discussed in Chapter 4, pages 347 to 350, these lesions can prove to be very complex, and caution is recommended in selecting the proper surgical procedure in the individual case. The procedures are described in Chapter 4, pages 350 to 355.

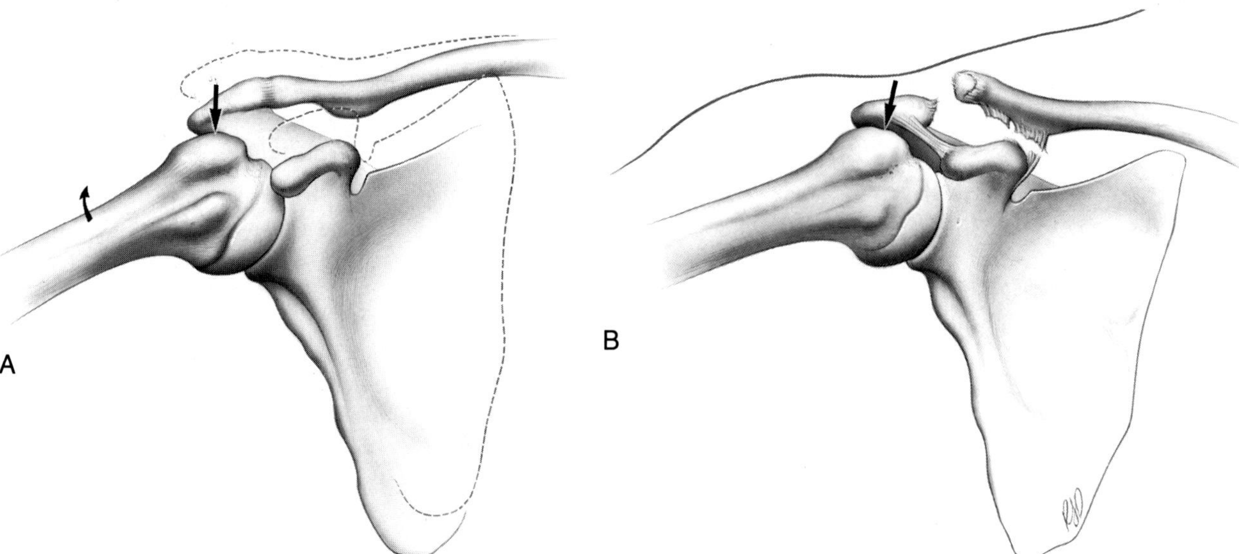

Figure 2–10. Loss of the suspensory mechanism may cause non-outlet impingement by impairment of scapular rotation as normally occurs when the arm is raised. This can be due to paralysis of the trapezius muscle (A) or to a dislocation of the acromioclavicular joint with tearing of the coracoclavicular ligaments (B).

Lesions of the Acromion

Examples of pathological conditions of the acromion that may cause impingement and require special surgical measures other than anterior acromioplasty include unfused acromial epiphysis, malunion and nonunion of the acromion, and Erb's palsy.

I first recognized *unfused anterior acromial epiphysis* as a potential cause of impingement and cuff tears a number of years ago.[62–64] The acromial epiphyses usually fuse by age 25 years; however, Grant[14] found unfused epiphyses at this site in 7 percent of 319 cadavers after the age of 30 years. Unfused acromial epiphyses can best be identified roentgenographically in the axillary view, which has become routine in the pre-operative evaluation of patients with tears of the rotator cuff (see Fig. 2–28). Four levels of fusion failure are seen—pre-acromial, meso-acromial, meta-acromial, and basi-acromial—as illustrated in Figure 2–55. If the unfused segment of the acromion is moveable, as illustrated in Figure 2–11A, it may cause impingement but preclude a routine type of anterior acromioplasty. If the ossification center is small, it may be excised. More commonly, the failure of closure of the epiphysis occurs in the middle of the acromion and in this case epiphysiodesis is performed—otherwise, too much acromion would be removed, weakening the deltoid muscle. It is difficult to accomplish an epiphysiodesis in this location and maintain the movement of the glenohumeral joint necessary to prevent subacromial adhesions. The technique is discussed on page 139 and in Figure 2–56.

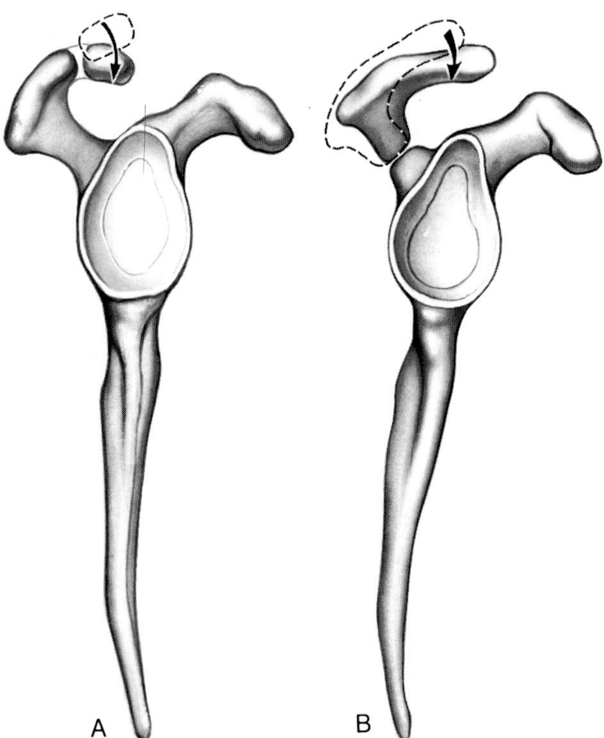

Figure 2–11. Lesions of the acromion may cause non-outlet impingement. A persistent unfused anterior acromial epiphysis may cause impingement and lead to a tear of the rotator cuff (A) in later life. It makes it impossible to do the usual anterior acromioplasty; therefore, it should be identified with axillary view x-ray films prior to rotator cuff repairs. Nonunion of the acromion (B) may cause non-outlet impingement. It requires repair of the nonunion rather than acromioplasty (p. 416).

Malunion and *nonunion of the acromion* may cause impingement. Fractures of the acromion usually occur near its base and if depressed may cause impingement (Fig. 2–11B). Reconstruction after malunion or nonunion of the acromion entails extensive soft-tissue release of adhesions, both subacromial and around the upper humerus, as well as re-positioning the acromion and securing fixation to hold the acromion out of the impingement position until the bone heals. Unless sufficient internal fixation is obtained to allow passive motion during the healing period, adhesions will recur, requiring later operative release. The technique of this repair is discussed on page 416 and in Figure 2–57.

In *Erb's palsy deformity*, an overhanging acromion and coracoid develop. This type of acromial impingement is rarely associated with adhesions. In mild cases, it can be corrected by excision of the undersurface of the acromion leaving most of the deltoid origin intact (see Chapter 6). Glenohumeral arthroplasty for long-standing problems is described in Chapter 3.

Thickened Bursa or Cuff

Thickening of the subacromial bursa in chronic bursitis or thickening of a portion of the rotator cuff as a result of a large, chronic calcium deposit may cause impingement. The most common cause of thickening of the subacromial bursa is Stage II impingement. Calcium deposits are not considered to be due to impingement. The treatment for chronic symptomatic bursitis is bursectomy (rather than acromioplasty). Large, impinging calcium deposits may require removal, as discussed further in Chapter 6.

Loss of the Lower Extremities

Loss of the lower extremities can be brought on by paralysis, amputation, and severe lower extremity arthritis. Symptoms may develop as a result of stress and wear on the shoulders, which differ from those of outlet impingement. The

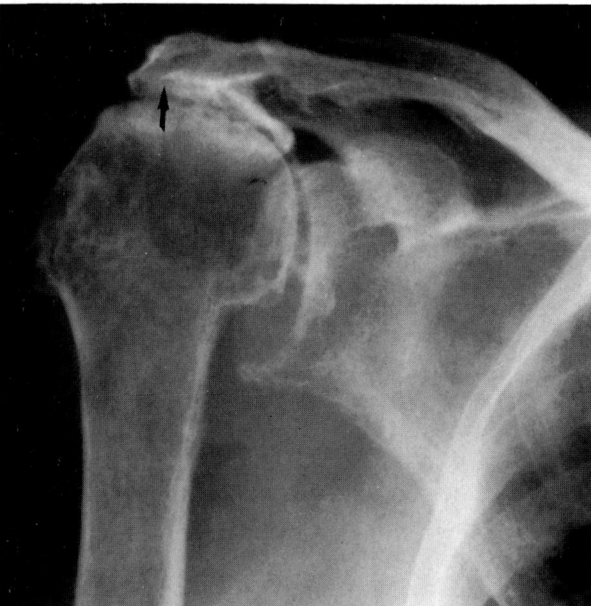

Figure 2–12. Loss of the lower extremities because of paraplegia, amputations, or arthritis can cause non-outlet impingement, as illustrated in this anterior-posterior film of a 48 year old man who has used crutches since he was 11 years old because of post-poliomyelitis paralysis of both legs. The area of impingement (arrow), shown by the sclerosis and spur on the undersurface of the acromion, is slightly lateral to the usual area seen in outlet impingement. The patient has a massive cuff tear, as discussed on page 533.

greater tuberosity is driven against the acromion in using crutches or making transfers from bed to chair. Wear on the undersurface of the acromion tends to occur more laterally than in outlet impingement (Fig. 2–12).

PATHOLOGY OF OUTLET IMPINGEMENT

Let us consider in more detail the pathology of supraspinatus outlet impingement and the evidence that it occurs anteriorly rather than laterally. The alterations resulting from this type of impingement are remarkably constant. In the later stages, wear can be seen to occur against the anterior edge and undersurface of the anterior third of the acromion (see Fig. 2–14) and acromioclavicular joint (see Fig. 2–15). On the humeral side, wear is centered on the supraspinatus tendon (see Fig. 2–16). The posterior half of the acromion is spared until the end stages, by which time the biceps and infraspinatus are also involved. The progression of changes is as expected, since the position in which the shoulder is most often used in ordinary activities is forward and not lateral (see Fig. 2–3).

Three Stages of Outlet Impingement

To understand the pathology and interpret clinical problems, it is helpful to think of impingement lesions as developing in three progressive stages.[27] The pathology, diagnostic problem, and clinical implications of the various stages of outlet impingement are outlined in Figure 2–13.

Stage I

In Stage I, there is edema and hemorrhage characteristically caused by overuse with the arm above the horizontal. This lesion is reversible with rest, with the tissues becoming normal. A typical example is a young baseball pitcher or tennis player, but it occurs at any age, such as in a middle-aged, weekend hedge clipper. A similar lesion can be produced by a single injury if impaction of the humerus against the acromion produces edema and

Stage I: **Edema and Hemorrhage**

typical age	<25
diff. diagnosis	subluxation, A/C arthritis
clinical course	reversible
treatment	conservative

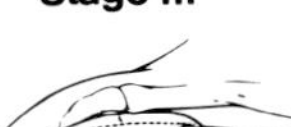

Stage II: **Fibrosis and Tendinitis**

typical age	25–40
diff. diagnosis	frozen shoulder, calcium
clinical course	recurrent pain with activity
treatment	consider bursectomy; C/A ligament division

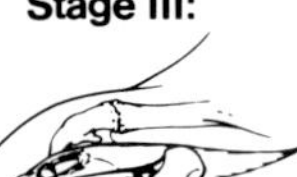

Stage III: **Bone Spurs and Tendon Rupture**

typical age	>40
diff. diagnosis	cervical radiculitis; neoplasm
clinical course	progressive disability
treatment	anterior acromioplasty; rotator cuff repair

Figure 2–13. Classification of the progressive stages of impingement. It is helpful in interpreting clinical problems to think of impingement lesions as developing in three progressive stages, as outlined in this classification. A Stage I or Stage II lesion may occur at any age—for example, in a middle-aged individual clipping hedges on the weekend. Stage III lesions with bone changes and ruptures of the rotator cuff or long head of the biceps occur almost entirely after age 40 years. A/C = acromioclavicular; C/A = coracoacromial. (From Neer, C. S. II: Impingement lesions. Clin. Orthop. 173:70, 1983.)

hemorrhage in the bursa. In this text, the term "acute traumatic subacromial bursitis" will be used for this condition[51] (see p. 81). Both of these lesions give symptoms and signs almost identical to those of a tear of the rotator cuff. Both are frequently misdiagnosed as tears of the rotator cuff, and when, after a period of rest, the pain permanently disappears, the lesion is easily misinterpreted to be a cuff tear that healed spontaneously. This has caused much of the confusion in the literature of the past regarding the indications for repairing rotator cuff tears.

Positive differentiation of these lesions from tears of the rotator cuff requires arthrography; arthroscopy; or, if it becomes perfected, imaging (see p. 89). The treatment for these lesions is conservative, as described on page 93.

Stage II

At Stage II, repeated mechanical insults have led to fibrosis and thickening of the subacromial bursa. The shoulder is comfortable and functions satisfactorily at the side with light activities, but becomes painful with vigorous use above the horizontal. These lesions are less common. They are typically found in an aging athlete between 25 and 40 years of age.

Removal of the thickened bursa and division of the coracoacromial ligament are logical steps when, despite conservative treatment, the disability has persisted for a long time. The results of this procedure have been less satisfying than those with acromioplasty because there has been less pain pre-operatively (the patient being pain-free between activities) and because the recovery time is often several months (while a new bursa is formed). Therefore, I insist on a minimum 18 month period of disability despite conservative treatment before considering this procedure, to give those with Stage I impingement lesions or acute hemorrhagic subacromial bursitis a chance to recover and to make sure there has been enough pain and disability to warrant the procedure.

I very rarely perform an acromioplasty on a patient under 30 years of age because the acromial epiphysis normally remains open until near that time. However, if, when performing a coracoacromial ligament division and bursectomy, a prominence or overhang of the undersurface of the anterior acromion or acromioclavicular joint is found, an anterior acromioplasty is performed even in this younger age group.

Arthroscopic removal of bursal tissue and division of the coracoacromial ligament have become a frequent operation for what is usually referred to as a Stage II impingement lesion. Most of the published series of this procedure contain a high percentage of young patients who have had injuries and have had less than six months disability. In my experience, most patients of this type will recover spontaneously if given time.

Stage III

Stage III is characterized by partial or complete impingement tears of the rotator cuff, biceps ruptures, and the bone changes of impingement. These lesions are extremely rare in patients under 40 years of age, but develop in at least 10 percent of the population subsequent to that age.

I believe, as shown in Table 2–2, that the majority of cuff tears are of the outlet impingement type. In the United States, during recent years, cuff tears in athletes under 40 years of age have been given a great deal of publicity. This has been misleading, since in a typical cross-section of the population, less than 5 percent of cuff tears occur in this younger age group.

Effect of Outlet Impingement on the Acromion

Anterior Acromial Spur

Whether the coracoacromial ligament has a significant function has long been disputed. The pathology of impingement leaves no doubt that it does have the function of acting as a buffer to cushion against the ascent of the humerus. Chronic impact of the humerus against this ligament explains the etiology of anterior acromial spurs, as described in 1972 and illustrated in Figure 2–14. These spurs are the earliest grossly visible alterations on the acromion caused by impingement.[27, 28]

I consider anterior acromial spurs to be traction osteophytes. There are several reasons for this opinion:

1. They are formed within the substance of this ligament.
2. They are separate and apart from the acromioclavicular joint and are not acromioclavicular osteophytes.
3. They are frequently present in patients with other impingement lesions such as cuff tears.

These spurs are thought to be analogous to the spurs on the plantar surface of the os calcis that develop from traction by the plantar fascia.

The old orthopaedic adage "The coracoacromial ligament should be cut whenever it can be seen at surgery" must be incorrect. Because there is convincing evidence that the coracoacromial ligament

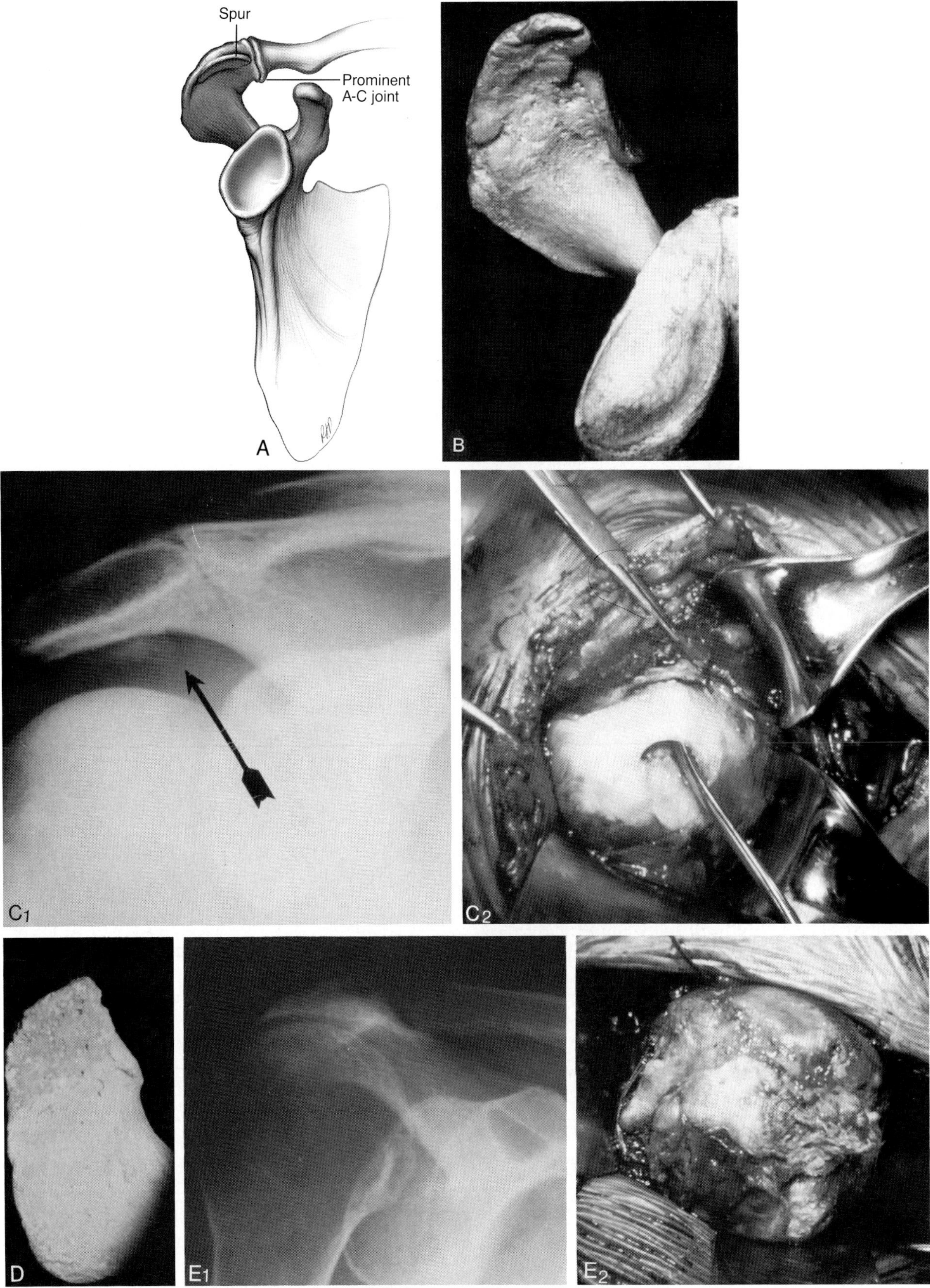

Figure 2–14 *See legend on opposite page*

has a function, it is logical that this ligament should be preserved unless there is a clear indication otherwise. It is sacrificed only for specific impingement problems.

Late Erosion of the Acromion

When there has been long-standing impingement, the undersurface of the anterior third of the acromion may become worn away with disappearance of the spur, leaving an area of erosion and eburnation as seen in Figure 2–13. Erosion may eventually extend to the undersurface of the acromioclavicular joint. In the final stages, as in some patients with cuff-tear arthropathy, the acromion is worn all the way through, producing a "flail acromion" (see Fig. 2–47), which has abnormal motion like that of an unfused acromial epiphysis.

Effect of Outlet Impingement on the Acromioclavicular Joint

There is good evidence to prove that the acromioclavicular joint may contribute to impingement. The supraspinatus tendon lies directly beneath it, and when the arm is raised above 70 degrees, the greater tuberosity passes under the acromioclavicular joint, where it may impinge. Radiographically, the acromioclavicular joint may be seen to encroach on the outlet for the supraspinatus in lateral views ("outlet view") (see Figs. 2–6 and 2–28). Evidence of impingement against the undersurface of the acromioclavicular joint includes the "geyser sign" and false acromioclavicular ganglion.

"Geyser Sign"

In long-standing impingement, the anterior acromion is worn away and replaced by an area of eburnation and sclerosis (see Fig. 2–14). Impingement wear may continue until it perforates the acromioclavicular joint. By this time, there is almost invariably an impingement tear of the rotator cuff. When there is a concomitant perforation of the acromioclavicular joint and tear of the rotator cuff, fluid injected into the glenohumeral joint for an arthrogram enters the acromioclavicular joint—the "geyser sign" (Fig. 2–15).

False Acromioclavicular Ganglion

The coexistence of a cuff tear and perforation of the acromioclavicular joint may be associated with distension of the acromioclavicular joint by joint fluid. Distension of the surface of this joint may come to resemble a ganglion (Fig. 2–15). Unwitting attempts to excise this as a ganglion usually result in a joint sinus.

Direction of Impingement Erosion

In some individuals, the acromioclavicular joint causes impingement before the anterior acromion because of marginal osteophytes at the acromioclavicular joint or the anatomical configuration of the deep surface of this joint. More often, the anterior acromion is involved first and the erosion extends later to involve the acromioclavicular joint.

In the end stages of the impingement process, as in cuff-tear arthropathy, there is erosion of the undersurface of the acromion, the acromioclavicular joint, the outer clavicle, and the coracoid process (see Figs. 2–18, 2–36, and 2–47). The type of erosion seen in the end stages proves that the pathway of impingement is directed anteriorly and toward the acromioclavicular joint rather than against the lateral acromion.

Effect of Outlet Impingement on the Supraspinatus Tendon

Theories on the etiology of cuff tears are discussed on pages 64 to 70. It seems important to disagree with any theory that lacks appreciation for the frequent role of impingement and the frequent need for decompression of the supraspinatus by an anterior acromioplasty when repairing these lesions (Table 2–2).

Figure 2–14. Effect of outlet impingement on the acromion. Drawing of an anterior acromial spur (A), similar to that seen in a dried specimen (B) and in the x-rays of a 44 year old woman who had a small tear of the rotator cuff (C). Note that the spur occurs in the coracoacromial ligament (which attaches on the undersurface of the acromion) and is not an osteophyte of the acromioclavicular joint because it does not reach the joint margin. The spur is considered to be a traction osteophyte. The photograph of the undersurface of the acromion (D) shows eburnation and erosion of the anterior one-third of the acromion extending into the acromioclavicular joint, characteristic of a later stage of impingement similar to what is seen in the x-ray of a 70 year old man (E1) who had a massive cuff tear (E2).

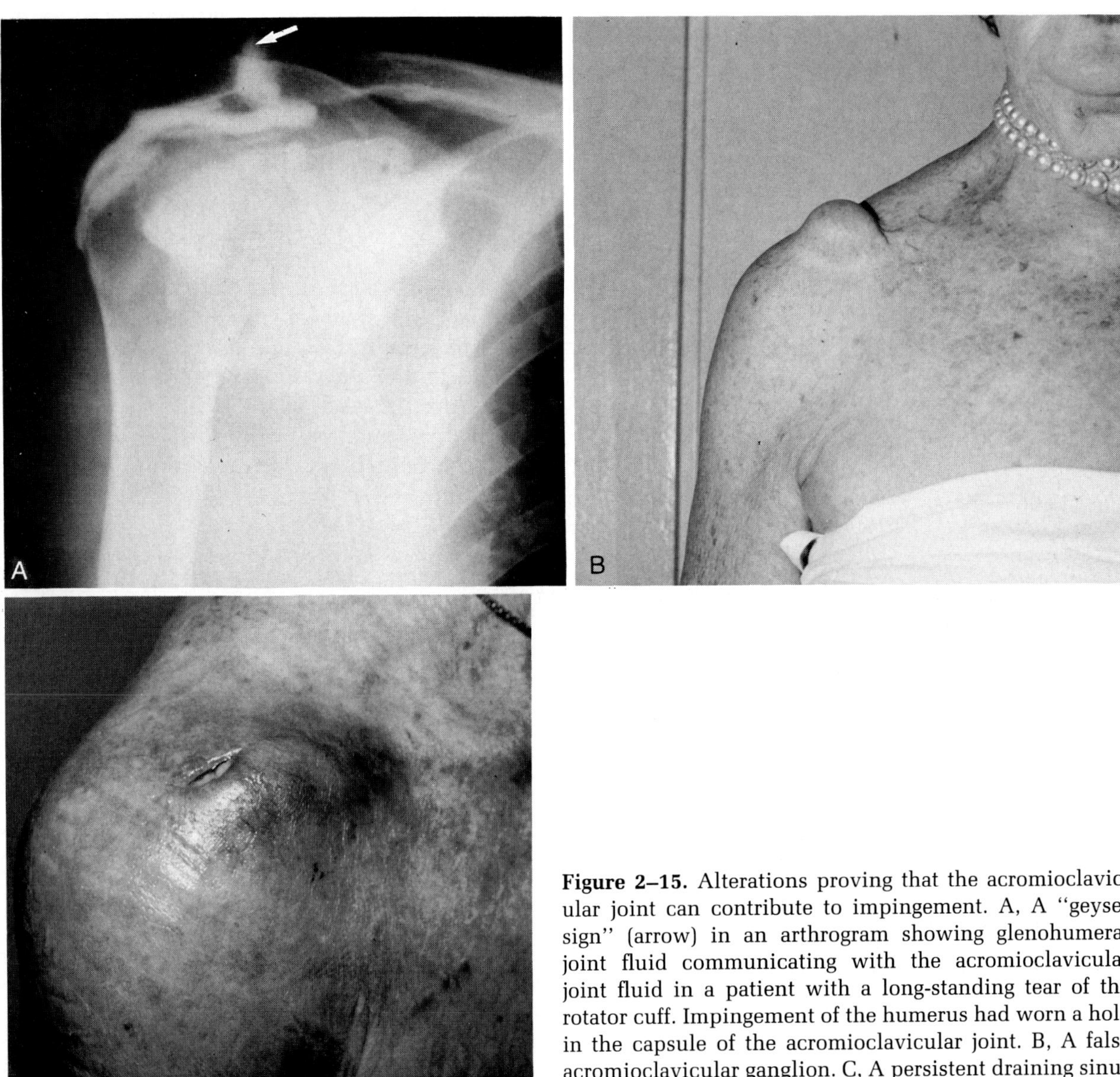

Figure 2–15. Alterations proving that the acromioclavicular joint can contribute to impingement. A, A "geyser sign" (arrow) in an arthrogram showing glenohumeral joint fluid communicating with the acromioclavicular joint fluid in a patient with a long-standing tear of the rotator cuff. Impingement of the humerus had worn a hole in the capsule of the acromioclavicular joint. B, A false acromioclavicular ganglion. C, A persistent draining sinus after an unwary surgeon had attempted to excise a false ganglion of this type.

Table 2–2. CLASSIFICATION OF TEARS OF THE ROTATOR CUFF

MECHANISM	% OF ALL TEARS	AGE OF PATIENT (YEARS)	PATHOLOGY	PROGNOSIS	TREATMENT
"Impingement Tears" Due to outlet impingement No injury in 50%	95	Over 40	Centered on the supraspinatus. May be suddenly enlarged by a trivial injury ("acute extension")	Tend to progress slowly unless "acute extension"	Anterior acromioplasty and cuff repair
Traumatic Tears Single injury	Under 5 Rare (without fractures)	Under 40	Usually incomplete supraspinatus tears	Tend to heal	Conservative
Repetitive microtrauma	For example, baseball pitchers	Under 40	Usually incomplete supraspinatus tears	Tend to heal	Rest. Later change style or use
Supreme violence	Traction injury or "superior dislocation"	Any age	Massive cuff avulsion, often with nerve injuries	Guarded	Early recognition and surgical repair
"Rotator Interval Tears" Enlarged rotator interval of acquired multidirectional dislocations	Under 5	Under 40	"Cleft" enlargement with instability. Arthrogram usually shows ballooning rather than leak	Recurrent dislocations Chronic disability	Repair interval and repair instability— e.g., inferior capsular shift (see Chapter 4)
Acute glenohumeral dislocations after age 40 years		Over 40	Interval and subscapularis tendon torn	Might heal	Observe initially

Wear on the Supraspinatus

On the humeral side, impingement wear is centered on the facet for the insertion of the supraspinatus tendon (Figs. 2–1 and 2–16). When the arm is at the side in neutral rotation, most of the rotation of the supraspinatus is anterior to the acromion (see Fig. 2–3). With internal rotation, the insertion of the supraspinatus is brought even more anterior. With external rotation, the facet for the insertion of the supraspinatus lies just lateral to the anterior third of the acromion. The reader can palpate his or her shoulder to confirm these points. With elevation of the arm, the insertion of the supraspinatus passes under the anterior acromion, coracoacromial ligament, and acromioclavicular joint. When there is a prominence of the undersurface of the acromion or acromioclavicular joint causing impingement, repetitive motion leads to outlet impingement tears that consistently start at the supraspinatus tendon.

Impingement tears begin with fibrillation followed by detachment of the superficial layers, the deep layers, or the intratendinous fibers of the supraspinatus (Figs. 2–16 and 2–42). These are termed "incomplete tears." If the tear enlarges with perforation of the full thickness of the tendon, it becomes a "complete tear" (Fig. 2–16B through G). With further enlargement of the tear, the area of fibrillation and inflammation may extend to include the anterior part of the infraspinatus and the long head of the biceps. Occasionally, the subscapularis tendon is involved before the infraspinatus, but this is unusual. When a tear involves two tendons, as shown in Figure 2–16G, it is termed "massive."

"Acute Extension"

The edges of impingement tears are usually smooth and falciform, and there is often an area of sclerosis on the greater tuberosity where the supraspinatus had inserted. Trauma may suddenly enlarge an impingement tear. In this text, this is termed "acute extension." An acute extension is characterized by irregularly torn edges extending from the area of scarred tendon and by a plaque of sclerotic bone on the greatest tuberosity (Fig. 2–16H).

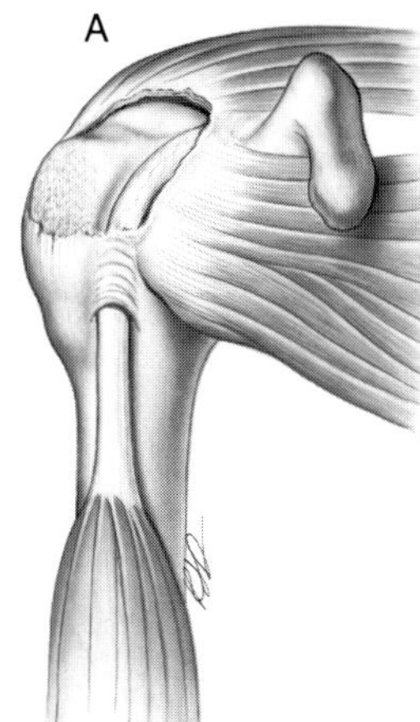

Figure 2–16. "Impingement tears" showing the effect of outlet impingement on the supraspinatus tendon. A drawing of a typical well-established impingement tear with complete disruption of the supraspinatus tendon, an excrescence on the greater tuberosity posterior to the biceps groove, and a rounded falciform edge at the tear, showing it has been there for some time.

B to G are photographs in the operating room of impingement cuff tears, progressing in size from B, an incomplete bursal side tear; to G, a massive, long-standing tear with early trophic changes of the articular surface and a rupture of the long head of the biceps.

B, "Deep surface blister." C, 1.5 cm. tear in the supraspinatus with a falciform edge. D, All of the supraspinatus tendon is torn. E, All of the supraspinatus tendon and the anterior part of the infraspinatus tendon are torn.

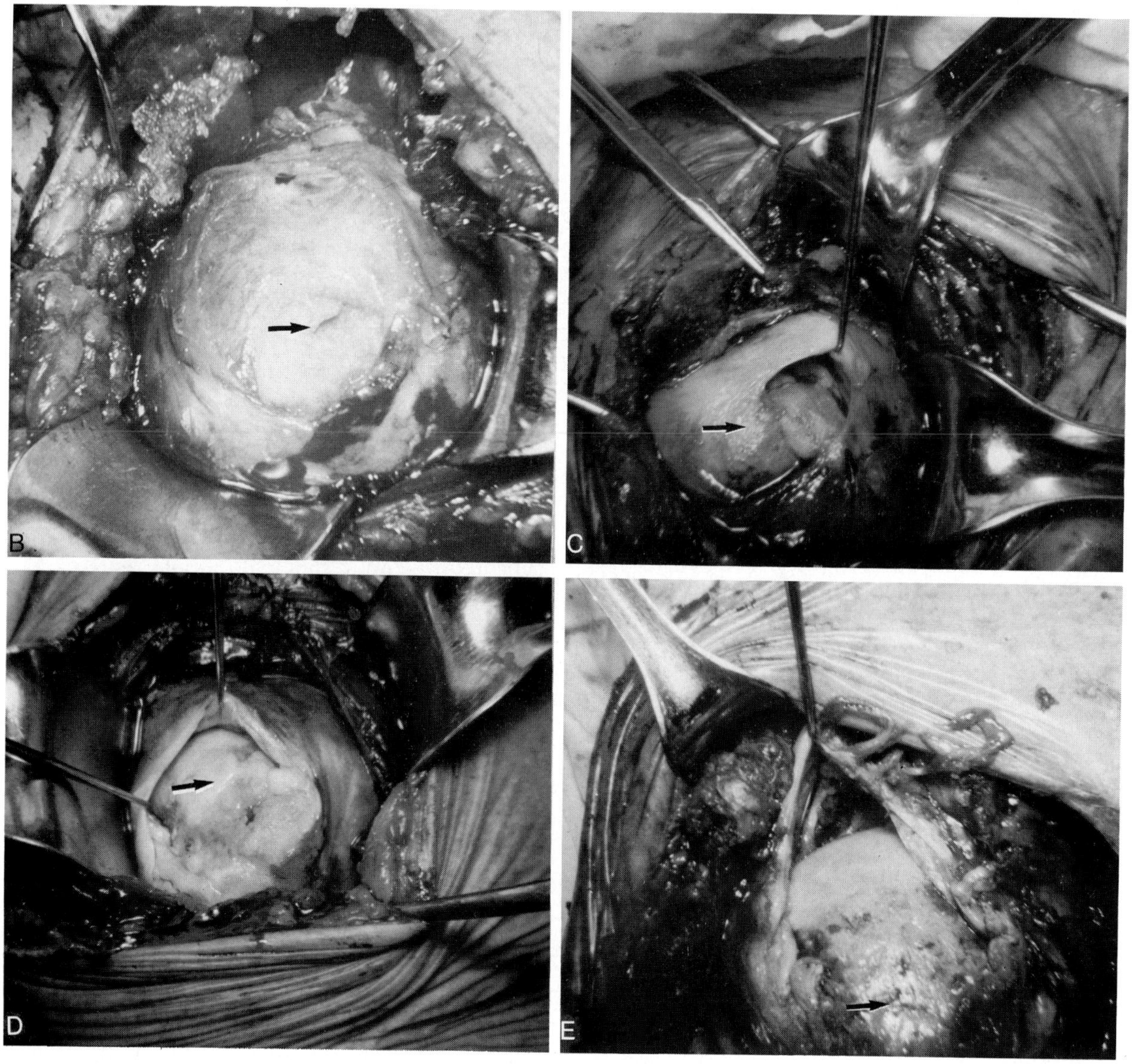

B

C

D

E

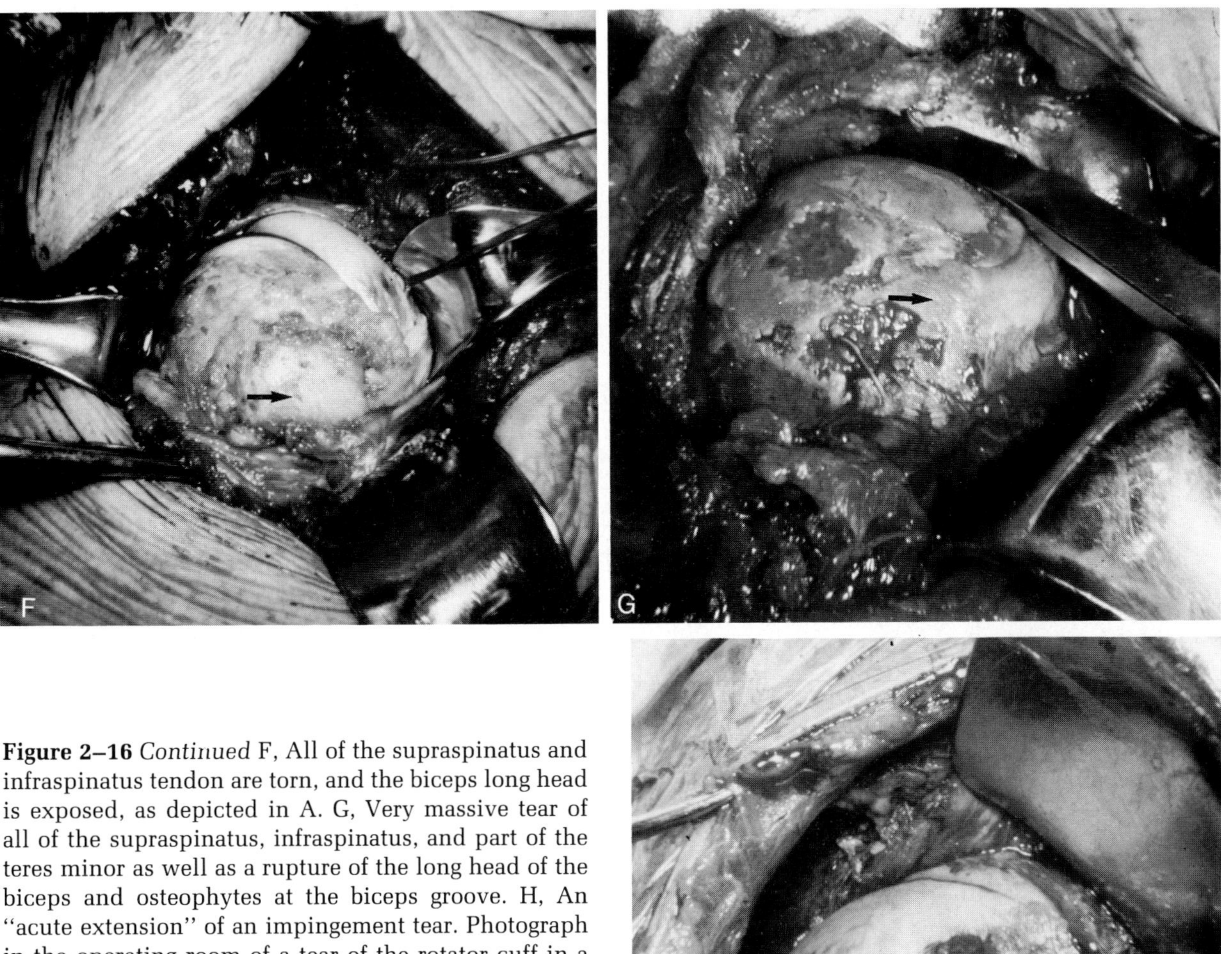

Figure 2–16 *Continued* F, All of the supraspinatus and infraspinatus tendon are torn, and the biceps long head is exposed, as depicted in A. G, Very massive tear of all of the supraspinatus, infraspinatus, and part of the teres minor as well as a rupture of the long head of the biceps and osteophytes at the biceps groove. H, An "acute extension" of an impingement tear. Photograph in the operating room of a tear of the rotator cuff in a 60 year old man showing a small area of sclerosis (arrow) where impingement wear had occurred and behind it irregular, recently torn tendon was seen. Wear had occurred prior to a trivial injury (starting a lawn mower), which tore through the remains of the supraspinatus and into the infraspinatus tendon and caused sudden weakness of external rotation and inability to raise the arm.

Effect of Outlet Impingement on the Biceps

The frequent finding of fraying or rupture of the long head of the biceps concomitantly with the larger tears of the supraspinatus tendon (see p. 74) is strong evidence that most cuff tears are caused by impingement rather than by deficient circulation in the supraspinatus tendon. Impaired blood supply in the supraspinatus would not cause ruptures of the biceps. Conversely, this finding indicates that most biceps lesions are also caused by impingement.

Many anatomists thought biceps lesions were caused by skeletal abnormalities in the slope and depth of the groove. I believe that impingement produces these skeletal abnormalities by causing bone proliferation and excrescences that cause narrowing of the groove, which have been misinterpreted as congenital defects (e.g., termed "supratubercular ridge," Fig. 2–17). When deformity of the groove develops, it may contribute to ruptures of the biceps; however, I believe that this contribution is less than the trauma of impingement directly on the biceps tendon. Excrescences at the bicipital groove are often present in glenohumeral osteoarthritis (see Chapter 3), but biceps ruptures very rarely occur in this condition,[2, 68] probably because there is no impingement with osteoarthritis.

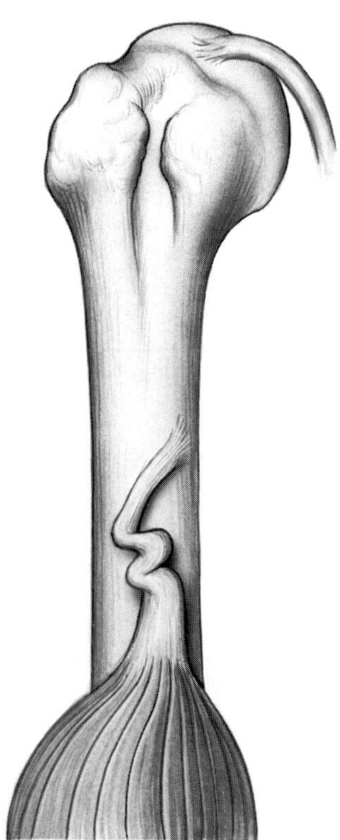

Figure 2–17. Effect of outlet impingement on the biceps. Chronic impingement can cause excrescences and narrowing of the bicipital groove and eventually rupture of the long head. These alterations have in the past been mistaken as developmental variants and termed "supratubercular ridge." Eventually, impingement can cause rounding of the tuberosities and flattening of the groove, as shown in Figure 2–18, with attenuation of the soft tissue bridging the groove, which in some patients who escape rupture is associated with a dislocation of the long head.

Collagen disorders, such as rheumatoid arthritis, proximal humeral fractures, and other conditions, may destroy the long head, but this is not germane to this discussion of biceps ruptures in healthy patients. In these conditions, the type of impingement that occurs when the articular surfaces of the glenohumeral joint are destroyed and the humerus translocates upward may become a factor in the destruction of the biceps.

Why the long head of the biceps occasionally ruptures before the supraspinatus can be explained by a more laterally located bicipital groove (see Fig. 2–25). Normally the bicipital groove is located on the humerus from 10 to 15 degrees lateral to straight ahead when the arm is held in the anatomical position. If this groove is located a little more laterally, nearer the usual location for the facet for the insertion of the supraspinatus tendon, impingement is then centered on the biceps groove rather than on the supraspinatus insertion. To date, this point of anatomy has not been proved because the few individuals who are seen with ruptures of the long head and an intact supraspinatus by arthrogram are infrequently explored and have not been studied with CT scans to determine the version of the groove.

The concept that most biceps lesions are caused by impingement is of great practical importance in the clinical evaluation and treatment of these lesions. Impingement lesions of the biceps include biceps tenosynovitis, fraying, splitting, flattening, ruptures, and dislocation (Table 2–3). The diagnostic implications are outlined in Table 2–7, and treatment is reviewed on page 91.

Table 2–3. CLASSIFICATION OF BICEPS LESIONS

I. *IMPINGEMENT LESIONS OF LONG HEAD*
   - A. Tendinitis and tenosynovitis
   - B. Rupture in the groove ("high rupture")
     1. Retracted
     2. Self-attaching
     3. Partial re-attachment
   - C. Subluxations and dislocations with large cuff tears

II. *NON-IMPINGEMENT LESIONS**
   - A. Rupture at the musculotendinous junction ("low rupture")
   - B. Rupture of the short head*

*Have not been encountered by the author.

Effect of Outlet Impingement on the Proximal Humerus

Excrescences

In the earlier stages of impingement—Stage I, Stage II, and early Stage III (see Fig. 2–35)—there are no definite roentgen evidences to indicate the presence of impingement. Later in Stage III, skeletal alterations appear. The first roentgen evidence of impingement is usually at the greater tuberosity rather than on the acromial side. An excrescence with squaring of the greater tuberosity at the site of insertion of the supraspinatus tendon is usually the first visible change (Figs. 2–18 and 2–35). This develops because of friction. An anterior acromial spur may appear next. Decalcification occurring beneath the area of impingement on the greater tuberosity soon develops because of disuse. Decalcification in the greater tuberosity can become intense, resembling a lytic neoplasm in x-ray films. This has been biopsied in error. Gradually, loss of the acromiohumeral distance occurs. Later, the excrescence on the greater tuberosity becomes worn away and a sclerotic plaque appears. The anterior acromial spur is usually worn away at the same time, and a corresponding sclerotic plaque develops on the undersurface of the acromion.

Rounding of the Greater Tuberosity

In the advanced stage of impingement, the greater tuberosity is rounded and the sulcus between the articular surface and the tuberosity is lost (Figs. 2–18 and 2–47). At this stage, it is difficult to distinguish where the margin of the articular surface begins and ends, and the bicipital groove may become obliterated. Rounding of the greater tuberosity in the late stage corresponds to what E. A. Codman[6] termed "recession of the tuberosity." He thought that this was due to disuse atrophy and that the loss of the greater tuberosity occurred because the rotator tendons were no longer exerting traction on the tuberosity. It seems important to disagree with this explanation because it implies that there is no need for anterior acromioplasty when repairing cuff tears. Rounding of the greater tuberosity is due to subacromial impingement, as proved by the consistent finding of a corresponding area of bone reaction or erosion on the undersurface of the acromion. Certainly, this would not have occurred if the loss of the greater tuberosity had been due to disuse atrophy rather than to wear.

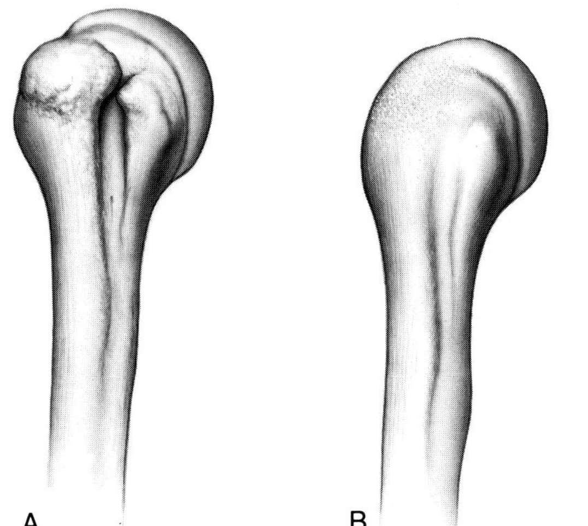

Figure 2–18. Effect of outlet impingement on the proximal humerus. A, The earlier skeletal changes consist of excrescences formed at the greater tuberosity and bicipital groove. B, In the late stages, the greater tuberosity becomes rounded and the bicipital groove is obliterated.

Cuff-Tear Arthropathy

This condition is discussed in detail on pages 124 to 134. "Cuff-tear arthropathy" is a term introduced in 1975[20–24] to denote a new entity recognized to be the end result of some cuff tears. It is characterized by extreme skeletal alterations (Figs. 2–36 and 2–47). Fortunately, not over 5 percent of cuff tears progress this far. The term denotes rounding of the greater tuberosity, retraction of the rotator tendons, rupture or dislocation of the long head of the biceps, and also distortion and incongruity of the articular surfaces of the humeral head and glenoid. Distortion of the articular surfaces is essential for making this diagnosis.

This condition has important physiological and therapeutic connotations. It demonstrates a third function for the rotator cuff. The rotator cuff is important not only for (1) movement of the glenohumeral joint and (2) stability, but also for (3) nourishment of the articular surfaces of the glenohumeral joint. Cuff-tear arthropathy also demonstrates the direction of the forces in outlet impingement. It is difficult to treat.

TEARS OF THE ROTATOR CUFF

Cuff-Tear Terminology

If you would speak to me, first define your terms.
Voltaire

"Partial Tear." This is the same as "incomplete tear" and indicates that it does not extend through the complete thickness of the tendon. Three types are recognized: superficial surface, deep surface, and intratendinous, as illustrated in Figure 2–16B.

"Complete Tear." Extends through the complete thickness of the tendon.

"Massive Tear." More than one rotator cuff tendon is torn.

"Degenerative Tears." This term is too vague to use. It could indicate nutritional or metabolic factors rather than wear or injury. If impaired circulation in the supraspinatus tendon is present, it is considered to be secondary to the scarring caused by impingement rather than the primary cause of the tear.

"Traumatic Tear." Implies an injury tearing a healthy tendon (see Table 2–2). (Cuff tears associated with fractures of the tuberosities are considered in Chapters 3 and 5, and are not included in this discussion.)

"Acute Extension." Implies an injury suddenly enlarging an impingement tear. The injury is often trivial.

Etiology of Cuff Tears

Smith (1834) is credited with the first description of a rupture of the supraspinatus tendon.[56] That lesion was thought to be due to an injury. Codman (1931 and 1934) also considered ruptures of the supraspinatus tendon to be primarily due to *trauma* and emphasized its importance in industrial workers.[6, 43] The anatomist Meyer (1931 and 1937) thought that supraspinatus tendon ruptures as well as ruptures of the long tendon of the biceps were due to attrition and *overuse*.[44, 45] However, Keyes (1935), in post-mortem studies, thought age and trauma to be factors and found no evidence of inflammation.[57] He favored the hypothesis of Meyer, that protracted use is the most important factor. Some investigators proposed *inflammation* that was due to toxin or a virus as a precursor to cuff tears. Olsson (1953) considered *curvature of the head of the humerus* to cause ischemia of the rotator cuff and biceps.[58] The hypothesis of *inadequate blood supply to the supraspinatus* tendon was also proposed by others. Rathbun and MacNab (1970), in microvascular studies, found an avascular area in the supraspinatus tendon and a similar avascular area in the long head of the biceps where these tendons cross over the head of the humerus.[33] They too thought inadequate blood supply to the tendons to be the main factor. However, Goldie and Moseley (1963) and others showed the "critical zone" in the supraspinatus tendon to be well vascularized throughout life.[49, 50] In 1972, I proposed *impingement* beneath the anterior acromion and acromioclavicular joint to be the most frequent cause.[28] Individual variations in the shape and slope of the acromion and the shape of the undersurface of the acromioclavicular joint better explained the consistent pathology and the variable lifestyle of patients and the frequent absence of an injury. The dissection studies of Peterssen (1983) confirmed my impingement theory.[53] He agreed that the impingement could come from either the anterior acromion or the undersurface of the acromioclavicular joint and concurred the validity of anterior acromioplasty at the time of repairing tears of the rotator cuff. He found osteophytes on the undersurface of the acromioclavicular joint more frequently than anterior acromial osteophytes. Subsequent dissection studies of other investigators also confirm impingement to be the most important etiological factor and confirm the logic of anterior acromioplasty in treatment.[52, 82–85, 115]

Table 2–2 summarizes the *author's opinion* on the etiology of cuff tears. The existence of traumatic tears and tears resulting from repetitive microtrauma is recognized, but these lesions are infrequent and are usually quite small. They are treated conservatively. The theory of inadequate blood supply in the "critical zone" of the supraspinatus tendon is explained by the scarring in the tendon resulting from chronic impingement. The theory of cuff tears being caused by the normal degeneration in the process of aging does not explain why most of the population never develops cuff tears. The theory of excessive use[44, 45, 57] in occupations and activities does not explain why, with improved methods of diagnosis, cuff tears are seen with greater frequency in sedentary individuals who have never done heavy labor, often in the nondominant shoulder, frequently in both shoulders of the same individual, and often in women. The theory of trauma as the primary cause cannot explain why many patients with complete tears of the rotator cuff are unable to recall ever having a definite injury. The theory of impingement explains the pathology and explains the variations in the types of patients involved.

Classification of Cuff Tears

The types of cuff tears I have seen are summarized in Table 2–2 according to etiology, incidence, typical age of the patient at the time of diagnosis, pathology, clinical behavior, and recommended treatment. We will consider each separately but with emphasis on impingement tears because they are far more important in everyday life. The different types of cuff tears are illustrated in Figure 2–19.

Traumatic Tears

Two types of traumatic tears are seen. Both are rare. One results from a single violent injury, and the other occurs from repeated microtrauma with a gradual breakdown of an area within the tendon.

Traumatic Tears from a Single Injury

The tendons of the cuff in younger individuals (under 40 years of age) are so thick and strong that they usually avulse part of the tuberosity rather than tear. In older patients, an impingement tear may be enlarged by the injury, but this is classified with impingement tears as an "acute extension" rather than with traumatic tears. Thus, a true traumatic tear resulting from a single violent event is extremely rare.

Of 340 tears of Series II (see p. 75), only eight occurred in patients under 40 years of age and only two as a result of a single violent injury (without avulsing fragments of bone). The rarity of complete traumatic tears can be appreciated by considering the findings in the hundreds of shoulders treated surgically for recurrent anterior dislocations in patients who are between 18 and 25 years of age without finding a single complete tear of the rotator cuff.

Patients with recurrent anterior dislocations may have arthrographic or arthroscopic evidence of incomplete deep surface tears near the site of the Hill-Sachs[162] defect in the insertion of the infraspinatus tendon; however, this type of tear is of no consequence. It is not seen during the repair of recurrently dislocating shoulders and causes no symptoms subsequent to the repair.

Other incomplete traumatic tears are occasionally seen after a single injury such as a hard fall

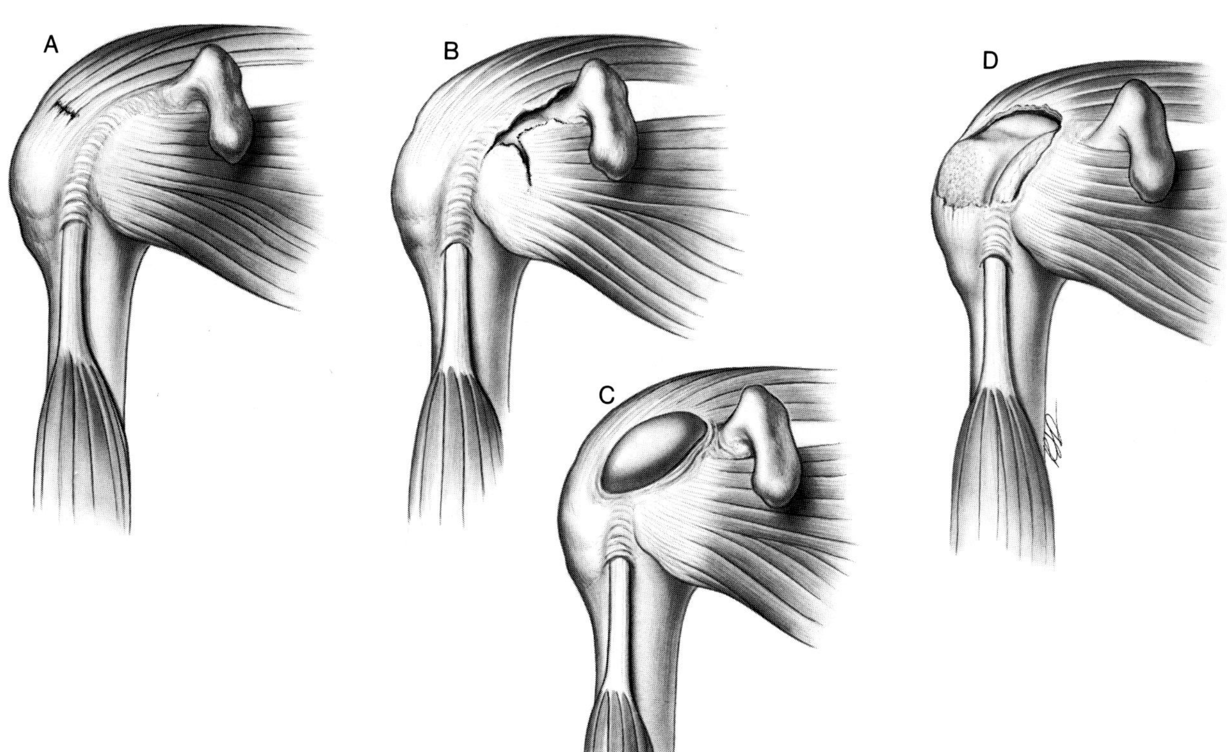

Figure 2–19. Classification of Cuff Tears. A, "Traumatic tear" as occasionally seen in the under 35 year old athlete. B, "Rotator interval tear" with or without an extension into the subscapularis tendon, as occurs at times in the over 40 year old age group who have acute glenohumeral dislocations when there has been no impingement wear to weaken the supraspinatus tendon. C, Rotator interval tear associated with multidirectional dislocations as caused by repetitive trauma in the under 35 year old age group. D, "Impingement tear" with wear centered on the supraspinatus as seen in the over 40 year old age group, which composes 90 percent of tears of the rotator cuff.

while skiing, as shown in Figure 2–20. These lesions are treated conservatively and, since there is no impingement to interfere with healing, can be seen to heal spontaneously when followed with arthrograms.

Treatment. My treatment of small traumatic tears following a single injury consists of reducing the activities of the patient temporarily (and prohibiting hard throwing, lifting, and impact loads for one year). Arthroscopic debridement of the edges of these tears has not been proved to hasten or enhance spontaneous healing. However, arthroscopic examination for purposes of determining the size of the tear and following the course of healing might yield useful information. The arthrogram is repeated 9 to 12 months after the injury to demonstrate healing of the tear. At that time, full activities are allowed.

Traumatic Tears Due to Repetitive Microtrauma

Breakdown of the fibers within the tendons of the rotator cuff as a result of repetitive microtrauma is seen only in a few activities that place unusual stress on the shoulder, such as baseball pitching. Jobe and Tibone have classified the mechanism of these tears in baseball pitchers.[55, 70] Repeated, hard stress on tendons augmented by an unnatural excursion of the shoulder occurs in this activity. The external rotation and extension of the shoulder cause some impingement of the rotator cuff against the acromion. This is a secondary factor that together with the abnormal force on the tendon, causes microdegeneration of some of the tendon fibers. The area of microdegeneration may enlarge to eventually become a defect visible in an arthrogram. This type of cuff tear is usually incomplete, and if complete, is usually small compared with the average impingement tears.

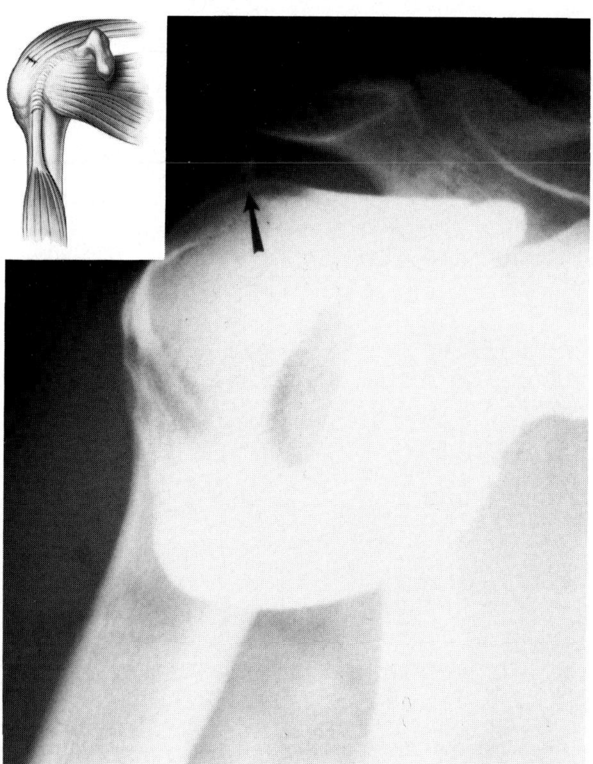

Figure 2–20. Traumatic tear in young athlete. Arthrogram showing a small tear (arrow, and as depicted in the inset), in a 28 year old man who had a hard fall while skiing. This healed spontaneously, and the arthrogram was negative 9 months later.

The pathomechanics of this type of tear differs from that of outlet impingement tears in that in this injury the impingement factor as well as the stress component can be eliminated by discontinuing the unnatural use of the shoulder. In contrast, outlet impingement may continue in everyday activities.

Treatment. Spontaneous healing of tears that are due to repetitive microtrauma can occur if throwing is discontinued. I have observed spontaneous healing of these lesions in arthrograms. Healing may also be seen by arthroscopy. Debriding the edges of this type of tear has not been proved to expedite or benefit the quality of the healing. After healing of the tendon has occurred, the style of throwing should be corrected and the arm carefully reconditioned before resuming play. Following this regimen a pitcher may eventually be able to resume pitching without recurrence of the tear. Jobe and Tibone, who have had the largest experience with this type of tear in baseball players, advise that the initial treatment should be conservative. Anterior acromioplasty to relieve impingement caused by the abnormal excursion of motion of the shoulder in this sport may eventually be considered in some patients who have chronic disability; however, since the supraspinatus outlet is normal, this procedure is less logical. Anterior acromioplasty makes more room to permit the abnormal excursion of motion without impingement; however, this should not be considered unless the disability has continued for at least one year. It is then advised only after making sure that there is no problem of glenohumeral instability, calcium deposit, frozen shoulder, or other lesion contributing to the disability. Repeated re-examinations are important in making this decision. The variable period before complete recovery following anterior acromioplasty, as described on page 106, must be emphasized pre-operatively, and the patient should be aware that the prognosis is guarded for his return to professional level pitching. The need for guarding the prognosis for return to such abnormal stress on the shoulder is obvious if one considers that it was this type of stress that caused the problem in the first place and that the lesion developed because of this activity in a normal individual with a normal supraspinatus outlet without a previous problem.

Rotator Interval Tears

The rotator interval is described on page 35 and Figure 1–27; it is the space between the supraspinatus and subscapularis tendons. Enlargement or disruption of this interval differs from impingement tears. There is no tendon at this site, and generally no ongoing impingement wear. Two types of rotator interval tears are seen. Both are associated with glenohumeral dislocations. First, in the under 40 year age group, a ballooning-out enlargement of this interval may be seen in patients with anterior and multidirectional glenohumeral laxity that has been acquired because of more violent repetitive trauma, as in javelin throwing (see Fig. 2–21 and Chapter 4). A second type of rotator interval tear is seen in patients over 40 years of age, which occurs with an acute anterior glenohumeral dislocation. In this type of tear, there is a longitudinal tear in the rotator interval that may be associated with some detachment of the upper part of the subscapularis tendon, as shown in Figure 2–19.

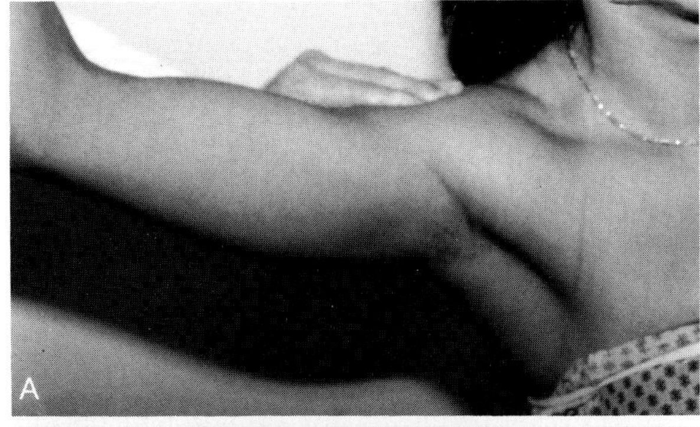

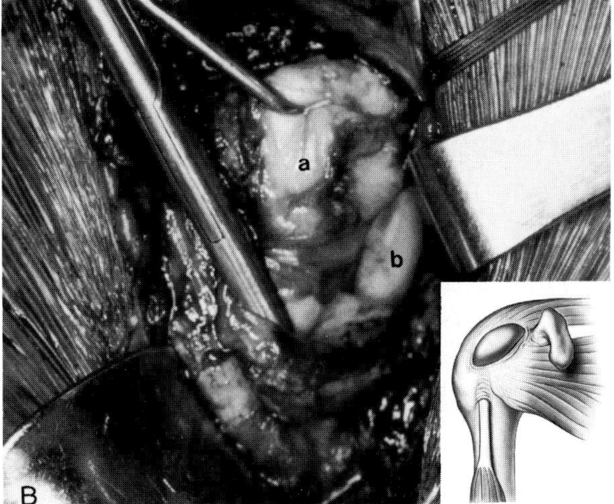

Figure 2–21. Rotator interval tear in a 29 year old javelin thrower (as depicted in the inset) who had developed multidirectional dislocations. A, Pre-operatively, the shoulder could be dislocated while doing an anterior apprehension test. B, Photograph in the operating room showing the opening between the supraspinatus tendon (a) and the subscapularis tendon (b).

Enlarged Rotator Interval in Acquired Glenohumeral Dislocations

Enlargement of the rotator interval in patients under 40 usually results from repeated violent forces on the capsule. Activities such as gymnastics, butterfly and backstroke swimming, and other less violent sports may lead to multidirectional instability, often with spreading of the "cleft" between the superior and middle glenohumeral ligaments[13] (see Fig. 1–9 and Chapter 4) but without enlargement of the rotator interval. Heavier activities, such as javelin throwing and weight lifting, may cause further enlargement of this opening between the ligaments until spreading and thinning of the tissue at the rotator interval occur. This lesion is usually seen in an arthrogram as a ballooning rather than a leak of dye into the bursa. In extreme cases, there is spreading and an opening in the rotator interval, as depicted in Figure 2–21, without tearing of a tendon.

Treatment. It is important to recognize that this lesion can occur and, if present, almost always exists with concomitant glenohumeral instability. If instability is present, closure of the rotator interval alone is insufficient treatment. Adequate surgical treatment involves repair of the dislocations by reconstruction of the capsule and ligaments in addition to the closure of the rotator interval, as discussed in Chapter 4, page 303 and Fig. 4–31E.

Interval Tears with Acute Dislocations

The only tears occurring with acute dislocations in the younger age group have been either incomplete deep surface tears of the infraspinatus tendon adjacent to a posterior head defect (Hill-Sachs defect) in patients with recurrent anterior dislocations or rotator interval enlargement, as has just been discussed. The exception to this is a special type of extensive tear that occurs only occasionally without a fracture from supreme violence. It is usually associated with nerve injuries (see Fig. 2–24). It occurs in the younger age group as well as after age 40 years, and is discussed on page 69. After age 40, cuff tears occurring with acute dislocations are common. In this group, the tear may extend from a pre-existing impingement tear in the supraspinatus, or it may be a longitudinal tear in the rotator interval extending into the subscapularis tendon. The latter type could heal spontaneously, whereas it is unlikely that the tear extending from an impingement lesion could heal satisfactorily without repair. In elderly patients, the extension of an impingement tear is often quite massive, leading to marked instability through the "posterior mechanism" (see Fig. 2–23A).

Treatment. Tears as indicated by a positive arthrogram following a dislocation in patients over 40 years of age are treated by four to six weeks of immobilization followed by gradual resumption of activities. If the tear is through the rotator interval rather than an enlargement of an impingement tear, there should be a good chance it will heal. If symptoms persist or recurrent dislocations occur, as depicted in Figure 2–22, surgical repair is advised. If surgery is performed, the labrum is inspected through the cuff defect prior to closing it. There may be, in addition to the cuff tear ("posterior mechanism"), a detachment of the anterior labrum ("anterior mechanism"), as in Figure 2–23B. In this case, the labrum is re-attached to the scapula before closing the cuff tear. This can be accomplished through the tear with the anterior acromioplasty approach (Fig. 2–23B), provided that the arm is maintained in forward flexion during the repair. Aftercare varies from the usual repair for recurrent anterior dislocations in that pendulum exercises and passive elevation to prevent adhesions around the cuff repair are started early, but external rotation is not allowed for several weeks to allow the labrum to re-attach.

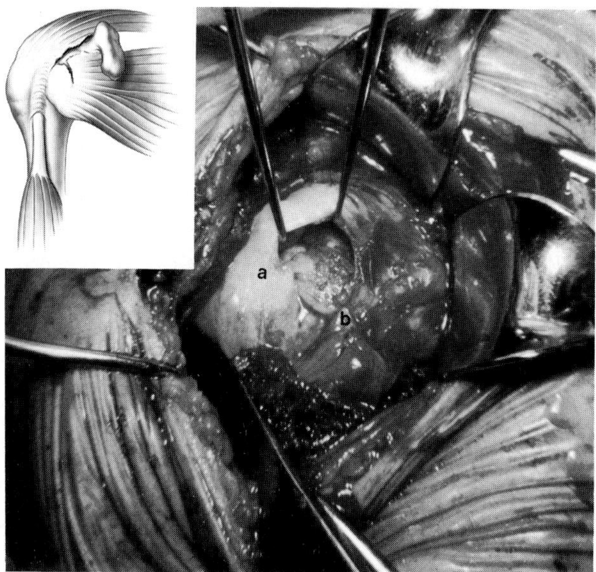

Figure 2–22. Rotator interval tear (between the supraspinatus tendon [a] and the subscapularis tendon [b] and extending down into the subscapularis tendon), as shown in the inset, in a 56 year old woman who had fallen down the stairs and sustained an acute anterior glenohumeral dislocation 3 months previously.

"Posterior Mechanism"

The term "posterior mechanism" refers to detachment of the rotator cuff from the humerus permitting the dislocation to occur rather than detachment of the anterior labrum or elongation of the capsule and ligaments. A displaced fracture of the greater tuberosity with anterior dislocation, although not included in this discussion of cuff tears without fractures, illustrates how the posterior mechanism works. This fracture is associated with a longitudinal tear of the rotator cuff that allows the dislocation to occur. When the dislocation is reduced, the displaced greater tuberosity usually falls back into good position with adequate approximation of the torn edges of the tendon. Spontaneous healing of the tear usually occurs without residual instability. This same type of healing can occur also in traumatic longitudinal tears of the rotator interval without fractures. However, an acute extension of an impingement tear occurring at the time of dislocation cannot be expected to heal without surgical repair. These points establish the logic for the treatment.

Initial Dislocation After Age 40 Without a Cuff Tear

Although it is important to know of the "posterior mechanism" and of the possibility of cuff tears occurring with dislocations after middle age, at the same time it should be clarified that the majority of patients who dislocate their shoulders for the first time after age 40 do not tear the rotator cuff. In one personal series of 17 patients who experienced dislocations for the first time after age 40 and were subsequently explored surgically, only 5 (30 percent) showed evidence of ever having sustained a tear of the rotator cuff. Those without tears have similar pathology to younger patients with dislocations—i.e., anterior labrum detachment or elongation of the glenohumeral ligaments, as discussed in Chapter 4. A patient who dislocates the shoulder for the first time after age 40 and has an intact cuff is treated with a period of immobilization in the same way as a young patient with a first dislocation.

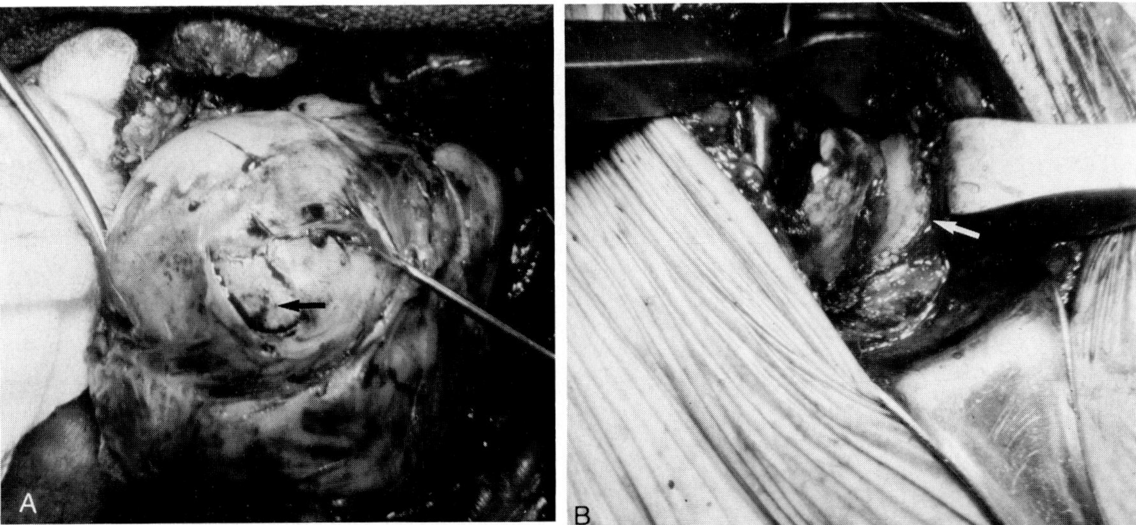

Figure 2–23. Anterior acromioplasty exposures photographed in the operating room of two types of pathology causing recurrent dislocations in patients who had their initial dislocation after 40 years of age. A, Very unstable shoulder in an 82 year old woman who at the time of her dislocation had a massive extension of an impingement tear. The arrow points to a small impression fracture in the facet for insertion of the infraspinatus tendon just behind an area of sclerosis on the facet for the supraspinatus. B, Detachment of the anterior glenoid labrum (arrow) combined with a tear of the rotator cuff in a 55 year old man who had been having recurrent anterior dislocations since falling 1 year previously, at which time he had dislocated his shoulder. The labrum was re-attached and the cuff repaired through this anterior acromioplasty approach.

Recurrent Dislocation After Age 40

Whether recurrent dislocations have been present for many years or have developed recently, if the patient is in good health and has a reasonable life expectancy, surgical repair is recommended. The possibility of a cuff tear, a detachment of the labrum, or both combined should be anticipated. An arthrogram is advisable pre-operatively to determine the approach and nature of aftercare. If a cuff tear is present, an anterior acromioplasty approach is preferred (Fig. 2–23B), rather than the anterior axillary approach ordinarily used for repairing anterior dislocations. Passive elevation is begun early after surgery to avoid adhesions. If the anterior labrum is detached, it is re-attached to the scapula through the cuff tear using the anterior acromioplasty approach with the arm supported in forward flexion on an armboard to take the stress away from the split in the deltoid muscle (see Fig. 4–27).

Extreme Violence with Dislocation, Cuff Avulsion, and Nerve Injuries

Occasionally, with an extremely violent traction and twisting injury, the shoulder is dislocated and literally torn out of its socket with extensive disruption of most of the joint capsule and cuff as well as nerve injuries. In addition to axillary nerve palsy, there is often involvement of most of the other nerve components to the upper extremity, as shown in Figure 2–24. Two of my patients were in their early twenties. Because there are no fractures, routine x-rays do not suggest the extent of the damage, which is often unrecognized initially. Arthrogram and serial electromyograms and myelograms to exclude root avulsions are helpful in evaluating these injuries.

If the nerve injuries are infraclavicular, rather than root avulsion, the prognosis is good for spontaneous recovery, but it may take a long time. The patient illustrated in Figure 2–24 required two years for recovery of the axillary nerve.

When there is a massive tear of the rotator cuff combined with the axillary nerve palsy, I advise repair of the rotator cuff without waiting for the axillary nerve to recover. Special care is taken to avoid injury to the deltoid muscle during this procedure. However, I believe that the deltoid recovers better and is more responsive to the rehabilitation program after the cuff has been repaired. Repairing the cuff seems to help by stabilizing and restoring the fulcrum for the deltoid to work against.

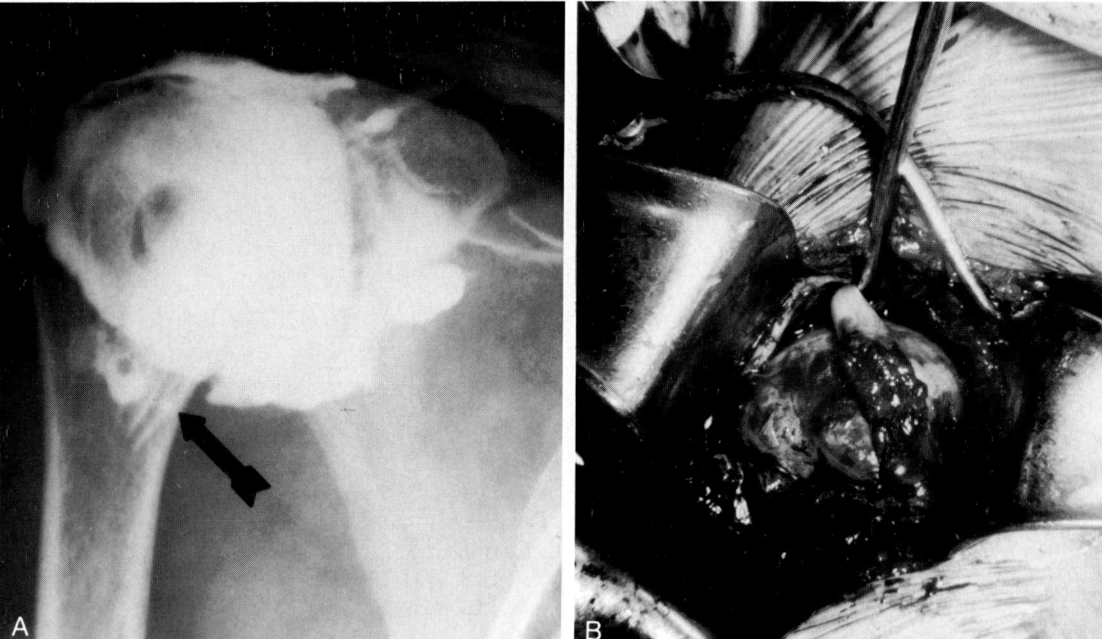

Figure 2–24. Massive avulsion of all of the rotator cuff, dislocation of the long head of the biceps, and paralysis of the axillary nerve seen 8 months after an extremely violent twisting and traction injury of the shoulder in a 60 year old woman. The arthrogram (A) shows the dislocated biceps (arrow) and a tear of the rotator cuff, but because of scarring of the bursa does not show the extent of the cuff tear as seen in the operating room (B). Through an anterior acromioplasty approach, the dislocated biceps was incorporated in the cuff repair. A brace, passive motion, and electrical stimulation were used, with eventual recovery of the axillary nerve.

Outlet Impingement Tears

Outlet impingement tears compose over 90 percent of the cuff tears seen in everyday practice and are by far the most important. We have considered the pathology of these lesions (see p. 57 and Fig. 2–16) and defined "acute extension" (see p. 59 and Fig. 2–16). Most of the remainder of this part of the book is devoted to the diagnosis and treatment of these lesions. First, however, consider in more depth the pathology of impingement lesions of the biceps.

PATHOLOGY OF IMPINGEMENT LESIONS OF THE BICEPS

The evidence showing that most biceps lesions are caused by outlet impingement is discussed on page 62 and in Figure 2–17. Much of the confusion about the treatment of biceps lesions has been because they have been considered separately rather than related to impingement. The etiology of tenosynovitis and rupture has been considered to be trauma, occupation and use, degeneration and aging, and congenital variations such as a "supratubercular ridge" or variations in the shape or slope of the bicipital groove.[65, 66] Most of the literature on rupture of the long head of the biceps was concerned with whether it weakened elbow flexion and supination and whether the long head should be re-attached, and if so, where. Sites preferred for re-attachment by various authors included the coracoid process, the bicipital groove, the deltoid insertion, the shaft of the humerus, and the insertion of the pectoralis major. In the 1940s, bicipital tenosynovitis was accorded a very important role in causing chronic shoulder pain, and many surgeons recommended biceps tenodesis for inflammation of the biceps sheath. This became a frequently performed operation. No one indicated concern over the possibility of an associated tear of the rotator cuff occurring with a biceps rupture.

Patients referred to me because of continuing pain after biceps tenodesis for biceps tendinitis, and other patients referred with huge tears of the rotator cuff following biceps ruptures stimulated a study presented to the American Academy of Orthopaedic Surgeons in 1977.[26] I had previously discussed the relationship between biceps inflammation and rupture and impingement in the article of 1972.[28] This further study emphasized the clinical importance of biceps ruptures in diagnosis, as outlined in Table 2–7, and the potential adverse effect on an impingement tear of the supraspinatus tendon.

My classification of biceps lesions caused by impingement is shown in Table 2–3. The vast majority of these develop insidiously in patients over 40 years of age without significant injury. Loss of the long head either by surgical tenodesis or by rupture often escalates impingement.

Biceps Tendinitis and Tenosynovitis

The earliest impingement lesion of the biceps is tendinitis. This is usually associated with a supraspinatus tear or tendinitis and subacromial bursitis rather than an isolated lesion.

Yergeson's sign,[72] the supination test, is not specific for biceps tendinitis. Supination does not cause the long head to move in its groove. Movements of the humerus inadvertently occurring with this test might irritate the biceps but this is not specific for the biceps because at the same time the humerus is moving in relation to the acromion. Furthermore, an associated tear of the rotator cuff may confuse the examination by causing pain referred to the biceps region and weakness of external rotation that can be interpreted as weakness of supination (Fig. 2–25).

The logical treatment of persistent biceps tendinitis caused by impingement is anterior acromioplasty rather than biceps tenodesis. Biceps tenodesis removes the action of the biceps to stabilize the humeral head from ascent and may intensify impingement by removing this action. Biceps tenodesis for tendinitis has been a frequent cause of patient dissatisfaction following shoulder surgery. The finding of redness and edema of the biceps sheath in association with tears of the rotator cuff or other impingement problems should not be considered an indication for biceps tenodesis unless there is so much fraying and deformity of the long head that it no longer moves well and no longer functions as a head depressor. Relieving impingement by anterior acromioplasty has proved to be effective at long term follow-up against inflammation of the biceps.

Flattening and Fraying of the Long Head

Codman considered flattening of the long head in the presence of a tear of the rotator cuff to be due to hypertrophy caused by the increased load on the biceps because of the loss of the supraspinatus.[6] I believe that the flattening is due to impingement and should be treated by anterior acromioplasty to relieve impingement without tenodesis, provided that the tendon moves in its groove and functions as a head depressor. If the flattened long head is too distorted in shape to function or is subluxed from its groove, it is tenodesed as described on page 134 and, at times, it is incorporated in a rotator cuff repair[81] (see Fig. 2–43L).

Rupture of the Long Head

With the understanding of the role of impingement in the production of biceps ruptures, the need for a new classification of biceps ruptures became obvious. This classification is shown in

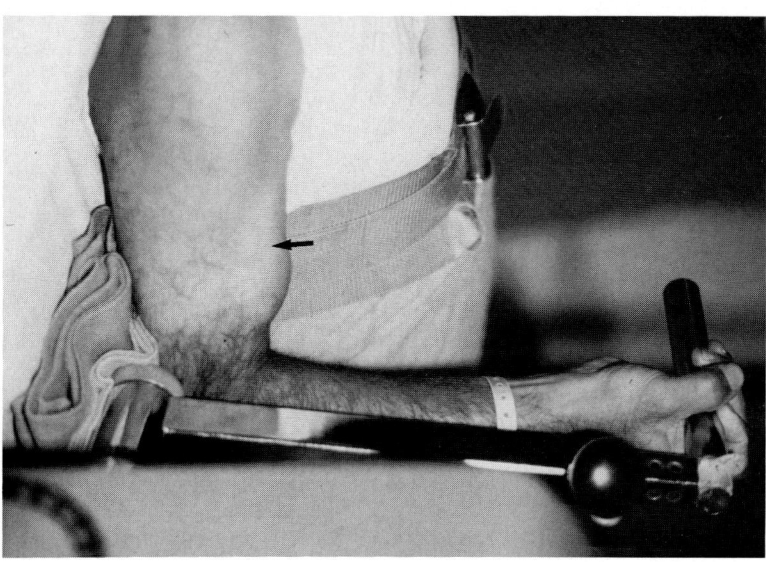

Figure 2–25. Attempts to measure strength after a rupture of the long head of the biceps (arrow) have been inaccurate because of frequently associated tears of the rotator cuff.

Figure 2–26. It is more accurate and descriptive of the pathology and true clinical findings. Previous literature referred to a "high" rupture (at the top of the groove), a "low" rupture (at the musculotendinous junction), and a rupture of the short head. I have never seen a pure rupture at the musculotendinous junction and cannot recall seeing a rupture at the short head. If these lesions occur, they are too rare to provide a meaningful discussion. The types of biceps ruptures I see are illustrated in Figure 2–26. They occur at the top of the groove in patients over 40 years of age. If one becomes aware of the self-attaching type and the partially retracted type, they are seen much more frequently than expected.

The *rupture with retraction* is easily recognized because of the characteristic lump that suddenly appears in the arm. It is the one usually discussed in the literature.

Rupture with partial recession and re-attachment is perhaps more frequent but is more subtle in presentation. If one looks closely at the arms of middle-aged and older patients who have chronic shoulder pain, an asymmetry and indentation indicative of this lesion can often be detected, which is extremely helpful diagnostically.

Self-attaching long head ruptures without retraction cannot be identified on physical examination. There is no deformity of the biceps muscle. These lesions are found at the time of surgery when repairing tears of the rotator cuff. Nevertheless, they are important because they make a successful cuff repair more difficult. Having a healthy biceps running in its groove to assist the supraspinatus as a head depressor after a cuff repair, or even a deformed biceps to incorporate in a difficult repair, is much better than no biceps.

The therapeutic implications for ruptures of

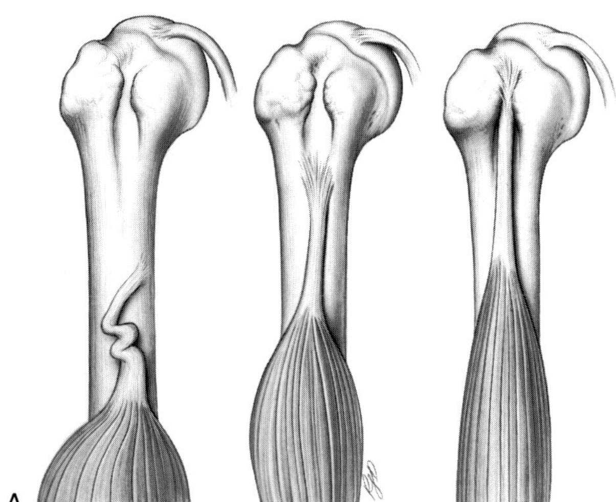

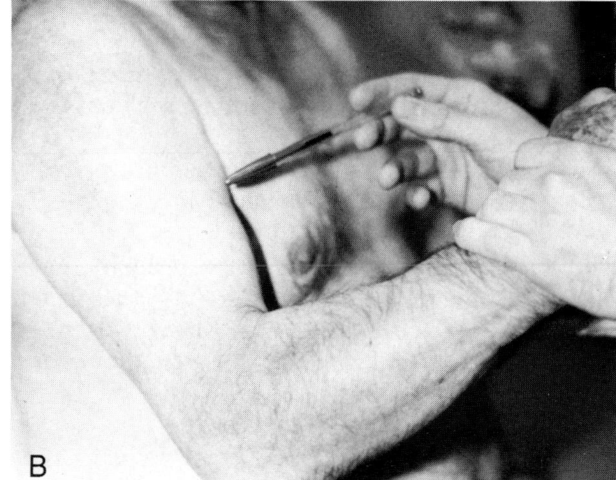

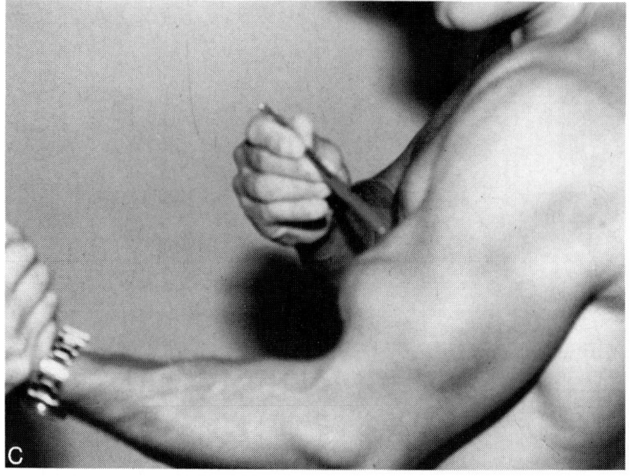

Figure 2–26. A, Classification of biceps ruptures. The only type of biceps ruptures I have seen have occurred near the top of the groove in patients who are over 35 years of age. Ruptures at the musculotendinous junction are said to occur in younger patients with violent trauma; however, they are so rare I have never seen a pure example and will not include it in this classification. It is of clinical importance to recognize three types of long head ruptures (A): 1, rupture with retraction (easily diagnosed); 2, rupture with partial recession (subtle but helpful in diagnosis); 3, self-attaching without retraction (cannot be diagnosed pre-operatively but may complicate a rotator cuff repair). B and C, Comparing a biceps with partial recession to one with retraction. The long head rupture with partial recession (B) has the same diagnostic implications as the obvious long head rupture with retraction (C). Recognizing long head ruptures with partial recession more than doubles the number of long head ruptures seen and greatly helps in the diagnosis of impingement cuff tears.

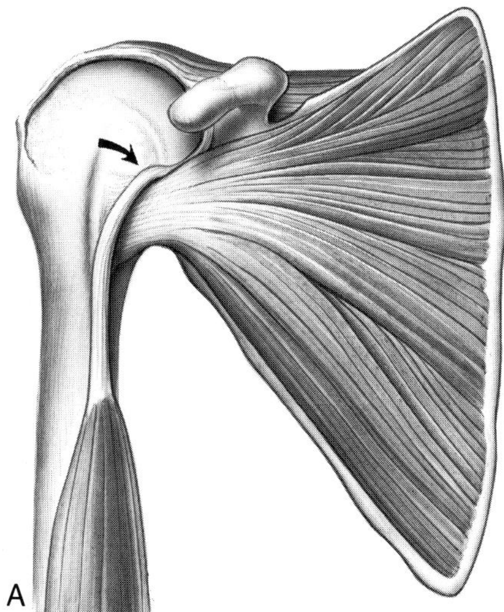

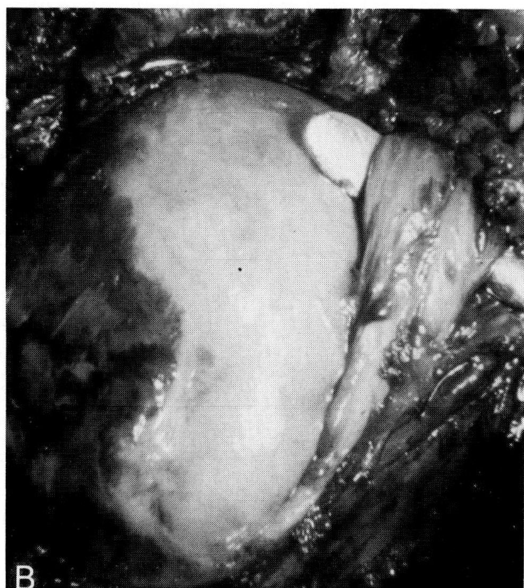

Figure 2–27A and B. Dislocation of the long head of the biceps is almost never seen except in association with a tear of the rotator cuff. Notice the rounding of the greater tuberosity, flattening of the biceps groove, and absence of the transverse humeral ligament, which are indicative of long-standing wear.

the long head are outlined in Table 2–7. The technique for biceps tenodesis is described on page 136.

Biceps Subluxation and Dislocation

Although there has been considerable literature on biceps subluxations and dislocations in young athletes, these lesions must be extremely rare. We see it in older patients when repairing large tears of the rotator cuff (Figs. 2–17 and 2–27). I have not seen dislocation or subluxation of the biceps in patients under 40 years of age except in association with fractures.

When these lesions are seen at surgery on large cuff tears, they are always associated with impingement wear on the proximal humerus with attenuation of the transverse humeral ligament. The long head slips anteriorly inside the joint (Fig. 2–27). It is important when repairing cuff tears to find the long head and make sure that it is in proper alignment before closing the cuff (see p. 117).

AUTHOR'S ANATOMICAL AND SURGICAL DATA

A common, erroneous teaching has been the assumption from the finding of cuff tears in cadavers, as shown in Table 2–4A, that a high portion of the active, living population has symptomless, unrecognized tears; therefore, it is unimportant to repair cuff tears. It is not possible to make this assumption. Published reports often lack the age of the specimen at the time of death, criteria for the diagnosis of an incomplete thickness tear in a cadaver, and the incidence of bilateral lesions. Figures vary depending on whether one is basing the incidence on the number of cadavers or on the number of shoulders. The age of cadavers at the

Table 2–4A. INCIDENCE OF COMPLETE CUFF TEARS IN CADAVERS

AUTHOR	NUMBER OF SHOULDERS	MALES/FEMALES	AGE (YEARS)	FULL-THICKNESS RUPTURES (%)	AGE OF YOUNGEST WITH FULL-THICKNESS RUPTURES
Codman and Ackerson[6] (1934)	200	72/28	46 to over 80	16.5	—
Skinner[41] (1937)	100	—	—	6	55
Grant and Smith[59] (1948)	190	85/10	17–86	19	47
DePalma[17] (1950)	96	36/14	18–74	9	40–50
Olsson[58] (1953)	106	28/25	25–88	8	57
Petersson[53] (1983)	250	69–57	18–93	14.5	60
Fukuda[52] (1986)	249	—	—	7	—
Neer (unpublished) (1965, 1973)	212	—	40–85	7	40–50
Satterlee and Dalsey[59] (unpublished) (1988)	62	—	—	9	—

time of death is, in general, much older than the average age of patients seen in practice. The incidence of cuff tears at the end of life is much greater than in the general population. In one recent study in our anatomy laboratory, the average age of the cadavers with complete cuff tears was over 89 years at the time of death. The incidence of cuff tears in this age group is much greater than in active patients seen in practice.

One almost never unexpectedly encounters a cuff tear during shoulder surgery on patients under 75 years of age during surgery for osteoarthritis or a fracture. Judging from my surgical findings, I estimate that not over 10 percent of the population between 40 and 75 years of age develop full thickness impingement tears of the rotator cuff prior to age 75 years. Approximately one-third of these tears occur in both shoulders of one individual, reducing the incidence of complete tears to about 7 percent per individual under 75 years of age. The incidence of complete tears in patients under 40 years of age is very low. In all of the cadaver studies listed in Table 2–4, no tear was seen in a specimen under 40 years of age at the time of death. As the age of cadavers at the time of death increases into the eighties and nineties, the percentage of tears also increases. The incidence of complete tears in very old female cadavers generally equals that of very old male cadavers.

Incomplete thickness tears have undoubtedly caused variations in the statistics, because there has been no universal agreement among surgeons and anatomists as to the amount of fraying or alteration in the tendon required to make the classification of "incomplete tear." Fukuda,[52, 85] in a careful study of 249 cadaver shoulders, classified 14 percent as having incomplete tears, whereas 7 percent had complete tears. These statistics are similar to those in one of my dissection studies in an unpublished series of 212 shoulders in which the incidence of full thickness tears was 7 percent. Incomplete tears were probably slightly more common.

Regarding the incidence of biceps ruptures in the anatomy laboratory, complete ruptures are more frequent as the age of the cadavers at the time of death increases. In one of our series the incidence of complete rupture of the long head was 1 percent, whereas in another older series it was 7 percent. Our data confirmed what other studies have shown,[17, 53] that the incidence of long head ruptures increases with the ages of the anatomical subjects. It has never been adequately emphasized that virtually all cadaver shoulders with ruptures of the long head of the biceps have a concomitant tear of the supraspinatus tendon. This indicates that most patients with biceps ruptures either have an accompanying supraspinatus rupture at the time of rupturing the biceps or will develop a supraspinatus rupture by the time of death. This is very germane to the discussion of the clinical significance and implications of the long head ruptures described in Table 2–7. It is further evidence that an impingement problem may increase following a long head rupture.

Personal Operative Series of Cuff Tears

Studies have been completed on two personal series of rotator cuff tears treated surgically by the author (Table 2–4B). Patients with fractures or arthritis were excluded. In addition, a series of 66 re-operations for failed cuff repairs will be described.

Series I: 1965–1970

Series I was published in 1972 with the original description of anterior acromioplasty and acro-

Table 2–4B. PERSONAL OPERATIVE SERIES OF CUFF TEARS*

	NUMBER OF SHOULDERS	DOMINANT SIDE	PRIOR SURGERY ELSEWHERE	AGE OF PATIENT (YEARS)	MALE/ FEMALE	HISTORY OF DEFINITIVE INJURY
SERIES I [28] (1965–1970)	50	66% (4 bilateral)	11	42–73 (avg. 58 for complete tears) None under 35 years of age	61% male 39% female	Less than 50%
SERIES II [107, 108] (1974–1986)	340	61% (26 bilateral)	66	22–83 (avg. 59 for complete tears) Only 2 under 35 years of age	69% male 31% female	Severe injury 5% Trivial injury 35% No injury 60%

*Tears with fractures, arthroplasties, arthritis, and those treated nonoperatively are excluded.

mioclavicular arthroplasty for impingement.[28] Fifty shoulders in 46 patients were analyzed. Partial tears of the supraspinatus tendon were present in 19 shoulders and complete tears in 31, of which 11 had failed, previous repairs through lateral acromionectomies and had residual impingement. The right shoulder was involved twice as often as the left. The age of the patients ranged from 42 years to 73 years, and averaged 51.5 years for those with incomplete tears and 58.1 years for those with complete tears. Approximately 40 percent of this series of patients were women (18 women and 28 men). Over 50 percent were unable to recall a definite injury. All were treated surgically by anterior acromioplasty, which included removal of the distal clavicle as necessary for prominences at the undersurface of the acromioclavicular joint. If the cuff was torn, it was repaired.

There were no post-operative infections. Five patients had subcutaneous hematomas that resolved spontaneously; there were no joint sinuses. The scars healed well. Excessive, unwanted new bone formation, which had been described as a serious problem following partial lateral acromionectomy, did not occur in this series. Because only a very small amount of the origin of the anterior deltoid was detached and the remainder of the deltoid remained intact, the shoulder responded to rehabilitation with excellent recovery of strength, in contrast to the high incidence of unsatisfactory results in patients previously treated with lateral acromionectomies. Forty-seven of the 50 shoulders were followed adequately. Only one of 16 patients who had incomplete tears was rated as having an unsatisfactory result. That patient had cervical arthritis as well as acromioclavicular arthritis and various other joint symptoms. One of the patients with complete cuff tears was rated as having an unsatisfactory result, and that patient had seizures and had subsequently damaged the shoulder. On the other hand, of the 11 individuals who had re-operations for failed lateral acromionectomies and failed cuff repairs, 7 were rated as having an unsatisfactory result, generally because of persistent weakness and fatigue pain.

Series II: 1974–1986

Series II was presented at the Annual Meeting of the American Academy of Orthopaedic Surgeons and the Open Meeting of the American Shoulder and Elbow Surgeons in 1988.[107] This was a prospective study of 340 tears of the rotator cuff treated operatively by the author during this time period. Tears with fractures, rheumatoid arthritis, and cuff-tear arthropathy were not included. Forty-one patients were followed less than one year after repair and were not considered in this series. Sixty-six patients had previous failed attempts to repair the rotator cuff, and they were analyzed separately.[108]

Primary Repairs

At the time of this writing, a minimum of 1 year follow-up had been obtained on 233 primary repairs.[107] Follow-up was from 1 to 13 years and averaged 4.6 years. These 233 tears occurred in 215 patients, 160 in the right shoulder and 73 in the left shoulder; there were 18 bilateral repairs. There were 154 men and 61 women. Their ages ranged from 22 years to 83 years, averaging 59 years; however, only eight patients were under 40 years of age and only two were under 35 years of age, both of whom had such violent trauma that it had torn the humerus out of the socket, as shown in Figure 2–24. With the exception of these two individuals, all had pain of varying duration which was generally worse at night and with use; however, 55 percent had no history of injury and the injuries in the remaining 45 percent were characteristically trivial.

Outlet impingement appeared to be the primary etiological factor in 229 tears, trauma in 3, and attenuation of the tendon by a large calcium deposit (see p. 142) in 1. Occupation and use may have been secondary factors in a few individuals, but could not explain why 70 percent of these patients were sedentary or did light work, rather than heavy labor, and why nearly one-third of these lesions were in women and in the nondominant arm. If impaired blood supply in the supraspinatus was present, it was thought it was due to the scarring and fibrosis caused by impingement rather than the primary cause of the tear.

There were 30 incomplete tears, 58 complete supraspinatus tears, and 145 massive tears involving multiple tendons. Physical signs included increased subacromial crepitus and the impingement sign (see Fig. 2–30). A painful arc of active motion was less reliable and pain could cause the patient to let go, mimicking weakness of external rotation. The patients were usually able to raise the arm overhead. Those with massive tears often had one or more of the following signs: fluid sign, spinatus atrophy, biceps rupture, and weakness of external rotation. X-ray findings were usually negative in the early stages, but loss of the acromiohumeral distance and the typical skeletal changes (see Figs. 2–18 and 2–35) were seen in those with long-standing tears. Although it has been said that stiffness of the shoulder does not occur with complete cuff tears, stiffness was present in 32 (14 percent) of these patients, in whom 10 tears were massive. Arthrograms were used routinely to confirm the diagnosis.

The indication for repair was a positive arthrogram for a tear in a motivated patient who was in good health and had good life expectancy. There was no fixed age limit. Because outlet impingement appeared to be the primary etiological factor, anterior acromioplasty was performed in all but two patients at the time of mobilizing and repairing the cuff. This was modified in ten patients who had an unfused anterior acromial epiphysis, corrected by epiphysiodesis in four patients and by excision in six (see p. 139).

Data were collected on the examination sheet (see Fig. 1–13), which is similar to that now used by the American Shoulder and Elbow Surgeons. For an "excellent" rating, the shoulder had essentially normal range, strength, and activities and the patient was free of pain and pleased with the result. For a "satisfactory" rating, active elevation was above the horizontal but with some residual weakness, no pain other than occasional fatigue or weather-ache was noted, and the patient was satisfied with the result. If there was less active elevation or more pain, the result was rated "unsatisfactory." Using these criteria, 180 (77 percent) of the 233 repairs were rated "excellent," 32 (14 percent) were rated "satisfactory," and 21 (9 percent) were rated "unsatisfactory."

Of the unsatisfactory ratings, 9 were in patients with massive, long-standing tears and 12 were in individuals who lacked compliance with the rehabilitation regimen, sustained new injuries, and disregarded the exercise program. These patients were generally free of significant pain but were weak and unable to elevate above the horizontal. Only four of the patients with unsatisfactory ratings had enough pain to be offered a further attempt at surgical repair.

Roentgen follow-up was obtained for from one to ten years (average 3.3 years) on 50 unselected shoulders. None had evidence of re-growth of bone at the site of the acromioplasty; however, it should be emphasized that careful removal of all fragments of bone at surgery had been considered to be an important step.

It was a policy to defer arthrograms following surgery for at least one year because all shoulders had been decompressed from impingement by anterior acromioplasty and it was thought that even if a leak of the dye and a residual defect or new tear were present, it might now heal spontaneously if given time. Of the 12 patients with new injuries, six had evidence of tears. Unfortunately, routine follow-up arthrograms were not possible for several reasons, but especially because those with symptomless shoulders were hesitant to have this test repeated. At the time of this writing, no noninvasive scanning technique is adequate for accurate assessment of the repair.

It was concluded the clinical results of anterior acromioplasty and primary repair using the technique described in this book were "excellent" or "satisfactory" in 91 percent of cases and did not deteriorate with time.

Re-operation for Failed Cuff Repairs

A separate prospective study was made of 66 shoulders in 65 patients re-operated upon by the author for persistent pain and unacceptable function following repairs of the rotator cuff.[108] Again, tears with fractures or rheumatoid arthritis were not included; however, 10 patients who developed cuff-tear arthropathy after failed repairs were included but were considered separately. Also, 30 shoulders with complete or lateral acromionectomies and 4 shoulders with multiple, complicated failed repairs were considered separately. The operative findings, steps at re-operation, and results were analyzed.

These shoulders had from 1 to 11 prior operations and averaged 1.9 operations. Initial surgery had been performed in our hospital in 4 shoulders, and elsewhere in 62. The age of the patients was from 19 to 75 years and averaged 57 years. Only three patients were under 35 years of age; two of these patients, described previously, had violent injuries with superior dislocations and massive avulsions of the cuff and capsule, whereas the third had no evidence of a tear at the time of re-operation.

Operative findings included complete cuff tears in 51 shoulders (36 massive), nonfunctional biceps in 30 (12 ruptured, 3 dislocated, and 15 tenodesed), residual outlet impingement in 44, deltoid retraction in 24, cuff-tear arthropathy in 10, and adhesions in all. For clarity in the analysis of the problem and results, it was necessary to create four subgroups. The results were graded as described previously for primary repairs.

Group I: Deltoid and Glenohumeral Joint Intact

Of the 22 shoulders in this group, 19 had complete tears (12 massive), 7 had nonfunctioning biceps, 17 had residual impingement, 1 had prior infection, 1 had partial axillary nerve palsy, and 2 had partial C5–C6 root palsies. "Excellent" or "satisfactory" results were obtained in 17 shoulders (78 percent) of this group. The 5 "unsatisfactory" ratings were all in patients with massive tears, three of whom had partial deltoid palsies and one of whom had previously been infected and had extensive scars.

Group II: Complete or Lateral Acromionectomy

Of the 30 shoulders in this group, there were 20 with complete cuff tears (13 massive), 14 with nonfunctional biceps, 21 with residual impingement, and 24 with retracted deltoid muscles. Electromyograms showed partial denervation of the deltoid in 8, and 5 had previously been infected. Retraction and adherence of the deltoid origin to the humerus posed a formidable problem. The anterior acromion and acromioclavicular joint remained to cause residual impingement in those with lateral acromionectomies. Nevertheless, the results of re-operation in this group were "excellent" in 16 shoulders (53 percent), "satisfactory" in 2, and "unsatisfactory" in 12.

Group III: Cuff-Tear Arthropathy

Of the 10 patients who developed cuff-tear arthropathy after attempted repairs of the rotator cuff, only one had complete healing of the rotator cuff and the other nine had massive residual tears. All patients required total shoulder arthroplasties, resulting in two "excellent," one "satisfactory," and seven "limited goals" results (see Chapter 3, p. 238).

Group IV: Multiple, Complex Procedures

The four shoulders in this group had had 24 previous procedures, including three acromionectomies; three total glenohumeral arthroplasties, of which two were constrained; one failed glenohumeral arthrodesis; and two multiple procedures for infection. Re-operations consisted of two cleanouts to control infection, eventually followed by glenohumeral arthrodesis; one uncemented humeral head replacement arthroplasty; and one total glenohumeral arthroplasty.

Summary of Study of Failed Repairs

This experience established the technique as discussed on page 120 for re-repairing failed repairs, of seeking four types of anatomical defects and, if present, correcting them: i.e., (1) remove residual impingement by anterior acromioplasty, (2) release adhesions, (3) mobilize and close residual cuff tears, and (4) re-attach and free a retracted deltoid muscle.

The results of second cuff repairs when the deltoid muscle was of good quality were generally adequate but were inferior to those of primary repairs. Satisfactory or excellent ratings were obtained in 78 percent of Group I, 60 percent of Group II, 30 percent of Group III, and none of Group IV.

Factors in the unsatisfactory ratings were long-standing, massive tears; nonfunctional biceps; acromionectomy; cuff-tear arthropathy; prior infection; and nerve deficits.

DIAGNOSIS OF OUTLET IMPINGEMENT CUFF TEARS AND BICEPS LESIONS

The physical signs and symptoms can be identical in all three stages of impingement (see Fig. 2–13). This has caused much confusion in the diagnosis and treatment of cuff tears. Overuse of the shoulder with the development of edema and swelling (Stage I) can produce the same clinical picture as a tear of the rotator cuff. Later, when the edema subsides and there is complete and permanent recovery, this Stage I lesion is easily mistaken for a tear of the rotator cuff that healed. Roentgenograms are negative and of little help until late in Stage III.

It is important in diagnosis to separate impingement lesions as a group from other causes of shoulder pain and then identify the stage of impingement present.

Separating Impingement Lesions from Other Causes of Chronic Shoulder Pain

Laboratory Routines for Impingement Lesions

Because the physical signs characteristic of impingement can be mimicked by arthritis, neoplasms, old fractures, and any condition causing frozen shoulder, it is essential to exclude systemic disease by obtaining appropriate blood and x-ray studies before attempting to interpret physical signs. A system must be developed for evaluating chronic shoulder pain, such as depicted in Table 1–1 and Figures 1–10 and 1–11. Initial x-rays for evaluating impingement problems should include anterior-posterior views in the scapular plane made with the arm in internal rotation, external rotation, and neutral rotation; and an axillary view showing the acromion, humeral head, and glenoid (see Fig. 1–12). These views are essential for excluding calcium deposits, glenohumeral arthritis, acromioclavicular arthritis, an unfused acromial epiphysis, and other skeletal abnormalities (Fig. 2–28). The "outlet view," a lateral of the erect scapula with 10 degrees downward tilt (see Fig. 1–12), may be helpful. Blood studies, including a complete blood count, serum uric acid, rheumatoid factor, sedimentation rate, and chemical profile, are essential for excluding systemic disoders.

An arthrogram is the most reliable method for identifying full thickness cuff tears (see p. 89), but it is not performed until after these routine tests have been obtained and one of the indications listed in Table 2–6 is present.

Signs Common to All Stages of Impingement

The following signs are useful in separating impingement lesions from other types of shoulder pain; however, the most reliable is the impingement injection test (see Fig. 2–30). The other signs are less consistent and less specific.

Arc of Pain

In this test, the arm is raised from the side and lowered from overhead in various positions of rotation. Maximum joint reaction force and tension on the rotator cuff occur as the arm passes between 70 degrees and 120 degrees (Fig. 2–29A). If pain occurs as the arm passes through these levels, the patient is said to have an "arc of pain." In my experience, this sign is not always present, even when there is a tear of the rotator cuff. It has not been as reliable as the impingement sign (see Fig. 2–30). Some investigators have attempted to determine which part of the rotator cuff is involved by changing the position of rotation of the arm during the arc of pain test, noting where the maximum discomfort is experienced. Unfortunately, this is not accurate.

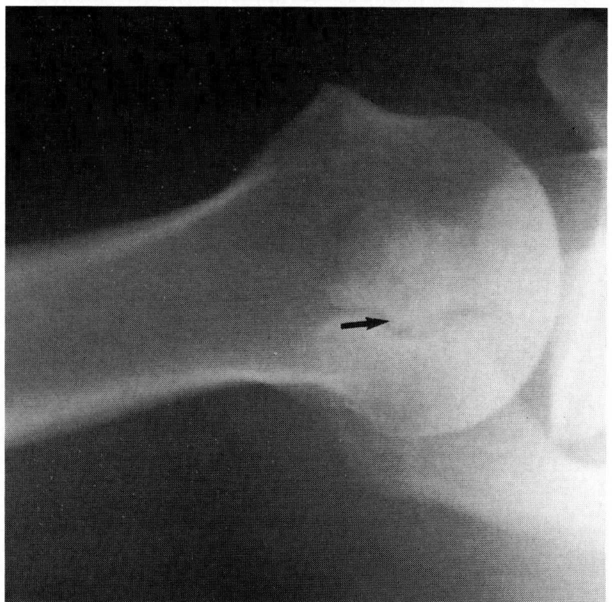

Figure 2–28. An axillary view showing an unfused anterior acromial epiphysis (arrow) in a 65 year old man with a tear of the rotator cuff. An axillary view is routine in the evaluation of impingement lesions (see Fig. 1–12A).

Crepitus

The examiner stands behind the patient, grasps the front and back edges of the acromion, and moves the palpating index finger anterior to the acromion to elicit crepitus as the humerus is rotated with the opposite hand. Crepitus is more marked in Stage III lesions, especially when there is a complete tear of the rotator cuff; however, it is present to some degree in all stages. Snapping noises may be heard with a stethoscope on the shoulder in any stage of impingement and do not necessarily indicate a complete tear of the rotator cuff. *Palpation of the defect in the cuff has been described as a method for identifying a tear; however, this is not reliable because a thickening of the subacromial bursa or soft tissue, as present in Stage II, can duplicate the sensation of a torn cuff.*

Varying Weakness

Some authors indicate that subtle weakness of abduction and external rotation is the most reliable early sign for a tear of the rotator cuff. Unfortunately, pain at any stage of impingement causes the patient to "let go," with the appearance of weakness. Conversely, many patients with complete cuff tears are remarkably strong during intervals when they are free of pain. Therefore, loss of strength is not a reliable sign for a cuff tear in the earlier stages. However, marked weakness in the later stages is indicative of a large tear.

"Impingement Sign" and "Impingement Injection Test"

A description of this sign and test was published in 1983.[27] I find it to be the most valuable method for separating impingement lesions from other causes of chronic shoulder pain.

To elicit the *impingement sign,* the humerus is elevated as the scapula is depressed with the opposite hand (Figs. 2–29C and 2–30A) so that the greater tuberosity is compressed against the anterior acromion. This almost invariably produces pain if an impingement lesion is present. This maneuver also produces pain when many other conditions are present, such as frozen shoulder, glenohumeral instability, acromioclavicular arthri-

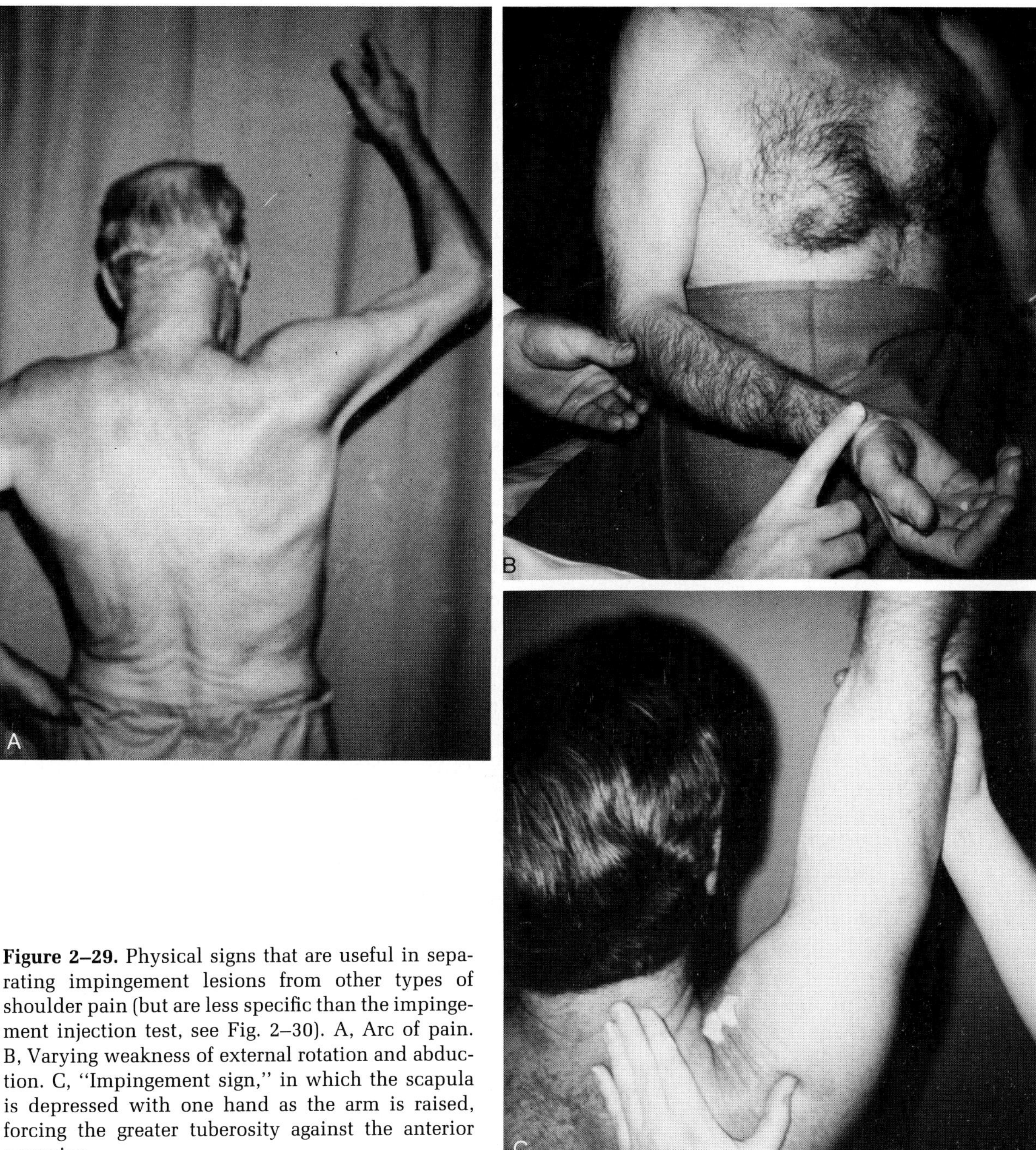

Figure 2–29. Physical signs that are useful in separating impingement lesions from other types of shoulder pain (but are less specific than the impingement injection test, see Fig. 2–30). A, Arc of pain. B, Varying weakness of external rotation and abduction. C, "Impingement sign," in which the scapula is depressed with one hand as the arm is raised, forcing the greater tuberosity against the anterior acromion.

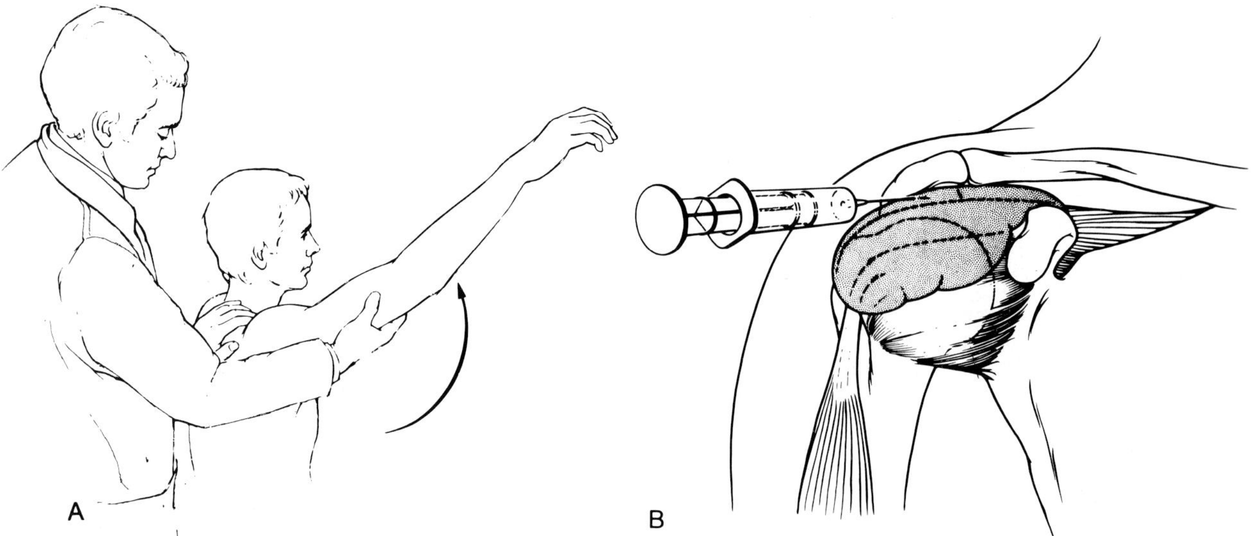

Figure 2–30. Impingement injection test: complete relief of pain on forced forward elevation of the humerus against the acromion as the examiner's opposite hand depresses the scapula (A) (the "impingement sign") after the injection of 10 cc. of lidocaine (Xylocaine) into the subacromial space (B). This indicates that the pain is from the subacromial mechanism. Failure to relieve the pain indicates some cause other than impingement.

Proper placement of the needle is facilitated by inserting the needle against the undersurface of the acromion as the assistant applies traction on the arm (with the patient supine) to distract the subacromial space. (From Neer, C.S., II: Impingement lesions. Clin. Orthop. 173:70, 1983.)

tis, a metastatic tumor in the greater tuberosity, or a calcium deposit in the rotator cuff tendons. Because frozen shoulder is a nonspecific lesion caused by many conditions (see Chapter 6), there are an infinite number of local and systemic problems that could cause a positive impingement sign. Therefore, the impingement injection test (Fig. 2–30B) is needed to exclude these other conditions.

In interpreting the *impingement injection test*, complete temporary relief of pain is almost specific evidence of the presence of an impingement lesion. The range of motion of the shoulder is recorded (see p. 7) before and after the injection to give more objective evidence of the degree of pain relief and the presence or absence of stiffness of the glenohumeral joint. The patient is asked to describe subjectively the amount of pain relief on a scale of "0" to "10," with 10 being complete relief. If pain relief is only partial and the acromioclavicular joint is tender, a second Xylocaine injection is made into the acromioclavicular joint. If this completely relieves all remaining discomfort, the diagnosis of impingement combined with acromioclavicular arthritis is made. If the relief of pain is incomplete, another diagnosis should be suspected. If the range of motion remains restricted, conservative treatment as for a frozen shoulder is advised and reevaluation should be performed later. In very advanced impingement lesions with bone-on-bone impingement or with joint changes such as cuff-tear arthropathy (see p. 124), the subacromial injection test may not completely eliminate impingement pain. In these cases, however, the diagnosis should easily be made on the basis of the marked x-ray findings and negative laboratory studies. Calcium deposits in the rotator cuff can produce a positive impingement sign, which may be temporarily eliminated by the subacromial injection test. These lesions are usually seen in x-ray films. Small "hidden deposits" can cause confusion. Inspection of the rotator cuff for hidden calcium deposits or incomplete tears is routine at the time of any exploration for chronic pain.

Identifying Stage I: Edema and Hemorrhage

Edema and hemorrhage from overuse are seen in patients of all ages. Typically, the shoulder pain is precipitated by overuse of the arm above the horizontal, such as in a young athlete with a sore shoulder after pitching a baseball game or tennis tournament; or a middle-aged, weekend hedge clipper or do-it-yourself house painter.

On examination, there may be signs indistinguishable from those of a cuff tear including the impingement sign, arc of pain, and crepitus, and because of pain, the patient may appear to have lost strength. X-ray findings are negative. A subacromial Xylocaine injection relieves the pain. The differential diagnosis is discussed further and in Table 1–2.

Treatment is conservative (see p. 93), with an excellent prognosis for complete and permanent recovery; however, months may be required before the patient can resume activities without recurrence.

Acute, Traumatic Subacromial Bursitis

This lesion differs from Stage I impingement only in that a single injury causes edema and hemorrhage rather than overuse.[51] It is of great diagnostic importance but has never received attention. It is seen in contact sports and after hard falls. The differential diagnosis includes spontaneously reduced glenohumeral dislocations in younger patients and tears of the rotator cuff in older patients. Roentgenograms are negative. Arthrograms or imaging may be indicated to be sure that the cuff is intact.

Treatment is conservative and similar to that of Stage I impingement (see p. 93). Several months are required for complete resolution.

Identifying Stage II: Fibrosis

Fibrosis is usually seen in patients 30 to 40 years of age who use the arm overhead in athletics or work. With repeated mechanical insults, the subacromial bursa becomes fibrotic and thickened. The thickened bursa occupies room reducing the subacromial space and making the shoulder susceptible to attacks of impingement pain. Very little edema and swelling are needed to precipitate the symptoms in the already tight space. Typically, the shoulder is comfortable between activities and pain lasting several days is exacerbated by use of the arm overhead.

The physical signs are similar to those of other stages of impingement. An injection of Xylocaine into the subacromial space temporarily relieves the pain. X-ray findings are negative.

Treatment is conservative, as outlined on page 93, including changing the style of use of the arm to avoid subacromial irritation. Usually there is a transition from Stage I (edema) to a mixture of edema and fibrosis. A vicious cycle may develop with the already thickened bursa becoming more thickened and fibrotic with each attack and with less activity producing an attack. However, only late in Stage II is there enough fibrosis and permanent thickening to consider bursectomy and resection of the coracoacromial ligament (see p. 94). This procedure is advised only after conservative treatment has failed and the patient has been disabled for at least 18 months.

Differential Diagnosis of Stage I and Stage II

Some frequently used practical points in the differential diagnosis of chronic shoulder pain are outlined in Table 1–2. The most important lesion to differentiate from Stage I in patients over 40 years of age is a *tear of the rotator cuff (Stage III)*. The signs and symptoms can be identical. Until imaging is perfected, an arthrogram is the only sure method for distinguishing tears. The indications for arthrography are discussed on page 89 and Table 2–6.

In younger patients, *anterior glenohumeral instability (subluxation or dislocation)* is the most important lesion in the differential diagnosis. Discomfort is aggravated in both conditions by overhead activities, and the impingement sign (see Fig. 2–30) and the anterior apprehension sign (see Fig. 4–9) are usually positive in both conditions. The impingement injection test (see Fig. 2–30) is of particular value in differentiating these two conditions. X-ray evidence of instability (see Fig. 1–12D and Figs. 4–10 to 4–12) may identify a dislocation, but this is not always present. Examination of the patient under anesthesia with or without arthroscopy may be required to make the differential diagnosis in some instances. As shown in Figure 2–31A, multidirectional glenohumeral instability can be a cause of impingement. This type of impingement is treated by repair of the instability rather than by coracoacromial ligament resection or acromioplasty.

Because irritation and edema of the biceps long head may occur in any stage of impingement, *biceps tendinitis* has been a common misdiagnosis too frequently treated in error by tenodesis.[26, 27] Tenodesis of the long head may make the symptoms worse if the pathology is an impingement lesion (Fig. 2–31B).

Acromioclavicular arthritis, as in "weightlifter's shoulder" (see Chapter 6), may give a positive impingement sign and pain on activities, suggesting subacromial pathology. The "horizontal adduction test" (see Chapter 6) has been said to be specific for acromioclavicular arthritis, but unfortunately is not specific. This maneuver causes pain when there is a subacromial impingement lesion. Xylocaine injected into the acromioclavicular joint is the most specific test for distinguishing pain emanating from this joint.

A slightly *frozen shoulder* (see Chapter 6) is easily confused with impingement because it produces an impingement sign as well as an anterior apprehension sign. Also, pain is made worse in

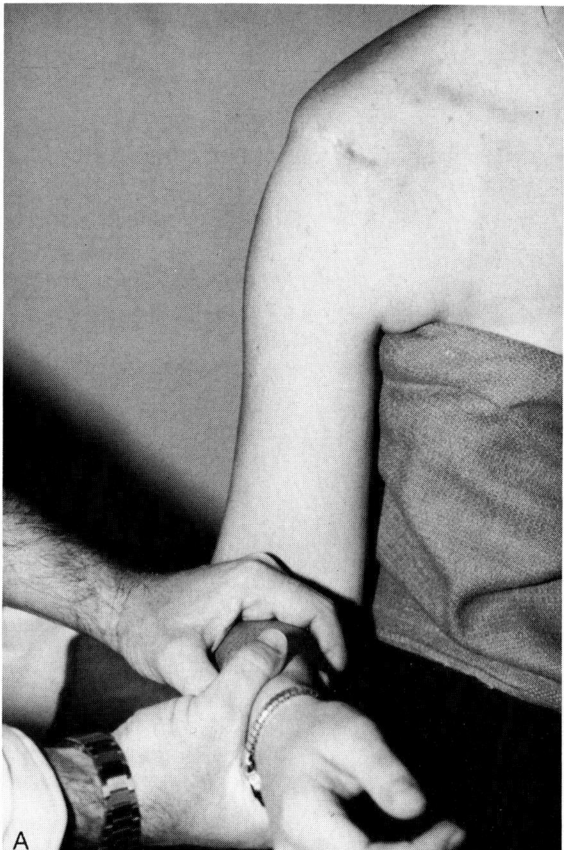

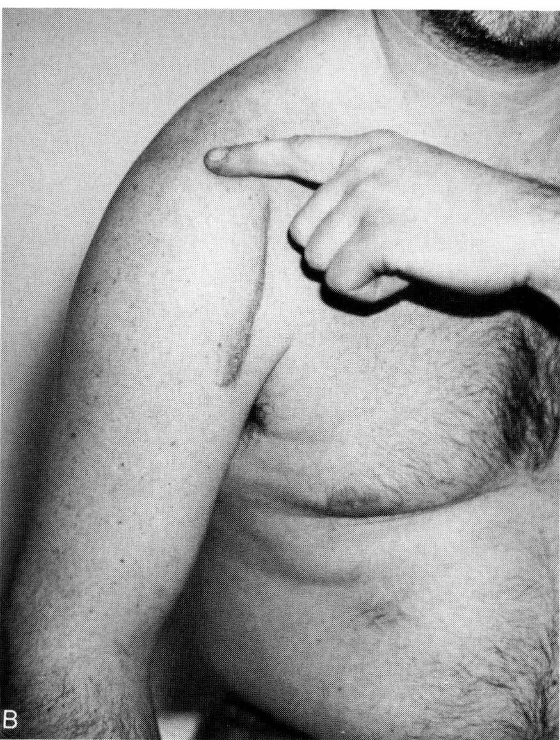

Figure 2–31. Important points in the differential diagnosis of impingement lesions. A, Failed anterior acromioplasty in a 23 year old woman whose impingement problem was due to multidirectional glenohumeral instability and required stabilization with an inferior capsular shift (see p. 316) rather than an anterior acromioplasty. B, Failed biceps tenodesis in a 44 year old man who had outlet impingement that had caused an incomplete rotator cuff tear and biceps tenosynovitis. His pain was made worse by the biceps tenodesis, which had removed the normal action of the long head of the biceps to stabilize and depress the humeral head against impingement. An anterior acromioplasty was required to relieve his pain.

both conditions by overhead activities. A subacromial injection test does not relieve this pain, caused by stiffness of the glenohumeral joint. Because the pain of a frozen shoulder is often relieved by stretching exercises, a therapeutic trial of heat and exercises usually confirms the diagnosis.

Calcium deposits in the rotator cuff (see Chapter 6) can cause signs and symptoms similar to those of impingement—i.e., a positive impingement sign that may be temporarily relieved by a subacromial injection test and pain made worse by use and relieved by inactivity. However, adequate x-rays usually show calcium deposits. Small "hidden deposits" that are not visible on x-ray films may be recognized only at the time of inspection of the rotator cuff during surgery.

Diagnosis of Cuff Tears

Age of Patients with Cuff Tears

The age of the patient is of greatest importance in the diagnosis of outlet impingement lesions. Cuff tears are common after age 50 years, but they are very rare prior to age 40 years. Patients with complete impingement tears average 59 years of age and those with incomplete impingement tears average 52 years of age at the time of surgery.

Onset of Impingement Cuff Tears

A *history of injury is not a pre-requisite* for the diagnosis of a cuff tear. Half of our patients with complete tears have had no history of injury; in the others, the amount of trauma required to complete a tear is generally less than that capable of tearing a normal tendon. Characteristic injuries include pulling a cable to start a lawn mower, lifting a suitcase up onto a shelf, and serving in tennis. A few patients have a significant injury such as a hard fall down stairs or slipping on the ice.

Pain often begins as "intermittent bursitis" that gradually becomes more steady and severe.

Patients usually forget to mention it unless specifically asked, and even then they may not have been impressed enough to remember all past episodes of intermittent pain. This pain probably corresponds to episodes of impingement wear. Eventually the pain becomes more consistent, usually worse at night and with activities. Initially those who stop using the arm find the pain diminishing and think they are getting better, but later the pain recurs when they resume the previous level of activity. Eventually, the pain may become constant and unbearable. Thus, the pain of a patient with a cuff tear varies from mild and intermittent to constant and unbearable. Typically, there is more pain in recumbency because there is more impingement in this position, whether lying on the back, on the "good" side, or on the involved side. Supporting the arm on pillows may help relieve the strain of recumbency, but eventually the patient may choose to sleep sitting up.

Weakness and popping noises are other common complaints. Some patients cannot raise the arm or lift a cup of tea. Others have no noticeable weakness. Some patients who are seen at surgery to have tears as large as 6.0 cm. were able to raise the arm overhead pre-operatively. On the other hand, some with small tears appeared to be very weak because of pain. Pain forces these patients to "let go" when they are tested for strength. Pain makes accurate determinations of strength impossible; however, with careful testing of those with complete tears, some weakness in external rotation and abduction can usually be detected (Fig. 2–32).

Physical Signs

The physical signs in patients with tears of the rotator cuff can be listed in approximately the order of their appearance as the size of the tear increases (Table 2–5). The signs common to all impingement lesions are seen early. These include the impingement sign, arc of pain, varying crepitus, and subtle weakness (see Fig. 2–29).

With time, when the infraspinatus tendon becomes involved, *spinatus atrophy* (Fig. 2–32) and weakness of external rotation appear. It is important when testing for weakness of external rotation to perform the test with the arm at the side rather than in abduction because although the infraspi-

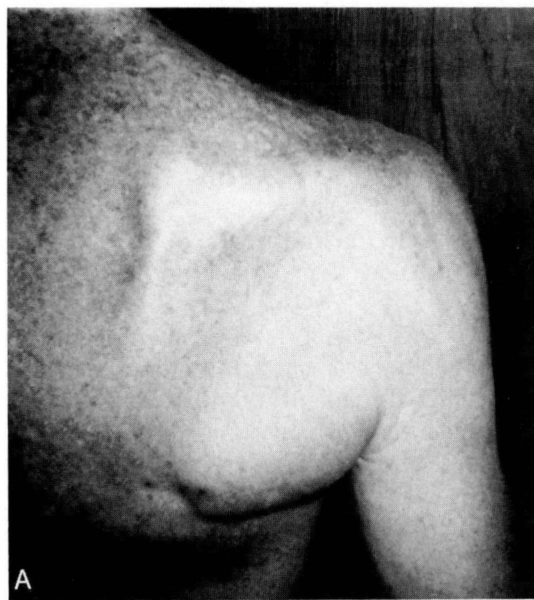

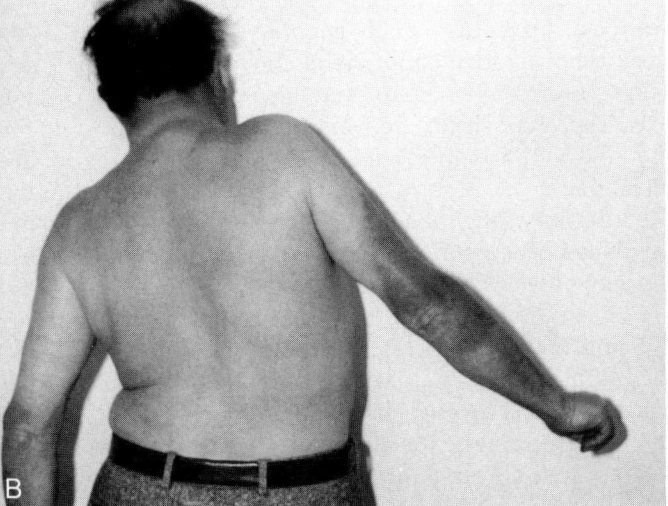

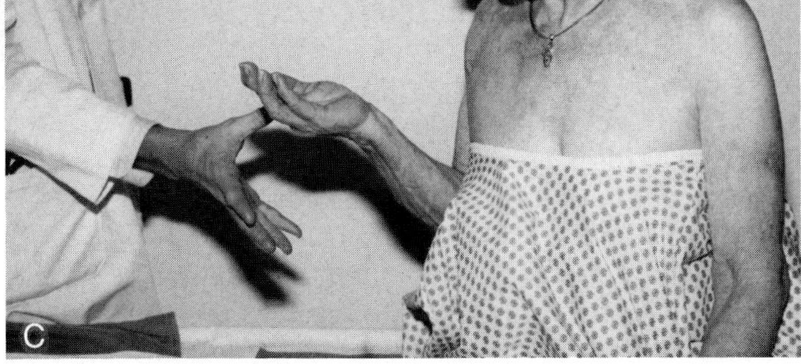

Figure 2–32. Progressive grades of weakness caused by rotator cuff tears. Initially there is subtle weakness that is difficult to evaluate, as shown in Figure 2–29B. This may be followed by A, "spinatus atrophy;" B, "shrugging sign;" and, later, C, the "dropping sign." (In the "dropping sign," the examiner fully externally rotates the arm with the elbow bent 90 degrees and then lets go. If the external rotators are weak, the hand falls helplessly to the side.)

Table 2–5. PROGRESSIVE SIGNS OF ROTATOR CUFF TEARS (STAGE III)

PHYSICAL SIGNS	ROENTGEN SIGNS
Impingement sign	Greater tuberosity excrescence
Arc of pain	Anterior acromial spur
Crepitus (subacromial)	Decrease in acromiohumeral distance
Subtle weakness	Greater tuberosity osteopenia
Biceps rupture*	Break in calcar line
"Shrugging sign"	
"Fluid sign"	
"Dropping sign"	
Acromioclavicular "ganglion"	Erosion of acromioclavicular joint and acromion
Ecchymosis	
Glenohumeral instability	
Painful glenohumeral motion†	Sclerosis or fragmentation of the glenohumeral joint†

*Partial recession or retracted. May also be contralateral.
†Cuff-tear arthropathy.

natus supplies approximately 90 percent of the power of external rotation with the arm at the side, the posterior deltoid gives some power for external rotation when the arm is held in abduction.

Preservation of passive motion and the absence of a frozen shoulder are, in general, characteristic of complete cuff tears. This is helpful in diagnosis (see Table 1–2). Joint fluid within the bursal sac is thought to be responsible for preserving motion. Those patients with incomplete thickness tears have a greater tendency to develop a frozen shoulder. It is typical for shoulders with complete tears to remain mobile; nevertheless, those who avoid glenohumeral movements for a long time because of pain may also develop stiffness. Therefore, it has become routine to manipulate all shoulders under anesthesia at the time of cuff repairs.

Rupture of the long head of the biceps suggests the presence of a cuff tear and is usually indicative of a large tear. When the rupture occurs gradually and is self-attaching, the signs can be quite subtle and minimal (Fig. 2–33). Dislocation of the long head is also associated with only subtle physical signs. A biceps rupture or recession may be found on the contralateral side and helps in the diagnosis of a cuff tear on the painful side.

The *shrugging sign* (see Fig. 2–32) appears when weakness or pain precludes active glenohumeral elevation. Later, when the infraspinatus tendon is involved, the "dropping sign" may appear, which is due to loss of active external rotation (see Fig. 2–32). This sign is elicited by the examiner holding the arm with the elbow bent at the side in external rotation, and asking the patient to maintain that position after the examiner lets go. Dropping of the arm helplessly into internal rotation indicates either a large tear involving the infraspinatus or paralysis of the C5–C6 nerve root (see Fig. 2–37). It is well to remember that an injury can produce an acute extension of an impingement tear, but also may, by jarring the cervical spine, cause cervical root edema and paralysis. It is easy to mistake a cuff tear for a neurological problem or a C5–C6 root problem for a cuff tear.

The *fluid sign* (Fig. 2–34), as described by Codman,[6] can be helpful in diagnosing complete tears. Joint fluid may communicate with and distend the bursa, causing increased thickness of the shoulder when compared with the opposite side.

Although *ecchymosis* is not a characteristic finding of tears of the rotator cuff, it can appear when there has been an injury with sudden enlargement of a tear, or in the later stages when there is bone-on-bone impingement between the greater tuberosity and the acromion. In both of these situations, a "hemarthrosis" as a result of bloody fluid from the bursa passing into the glenohumeral joint may also be present (see Fig. 2–34).

In advanced Stage III lesions when the capsule of the undersurface of the acromioclavicular joint has been worn through, the fluid may distend the acromioclavicular joint, giving the appearance of a *ganglion of the acromioclavicular joint* (see Fig. 2–15).

Patients who are unlucky and develop cuff-tear arthropathy have pain on movements of the humerus against the glenoid and may have palpable glenohumeral subluxations or dislocations.

X-ray Changes with Cuff Tears

There are no positive x-ray findings in Stage I and Stage II and in early Stage III. The arthrogram is the most reliable roentgen method for the early diagnosis of complete tears. However, eventually in Stage III, bone changes appear, which are often

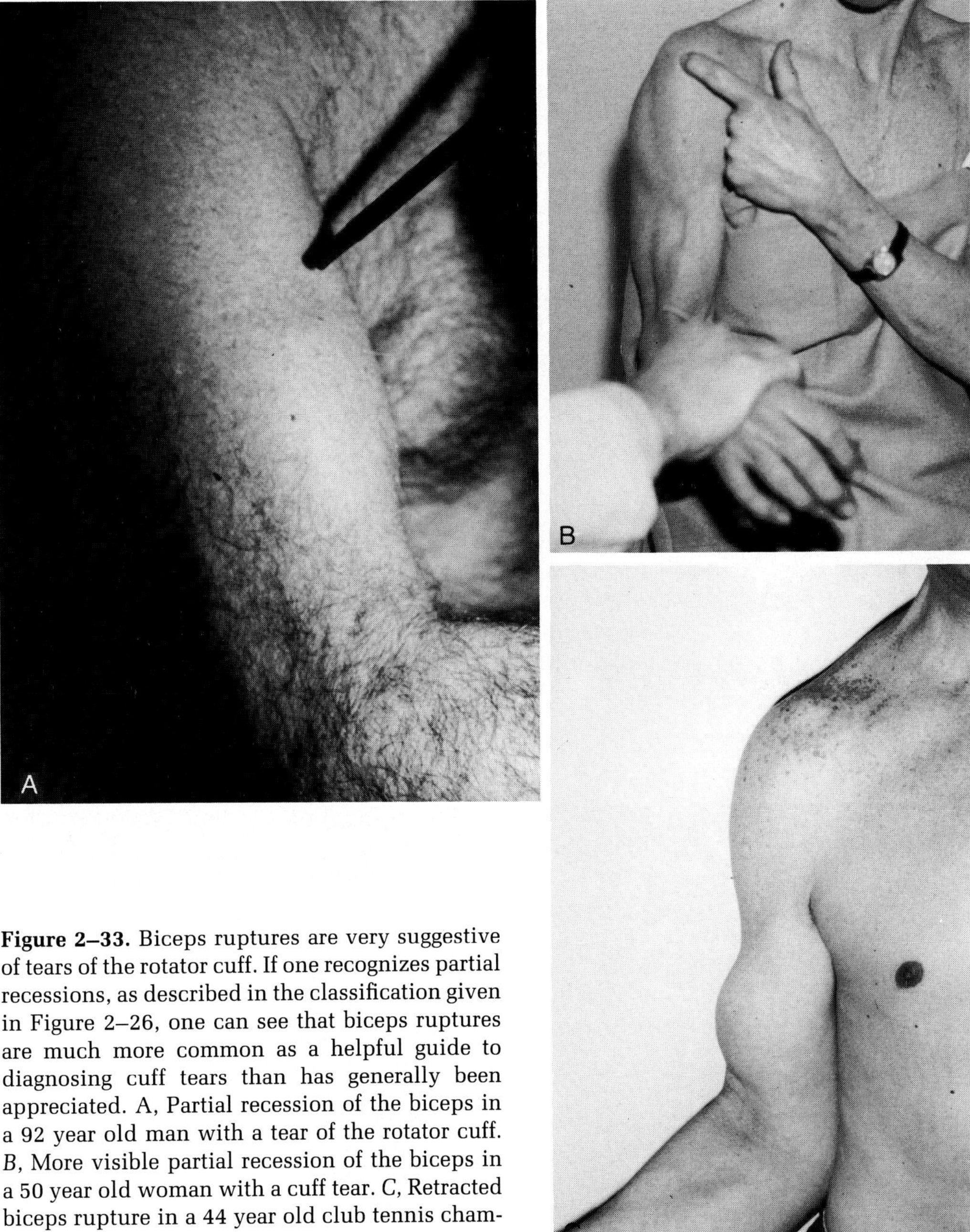

Figure 2–33. Biceps ruptures are very suggestive of tears of the rotator cuff. If one recognizes partial recessions, as described in the classification given in Figure 2–26, one can see that biceps ruptures are much more common as a helpful guide to diagnosing cuff tears than has generally been appreciated. A, Partial recession of the biceps in a 92 year old man with a tear of the rotator cuff. B, More visible partial recession of the biceps in a 50 year old woman with a cuff tear. C, Retracted biceps rupture in a 44 year old club tennis champion who had a cuff tear.

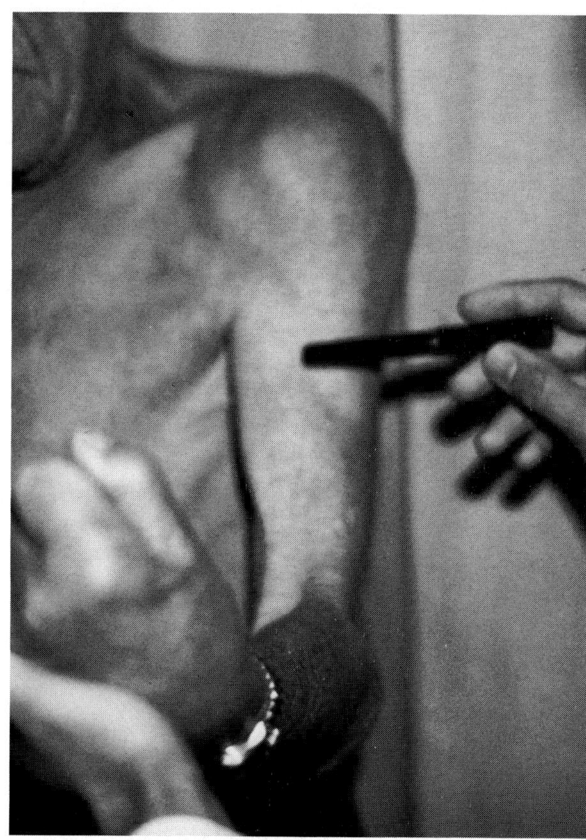

Figure 2–34. Evidence of a massive cuff tear includes "fluid sign;" biceps rupture; weakness of external rotation; and, in this 80 year old man, ecchymosis about the shoulder and hemarthrosis from bone-on-bone impingement.

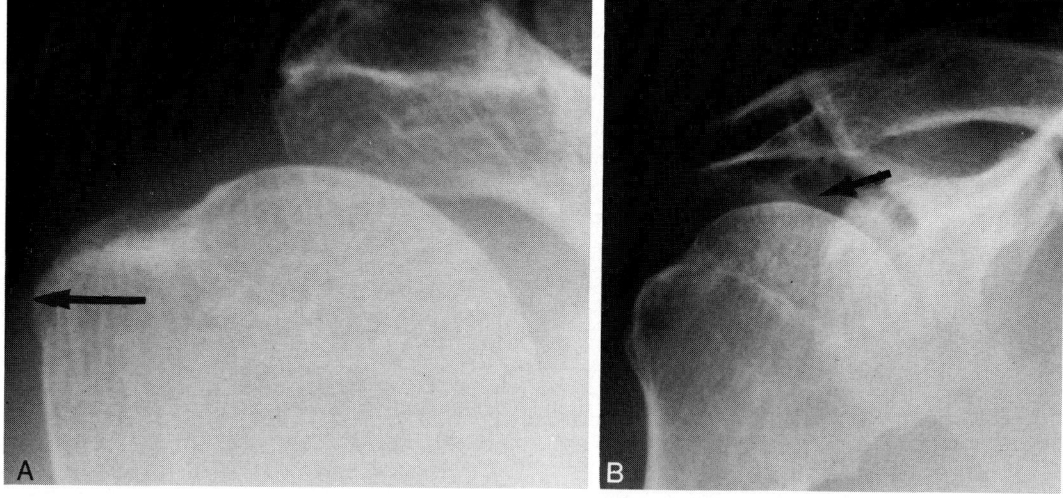

Figure 2–35. Progressive roentgen changes that may appear in Stage III. A, Prominence or exostosis of the greater tuberosity at the facet for the supraspinatus insertion. B, Anterior acromial spur.

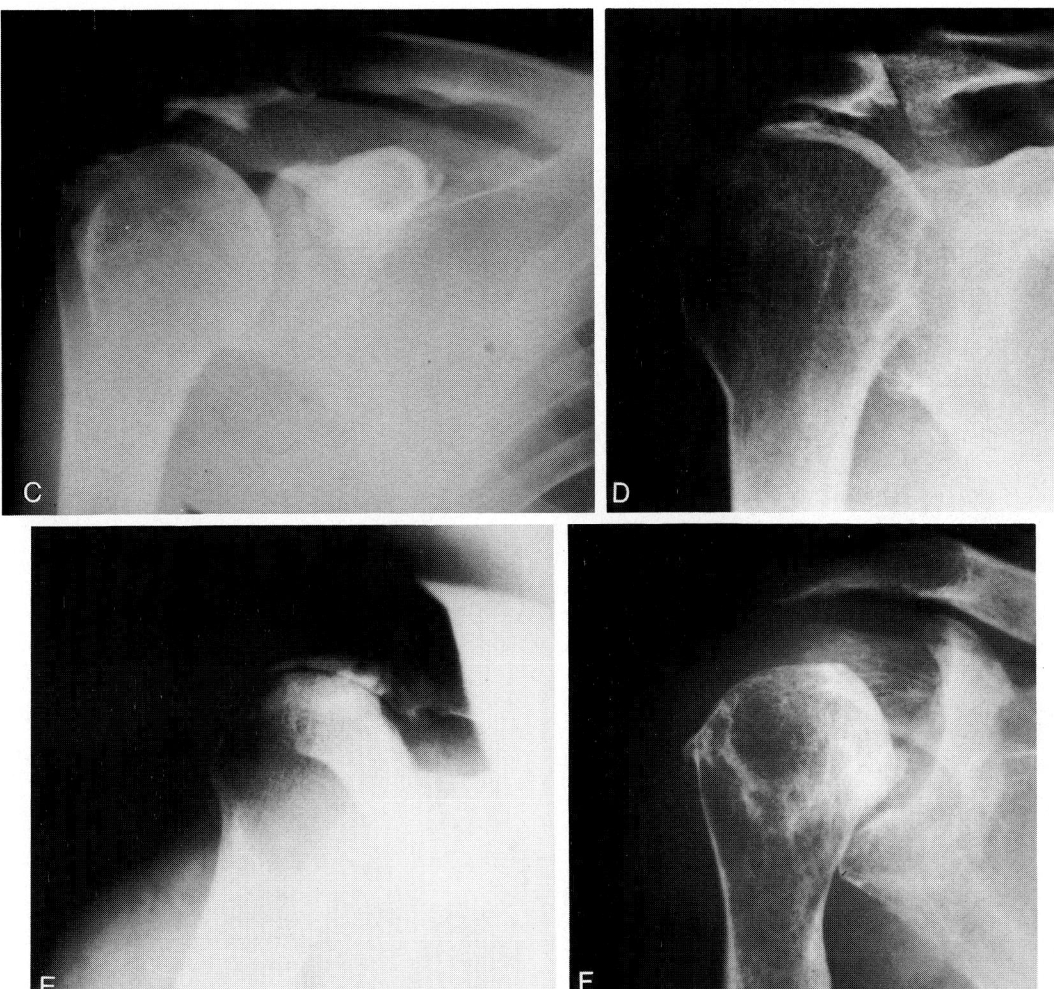

Figure 2–35 *Continued* C, Larger excrescence at the greater tuberosity and sclerosis of the undersurface of the acromion. D, Loss of the acromiohumeral distance, prominent undersurface of the acromioclavicular joint, wear of the anterior acromial spur, break in the calcar line, and decalcification of the greater tuberosity. E, Eburnation and erosion of the anterior acromion, acromioclavicular joint encroachment, and rounding of the greater tuberosity. F, End-stage erosion of the coracoid, glenohumeral joint, and undersurface of the acromioclavicular joint; further rounding of the greater tuberosity; instability; and beginning irregularity of the humeral head, which, with the erosion of the glenoid, qualifies this lesion as cuff-tear arthropathy.

very helpful, as shown in Figures 2–4 and 2–35. Consider these roentgen signs in the approximate order of appearance (see Table 2–5).

First Roentgen Evidence

1. *Prominence (squaring), eburnation, or exostosis of the greater tuberosity.* This occurs at the facet for the insertion of the supraspinatus tendon on the greater tuberosity at the spot where the tuberosity impinges on the acromion.

2. *Anterior acromial spur.* As described on page 55, I consider this to be a traction spur forming within the coracoacromial ligament. It is the earliest skeletal alteration seen on the acromion. In usual anterior-posterior roentgen views, the spur is superimposed on the base of the acromion and is not as evident as in the outlet view (lateral scapula view, Figs. 2–4 and 2–14). The spur is not diagnostic of a cuff tear and may be seen in patients who have no shoulder symptoms. Conversely, patients with complete tears may have no spur. Nevertheless, the presence of the spur should suggest the diagnosis of impingement in patients who have chronic shoulder pain.

3. *Prominent undersurface of acromioclavicular joint.* Narrowing of the outlet for the supraspinatus tendon can be caused by marginal excrescences or enlargement of this joint (see Fig. 2–6).

Moderately Advanced Changes

4. *Loss of the acromiohumeral distance.* It is important to measure the distance between the greater tuberosity and the acromion when suspecting the possibility of an impingement tear. A more

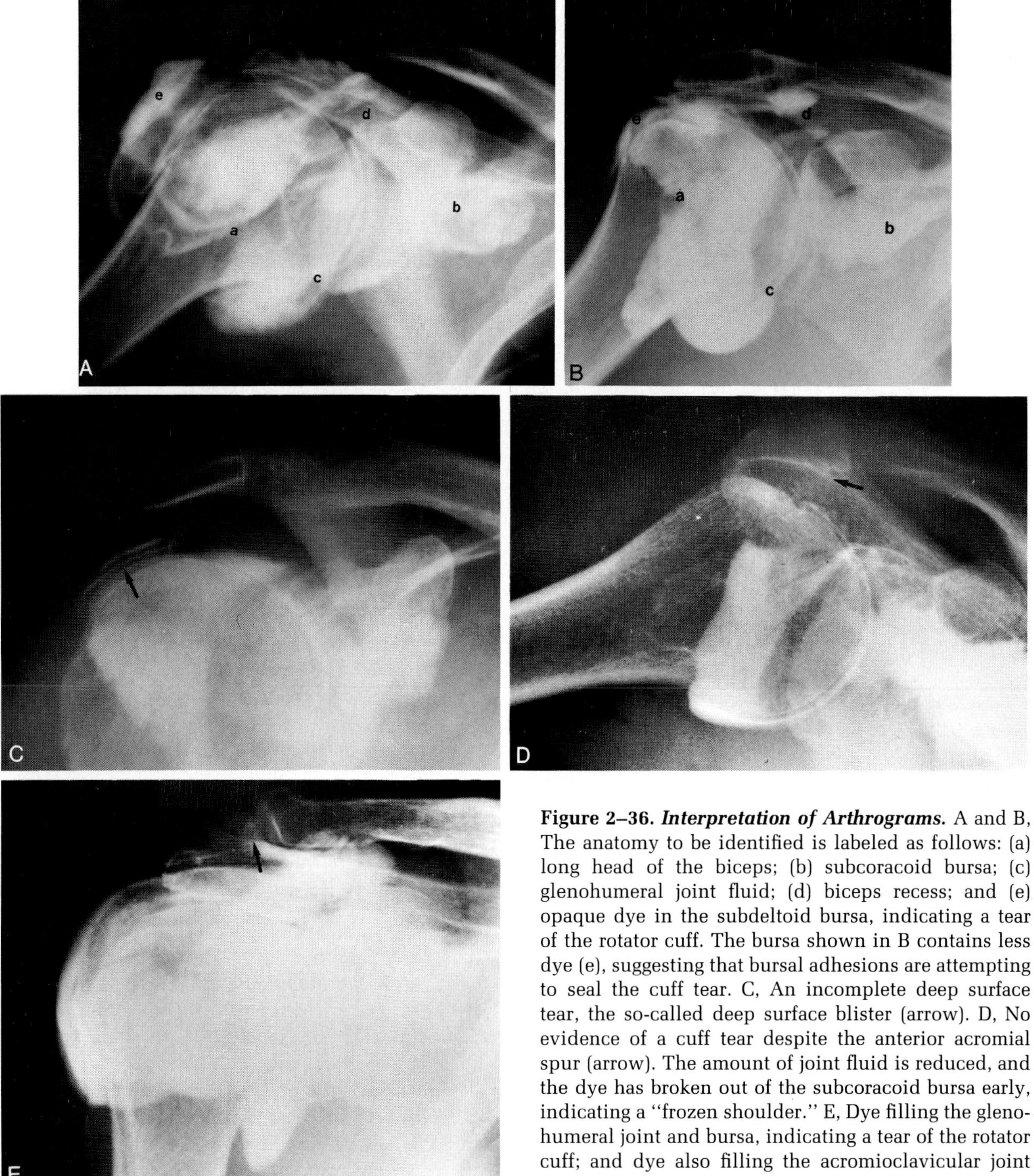

Figure 2–36. ***Interpretation of Arthrograms.*** A and B, The anatomy to be identified is labeled as follows: (a) long head of the biceps; (b) subcoracoid bursa; (c) glenohumeral joint fluid; (d) biceps recess; and (e) opaque dye in the subdeltoid bursa, indicating a tear of the rotator cuff. The bursa shown in B contains less dye (e), suggesting that bursal adhesions are attempting to seal the cuff tear. C, An incomplete deep surface tear, the so-called deep surface blister (arrow). D, No evidence of a cuff tear despite the anterior acromial spur (arrow). The amount of joint fluid is reduced, and the dye has broken out of the subcoracoid bursa early, indicating a "frozen shoulder." E, Dye filling the glenohumeral joint and bursa, indicating a tear of the rotator cuff; and dye also filling the acromioclavicular joint (= "geyser sign") (arrow), suggesting a large cuff tear.

accurate measurement of the distance can be made on a true lateral view ("outlet view")[32] (see Figs. 1–12 and 2–2) than in the anterior-posterior view because the distortion from a curved or sloping acromion or from projection is largely eliminated.

5. *Break in the "calcar line."* This is reliable evidence of ascent of the humerus. It is important to recognize, especially in rheumatoid arthritis, that the ascent may be due to loss of the articular surfaces rather than a tear of the rotator cuff.

6. *Decalcification of the greater tuberosity.* With disuse atrophy of the bone because of pain and weakness, decalcification of the greater tuberosity occurs beneath the sclerotic plaque on the surface caused by impingement. This can be quite striking, and I have seen biopsies performed on it more than once with the erroneous diagnosis of metastatic tumor.

Advanced Changes

7. *Eburnation and erosion of the anterior acromion.* With time, the undersurface of the anterior acromion becomes contoured to match the shape of the greater tuberosity and the worn surfaces become sclerotic and eburnated. Erosion may extend into the acromioclavicular joint but does not involve the posterior acromion until late in the final stages.

8. *Acromioclavicular joint encroachment.* Eventually, erosion extending from the acromion and undersurface of the acromioclavicular joint becomes evident by x-ray. When erosion perforates the capsule of the acromioclavicular joint, the "geyser sign" (see Figs. 2–15 and 2–36) is seen in the arthrogram.

9. *Rounding of the greater tuberosity.* Longstanding impingement wear causes sclerosis and rounding of the greater tuberosity with loss of the bicipital groove and loss of the delineation between the articular surface and the greater tuberosity (see Fig. 2–18).

End Stage

10. *Erosion of the coracoid and acromioclavicular joint.* In the end stages of impingement, there is erosion of the superior part of the glenoid, the coracoid, and the undersurface of the clavicle and acromion (see Figs. 2–35 and 2–47).

11. *Glenohumeral instability.* With massive tears of rotator cuff, the humeral head can be displaced anteriorly and posteriorly because of the lack of support of the rotator tendons. This is the "posterior mechanism" of dislocation (see p. 68). Dislocations of this type are considered to be a prerequisite for the deformation of the humeral head seen in cuff-tear arthropathy.

12. *Head deformity.* I estimate that approximately 4 percent of those with tears of the rotator cuff eventually develop the deformity of the head required for the diagnosis of cuff-tear arthropathy (see p. 124).

13. *Flail acromion.* With extreme erosion of the acromion, it may break in the middle. A persistent acromial epiphysis with end-stage erosion gives the same picture.[24, 109] In either case, the anterior acromion falls down on the humerus, blocking elevation and weakening the anterior deltoid because its origin has been rendered unstable.

Arthrograms

Indications for Arthrography

Neither the physical signs nor the roentgen findings of a cuff tear are diagnostic until the end stages. Arthrography is the most practical and reliable method for determining the presence of a complete cuff tear. Arthroscopy[60, 69, 79] has been used by some surgeons for diagnosing and estimating the size of tears. Ultrasonography is used by some investigators for diagnosing incomplete tears; however, it is, in its present stage of development, less accurate and cannot be relied upon for diagnosing incomplete tears that are not visible in arthrograms.[85] There has been some progress with magnetic resonance imaging (MRI) for identifying cuff defects. However, because of difficulty in interpreting ultrasonograms and MRIs and because arthroscopy is more invasive, arthrography remains the most reliable method for identifying complete tears.

My indications for arthrography in patients over 40 years of age (Table 2–6) are as follows:

1. Clinical findings suggesting the possibility of a cuff tear with failure to respond to conservative treatment for three months. Patients who are seen after they have had more than one year of disability and adequate conservative treatment elsewhere

Table 2–6. INDICATIONS FOR AN ARTHROGRAM*

After age 40: frequently indicated
1. Clinical signs of impingement and failure of conservative treatment for three months
2. Injury with sudden loss of strength (negative x-rays and negative neurological examination)
3. Rupture of long head of the biceps and chronic shoulder pain
4. Glenohumeral dislocation followed by persistent shoulder pain

*Under age 40, arthrogram is rarely indicated (see p. 65).

may be treated by anterior acromioplasty and exploration of the cuff, rather than undergoing arthrography, provided that their pain is relieved by the impingement injection test. This is done with the understanding that if a cuff tear is found it will be repaired. Arthroscopy appears to have only a limited place in the diagnosis and evaluation of impingement tears (see below).

2. Arthrography is recommended immediately when there has been an injury with sudden loss of strength and clinical findings suggest the possibility of an acute extension of an impingement tear.

3. Arthrography is advised for patients who have a rupture of the long head of the biceps with a history of previous shoulder pain or lingering shoulder pain after the biceps rupture (see p. 91 and Table 2–7).

4. Arthrography is advised when there has been an acute glenohumeral dislocation with persistent shoulder pain (see Chapter 4).

In patients under 40 years of age, the indications for arthrography are much less frequent. A careful search of plain films for fracture fragments or evidence of instability usually makes it unnecessary to obtain an arthrogram. An arthrogram is helpful for identifying traumatic tears in those patients with violent injuries and hard pain who have no roentgen evidence of fractures and in a few with long-standing, undiagnosed pain.

Technique of Arthrography

Prior to the recommendation of an arthrogram, a history of freedom from allergy to the dye is obtained and an erythrocyte sedimentation rate determination and blood count are performed to exclude the possibility of a low-grade infection in the glenohumeral joint from previous injections. If abnormal fluid is encountered during arthrography, the fluid is cultured and the test is abandoned. Scrupulous asepsis is observed. Adequate pre-medication is important for nervous patients because it is difficult to enter the joint if there is guarding and pulling away from the needle.

Double-contrast studies (opaque dye and air) with and without tomograms have been used in an effort to demonstrate the size of the tear. This technique entails less constrast media and can be confusing unless performed by someone especially experienced. A single-contrast method is more satisfactory for most surgeons. Other parameters (see Table 2–5 and p. 84) are used to estimate the size of the tear.

More can be learned if the test is performed with fluoroscopic control using the image intensifier and recording the events with spot films. When there is a large tear, the dye leaks out rapidly unless the opening has been partially sealed by scarred bursa. Finding the edge of the tendon in films made in internal and external rotation and in neutral position may be helpful in estimating the size of the tear.[112] No arthrogram should be considered negative unless the shoulder has been moved while the dye is in the joint to bring out incomplete and smaller tears. Spot films of the biceps groove may be beneficial in evaluating associated lesions of the long head. The interpretation of arthrograms is illustrated in Figure 2–36.

Alternatives to Arthrography

Bursagram. Bursagrams have been used to identify complete tears but were less informative than arthrograms. Fukuda[52, 85] has perfected a technique of bursography to show incomplete tears on the bursal side, but this requires experience for intrepretation and, of course, does not show deep surface or intratendinous tears.

Ultrasonography. Matsen[86] first suggested sonographic imaging for diagnosing rotator cuff lesions. This technique is appealing because it is noninvasive and has the potential, although not yet achieved, of showing incomplete tears regardless of whether they are superficial, deep, or intratendinous. Although improvements in the technique are being made, to date, the interpretation of the sonographic images remains difficult.[87, 88, 88a]

Magnetic Resonance Imaging. Nuclear magnetic resonance in its present state is of value in showing soft-tissue masses, but is less reliable at the tendon-bone insertions. As of this writing, it has not been perfected sufficiently and lacks the accuracy of arthrograms for the diagnosis of rotator cuff tears.

Diagnostic Arthroscopy. Arthroscopy requires anesthesia and is a much more involved procedure than arthrography. It may be of some value in special circumstances for diagnosis and for evaluating the size of tears.[60, 69, 79] However, I discontinued using it in impingement tears because if a cuff tear is found, it cannot be adequately repaired arthroscopically; and open acromioplasty seems to be of better quality than arthroscopic acromioplasty. Arthroscopic exploration may be of value for some small traumatic tears in the under age 35 group, but this is not always true because some of these tears are demonstrated in an arthrogram, they tend to heal spontaneously, and debriding the edges of these tears has not been proved to enhance healing.

Diagnosing Incomplete Tears

The diagnosis of incomplete tears can be difficult. Arthrograms may show tears on the deep surface (see Fig. 2–36C), but not intratendinous tears or those on the superficial surface. It is hoped that ultrasonography may one day be reliable for diagnosing incomplete tears; however, at present the diagnosis is often uncertain until the lesion is seen at the time of anterior acromioplasty. The indications for anterior acromioplasty are listed in Table 2–8.

Diagnostic and Therapeutic Implications of Biceps Ruptures

Patients are referred to me with recent retracted ruptures of the long head of the biceps who have received conflicting advice. Usually, one or two surgeons have recommended surgical re-attachment of the tendon and an equal number advised no treatment. Another group of patients with ruptures of the long head of biceps have been referred with inability to raise the arm as a result of massive, long-standing tears of the rotator cuff. As mentioned previously, it became apparent to me that long-standing cuff tears that were the most difficult to repair had associated biceps ruptures. These clinical problems precipitated a study of biceps lesions in the mid-1970s, the conclusions of which are summarized in Table 2–7.

The study on the clinical behavior of patients with ruptures of the long head of the biceps confirmed that the loss of the long head as a depressor of the humerus could escalate impingement and lead to the most devastating types of tears of the rotator cuff.[26] Therefore, rather than showing concern for the disputed role of the biceps in strength and function of the elbow, we emphasized the importance of evaluating the patient for a possible concomitant tear of the rotator cuff because it might more rapidly deteriorate following the biceps rupture. Previous literature on biceps ruptures seemed to have overlooked this important clinical point.

A history of shoulder pain before and after a biceps rupture should be obtained and the shoulder examined for evidence of a cuff tear. The clinical possibilities and the implications of each are given in Table 2–7, as follows:

1. If the patient is an active individual with a history of shoulder pain preceding the biceps rupture, an arthrogram is recommended. If the arthrogram shows a tear of the rotator cuff, anterior acromioplasty, repair of the rotator cuff, and re-attachment of the long head to the humerus (see Fig. 2–54) are advised. If the arthrogram is negative and the patient prefers the lump caused by the biceps rather than an operation, observation is advised. The patient is advised to return if shoulder pain continues or increases. This may occur because the depressor function of the long head has been lost and there is the distinct possibility of future development of a tear of the rotator cuff.

2. If there has been no previous shoulder pain and the patient prefers the lump to the surgery, the arthrogram is deferred and observation is recommended, but with the advice to return if shoulder pain develops for further evaluation of the rotator cuff.

3. If the patient is unwilling to accept the lump or the possiblity of slight weakness at the elbow and requests surgery, the long head is re-attached to the humerus, at which time an anterior acromioplasty with inspection of the rotator cuff is performed. An arthrogram is unnecessary because the rotator cuff is visualized at surgery.

Occasionally, a patient is seen who has a retracted rupture of the long head of the biceps that has been present for years without shoulder pain. However, the majority of patients with ruptures of the long head of the biceps either already have or will develop an associated tear of the supraspinatus tendon, as shown in our studies of biceps ruptures in cadavers (see p. 74). Virtually every specimen with a rupture of the long head of the biceps also had a tear of the rotator cuff. Therefore, it seems safe to assume that the majority of those who sustain a biceps rupture will eventually, by the end of life, have a rupture of the supraspinatus tendon as well. Apparently, in a few individuals the supraspinatus rupture occurs late in life.

Table 2–7. DIAGNOSTIC AND THERAPEUTIC IMPLICATIONS OF ACUTE* BICEPS RUPTURES

PREVIOUS SHOULDER PAIN	PATIENT "ACCEPTS BULGE"	ARTHROGRAM	TREATMENT RECOMMENDED
No	Yes	DEFER	OBSERVE
Yes	Yes	If *positive* for a tear:	Anterior acromioplasty, repair cuff, and re-attach biceps
		If *negative*:	OBSERVE
Yes or no	No	Not obtained	Anterior acromioplasty, re-attach biceps, and inspect cuff (repair cuff if torn)

*This table refers to recent biceps ruptures with retraction. Long-standing ruptures and those with partial recession are discussed elsewhere in the text.

If healthy and active patients with ruptures of the biceps are treated according to the recommendations in Table 2–7, many serious rotator cuff problems can be avoided and rather than being confused by conflicting advice, the patients are reassured they are receiving logical treatment. Self-attaching biceps ruptures (see Figs. 2–26 and 2–33) have the same diagnostic significance and should be treated with equal respect.

Estimating the Size of Cuff Tears

Neither arthrograms nor scans are completely reliable for showing the size of a cuff tear. Clinical evidence is more important. Physical signs suggestive of a large tear include the "dropping sign," rupture of the long head of the biceps, spinatus atrophy, and marked weakness. Earlier roentgen evidences of a large tear include a break in the calcar line and narrowing of the acromiohumeral distance. Of course, when the advanced skeletal changes seen in some long-standing tears are present, it is obvious that the tear is large.

Differential Diagnosis of Cuff Tears

The differential diagnosis of cuff tears is outlined in Table 2–5. *Stage I and Stage II impingement* can give signs exactly like those of tears of the rotator cuff and may require arthrograms for clarification. Because impingement is the most frequent cause of *biceps tendinitis*, a common error in the past has been a biceps tenodesis on an impingement lesion with the disastrous results of causing the humerus to ascend, aggravating impingement.

Acute hemorrhagic subacromial bursitis is another common and important lesion, as discussed on page 81.

Paralysis of the C5–C6 root can give a picture much like a tear of the rotator cuff when there is weakness of the supraspinatus, infraspinatus, and deltoid muscle. I have found the associated weakness of the biceps and usually (not always) exacerbation of pain on extension and tilting of the neck toward the involved side to be very helpful in distinguishing this from tears of the rotator cuff (Fig. 2–37). There is no weakness of the biceps

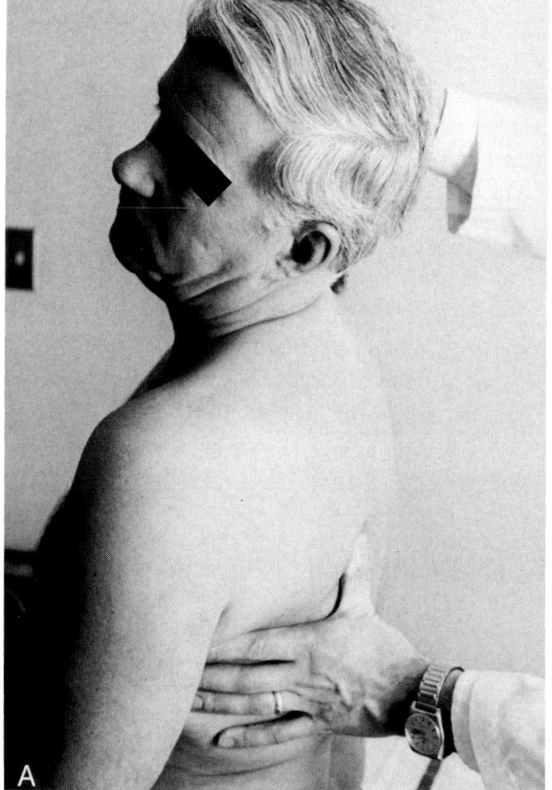

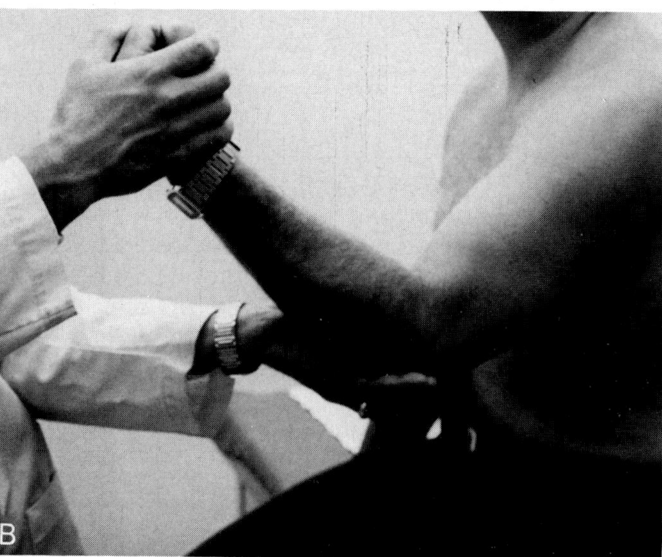

Figure 2–37. Important clinical tests to distinguish weakness of shoulder external rotation and elevation as a result of a C5–C6 nerve root lesion from that due to a rotator cuff tear. These two tests are routine in every initial examination of the shoulder (see Fig. 1–12). A, Extension and tilting of the neck toward the involved side reduce the space in the neural foramen and often cause a temporary exacerbation of arm symptoms that are due to a C5–C6 problem. B, A C5–C6 lesion often causes weakness of elbow flexion, which is not seen with a tear of the rotating cuff.

associated with rotator cuff tears. Negative arthrographic findings, cervical spine x-rays, and electromyographic studies confirm the diagnosis.

As discussed in Chapter 6, p. 448, *suprascapular nerve paralysis* has too often been posed as a diagnosis when actually the problem is a tear of the rotator cuff. Weakness of external rotation and abduction is common to both; however, as discussed, in my experience suprascapular nerve syndrome is extremely rare and unlikely, and an arthrogram should readily make the diagnosis.

Patients with *other neurological conditions*, including syringomyelia, amyotrophic lateral sclerosis, and polymyositis, have been referred with a mistaken diagnosis of a tear of the rotator cuff. One must be alert to these possibilities and examine every new patient carefully for deficits requiring more detailed neurological work-up.

TREATMENT OF IMPINGEMENT LESIONS

This discussion of surgical indications for impingement lesions considers only active patients who are well motivated, without undue anesthesia risks, and who have reasonable life expectancy. The selection of treatment always considers both the anatomical problem and the general health of the patient; the chronological age is of less importance.

Except for recent injuries with sudden loss of strength and positive arthrograms, the initial treatment of impingement lesions is conservative. The indications for arthrograms are listed in Table 2–6.

Conservative Treatment

Cold or Heat? Rest or Exercise?

Conservative treatment is based on heat and "rest." Cold applications are used only when there has been an injury or overuse and then only during the initial 24 hours. Use of the arm above the horizontal is avoided, but the patient is taught to stretch the shoulder passively through a full range of motion each day to avoid stiffening.

Medications and Injections

Oral anti-inflammatory medications can at times be helpful to reduce the edema in Stage I lesions and to avoid the possible side effect of weakening the tendons that is said to result from steroid injections.

Injections are deferred until appropriate laboratory studies have been obtained. The impingement injection test (see Fig. 2–30) with Xylocaine is helpful and may have some therapeutic effect. Although some patients tolerate many steroid injections without apparent adverse effect on the tendons, others seem to be sensitive to local steroid injections, as evidenced by the disappearance of subcutaneous tissue occasionally seen following a single injection of steroids at the lateral epicondyle of the elbow. Also, it is thought that a steroid injection in this type of patient might weaken the rotator cuff tendons. Because there is no way of knowing what type of reaction may follow, it seems best to avoid steroid injections in patients under 40 years of age and to limit their use in older patients.

Exercises for Impingement

As mentioned previously, the patient is taught to stretch the shoulder through a full range of motion each day to avoid stiffening, but is cautioned to avoid use of the arm overhead. When the acute inflammation has subsided, resistive, strengthening exercises below the horizontal are progressed. The lower part of the subscapularis, teres major, latissimus dorsi, and sternal head of the pectoralis major are strengthened by resistive internal rotation. Resistive external rotation, also with the arm at the side, strengthens the infraspinatus and teres minor. Isometrics against raising the arm in abduction strengthens the supraspinatus. The biceps and supraspinatus are strengthened by the "upper-cut" exercise (see Fig. 7–13). Strengthening exercises should be followed by periods of rest to allow recovery; therefore, these exercises are performed only once a day.

Prior to resuming activities, the patient, athletic or otherwise, should have recovered protective muscle tone against impingement and know how to do stretching and warm-up exercises prior to the activity. Repetitive movements are eliminated whenever possible by modifying the position of the arm at work or in sports.

Surgery for Impingement

Anterior acromioplasty, as will be described in detail, is used for all impingement problems in patients over 40 years of age and in the few under that age with demonstrable skeletal prominences at the undersurface of the acromion or acromioclavicular joint. The procedure of bursectomy and coracoacromial ligament section is considered for very few patients. These patients are in the younger age group, have chronic Stage II symptoms persisting over one year, and have no evidence of skeletal impingement.

Resection of the Coracoacromial Ligament and Bursectomy

Indications

Stage II impingement symptoms occur following activities and disappear within a few days with rest. This makes the pre-operative evaluation more difficult and also makes for less dramatic improvement following the surgery. I find it more gratifying to operate on a patient with more constant pain that is promptly relieved by an operation.

The few patients considered for this procedure are in the under 40 age group. I require a full year of conservative treatment before considering this procedure. This time is needed to exclude the possibility of a Stage I lesion that would resolve spontaneously if given time. Care is taken to exclude subluxations and dislocations, frozen shoulder, and other conditions discussed in the differential diagnosis of Stage I and II lesions (see p. 81).

Pre-operative evaluation usually requires the patient to return after activities when the shoulder is painful in order to perform an impingement injection test (see Fig. 2–30). Because the pain preoperatively is present only after activities, the patient is warned that the discomfort following surgery is often greater than it was pre-operatively until a new bursa forms, which may require several months. I insist that the patient understand this, agrees to be diligent in the post-operative exercise program, and does not expect maximum recovery until after six months or a year. With these requirements, very few patients qualify for this procedure, but it is helpful for the occasional patient in the younger age group who has long-standing disability and does not require an anterior acromioplasty, as specified in Table 2–8 and on p. 98. With these criteria, I perform this operation less frequently than once a year.

Table 2–8. INDICATIONS FOR ANTERIOR ACROMIOPLASTY

1. When repairing an impingement tear
2. Pain over one year and negative arthrogram with positive "impingement injection test"
3. Occasional Stage II impingement lesion with demonstrable bone prominence at the undersurface of anterior acromion or acromioclavicular joint
4. Concomitantly with other procedures in selected non-outlet impingement lesions—e.g., malunited greater tuberosity; rupture of long head of biceps; cuff tears; old, stable acromioclavicular dislocations

Bursectomy with or without division of the coracoacromial ligament, a "soft-tissue decompression," can be performed arthroscopically. I believe this is perhaps the best arthroscopic operation in the shoulder; however, the indications for it should be the same outlined previously. The advantages of an open procedure over an arthroscopic soft-tissue decompression are better visualization for excision of the bursa and ligament, the ability to control bleeding from the acromial branch of the thoracoacromial artery should it occur, and the ability to repair a tear of the rotator cuff if it should be unexpectedly encountered. The advantage of an arthroscopic soft-tissue decompression is the small skin incision and less invasion of the deltoid muscle (although the open procedure is performed through a two-inch muscle-split without detachment of any deltoid origin).

Technique of Open Coracoacromial Ligament Resection and Bursectomy

The patient is positioned in the beachchair position (see Figs. 1–28A, 2–41, and 2–43) with the head of the table raised about 35 degrees and the knees gatched sufficiently to prevent sliding down. Folded towels are placed under the scapula to hold it forward, and the shoulder protrudes over the corner of the table sufficiently so that its posterior aspect is exposed. The arm is draped free so that it can be moved. The operation can be performed with local, regional, or general anesthesia.

Prior to the skin preparation, the arm is manipulated through a full range of motion. If adhesions are broken to gain this amount of movement, the diagnosis of frozen shoulder is added and special attention will be given in the post-operative exercise program. If full motion is present, the shoulder is manipulated to exclude the possibility of unrecognized instability.

A 5.0 cm. skin incision is made in Langer's lines starting just lateral to the anterior acromion and directed forward toward a point a fingerbreadth's lateral to the coracoid (Fig. 2–38). The subcutaneous tissue is elevated from the deep fascia, and the deep fascia is incised in the direction of the deltoid fibers from the tip of the anterior acromion downward 5.0 cm. Using two dissecting elevators, the surgeon splits the deltoid 5.0 cm. from above downward, avoiding injury to the intramuscular branches of the axillary nerve by further splitting (see Fig. 1–28B). By sharp dissection, the clavipectoral fascia, which is a continuation of the coracoacromial ligament and overlies the subacromial bursa, is incised, exposing the bursa. The

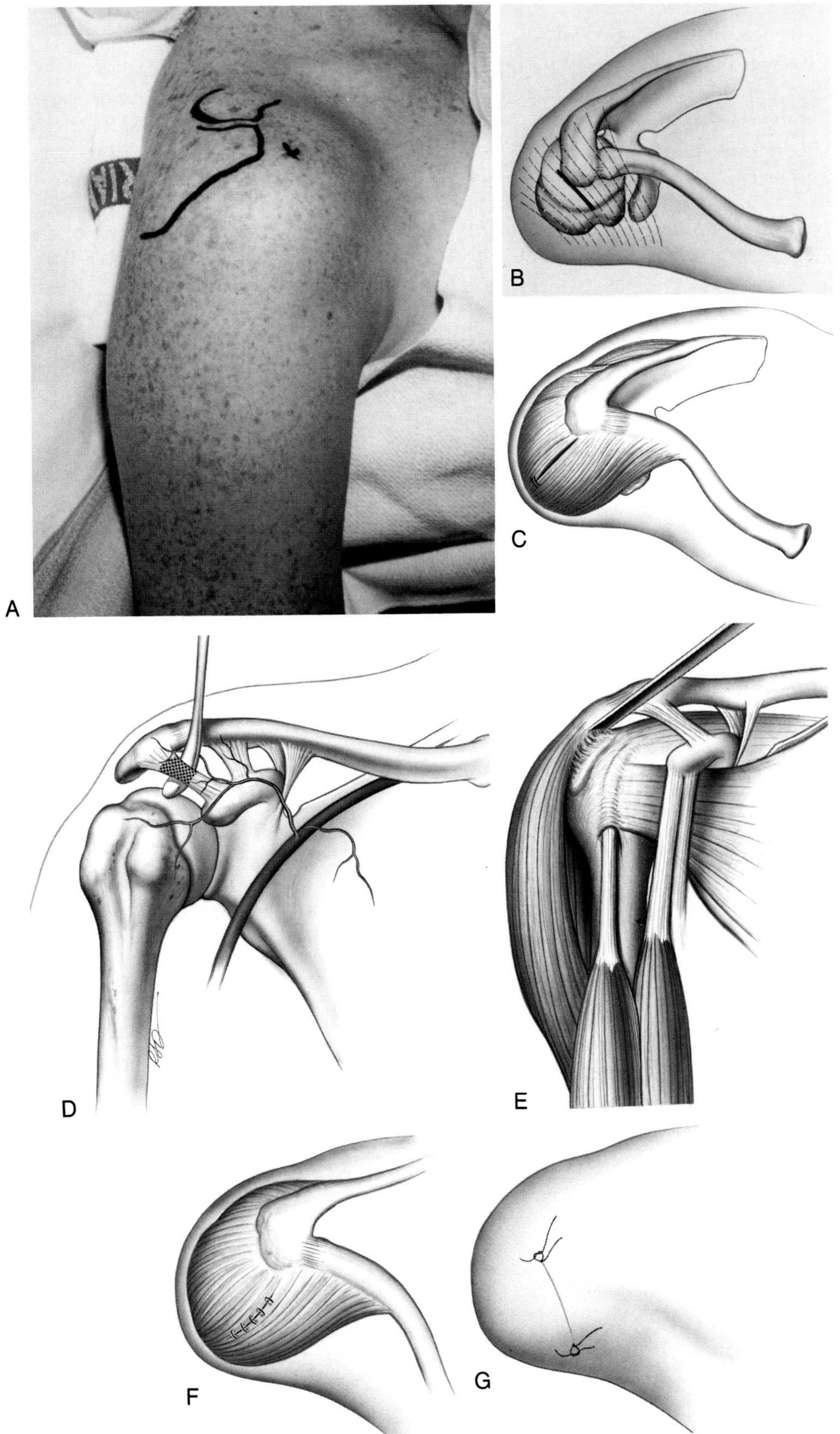

Figure 2–38. *Technique for Coracoacromial Ligament Resection and Bursectomy*

A, Position is 30 degree beachchair. B, Skin incision 2.0 cm. or less. C, Split in the deltoid muscle. D, Surgeon anticipates the artery on the ligament before resecting 1.0 cm of the ligament. E, Bursectomy removing the thickened and adherent part of the bursa. F, Closure of the deltoid with two or three interrupted fascial sutures with buried knots. G, Skin closure with a removable subcuticular stitch.

coracoacromial ligament is then exposed by pushing the acromial branch of the thoracoacromial artery medially off of its superficial surface and placing a blunt elevator behind it to expose its full width. The ligament is then cut across, and a 1.0 cm. segment of the full width of the ligament is removed to prevent its re-uniting. Its medial aspect is palpated to make sure it has been completely sectioned all the way across.

The thickened portion of the bursa is then excised with scissors. The entire rotator cuff can then be inspected for hidden calcium deposits or other abnormalities. This requires positioning the humerus correctly in the small wound to bring the tendons individually into view. The subscapularis tendon is exposed by holding the humerus in a flexed and externally rotated position. The supraspinatus tendon is seen in neutral rotation. The infraspinatus and teres minor are exposed by internally rotating the humerus and extension.

The split in the deltoid muscle is closed with interrupted sutures through the superficial fascia with buried knots. The skin is closed with a subcuticular pull-out suture. A sling and swathe is applied for comfort during transportation from the operating room.

Aftercare

No muscle is detached during this procedure; therefore, the exercise program can be advanced as rapidly as pain permits. The patient is ambulatory on the day of surgery. Pendulum and passive elevation[89] (see Fig. 7–7) by the surgeon and therapist is started within 24 to 48 hours after surgery, at which time the sling is discarded. The initial emphasis is on passive exercises for range of motion, which are soon advanced to the full self-assistive exercise regimen (see Fig. 7–8). The patient is discharged from the hospital as soon as he or she has achieved a near-normal passive range. Analgesics on a regular basis and low heat may be used in stubborn cases, but this amount of motion is usually obtained within 48 hours.

The subcuticular skin suture is removed at 10 days following surgery (if removed earlier, adherent strips are applied to protect against the stress of the exercise program), at which time strengthening exercises are progressed, beginning with isometrics and advancing (see Fig. 7–10) as tolerated. Motion is recorded at each visit, and the exercises are continued until there is normal motion and strength.

Result to Be Expected

Patients who had complete relief of pain with the impingement injection test pre-operatively can be expected to eventually be pleased with the result and achieve normal motion and function. As discussed previously, the recovery period may be longer than expected, and during this time strenuous activities associated with pain are avoided. Although some patients recover faster, it is important that the patient know pre-operatively that some individuals require a full year. Unless the latter group has been forewarned, they will be apprehensive about the outcome during the recovery period.

Causes of failure include incomplete section of the coracoacromial ligament, residual impingement from unrecognized bony prominences, residual frozen shoulder because of inadequate manipulation during the procedure, unrecognized glenohumeral subluxations and dislocations, and the development of adhesions because of inadequate aftercare. It is especially important in young athletic patients to have excluded the possibility of acromioclavicular joint symptoms, such as caused by traumatic osteolysis of the distal clavicle in "weightlifter's shoulder" (see Fig. 6–6), or glenohumeral subluxations and dislocations. Symptomatology in the acromioclavicular joint has to be determined pre-operatively with a Xylocaine injection into this joint. At the time of this procedure, I routinely manipulate the glenohumeral joint to exclude the possibility of instability or frozen shoulder.

Anterior Acromioplasty

The objective of anterior acromioplasty is to establish a tunnel beneath the anterior acromion and the acromioclavicular joint to free the supraspinatus tendon by enlarging the "supraspinatus outlet" (see Fig. 2–2). The origin of the deltoid muscle is preserved.

Background of Anterior Acromioplasty

Codman[6] thought cuff tears were primarily caused by injuries but interestingly wrote in 1934, regarding repairing the cuff, "Assuming the operation is done soon after the accident . . . it seems to me this immediate operation would be easy . . . but I have not been able to operate on one of these cases in an early stage." Earlier in his experience, he repaired cuff tears through what he termed the "sabre-cutting" approach, which he credited Gill for describing in connection with shoulder fusions.[233] This approach went through the acromioclavicular joint and divided the base of the acromion. Codman discontinued using this approach in favor of a simple, two inch deltoid-splitting approach for cuff repairs, even though it was "more cramped." Later in the 1930s, impingement was

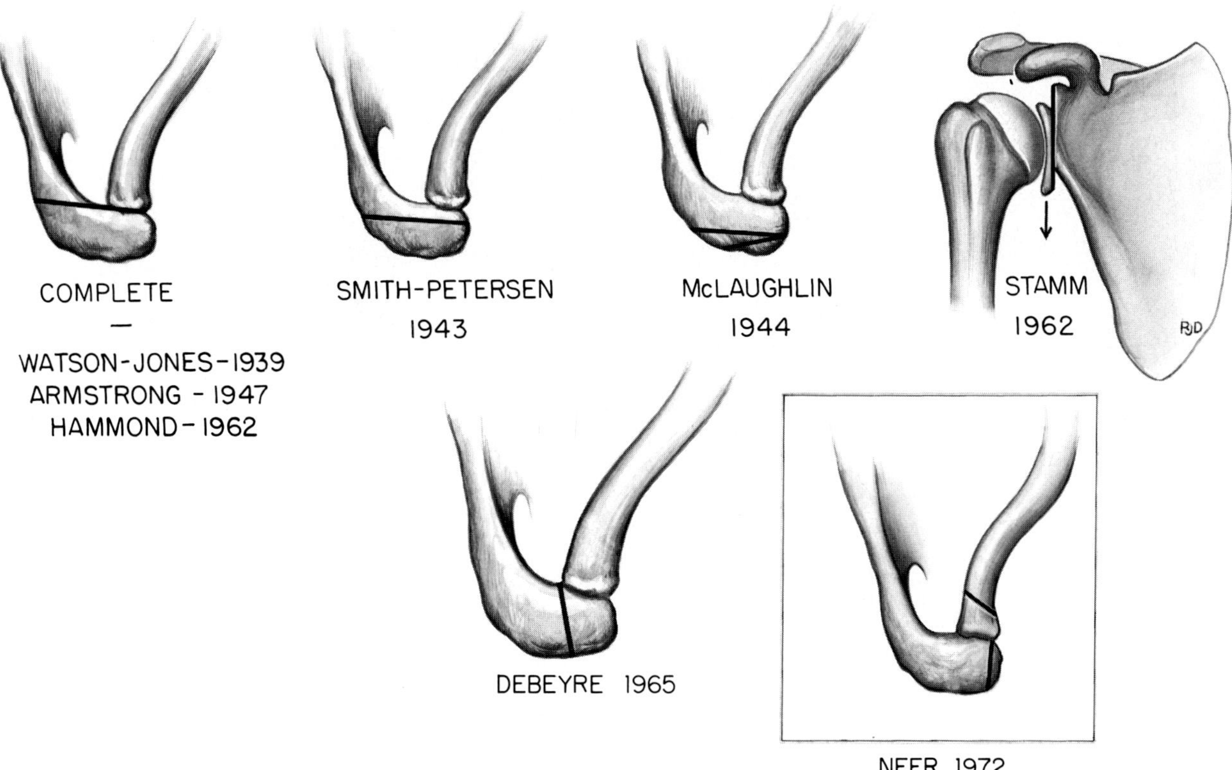

Figure 2–39. History of operations for impingement.

recognized by Armstrong and others as a source of chronic shoulder pain, but these investigators did not relate impingement to rotator cuff tears. Impingement was thought to occur against the lateral edge of the acromion rather than against the anterior acromion and acromioclavicular joint. Complete acromionectomy[35–37] and lateral acromionectomy[38, 40] (Fig. 2–39) were advised. Both of these procedures weakened the deltoid, led to wound complications, and impaired shoulder function[29] (Fig. 2–46). Stamm (1962) suggested an osteotomy of the glenoid to shift the glenohumeral joint downward away from the acromion to relieve impingement.[92] This was not intended for cuff repairs. Debeyre (1965) described the transacromial approach for repairing tears of the rotator cuff.[34] This gave adequate exposure of the rotator cuff with preservation of the deltoid origin but was not intended to relieve impingement. Disappointment with the lateral approaches, with or without acromionectomy (because of weakening the deltoid), and disappointment with the transacromial approach (because of residual impingement) caused me in the 1960s to develop the anterior acromioplasty approach, a report of which was published in 1972.[28]

Anterior acromioplasty emphasizes three points: (1) preservation of the origin of the deltoid muscle, (2) adequate exposure of the rotator cuff, and (3) decompression of impingement. The superficial surface of the acromioclavicular joint is left intact to preserve the attachments for the deltoid origin, and resection of the outer clavicle is performed in only a few patients with specific indications—e.g., for exposure of the supraspinatus or painful acromioclavicular arthritis (see p. 98).

In 1985, Ellman described how to perform an anterior acromioplasty with an arthroscope.[60] To date, the quality of arthroscopic anterior acromioplasty has been inferior to that of open anterior acromioplasty (Fig. 2–40), and if a cuff tear is encountered, it cannot be repaired arthroscopically. Arthroscopic anterior acromioplasty remains developmental. It should be remembered that an arthroscope is an instrument and does not alter the indications or anatomical objectives of anterior acromioplasty.

Anterior acromioplasty has given adequate exposure for repairing all 390 cuff tears in Series I and Series II. Complete excision of the distal end of the clavicle for exposure (see Fig. 2–43) was rarely required, and detachment of the posterior deltoid for mobilizing the infraspinatus (Fig. 2–43) was performed in only five shoulders in this series of primary repairs, even though 60 percent of patients had massive tears. There was almost no

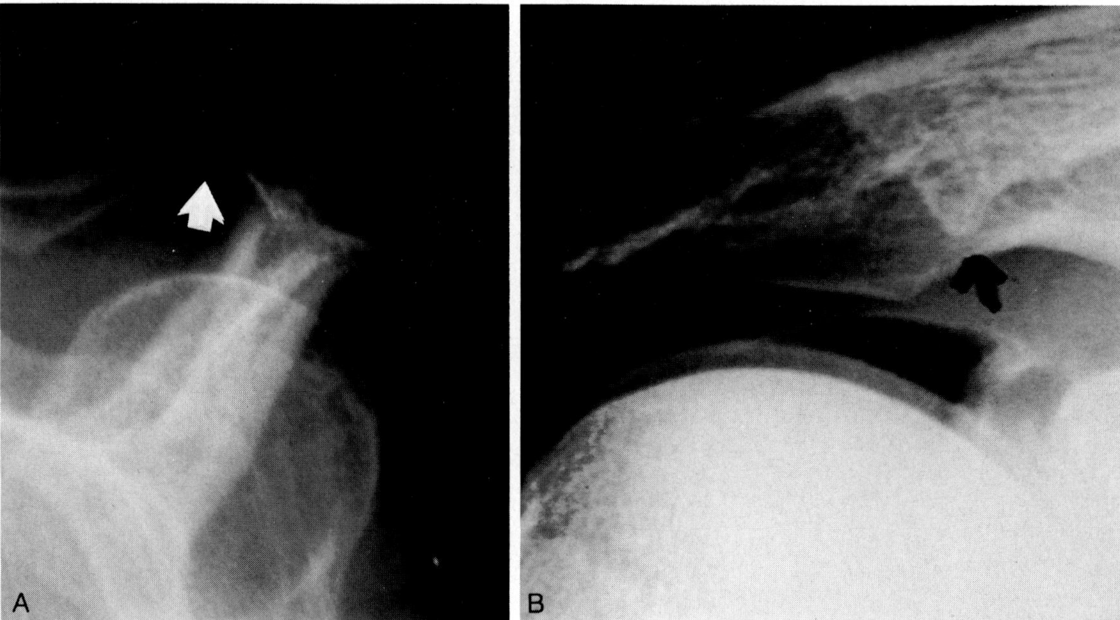

Figure 2–40. Open compared with arthroscopic anterior acromioplasty. A, Outlet view made 8 years after surgical anterior acromioplasty showing an excellent tunnel (arrow) for the supraspinatus tendon without regrowth of bone. B, Anterior-posterior view made 1 year after a failed arthroscopic anterior acromioplasty showing inadequate removal of clavicle (arrow) and bone debris. To date, the quality of anterior acromioplasty achieved with an arthroscope has been inferior to that of open anterior acromioplasty (see p. 137).

problem of weakening the deltoid, wound healing, or re-growth of bone (see pp. 74 to 76). Exposure of the supraspinatus through this anterior approach was better than through lateral approaches because the insertion of the supraspinatus on the greater tuberosity naturally protrudes anterior to the acromion when the patient is positioned for a cuff repair as shown in Figure 2–43. Anterior acromioplasty is the only approach I use for repairing cuff tears.

Indications for Anterior Acromioplasty

The indications for anterior acromioplasty are listed in Table 2–8. This frequently performed procedure is performed routinely for cuff repairs; for persistent disability that is due to chronic outlet impingement even when the arthrogram is negative; and in conjunction with various other surgical procedures. It may be required for non-outlet impingement, for example, when re-attaching a ruptured biceps or with revision arthroplasty or arthroplasty for old trauma; or in outlet impingement, e.g., when encountering bone proliferation at the acromion or acromioclavicular joint.

In those patients with outlet impingement and a negative arthrogram for a tear of the rotator cuff, anterior acromioplasty is considered only after symptoms have persisted despite adequate conservative treatment for at least one year and the pain is temporarily relieved by the impingement injection test (see Fig. 2–30). Sonography is still developmental, and does not give reliable evidence of incomplete tears at this time.

Anterior acromioplasty is very rarely performed in patients who are under 25 years of age because the anterior acromial epiphyses are normally open until that age. Unless there is an obvious skeletal abnormality, the soft-tissue decompression by coracoacromial ligament section and bursectomy would seem preferable.

Non-outlet impingement (see p. 48 and p. 138) is generally treated by some other procedure, often without anterior acromioplasty.

Indications to Resect the Acromioclavicular Joint During Anterior Acromioplasty

Complete resection of the distal 2.0 cm. of clavicle is performed as a step in anterior acromioplasty in only two specific indications: (1) if during the pre-operative examination this joint is found to be painful and tender as a result of arthritis, and (2) if during surgery more exposure of the supraspinatus is needed to repair a large rotator cuff tear.

For a prominent acromioclavicular joint contributing to impingement, only the undersurface of the distal clavicle and adjacent acromion are removed. This leaves the superficial surface intact to provide a secure anchorage for the deltoid origin.

Anterior Acromioplasty Under Age 40

A few individuals who use their shoulders strenuously throughout their early years come to anterior acromioplasty in their thirties, with shoulders that appear at least ten years older than their chronological age. The acromial epiphysis is normally open until age 25 years, and anterior acromioplasty is rarely performed before that age and is performed infrequently in patients under 40 years of age. However, it is indicated occasionally in this younger age group when there is a definite skeletal deformity of the acromion, as shown in Figure 4–23.

Anterior acromioplasty may have a role in creating more room for the supraspinatus tendon in those who subject the supraspinatus to impingement because of using the arm in an extraordinary excursion of motion with extreme violence, such as a baseball pitcher. The procedure is not advised unless conservative treatment has failed for a period of one year and the impingement injection test temporarily relieves the pain completely. The prognosis for returning to the same strenuous activity must be guarded, because it was the strenuous sport that caused the problem in the first place.

For reasons discussed on p. 142, I do not perform anterior acromioplasty at the time of excision of a calcium deposit and believe it prolongs the recovery.

Technique of Anterior Acromioplasty

The patient is placed high on the table with the head on a headrest, avoiding hyperextension of the neck that might compromise the cervical nerve roots (see Fig. 1–18A). The point of the affected shoulder protrudes over the corner of the table to give a wide field for skin preparation and to give access to the back of the shoulder (see Fig. 2–43A). The table is adjusted to the beachchair position so that the head is raised 35 degrees, and the knees are bent sufficiently to prevent sliding down. This brings the acromion perpendicular to the floor and parallel to the wall (Fig. 2–41A). In this position, the humeral head can be palpated anterior to the acromion. The arm is draped free so that it can be fully extended and rotated off the side of the table without interference. This is important because the humerus must be moved in various directions in order to see all of the rotator cuff through such a small opening. The edge of the operating table is padded by sliding the mattress over to cover it to prevent contusing the ulnar nerve. General or regional (scalene block) anesthesia is used.

After the anesthesia has been established and just prior to beginning the skin preparation, the shoulder is manipulated through a full range of motion to eliminate adhesions and to make sure that a full range of elevation, external rotation, and internal rotation has been re-established (Fig. 2–41B), as discussed on page 425. Despite the efforts to eliminate stiffness during conservative treatment before surgery, there may be some residual limitation of motion that would interfere with recovery following surgery.

I prefer an incision about 7.5 cm. long (shorter in small individuals, and slightly longer in large men) made obliquely in Langer's lines extending from just lateral to the anterior acromion forward in a direction toward a point one fingerbreadth lateral to the coracoid (Fig. 2–41C). This incision is between the branches of the suprascapular and axillary sensory fibers and creates no anesthetic area. An alternate skin incision, used for larger cuff tears and when complete excision of the distal clavicle is anticipated, extends from the acromioclavicular joint downward in the direction of the deltoid muscle fibers (Fig. 2–43A). In either case, the subcutaneous tissue is mobilized as required and a split is made by blunt dissection in the deltoid muscle extending from the acromioclavicular joint capsule downward 5 cm. Further splitting jeopardizes the axillary nerve (see Fig. 1–28B). The distal end of this split in the deltoid is secured with a stay suture to prevent further splitting by retractors (Fig. 2–41D). With sharp dissection, the anterior part of the acromioclavicular joint capsule is incised and the acromial side of the capsule with attached periosteum is raised off the surface of the acromion with a scalpel, staying as close to bone as possible to keep the tendinous origin of the deltoid muscle intact and to expose about 1.0 cm. of the anterior edge of the acromion. This exposes the coracoacromial ligament, which attaches on the undersurface of the anterior acromion. Anticipating and elevating the acromial branch of the thoracoacromial artery (Fig. 2–41E), this ligament is detached from the undersurface of the acromion and removed to facilitate exposure of the anterior acromion.

All adherent soft tissue is elevated from the undersurface of the acromion (see Figs. 2–41F and 2–43C), and a flat (Darrach) elevator is placed under the acromion (Fig. 2–41G1). With traction on the arm and depression of the Darrach elevator to bring the humeral head out of the way, the undersurface of the anterior acromion can then be inspected and palpated for sharp edges and osteophytes and to determine the thickness of the acromion. A thin, 22 mm. osteotome that is beveled on one side (AO osteotome) is placed with the bevel

Text continued on page 105

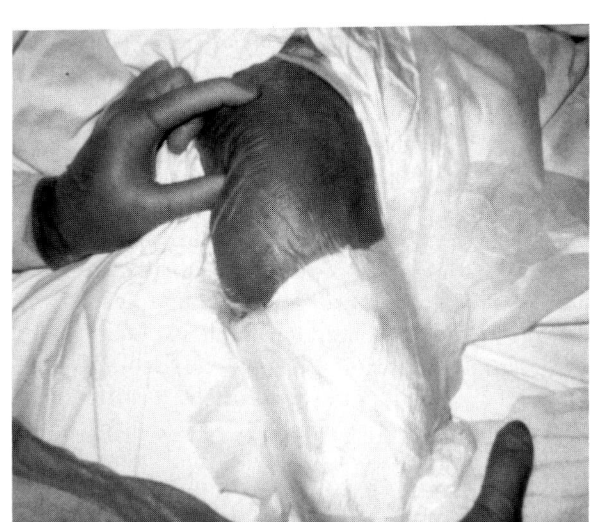

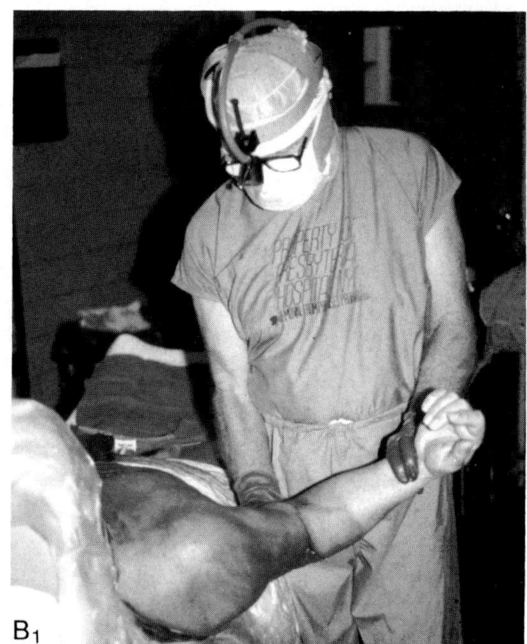

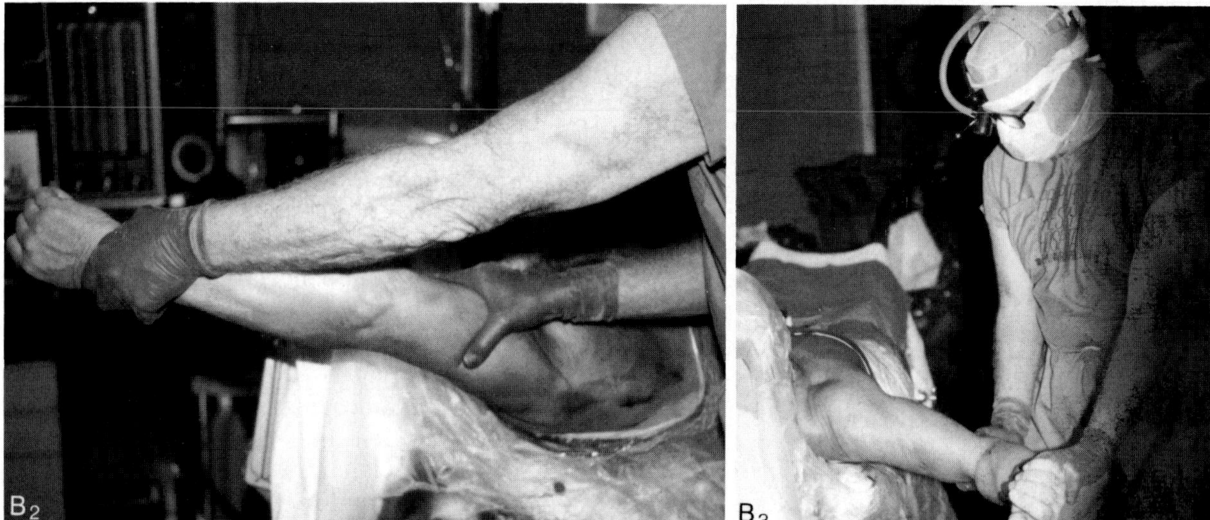

Figure 2–41. ***Technique of Anterior Acromioplasty***

A. Position of the patient places acromion perpendicular to the floor, and the humeral head is anterior to the acromion.

B. Manipulation with two fingers' pressure in (1) external rotation, (2) elevation, and (3) with the arm at 90 degrees of abduction in internal and external rotation.

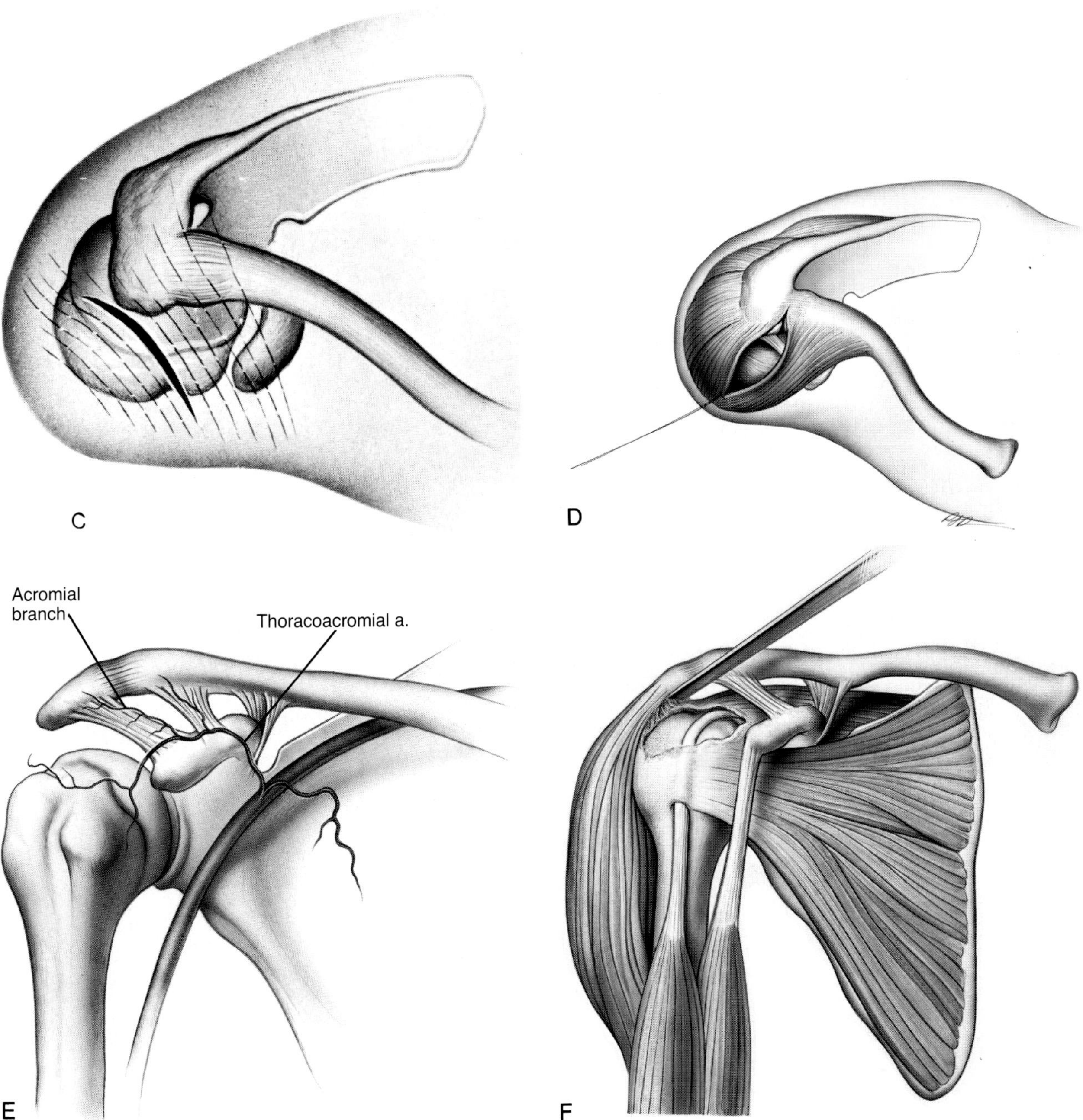

Figure 2–41 *Continued*
C. Incision.
D. Muscle split with anterior capsule open.
E. Elevation of artery from the coracohumeral ligament.
F. Surgeon divides adhesions and denudes the undersurface of the acromion to free the rotator cuff.

Illustration continued on following page

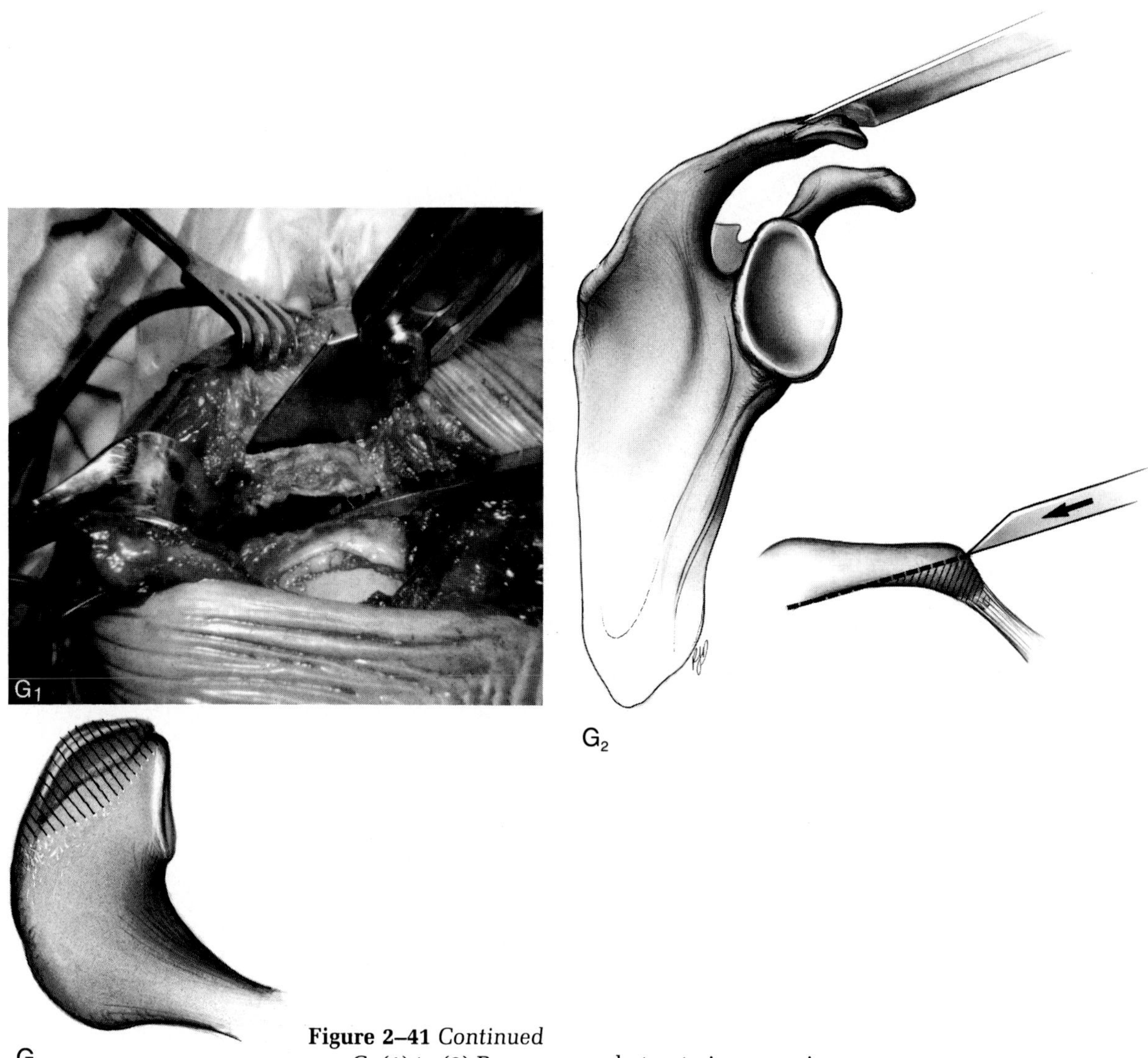

Figure 2–41 *Continued*
G. (1) to (3) Bone removed at anterior acromion.

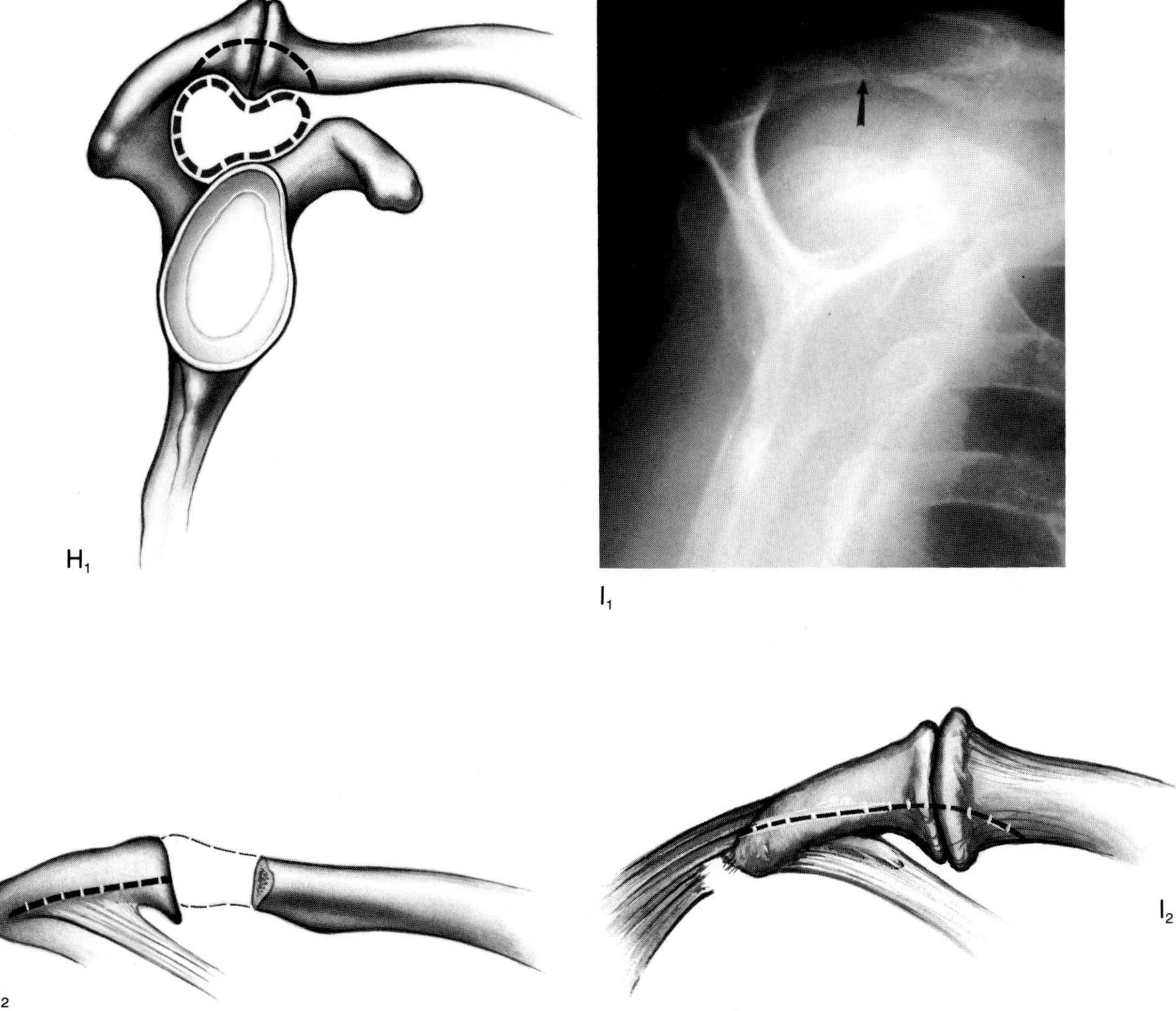

Figure 2–41 *Continued*

H. Bone removed at acromiocalvicular joint for (1) impingement and (2) resection if there was painful acromioclavicular arthritis pre-operatively. The trapezius muscle is marked with a stay suture and later approximated to the deltoid muscle in the closure, as in Fig. 6–8C.

I. (1) and (2) Final appearance of usual anterior acromioplasty.

Illustration continued on following page

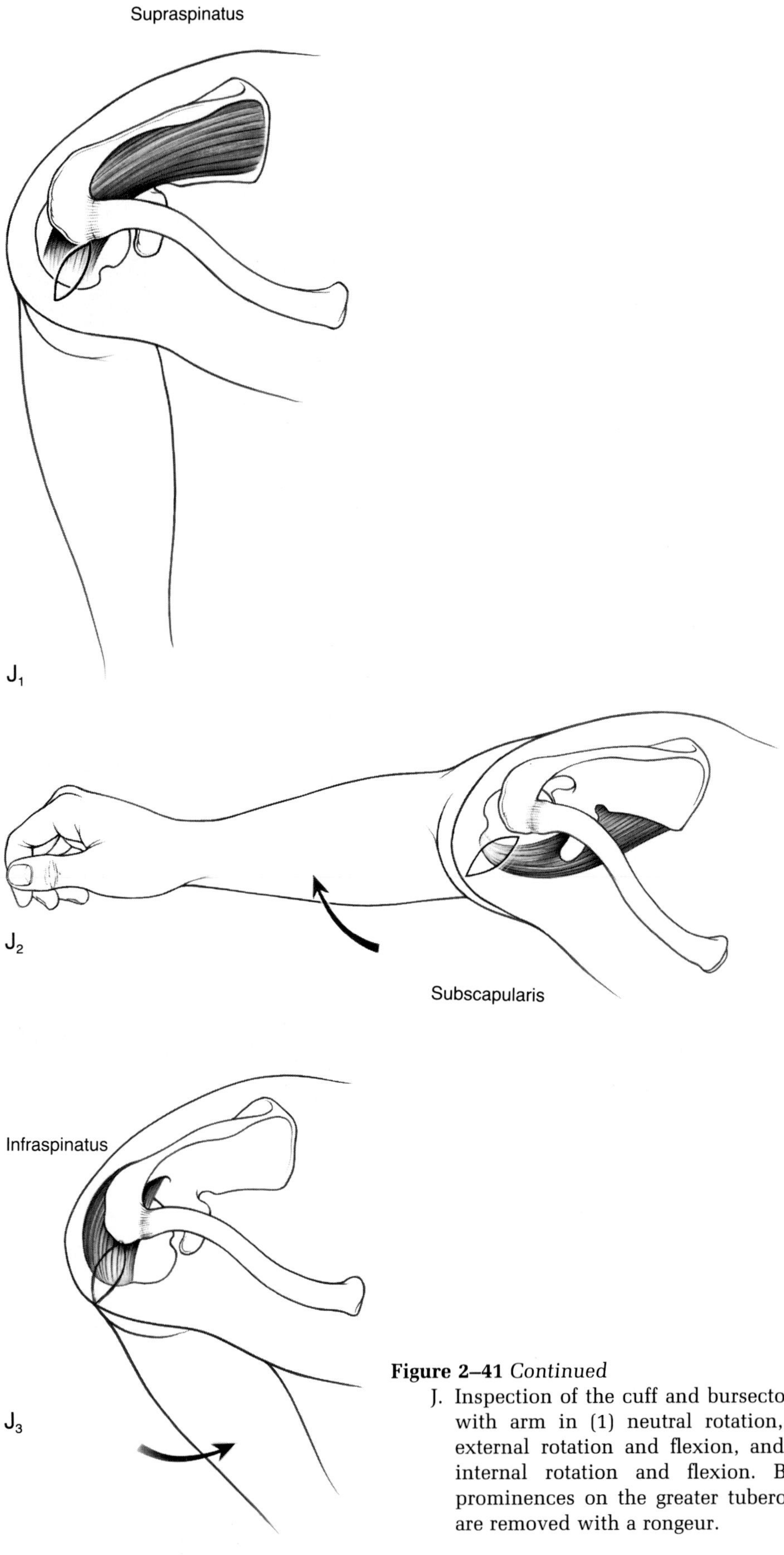

Supraspinatus

J1

J2

Subscapularis

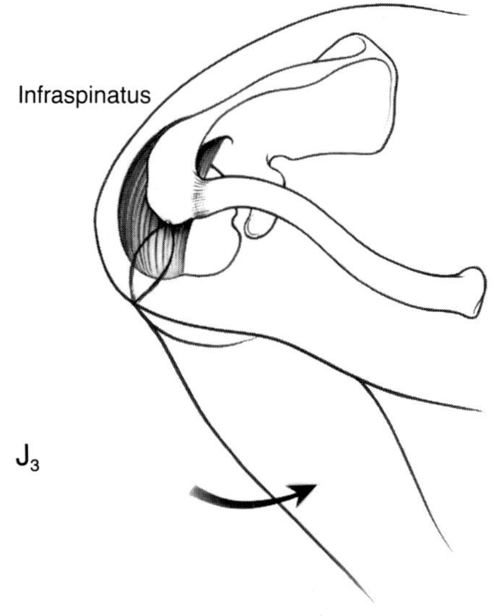

Figure 2–41 *Continued*

J. Inspection of the cuff and bursectomy, with arm in (1) neutral rotation, (2) external rotation and flexion, and (3) internal rotation and flexion. Bone prominences on the greater tuberosity are removed with a rongeur.

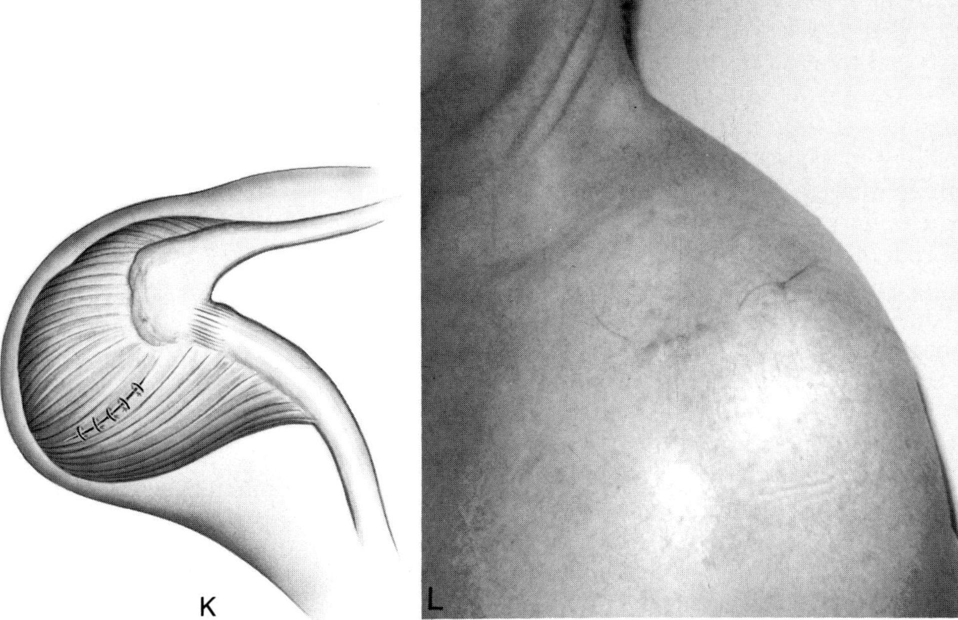

Figure 2–41 *Continued*

K. Closure of the deltoid. If the distal clavicle had been resected, the deltoid is approximated to the trapezius muscle (as shown in Fig. 6–8C).

L. Skin closure with removable subcuticular suture (as shown in Fig. 2–38G). Subcutaneous sutures are avoided.

cephalically to remove only that amount of acromion that protrudes anterior to the clavicle and to bevel the undersurface of the anterior third of the acromion so that there is no overhanging edge. The normal length of the acromion is maintained, but overhanging prominences are eliminated so that the undersurface is made straight and flat (Fig. 2–41G2). To avoid fracturing the acromion during this step, the operator holds the osteotome with one hand and places the index finger of the other hand on the dorsum of the acromion to determine the depth and proper direction of the blade while the assistant strikes the osteotome with a mallet. The cephalically placed beveled edge of the osteotome carries the blade out of the undersurface of the acromion rather than deeper into the acromion. Care is taken to remove the undersurface of the lateral edge of the acromion cleanly without leaving a ridge of bone or fragments attached to deltoid (Fig. 2–41G3 and 2–41I2). More than one cut is usually required to remove a wedge-shaped piece of bone that is approximately 0.9 cm. thick anteriorly (depending on the thickness of the acromion) and 2.0 cm. long. This includes the entire acromial attachment of the coracoacromial ligament. Residual ridges of bony prominences are removed with a rongeur. It is important to remove all particles of loose bone from the subacromial space or fragments attached to deltoid muscle, which might later form undesirable spikes of bone. In this regard, a power burr or hand rasp is considered unsuited for this step because they scatter bone.

When the acromial part of the acromioplasty has been completed, the undersurface is straight without overhang anteriorly or a lateral ridge. The undersurface of the acromioclavicular joint is then palpated, and osteophytes and prominences are removed on each side of the joint to create a tunnel for the supraspinatus (Fig. 2–41H and I). The distal clavicle is excised when it has been determined pre-operatively that the acromioclavicular joint is arthritic and painful or if more exposure is needed for repairing a cuff tear. In this case, approximately 1.5 to 2.0 cm. of distal clavicle is removed, preserving the attachments of the coracoclavicular ligaments and removing more clavicle posteriorly than anteriorly (in order to prevent the scapula from striking against the posterior edge of the stump of clavicle), and more superiorly than inferiorly (in order to maintain the coracoclavicular ligaments intact) (Fig. 2–41H2). When the outer clavicle is excised, the trapezius muscle is tagged with a stay suture to facilitate the approximation of this muscle to the deltoid during closure.

Because of the normal slope of the acromion and position of the humerus anterior to it, this approach places the supraspinatus tendon in the center of the field, giving much better exposure for repairing the rotator cuff than would be expected. Thickened bursa is then excised, and the rotator cuff is routinely inspected for tears or calcium deposits. Even if the arthrogram was negative preoperatively, incomplete thickness tears may be identified at this time, and in some cases, a full thickness tear might have developed subsequent to the arthrogram. The subscapularis is exposed by flexion and external rotation of the humerus (Fig. 2–41J2). The infraspinatus and teres minor are exposed by hyperextension and internal rotation (Fig. 2–41J3). The supraspinatus is seen when the arm is in neutral rotation (Fig. 2–41J1). This exposure is adequate for repairing at least 95 percent of tears of the rotator cuff. The steps for repairing torn rotator tendons are outlined on pages 107 to 119. Very few massive tears require extending the skin incision backward so the posterior deltoid can be detached from the spine of the scapula for mobilization of the infraspinatus (see Fig. 2–43).

The treatment of the long head of the biceps is discussed on pages 134 to 137. Tenodesis is considered only if this tendon does not move properly in its groove because of flattening, splitting, or dislocation. Otherwise, it is left intact to remain as a depressor of the humeral head. Inflammation of the biceps alone is not an indication for tenodesis.

The repair of the deltoid is important (Fig. 2–41G). The deltoid origin is carefully sutured to the flap of periosteum and capsule that had been reflected from the top of the acromion, and the capsule of the acromioclavicular joint is closed. When the distal clavicle has been excised, the trapezius is pulled forward and sutured to the deltoid to eliminate dead space against hematoma or unwanted bone formation and to cover the stump of the clavicle.

No skin scar in orthopaedic surgery is noticed more by the patient than one on the front of the shoulder. A removeable, nonabsorbablable subcuticular stitch is used. Subcutaneous sutures are avoided because they tend to cause local tissue reaction, probably owing to the great excursion of movements of this joint.

Aftercare

The post-operative exercise regimen following anterior acromioplasty and repair of the rotator cuff is determined by the strength of the cuff repair. When the rotator cuff is intact, the exercise program can be advanced as rapidly as pain allows. Strenuous forward active elevation is avoided for about two weeks to allow the anterior deltoid to recover.

The typical regimen when the cuff is intact is pendulum and early passive motion[89] (see Fig. 7–7) begun on the first or second day after surgery. Self-assistive exercises (see Fig. 7–8) are added progressively, beginning with supine elevation, external rotation with a stick, the pulley, and advancing on to the stretching and strengthening exercises as soon as tolerated. The subcuticular skin suture is removed between the tenth and fourteenth day. Although it is anticipated that a number of weeks will be required for the re-formation of the bursa, full activities are permitted as desired after three weeks. Some patients have discomfort for several months.

Result of Anterior Acromioplasty to Be Expected When the Cuff Is Intact

There is considerable variation in the rate of disappearance of pain and the recovery of function after simple anterior acromioplasty with an intact cuff. Some patients are relieved of pain and want to go on to full use almost immediately, whereas others, particularly those who had a frozen shoulder prior to the operation and required manipulation at the time of surgery, are unexpectedly slow. The latter group may have lingering complaints for months before they appreciate the results of the procedure. All patients are warned pre-operatively to expect some discomfort for the first five or six months. Re-operation should not be considered unless every trace of frozen shoulder has been eliminated with stretching exercises and at least a year has been allowed for the re-formation of the bursa and the protective muscles to become normal.

Eventually, over 95 percent of our series of patients became completely and permanently free of pain. Some have been followed over 20 years without re-growth of spurs. A few have been referred with what seemed to be incomplete removal of bone fragments. In Series II (see p. 75), in roentgen follow-up averaging 3.3 years, there was no re-growth of bone.

The impingement injection test (see Fig. 2–30) is very helpful in patient selection. Virtually all who had complete relief of pain with this test became entirely relieved by acromioplasty without recurrence of pain.

Repair of Tears of the Rotator Cuff

Indications for Cuff Repair

A few traumatic tears in younger patients and tears following dislocations are treated conservatively initially (see pp. 65 to 67). The vast majority are outlet impingement tears and are expected to persist or advance unless decompressed and repaired. Authors of books and articles advocating conservative treatment for complete impingement tears will have to produce a sizeable series of tears documented with a positive arthrogram and followed a minimum of ten years before I can consider that point of view. I have seen a number of such patients who did not do well and advise an active, healthy patient over 40 years of age with a positive arthrogram to have an anterior acromioplasty and repair.

An incomplete, deep surface impingement tear may be identified in an arthrogram; however, most incomplete tears are diagnosed during exploration. When the incomplete tear is small and sufficient strong tendon remains intact, anterior acromioplasty alone may suffice; otherwise, the tear is repaired (see Fig. 2–43L).

Very large, long-standing tears have been treated by anterior acromioplasty and debridement of the cuff. I must disagree with those who have advocated this procedure.[80] I believe that the results are more predictable and lasting if the defect in the tendon is closed. Sealing the opening is logical for the nutrition of the articular cartilage. French surgeons[90, 91] debrided the cuff for large tears in the early 1970s, and have since reported deterioration of the glenohumeral joint late after debridement of large tears without closure. They have discontinued debriding large tears and strive to close the opening to prevent deterioration using a portion of the deltoid muscle to fill the defect when necessary.

Four Major Objectives in Surgery for Impingement Tears

There are four major objectives in repairing impingement tears of the rotator cuff: (1) closure of the cuff defect, (2) eliminating impingement, (3) preserving the origin of the deltoid muscle, and (4) preventing adhesions post-operatively without disrupting the repair by a careful exercise program.

Why Close the Cuff Defect? The rotator cuff has three important functions: (1) strength (especially for external rotation and for the efficient action of the deltoid muscle), (2) stability (against subluxation and dislocation), and (3) nutrition of the articular surfaces. As discussed previously, it is logical to repair impingement tears of the rotator cuff unless the general health and life expectancy of the patient precludes.

Eliminate Subacromial Impingement. Impingement is the major source of pain in patients who develop impingement cuff tears. Furthermore, because impingement was the main cause of the lesion and when a complete tear of the cuff occurs, it weakens the head-depressing action of the cuff and may escalate impingement. Therefore, the tear is expected to continue and often slowly progress unless the impingement is removed. Anterior acromioplasty is a logical routine when repairing impingement tears because residual impingement may cause failure because of continuing pain or continuing wear and re-rupture of the tendons.

Preserve the Origin of the Deltoid Muscle. The deltoid is the prime motor of the glenohumeral joint, and if it is weakened, especially in the face of an already weakened rotator cuff muscle, the shoulder will be rendered even less functional than before surgery. Detaching the origin of the deltoid, even if accurately re-attached, permanently weakens this muscle more than would be expected. Radical acromionectomy introduces many problems (see Fig. 2–46), and is avoided.

Rehabilitation Preventing Adhesions but Maintaining the Repair Intact. Every repair of the rotator cuff initiates a conflict between rest and movement. Rest will cause failure by allowing adhesions to form around the repair. Movement may re-tear the repair. If mature adhesions form, further surgery is necessary to release them because late exercises alone are unlikely to succeed and closed manipulation will surely re-tear the rotator cuff. Because of this conflict between rest and motion, the surgeon should supervise the patient and therapist in the progression of exercises and activities. No one else knows the size of the lesion and the strength of the repair.

Predictable Patterns of Impingement Tears

The patterns of impingement tears are remarkably constant. They consistently begin at the insertion of the supraspinatus tendon as incomplete lesions and may progress to complete or massive tears. The pattern varies only according to the duration of the tear, subsequent trauma, and the three directional forces exerted by the pull of the rotator cuff muscles (Fig. 2–42). An understanding of these principles is of tremendous help in mobilizing and repairing cuff tears.

System for Repairing Cuff Tears

If the diagnosis could always be made early and surgical repair performed within a few months, the extensive measures needed for the larger tears would become obsolete. Unfortunately, because of delays in seeking medical help or delays in diagnosis, there will probably always be larger tears. Thus, the surgeon should know a system for mobilizing and repairing tears of all sizes. The system I use is shown step by step in Figure 2–43 and Table 2–9.

Pre-operatively, the patient is made aware of the long healing time of the tendons after repair and of the necessity of the post-operative exercise program. Starting about five days before surgery, antiseptic soap is applied to the shoulder and axilla during the daily shower to reduce the bacterial count of the skin.

Text continued on page 115

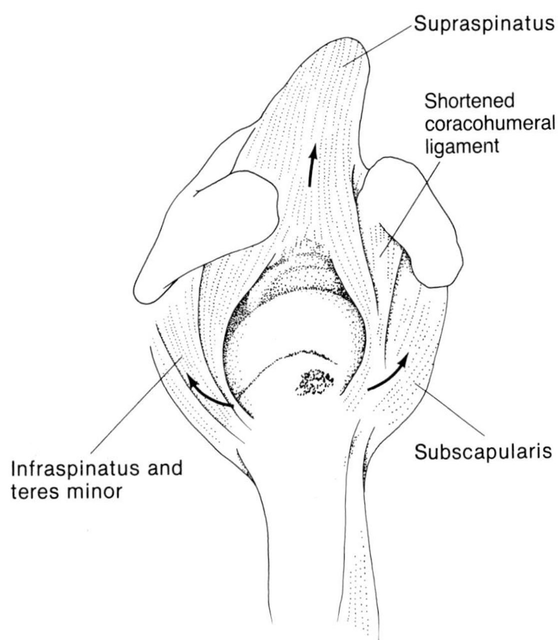

Figure 2–42. ***Patterns of Impingement Tears Are Predictable.*** The tear begins in the supraspinatus tendon, and the edges of the tear are smooth unless suddenly enlarged by an injury. The forces determining the pattern of the tear are as follows: (a) the subscapularis pulls part of the remains of the supraspinatus anteriorly, (b) the infraspinatus and teres minor pull the posterior part of the supraspinatus tendon posteriorly, and (c) the supraspinatus muscle exerts a medial force on the apex of the tear. The coracohumeral ligament becomes shortened. The exact pattern varies slightly, depending upon whether the bulk of the supraspinatus tendon is attached to the subscapularis or is attached to the infraspinatus and depending upon whether an injury enlarges the tear; however, the basic pattern can easily be understood. This is a great help in mobilizing the tendons for repair.

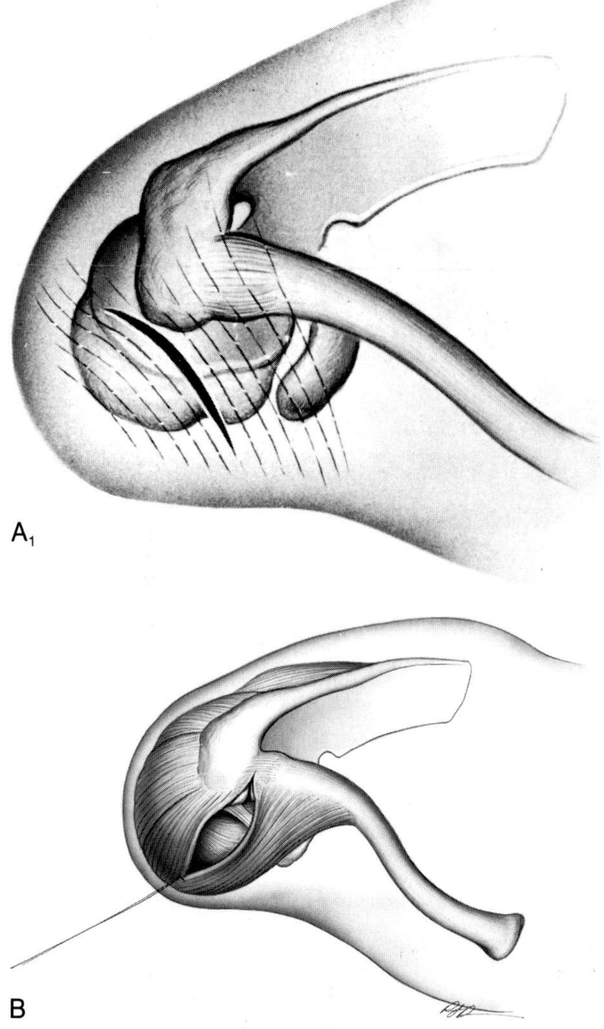

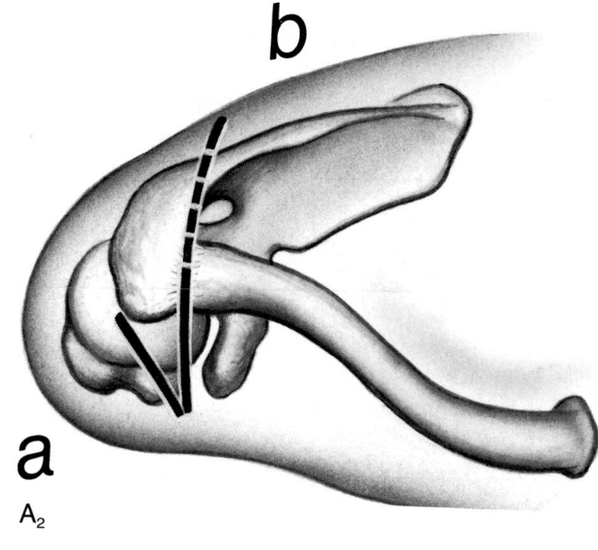

Figure 2–43. ***Systems for Repairing Cuff Tears.*** The position of the patient and the routine manipulation of the shoulder prior to the skin preparation are the same as described in Figure 1–41A and 2–41B.

A. Skin incisions. (1) The incision usually used is the same as for anterior acromioplasty (see Fig. 2–41C). (2) Occasionally, usually in problem reoperations, the incision shown in "b" is used.
B. Deltoid split and elevation of deltoid origin from the acromion.

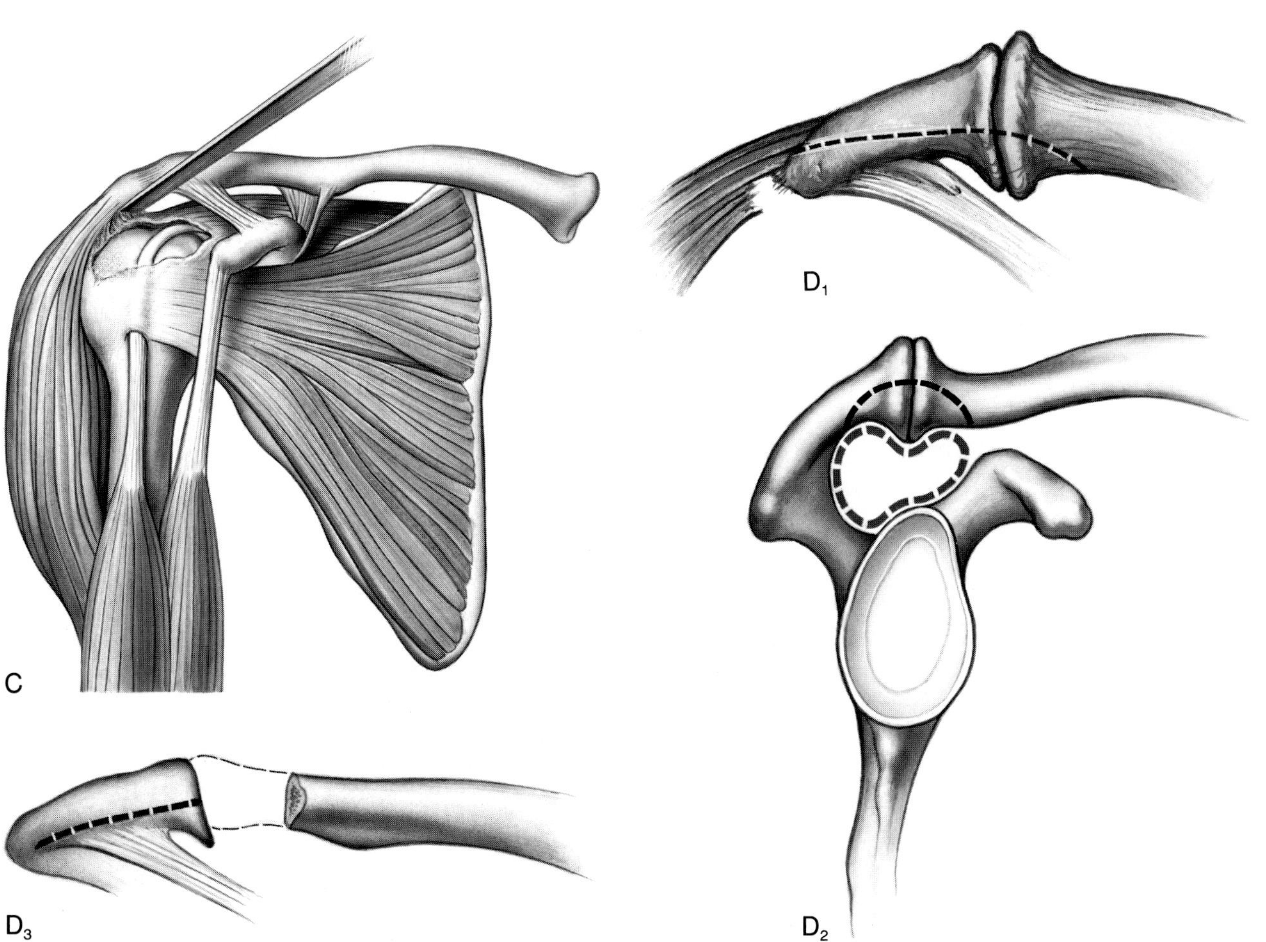

Figure 2–43 *Continued*

C. Surgeon frees the undersurface of the acromion of soft tissue prior to the acromioplasty to save as much cuff as possible and to identify the interval between the deltoid and the rotator cuff.

D. Anterior acromioplasty preserving the superficial surface with the attached deltoid origin (1 and 2). The distal clavicle is resected (3) only if painful acromioclavicular arthritis had been noted pre-operatively.

Illustration continued on following page

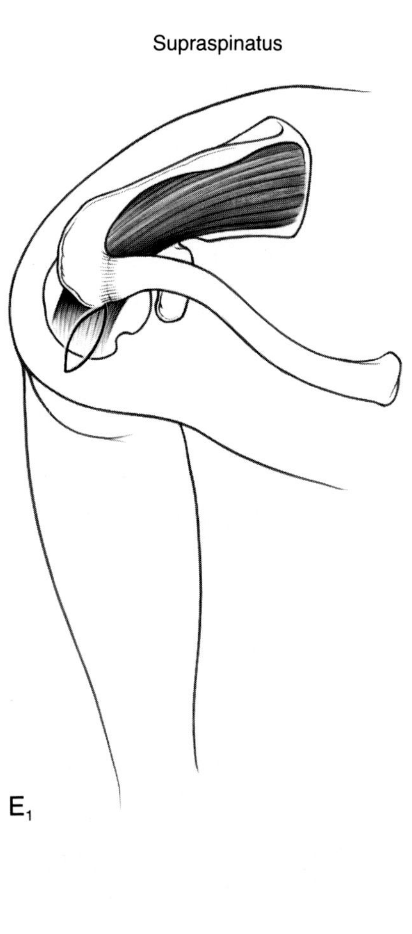

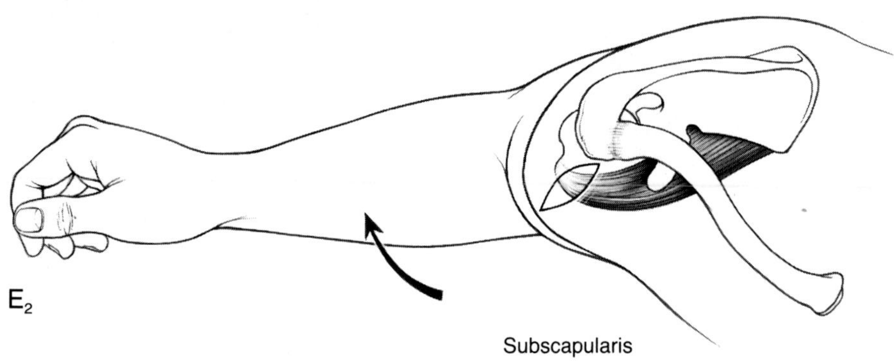

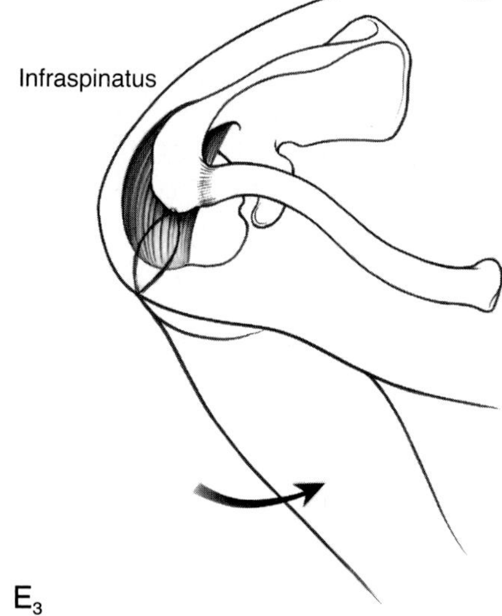

Figure 2–43 *Continued*

E. Adhesions are released from the superficial surface of the rotator cuff with the shoulder in (1) neutral rotation to expose the supraspinatus tendon, (2) flexion and external rotation for the subscapularis, and (3) extension and internal rotation to expose the infraspinatus and teres minor insertions.

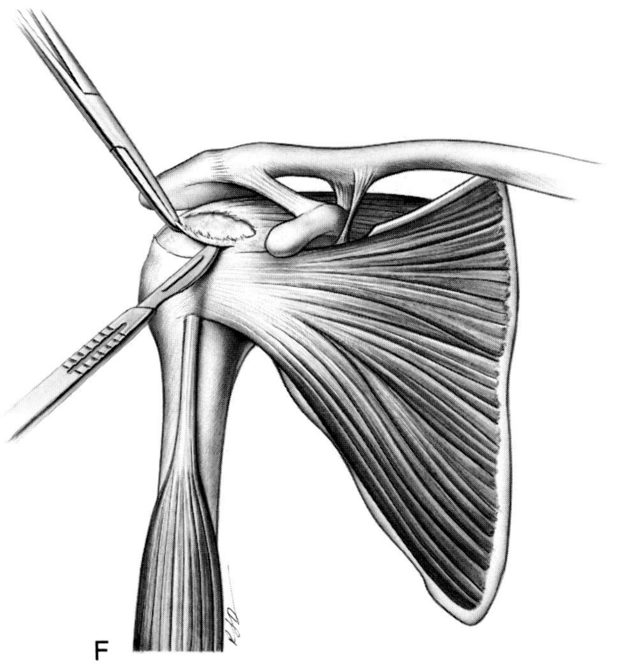

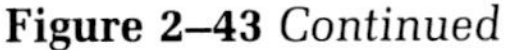

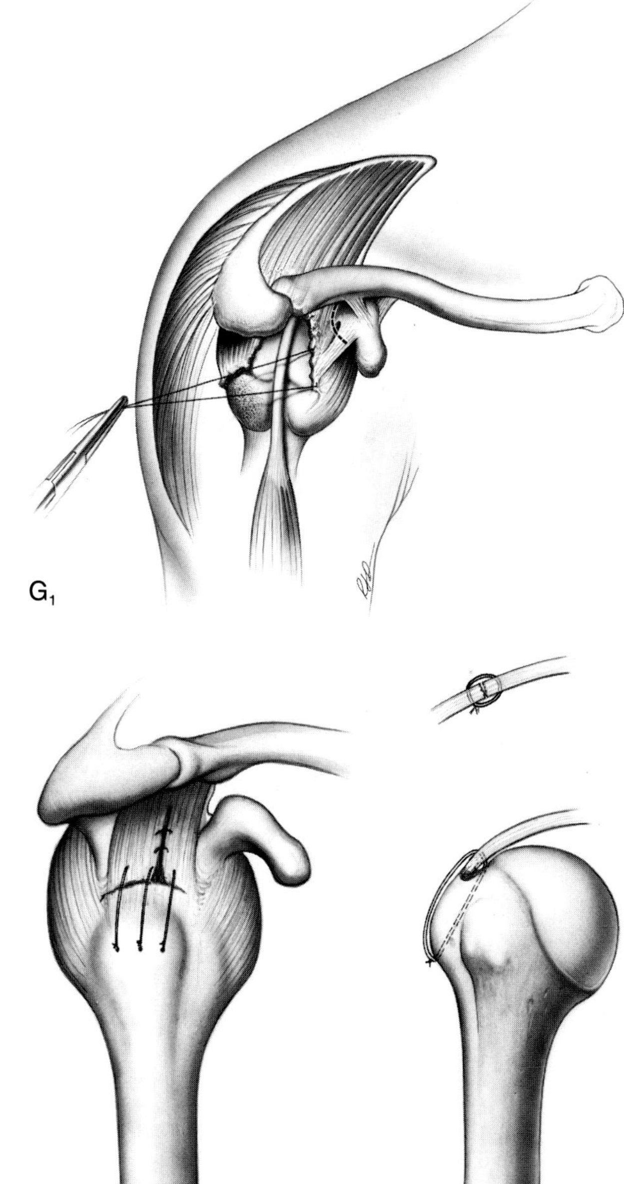

Figure 2–43 *Continued*

F. Surgeon freshens the edges of the tear, saving as much tendon as possible.

In the majority of primary repairs, the cuff can be closed at this time by one or all of the steps shown in G.

G. (1) Traction sutures are inserted for mobilizing the cuff, pulling in the reverse directions from the forces shown in Figure 1–42, dividing the coracohumeral ligament and, when necessary, dividing the capsule inside the joint. (2) Reattachment is to the shallow slot on the greater tuberosity with knots tied on the humerus or buried in the tendon.

If more mobilization is required, the procedures shown in H and I (together or separately) will allow closure of almost all other primary repairs.

Illustration continued on following page

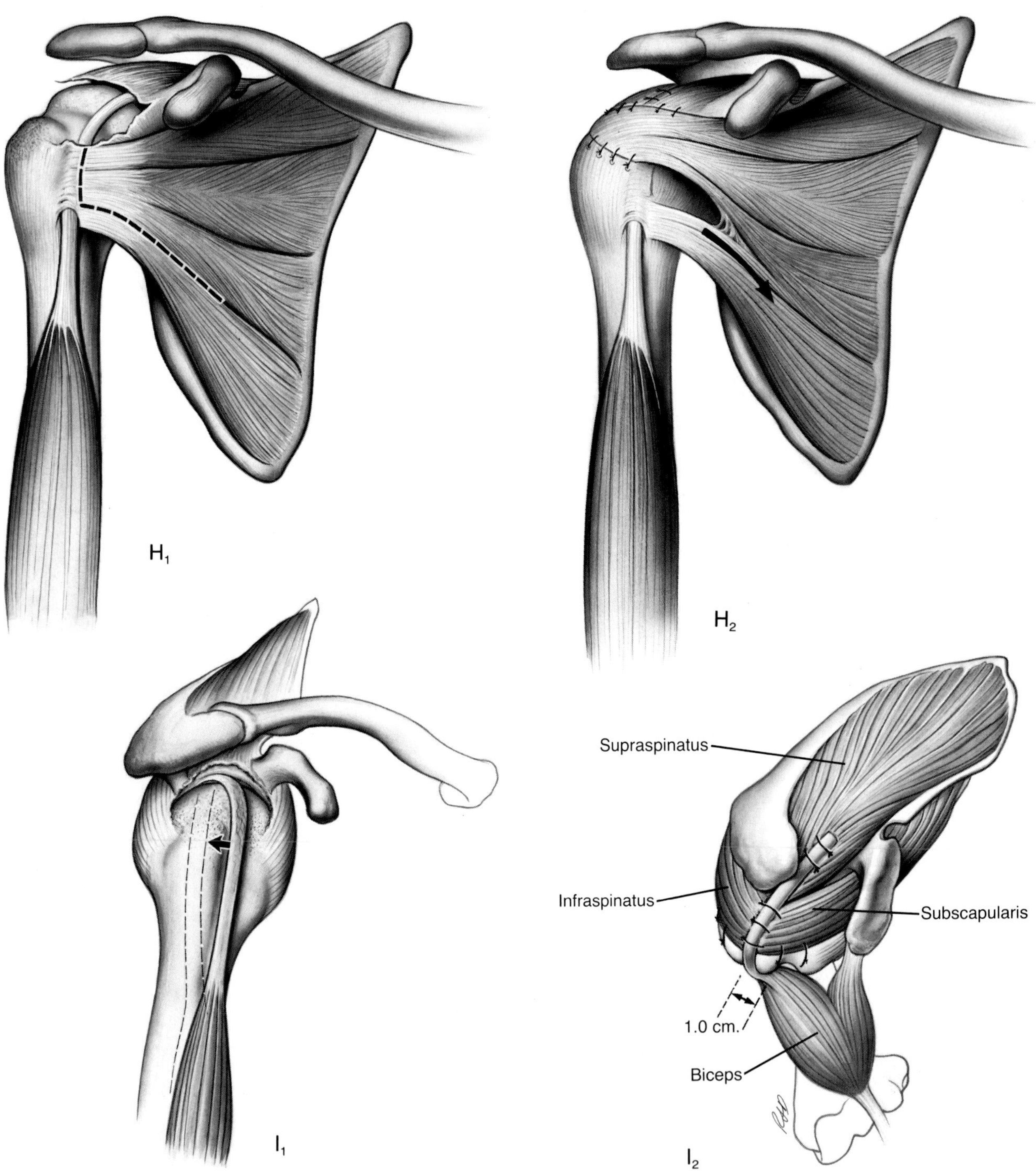

Figure 2–43 *Continued*

H. Surgeon transfers 70 percent of the subscapularis for the supraspinatus. (1) Detachment of the longest possible flap of subscapularis from the underlying capsule, avoiding the injury to the axillary nerve. (2) Flap is sutured to the greater tuberosity, infraspinatus, and stump of supraspinatus, leaving the capsule intact to stabilize the head.

I. (1) If the biceps is flattened and split or dislocated, it is realigned and tenodesed in a groove 1.0 cm. posterior to the bicipital groove. (2) It is then incorporated in the repair (between subscapularis and infraspinatus), and either it is detached from the glenoid and sutured into the supraspinatus (shown) or infraspinatus; or it is left attached to the glenoid, in which case no sutures are placed in it near the glenoid because they would anchor the cuff to the scapula.

Very rarely, usually in re-operations rather than during primary repairs, the procedures shown in J and K may be required.

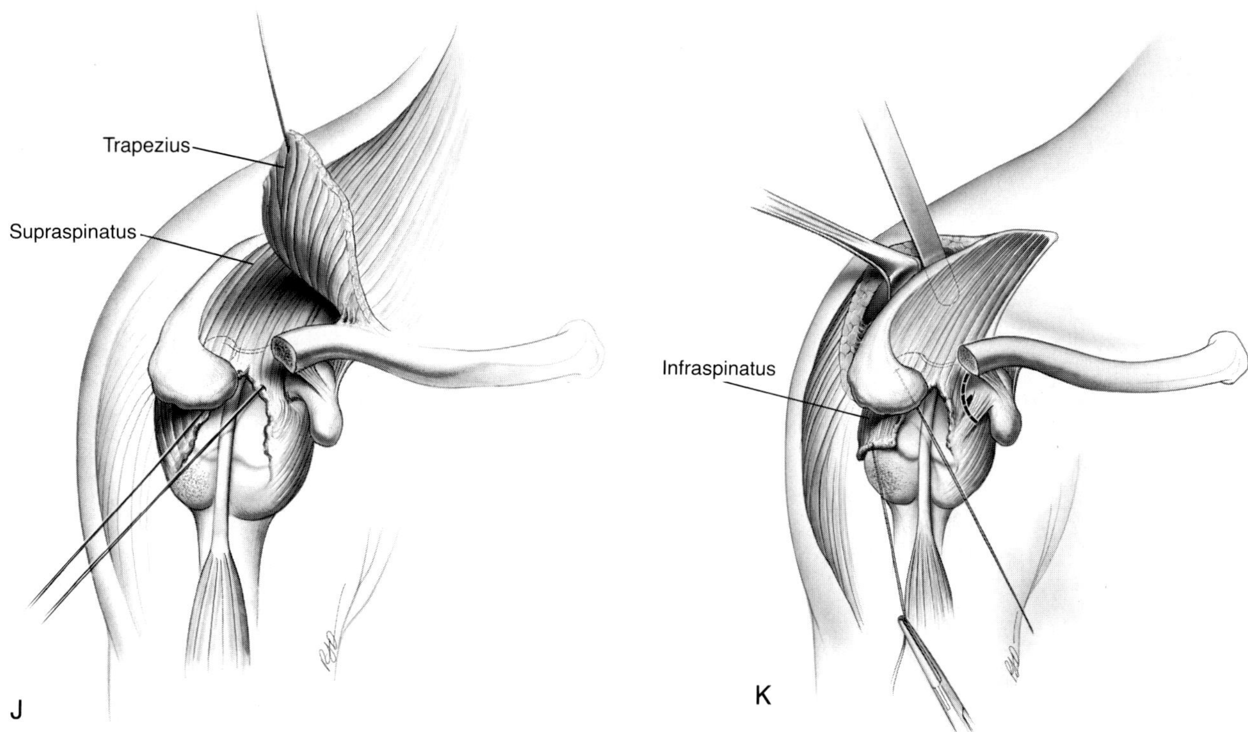

Figure 2–43 *Continued*

J. Surgeon resects the distal clavicle for mobilization of the supraspinatus.

K. Detachment of the posterior deltoid origin for mobilization of the infraspinatus.

Illustration continued on following page

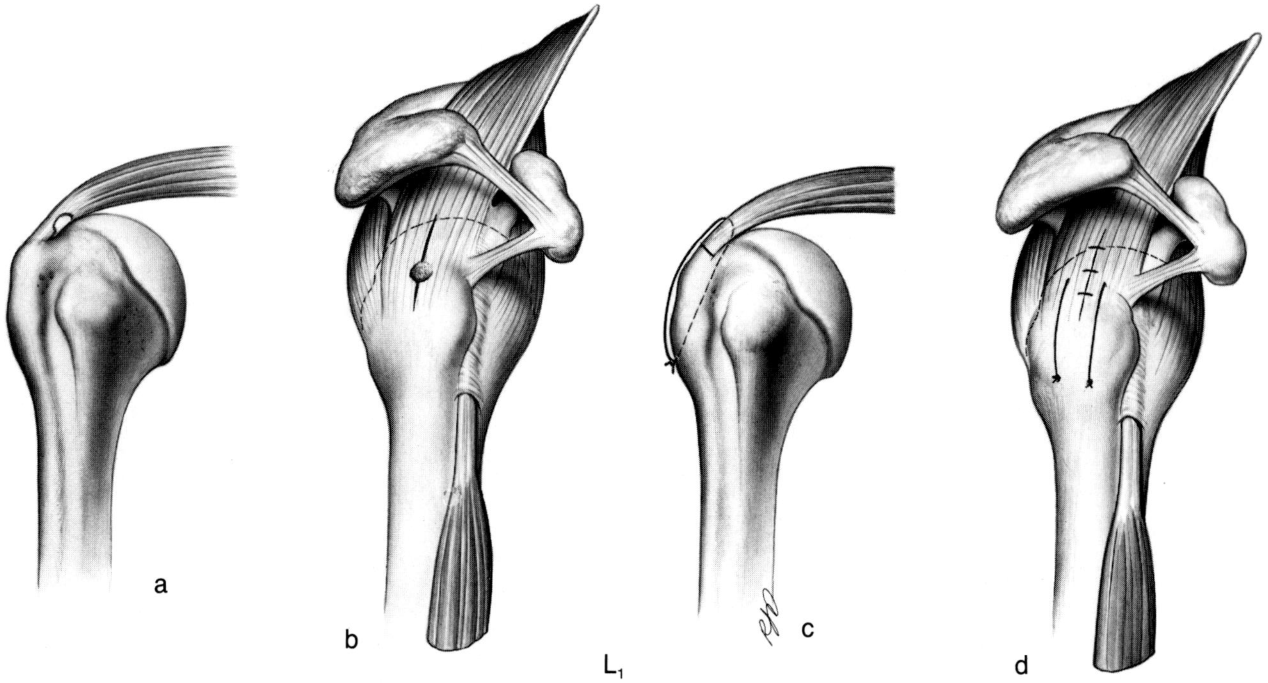

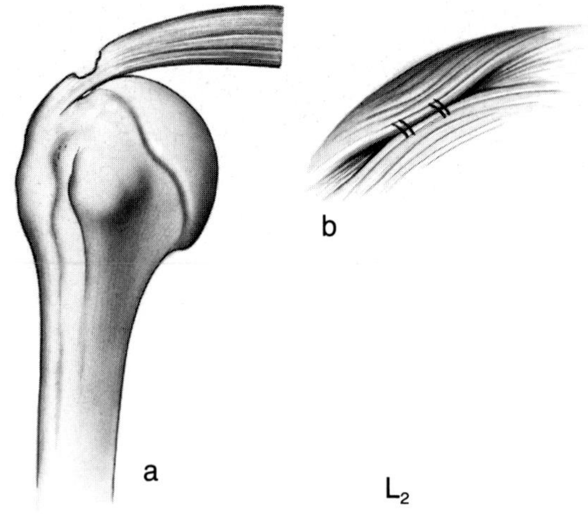

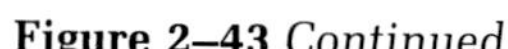

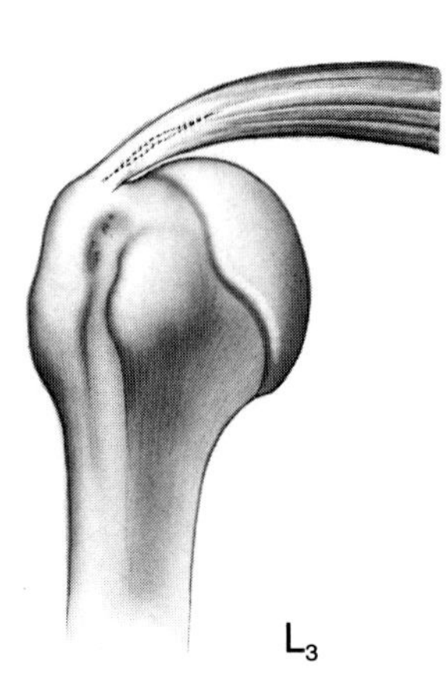

Figure 2–43 *Continued*

Incomplete tears of the rotator cuff are treated with anterior acromioplasty alone unless the tendon is thin, threatening complete rupture, in which case the procedures shown in L(1) through L(3) are considered.

L. Part 1a depicts a deep surface incomplete tear ("deep surface blister"). Large lesions are treated by incising the tear longitudinally, freshening the edges of the tear (1b), and sewing the tendon to a slot on the greater tuberosity (using awl holes) and approximating full thickness edges of tendon (1c and 1d). Part 2a depicts a superficial ("bursal-side") incomplete tear. Large lesions of this type with thin areas are treated by imbrication with double-looping sutures (2b). As shown in Part 3, intratendinous incomplete tears cannot be seen and are not treated.

The long head of the biceps should be inspected in all repairs of complete tears. The deltoid muscle and the skin closures are important. As discussed in the text, more desperate measures have not been required for primary repairs.

Table 2–9. SYSTEM FOR REPAIRING IMPINGEMENT TEARS

1. *DECOMPRESS IMPINGEMENT BY ANTERIOR ACROMIOPLASTY*
   a. Bevel undersurface of anterior acromion and acromioclavicular (AC) joint
   b. Distal clavicle resected in two situations:
      (1) Painful arthritis of AC joint (determined preoperatively)
      (2) When more exposure of the supraspinatus is needed to mobilize a large tension tear
2. *MOBILIZE THE ROTATOR CUFF TO AVOID TENSION ON THE REPAIR SO THAT THE CUFF MUSCLES CAN "PULL"*
   a. Freshen edges of the tear and place traction sutures
   b. Excise thickened bursa and free superficial surface of the cuff
   c. Divide coracohumeral ligament and clear the base of the coracoid
   d. Detach glenohumeral joint capsule from inside of the joint
   e. or f. Transfer 70% of the subscapularis tendon cephalically or re-align and tenodese the biceps
   g. Resect outer 2.0 cm. of clavicle to mobilize the supraspinatus
   h. Detach the posterior deltoid to mobilize the infraspinatus
   i. Steps g. and h. have rarely been needed in primary repairs, and more desperate measures have not been required for impingement tears
3. *CLOSING THE CUFF SO THAT THE ARM CAN BE BROUGHT TO THE SIDE*
   a. Small tears: direct suture
   b. Supraspinatus tears: Direct suture after dividing coracohumeral ligament and clearing the cuff
   c. Massive tears: 70% subscapularis transfer or biceps realignment and incorporation
4. *REPAIR OF DELTOID MUSCLE IS IMPORTANT FOR STRENGTH*
5. *SKIN CLOSURE IS IMPORTANT FOR OPTIMUM RECOVERY*
6. *BRACE (4–6 WEEKS) IN 20%*
   a. If tenuous repair
   b. Re-operations when deltoid muscle retracted and extensive adhesions

The patient is positioned in the beachchair position with the head of the table raised 35 degrees and the knees broken to prevent sliding down. General anesthesia is usually used but scalene block may be advantageous in special cases. Because many patients with cuff tears have degenerative changes in the cervical spine, the patient's head is carefully supported to avoid hyperextension of the neck that might compromise the cervical nerve roots. A pad is placed beneath the scapula to hold it forward to expose the back of the shoulder to support the scapula for the acromioplasty, and the shoulder protrudes over the corner of the table to allow access posteriorly (Fig. 2–43A). The side of the table is padded by sliding the mattress over it to permit free movements of the arm without contusing the ulnar nerve. An antibiotic is used intravenously during the procedure.

It is routine to check the range of glenohumeral motion when the patient is under anesthesia and prior to beginning the preparation of the skin. Restricted movement is eliminated at this time by closed manipulation as described for a frozen shoulder (see Fig. 2–41B and p. 425). Although complete cuff tears have less tendency to cause shoulder stiffness than many other conditions, restriction of motion is not rare, and unless eliminated at the time of surgery, it will make the postoperative exercise program extremely difficult. It is essential to have the arm draped free so that all of the rotator tendons can be visualized through a small opening by moving the arm in appropriate positions.

ANTERIOR ACROMIOPLASTY APPROACH

The anterior acromioplasty approach (see Fig. 2–41) is used for all cuff repairs. It is performed with the least possible detachment of deltoid origin and with careful decompression of the supraspinatus from impingement. These precautions are considered essential for prompt relief of pain and for the durability of the cuff repair. If the acromioclavicular joint is arthritic with pain on the horizontal adduction test (see Fig. 4–63D) and tender preoperatively, the distal clavicle is excised first; otherwise, its superficial surface is preserved to maintain the deltoid origin intact. The undersurface of the acromion is carefully cleared of adherent rotator tendons. This is a key step in identifying the interval between the rotator cuff and the deltoid muscle. The supraspinatus outlet is enlarged by beveling the anterior edge and undersurface of the anterior third of the acromion and by creating a tunnel for the supraspinatus (see Fig. 2–41). It is important to remove all fragments of bone.

Having completed the anterior acromioplasty, the surgeon freshens the edge of the tear by sharp dissection, removing only a thin margin. This differs from the policy of some surgeons, who excise "back to healthy tendon" before attempting the repair. Scarred, worn, and fibrillated tendon can revert back to strong tendon if it has been decompressed from impingement and incorporated into the repair.

STEPS IN MOBILIZING THE CUFF

After freeing the undersurface of the acromion (Fig. 2–43C), identifying the interval between the deltoid and the rotator cuff, and freshening the bare edges of the tear, the surgeon places stay sutures in the tendons for traction to avoid crushing the tendons with clamps (Fig. 2–43G).

The superficial surfaces of all of the tendons of the rotator cuff are cleared of adhesions and thickened bursa. The subscapularis is exposed by holding the arm in a flexed and externally rotated position (Fig. 2–43E2). The infraspinatus and teres minor are exposed by holding the arm in internal rotation and extension, and the supraspinatus is seen with the arm in the neutral position (Fig. 2–43E3). Care is taken to avoid injury to the axillary nerve, which lies on the front of the subscapularis (Fig. 2–43D). This is usually sufficient mobilization to repair smaller tears.

If there continues to be resistance to approximation of the tendon to the greater tuberosity when the arm is at the side, the next step is division of the coracohumeral ligament and detachment of adherent supraspinatus tendon from the base of the coracoid (Fig. 2–43G). All of the soft tissue is detached from the base of the coracoid anteriorly, laterally, and posteriorly; however, the dissection does not go medial to the coracoid because the suprascapular nerve might be injured where it is anchored in the suprascapular notch. A blunt elevator is then placed between the coracoid and the soft tissue to forcibly displace the remains of supraspinatus laterally and cephalically. This extremely helpful step has never been mentioned in the literature, and yet contracture of the coracohumeral ligament prevents recovering external rotation and prevents adequate mobilization of the supraspinatus tendon.

If more length is needed, the glenohumeral joint capsule is detached from the glenoid by sharp dissection, working through the opening provided by the tear in the rotator cuff (Fig. 2–43F). The capsule is divided posteriorly under the infraspinatus tendon, superiorly under the supraspinatus tendon, and anteriorly under the subscapularis with a scalpel; however, care should be taken to avoid detachment of the long head of the biceps from the glenoid. The detached capsule is then forcibly displaced cephalically and laterally from the glenoid with a blunt instrument placed inside the joint, levering the capsule with its attached cuff from inside the joint. This maneuver with traction on the stay sutures will often close the defect.

If the tendons cannot be brought together, the choice is then made between transfer of the upper 70 percent of the subscapularis tendon (Fig. 2–43H) or re-alignment and incorporation of the long head of the biceps (Fig. 2–43I). If the long head of the biceps is of normal shape and is running well in its groove, even if inflamed, it is preserved and the subscapularis transfer is performed.[81] If the biceps is flattened, split, or subluxated, it is re-aligned first before a decision is made as to whether it will be necessary to transfer the upper subscapularis as well. In the transfer of the subscapularis, the glenohumeral joint capsule remains intact for coverage and stability and the lower 30 percent of subscapularis is intact to function as a head depressor as the arm is elevated (see Fig. 1–19). The upper 70 percent of the subscapularis is brought cephalically over the humeral head and is attached to the infraspinatus, remains of supraspinatus, and the greater tuberosity. If the long head of the biceps is incorporated in the repair, it is tenodesed in a slot about 1 cm. posterior to the bicipital groove, where the supraspinatus tendon is normally located. The subscapularis and infraspinatus tendons are then sewn to it. The proximal end of the long head can be left attached to the scapula or may be detached from the scapula and sewn into the supraspinatus or infraspinatus muscle, as illustrated in Figure 2–43I2, in an effort to make it contribute an active force.

The preceding steps have been adequate to repair the cuff in 95 percent of the over 300 primary repairs in my current personal series; however, if these maneuvers have been inadequate, the next step is resection of the distal clavicle for more extensive mobilization of the supraspinatus tendon (Fig. 2–43J). With the distal clavicle resected and the trapezius muscle detached from the clavicle and acromion, the entire supraspinatus can be exposed. A slide* of this muscle could be made, as has been advocated by some investigators; however, I would reserve a slide for the most desperate situations because it permanently weakens the muscle by reducing the length of contractile tissue and have not found it necessary in my primary cuff repairs.

If more extensive mobilization of the infraspinatus tendon is needed, the skin incision is next extended posteriorly (Fig. 2–43K). The posterior deltoid origin is detached as necessary to place traction sutures in the infraspinatus, pass them under the acromion, and apply traction to tendon as it is carefully elevated from the scapula with care to avoid injury to the suprascapular nerve. The aim is to displace the infraspinatus cephalically more than laterally. The teres minor is left intact (to stabilize the head and function as a head depressor when the arm is in abduction). A slide* of the infraspinatus would be attempted only as a last resort and was not necessary for primary cuff repairs.

CLOSING THE CUFF DEFECT

When the objective in mobilizing the tendons has been reached, i.e., establishing free excursion without adhesions that interfere with "pull" when the muscle contracts and making it possible to approximate the tendons to the greater tuberosity without undue tension when the arm is at the side, the tendons are sutured. According to the size of the tear, a shallow slot 0.5 cm. wide is made on the greater tuberosity where the tendons had been detached. Holes for passing the sutures are made with an awl and a small, angulated curette to avoid leaving bone particles. The cuff is attached to the bone first using double-looping su-

*A "slide" refers to moving the origin of either the supraspinatus or the infraspinatus laterally.

tures through the holes and placing the knots on the bone rather than on the tendons (Fig. 2–43G2). Longitudinal defects in the cuff are closed with double-looping sutures with buried knots. Everting sutures are avoided. I prefer 0 or 00 nonabsorbable sutures for closing the cuff.

Closing Incomplete Tears

Smaller incomplete tears require no closure and are treated by anterior acromioplasty alone. One small lesion of this type treated by acromioplasty alone was seen on re-exploration later to have reverted back to normal-appearing tendon.

Larger incomplete tears on the *superficial surface* may require imbrication to make a thin area of tendon thicker (Fig. 2–43L2). Only the surface of the tear is freshened by scraping with a knife prior to suturing.

Larger incomplete tears on the *deep surface* that have a thin, weak area are treated by incising longitudinally in the direction of the fibers, freshening the edges of the "blister," and freshening an area of bone on the greater tuberosity for re-attaching the tendon (Fig. 2–43L1).

Intratendinous tears are not seen except in anatomical specimens, and although their existence in the living may be suggested by sonograms, no attempt is made to close them. Anterior acromioplasty alone should be adequate.

Closing Complete Supraspinatus Tears

Small full thickness tears are just a step beyond the larger incomplete tears, and they are treated in a similar fashion by trimming the bare edges of the tear and re-attaching the tendon to the greater tuberosity by direct suture. These small lesions can be closed without tension after Step 2b, Table 2–9, i.e., after freeing the superficial surface of the rotator cuff front and back by removing the thickened bursa. Larger supraspinatus tears require division of the coracoacromial ligament and clearing the base of the coracoid (see Step 2C, Table 2–9). The freshened edges of the supraspinatus tendon are secured to the groove on the greater tuberosity and are approximated to each other with double-looping, nonabsorbable suture, as shown in Figure 2–43K.

Closing Massive Tears

Large tears require release of the capsule inside the joint and may require transfer of the upper 70 percent of the subscapularis or alignment and incorporation of the biceps (see Step 2e or 2f, Table 2–9; Fig. 2–43L and M). It is important in repairing all complete cuff tears to find the long head of the biceps to see if it is deformed or displaced. If the long head of the biceps is flattened, split, or subluxated and is not running in its groove, it is re-aligned to reinforce the repair before deciding whether or not the subscapularis will require transfer. Otherwise, the biceps is left intact and the subscapularis is transferred first. Steps 2g and 2h, Table 2–9, are rarely required. Desperate measures are discussed below. They are almost never needed in primary repair of impingement tears. They are considered occasionally in revision replacement arthroplasties (see Chapter 3, p. 255), for old trauma, and when there has been resection of the cuff.

The long head of the biceps must be visualized prior to closing all full thickness tears to make sure that it is not dislocated or deformed. If it is in good condition, care is taken to avoid incorporating it in the repair.

The deltoid closure is important. The deltoid is approximated anatomically by closing the flaps of acromioclavicular joint capsule on the acromion. If the distal clavicle has been excised, the trapezius muscle and deltoid are sutured together (Fig. 2–43N). Drainage tubes are avoided in cuff repairs because of the risk of creating a joint sinus.

A careful skin closure is important for two reasons. The patient sees these incisions frequently, so they are cosmetically important. Beyond this, prompt skin healing together with a good deltoid closure avoids joint sinuses and wound complications. No buried subcutaneous sutures are used because they too frequently migrate and cause irritation during the exercise period. The skin is closed with subcuticular pull-out sutures (Fig. 2–43O). This eliminates the need of buried subcutaneous sutures and eliminates the "cross-hatching" that occurs when interrupted skin sutures or skin staples are used.

Although the cuff is always re-attached so that the arm can be brought to the side without disrupting the repair, a brace is used initially following surgery in about 20 percent of my patients. A sling and swathe is applied in the others. An abduction brace is preferred when the tear is large and the repair tenuous and in re-operations when there has been extensive detachment of the deltoid requiring deltoidplasty (see Fig. 3–32 and Chapter 7).

Desperate Measures. Desperate measures such as slides of the supraspinatus or infraspinatus muscles, grafts, and transfers other than as shown in Figure 2–43 were not required in Series I or Series II (see p. 74). They might be needed in connection with revision arthroplasties, long-standing rheumatoid arthritis,[104] and failed surgery, as discussed in Chapter 3 and Figure 3–31.

"Slides"[96] (moving the origin of either the supraspinatus or infraspinatus laterally) weaken the muscle and have not been used in recent years. Transfer of the trapezius tendon to the greater tuberosity to replace the supraspinatus is unsatisfactory because the trapezius pulls the humerus upward, rather than depressing the head. I have on occasion used the trapezius as an extension of the stump of the supraspinatus tendon in difficult glenohumeral arthroplasties (see Chapter 3, Fig. 3–31D and p. 189). This is done by detaching the trapezius from the clavicle and acromion and by sewing the stump of the supraspinatus into the undersurface of the trapezius. The trapezius tendon is then attached to the greater tuberosity. Although this covers the head and interposes some tissue between it and the acromion, it has not given overhead function.

Transfer of the latissimus dorsi for infraspinatus (see Fig. 3–31) is a very logical procedure. It is a powerful muscle, is aligned to act as a head depressor, and it would seem especially valuable to be able to compensate for the infraspinatus because it normally supplies most of the power for external rotation. Although I have used the latissimus dorsi for Erb's palsy in children (see Chapter 6, Fig. 3–31E and p. 452), a modification of the L'Episcopo procedure,[255] I have not yet needed to use it for impingement tears. To date, we have been able to close the defect by the steps described in Figure 2–43. The few patients we have seen with massive, long-standing impingement tears who might have been considered for this procedure have been rather frail and elderly and did not seem suitable for the more extensive dissection required. Gerber[105] has recently carried out this procedure in a few patients but without their recovering use of the arm overhead.

Other transfers that have been used in connection with arthroplasties, trauma, or failed surgery are discussed in Chapter 3, Figure 3–31B and C, p. 188, and include transfer of the sternal head of the pectoralis major using a local soft-tissue extension to the lesser and greater tuberosities, and transfer of the pectoralis minor using local tissue for an extension.

Debridement of the tendons at the edges of massive tears was once advocated by Apoil in France[90] and more recently by Rockwood.[80] Apoil later discontinued this procedure in favor of transfer of a piece of the posterior deltoid to fill the defect in the rotator cuff, as had been recommended by Takagishi,[106] in hopes of averting the degenerative changes of the head that he had seen late in some of these cases. Mansat[91] also abandoned debridement of the cuff because of late degenerative changes in the glenohumeral joint. As discussed previously, I cannot agree with the principle of debridement of massive cuff tears. It disregards the function of the rotator cuff not only as a stabilizer of the head against ascent but also in the nutrition of the glenohumeral joint.

I have not used a fascial graft in a cuff repair for over 15 years and have never found it necessary to use a synthetic graft.

Aftercare Following Cuff Tears

The exercise program is determined by the size of the tear and the strength of the repair. No one knows this as well as the surgeon. As discussed in Chapter 7, for optimum results, the surgeon should supervise the aftercare program. He or she must inform both the patient and the therapist of the limitations imposed by the tear, and later, as healing occurs, of the changing objectives of the exercise program. Confusion among the patient, therapist, and surgeon can be disastrous. A well-informed patient not only achieves the maximum return of function but also is happy, confident, and proud of the accomplishments. The patient should be made aware of this program before surgery and also of the possibility of a brace following surgery. I find it helpful to explain to the patient preoperatively that 12 months will be required for mature healing of the tendons and the re-formation of a bursa for the "lubricating system" and during this time activities are advanced as instructed.

Post-operative Regimen for Incomplete Tears. The aftercare for small incomplete tears is as outlined in Chapter 7 (when the cuff is intact). The aftercare for incomplete tears that have been repaired with sutures is similar to that outlined in the following section for supraspinatus tears, but activities such as golf or tennis are allowed sooner.

Post-operative Regimen for Supraspinatus Tears. Complete tears of the supraspinatus are associated with good quality tissue that can be closed without tension. A sling and swathe is used during the first few days for comfort and for six weeks at night for protection. Pendulum exercises are begun after 48 hours, at which time the arm is passively elevated by the surgeon and the therapist (see Fig. 7–7). Soon after this, the sling is discarded during the daytime and by the fifth day, the self-assistive program is under way, including external rotation with a stick (see Fig. 7–8), extension with a stick, and use of the pulley.[74] When it is clear that the wound is in good condition and the patient is able with self-assistive exercises to maintain at least 150 degrees elevation and 40 degrees external rotation, the patient is discharged from the hospital. The pull-out, subcuticular skin suture is removed about the tenth day following surgery (if removed earlier, adherent strips are applied to protect against the stress of the exercise program). The patient is warned against leaning on the arm, carrying more than 5 pounds of weight, or trying to raise the arm overhead until instructed to do so.

Six weeks following surgery, the patient is

examined again and more self-assistive exercises are added. These include supine elevation powered with the "good" arm (see Fig. 7–8E); internal rotation (see Fig. 7–8F); and the "abduction" movement, accomplished by placing the hands in back of the head (see Fig. 7–8G). If motion seems restricted at this time, some additional stretching exercises (see Fig. 7–9) are added and supervision with the therapist is considered.

For supraspinatus tears at three months following surgery, I begin isometric exercises against the opposite hand (see Fig. 7–10) and later progress to a light strength of rubber (see Fig. 7–11). Holding the arm overhead with a stick (see Fig. 7–12: i.e., learning how to raise the arm overhead) is deferred until such time as the surgeon is confident with the strength of the repair. I advise patients who had complete tears of the supraspinatus tendon to avoid carrying more than 15 pounds of weight in the operated hand during the first year; however, light activities are advanced throughout this period. Swimming is allowed after five months. Overheads and serves in tennis are permitted after nine to twelve months. Skiing is forbidden during the first year. Work requiring lifting more than 15 pounds is done with the opposite arm during the first year, after which full activities are usually allowed.

Many patients with rotator cuff tears are very active people and want to do too much during the first twelve months after surgery. Some become frightened a few months after surgery because of pain precipitated by these activities and they return to the surgeon expecting to require re-operation to re-attach the rotator cuff. Unless there has been severe trauma, I restrict their activities and advise that even if the cuff has been re-torn, because the impingement has been removed by the anterior acromioplasty, it is quite possible that the tear may heal spontaneously if they restrict activities and discontinue active use but maintain motion by occasional passive exercises. The vast majority of these patients completely recover. A further arthrogram is deferred unless the patient is having persistent symptoms after one year. One patient who lifted a heavy bag of charcoal four months after surgery and another who had a hard fall did not regain strength or comfort and required further arthrograms and surgery.

Post-operative Regimen for Massive Tears. In those with massive tears, previous surgery, deltoidplasty, or a tenuous repair, although the repair of the rotator cuff is performed with the arm at the side, the arm is maintained in 90 degrees of elevation with a brace during the first four to eight weeks following the repair (see Fig. 7–15). Two to five days following surgery, the arm is passively elevated off of the brace to the overhead position daily by the surgeon or therapist. After the patient is discharged from the hospital, daily passive elevation is continued by a relative or friend.

About one week before the brace is to be discarded, the patient begins pendulum exercises off of the brace and begins letting the arm come down to the side in preparation for discarding the brace. A sling with a pad between it and the body to maintain moderate abduction is used for a day or two until the arm accommodates for being at the side. The same exercise regimen as outlined previously for supraspinatus tears is then followed. The initial four exercises, consisting of pendulum, external rotation with a stick, extension with a stick, and the pulley (see Fig. 7–9), are begun and then advanced later. Isometrics and strengthening exercises are usually deferred until after the fifth month following surgery. Active exercises overhead are deferred longer. The patient is made aware that improvement in strength overhead can occur throughout the first year. Some patients are discouraged by the weakness at this time. It has been my policy to defer an arthrogram or further consideration of surgery for at least a full year after repair because the cuff has been decompressed by the acromioplasty, which may permit even poor quality tendons to heal and strengthen if given time.

Result to Be Expected of Primary Repairs

The results of Series I and Series II are detailed on pages 74 to 76. In the more recent series of 233 primary repairs followed an average of 4.6 years, "excellent" results (essentially normal shoulders, as in Figure 2–44) were obtained in 77 percent, "satisfactory" results (some weakness but good function and no significant pain) were achieved in 14 percent, and "unsatisfactory" results occurred in 9 percent. Massive tears were found at the time of surgery in 145 shoulders, of which 47 had transfers of 70 percent of the subscapularis, 45 had re-alignment and incorporation of the long head of the biceps, and all were closed according to the principles above.

The unsatisfactory ratings were usually due to lack of compliance with the exercise program or new injuries. A few were because of very large, long-standing tears with weak, retracted rotator cuff muscles.

Bilateral Cuff Tears

The incidence of bilateral cuff tears in those who have a documented complete tear on one side varies with the age of the patient. Nearly all patients with cuff-tear arthropathy in one shoulder

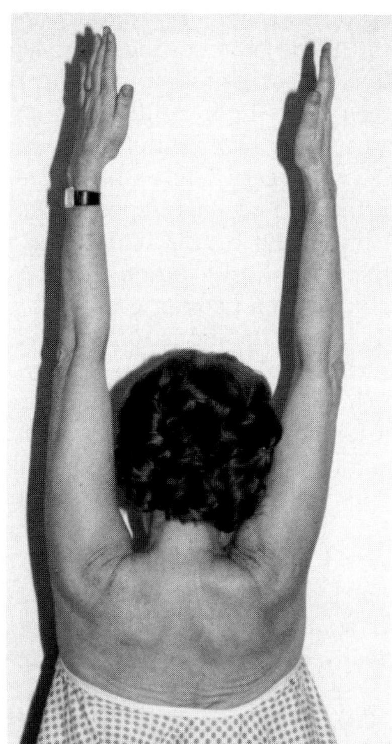

Figure 2–44. Illustrating an "excellent" five year result of anterior acromioplasty and repair of the rotator cuff in the left shoulder of a 60 year old woman who had a massive tear treated by transfer of 70 percent of the subscapularis, re-alignment and incorporation of the long head of the biceps, and a brace for 6 weeks after surgery. Note the absence of spinatus atrophy and how well her deltoid muscle has been preserved.

have a cuff tear in the opposite shoulder as well. This is a point in favor of the hypothesis that individual variations in the shape and slope of the acromion with impingement account for the majority of tears in the over 40 age group.

Bilateral arthrograms can be performed during the same session without very much inconvenience to the patient. When it is known that bilateral complete cuff tears are present, I prefer to repair the more symptomatic side first and defer surgery on the other side for at least four months until the operated arm can assist in some of the exercises.

Treatment of Cuff Tears in Paraplegics

Patients with long-standing paraplegia, from poliomyelitis or spinal injuries, are prone to develop tears of the rotator cuff because they use their arms for transfers and crutch walking (see Fig. 2–12). Because they are more dependent on their arms, they have an inherent fear of surgery. They fear becoming even more disabled. Beyond this, they have a special aftercare problem. The rehabilitation program must be designed to avoid using their arms for transfers. Nevertheless, repair and decompression of the cuff are often worthwhile because the general health and expectancy of most of these patients are good.

Pre-operatively, a physical medicine consultation is obtained to give special training to enable the patient to carry out necessary activities using a one-armed wheelchair and a sliding board for making transfers, as illustrated in Figure 7–16. If the patient is unwilling to accept this regimen without weight on the involved shoulder for at least six months or a year, it is unwise to attempt repairing the cuff. One of my patients re-tore her rotator cuff four months after repair by disregarding this advice. She was doing well up until the time she began transfers on her own. As in other patients, when the tear is very large, a brace is required post-operatively. This can be especially difficult for a paraplegic.

After surgery, when healing of the rotator cuff has advanced sufficiently, these patients can easily participate in the self-assistive exercise program. They can perform many exercises supine, and many others sitting in the wheelchair. If the paraplegic patient is cooperative with this exercise program and respects the warning that more than a year following repair is required for mature healing of the cuff, the end result can be good and comparable with that of other patients.

Re-repairing Failed Repairs

When evaluating a shoulder with a failed cuff repair, I look for four causes of failure: (1) persistent impingement, (2) adhesions from inadequate aftercare, (3) tear of the rotator cuff, and (4) damaged deltoid muscle. Each of these causes of failure can be considered individually, although they frequently occur in combination. Failures because of post-operative infection or radical acromionectomy are special problems and are considered separately (see p. 122, Fig. 2–46).

Residual Impingement

Residual impingement may cause adhesions because pain may make it impossible for the patient to move the shoulder properly. Residual impingement may also cause a re-tear of the rotator cuff. To correct these two problems, the first step is an adequate anterior acromioplasty followed by release of adhesions and manipulation of the shoulder to recover full passive motion.

Adhesions

Adhesions are present in almost all failed cuff repairs. If one attempts closed manipulation to overcome them, the cuff will almost certainly be

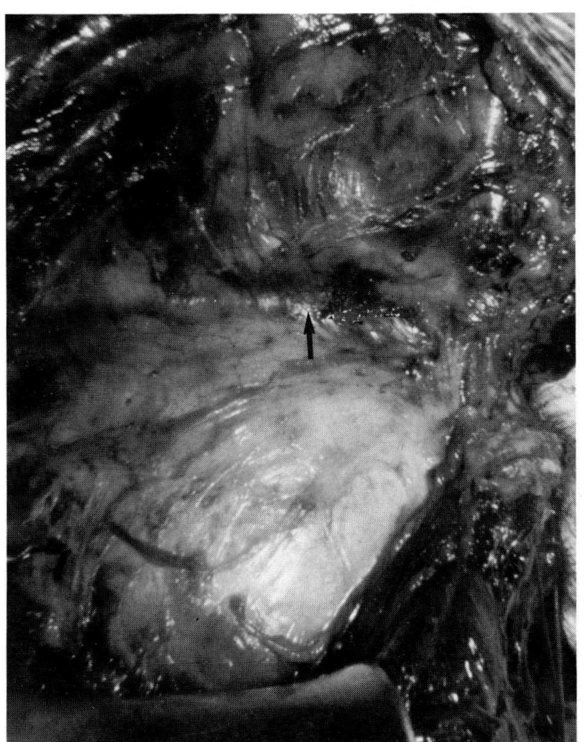

Figure 2–45. Failed cuff repair because of adhesions seen 18 months after surgery. The arrow points to dense adhesions between the intact rotator cuff and the deltoid muscle.

re-torn. Initial treatment is nonoperative, consisting of heat and stretching exercises. These are continued so long as improvement is occurring. When there has been no improvement during a four month period, open release is considered. The release is performed through the anterior acromioplasty approach, as seen in Figure 2–45. Subacromial and bursal adhesions are excised; the coracohumeral ligament is divided at the base of the coracoid; and after obtaining full passive motion, the shoulder is then inspected for residual impingement or cuff tear. When the cuff is intact, the exercise program can be advanced as rapidly as possible and the results are usually quite good.

Re-tear of the Cuff

It is natural to think of dehiscence of the cuff repair as the cause of failure. This may be the case; however, it was of interest to find in 66 failed repairs, 64 referred from other hospitals, that the cuff was intact in 23 percent (see p. 76). If subacromial impingement has been relieved at the time of repair so that it no longer interrupts healing, further healing of the tendon can occur over a number of months. For example, one patient who was referred from another hospital for re-operation because of a positive arthrogram made four months after an initial anterior acromioplasty and repair was advised to continue conservative treatment and to have another arthrogram in nine months. The repeated arthrogram showed healing of the cuff, and no further surgery was ever performed.

When re-operation is undertaken for a residual cuff defect, the rotator tendons must be carefully separated from the acromion and deltoid muscle, preserving both the deltoid and the rotator tendons as much as possible. This can be a very difficult step. It is best first to identify the superficial surface of the rotator cuff under the acromion. Dissection can then be carried out under the deltoid in proper planes posteriorly and laterally. Anteriorly, the plane of the coracoid and coracoacromial ligament is followed to identify the subscapularis. The rotator tendons are then mobilized in accordance with the principles given elsewhere (see pp. 106 to 119, Fig. 2–43), in order to increase their "pull" and excursion. The edges are freshened, and the tear is closed in the usual way.

Damaged Deltoid Muscle

An approach that detaches the deltoid origin has a peculiar detrimental effect on this muscle. The deltoid is weakened even though it has been carefully re-attached. If some of its origin pulls away from the acromion, it adheres to the underlying rotator cuff and humerus where it blocks motion. The retracted portion of deltoid becomes permanently shortened by scar tissue.

If the deltoid is retracted and scarred, it is never completely possible to restore its strength. Nevertheless, an effort to repair it should be made. If there is severe retraction, "deltoidplasty" entails freeing it from the overlying skin as well as from the humerus and rotator cuff before attempting to re-attach it back up on the acromion. I make an effort to pull the deltoid all the way up to the top of the acromion, suturing it to the trapezius tendon, rather than to the side of the acromion. A brace is used post-operatively for six weeks, during which time the arm is elevated and rotated passively each day to prevent the re-formation of adhesions between the deltoid and rotator cuff (see Fig. 7–15). After removing the brace, self-assistive exercises are continued for at least three months before attempting to raise the arm.

Special techniques in dealing with damaged deltoids are discussed with arthroplasties (see Chapter 2). They include transfer of the posterior deltoid anteriorly, transfer of the pectoralis major, and rotation of latissimus dorsi. None of these procedures has been completely successful. The treatment of radical acromionectomy is considered further on page 122, and in Figure 2–46.

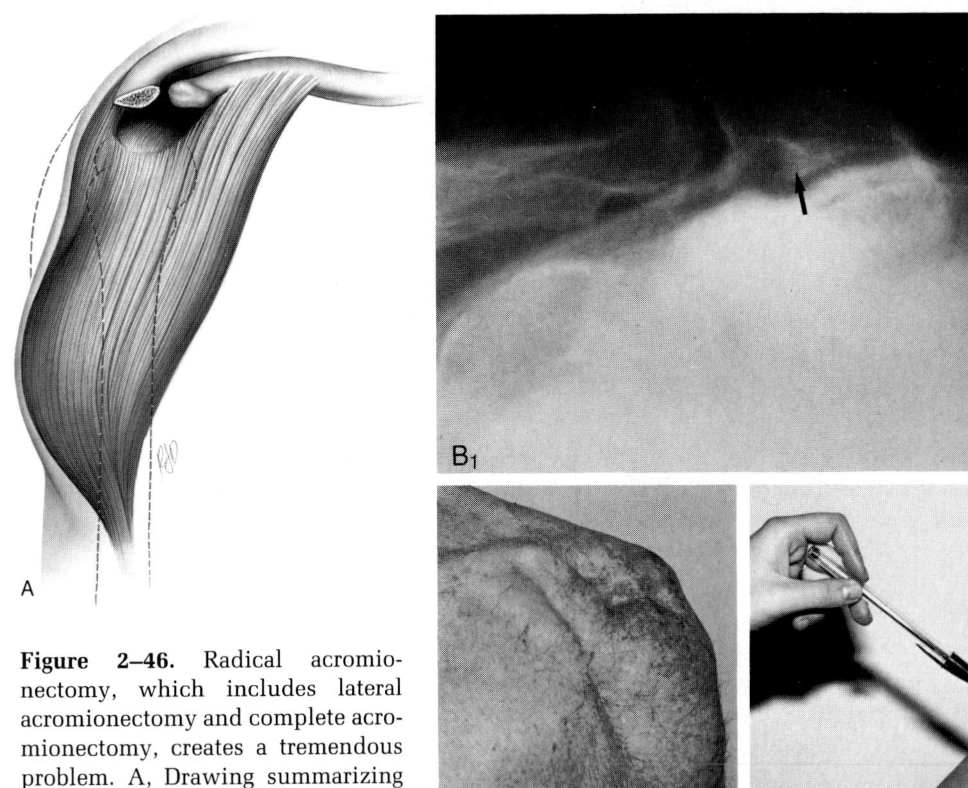

Figure 2–46. Radical acromionectomy, which includes lateral acromionectomy and complete acromionectomy, creates a tremendous problem. A, Drawing summarizing the devastating effect of complete acromionectomy, which is due to loss of the lever arm and weakening of the deltoid muscle, extensive adhesions between the retracted deltoid muscle and the humerus, and capsular adhesions. Lateral acromionectomy has a similar effect, but in addition leaves residual impingement. B1, Arthrogram of a patient showing residual impingement as a result of an anterior acromial spur (arrow) and excrescences at the acromioclavicular joint (just left of the arrow) with recurrence of the cuff tear. B2, Appearance of the shoulder of the patient shown in B1 after a lateral acromionectomy followed by four failed rotator cuff repairs. C, A failed complete acromionectomy and cuff repair, which was followed by a draining sinus that communicated with the glenohumeral joint for many months and eventually became infected. Note the retracted deltoid and scar from the previous sinus. (A from Neer, C. S., II, and Marberry, T. A.: On the disadvantages of radical acromionectomy. J. Bone Joint Surg. 63-A:416, 1981.)

Results to Be Expected After Failed Cuff Repairs

In Cofield's[97] series, the results after failed repair were generally adequate for relief of pain but recovery of strength was less certain. He emphasized the importance of a good initial repair. My experience confirms this. The prognosis should be guarded. Adequate strength for use of the arm overhead cannot be restored if the deltoid or cuff is permanently shortened by scar tissue. However, in our series, if we considered only the 17 reoperations in patients with good deltoid muscles, the adhesions and impingement could be eliminated and the tendons repaired sufficiently for an excellent result in 15 and a satisfactory result in 2.[108] Of the 49 patients with problems reducing either deltoid power or the efficiency of the glenohumeral joint, such as axillary nerve injuries, acromionectomies, cuff-tear arthropathy, and repeated failed surgery, all but 19 were relieved of pain; and 28 were unable to use the arm overhead.[108]

Reconstruction After Radical Acromionectomy

In reviewing 30 consecutive patients we saw who were treated with radical acromionectomies performed elsewhere for various diagnoses, the following conclusions were made:

1. Radical acromionectomy for cuff tears did not relieve pain, and because the shoulder was already weakened by the cuff tear, it was made worse.
2. Radical acromionectomy for malunited greater tuberosity fractures did not relieve pain because the tuberosity continued to impinge against the glenoid and because these shoulders were made weak.
3. Radical acromionectomy for rheumatoid arthritis did not relieve the pain because of the incongruity between the articular surfaces of the glenohumeral joint, and these shoulders were made weaker. It was concluded that other than for en bloc resection of a malignant tumor, there was no indication for radical acromionectomy and the procedure should be abandoned.[29]

Radical acromionectomy includes lateral acromionectomy and complete acromionectomy. The devastating effect of these procedures is summarized in Figure 2–46A. The deltoid retracts, adheres to the underlying humerus and rotator cuff, and is permanently weakened. Weakening the deltoid is especially disabling when there is a weak cuff. Adherence of the deltoid to the humerus blocks motion. This restriction of motion leads to capsular and extra-articular adhesions at the glenohumeral joint. The stiffening of the shoulder causes pain similar to that of a frozen shoulder (see Chapter 6). Lateral acromionectomy causes a similar degree of deltoid retraction and a similar problem of adhesions, and, in addition, leaves residual impingement. Although complete acromionectomy removes impingement, the extensive loss of skeletal support for the deltoid origin makes reconstruction even more difficult. Both lateral and complete acromionectomy invite wound complications.

Reconstruction After Failed Lateral Acromionectomy

The original skin incision is used and an anterior acromioplasty is performed to create a tunnel for the free excursion of the supraspinatus. The rotator tendons are freed beneath the acromion and dissected free from under the deltoid, staying in this same plane. The undersurfaces of the coracoacromial ligament and coracoid serve to define a definite point of separation anteriorly between the deltoid and the rotator cuff. If the deltoid has become retracted, it must be freed superficially from the skin before it can be brought up to maximum length (see Fig. 3–32). Adhesions are freed inside the joint through the cuff tear, and the coracohumeral ligament is divided. When the cuff has been completely mobilized, according to the principles outlined on pages 106 to 119, it is finally closed. The deltoid origin is then re-attached to the superficial surface of the acromion and to the trapezius tendon. A brace is worn for six weeks, with daily passive elevation and rotation before advancing to the self-assistive program (see Fig. 7–15).

Reconstruction After Complete Acromionectomy

It is even more difficult to define the plane between the rotator cuff and the adherent deltoid muscle when the entire acromion has been excised. Removal of the acromion causes the rotator cuff to lie just beneath the skin (Fig. 2–46A). The spine of the scapula and the coracoid are good bony landmarks to help in separating the deltoid from the cuff. After an extensive release of adhesions and manual manipulation of the glenohumeral joint to re-establish motion and after mobilizing and repairing the cuff as described previously, the deltoid is re-attached to the stump of the clavicle and base of the acromion. Because one of the problems with reconstruction after complete acromionectomies is the loss of the lever arm for re-attaching the deltoid origin, a bone graft can be considered to create a new acromion (see Fig. 3–32). This can be performed by osteotomizing and sliding the spine of the scapula laterally and internally fixing it with screws. Iliac grafts have also been used. After re-attachment of the deltoid, a brace is used for six weeks, during which time passive elevation and rotation are given before progressing the exercises. A very long recovery period should be anticipated, stressing preservation of motion with passive exercises and gradually strengthening the cuff and deltoid.

Results of Surgery for Radical Acromionectomy

Repair of 20 such shoulders in patients referred with failed radical acromionectomies was reported in 1981.[29] All patients had their original surgery for cuff tears. A tear of the rotator cuff persisted in 15 shoulders, and the cuff was found intact in 5. Extensive retraction of the deltoid and adhesions around the joint were found in all cases.

At surgery, an effort was made to follow the principles outlined previously. A new acromion was created in one patient by sliding the spine of the scapula laterally and internally fixing it with screws; however, this patient did not return for adequate aftercare and a great deal of shoulder stiffness developed, which was never overcome. At late follow-up, only 6 of the 20 patients could raise their arm above the horizontal and the majority continued to have some discomfort. Arthrodesis was eventually performed in two patients and total shoulder arthroplasty in two others, with relief of pain but without restoring use above the horizontal. We concluded that it might be justified to attempt reconstruction after failed radical acromionectomy; however, the prognosis should be extremely guarded.

Treatment After Infected Cuff Repairs

Only after all evidence of active infection has disappeared and the erythrocyte sedimentation rate has returned to normal is a re-repair considered. I wait at least one year. It is important to know the organisms and sensitivities of all previous cultures. Appropriate antibiotic coverage is essential. Some of the sutures and devitalized tissue are sent for further cultures at the time of surgery; and at surgery, if there is any evidence of residual infection, only a "clean-out" is performed. The clean-out aims at the removal of all sutures and necrotic tissue and copious antibiotic irrigation. In some cases, a second clean-out is required before attempting repair.

The objectives in the re-repair are the same as those discussed for clean cases and failed cuff repair—decompression of residual impingement, release of adhesions, mobilization and closure of the cuff, and repair of the deltoid. Resorbable sutures may be used for repairing the cuff, but in some cases I have used nonabsorbable sutures, as in other repairs, but conserve on the number of sutures.

All patients are warned pre-operatively of the special risks of igniting another infection and of the special need for their cooperation during the long exercise program to follow. The aftercare program is determined by the size of the cuff defect.

Glenohumeral arthrodesis is considered when the infection has destroyed the articular surfaces and in selected, especially active patients (such as a farmer) who have too much damage by retraction or excision to both the deltoid and the cuff to expect adequate recovery of function.

Cuff-Tear Arthropathy

Cuff-tear arthropathy is a new clinical entity that I recognized in the early 1970s. It consists of severe glenohumeral joint disorganization and collapse of the humeral head developing with massive tears of the rotator cuff in the absence of other known etiological factors. In an intensive search of the literature, no good description of this lesion could be found, and yet it has important physiological and therapeutic connotations. I introduced the term "cuff-tear arthropathy" in 1975.[20–24] Later, in 1981, the "Milwaukee shoulder" was reported,[25] which is undoubtedly the same condition, although one of the eight cases in that series did not have a cuff tear and the authors thought it was a biochemical phenomenon. I believe this problem is peculiar to the shoulder because no other joint has a rotator cuff. Also, I believe whatever biochemical alterations occur are secondary to the effect of the patient having lost the function of the rotator cuff and are not of primary etiological importance.

Theory of Pathomechanics and Etiology

My theory on the etiology of cuff-tear arthropathy is illustrated in Figures 2–47 to 2–52. There are both nutritional and mechanical factors. The *nutrition of the articular cartilage* is dependent on

Text continued on page 131

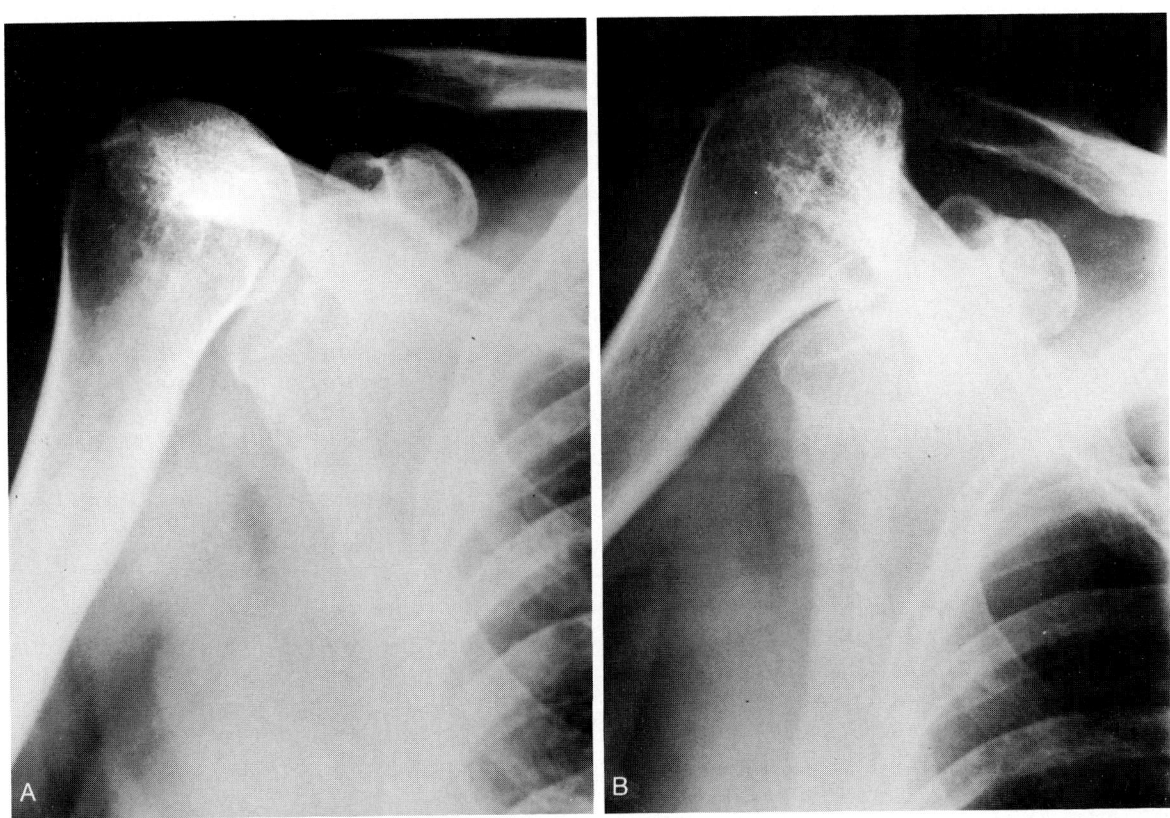

Figures 2–47 through 2–52. ***Cuff-tear Arthropathy***

Figure 2–47. Progressive roentgen changes in a 63 year old woman who presented in 1975 with several years of shoulder pain without an injury. An x-ray film (A) was taken at that time and an arthrogram made, which showed a tear of the rotator cuff. She refused surgical treatment. Two years later, in 1977, an x-ray film (B) was obtained and showed disintegration and distortion of the articular surface of the humeral head and glenoid.

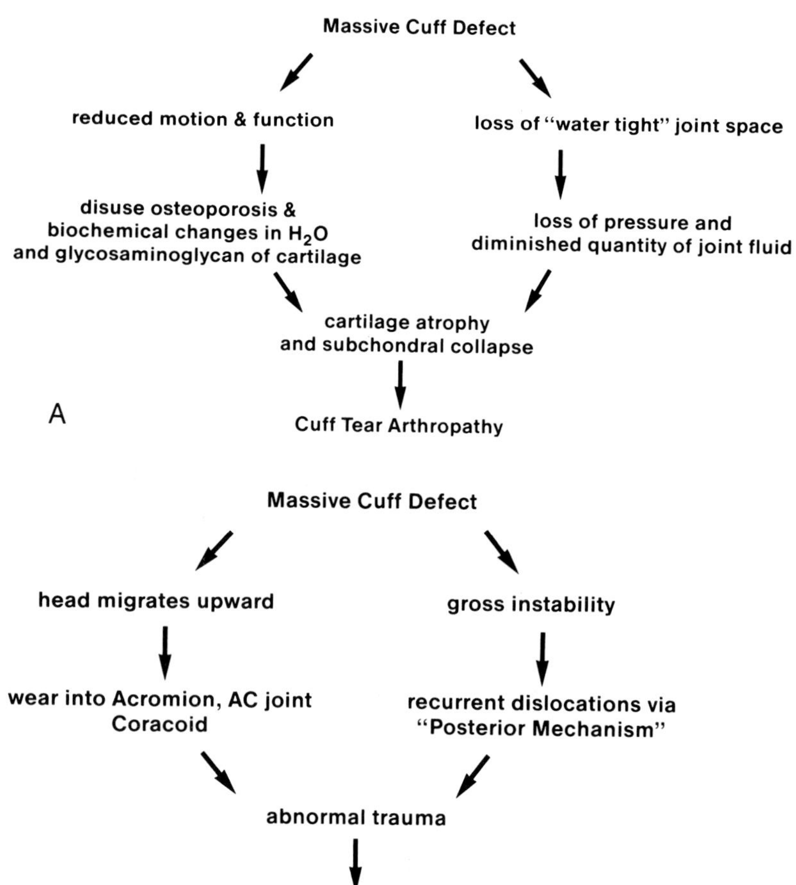

Figure 2–48. The author's theory on the etiology of cuff-tear arthropathy. There are both nutritional factors (A) and mechanical factors (B). (From Neer, C.S., II, Craig, E.V., and Fukuda, H.: Cuff-tear arthropathy. J. Bone Joint Surg. 65-A: 1232, 1983.)

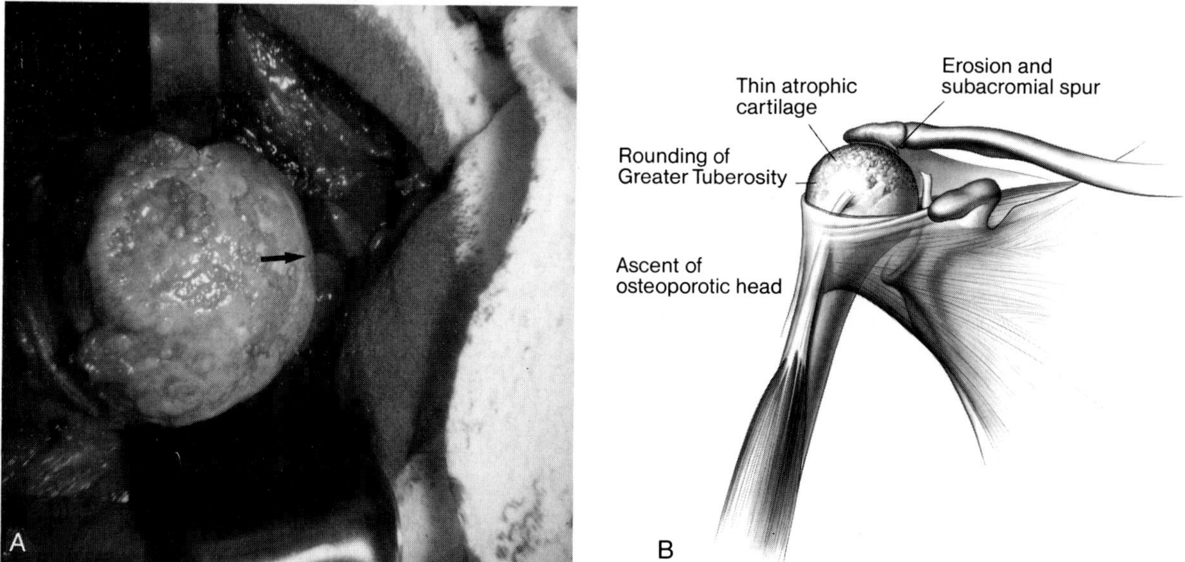

Figure 2–49. Stage of pre-collapse before cuff-tear arthropathy. A, Photograph in the operating room of a 57 year old man who had a massive tear of the rotator cuff. B, Depicts the anatomical problem. At this stage (prior to cuff-tear arthropathy), when the articular surface retains its normal shape and there is some articular cartilage (arrow in A), a total shoulder arthroplasty is not performed. (From Neer, C.S., II, Craig, E.V., and Fukuda, H.: Cuff-tear arthropathy. J. Bone Joint Surg. 65-A:1232, 1983.)

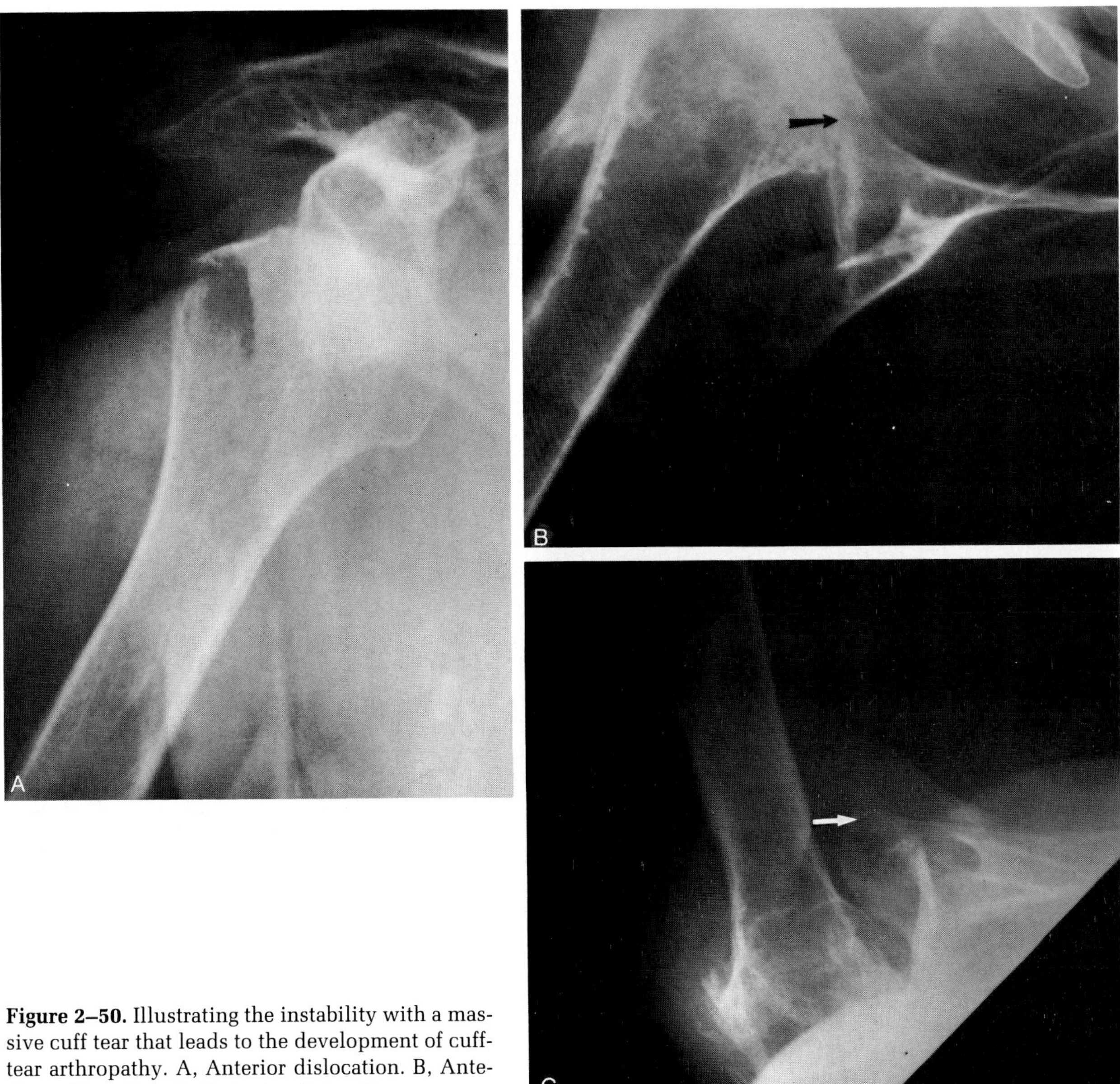

Figure 2–50. Illustrating the instability with a massive cuff tear that leads to the development of cuff-tear arthropathy. A, Anterior dislocation. B, Anterior subluxation. C, Posterior dislocation.

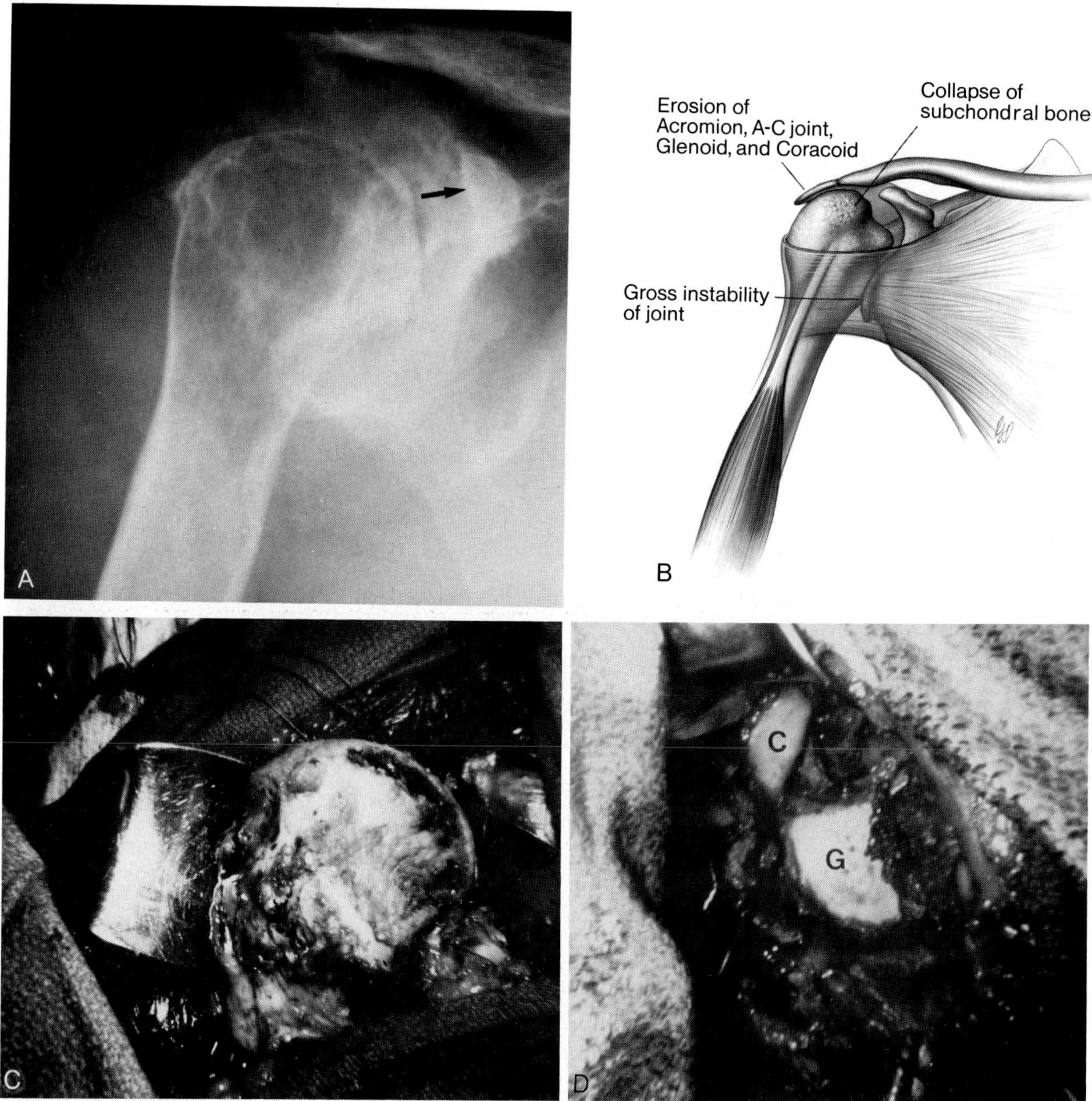

Figure 2–51. ***The Gross Pathology of Cuff-tear Arthropathy.*** A, Roentgenogram showing erosion half way through the coracoid (arrow) and clavicle, marked distortion of the head, erosion of the clavicle, impingement wear causing a fracture through the acromion, and other changes depicted in B (A-C= clavicular). There are bone fragments outside the joint, showing the gross instability. C, The appearance of the head at surgery, showing sclerotic areas and soft areas. D, The appearance of the glenoid (G) and coracoid (C) at surgery, confirming deep wear and erosion and making it extremely difficult to implant a glenoid component. (From Neer, C.S., II, Craig, E.V., and Fukuda, H.: Cuff-tear arthropathy. J. Bone Joint Surg. 65-A:1232, 1983.)

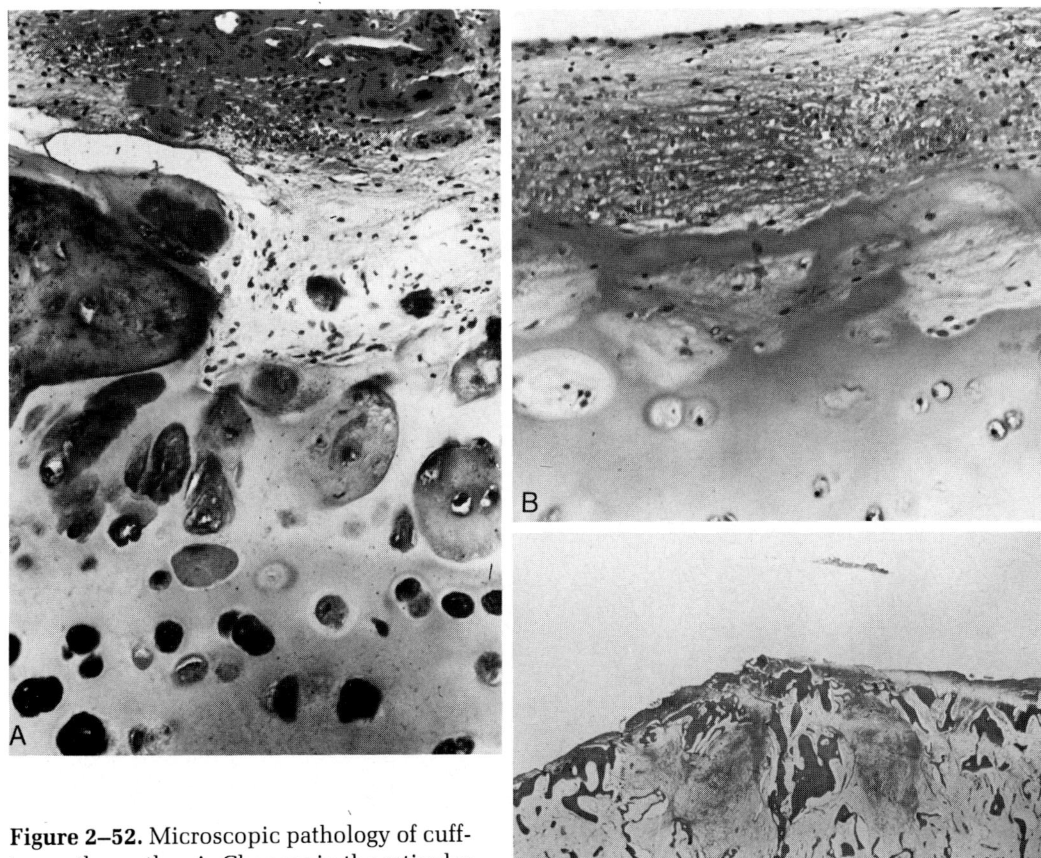

Figure 2–52. Microscopic pathology of cuff-tear arthropathy. A, Changes in the articular cartilage of the humeral head and subsynovial fragments of cartilage. B, Fibrous pannus and cartilage changes as in disuse atrophy. C, Avascular scar replacing articular cartilage.

Illustration continued on following page

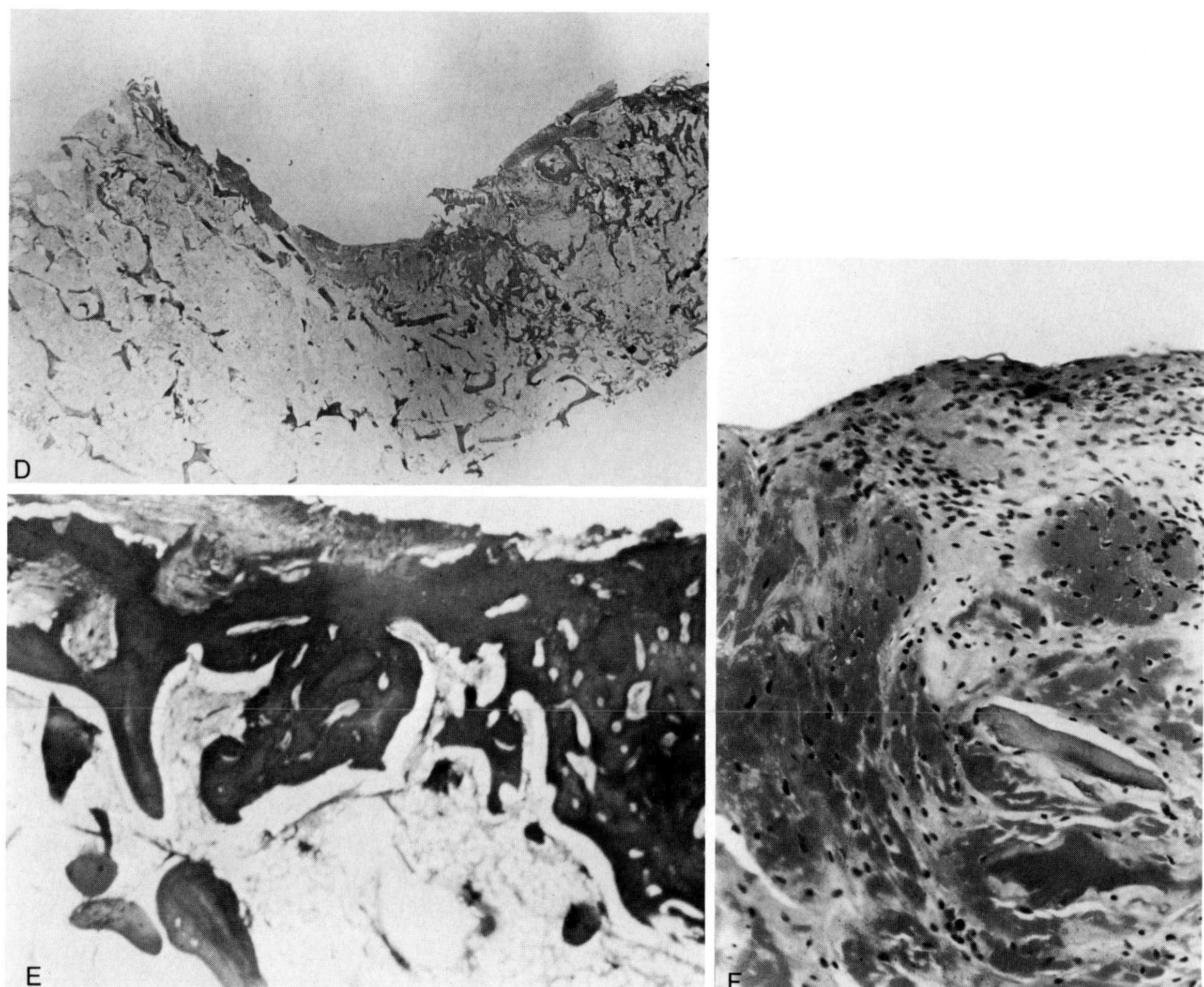

Figure 2–52 *Continued* D, Changes in the bone of the humeral head are those of osteoporosis and articular fractures. E, Sclerosis of the head at a point of fixed contact with the glenoid. F, Subsynovial fragments of bone and cartilage thought to be a result of repeated dislocations. (From Neer, C. S. II, Craig, E. V., and Fukuda, H.: Cuff-tear arthropathy. J. Bone Joint Surg. 65-A:1232, 1983.)

the quality of the synovial fluid and on joint motion. When there is a large tear of the rotator cuff, both the chemistry and the pressure of the joint fluid are altered. There are changes in the water content and in the glycosaminoglycan of cartilage associated with the loss of the "watertight joint space" and inactivity. *Mechanically*, the joint is used less than normally, leading to disuse osteoporosis of the subchondral bone of the humeral head and glenoid as well as atrophy of the cartilage of their articular surfaces. Another mechanical factor is the instability of the glenohumeral joint, which develops with a large cuff tear through the posterior mechanism (see Chapter 4). The subluxations and dislocations subject the articular surface to unusual wear and trauma. The collapse of subchondral bone and the bizarre distortion of the head characteristic of cuff-tear arthropathy probably do not occur until dislocations or subluxations develop.

With time, the irregular head wears into the glenoid, coracoid, and acromioclavicular joint (Fig. 2–47). These advanced impingement lesions show the direction of force and wear in outlet impingement. All of the alterations of impingement discussed on pages 54 to 63 occur, beginning with spur formation and then on to deep erosion of the undersurface of the acomion and acromioclavicular joint until the acromion is worn through.[109] Impingement wear eventually leads to the rounding and loss of the greater tuberosity. This, together with the atrophy of the articular cartilage, makes it difficult for the surgeon to distinguish where the articular surface of the head begins and ends. Eventually, impingement ruptures the long head of the biceps or loosens the transverse humeral ligaments, so the long head dislocates from its groove. When this occurs, the stabilizing function of the biceps against upward migration of the humeral head is lost and impingement is probably further escalated.[26] When the impinging tuberosity erodes through the acromioclavicular joint capsule, glenohumeral joint fluid communicates with the acromioclavicular joint and a swelling of the acromioclavicular joint can occur that clinically resembles a ganglion. At this stage, arthrograms show dye entering the glenohumeral joint as the "geyser sign" (see Figs. 2–15, 2–35, and 2–47 to 2–52).

The term "cuff-tear arthropathy" is used only after collapse of the osteoporotic subchondral bone of the head with distortion of the shape of its articular surfaces. At this stage, there is usually gross instability of the glenohumeral joint often both anteriorly and posteriorly as well as uncontrolled upward displacement of the head. The incongruous, unstable head erodes the glenoid, coracoid, acromion, and acromioclavicular joint, as discussed previously. Eventually, the distorted head usually becomes fixed in a dislocated position with disappearance of the instability. When this occurs, the bone at the point of contact between the humerus and the scapula becomes eburnated, while the surrounding bone becomes osteoporotic from disuse atrophy.

The fact that cuff-tear arthropathy does not develop in all untreated tears of the rotator cuff is thought to be best explained by the assumption that many tears never enlarge sufficiently and some become sealed with bursal scar. The abnormal trauma caused by recurrent dislocations associated with a massive tear is thought to be an essential etiological factor in the collapse and disintegration of the head required for this diagnosis. This type of collapse of articular surfaces is not seen in simple frozen shoulders in which there is disuse atrophy but the rotator cuff is intact and there is no instability.

Clinical Series

Although many more examples of this condition have been encountered, we limited the 1983 series to 17 patients I had explored surgically between 1975 and 1980 and followed post-operatively for a minimum period of two years.[24] Total shoulder replacement was performed in each patient. Five had bilateral cuff-tear arthropathy. Eleven of the patients were female, and six were male. Their ages ranged from 57 years to 87 years and averaged 69 years. The dominant arm was involved in 11 of the 17 patients.

History

These patients had long-standing, increasing pain, worse at night and made worse by use and activity. Pain averaged 9.8 years in duration. The patients also complained of inability to elevate the arm or externally rotate the shoulder. The cuff tears seemed to be due to progressive wear and impingement rather than to trauma. Eleven of the seventeen had no injury whatsoever, and the majority were female patients not engaged in heavy labor. Steroid injections did not seem to be an etiological factor, since five patients had no injections, three others had none until after the development of roentgen changes, and only four patients had more than three injections. Previous surgery had been performed in nine of the seventeen, one in our hospital and eight in other hospitals. The initial surgery consisted of biopsies and attempts to repair the rotator cuff, with complete acromionectomies in four patients. One patient had been operated on four times, and two were operated on twice. One patient had sustained a recent fracture of the humeral shaft during an attempt in another hospital to reduce the dislocated head by closed manipulation.

Physical Findings

Most of the physical signs typical of a massive tear of the rotator cuff were present, including swelling as a result of glenohumeral joint fluid distending the bursa ("fluid sign"), which at times communicated with the acromioclavicular joint causing a swelling that looked like a ganglion of this joint. There was atrophy of the supraspinatus and infraspinatus muscles and weakness of external rotation and abduction. The incongruity of the glenohumeral joint surfaces limited motion more than is usually seen with tears of the rotator cuff and caused almost all glenohumeral movements to be painful, making the usual physical signs for a torn rotator cuff, such as the arc of pain and the impingement sign, of no value. In some patients the humeral head could be dislocated both anteriorly and posteriorly, whereas in the majority the head had become fixed in a dislocated position with stiffness, limitation of motion, and without the instability that had once been present. Palpable crepitus and tenderness at the glenohumeral joint line posteriorly, as is characteristic of glenohumeral incongruity in arthritis or trauma (see Chapter 3, pp. 163 to 166) were usually present.

Laboratory Findings

Laboratory data were unremarkable. Two female patients had pre-operative erythrocyte sedimentation rates higher than 30 mm./hour, one with a urinary tract infection. Complete blood counts, uric acid determinations, albumin/globulin ratios, and latex fixation (or rheumatoid factor) tests were normal, with the exception of two patients who had weakly reactive latex fixation tests and who had no other joint symptoms. Electromyograms were performed in the upper extremities of five patients, which were normal in three and showed mild cervical radiculitis in two. Arthrograms showed a tear of the rotator cuff, usually with communication of the dye into the acromioclavicular joint. Seven patients had arthrograms of the opposite shoulder, all showing tears of the rotator cuff on the contralateral shoulder; however, only five of the seven had bilateral cuff-tear arthropathy.

Roentgen Findings

The x-ray findings are dramatic, as seen in Figures 2–17, 2–35, and 2–50. They will be considered separately for the humeral head, the acromion and acromioclavicular joint, and the glenoid. At the *proximal humerus*, an area of collapse of the articular surface was seen in all cases, which was a requirement for the diagnosis. Large osteophytes, as are characteristic of osteoarthritis, were not seen. Evidence of anterior and posterior dislocation or subluxation of the head was often demonstrated in routine rotation and axillary films. If the head became fixed in a dislocated position, it could easily be mistaken for an unrecognized traumatic dislocation. At the greater tuberosity, there was characteristically superficial reactive bone formation with sclerosis and often a prominence or excrescence as is caused by subacromial impingement. This was always centered at the facet for the insertion of the supraspinatus tendon. Beneath this, the bone was so osteoporotic that the radiologists often mentioned the possibility of a metastatic lesion. In the more advanced lesions, degenerative cysts developed beneath the sclerotic area on the greater tuberosity. In most cases, rounding off of the greater tuberosity with loss of the sulcus between it and the articular surface made it impossible to tell where the tuberosity ended and the articular surface began. Proximal migration of the humerus was evidenced by loss of the acromiohumeral distance and by a break in the normal smooth curve made by the neck of the humerus and the neck of the scapula. The acromiohumeral interval was 2.0 mm. or less in all but three patients. At the *acromion and acromioclavicular* joint, the roentgen evidences of impingement were seen, consisting of remnants of an anterior acromial spur within the coracoacromial ligament in 16 shoulders, associated with erosion of the undersurface of the acromion, acromioclavicular joint, and distal clavicle. An axillary view was helpful to determine the possible presence of an unfused anterior acromial epiphysis or the presence of such deep erosion that a pathological fracture of the acromion had occurred.

At the *glenoid*, erosion of the glenoid anteriorly and posteriorly was often seen in the axillary view and erosion of the cephalic portion of the articular surface into the coracoid was present in over half of the patients. In five patients, the glenoid was eroded so deeply that more than half of the coracoid was worn away.

Operative Findings

The findings described previously under pathomechanics were seen at surgery. Large, complete cuff tears were present in all patients, and the head was either fixed in a subluxed position or extremely unstable. Both the supraspinatus and infraspinatus tendons were completely ruptured in all but one patient. There was usually a profuse quantity of fluid that was often streaked with blood, apparently caused by the impact of the tuberosity against the acromion. Some patients had evidences of ecchymosis associated with these local hemorrhages. The long head of the biceps was ruptured in ten patients and was dislocated in two. The appearance of the atrophied, pebblestone cartilage and the collapsed articular surfaces was typical (Figs. 2–47 to 2–52). The head was usually soft and easily indented. When the head had become fixed in a dislocation position, the point of contact between the head and the scapula became sclerotic, but the remaining portion of the articular surface was soft. Varying degrees of erosion of the glenoid, acromioclavicular joint, acromion, and outer clavicle were easily visualized at surgery, and the proximal humerus was usually rounded off with loss of the greater tuberosity, so that it resembled a femoral head. In all cases, however, some vestige of the insertion of the teres minor and inferior part of the subscapularis remained. The remains of the supraspinatus were displaced medially and were adherent, whereas remains of the teres minor and subscapularis tended to be displaced toward the elbow.

Gross and Microscopic Pathology

I am indebted to Dr. Austin Johnston and Dr. May Parisien for their help as our pathologists in describing this entity. On gross examination, the head typically sectioned with decreased resistance, indicating osteoporosis. The articular cartilage was quite thin and irregular, and the soft subchondral bone allowed it to be indented on pressure. However, at points with fixed contact between the head and the scapula, the cartilage was completely worn away and the subchondral bone was sclerotic. The atrophied articular cartilage of the head usually became covered in large part with a disorderly fibrous membrane. This contained scattered histiocytes and occasional lymphocytes and plasma cells but was nothing like the inflammatory pannus of rheumatoid arthritis. The spongiosa of the head was osteoporotic, hypervascular, and often evidenced attempts at repair and reconstruction at the points of subchondral collapse. The subacromial bursa was markedly thickened and fibrotic, as in other patients with cuff tears.

Differential Diagnosis of Cuff-Tear Arthropathy

It is important to recognize cuff-tear arthropathy as a distinct clinical entity separate from other causes of glenohumeral joint destruction because of different treatment and prognosis. The differential diagnosis is summarized in Figures 2–47 to 2–52. In *osteoarthritis*, the articular surfaces are eburnated, the head is enlarged by marginal osteophytes, and the rotator cuff is intact. In *rheumatoid arthritis*, there is destruction by pannus erosion, polyarthritis, distinctive laboratory data, and the cuff may be attenuated but is usually intact. In *suppurative arthritis*, there is purulence, a positive culture, and the cuff is intact. In *metabolic diseases* with joint destruction, there are often distinctive crystals to aid in the differential between this and primary osteoarthritis and the cuff is intact. In *aseptic necrosis*, there is the characteristic subchondral collapse with preservation of a thick, loose cartilaginous covering until such time as secondary osteoarthritis appears, and the rotator cuff is intact. In *neuropathies*, the disorganization and fragmentation may resemble those seen in the type of cuff-tear arthropathy associated with marked instability; however, neuropathies usually have the neurological aura associated with syringomyelia or lues and the rotator cuff is always intact. *Villonodular synovitis* of the shoulder is extremely rare and has not been seen in my experience as a cause of glenohumeral joint destruction. If it does occur, the rotator cuff would be expected to be intact.

For the diagnosis of cuff-tear arthropathy to be made, there must be collapse and disintegration of the articular surfaces of the glenohumeral joint associated with a large cuff tear without other laboratory or systemic abnormalities. The diagnosis is made by exclusion of other conditions and by the gross appearance at surgery. In some patients with cuff-tear arthropathy, the articular surfaces are sclerotic and there is lipping reminiscent of osteoarthritis; however, there is a large rotator cuff tear. In these patients, there is erosion of the glenoid and the condition of the joint surfaces precludes an adequate result by repair of the rotator cuff alone. The distinction has been made, however, of "pre-collapse," in which the head retains its normal contour and although there may be some involvement of cartilage, sufficient cartilage remains for treatment by repair of the cuff alone without concern for the articular surfaces. I have illustrated this state of "pre-collapse" in Figure 2–49 to emphasize that the term cuff-tear arthropathy is not applied to these lesions.

Treatment of Cuff-Tear Arthropathy

The combination of destruction of the articular surfaces and a very large tear of the rotator cuff is a formidable problem. The indication for surgery is determined by the amount of pain and disability and by the general health of the patient. The average age of my patients at the time of surgery is 69 years. Some are seen who are too old for surgery; however, the majority seek and deserve relief from the unrelenting pain.

Arthrodesis can be considered, but it is usually contraindicated because of concomitant rotator cuff disease in the contralateral shoulder and because the aftercare program for a fusion is too arduous for many patients in this age group.

A constrained shoulder prosthesis is a logical procedure because of the extensive loss of the rotator cuff. The softening erosion of the scapula, however, makes a fixed fulcrum very likely to fail by pulling out of the bone or impossible to install.

Resection of the proximal humerus or resection of the glenoid cannot be relied upon to relieve pain. In my experience, these procedures leave the shoulder flail and render patients even more disabled than they were before surgery.[12]

The use of a subacromial spacer to prevent the impingement of the proximal humerus against the acromion has been suggested by several authors. However, this cannot be expected to be adequate in cuff-tear arthropathy, because the massive tear of the rotator cuff makes the proximal humerus too unstable for the humerus to remain in contact with the spacer and the spacer will not solve the problem of pain stemming from the incongruous glenohumeral joint.

A humeral component with a large head can be used alone without a glenoid component by placing it slightly high in hopes of eliminating impingement pain as well as that emanating from the articular surfaces. Unfortunately, this makes repair of the rotator cuff more difficult or impossible. My choice has generally been a nonconstrained total shoulder arthroplasty, usually with a glenoid component about the size of the normal glenoid but occasionally with a slightly oversized glenoid component and often using a shorter head to facilitate repair of the rotator cuff, as discussed in Chapter 3, pp. 234 to 239.

The objectives in total shoulder arthroplasty are to prevent painful contact between the proximal humerus and the articular surface of the glenoid and also against the acromion and undersurface of the acromioclavicular surface. The rotator cuff is repaired at least sufficiently to establish stability against anterior and posterior dislocations and usually sufficiently to cover the humeral component. The same principles are used as outlined in Figure 2–43. A hooded glenoid component with an articular surface 600 percent larger than the average glenoid was used developmentally in two patients in my series, but has been discarded because it interfered with closing the rotator cuff and was not associated with better active motion. A glenoid component with an articular surface approximately twice the size of the normal glenoid has been used occasionally when there is marked loss of bone, and this allows closure of the rotator cuff. More recently, however, the standard-sized glenoid component has generally been preferred because it allows better repair of the rotator cuff.

The technique of nonconstrained arthroplasty, the limited goals exercise program, and the results are discussed in Chapter 3, page 238. The technique of arthrodesis is discussed in Chapter 6, page 441.

TREATMENT OF IMPINGEMENT LESIONS OF THE BICEPS

The classification of biceps lesions is discussed on page 62 and in Table 2–3, and on pages 70 to 73; the diagnosis is reviewed on page 91.

Indications for Biceps Tenodesis

I believe nearly all of the ruptures of the long head and other biceps lesions are caused primarily by impingement (see p. 62; Figs 2–8, 2–17, 2–26, and 2–33). Tenodesis is never performed for inflammation of the long head unless the tendon has become flattened, split, or displaced, so that it no longer runs in its groove. I see three clinical types of long head ruptures (see Fig. 2–26); of these, reattachment is considered only in the retracted type and is, of course, unnecessary in the self-attaching types whether attaching in place or with partial retraction.

Indications to Re-attach Acute Biceps Ruptures with Retraction

My indications for surgical re-attachment of recent retracted ruptures of the long head of the biceps in active patients are summarized in Table 2–7. Some patients are definitely concerned about the appearance of the lump and wish to have it eliminated if possible. Others prefer to avoid surgery unless there is some serious interference with the strength of the arm without it. As has been previously discussed, most of the discomfort associated with biceps ruptures is from impingement and this will not be relieved by tenodesing the long head to the humerus. Tenodesing it to the coracoid tends to make the impingement worse.

Unfortunately, there is no effective technique for preserving the head depressor function of the long head by end-to-end tendon repair.

Table 2–7 can be briefly summarized as follows:

1. If the patient is unwilling to accept the lump in the arm and requests repair, the long head is tenodesed and an anterior acromioplasty is performed for decompression and inspection of the rotator cuff, which if torn is repaired.

2. If the patient has had no previous shoulder pain and prefers the lump to surgery, the shoulder is observed and an arthrogram is deferred unless there is persistent pain and signs suggesting the presence of a rotator cuff tear.

3. If the patient has had previous pain indicative of impingement, an arthrogram is advised; if the arthrogram is positive for a tear of the rotator cuff, an anterior acromioplasty, repair of the rotator cuff, and tenodesis of the long head to the humerus are advised.

Indications to Re-attach Old Biceps Ruptures

Because (1) scar and shortening of the muscle belly make the cosmetic improvement after re-attachment of old biceps ruptures less perfect, (2) ruptures of the long head per se rarely cause significant pain other than that associated with impingement, and (3) re-attachment of old ruptured biceps tendons has little if any effect on elbow strength, long-standing biceps ruptures are rarely re-attached. However, some patients who plan to have a repair of the rotator cuff request that the biceps also be repaired at the same procedure. In this instance, the limitations of the repair are discussed. I ask the patient to let us make the decision at surgery based on the difficulty of the cuff repair. If a difficult repair is encountered, an additional step to re-attach the biceps may seem to be unwise, especially since it could interfere with the rehabilitation program. On the other hand, when the decompression and repair of the cuff have been straightforward, the patient may appreciate the improved appearance of the arm associated with re-attaching the biceps at the same time. Several of my patients believe that re-attaching the biceps to the humerus eliminated the cramping sensations they were having in their arm; however, I suspect the discomfort had actually been referred pain from impingement that was relieved by the anterior acromioplasty rather than by re-attaching the biceps.

Treatment of Old Biceps Dislocations

I have not seen a dislocation of the long head in patients under the age of 40 other than those with fractures of the tuberosities (see Chapter 5). On the other hand, subluxation or dislocation of the biceps is not rare in older patients with large cuff tears (see Fig. 2–27). No satisfactory method of restoring the excursion of the long head in its groove has been developed. Deepening the groove and repairing the transverse humeral ligament are followed by adherence of the tendon. Tenodesis is more dependable. The tenodesed biceps is usually incorporated in the cuff repair.

Technique of Biceps Tenodesis

Although it would be desirable to restore the stabilizing functions of the biceps on the humeral head by repairing ruptures of the long head by end-to-end suture, a satisfactory method for accomplishing this has not been achieved and tenodesis to the humerus has been more reliable. However, anterior acromioplasty is performed routinely with this procedure, in an attempt to offset the loss of the long head against ascent of the humerus. Re-attachment of the biceps to the humerus is preferred over re-attachment to the coracoid because the latter would be expected to aggravate impingement further (see Fig. 1–22).

The anterior acromioplasty (see Fig. 2–41) is performed first, and if the biceps rupture is less than three weeks old, this may be the only incision required. If the retracted end of the biceps becomes adherent, a second incision will be necessary distally to mobilize the tendon. The acromioplasty is performed as usual, eliminating overhang and prominences on the undersurface of the anterior acromion and acromioclavicular joint.

In the case of *recent biceps ruptures*, when the acromioplasty has been completed and if the rotator cuff is torn, it is repaired according to the principles in Figure 2–43, the shoulder and elbow are both flexed, and the biceps muscle is squeezed in an effort to milk the stump of the tendon into the wound. A skin hook or long, narrow clamp may be used to pull the stump of the biceps up into its sheath, but one must bear in mind the proximity of the musculocutaneous nerve. If the long head can be retrieved in this way, it is anchored with nonabsorbable sutures to a window in the bone in the vicinity of the biceps groove (Fig. 2–53A). The proximal stump of the biceps may be excised if desired, although I have never seen it

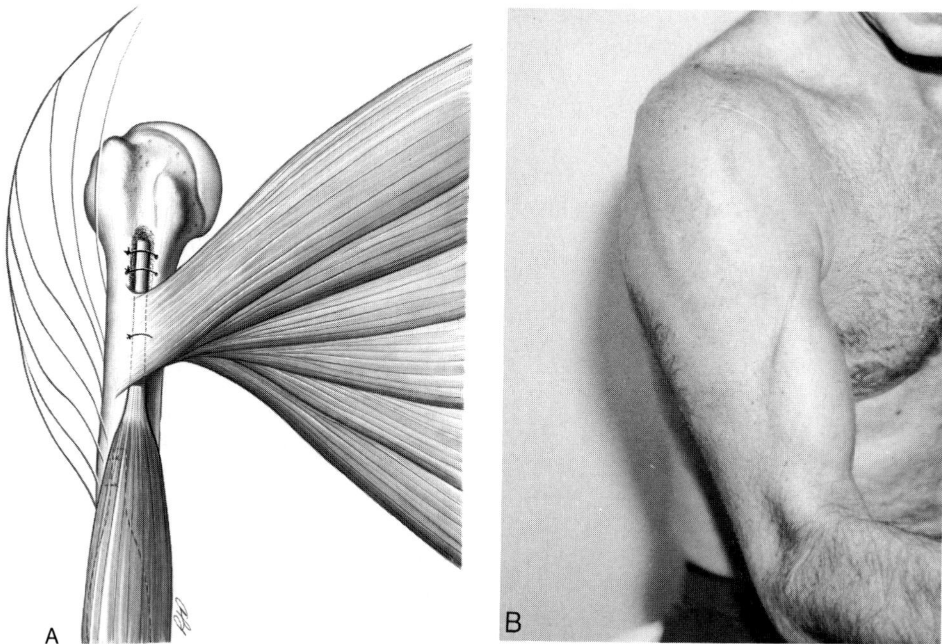

Figure 2–53. A, Re-attachment for retracted rupture of the long head of the biceps. B, Result 2 years after re-attachment of the long head of the biceps, which had been performed as shown in A at the time of anterior acromioplasty and repair of a torn rotator cuff. The biceps rupture had been present for 6 months at the time of re-attachment. The patient had no pain, was normally active, and was pleased with the result.

cause trouble if left undisturbed, or it may be used in repairing the large rotator cuff tears.

In repairing *old ruptures of the long head*, the distal end can be palpated buried in scar and coiled up in the retracted position. A second incision is made over the deltopectoral interval, approximately 7 cm. long. The pectoralis insertion is exposed and the long head palpated. With the surgeon taking care to avoid injury to the musculocutaneous nerve lying just deep to the pectoralis insertion and between the two heads of the biceps, the stump of the long head is dissected free from adhesions and is pulled up to as near normal length as possible before anchoring it to a window on the front of the humerus. I usually add additional nonabsorbable sutures to anchor the biceps to the deltoid insertion or the pectoralis insertion or both (Fig. 2–53A).

When there is a *dislocated long head of the biceps*, there is almost invariably a large tear of the rotator cuff and flattening of the bicipital groove (see Fig. 2–27). If the long head is to be incorporated in the cuff repair, it is best to deepen the groove or make a new groove about 1 cm. posterior to the biceps groove with a gouge and to tenodese the long head at this site on the humerus prior to suturing it in the cuff repair (see Fig. 2–43). However, it is important to note that the biceps should not be sutured in the cuff repair too near its insertion on the glenoid, or else it will anchor the supraspinatus to the scapula.

Post-operatively following biceps tenodesis for ruptures or dislocations, the elbow is allowed out of the sling or brace for light movements, but heavy resistance against elbow flexion is avoided for several weeks. Shoulder exercises are advanced as tolerated. If securely anchored, as described previously, the biceps repair should not significantly alter the exercise program for the freshly repaired rotator cuff.

Results of Biceps Re-attachment

Re-attachment of recent long head ruptures should give a near normal anatomical appearance, eliminating both the lump and medial deviation in the alignment of the biceps. In addition, there may be slightly improved power for supination. However, it is difficult to prove this point because what may have appeared to be weakness of supination was in fact due to an associated tear of the rotator cuff; and if the rotator cuff is repaired, there may well be improved power for turning a doorknob and turning a screwdriver, which could easily be misconstrued as improved power of supination.

In older long head ruptures, the anatomical appearance is usually improved but is not as good as that achieved in recent long head ruptures. Nevertheless, our patients with repairs of old biceps ruptures are usually satisfied with the appearance (Fig. 2–53A and B), and several believe that the re-attachment of the biceps improved the strength of the arm. However, the re-attachment of the biceps was always performed concomitantly with repair of the rotator cuff. Most of the preoperative discomfort in these patients is undoubtedly due to subacromial impingement, but because all types of shoulder pain are referred to the region of the deltoid insertion and long head of the biceps, patients often mistakenly believe that the ruptured biceps had been causing most of the pain when in fact the major pain relief probably came from the relief of impingement by the anterior acromioplasty. The improvement in strength and comfort following anterior acromioplasty and cuff repair without re-attaching the biceps has been about the same as that achieved by procedures that include long head re-attachment. Nevertheless, if a patient who is about to undergo a cuff repair requests re-attachment of the long head at the time of cuff repair, it may be best to comply with this request.

ARTHROSCOPY IN THE TREATMENT OF OUTLET IMPINGEMENT

The value of arthroscopy in the diagnosis of impingement lesions is discussed on page 90, Figure 2–40. For clarity in evaluating the role of arthroscopy in treatment, it is important to remember that an arthroscope is a tool with certain advantages and limitations. This tool does not alter the basic principles of anterior acromioplasty or its indications.

In considering the pros and cons of arthroscopic anterior acromioplasty, it eliminates the need for a skin incision and makes a much smaller opening in the deltoid muscle. This shortens the hospital stay and eliminates the need for pampering the anterior deltoid, as is usually done for two or three weeks after open acromioplasty. On the side of open anterior acromioplasty, it permits a more thorough subacromial decompression and evaluation of the rotator cuff. If a tear of the rotator cuff is encountered, it can be repaired, and this cannot be done through an arthroscope.

The arthroscope is currently being used by some surgeons for trimming the frayed edges of incomplete tears on the assumption that this might hasten the healing of the tear. No proof has been given that trimming the edges of incomplete traumatic tears has hastened or improved the quality of healing over that accomplished by simple rest. In the case of small traumatic tears (see p. 65), most of these lesions are capable of spontaneous healing without freshening the edges.

It is generally agreed that arthroscopy has little place in the treatment of complete tears of the rotator cuff. Ellman first described arthroscopic anterior acromioplasty. I had the privilege of discussing his initial paper in 1985[60] as well as his present (1988)[76] series of 169 "arthroscopic decompressions." In this last series, 39 patients had tears of the rotator cuff and 130 had no tear but had decompressions because of six to twelve months of persistent symptoms. Of the 39 cuff tears, 10 were incomplete. The longest follow-up was three years. Ellman's results were objectively reported and could be compared with our ongoing operative series.

First, regarding the group with an intact cuff, these patients were generally younger and were usually classified as having a chronic Stage II impingement lesion. They generally did well. Ellman has been more conservative in performing arthroscopic decompression in this group than most arthroscopists; however, as discussed on page 93 and page 98, I am even more conservative. I rarely perform any type of decompression in the under 40 age group because most of our patients recover on conservative treatment prior to the 12 months disability required for surgical bursectomy and coracoacromial ligament section. I very rarely perform an anterior acromioplasty in this younger age group because the acromial epiphysis may normally remain open until age 30 years, making anterior acromioplasty seemingly undesirable prior to that age unless there is a definite bony abnormality at the acromion. There appears to be a place for removing thickened bursa and scar with an arthroscope ("arthroscopic bursectomy") in the occasional patient in the younger age group who is truly disabled.

In comparing Dr. Ellman's results of arthroscopic debridement and anterior acromioplasty in 39 cuff tears with those of the 233 primary repairs in our Series II, the results of surgical anterior acromioplasty and primary repair were quite superior. The ages of the patients in the two series were similar: 37 to 84 years (average 65 years) in the Ellman series, and 22 to 83 years (average 59 years) in our Series II. In the arthroscopic series overall, only 1 result was "excellent," 9 of the 10 with incomplete tears were "satisfactory," and 15 (55 percent) of the 29 with complete tears were "satisfactory." Arthroscopic debridement and acromioplasty in 6 massive tears were of special interest to me because I hoped that this procedure might be of value for an elderly, poor operative risk group with intractable pain. At follow-up (which was short), Dr. Ellman found that these six patients had less pain but still had pain and neither range of motion nor strength was improved. Of the results in Series II, described on page 75, overall 81 percent were "excellent," all 30 with incomplete tears were "excellent," and 90 percent of those with complete tears (of which 145 were massive) were "excellent" or "satisfactory." Dr. Ellman obtained the overall results of arthroscopic anterior acromioplasty and cuff debridement of two other arthroscopists, and their combined results for complete tears were similar. Most investigators agree there is little place for the arthroscopic treatment of complete tears.

I prefer open anterior acromioplasty to arthroscopic anterior acromioplasty for three reasons. First, in its present state, arthroscopic acromioplasty is not a shorter or less difficult procedure. Second, it does not permit repair of the rotator cuff if a tear is encountered. Third, the quality of the decompression seems to be inferior, probably owing to difficulty in visualization; estimating depth; possible uncontrollable bleeding; and failure to remove fragments, bone dust, and debris (see Fig. 2–40).

TREATMENT OF NON-OUTLET IMPINGEMENT LESIONS

Treatment of Impingement Due to Prominence of the Greater Tuberosity

The treatment of impingement due to prominence of the greater tuberosity differs depending on whether there is malunion or nonunion of a retracted greater tuberosity fragment, a varus malunion at the surgical neck level, or low placement of the humeral component in an arthroplasty. All differ from outlet impingement, and acromioplasty alone is usually inadequate.

Surgery is indicated for persistent pain and disability when an adequate trial of conservative treatment based on stretching exercises has failed. The impingement injection test may help in the pre-operative assessment of these lesions. The procedure for malunion of the greater tuberosity, the procedure for varus malunion of the surgical neck, and the procedure for low placement of the humeral component are described in Chapter 5, page 397 and Figure 5–34.

Treatment of Loss of the Head Depressors

As has been discussed, the principal humeral head depressors are the rotator cuff and the long head of the biceps. Rupture of the rotator cuff allows the head to ascend, increasing the problem of impingement. Both the pain and the wear of the tendons may be escalated, and the logical treatment for this problem is a repair of the rotator cuff performed with adequate anterior acromioplasty (see Fig. 2–41). Rupture of the long head of the biceps may also escalate impingement; and because a repair of this tendon that is effective in stabilizing the humeral head cannot be achieved, the only treatment, to date, is anterior acromioplasty with or without tenodesis of the long head to the humerus.

Treatment of Impingement Due to Loss of the Fulcrum Action of the Glenohumeral Joint

Translocation of the humerus upward occurs when the articular surfaces of the humeral head or glenoid have been destroyed such as by rheumatoid arthritis, trauma, or surgical removal of the hu-

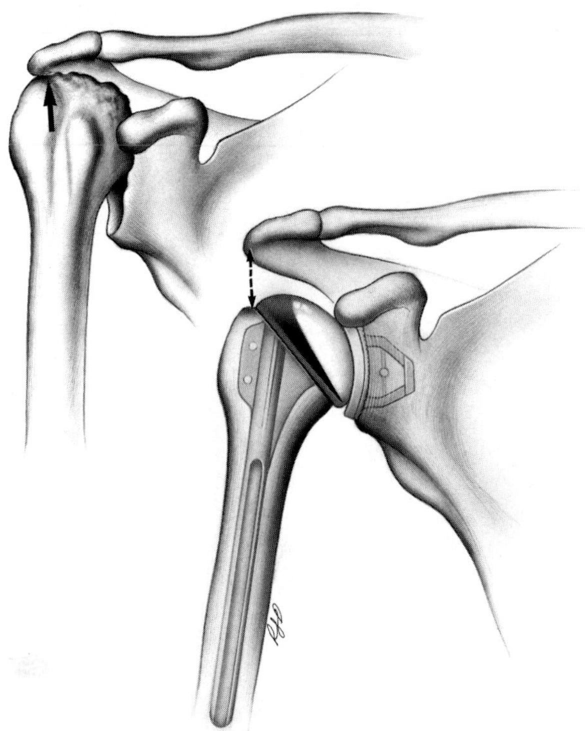

Figure 2–54. An example of "non-outlet impingement" (see Table 2–1) requiring treatment other than anterior acromioplasty. Impingement caused by loss of the humeral head is treated with a replacement arthroplasty rather than an anterior acromioplasty.

meral head. Restoration of the stability and fulcrum action of the glenohumeral joint is required to correct this type of impingement problem. This is done by positioning the prosthetic articular components so that the combination of the length and height of the head prevents upward displacement of the tuberosities, as described in Chapter 3, Figure 3–26; and illustrated in Figure 2–54.

The treatment of impingement caused by glenohumeral instability is elimination of the cause of the dislocations or subluxations, as described in Chapter 4; and not anterior acromioplasty (see Fig. 2–31).

Treatment of Impingement Caused by Loss of the Suspensory Mechanism

Abnormalities of the suspensory mechanism include complete acromioclavicular separations and paralysis of the trapezius muscle. Both can cause impingement as a result of impaired rotation of the scapula (see Figs. 1–1, 1–13, and 1–14; p. 449). Each patient should be carefully evaluated to determine which of several types of pain is present, as discussed on page 349 and in Figure 4–63.

Treatment of Old Acromioclavicular Dislocations

The surgical procedures for old acromioclavicular dislocations are discussed in detail in Chapter 4, pages 347 to 355.

Treatment of Impingement Due to Unfused Acromial Epiphysis

The axillary view, which is part of the preoperative x-ray routine study for cuff tears (see Fig. 2–28), is excellent for recognizing this lesion[24, 62–64] and for estimating its size. The possible configurations of the acromion are shown in Figure 2–55. The unfused epiphyseal center may be stable without symptoms and without impinging; however, when it is associated with a tear of the rotator cuff, it is usually moveable and flail. This makes a

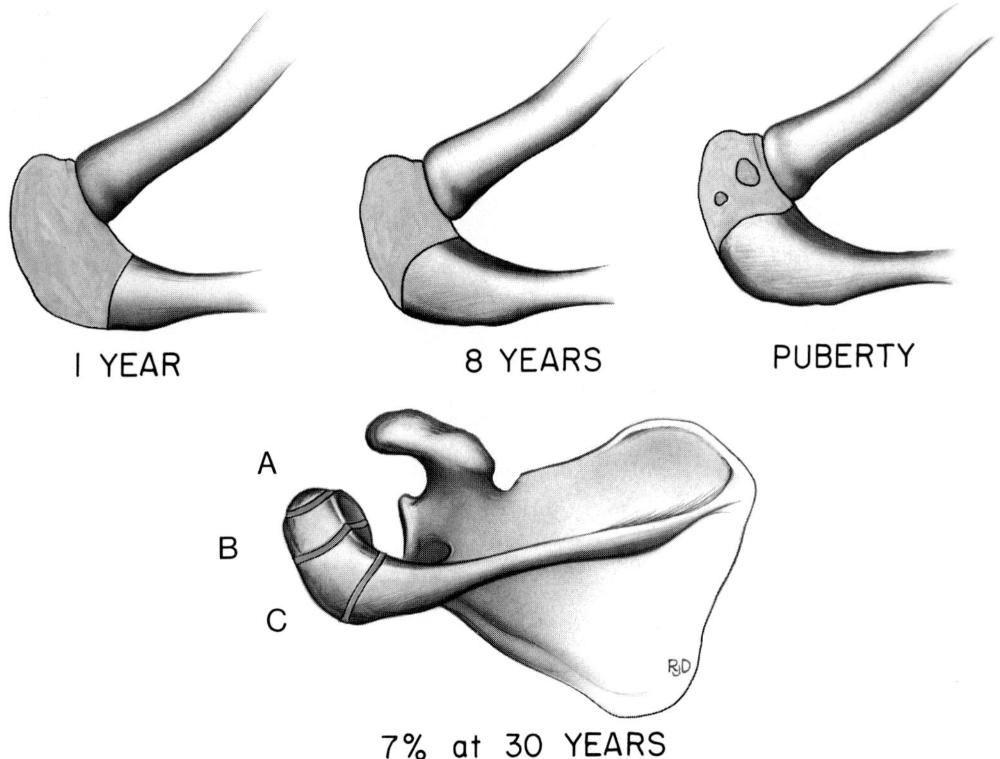

Figures 2–55 through 2–57. ***Treatment of Unfused Anterior Acromial Epiphysis***

Figure 2–55. Diagram of the development of the anterior acromion and the types of unfused ossification centers that may persist after age 30 years. A, Pre-acromion. B, Meso-acromion. C, Meta-acromion. Meso-acromion is the most common and requires epiphysiodesis. Pre-acromion is the second most common and may be treated by excision.

standard anterior acromioplasty impossible. The unfused center must be excised or stabilized to relieve impingement. This must be done in such a way as to preserve the origin of the deltoid and allow passive exercises soon after the operation to avoid adhesions. Small unfused segments may be excised, but larger centers require epiphysiodesis in a position that holds the unfused center cephalically so that it no longer impinges on the rotator cuff. Excision of a large unfused center would create the same problem as radical acromionectomy (see Fig. 2–46).

Surgical Technique

When the unfused center is *small*, as shown in Figure 2–56A, excision is carried out by sharp dissection, staying very close to bone to preserve the tendinous origin of the deltoid. The undersurface of the remaining acromion is then beveled to eliminate overhang, and the tendinous stump of the deltoid origin is sutured directly to the acromion. Alternatively, the epiphyseal plate may be excised and the small fragment sutured directly to the acromion, as in Figure 2–56B.

When there is a *large* unstable ossification center, as in Figure 2–57A, epiphysiodesis is required to hold the ossification center cephalically away from the rotator cuff. It is surprisingly difficult to obtain bone union across this epiphysis. The epiphyseal plate must be excised to raw bone on each side, and internal fixation must be carefully performed. Regardless of the type of fixation, it is important to have completed the cuff repair prior to attempting the fixation of the acromion. Fixation with smooth Steinmann pins usually fails. Compression screws are effective if there is sufficient bone; however, the fragments are usually too small and soft to permit this. Tension band technique using two smooth wires and a nonmetallic suture (Fig. 2–57B and C) may be considered when the bone is of poor quality. Bone grafts are taken locally to cross the epiphyseal plate.

The aftercare program is the same as that following other repairs of the rotator cuff but with more care taken to avoid forced elevation of the humerus against the anterior acromion until union across the epiphysis occurs. Rotation of the humerus does not disturb the epiphyseal repair as much as the extremes of elevation. The progress of healing is followed with axillary views and CT scans. Strengthening exercises are deferred until early bony union is present. The results of these procedures have been surprisingly disappointing.

Treatment of Impingement Caused by Malunion or Nonunion of the Acromion or Erb's Palsy Deformities of the Acromion

These lesions (see Fig. 2–11B) are considered separate from outlet impingement. Nonunion and

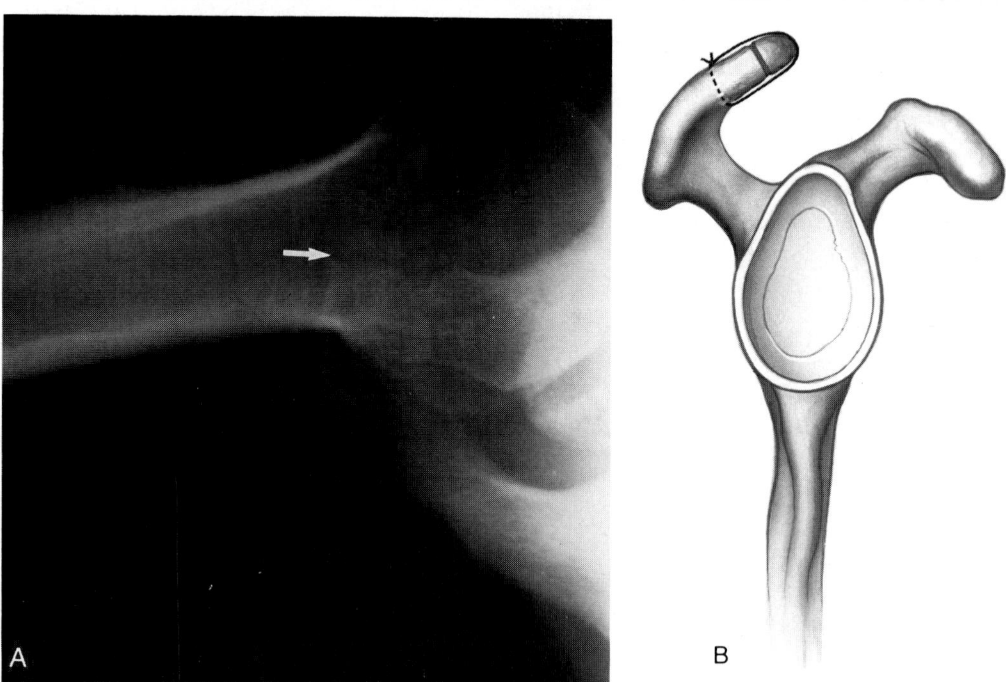

Figure 2–56. Axillary view (A) showing a small (pre-acromial) center (arrow), as is amenable to excision or epiphysiodesis by direct suture (B).

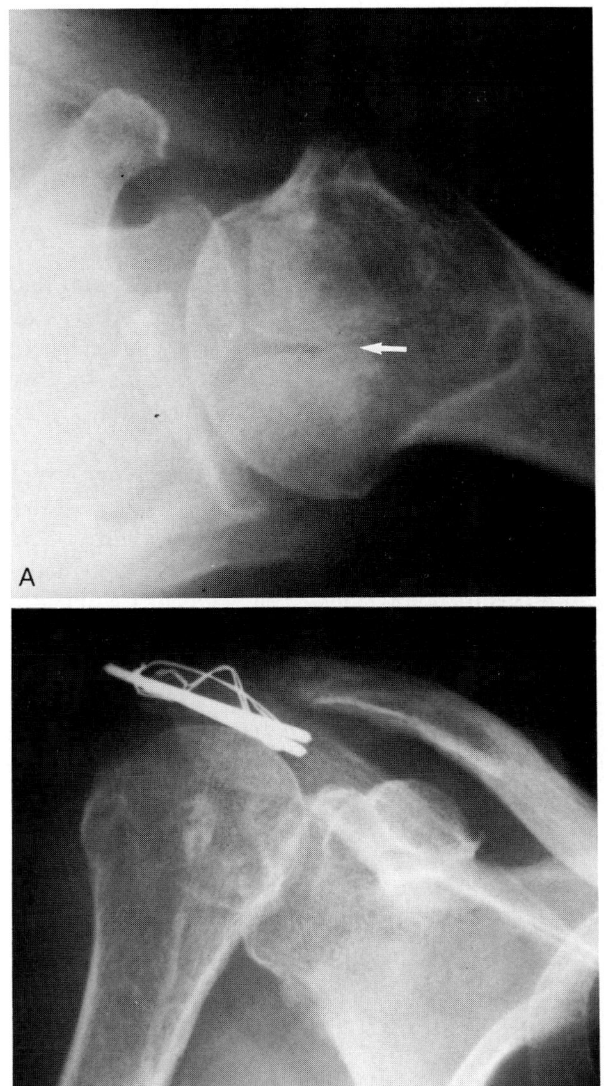

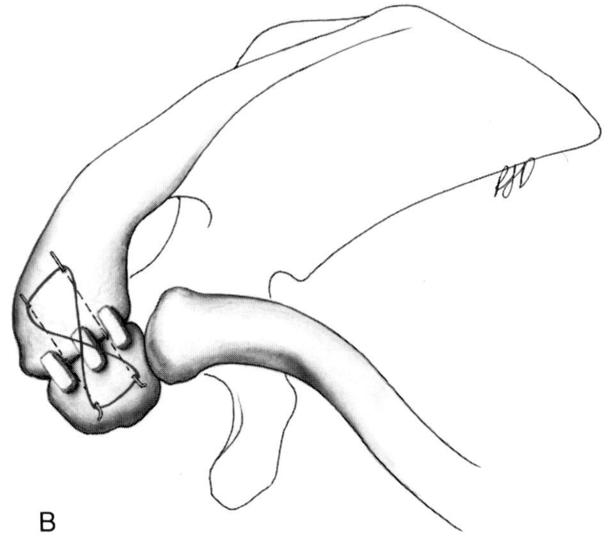

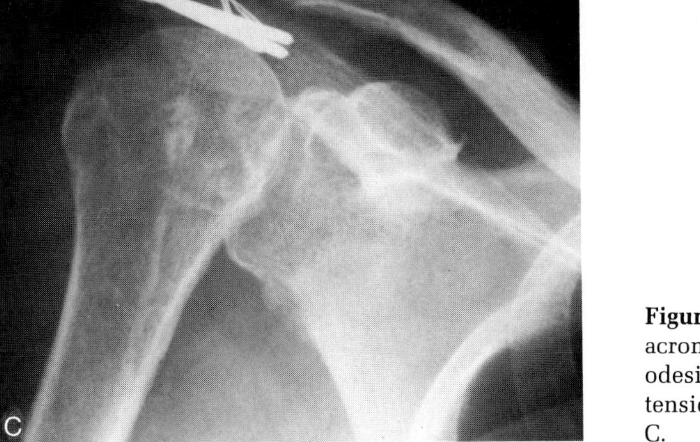

Figure 2–57. Axillary view (A) showing a large (meso-acromial) center (arrow), which requires epiphysiodesis rather than excision, as was attempted with a tension band and local bone grafts as shown in B and C.

malunion of the acromion are associated with soft tissue injury and scarring from trauma. Treatment is described in Chapter 5. The Erb's palsy deformity is associated with other skeletal deformities of the coracoid and proximal humerus as well as muscle deficits, and the procedures for it are described in Chapter 3 and Chapter 6.

CALCIUM DEPOSITS ARE *NOT* PRIMARILY IMPINGEMENT LESIONS

Calcium deposits in the rotator cuff are considered elsewhere (see Chapter 6, p. 427), rather than with impingement lesions, because they are believed to be due to an injury or localized vascular impairment within the tendon rather than to impingement. They are considered to be unrelated to impingement for the following reasons:

1. Calcium deposits more frequently occur in the middle-aged group (between 40 and 60 years of age) and are rare after age 65 rather than becoming more prevalent with aging.
2. They may involve any tendon of the rotator cuff, such as the subscapularis, teres minor, and infraspinatus. They are not restricted to the impingement area—i.e., the insertion of the supraspinatus tendon.
3. Deposits often disappear spontaneously or after "needling" without residual symptoms of impingement. If impingement had been present, symptoms would be expected to continue.
4. Calcium deposits are rarely associated with tears of rotator cuff or biceps lesions, as would be expected if impingement was present.

I believe calcium deposits are best explained by local injury of some type that causes impairment of circulation within the tendon with degeneration and altered chemistry precipitating a deposit of calcium soaps.

Anterior acromioplasty at the time of calcium removal has been tried sufficiently to convince me that it retards recovery rather than hastening it or enhancing the result. I do not believe that anterior acromioplasty has a role in the treatment of calcium deposits other than perhaps for the very rare lesion that is associated with an impingement tear of the rotator cuff.

Calcium Deposits with Cuff Tears

The coexistence of calcium deposits and cuff tears is surprisingly infrequent; however, it is an oversimplification to say that they never occur together. Some patients with calcium deposits have been denied arthrograms too long, resulting in excessive delay in the diagnosis of a cuff lesion. This does not happen very often, and the presence of a calcium deposit is generally evidence against a cuff tear being present; however, when the response to conservative treatment has been inadequate and the signs suggest the possibility of a cuff tear, an arthrogram is advised. One patient, an expert golfer, had a large calcium deposit in the infraspinatus tendon of the left shoulder that led to an infraspinatus tear. This tear was not diagnosed for years, resulting in permanent weakness of the infraspinatus.

3

GLENOHUMERAL ARTHROPLASTY

The most dramatic advance in shoulder surgery in the last half century has been the introduction of replacement arthroplasty. Codman, who did more than anyone before him to show the importance of ruptures of the supraspinatus tendon, thought that glenohumeral arthritis was insignificant. In 1934 he wrote:

> I doubt whether cartilage erosion occurs in the shoulder joint unless the supraspinatus has been damaged or when suppurative inflammation, which is rare in this joint, has occurred. . . . I have never seen a monarticular arthritis in this joint sufficiently severe to cause deformity.[6]

Since that time, many causes of glenohumeral incongruity have been delineated, and shoulder arthroplasty has now almost entirely eliminated glenohumeral arthrodesis and resection (see Table 3–1). Both the surgical technique and the aftercare of shoulder arthroplasty are made difficult by the peculiar anatomy of the rotator cuff; however, the results of properly performed shoulder arthroplasties are superior to those of arthroplasties of other joints, not only in range of motion and function but also in durability.

DESIGN

Background

When I was a resident in orthopaedic surgery at the New York Orthopaedic, Columbia-Presbyterian Medical Center, the only procedures used to treat problems of the glenohumeral joint were fusions or resections to manage tuberculosis, infections, and old injuries. I became interested in severely displaced fracture-dislocations of the proximal humerus and made a study of lesions of this type that had been treated by our Fracture Service with open reduction and internal fixation, closed reduction, and removal of the humeral head. The results were unsatisfactory.[12] Reduction was usually followed by avascular necrosis because the humeral head was devoid of soft-tissue attachments. Arthrodesis was made difficult by the associated fragmentation and displacement of the tuberosities. Excision of the humeral head, regardless of whether or not the tuberosities were attached to the shaft, resulted in a flail joint that lacked a fulcrum for rotation and caused the upper humerus to impinge against the acromion during attempts to raise the arm (Fig. 3–1). After resection of the humeral head, the shoulder characteristically remained uncomfortable for many months until ankylosis by fibrosis tissue or bone finally took place. Replacement of the articular surface with a prosthesis presented a logical solution. The initial prosthesis was designed for the treatment of injuries. This technique was encouraged by my Chief, Doctor William Darrach.

The original prosthesis for the articular surface of the proximal humerus was designed in 1951, (Fig. 3–2). I was very fortunate to obtain the help of the good people from Austinal Laboratories, who had made the molds according to my specifications obtained from measuring 50 dried, adult humeri. It was good fortune also that the prosthesis was made of cast cobalt-chrome alloy (Vitallium), which at that time was becoming recognized as a strong and inert material for the internal fixation of fractures. In a talk given at the New York Academy of Medicine, I explained that the criteria in selecting materials for joint replacement were (1) strength, (2) inertness, and (3) resiliency and elasticity approaching that of bone. The cast cobalt-chrome alloy had the first two qualities but had the disadvantage of stiffness. Nevertheless, it has since proved to be an outstanding material for joint replacement.

For historical completeness, I will briefly describe a recent translation from the French literature into English by an Italian surgeon (Lugli), which was published in 1978.[132] This article made me aware for the first time that a replacement of the entire proximal half of the humerus had been performed in France in 1893. This prosthesis had been designed and fabricated by a French dentist, Michaels, and had been implanted in an infected, draining tuberculous lesion of the upper humerus by Pean, a French surgeon. The infection and drainage continued after the operation, and after several further surgical procedures, the prosthesis was removed. This replacement of the upper half of the humerus, with anchorage to the scapula and without reconstruction of the muscles, was an effort to control infection and could not be considered an arthroplasty. Certainly, replacement of the upper humerus would not be considered for this indication today. Lugli thought this implant merited reporting because he believed it was the first

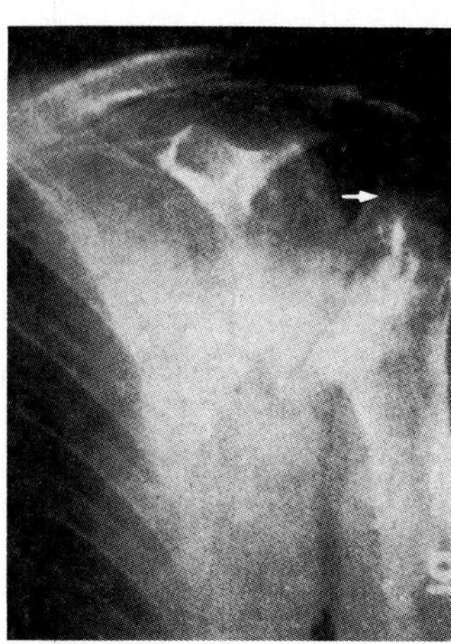

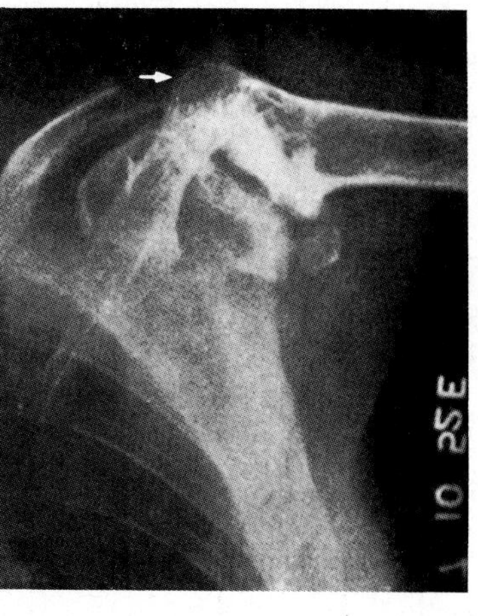

Figure 3–1. The original prosthesis as designed in 1951. A follow-up study of fracture-dislocations treated by removal of the humeral head showed that the shoulder lacked a fulcrum for motion and the greater tuberosity impinged against the acromion on attempts to raise the arm (arrows). (From Neer, C. S., II, Brown, T. H., Jr., and McLaughlin, H. L. Fractures of the humerus with dislocation of the head fragment. Am. J. Surg. 85:252, 1953.)

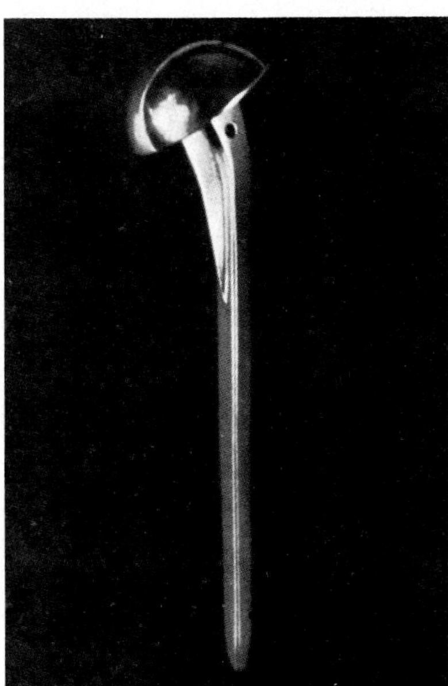

Figure 3–2. The initial prosthesis was designed to cope with this problem. (From Neer, C. S., II, Brown, T. H., Jr., and McLaughlin, H. L. Fractures of the humerus with dislocation of the head fragment. Am. J. Surg. *85*:252, 1953.)

implant of any kind to replace any part of the skeletal system or any other part of the body. He gave Michaels, the dentist, credit for the design and construction of the implant. Another dentist brought the implant to the United States, where it was on display at the Smithsonian Institution as an achievement of early dental science. I was unaware of the existence of this device until 1985.

Original Design

The initial shoulder prosthesis for replacing the proximal humeral surface is shown in Figure 3–2. The first clinical series was published in 1955[42, 48] and consisted of seven recent fracture-dislocations, five old fractures with malunion and avascular necrosis, and one case of degenerative arthritis (later [in 1961[68] and 1974[2]] identified as "primary osteoarthritis"). By that time the prosthesis had been modified with multiple diameters of the stem for better press-fit. Soon, holes were introduced in the flanges for ingrowth of bone (Fig. 3–3). Drill specifications were provided to assist in the preparation of the medullary canal to receive the implant.

It has always been my opinion that a joint replacement operation should retain as much of the normal anatomy as possible.[22, 47, 117, 125] The head of the prosthesis was designed with a 44 mm. radius of curve, which was the average of the measurements of the dried bones. The head of this prosthesis was made like an umbrella to fit over bone with minimal removal of bone and to permit adjustments in the length of the head (tuberosity-glenoid distance). The tuberosities and rotator cuff were left intact or, when fractured, were re-attached under the prosthesis to preserve normal anatomy. The initial head was flattened slightly on top to allow more space for the supraspinatus tendon.

I used this prosthesis during a 20-year period,

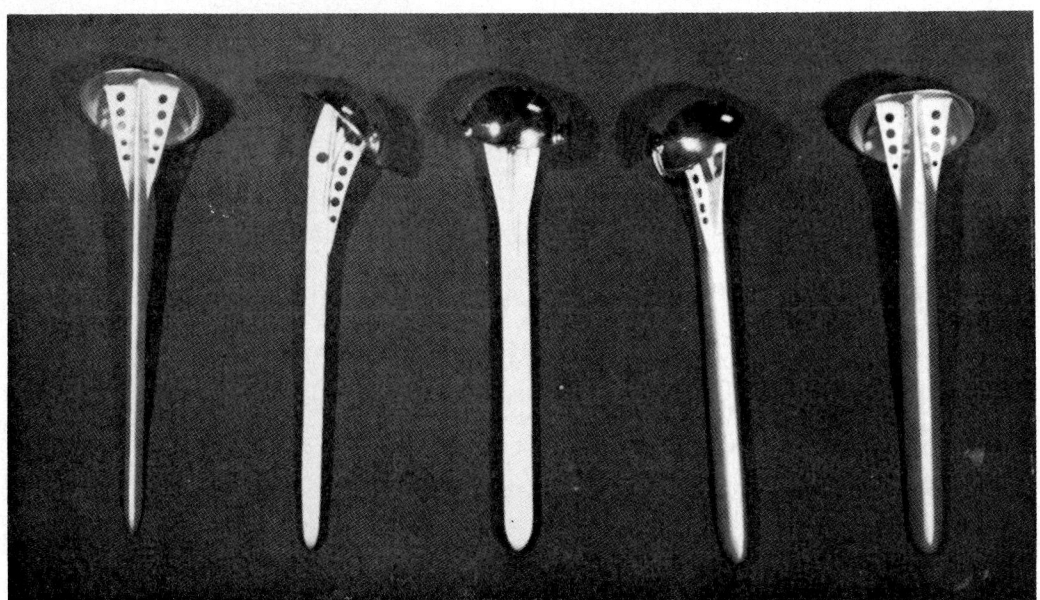

Figure 3–3. The initial prosthesis was modified within five years by adding multiple diameters of stem and fenestrations in the flanges. Thus, the Neer I system introduced to implant surgery (1) multiple diameters of stem for a better press-fit, and (2) holes for the ingrowth of bone. (Reproduced by permission from Sisk, T. D.: Fractures of shoulder girdle and upper extremity. *In* Crenshaw, A. H. (ed.): Campbell's Operative Orthopaedics, 7th ed. St. Louis, 1982, The C. V. Mosby Co.)

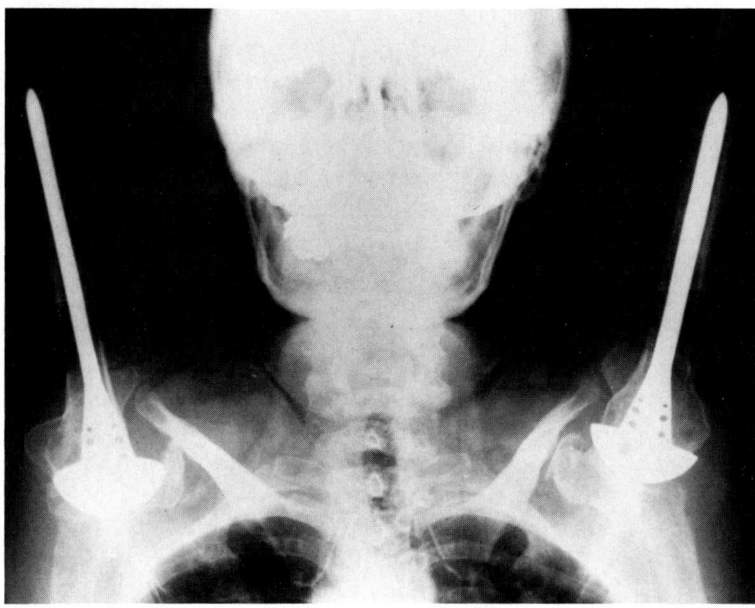

Figure 3–4. The Neer I system was durable (several implants have been in place for more than 30 years), and when there were good muscles and a good glenoid, an excellent functional result could be obtained.

until 1973, and it is still preferred by some surgeons. There was never a problem of loosening of the stem of this prosthesis provided it was set firmly in the medullary canal at the time of insertion. When there was a good rotator cuff, a good deltoid muscle, and a good rehabilitation regimen, an excellent result could be obtained (Fig. 3–4). Patients could engage in all types of activity, including farming and carpentry, without breakage, loosening, or painful glenoid erosion. Several of my patients have been followed for over 30 years, and I have never been required to convert any of these procedures to a total shoulder arthroplasty because of deterioration of the glenoid. Because of this experience, I continue to use the humeral component alone without a glenoid component when the articular surface of the glenoid is normal. Erosion of the glenoid does occur if the shoulder is stiff, causing the articular surfaces to bear constantly against each other in one area, and I have been required to perform conversion of this implant used by others because of stems that were loose at the time of insertion and because of glenoid erosion associated with stiffness and constant pressure of the prosthesis on the glenoid.

Fixed-Fulcrum Designs

The functional results of humeral head arthroplasty were not as good when either the rotator cuff or the deltoid muscle was inadequate or when the articular surface of the glenoid was abnormal. Therefore, in 1970 the use of acrylic cement to anchor prosthetic components as introduced by Charnley[266–268] was applied to the fixation of glenoid components. I chose initially to use a fixed-fulcrum design because it might eliminate the need for reconstruction of the rotator cuff and simplify the operation and its aftercare. I designed three types of fixed-fulcrum total shoulder implants with the help of Robert G. Averill (Figs. 3–5 through 3–8). In the first design, the ball was made oversized to allow more motion, but this was soon discarded

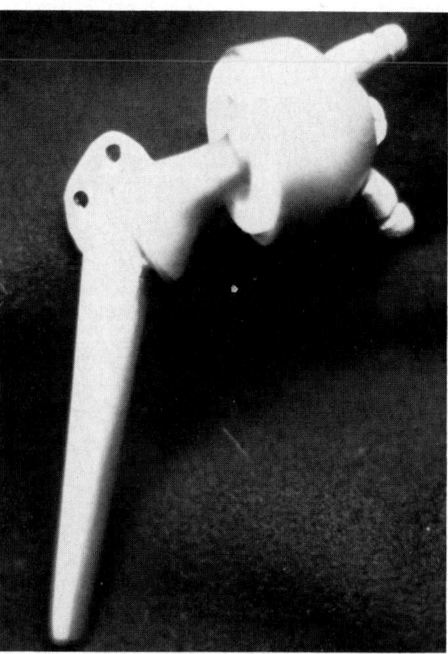

Figure 3–5. Several constrained, fixed-fulcrum implants (see also Figs. 3–6, 3–7, and 3–8) were developed between 1970 and 1973 in the hope that they would solve the problem of an inadequate rotator cuff or glenoid. Fixed-fulcrum implants were abandoned in 1974. This figure shows a 1970 prototype.

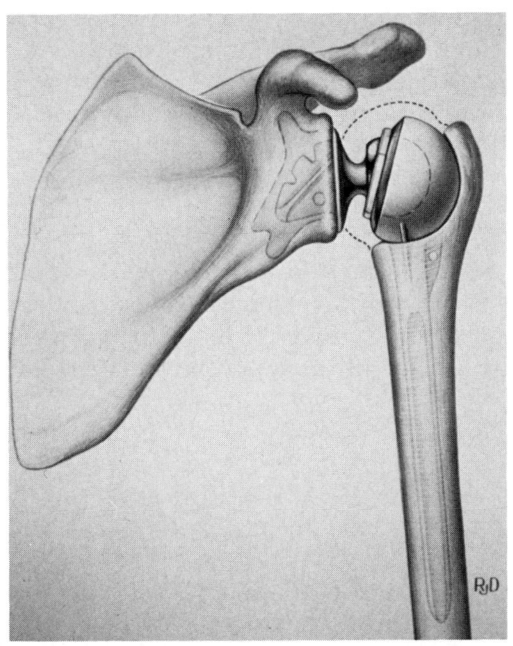

Figure 3–6. The Mark I system had a larger ball that allowed more motion, but the large head precluded re-attachment of the rotator cuff.

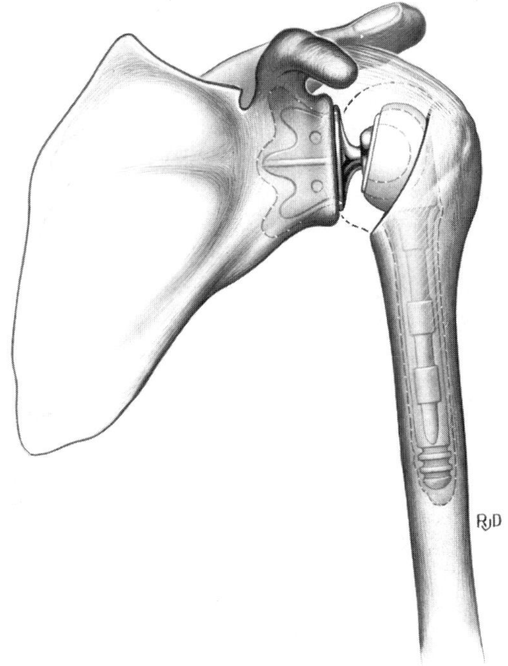

Figure 3–7. The Mark III system introduced the concept of axial rotation in the shaft of the humerus to eliminate rotary constraint and permit use of a small ball, allowing re-attachment of the rotator cuff.

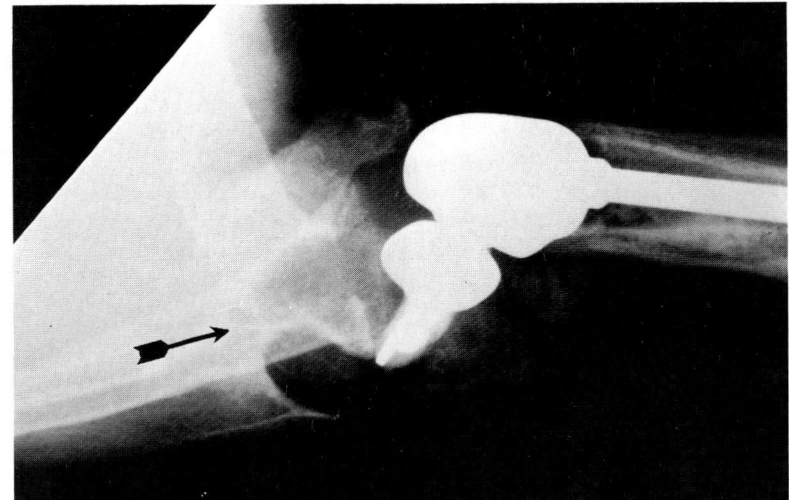

Figure 3–8. Axillary view showing how the last patient with a Mark III implant pulled the prosthesis out of the glenoid (arrow) when leaning on his arm to get out of bed. This accident occurred despite effective rotation without constraint provided by the polyethylene sleeve cemented in the shaft that allowed the metal stem to rotate inside the humerus.

because the large ball made it impossible to re-attach the rotator cuff to the humerus. A second design with a smaller ball allowed re-attachment of the cuff, but introduced a greater threat of mechanical failure because the small ball limited the excursion of movement. The third fixed-fulcrum design introduced axial rotation in the stem of the prosthesis, allowing rotation of the shaft of the humerus on the stem of the prosthesis. Despite this improvement, one of the patients soon dislodged the prosthesis from the scapula when leaning on the arm to get out of bed (Fig. 3–8).

Furthermore, these patients demonstrated that use of a fixed-fulcrum implant cannot eliminate the need for re-attaching the infraspinatus. The infraspinatus supplies 90 per cent of the power needed for external rotation; without it, active motion was disappointing (see Figs. 1–21 and 1–23). I concluded that because of the mechanical force applied to the frail scapula, the only safe fixed-fulcrum prosthesis was one buried in dense scar tissue to protect it from breakage and loosening, and second, that a fixed-fulcrum implant did not eliminate the need for re-attaching and rehabilitating the rotator cuff. Other surgeons agree.[100, 131] I have not used a constrained, fixed-fulcrum prosthesis since 1974.

The "Neer-II" System

In 1973 we re-designed the humeral component to conform to a glenoid component (Figs. 3–9 and 3–10). Kenmore[123] and Zippel[124] independently had already used polyethylene glenoid com-

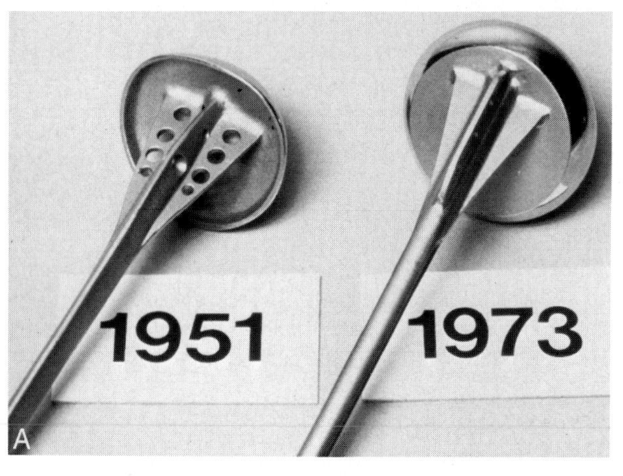

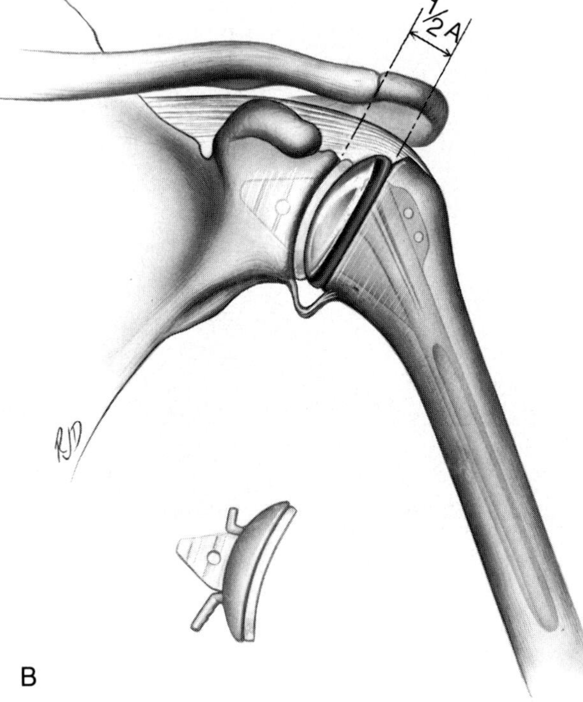

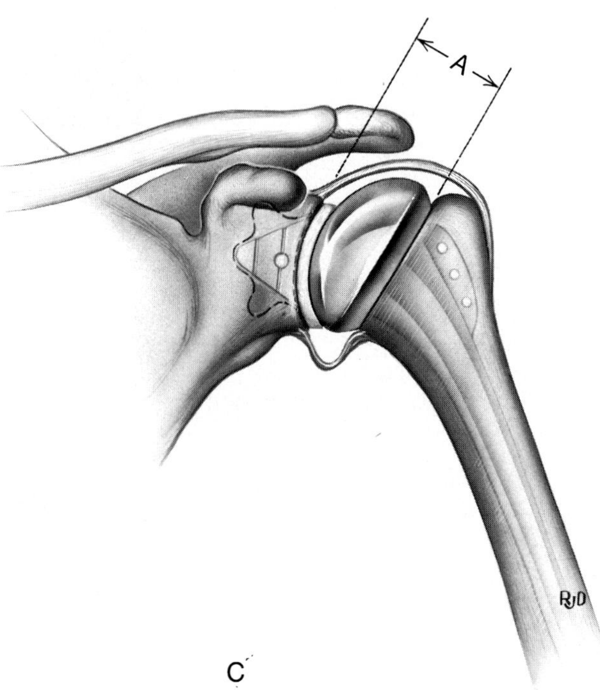

Figure 3–9A and B. Re-design of the humeral component in 1973. A, The humeral component was made to conform to a polyethylene glenoid component. B, The short head humeral component is shown in B with a 200 percent glenoid component that was used developmentally when the rotator cuff or superior part of the glenoid was deficient. C, The long head humeral component is shown with a standard polyethylene glenoid component.

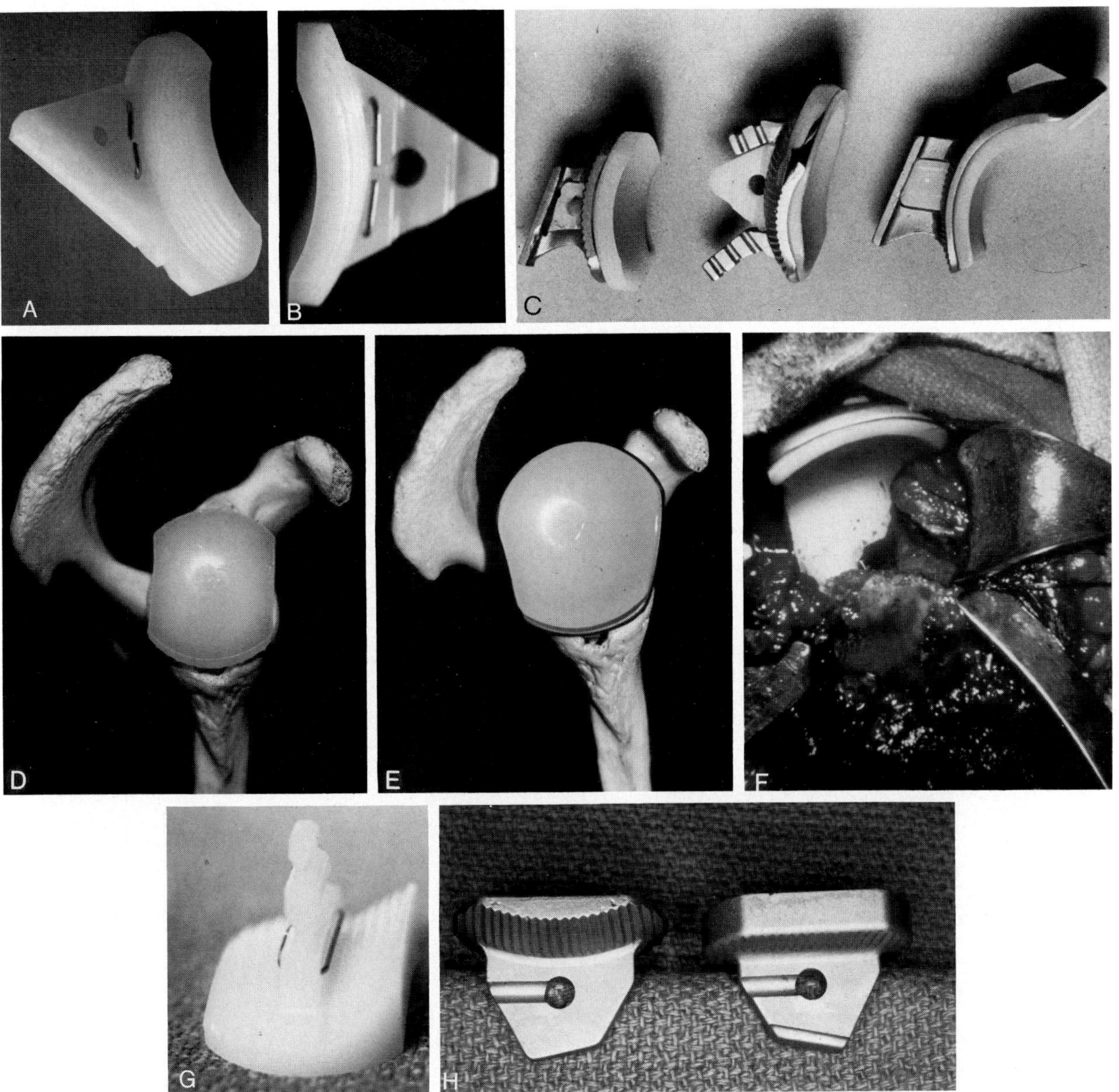

Figure 3–10A–H. Some of the glenoid components that led up to development of the present Neer II system (see Fig. 3–11).

A, The initial glenoid component required a one-quarter inch drill hole and slot, making it secure but difficult to implant.

B, The standard polyethylene component was used satisfactorily in many shoulders. It was recently modified by removing the proximal groove (see Fig. 3–11B).

C, Three early metal-backed glenoid components.

D, Standard metal-backed glenoid component, approximately the size of a normal glenoid. This was the preferred component.

E, Two hundred percent glenoid component (allows closing of the cuff). Anchoring device has been re-designed twice. Rarely used.

F, Six hundred percent glenoid component precluded reattaching the supraspinatus. Now abandoned.

G, Augmented polyethylene glenoid component was used successfully a few times in elderly, inactive patients, but it was never used in active younger patients.

H, Thin-keel metal-backed (left) and flat-back metal-backed (right) components were designed for special problems of deep wear or flattening of the glenoid.

ponents with my original humeral component. I thought it best to retain the normal, anatomical size of the humeral head with its 44 mm. radius of curve but to re-design it to eliminate the edges that might encroach on a glenoid component and to eliminate the flattened top. The stem of this component was re-designed to be used with cement. The radius of curve of the glenoid component was made to conform to that of the humeral head (unlike the larger radius of curve of a normal glenoid). Since the cup-like head had been used retaining various lengths of the humeral neck to determine the tuberosity–glenoid distance and was being eliminated because it might dig into the articular surface of the glenoid, the new humeral component was made with two lengths of head. The stem of the new humeral component was tapered slightly (smaller at the tip) to facilitate its removal from cement. Three diameters of stem were thought to be adequate because they could be used with cement (Fig. 3–11). This was named the "Neer II" system. The humeral component could be used without a glenoid component and, if a secure press-fit could be obtained, might be used without acrylic cement. The holding device of the initial glenoid component was difficult to insert and was soon changed. Several other types of glenoid components were used.

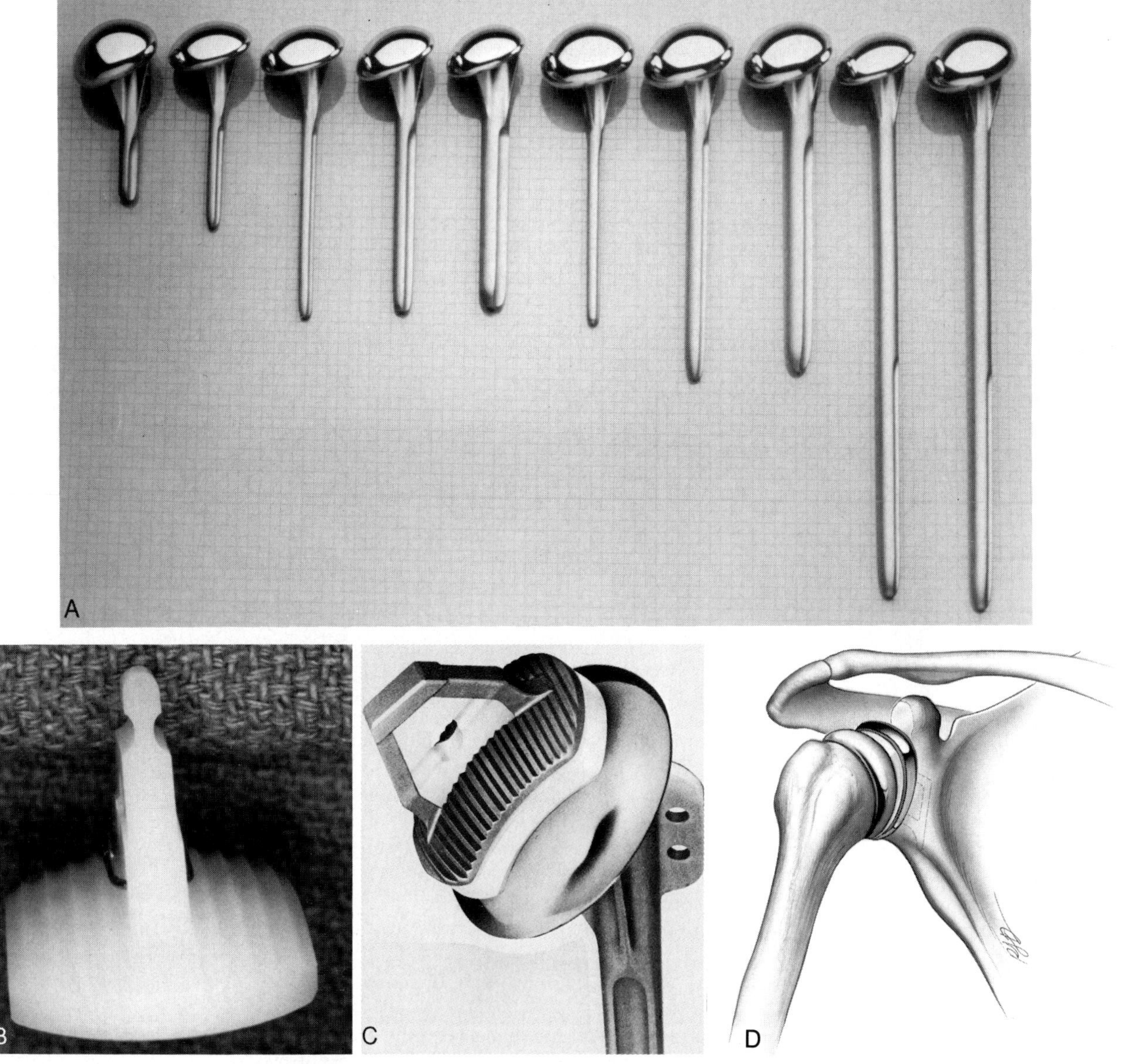

Figure 3–11. The current Neer II system (in general use).

A, Humeral components with two diameters of stem, two lengths of head, and three lengths of stem.

B, Standard polyethylene component.

C, Standard metal-backed component.

D, Revised 200 percent glenoid component.

A Food and Drug Administration field test of this implant was conducted for eight years before it was released for general use. Doctors Richard L. Cruess of Montreal, Clement B. Sledge of Boston, and Alan H. Wilde of Cleveland participated in this test. A preliminary report was made to the American Orthopaedic Association in 1977.[20] I made a detailed report to the American Academy of Orthopaedic Surgeons of my experience with this implant and five different glenoid components in 1981.[22] The standard humeral and glenoid components were made available for general use in 1982.

During the years 1973 to 1988, I used eleven different glenoid components developmentally (Fig. 3–10). Hooded glenoid components with a 200 per cent and 600 per cent overhang were designed, the objective being to give constraint against ascent of the head and yet allow the components to dislocate rather than pull out of the bone if a violent force, such as a hard fall, was applied. It was hoped that a glenoid component with overhang superiorly might give the desired constraint for special situations when the rotator cuff was severely deficient. I have concluded that too much overhang of the glenoid component precludes closure of the rotator cuff, creates a greater risk of mechanical failure because of constraint, and should not be used. I find it helpful to have available a slightly oversized glenoid component when there is severe bone loss, as in some patients with cuff-tear arthropathy, severe rheumatoid arthritis, or failed previous surgery (see Figs. 3–11D and 3–28E3). However, it is usually very difficult to implant even the standard-sized glenoid component when there is severe bone deficiency, and,

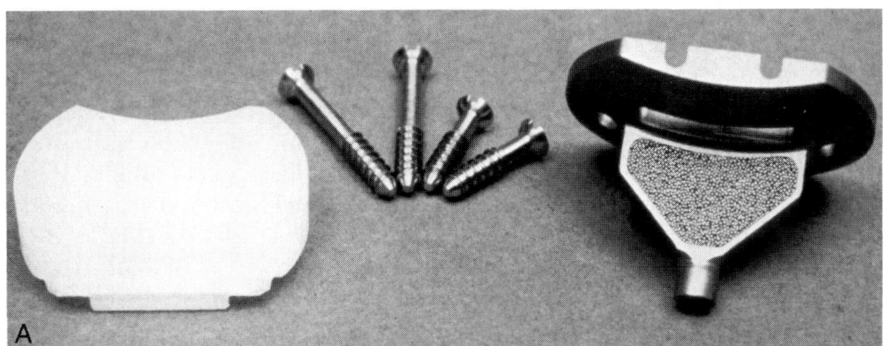

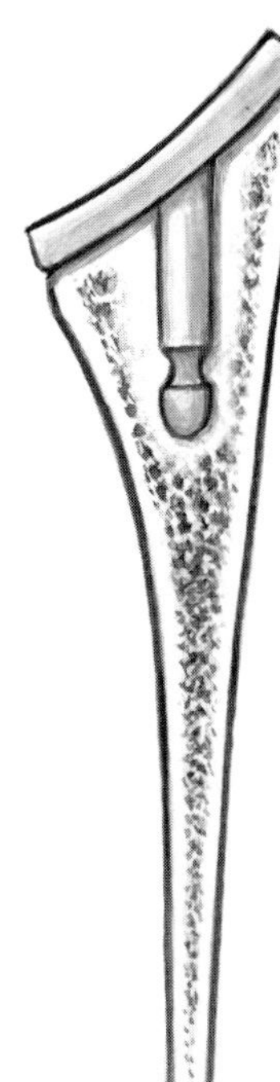

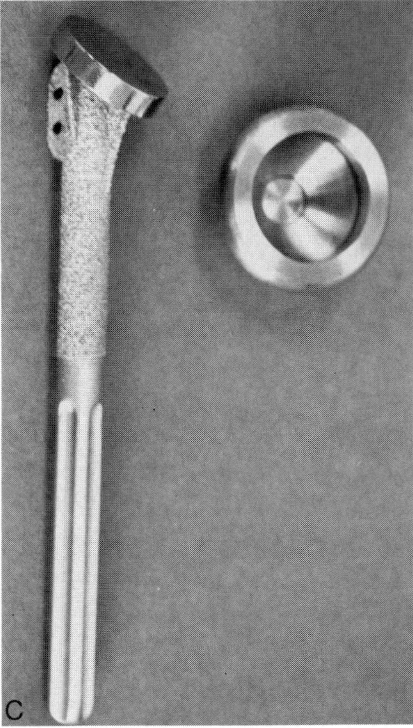

Figure 3–12. Current developmental components under consideration but untested.

A, Surface ingrowth glenoid component has been considered for developmental use for three years but has not yet been implanted.

B, Angulated stem for uneven glenoid bone loss (see Fig. 3–28).

C, Developmental modular humeral component, about which there are several reservations.

because an oversized glenoid component may interfere with repair of the rotator cuff, even a slightly oversized glenoid component is rarely used. I almost always prefer a glenoid component about the size of a normal glenoid because it does not interfere with cuff repair. If there is too much destruction of the rotator cuff or bone to allow a full exercise program, I use a "limited goals rehabilitation" program to obtain stability, as described in Figure 7–14. It must be remembered that scapular rotation usually occurs early when the rotator cuff is weak, making an overhanging glenoid component ineffective in preventing ascent of the head. Some current developmental components under consideration but untested are shown in Figure 3–12. Neither modular design nor surface ingrowth has been proved to be of value in the shoulder, as discussed later and in Figure 3–15.

Principles of Shoulder Design

As mentioned previously, the size and design of the articular surfaces should be aimed at restoring normal anatomy. I do not believe this objective should change with time. The shape and size of the stems of the components to be anchored in bone will be altered if materials are improved; however, current materials used as described in the following discussion are extremely effective for reconstructing the glenohumeral joint.

Mechanical Stress on the Implant

A number of surprisingly powerful forces act on an implant in the glenohumeral joint. They can be listed as follows.

Joint Reaction Force Equals Body Weight. When the arm is raised out to the side with the elbow straight, empty handed, the joint reaction force equals approximately body weight. This force is magnified if weight is added to the hand or if the arm is moved rapidly as in throwing. Thus, in simple everyday activities the forces on the implant are of "weight-bearing" proportions. The shoulder should not be considered a nonweight-bearing joint.

Impact Loads. Stress on the implant is greatly increased by impact loads (for example, hard falls, swinging an axe, and accidental injuries). To indicate the frequency of impact loads on this joint in everyday life, I have seen more than 100 fractures in the arm with the prosthesis (fractures at the elbow, humeral shaft, wrist, or clavicle; see Fig. 3–30) occur without apparent harm to the implant. Fracture of the implant out of the bone occurred in only three shoulders in my series (see later discussion of complications).

Forces in All Directions. Because the glenohumeral joint is capable of more motion and a greater variety of movements than other joints, forces are applied from more directions. This, and the fact that the scapula is a frail bone, makes this joint especially unsuited for a constrained implant.

Favorable Anatomical Features

Despite the gigantic forces acting on the prosthesis, the record of durability of an unconstrained shoulder arthroplasty is better than that of any other joint. This is true because of the following factors.

Maintenance of Compressive Forces. When the humerus is raised, the scapula rotates, causing the glenoid to be positioned in front of the humeral head. This maintains compressive forces between the humeral head and the glenoid with minimal shear force. Because there are individual variations in the complex synergistic movements between the scapula and the humerus, there are variations in the point where maximum shear force occurs; however, there is little doubt that compressive forces predominate throughout most shoulder movements, creating a very favorable environment for the survival of a glenoid component.

Scapula Has "Give." The scapula has "give" on impact because it is suspended in muscles. This reduces the impact load on the shoulder components compared to that at the hip because the pelvis is more rigid and fixed.

Glenoid Is Small. The articular surface of the glenoid is little more than one-quarter the size of the humeral head. This provides "low friction," making it unnecessary to consider a prosthesis with a small head to reduce friction.

Glenoid Radius of Curve Is Greater than that of the Head. The radius of curve of the articular surface of the normal glenoid is greater than that of the humeral head. This type of articular surface provides minimal constraint and minimal stability. In contrast, at the hip, where the acetabulum surrounds half of the femoral head, there is great constraint and stability. Much of the stability at the shoulder is dependent on the rotator cuff. If the articular surface of a glenoid component were made with a larger radius of curve than the head, in the exact proportions existing between the normal glenoid and the normal head, there would be even less constraint than that found in present glenoid components, which conform to the radius of curve of the prosthetic head. Although the articular surface of present glenoid components is made to conform to the radius of curve of the head, there is far less constraint than that found in the hip, where the acetabulum makes a half-circle around the femoral head, providing the advantage of great stability but the disadvantage that the forces of constraint tend to loosen the acetabular component. Successful arthroplasty is much more difficult at the shoulder than at the hip because it is necessary to preserve the rotator cuff; however, once this is achieved, the tendency for a glenoid component to fail mechanically should be much less than that of an acetabular component. If the glenoid components were prone to mechanical failure, it would be logical to increase the radius of curve of their articular surfaces. To date, however, this has not been done because a conforming glenoid surface provides some stability and has not seemed to be an important factor in loosening of glenoid components.

Head Supported by Bone. The undersurface of the head of the humeral component normally rests on bone at a 50-degree angle from that of the longitudinal axis of the stem. This support for the head eliminates rotary stress on the stem.

Good Cortical Bone. Although the medullary canal at the surgical neck is cone-shaped and the bone is mainly soft and cancellous, the shaft below this level has good cortical bone unless it has been weakened by disease or injury. The strong cortical bone in the shaft provides good support for the prosthesis. The stem of the prosthesis should be made to fit tightly in the shaft, and the stem must be made to diffuse the force over a large area of the shaft so that the bone interchange (of bone formation and bone resorption) is preserved at the interface.

Good Muscle Coverage. Finally, the glenohumeral joint has unusually good muscle coverage and blood supply that protects the implant. This is undoubtedly a major factor in the low rate of postoperative infection.

Design for Normal Anatomy

Because, as described previously, the normal anatomy of the shoulder is favorable for nonconstrained arthroplasty, the design of the prosthesis should mimic the normal anatomy of the scapula and humerus. Implants made with this principle in mind have provided the best function and durability.

Humeral Component

Radius of Curve. The articular surface of the humeral head has a radius of curve averaging approximately 44 mm. There is amazingly little variation in this measurement of normal humeral heads regardless of the size of the patient. Of course, in patients with osteoarthritis and other degenerative conditions with osteophyte formation, osteophytes may enlarge the head to as much as twice the normal size, causing the glenoid to flatten and enlarge to match the arthritic head.

The enlargement of the head in osteoarthritis has prompted several surgeons to suggest a larger prosthetic head be added to the system. To evaluate the possible need for this, Dr. Bigliani and I studied the x-rays made of ten very large male weightlifters who had asymptomatic and nonarthritic shoulders to determine the size of their humeral heads.[122] All of these men were over six feet tall and weighed more than 200 pounds. As shown in Figure 3–13, their humeral heads had the same average measurement of 44 mm. for the curve and 22 mm. in length as the measurements of the standard long prosthetic head; there was insufficient difference to justify the addition of a larger prosthetic head.

Dr. Fukuda thought Japanese humeral heads might be smaller than American humeral heads.[121] He made measurements in an anatomy laboratory in Japan but found surprisingly little difference. Subsequent studies in Japan suggested the humeral head was ellipsoidal rather than round; however, we have found the normal humeral head in the United States to be essentially round.

Because of a very small patient with juvenile rheumatoid arthritis, Dr. Cofield had some humeral and glenoid components made using the same proportions as Neer II components but one-half the size. Although I believe there may be exceptional cases, they must be rare because I have not yet encountered a patient requiring these smaller components.

Length of Head. There is a need for different lengths of head because of (1) wear and bone loss at the articular surfaces, (2) differences in the size of individual patients, and (3) tears of the rotator cuff that require a shorter head for closure. Two lengths of head have been found to be adequate, but the surgeon must implant the prosthesis at the proper height so that the head is somewhat higher than the greater tuberosity to avoid impingement (see Fig. 3–26A) and to preserve the desired distance between the greater tuberosity and the glenoid by maintaining the proper length of the head (see Fig. 3–26C). A longer head provides better leverage for the muscles and is preferable; however, a shorter head is necessary in some smaller patients and to facilitate closure of some very large rotator cuff tears.

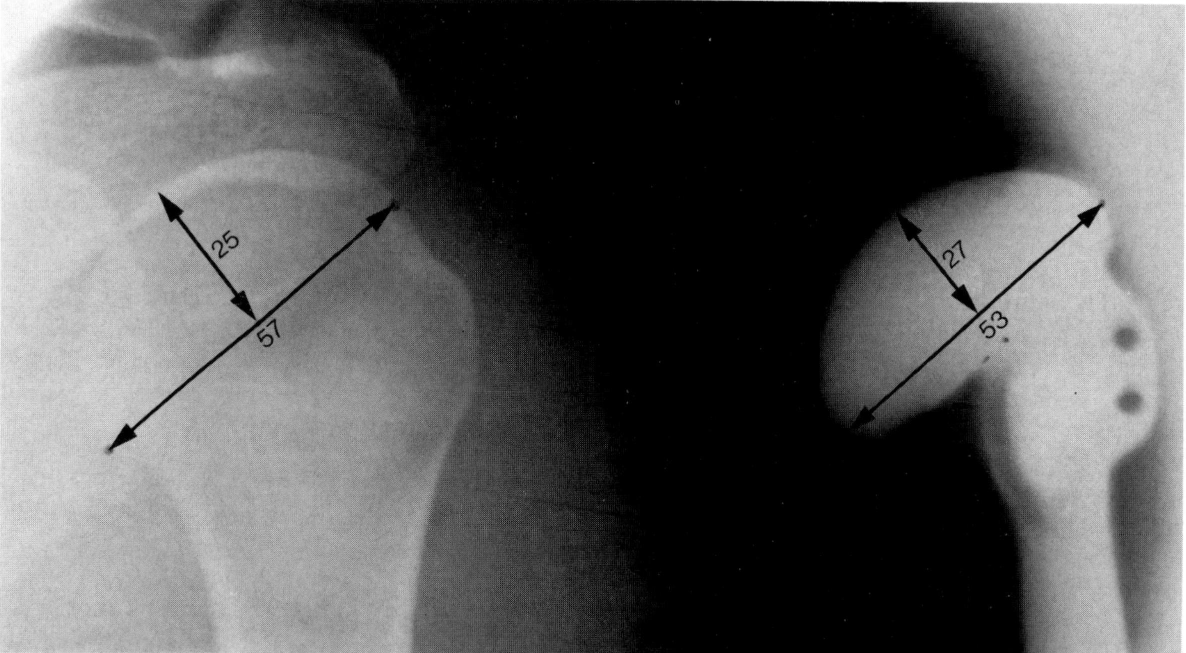

Figure 3–13. There is amazingly little variation in the size of normal humeral heads. Measurements of the diameter, length, and radius of curve of very large men (over 200-pound athletes) averaged the same as the measurements for the existing long-head humeral component.

Modular Humeral Head

The introduction of "modular heads" (removable and interchangeable heads [see Fig. 3–12C]) makes it possible to have a variety of head sizes; however, because the radius of curve of the head normally does not match that of the articular surface of the glenoid, it is unnecessary to match the prosthetic head to the articular surface of the glenoid with the same precision as required in a hip when a prosthetic femoral head is used without an acetabular component. The distance between the greater tuberosity and the glenoid can be varied by the amount of bone retained at the neck. Therefore, the availability of many humeral head sizes is less important. I believe it is an important principle in prosthetic design to avoid components with multiple parts when possible. Modular design seems to be more important in other joints.

Bipolar Humeral Head

An implant composed of a small ball within a larger ball seems logical for some conditions in the hip; however, it seems unnecessary in the shoulder. Because the socket of the shoulder is largely composed of soft tissue, movement and stability depend on retaining the rotator cuff. Wear on a normal glenoid has not been a significant problem. It seems unwise to use a humeral component with multiple movable parts without good reason.

Stem Diameter

The medullary canal of the proximal humerus is cone-shaped, making it difficult to obtain intimate contact between the humeral component and the bone. The cancellous bone beneath the tuberosities cannot be relied on for support, especially in the osteopenic bone characteristic of disuse and arthritis. Further down there is strong cortical bone, and good contact of the stem can be obtained.

At the surgical neck level, fins rather than a solid cone have the advantage of being adjustable by cutting slots in the bone, whereas a prosthesis with a solid neck, as in one American design, often splits the humerus like a wedge.

Below the surgical neck level, the diameter of the medullary canal in the shaft varies from 6.0 mm. to more than 14 mm. (if one includes osteopenic bone). Therefore, one should have available a variety of stem diameters to allow for press-fit, ongrowth press-fit, or surface ingrowth. When a good fit has been obtained in the humerus, there has rarely been a problem of loosening of the implant. A loose fit with motion may result in further resorption of the bone and further loosening. Unless a firm press fit is obtained, a grouting material, currently acrylic cement, should be added. The need for a variety of stem diameters was recognized in the Neer I system over 35 years ago (see Fig. 3–3). It is surprising that for so many years femoral components were made with only one diameter of stem, and many were undoubtedly loose at the time of insertion.

Stem Length

Using present materials, a stem length of approximately six times the diameter of the humerus has worked well. This length of stem diffuses the stress over a broad enough surface to allow exchange of bone resorption and bone formation at the bone-prosthesis interface. A firmly fitted stem of this length has been free of complications.

Gross motion of the stem within the medullary canal escalates bone resorption and is undesirable; however, slight motion at a fibrous interface after a good press-fit can be expected without pain or bone resorption. This thin fibrous interface is probably desirable to compensate for the difference in the modulus of elasticity (flexibility) between the bone and the stiffer stem of the implant.

Attempts have been made by others to shorten the stem of the humeral component. This change introduced problems of bone resorption and loosening. On the other hand, when there is a malunion of the shaft of the humerus or deformity of the proximal humerus, it may be desirable to use a shorter stem component to avoid having to osteotomize the shaft; therefore, shorter stem components are available (see Fig. 3–11).

Long stems produce an increased concentration of stress at the distal tip of the stiff stem. If materials are improved to provide sufficient strength against bending or breaking and yet have the same flexibility as bone, then a longer stem might be preferred. When most of the proximal humerus has been destroyed or removed, as in severe trauma and after en bloc resection of tumors (see Figs. 3–94 and 3–95), a long-stem prosthesis is required.

The Neer II system offered a better variety of lengths of stem than the original design (Figs. 3–3 and 3–4); however, it was designed with a smoother taper for use with acrylic cement and fewer diameters of stem.

Glenoid Component

Radius of Curve of the Glenoid Component

The curve of the articular surface of the glenoid is normally bigger than that of the humeral head. In the Neer II system, it seemed preferable to deviate from normal anatomy in this regard, however, and use a glenoid surface that conforms to the 44 mm. radius of curve of the head of the prosthesis. This design adds some constraint and provides a more efficient fulcrum that seems helpful in rehabilitating weak muscles. It was recognized that it might be necessary to increase the size of the radius of curve of the articular surface of the glenoid component if in clinical follow-up there was a significant rate of loosening that could be attributed to this cause. To date the rate of loosening has been low, and it seems unjustified to increase the radius of curve of the glenoid component.

Size of the Articular Surface

In clinical tests, an articular surface approximately the same size as a normal glenoid seems best for almost all situations. Glenoid components with larger articular surfaces interfere with repair of the rotator cuff and increase the risk of mechanical failure by adding friction and constraint (see Fig. 3–10). A slightly bigger articular surface that does not interfere with closing the rotator cuff may be helpful in the rare special circumstance of patients with selective bone loss but sparing of enough bone to support the implant or with extreme loss of rotator cuff associated with adequate bone (as in the rare cuff-tear arthropathy, revision, long-standing rheumatoid arthritis, or after cuff excision). However, as mentioned previously, in these few extreme situations the bone is usually inadequate to support a larger implant, and although the condition of the muscles forces reduced activity, a higher incidence of radiolucent lines occurs when an oversized glenoid component has been used. There seems to be no place for oversized or "hooded" (overhanging superior edge) glenoid components in routine shoulder arthroplasties.

Stem of the Glenoid Component

Because most of the scapula is paper-thin (Fig. 3–14), a fixation device for a glenoid component can be supported in only three areas: the glenoid, the coracoid, and the lateral margin of the scapula. The medullary canal of the glenoid is funnel-shaped, making it important to save the subchondral bone. This precludes a thick anchoring stem, which would require removal of the subchondral bone for its insertion. A slot-shaped opening the size of the base of the stem allows undercutting the subchondral bone to provide better anchorage. As shown in Figure 3–27, it is important to place the upper end of this slot at the level of the coracoid with anchorage extending into the coracoid and down the "lateral mass" of bone.

In addition to bone support within the scapula, it is essential that the surface of the glenoid provide bone support for the back of the articular surface of the glenoid component to eliminate tilting and rocking. Otherwise, strain on the anchoring device may in time cause loosening or breakage (see Fig.

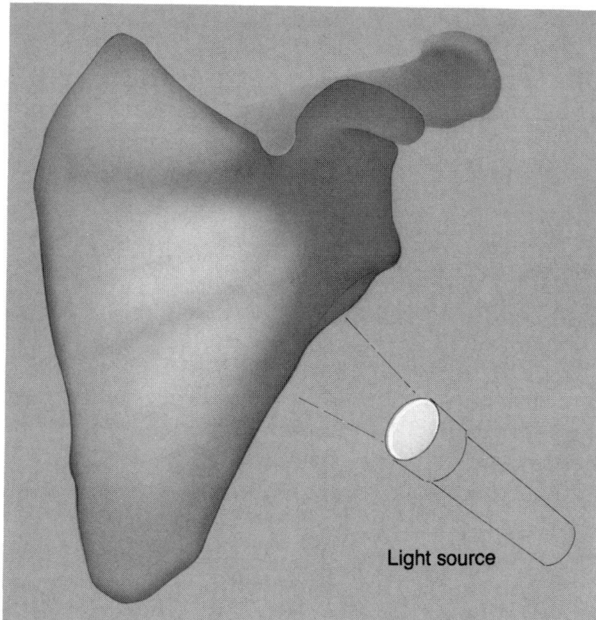

Figure 3–14. Most of the scapula is paper-thin and supports a fixation device in only three areas: the glenoid, the coracoid, and the lateral margin.

3–98G and H). Providing this support can be extremely difficult when there has been extreme loss of bone at the articular surface of the glenoid. Ways of compensating for glenoid bone loss are shown in Figure 3–28.

Subacromial Spacer

A prosthetic component beneath the acromion was first suggested by MacNab and was used by several surgeons both in the United States and abroad.[98, 102, 133] I have never implanted such a device but have seen several failures. This type of implant prevents ascent of the head and prevents contact between the head and the acromion. However, it fails in three respects:

1. It does not eliminate pain from glenohumeral incongruity.
2. It interferes with closure of the cuff.
3. It becomes dislocated unless there is sufficient cuff to provide stability for the glenohumeral joint.

The use of subacromial spacers has now been generally discontinued.[275]

Future Designs

In the future, improvements in materials will alter the method of anchoring components in bone (by altering the length and types of stems), but the basic design of the articular surfaces should remain the same as normal anatomy. No biomechanical theory can improve on an anatomical design. The principles of preserving and repairing the soft tissues around the implant will also endure. Optimum strength for active motion and shoulder function depends on these muscles rather than on altering the normal design of the implant.

During recent years, there has been interest in surface ingrowth of bone with the aim of more secure fixation and elimination of cement. In the case of the humerus, it should be remembered there has been virtually no problem of loosening of a press-fit (with some followed over 30 years) or cemented stem provided it was set firmly initially. At this time, with 15 to 20 years of follow-up, we do not know if the chemical and physical properties of implanted methylmethacrylate will change during the lifetime of younger patients. Therefore, in younger individuals who have thick, carrot-like bone and can be expected to use the prosthesis for half a century, the use of a surface ingrowth prosthesis has the most appeal. However, anchorage with surface ingrowth using present materials in the average implant patient has a number of disadvantages:

1. All metals have some surface ionization, which is being observed for tissue response. Porous surfaces increase the surface area by as much as 30 or 40 times, which introduces the potential of 30 or 40 times more ion release, with the possibility of increased biological reactions.
2. Porous coatings have the potential of causing stress risers that might lead to breakage of the stem because of defects in the surface of the metal.
3. The need for intimate contact at the bone-prosthesis interface requires cabinetmaker-like preparation of the bone. Although this may be possible in the bone of younger patients, it is impossible in the osteopenic bone of patients with rheumatoid arthritis or long-standing injuries and in other situations in which the quality of the bone precludes achieving this sort of contact.
4. Mechanical stabilization of the implant is required to prevent motion at the interface for a number of months until bone ingrowth occurs. Secure anchorage may be impossible in osteopenic bone and when there has been loss of bone. Unless the shoulder can be moved during the postoperative period, soft-tissue adhesions will form to spoil the result.
5. After ingrowth occurs, there can be damage to the humerus, either by stress-shielding, which leads to resorption of bone, or by making it impossible to revise the implant without severely breaking the bone.
6. Implanting an ingrowth prosthesis, even in bone of normal quality, requires a perfect fit and is technically more difficult.

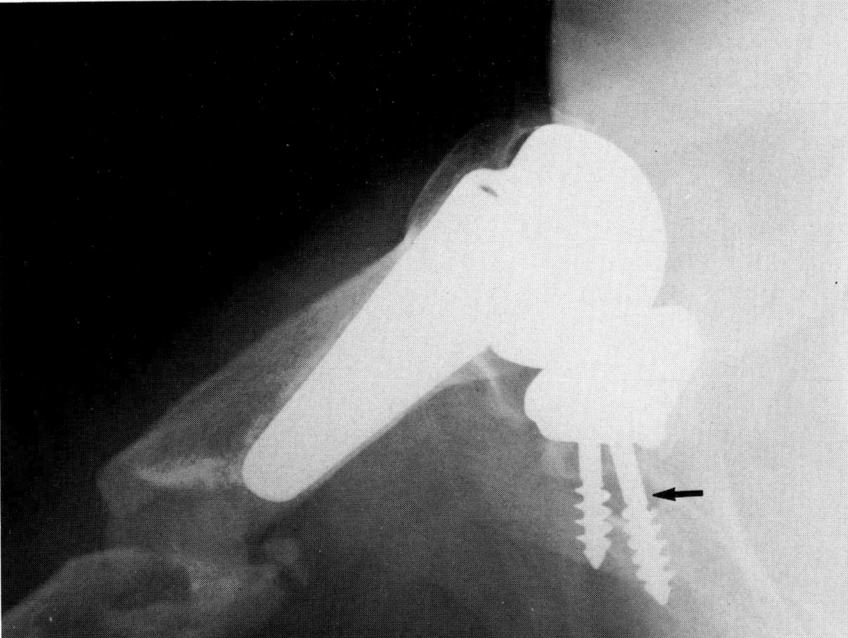

Figure 3–15. Revision arthroplasty demonstrates some problems five years after a surface ingrowth system in the shoulder (see also Figs. 3–16, 3–17, and 3–18). Pre-operative axillary view is shown. The reaming required for the introduction of the stem of the humeral component led to a fracture that went on to a nonunion. The screws used to immobilize the glenoid component until surface ingrowth occurred protruded from the frail scapula (arrow) and were loose.

7. Current studies show that true bony ingrowth occurs in only about 25 per cent of current surface ingrowth components.

Considering this list of disadvantages and some of the problems encountered with surface ingrowth (Figs. 3–15 to 3–18 and 3–97 to 3–99), and comparing the good results achieved to date using press-fit or cemented components, it seems unwise for a surgeon to commit himself to only one type of implant fixation. Despite the disadvan-

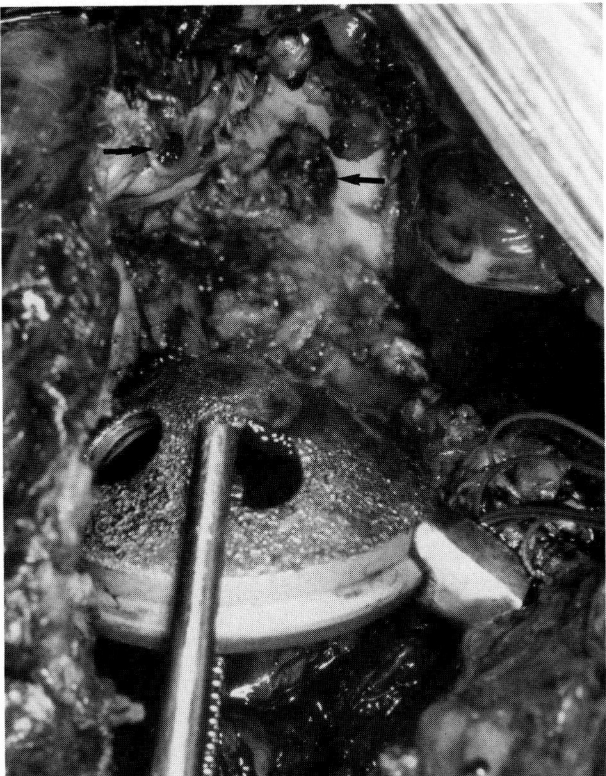

Figure 3–16. The glenoid component was loose with marked resorption of bone. The screw holes (arrows) were quite enlarged.

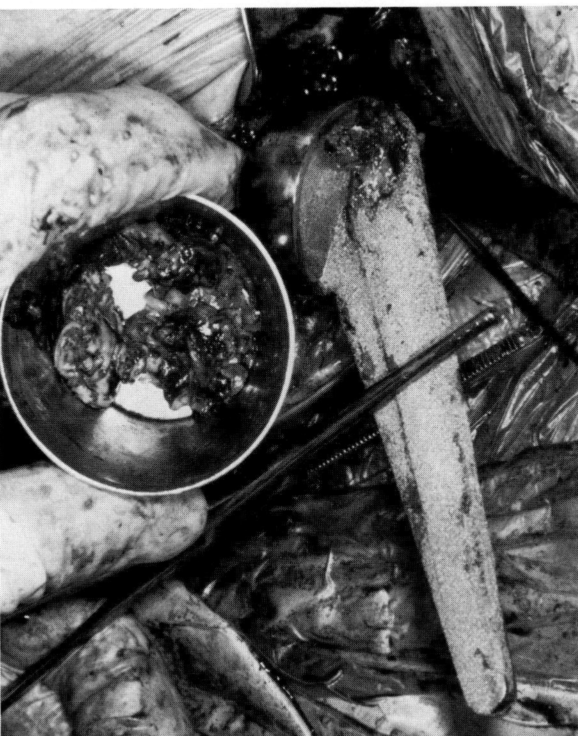

Figure 3–17. Removal of the humeral component was very traumatic to the thin, stress-shielded bone.

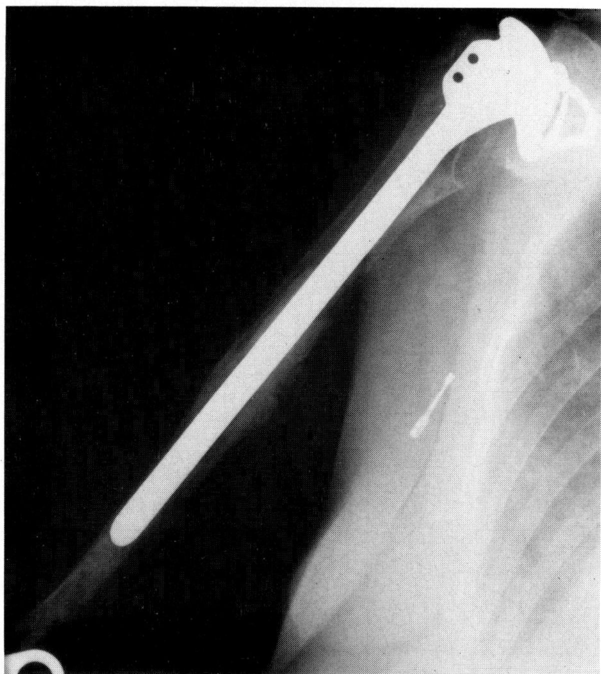

Figure 3–18. The repair made use of a Neer II cemented, long-stem humeral component with bone grafts and cemented glenoid components.

tages of porous coating fixation, controlled studies of this technique and its application by a few interested surgeons are justified.

Some new material will undoubtedly be developed that is stronger than polyethylene and has a better modulus of elasticity than present metals. In place of methylmethacrylate, perhaps a more biological grouting material will be created that can be replaced by bone. In the meantime, however, change for the sake of change should be avoided because the current system of nonconstrained shoulder arthroplasty is reliable and works extremely well.

CLINICAL ASSESSMENT OF SHOULDER ARTHROPLASTY

Indications

The indications for nonconstrained arthroplasty are listed in Table 3–1 according to diagnosis and the type of implant used.

Pain

The primary indication for a shoulder arthroplasty is pain due to incongruity of the glenohumeral joint. When both sides of the joint are incongruous, a total arthroplasty is usually performed.

Table 3–1. CURRENT PERSONAL SERIES OF 776 GLENOHUMERAL ARTHROPLASTIES*

INDICATIONS	HUMERAL HEAD ARTHROPLASTY	NONCONSTRAINED TSA†
Trauma		
Acute	75	
Old	37	120
Avascular necrosis	23	
Osteoarthritis (primary and secondary)	7	185
Arthritis of recurrent dislocations	9	52
Rheumatoid arthritis	3	145
Revision	3	63
Cuff-tear arthropathy		34
Miscellaneous fusion (neoplasm, dysplasia, etc.)	<4	16
	161	615

*1973–1988.
†TSA = total shoulder arthroplasty.

Functional Impairment

Improvement in range of shoulder motion and function are secondary objectives, but none of my patients have had this procedure for stiffness alone without pain. It is important, however, to make a detailed inquiry about specific activities that are frequently associated with pain rather than asking a brief question about the presence of pain. For example, patients with severe rheumatoid polyarthritis who are extremely eager to become independent of others for self-care and who have many generalized aches and pains place much more importance on the limitation of function and motion than on pain. Others often think that the doctor is asking about pain at the moment rather than pain on movement of the shoulder. One should ask specific questions such as the following: "Do you have pain at night?" "Can you sleep on that side?" "Do you have pain when you put on your overcoat?"

The presence of pain can also be demonstrated by eliciting tenderness over the posterior joint line and at the extremes of glenohumeral motion. Moving the humerus on the scapula helps estimate pain. Most patients, however, readily describe how the shoulder pain interferes with sleep and daily activities. The pain of arthritis is often more intolerable at the shoulder than at the hip or knee because shoulder pain is not alleviated by recumbency, but is made worse.

Modern shoulder arthroplasties aim at the restoration of near normal function and motion. Preoperatively, sports and hobbies have become impossible, and such activities as writing, turning keys, and everyday movements of personal care such as brushing the teeth, combing the hair, and dressing have become painful. Severely arthritic patients with bilateral shoulder involvement become totally dependent on others for bathroom functions and dressing. They are most appreciative of a "limited goals" functional result and independence.

Age and General Health

I set no chronological age limit, young or old, but require that the patient be a reasonable surgical risk and be well motivated.

Motivation

Because of the importance of the exercise program following shoulder arthroplasty, it is essential that the patient understands his or her role and wants to cooperate. Patients should know that the arthroplasty simply sets the stage for them to do the exercises required to achieve the pain relief, motion, and function desired. Severe alcoholism or a paranoid personality should be at least a temporary contraindication for shoulder arthroplasty.

Radiographic Destruction of the Glenohumeral Joint

Loss of the joint space and bone destruction is usually obvious in plain films. The axillary view is very helpful in estimating loss of joint space and subluxation of the head. Anterior-posterior tomograms are helpful in revealing defects in bone, and when necessary they can be supplemented with magnetic resonance imaging (MRI). CT (computerized tomography) scans are helpful in showing the joint space in borderline cases of arthritis and fractures and in estimating the slope of the glenoid.

Failure to Respond to Conservative Treatment

Most patients referred for shoulder arthroplasty have tried various medications and exercises without experiencing relief of pain. If not, or if they have milder symptomatology, a period of conservative treatment is indicated.

Contraindications

Contraindications to shoulder arthroplasty are as follows:

1. Active infection
2. Paralysis or destruction of both the rotator cuff and the deltoid muscles
3. A neurotrophic shoulder (e.g., syringomyelia [Chapter 6, p. 457])
4. Inappropriate motivation (unrealistic physical demands, lack of cooperation in aftercare)

Loss of bone is *rarely a contraindication* to nonconstrained shoulder arthroplasty. The humerus may be destroyed by trauma (see Figs. 3–94, 3–95, and 3–99) or excised as for a neoplasm (see Figs. 3–94 and 3–95) and yet be satisfactorily treated with a nonconstrained arthroplasty. Glenoid deficiencies are usually compensated for as shown in Figure 3–28; however, extensive loss of the glenoid may make it unwise to use a glenoid component. Tears of the rotator cuff are not considered a contraindication to nonconstrained shoulder arthroplasty. Cuff tears are almost always repaired according to the principles outlined in Figure 3–28. However, patients with a large amount of bone loss and massive cuff tears are generally treated with "limited goals" rehabilitation (see Fig. 7–14).

ALTERNATIVES TO REPLACEMENT ARTHROPLASTY

Conservative Treatment

Although much research continues on the cause, prevention, and cure for osteoarthritis and rheumatoid arthritis, to date there is no specific treatment. Conservative treatment, consisting of exercises, heat, and nonaddicting medications, should be given a thorough trial before advising shoulder arthroplasty, as in the treatment of arthritis of other joints. Exercises are gentle and assistive with the goal of maintaining motion without causing too much pain. Exercises must be discontinued if they are associated with too much discomfort. Activity can be modified. If x-rays show real incongruity and exercises make the symptoms worse, they are discontinued. As symptoms progress, pain is usually too intense to be helped by ordinary medications, in which case it is considered more conservative to advise an arthroplasty than to prescribe medications that lead to gastric hemorrhage or addiction.

Occasionally one sees a shoulder with rather advanced glenohumeral arthritis that is associated with few symptoms and little pain. In this case, conservative treatment is continued.

Fusion

Glenohumeral arthrodesis is considered in two situations: (1) low-grade infection, and (2) loss of both the rotator cuff and the deltoid muscles (from paralysis or extensive injuries) (see Chapter 6, p. 438). The difference in function compared with an arthroplasty is shown in Figure 3–19.

Synovectomy

Synovectomy for rheumatoid arthritis of the glenohumeral joint has given disappointing results,[21, 39, 52] with one exception. This is the rare situation in which there is mainly a rheumatoid subacromial bursitis (which may be quite extensive with rice bodies) and acromioclavicular joint destruction but no involvement of the articular surfaces of the glenohumeral joint (see Fig. 3–53).

Resection

Resection of the humerus and glenoid for arthritis or fractures has given unsatisfactory results (Figs. 3–1, 3–2, and 3–20A). These procedures are considered only for control of infection or when the nerves and muscles have been destroyed, precluding prosthetic reconstruction (see Chapter 6, p. 442).

Debridement

Glenohumeral "cheilotomy" (removal of spurs, loose bodies, or frayed surfaces with or without drilling holes in areas of sclerosis and wear) has been performed both surgically and arthroscopically for glenohumeral osteoarthritis. Because the glenoid is small and tends to be distracted by gravity, one might expect such a procedure to produce better results in the shoulder than in other joints. This has not been the case. All four open debridements I performed progressed to dismal failure.[2] A number of patients have been referred after unsuccessful open or arthroscopic debridements. In some individuals, the pain and stiffness had been made worse. I cannot recommend this procedure.

Osteotomies

Various types of osteotomies and double osteotomies have been used for glenohumeral arthritis. I believe these procedures have now been abandoned. One has only to view the incongruous joint surfaces in patients with established arthritis to realize how futile it is to expect these procedures to relieve pain or improve motion. The only situation in which I have performed osteotomies is a

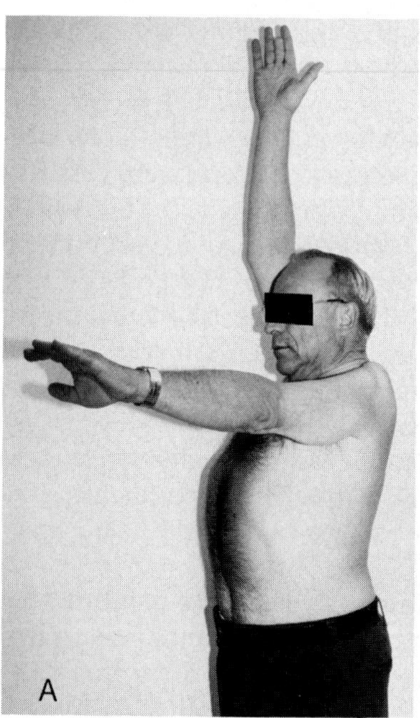

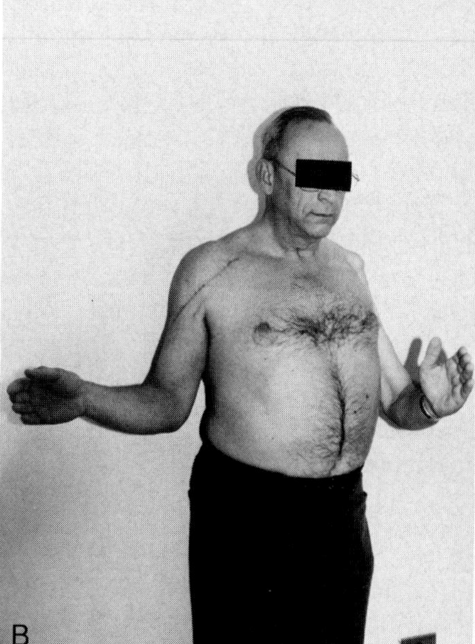

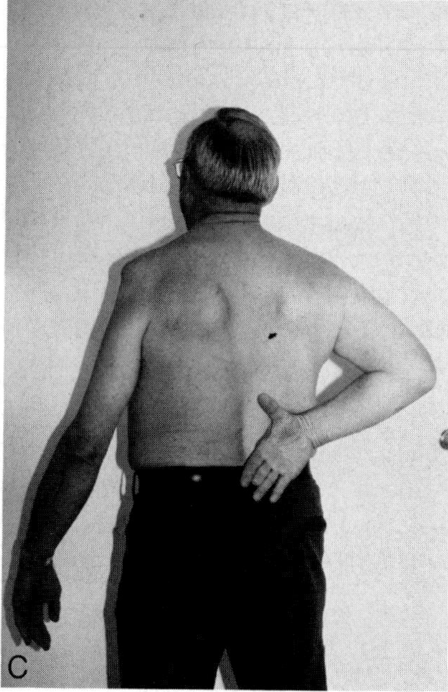

Figure 3–19. Comparison of function after glenohumeral arthrodesis of the left shoulder five years previously and total shoulder arthroplasty of the right shoulder five months previously. Both operations were performed for glenohumeral osteoarthritis.

A, Maximum elevation of both sides.

B, Maximum external rotation.

C, Maximum internal rotation.

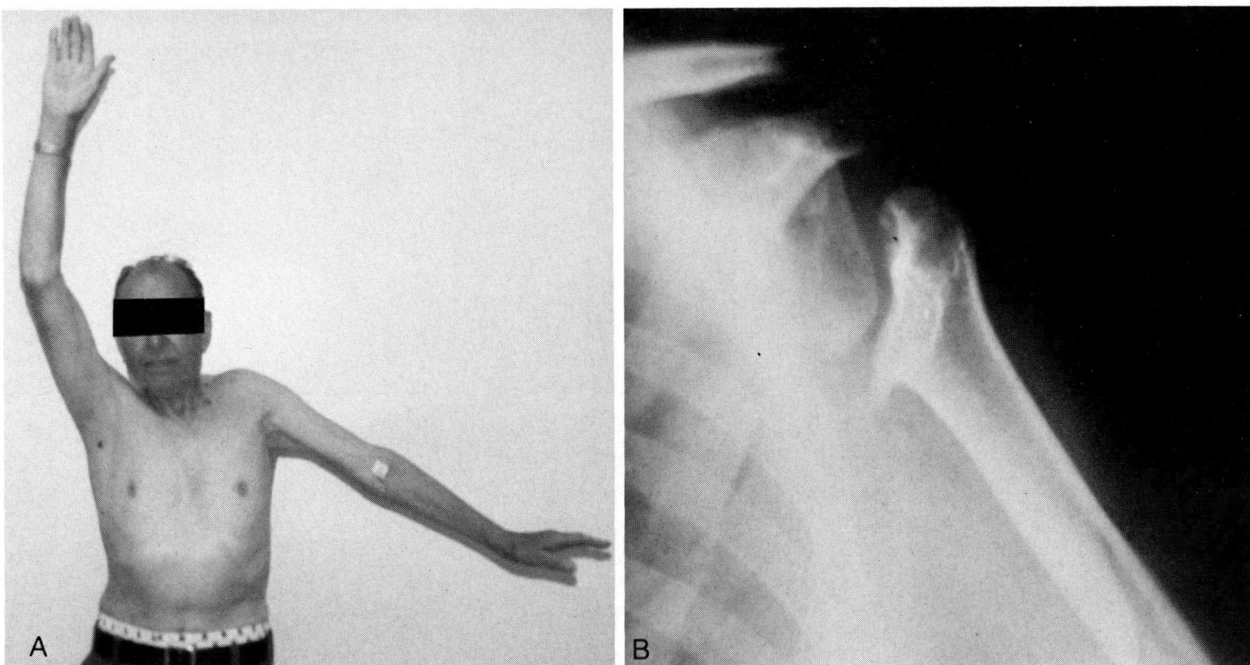

Figure 3–20A and B. Pain, weakness, and loss of active motion two years after resection of the humeral head.

severely deformed or dislocated shoulder that is free of pain, is paralyzed or spastic, and is fixed in an internally rotated position that precludes using a walker. These osteotomies were not expected to relieve pain or improve motion but to achieve neutral rotation or improved function (see Chapter 6 and Fig. 6–15).

Osteochondral Allografts

Transplanting articular cartilage or whole joints is not a new idea. It has never been practical in the shoulder because of the high incidence of avascular necrosis of the humeral head,[120] the scarring and adhesions of the rotator cuff caused by prolonged immobilization, and other complications inherent in the transplantation of this amount of foreign protein.[139] Parrish[129] found that the incidence of avascular necrosis of the humeral head following proximal humeral allografts after en bloc resection of tumors was so high that he used my original humeral head prosthesis to replace the articular surface of the allograft.[130] I have preferred to reconstruct the proximal humerus after extensive trauma or tumor resection by using a long-stem humeral component with autogenous fibular grafts (see Figs. 3–94 and 3–95).

Vascularized Upper Humerus or Shoulder Transplants

Vascularized transplants of the upper humerus or shoulder may one day be a solution after en bloc resections for neoplasms, but currently there are problems. These include adhesions because of inadequate fixation of the transplant to allow movement of the joint and inadequate circulation to the humeral head.

APPRAISAL OF GLENOHUMERAL ARTHRITIS

When the laboratory routines, as listed in Figures 1–10 to 1–12, are negative, the diagnosis is confirmed and the severity of involvement determined by the following tests.

Limited Motion

A key point in differentiating shoulders with glenohumeral arthritis from those with tears of the rotator cuff is loss of motion (see Table 1–2). The typical shoulder with a tear of the rotator cuff retains full passive motion even though active motion and strength may be impaired. In the early stages of glenohumeral arthritis, the amount of impairment of movement may be so small that very careful measurements with the patient supine are required, as illustrated in Figures 1–5 to 1–9, to detect true differences in external rotation and elevation compared with the normal side. Later, shoulder motion gradually becomes restricted to essentially scapular movement. Because scapular movement does not contribute very much to rotation, limitation of external rotation is a more sen-

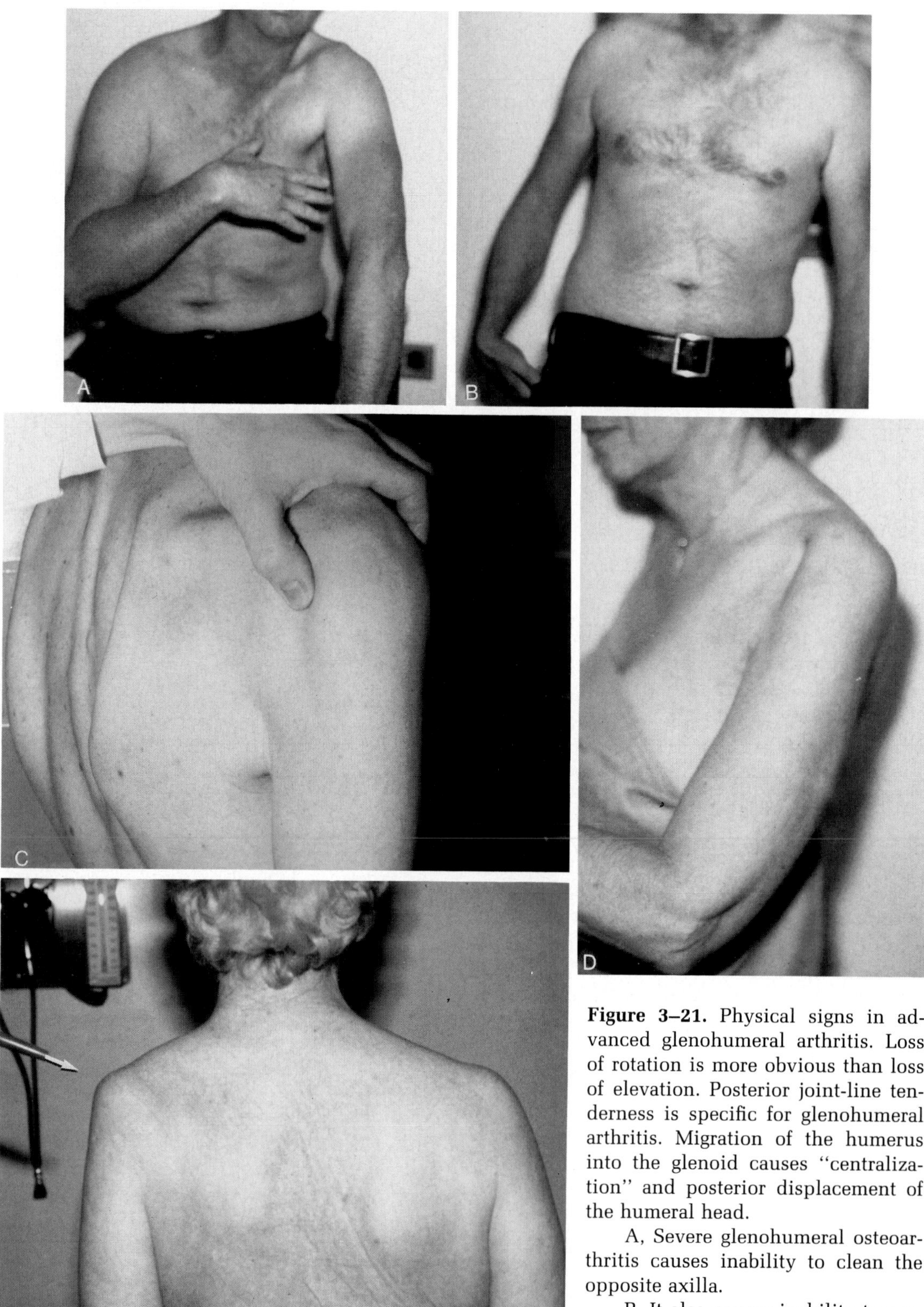

Figure 3–21. Physical signs in advanced glenohumeral arthritis. Loss of rotation is more obvious than loss of elevation. Posterior joint-line tenderness is specific for glenohumeral arthritis. Migration of the humerus into the glenoid causes "centralization" and posterior displacement of the humeral head.

A, Severe glenohumeral osteoarthritis causes inability to clean the opposite axilla.

B, It also causes inability to perform self-care at the toilet.

C, Posterior joint-line tenderness (a most useful sign).

D, Posterior migration of the head gives the appearance of a posterior dislocation, the axis of the arm pointing posteriorly rather than toward the anterior acromion.

E, Centralization of the head with loss of the width of the shoulder. (This sign is a warning of probable severe glenoid destruction in patients with rheumatoid arthritis.)

sitive physical sign than loss of elevation (Fig. 3–21A and B).

Posterior Joint Line Tenderness

A "frozen shoulder" (see Chapter 6, p. 422) from any source can limit motion, and therefore tenderness over the posterior joint line is a helpful sign because it is more specific for glenohumeral arthritis (Fig. 3–21C). Tenderness superiorly, over the rotator cuff or bursa or in front over the biceps, is present in impingement lesions, calcium deposits, and any type of bursitis. However, tenderness over the posterior joint line is specific for glenohumeral arthritis, especially if posterior osteophytes and spurs are palpated as the tenderness is elicited.

Catching and Squeaking

In advanced osteoarthritis, movements of the humerus on the glenoid can cause a squeaking noise that at times can be heard across the room. Incongruity may cause catching sensations, which often cause the patient to think the shoulder is dislocating. In many patients, however, these signs are more subtle and are detected only over the posterior joint line as the humerus is rotated on the glenoid.

Pain When Rotating the Humerus on the Glenoid

Using one hand to stabilize the scapula while the other rotates and compresses the humerus against the glenoid elicits the pain of glenohumeral incongruity. Grinding sensations may be palpable. The pain is often referred to the deltoid insertion or to the elbow. It is this pain on movements of the humerus on the glenoid that becomes intolerable in advanced glenohumeral arthritis. It interferes with sleep because when the patient is recumbent the humerus normally falls in stressful positions whether the patient is lying on the back, the good side, or the painful side. In advanced stages of disease the patient often sleeps sitting up and is unable to use the involved arm for cleanliness and self-care.

Thickening and Fluid

If one stands behind the patient and grasps both shoulders between the thumbs and index fingers, as in Figure 3–21C, the thickness of the two shoulders can be compared, and marginal osteophytes and fluid can often be palpated on the painful side. This is a reassuring test for confirmation of the diagnosis. In some cases the fluid makes a bulge, usually at the anterior axillary line, causing less experienced surgeons to make a diagnosis of a tumor and misleading them into doing a biopsy (see Fig. 3–44).

Roentgen Assessment

Anterior-posterior views can be misleading in estimating the amount of joint space because the glenohumeral joint is in the scapular plane rather than in the coronal or sagittal plane. A better estimate can be made from anterior-posterior views made in the scapular plane; however, the axillary view is the most valuable for evaluating the joint surfaces (Figs. 1–12 and 3–22). These views are routine for estimating the amount of erosion of the glenoid and subluxation of the head. Tomograms and MRI are valuable for assessing involvement of the humeral head in patients with avascular necrosis, tumors, or infections. CT scans are also helpful in detecting subtle tumors and bone lesions as well as for showing the amount of bone loss at the glenoid or head when planning an arthroplasty (Fig. 3–23).

Petersson[128] made an interesting study of the normal glenohumeral joint space in healthy patients of different ages. Studying the thickness of the glenohumeral joint space in patients ranging in age from 10 to 90 years, he concluded that this joint space does not normally decrease with age. I believe it is important to obtain axillary views of both shoulders for a comparison before making the assumption that narrowing of a glenohumeral joint space should be expected because of the patient's age. Of course, as joint destruction advances it becomes evident that the condition is abnormal. When the arthritic process becomes well established, the roentgen appearance of each of the many types of pathology is diagnostic, as will be discussed with each category of disease. The sclerosis and marginal osteophytes of osteoarthritis, the marginal erosion of rheumatoid arthritis, the uneven wear and large glenoid osteophytes of the arthritis of dislocations, the sparing of the glenoid with avascular necrosis, and the fragmentation of the head in neurotrophic disorders are some examples of the ways in which routine x-ray films can be helpful in making the specific diagnosis and planning the arthroplasty.

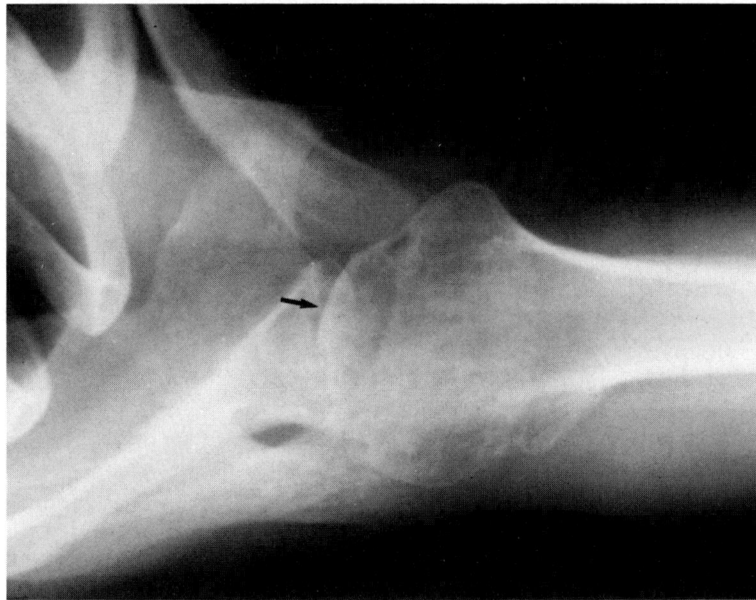

Figure 3–22. Roentgen assessment of glenohumeral arthritis. A better estimate of the amount of joint destruction is obtained from the axillary view than from anterior-posterior views. This axillary view shows posterior glenoid destruction with posterior subluxation of the head in a rheumatoid shoulder, suggesting that further nonoperative treatment is hopeless. The arrow shows the beginning of posterior glenoid destruction with the normal level of the articular surface of the glenoid visible anterior to this point.

Ancillary Tests

Neck Extension Test and Neurological Examination

The neck extension (see Figs. 1–10 to 1–12 and 2–37) is an important maneuver in eliciting the presence of painful conditions of the cervical spine and cervical radiculitis. A brief neurological examination is routine, looking for weakness of the biceps (which might indicate a C5–C6 cervical root involvement) and weakness or loss of sensation. The possibility of syringomyelia should be kept in mind, and we, as shoulder surgeons, often make this diagnosis for the first time using a simple pinprick, cotton, and test tubes with hot and cold water (see Chapter 6 and Fig. 6–22).

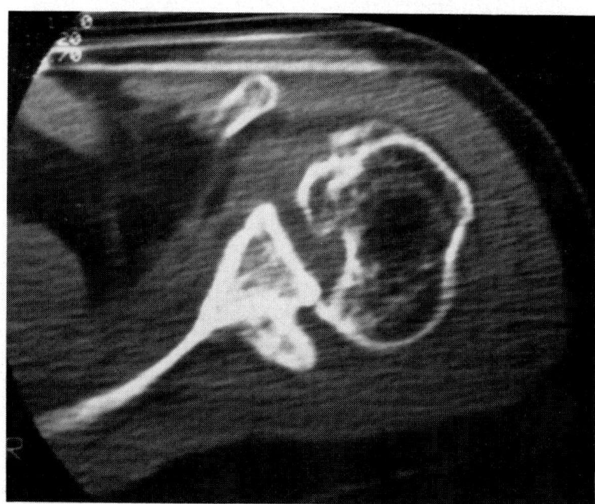

Figure 3–23. Computerized tomography can help in assessing glenoid bone stock in patients with arthritis, as in this old posterior fracture-dislocation.

Exclude Infection

Many patients with painful glenohumeral joints have had repeated injections or previous surgery. The routine blood count and sedimentation rate is helpful in signaling the possibility of infection, and it is important to aspirate the joint to acquire material for cultures if the blood tests, history, and examination raise doubts.

Evaluate the Acromioclavicular Joint

A painful acromioclavicular joint can spoil a perfect glenohumeral arthroplasty by interfering with the rehabilitation program. Such a possibility must be excluded preoperatively rather than at surgery, and if this joint is tender compared with the opposite side, a lidocaine (Xylocaine) injection test is indicated (see Chapter 6, p. 434). If it is established that this joint is painful, an acromioclavicular excisional arthroplasty is indicated at the time of the glenohumeral arthroplasty.

Rotator Cuff

Preoperative arthrograms are rarely obtained because the rotator cuff will be examined at the time of arthroplasty. If the tendons are torn they will have to be repaired. However, as will be discussed in the section on pathology in each diagnostic category, one can usually estimate preoperatively the probable condition of the rotator cuff.

Timing of Shoulder Arthroplasty

The timing and priority of shoulder arthroplasty will be considered when one shoulder is involved or both shoulders are involved, and in relation to hip, knee, elbow, or hand procedures.

One Shoulder Involved

Patients with one shoulder involved often ask if there is harm in delaying the procedure. Because the pathologic condition has been developing over a period of years, there should be little harm in a reasonable delay. However, once severe pain due to incongruity is established, it is advantageous to perform the arthroplasty in a rheumatoid shoulder before there is needless damage to the rotator cuff or excessive destruction of the glenoid (see Figs. 2–54 and 3–49A through 3–49F). In patients with osteoarthritis, arthritis of dislocations, old injuries, and any situation in which the head is out of alignment and is causing uneven wear of the glenoid, the patient should be advised of the value of having the procedure done within a few months rather than waiting years.

Bilateral Shoulder Involvement

Bilateral shoulder involvement is more frequent in patients with rheumatoid arthritis than with other conditions but also occurs in patients with osteoarthritis and trauma. When the two shoulders are about equally disabling and painful, the arthroplasty on the second shoulder can be done as soon as ten days after the first if all is going well. To date, I have not performed arthroplasties on both shoulders during the same operation. However, when both shoulders are sufficiently painful to interfere with the patient's sleep and work, it has been found better to proceed with the second shoulder procedure during the same hospitalization so that the final rehabilitation and exercise program can be organized for both sides when the patient leaves the hospital.

When one shoulder is much less painful than the other, I prefer to discharge the patient from the hospital after the first arthroplasty, advising him or her that in some cases, when an arthroplasty has relieved the pain and restored function in the bad shoulder, the less painful side is better tolerated because the operated side will assume most of the functional demands. If pain in the unoperated side continues or increases, an arthroplasty on the contralateral side is done when the patient requests it.

Priority When Multiple Joints are Involved

Multiple joint involvement is more common in rheumatoid arthritis than in other conditions. In rheumatoid patients, there has been some confusion about the priority of shoulder arthroplasty compared with the elbow and hand in the upper extremity and lower extremity procedures. My opinion is outlined in Table 3–2a.

Regarding the elbow and hand, I believe the shoulder should have priority. Pain from the shoulder is often referred to the elbow, and relieving shoulder pain may have a beneficial effect on the hand and elbow. Re-establishing shoulder rotation relieves some of the mechanical stress at the elbow. Post-operative infections and other complications are more frequent following elbow arthroplasties and may burn bridges, so that shoulder arthroplasty may never be feasible. Finally, and most important, the rotator cuff becomes damaged with delay, making both the operation and recovery much more difficult.

An old teaching among some hand surgeons was to restore the hands to as near perfect condition as possible prior to reconstructing other joints. The hand in upper extremity functions was thought to be so important that it was useless to perform other arthroplasties until the hands had been restored. However, aside from a few conditions in which there is a threat of tendon ruptures, there is little urgency in performing hand procedures because the hands are usually much less painful. Therefore, because of the threat of rotator cuff involvement and the possible benefits of the shoulder arthroplasty on the hand, the shoulder has priority.

In regard to the hips, knees, and feet, if the arthritic patient is nonambulatory because of lower extremity involvement, it seems preferable to perform the necessary lower extremity procedures first to free the shoulders from the stress of transfers and crutches. When one or two lower extremity joints are equally painful but the patient remains ambulatory, the shoulder has priority if the patient accepts delaying any lower extremity procedure requiring crutches for at least six months to allow healing of the rotator cuff. Crutches can be used without adverse effects following shoulder arthroplasty after the rotator cuff has healed; however, disruption of the rotator interval or tendons has occurred because of too early use of crutches (see

Table 3–2a. PRIORITY FOR ARTHROPLASTY OF RHEUMATOID SHOULDERS (PAIN EQUAL)

1. Total shoulder arthroplasty before elbow arthroplasty because:
   a. Complications greater at elbow than at other joints
   b. Elbow implant mechanically stressed if shoulder rotation limited
   c. Referred pain from the shoulder to the elbow is relieved by total shoulder arthroplasty
   d. Rotator cuff threatened by delay of shoulder arthroplasty
2. Total shoulder arthroplasty before lower extremity arthroplasties if the patient is ambulatory
3. Lower extremity procedures before shoulder arthroplasty if these procedures make the patient ambulatory

pp. 120, 199, 206, 492; Figs. 3–37 and 7–16). Some judgment and flexibility are required in planning the order of procedures in a severely arthritic patient; however, it is distinctly wrong to defer shoulder arthroplasty to perform multiple other procedures while the disease process is destroying the rotator cuff and glenoid.

SELECTION OF IMPLANT

Overall Design

This section on design will be summarized here (and in Table 3–2b) as follows. I described my experience with a fixed-fulcrum, constrained total shoulder prosthesis and the reasons why I have not used one since the early 1970's. With more experience in obtaining stability of nonconstrained components by restoring the proper length of the humeral head for tension on the posterior capsule and restoring the proper length of shaft for tension on the myofascial sleeve, along with proper version of the humeral component (see Fig. 3–26), I now see no indication for a completely constrained, fixed-fulcrum prosthesis.

An oversized glenoid component increases friction and constraint, creating a greater risk of mechanical failure. A large amount of overhang of the superior rim of the glenoid component makes it difficult or impossible to repair the rotator cuff. I prefer a normal sized glenoid component. Very rarely, when there is bone loss from trauma, cuff-tear arthropathy, or at revision, the slightly larger glenoid component is helpful provided it does not interfere with repair of the rotator cuff. I have not used a significantly larger glenoid component such as the "600 per cent" component (see Fig. 3–10F) for a number of years.

During recent years, some surgeons have used a slightly "hooded" (overhanging superior edge) glenoid component routinely. This fails to consider the normal rotation of the scapula that occurs when the arm is raised, rendering the overhang ineffective. The glenoid component that I prefer to use has a radius of curve that corresponds to the 44 mm. curve of the articular surface of the humeral head. Although the articular surface of the normal glenoid has a larger radius of curve than the head, to date this deviation from normal anatomy has not seemed to contribute to loosening of the glenoid component, and the small amount of constraint provided by the slightly increased curvature offers a better fulcrum than would be possible if the articular surface of the glenoid component were flattened.

Regarding the humeral component, regardless of future improvements in materials that might allow changes in the design of the bone–prosthesis interface, the prosthetic head should remain anatomical in design and near the 44 mm. radius of curve. The length of the head can be adjusted by the placement of the prosthesis in relation to the neck of the humerus; however, a shorter length of head is desirable for occasions when there are problems with the rotator cuff and for smaller patients. There must be sufficient length of stem to diffuse stress over a wide area and enough variation in the diameter of the stem to permit use in both small and large bones. It is best to have stems designed to be press-fit as well as for use with cement. Modular humeral components (with interchangeable heads) present both advantages and disadvantages, as does surface ingrowth at the stems of the components.

Table 3–2b. SELECTION OF IMPLANT

A. *Humeral component is used without a glenoid component when the glenoid is in good condition*
   1. Avascular necrosis (see Fig. 3–34 to 3–39), before glenoid changes
   2. Recent four-part and head-splitting fractures (see Fig. 5–23)
   3. Recent greater tuberosity three-part fractures in the elderly (see Fig. 5–14A and B)
   4. Some proximal humeral neoplasms
   5. Some cases of old trauma

B. *When the glenoid is too destroyed for the usual implantation of the glenoid component, the choice is between altering the version of the components, glenoid bone graft, or humeral component alone* (see Fig. 3–28), as seen in:
   1. Long-standing rheumatoid arthritis (see Figs. 3–48 to 3–56—granulation erosion and osteopenia)
   2. Congenital defects (see Figs. 3–83 to 3–86—glenoid hypoplasia and multiple epiphyseal dysplasia)
   3. Long-standing dislocation (see Figs. 3–57 to 3–63—pressure erosion)
   4. Severe trauma, e.g., gunshot wounds (see Chapter 5)
   5. Revision arthroplasty (see Figs. 3–97 to 3–99—bone loss)
   6. Arthritis of recurrent dislocations (see Figs. 3–46 and 3–47—uneven wear)
   7. Cuff-tear arthropathy (see Figs. 3–72 to 3–82—Charcot-like instability)
   8. Long-standing osteoarthritis (see Figs. 3–40 and 3–45—uneven wear)
   9. Erb's palsy deformity (see Figs. 3–87 to 3–89—old posterior dislocation, abnormal version, and short external rotators)

Current Personal Series

My personal series using the Neer II System is shown in Table 3–1. The diagnosis and components used are listed there also.

The humeral component is used without a glenoid component when the articular surface of the glenoid is in good condition and also in a few situations when glenoid bone loss is so severe that it is unwise to attempt to implant a glenoid component, as listed in Table 3–2b. In some situations severe bone loss is compensated by altering the version of the components or by using glenoid bone grafts (see Figs. 3–26 and 3–28).

The longer humeral head component gives more leverage for the muscles and is preferred except in small patients and when it is difficult to repair the rotator cuff. In the Neer II System, acrylic cement grouting is used routinely for the humeral component in patients with fractures (see Chapter 5) (because the broken tuberosities fail to prevent rotation), in rheumatoid arthritis (because of osteopenia), and in any situation when a secure press-fit of the stem cannot be obtained. Using this system, the glenoid component requires acrylic cement.

Surface ingrowth on the stems of the humeral and glenoid components is at the time of this writing developmental.

Previous infection is considered a contraindication to shoulder arthroplasty with the few exceptions discussed on page 245.

TECHNIQUE ACCORDING TO PATHOLOGY

Shoulder arthroplasty, more than arthroplasties of other joints, demands the preservation and rehabilitation of the soft tissue. Treatment of the soft tissue is as important as the orientation and fixation of the components. The rotator cuff makes this the most difficult of all joints to obtain a good functional result. Active motion depends on (1) the rotator cuff and deltoid muscles, (2) freedom from adhesions, and (3) a stable implant. Durability depends not only on design and materials but equally on the quality of the bone and surgical technique (which can optimize the orientation of the components for bone support).

Because details of the procedure vary with the pathologic condition, it is more explicit to discuss the problems and special steps under each diagnostic category. However, we will first consider the aspects of the procedure that are common to all.

Aspects of the Procedure Common to All Diagnostic Categories

Pre-operative Care

1. Before the operation details of the procedure and aftercare are explained to the patient, emphasizing the need for patient participation in the exercise program not only in the hospital but also in the months to follow. It is important for the patient to understand how the muscles have been weakened by years of arthritis or the scars of injuries. Models, photographs, exercise sheets, and drawings are helpful in giving the patient the desire to cooperate as part of a team.

2. Because many patients with shoulder arthritis or injuries have disorders of the cervical spine, preoperative neck x-rays are routine along with those of the chest and opposite shoulder. Electromyograms are obtained before surgery if a neurological deficit is suspected. The acromioclavicular joint is routinely examined; if found to be tender and painful, it is excised during the arthroplasty. The decision about the acromioclavicular joint must be made and recorded prior to giving the anesthesia.

3. Iron, vitamins, and calcium are given while the patient is awaiting admission to the hospital. Starting about one week before admission, the patient applies a long-acting antiseptic soap on the shoulder and the axilla during the daily shower to reduce the bacteria count of the skin. It is helpful if the therapist who will be treating the patient meets him or her and gives instruction in the exercise program prior to surgery. Of course, the exercises are individualized depending on the condition of the muscles, and therefore, the therapist must be made aware of expected restrictions.

4. Antibiotics are given routinely because large foreign bodies are implanted, the soft tissues are subjected to a large excursion of motion soon after surgery, and tissue contamination by previous injections or shoulder surgery is possible. I continue antibiotic coverage until results of the final cultures taken at surgery, both anaerobic and aerobic, have been reported. This usually requires ten days. If the patient is receiving steroids or immunosuppressants, antibiotics are routinely continued for three weeks following surgery. If the results of cultures taken at surgery are positive, antibiotics are continued longer, usually for from 6 to 12 weeks.

5. On the day before surgery, a hairclipper is used on the upper extremity and across the body to the midline front and back from the jaw to the waist. Bactericidal soap is applied to this area. Just prior to administration of anesthesia the shoulder is covered with a sterile towel to protect it from saliva during intubation. Shaving is deferred until the patient is under anesthesia because scratches made the night before might grow bacteria and because the shoulder is usually too painful to allow proper shaving of the axilla.

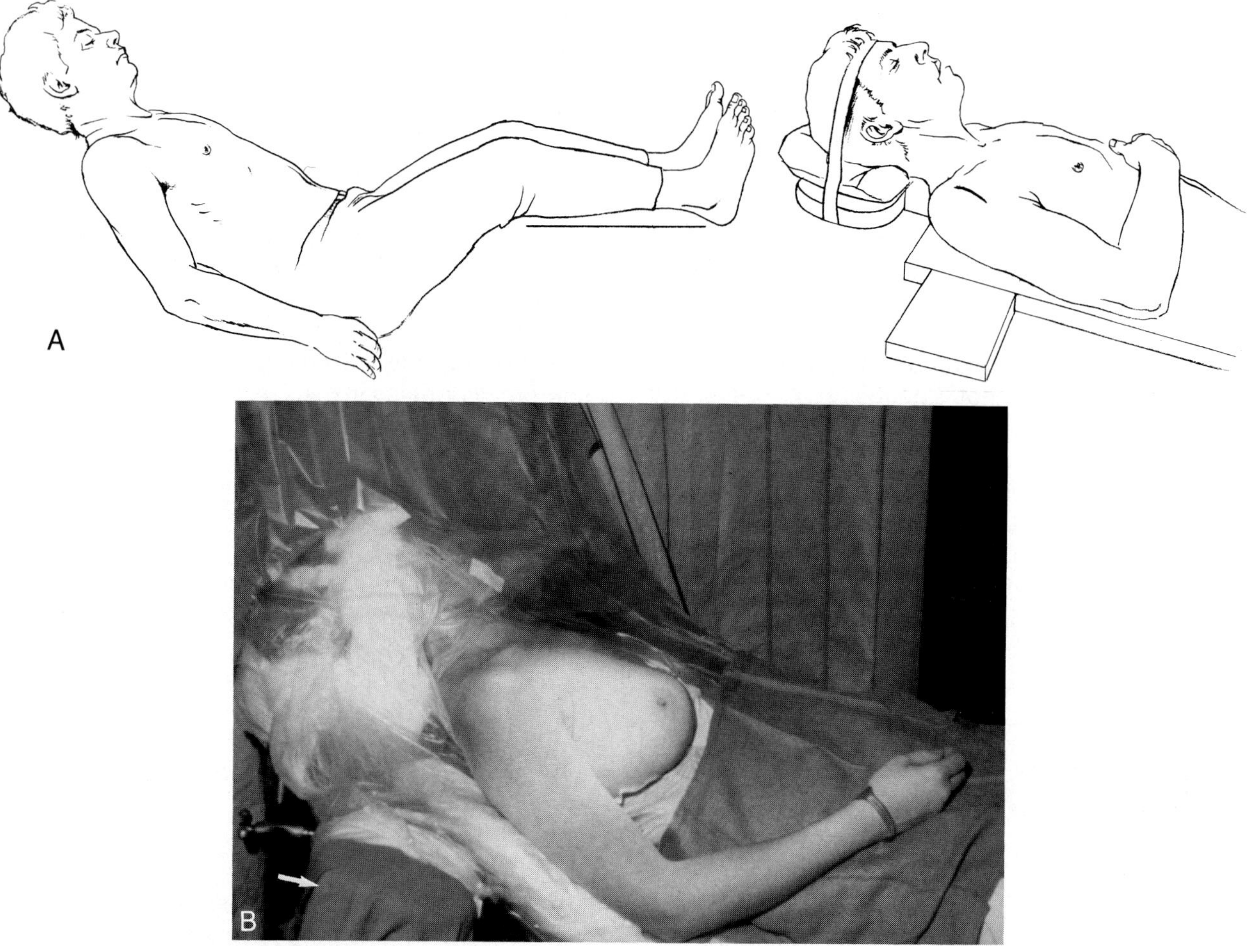

Figure 3–24. ***Technique of Shoulder Arthroplasty.*** Positioning and draping.

A, The semi-sitting, beachchair position is used with the head supported to prevent hyperextension of the neck and the legs parallel to the floor to avoid dependency.

B, Photograph made just prior to beginning the skin preparation to show how the shoulder is draped from the anesthesia team. The edge of the table is padded with the mattress, and, if a glenoid component is to be used, a padded, short armboard (arrow) or well-padded table is made available to support the arm when the glenoid is exposed. The arm is later draped free so that it can be moved, and the skin is covered with adherent plastic drapes.

Positioning and Draping

The beachchair, semi-sitting position with the point of the shoulder extending over the corner of the table is routine. The patient is placed high on the table in the supine position with a head rest that extends beyond the end of the table (Fig. 3–24). The head rest is positioned to prevent hyperextension of the neck that might compromise the cervical nerves by closing the neural foramen. The mattress is moved over the hard edge of the table to prevent contusion of the arm. Folded towels are placed under the ipsilateral scapula to hold it forward. The table is adjusted to the semi-sitting position with the upper part of the body raised 30 to 40 degrees and the knees raised sufficiently to prevent the patient from sliding down. The legs, from the knees down, are parallel to the floor rather than dependent. If it is expected that the procedure itself will last more than two hours, a retaining urinary catheter is inserted to prevent overdistention of the bladder.

If a glenoid component is to be used, it is important to have a support to maintain the involved arm abducted and externally rotated while the glenoid is exposed. I use a well-padded, short (8 inch) armboard (Fig. 3–24A). The short armboard is attached to the side of the table at the level of the shoulder, where it will allow hyperextension of the arm off the side of the table during preparation for the insertion of the humeral component. Alternatively, a small padded table can be brought in during the implantation of the glenoid component.

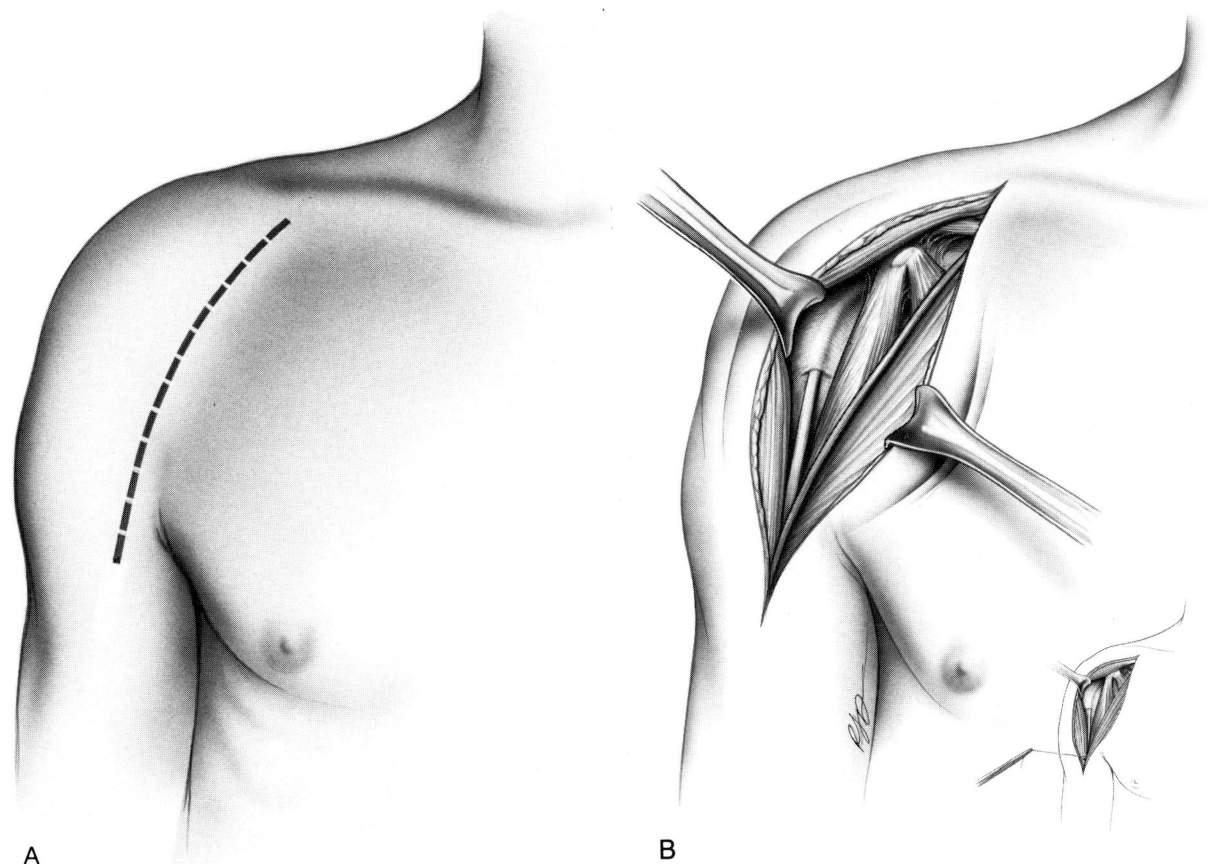

Figure 3–25. ***Technique of Shoulder Arthroplasty.*** Extended deltopectoral approach, saving a capsular flap for subscapularis length.

A, Incision begins near the clavicle at the deltopectoral interval, passes over the coracoid process, and ends at the level of the deltoid insertion.

B, After the surgeon divides the lateral branches of the cephalic vein, the deltoid is retracted laterally and the cephalic vein is retracted medially. The deltoid insertion is occasionally released (inset) when there is difficult, traumatic retraction of the deltoid muscle.

Illustration continued on following page

I prefer endotracheal general anesthesia although I request interscaline block anesthesia in the occasional patient with a special problem; however, it has disadvantages. After anesthesia has been established and shaving completed, the skin is meticulously cleaned, paying special attention to the axilla. The arm is draped free so it can be moved. Adherent, plastic drapes are applied to the skin (Fig. 3–24).

Extended Deltopectoral Approach

The "extended deltopectoral approach" is by far the best approach for shoulder arthroplasties (Fig. 3–25). The origin of the deltoid muscle is left intact.

The disadvantages of a posterior approach are discussed in Chapter 1, pages 33 to 35—i.e., the posterior acromion obstructs exposure, release of the internal rotation contracture is hazardous, and this approach detaches the important infraspinatus tendon unnecessarily.

A 17.0-cm. skin incision is made from the clavicle across the coracoid and down to the deltoid insertion. The cephalic vein is preserved and retracted medially because I believe there is less swelling of the hand in the immediate post-operative period if this vein is maintained intact. Its lateral tributaries are coagulated and divided far enough away to avoid injury to the vein. In revisions and injuries, the vein may be so scarred that it requires ligation. The deltoid muscle is retracted laterally. Slight abduction facilitates exposure at this point by relaxing the deltoid; however, more abduction may displace the axillary nerve upward, where it is more easily injured (see Fig. 1–31A and B). The clavipectoral fascia is divided from the coracoacromial ligament downward to the level of the deltoid insertion. If more exposure of the supra-

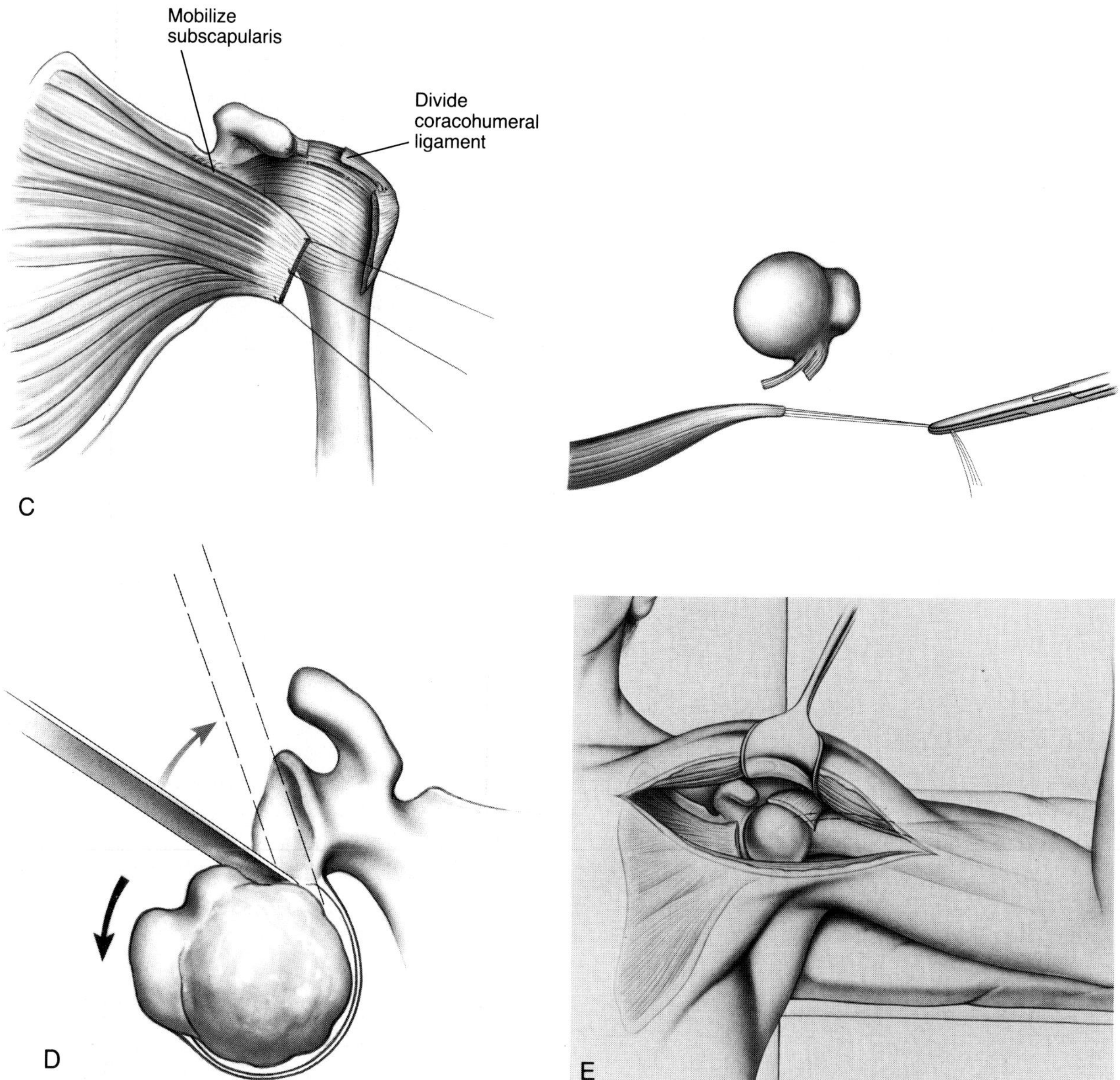

Figure 3–25 *Continued* C, The subscapularis tendon is divided transversely just medial to the lesser tuberosity, and the capsule is divided just lateral to the glenoid to create a flap of capsule attached to the humerus that can at closure be used to lengthen the subscapularis tendon (see Fig. 3–30). The subscapularis tendon and capsule are too thin to permit this step in shoulders with rheumatoid arthritis and congenital defects.

D, The head is dislocated with a Darrach elevator for leverage rather than with rotary force, which might fracture the shaft of the humerus.

E, Showing how the origin of the deltoid muscle is preserved, the subscapsularis is the only muscle detached, and the flap of capsule remains on the humerus. Abduction relaxes the deltoid muscle but places the axillary nerve in greater jeopardy (see Fig. 3–31).

spinatus tendon is needed, the coracoacromial ligament is divided; otherwise, it is maintained intact. A Darrach elevator is placed in the subacromial bursa under the acromion, exposing the upper end of the humerus. A second Darrach elevator is placed under the deltoid muscle just above its insertion (but below the level of the axillary nerve) to displace the deltoid laterally. When there is thickened subacromial bursa, it is removed as the humerus is rotated inward and outward and flexed. The humerus is externally rotated and adducted (to displace the axillary nerve out of harm's way), exposing the subscapularis tendon and the anterior circumflex vessels. Exposure of these vessels may require division of a small amount of the upper edge of the tendon of the sternal head of the pectoralis major. The axillary nerve is palpated in front of the subscapularis and also inferiorly beneath the glenohumeral joint capsule to make sure it is out of harm's way prior to coagulating and dividing the anterior circumflex vessels (see Fig. 1–31). Because the subscapularis muscle is often shortened, it is routine, when possible, to divide the subscapularis tendon transversely near the lesser tuberosity while the capsule beneath it is divided near the glenoid, as illustrated in Figure 3–25. In most rheumatoid shoulders the capsule is inadequate to permit this; however, the great majority of rheumatoid shoulders have an adequate length of subscapularis. Dividing the capsule at a point medial to the level where the subscapularis was divided also has the advantage of facilitating the closure of large cuff tears (see Fig. 3–30). The joint capsule is divided anteriorly up to the level of the long head of the biceps (avoiding injury to the biceps tendon); then, after placing a Darrach elevator next to the capsule inferiorly to protect the axillary nerve, the capsule is divided inferiorly sufficiently to allow the head to be dislocated anteriorly.

If there is a moderate tear of the rotator cuff, it is repaired at this time. Massive tears are mobilized after the humeral head has been removed and are re-attached to the greater tuberosity before implantation of the humeral component (Figs. 3–76 and 3–77).

The humeral head is then dislocated anteriorly into the wound by gentle external rotation (avoiding forceful external rotation, which might fracture the shaft of an osteopenic humerus) while a Darrach elevator is placed inside the joint to lever the head forward (Fig. 3–25). The elevator, not forceful twisting of the arm, applies the force that dislocates the head. When there has been long-standing subluxation of the head or when there is severe deformity of the head, this step can be quite difficult, as in patients with old trauma (see p. 222) or arthritis of dislocations (see Figs. 3–46 and 3–47).

Orientation of Trial Humeral Component

The humerus is then prepared to receive the trial humeral component. Osteophytes around the head are trimmed to identify the margin of the articular surface. During this step fragments of bone are carefully removed to prevent unwanted bone formation. Exuberant synovial tissue and loose bodies are also removed. The greater tuberosity is exposed so that the proper level of the silhouette or trial prosthesis can be visualized. The head of the silhouette or prosthesis is placed slightly higher than the top of the greater tuberosity, and, using these guides, the neck of the humerus is cut across with sharp osteotomes (Fig. 3–26). Ordinarily, unless some special version of the humeral component is required, the head is directed in 35 to 40 degrees of retroversion, as illustrated in Figure 3–26. However, in many cases the final version of the humeral component cannot be determined until after the glenoid component has been implanted. The version of the humeral component is calculated to make 40 degrees of total retroversion of both components combined (see Fig. 3–27).

A surprisingly small amount of bone is removed from the upper humerus—only the amount of bone remaining that had once been covered by articular cartilage. The superior part of the head is often worn, and this, combined with osteophyte formation inferiorly, makes it easy to remove too much of the neck (Fig. 3–26). Osteotomes are preferred for removing the head because they avoid the bone dust of saws or power tools. Care is taken to maintain the rotator cuff and long head of the biceps intact.

The medullary canal is then prepared with reamers, which have the same taper as the stems of the prosthesis. Drill points are available that can be used to enlarge the medullary canal when necessary. Fat and loose cancellous bone are removed from the canal, which is then irrigated with antibiotic solution. The trial humeral component is inserted with the arm extended off the side of the table, and the assistant supports the arm and pushes it upward to prevent stretch on the brachial plexus. The height of the head of the prosthesis above the greater tuberosity and the retroversion of the head is checked prior to reduction. After reducing the head into the joint, the length of the head can be compared to the available length of

Text continued on page 178

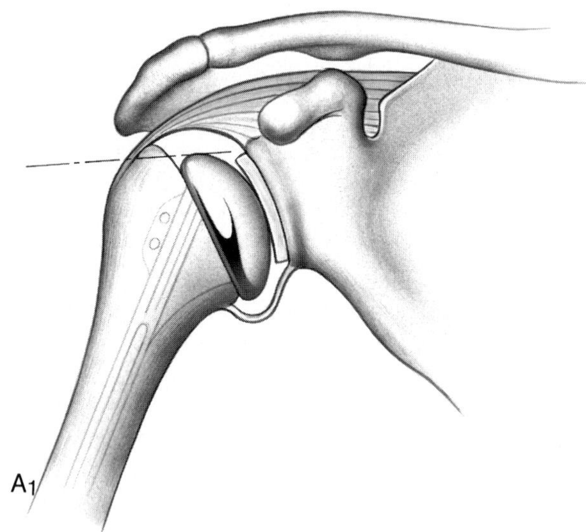

Figure 3–26. ***Technique of Shoulder Arthroplasty.*** Orientation of the humeral component. The following four criteria must be met.

A, Firstly, the articular surface of the prosthesis must be cephalad to the greater tuberosity to prevent impingement. (1) The error of low placement of the head, causing the greater tuberosity to impinge on the acromion. (2) Silhouette or trial prosthesis to mark the level, and drawing indicating the proper level. Note the inferior osteophytes remaining.

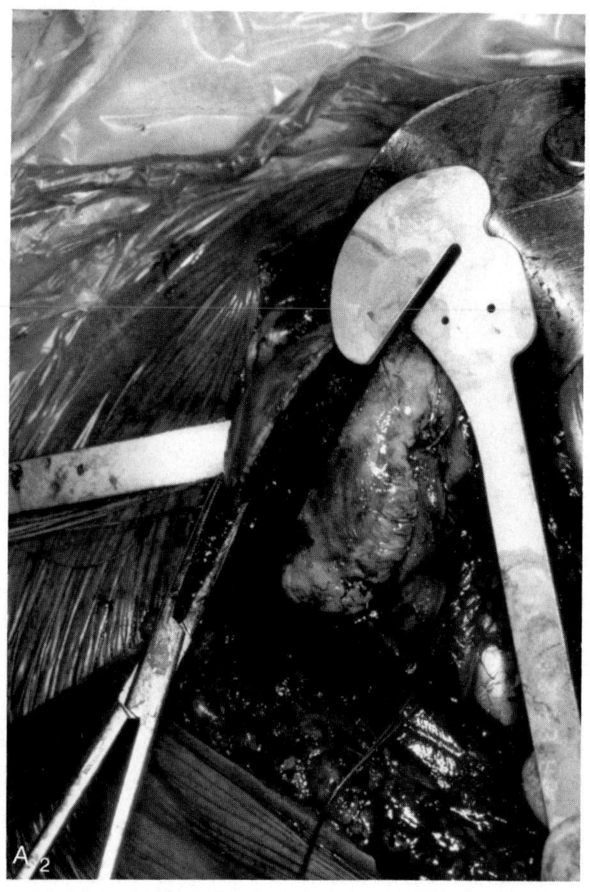

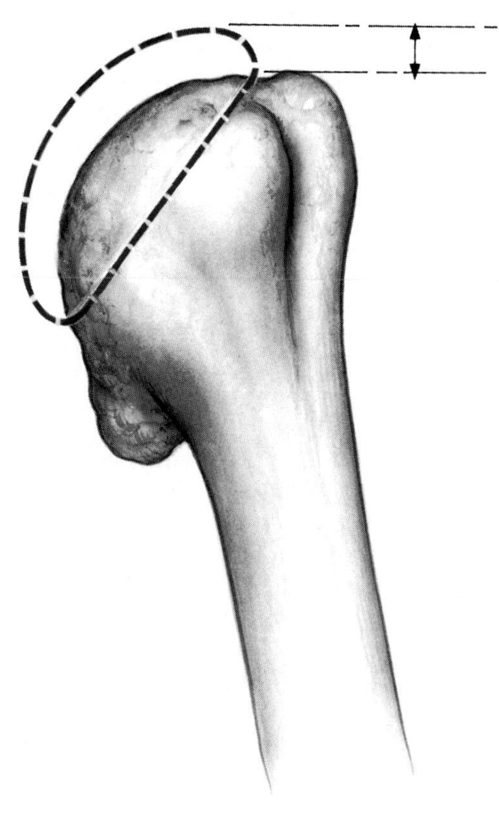

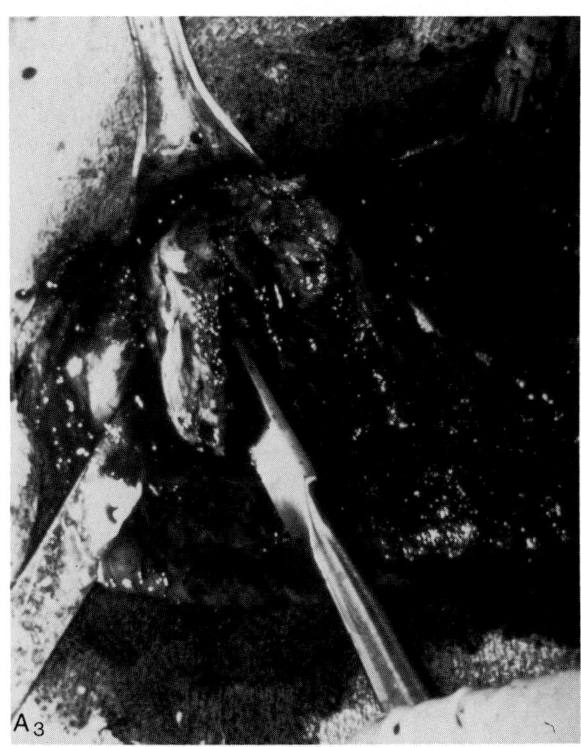

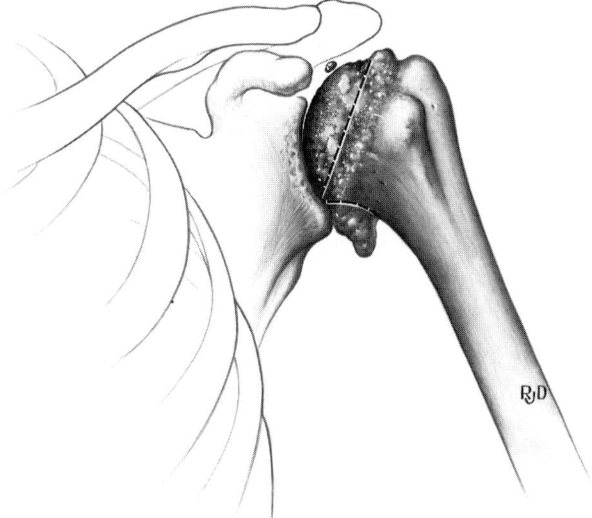

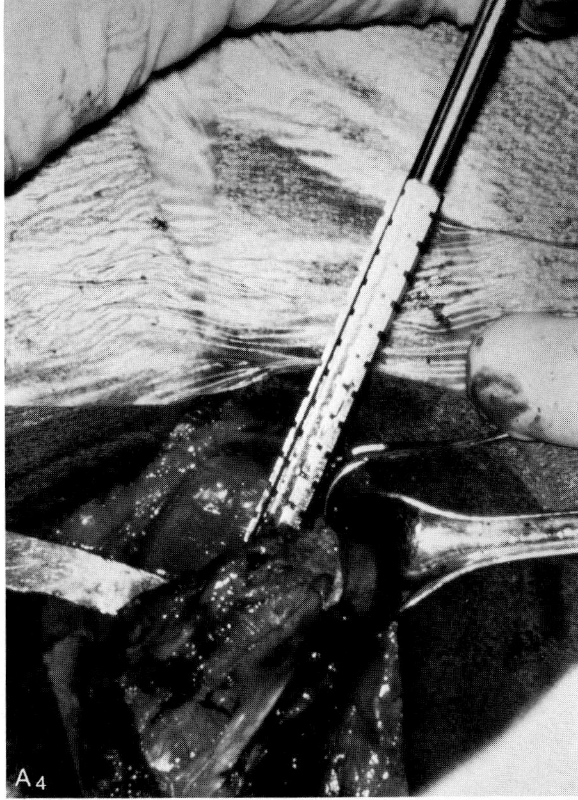

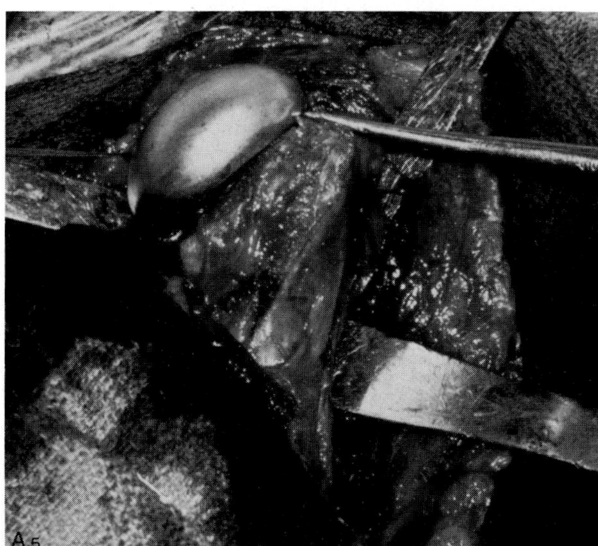

Figure 3–26A *Continued* (3) Osteotome removes only the bone normally covered with articular cartilage. The inferior osteophytes are later removed, as in the drawing. (4) Reaming the medullary canal to remove loose particles of bone. (5) Trial prosthesis in place at the proper level in relation to the top of the greater tuberosity. Osteophytes have been removed.

Illustration continued on following page

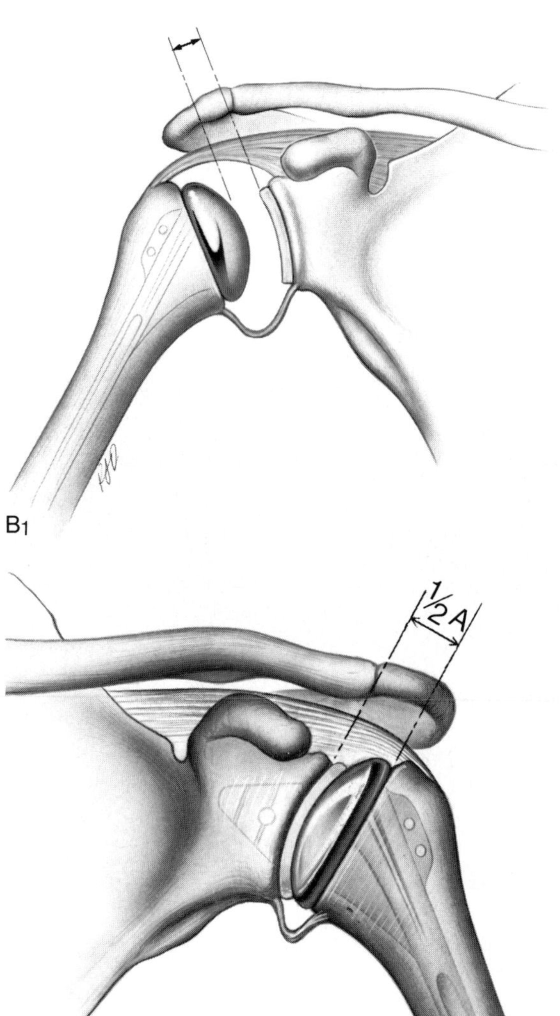

Figure 3–26 *Continued* B, Secondly, the head of the prosthesis must be long enough to fill the tuberosity glenoid space, or the components will be unstable. However, if the head is too long, it will interfere with closing the subscapularis tendon and, if the posterior capsule is contracted, it will prevent internal rotation of the shoulder in the end result, as illustrated in Figure 3–21A and B. (1) Showing the error of using a head that is too short, causing instability. (2) The length of head is selected by inserting trial prostheses. The prosthesis to be used can be cemented proud to make final adjustments (see Fig. 3–29).

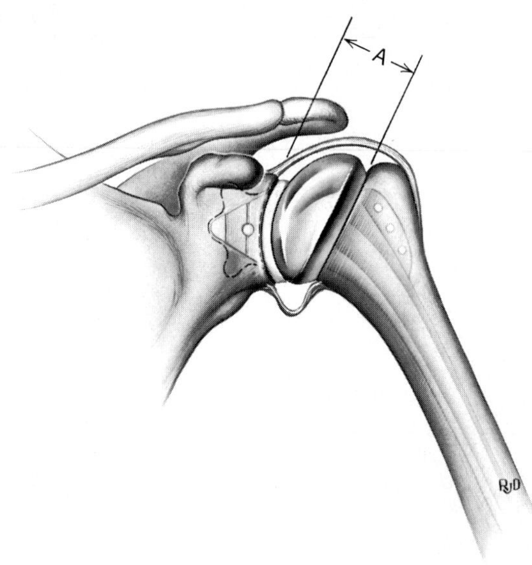

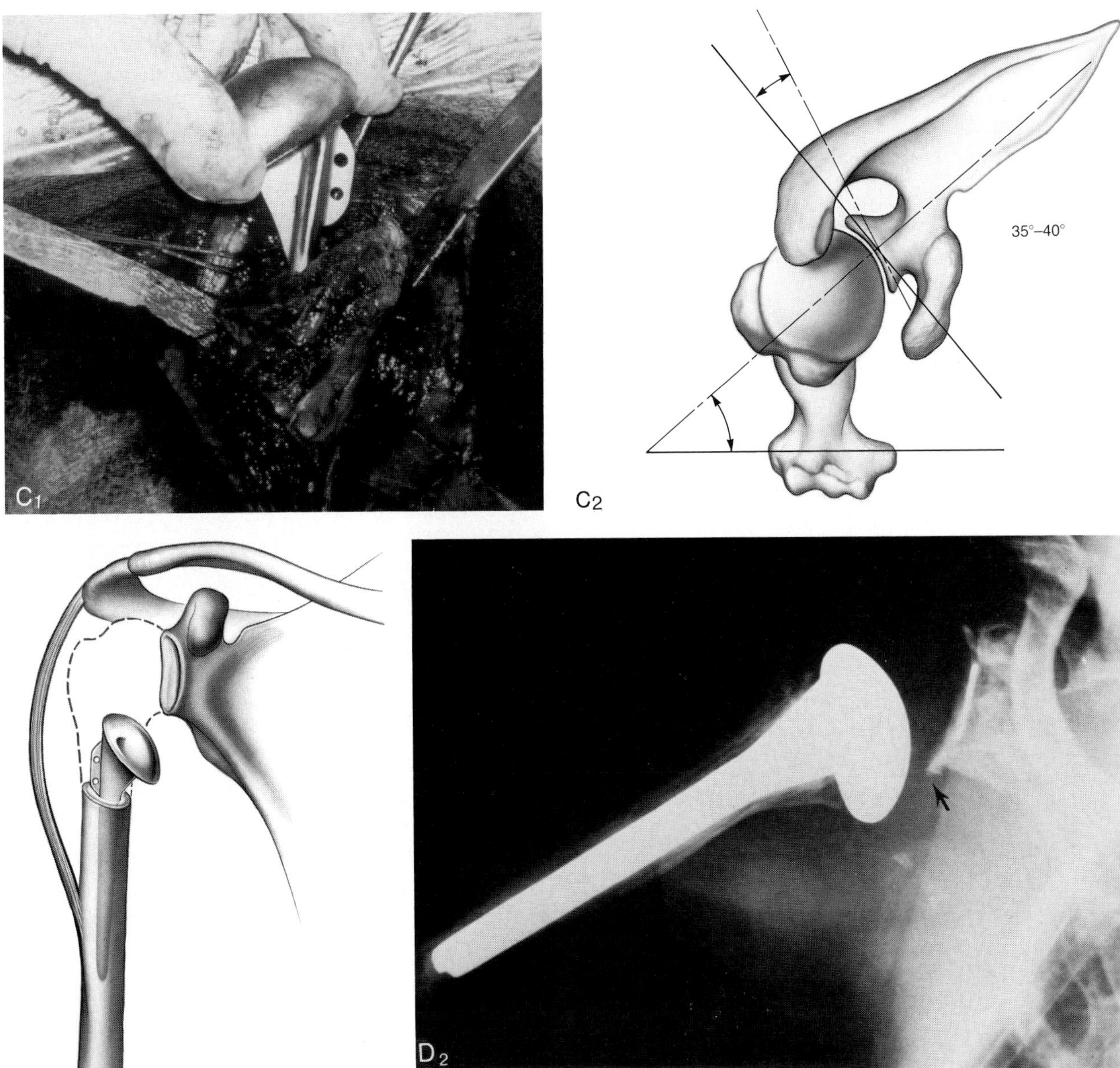

Figure 3–26 *Continued* C, Thirdly, unless the articular surface of the glenoid is deformed, the humeral component is seated in 35 to 40 degrees of retroversion. If the glenoid is retroverted or anteverted, adjustments are made so that the total retroversion of the two components combined is about 40 degrees (see Fig. 3–28D). If the joint capsule is enlarged because of the head having been subluxed or dislocated, adjustments are made in the version of the humeral component at the time of cementing (see Fig. 3–28D). (1) Trial prosthesis being placed in 40 degrees of retroversion. Its nne mark on the bone shows the rotary alignment in relation to the epicondyles and forearm. (2) The total retroversion of the humeral head and articular surface of the glenoid combined should be 35 to 40 degrees.

D, Fourthly, the length of the humerus must be preserved, or the prosthesis will be unstable (2) and the deltoid muscle will be slack and unable to raise the arm (1).

soft tissue of the rotator cuff by exerting traction on the stay sutures of the subscapularis tendon. Traction is applied to the arm while the position of the head relative to the glenoid is observed to make sure the proper length of the arm is maintained. The head of the trial prosthesis should be at the level of the glenoid when traction is applied. This indicates the level for final cementing of the humeral component. The trial prosthesis is then removed.

Implanting the Glenoid Component

Good technique and care in implanting the glenoid component are of key importance in eliminating radiolucent lines around the cement in postoperative films. Exposure of the glenoid is obtained by supporting the arm with a bolster placed on the short armboard (or side table) and placing the arm in abduction and external rotation. Abduction relaxes the deltoid, and external rotation relaxes the posterior capsule and reduces the tension on the axillary nerve. A Fukuda-Ogawa[127] ring retractor is placed behind the glenoid to hold the humerus posteriorly (Fig. 3–27). I prefer this retractor because the opening in the ring can be positioned so it does not press against the glenoid component, interfering with its insertion. The anterior labrum is excised, and the soft tissue is excised to expose the upper and lower margins of the articular surface of the glenoid and to allow palpation or visualization of the base of the coracoid. The inferior part of the posterior labrum is also excised, but because the long head of the biceps inserts into the posterior labrum, care must be taken in removing the posterior labrum so that

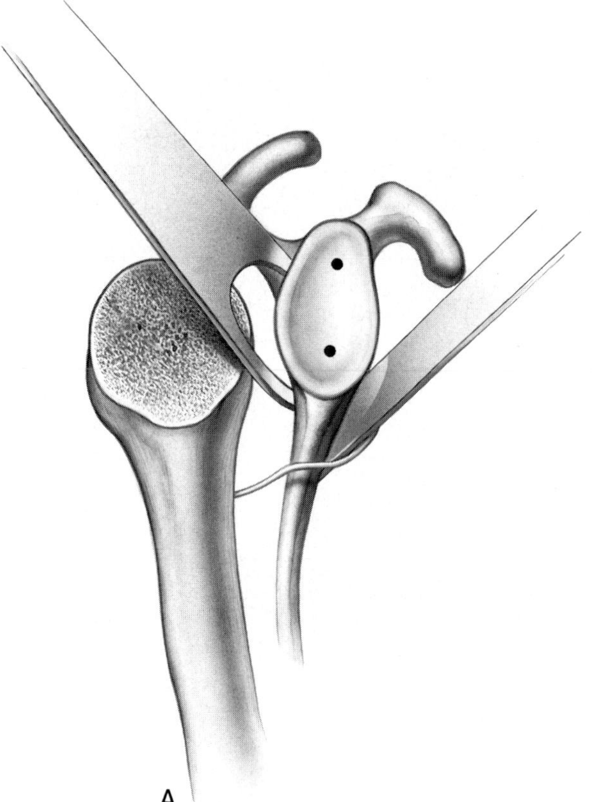

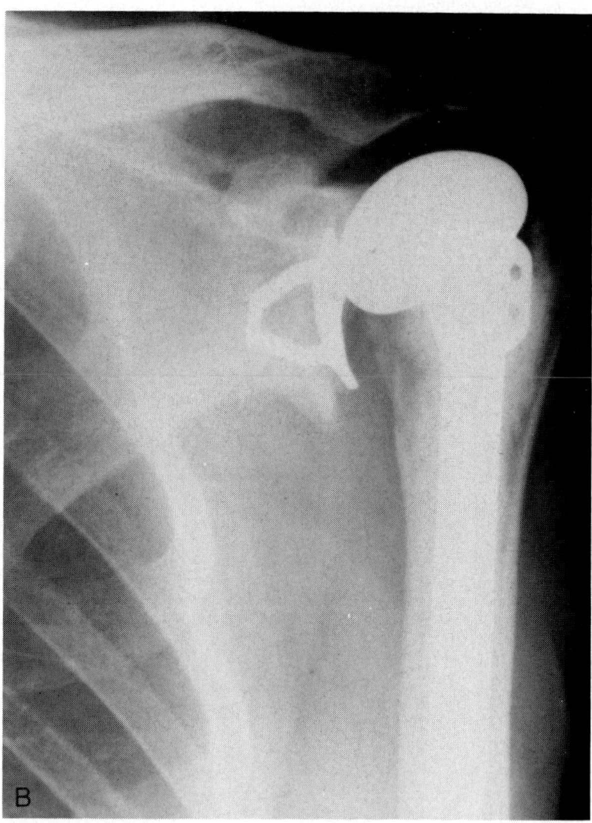

Figure 3–27. ***Technique of Total Shoulder Arthroplasty.*** Implanting the glenoid component. The arm is supported on a padded armboard or side table in the position of rotation that offers the best exposure of the glenoid.

A, A ring retractor is placed inside the joint behind the posterior rim of the glenoid to displace the humerus posteriorly. The anterior labrum is excised, and a Darrach elevator is placed subperiosteally in front of the glenoid to protect the axillary nerve. The posterior labrum is then excised for better exposure of the articular surface of the glenoid and to give the ring retractor better stability. Care is taken to preserve the attachment of the long head of the biceps on the scapula. Two awl holes are made to mark the location of the slot. The upper hole is made first near the top of the glenoid to avoid the error of low placement of the glenoid component.

B, Illustrating the error of low placement of the glenoid component. This is an easy mistake to make when the glenoid is enlarged by wear and osteophytes.

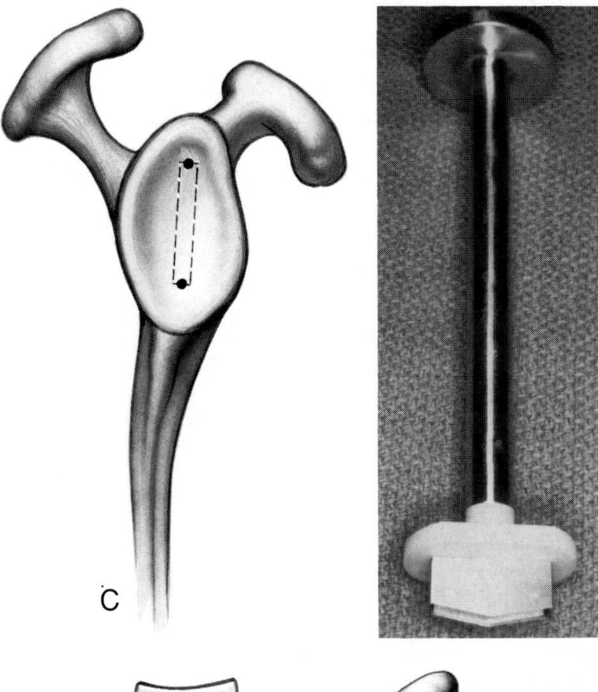

Figure 3–27 *Continued* C, The site of the slot for the keel of the glenoid component is outlined with a cookie-cutter (right) or osteotome. The subchondral bone is otherwise maintained intact.

D, The slot is undermined with curved curettes to remove loose cancellous bone and to create anchor holes for the cement in the coracoid process and along the lateral margin of the scapula. The slot is given its final shape, and its depth is tested with reamer-guides (right), which are the same shape as the keel of the glenoid components. Finally, the articular surface of the glenoid is contoured to support the back of the articular surface of the glenoid component on all sides.

Illustration continued on following page

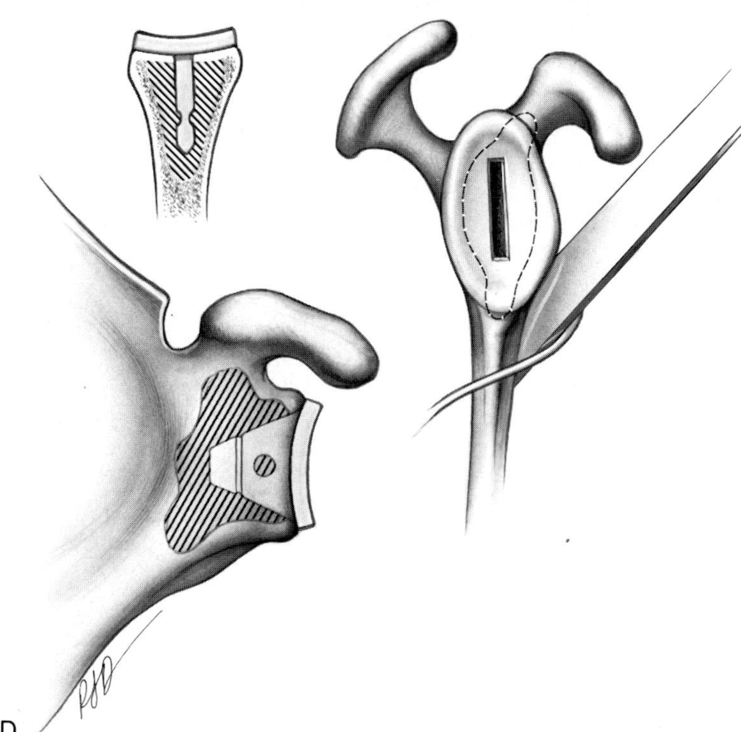

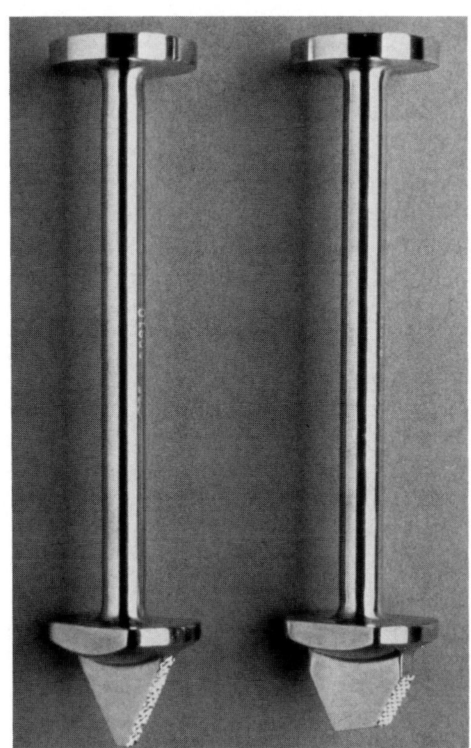

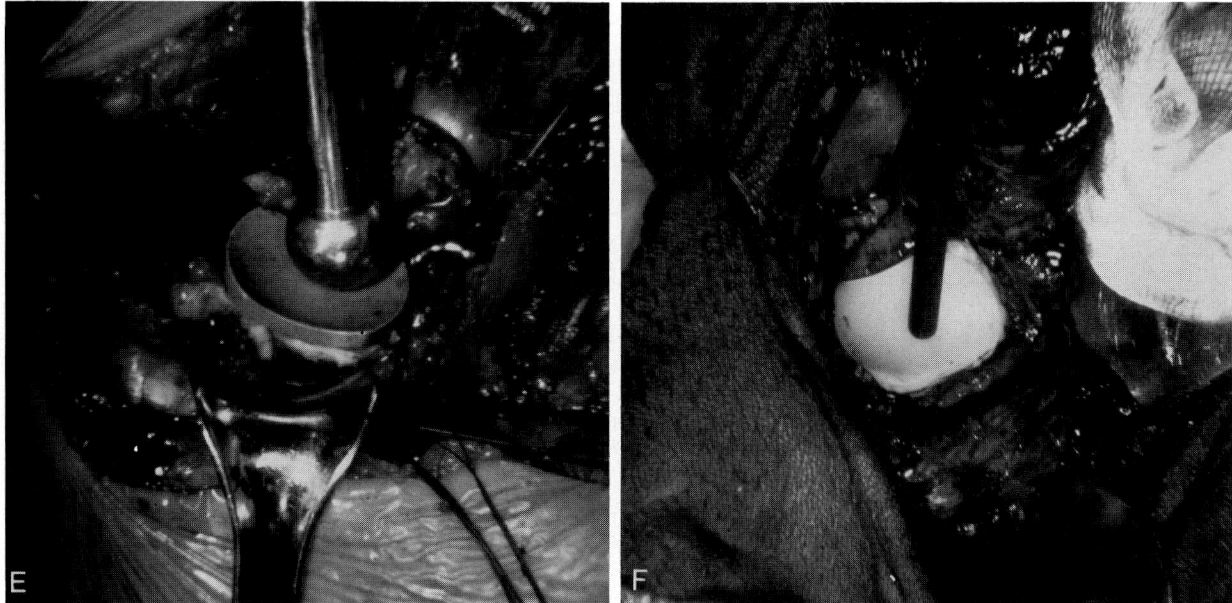

Figure 3–27 *Continued* E, A trial glenoid component is hammered into place with an impactor. When the trial glenoid component is firmly seated without tilting or rocking, the final glenoid component can be cemented in place.

F, Cementing the glenoid component. The glenoid cavity is thoroughly irrigated with antibiotic solution, and all particles of loose bone are removed. One batch of cement is introduced in two phases. The first plug of cement is forced into the finer openings with a sponge. The second plug (from the same batch of cement) is used to fill the glenoid cavity just prior to implanting the glenoid component. All visible cement is removed from around the component, and the component is held firmly in place until the cement hardens. The glenoid component is then stressed to make sure that there is no motion between it and the underlying bone before going on to the next step.

the insertion of the long head remains intact. The soft tissue is elevated in front of the scapula, and a Darrach elevator is placed against the bone to provide exposure of the glenoid and to protect the axillary nerve (Fig. 3–27).

The arm is then rotated into the position that offers the best view of the glenoid. The bolster is adjusted to support the weight of the arm in this position, eliminating leverage of the upper humerus against the retractors. This position of rotation must be maintained by the assistants, and the anesthesiologist must maintain muscle relaxation until the glenoid component has been implanted.

Scar and remnants of articular cartilage are removed from the surface of the glenoid with a large curette and a power burr. Subchondral bone is preserved. Osteophytes on the inferior edge of the glenoid may mislead the surgeon into placing the glenoid component too low. To avoid this error, the location of the slot on the articular surface of the glenoid is marked with an awl starting at the top of the glenoid (Fig. 3–27). The base of the coracoid is palpated, and the first mark is made in line with it just below the superior edge of the articular surface of the glenoid. The second awl mark is made below this in line with the lateral margin of the scapula. A cutting guide or osteotome is used to outline the exact length and width of a slot that will match the exact size of the base of the holding device of the glenoid component. A slot of this exact size is cut with a power drill, leaving the surrounding subchondral bone intact. Small angulated curettes are used to find the medullary canal and to undermine the subchondral and adjacent bone by removing loose cancellous bone under the subchondral plate, down the lateral border of the scapula, and into the coracoid process. Undermining the subchondral plate and creating these two anchor holes under the cortical bone will cause the cement to be locked inside the scapula. If perforations are accidentally made through the cortex of the scapula, they are closed with cancellous bone grafts or, if large, with wire cement restrictors. Metal guides are used to determine the length, width, depth, and direction of the opening for the stem of both of the standard glenoid components. After having made this opening, loose cancellous bone is removed with curettes, and the cavity is irrigated with antibiotic solution.

Next, the articular surface of the glenoid is contoured to fit the back of the articular surface of the glenoid component. This is of critical importance. The back of the glenoid component should be supported by bone on all sides to prevent tilting of the component. The articular surface of the glenoid must be shaped like a dish to conform to the shape of the back of the glenoid component to prevent rocking. A build-up of cement between the articular surface of the glenoid component and the articular surface of the glenoid is undesirable because the cement might break out, with loss of support (see Fig. 3–98G and H). A trial glenoid component is inserted and hammered into place using the "ball" impactor (see Fig. 3–24). I have used both flat-back and curved-back metal components but generally prefer the curved-back design. Unfortunately, when the articular surface of the glenoid has been worn and flattened, it is necessary to contour the sclerotic bone to fit the curved back of this component. Otherwise, the curved back on a flat surface allows rocking.

When the glenoid is worn or eroded, the stem of the component may be too long or too thick to fit inside the available bone. The polyethylene component has a thinner stem, which can easily be cut off and shortened at the operating table, so it is more adaptable when glenoid bone stock is deficient.

When motion and stability are satisfactory, the glenoid component is anchored with methylmethacrylate introduced in two stages. Loose cancellous bone and blood are removed, and the glenoid is thoroughly irrigated with antibiotic solution. Introducing the cement under pressure has been attempted but has been unsatisfactory because the soft cement tended to leak out into the surrounding tissue and tended to perforate the frail scapula. Therefore, the technique of inserting a preliminary plug of soft cement using finger pressure and a sponge (forcing the cement into the finer openings and controlling bleeding) followed by a second plug of firmer cement (from the same batch) is usually preferred. Occasionally the glenoid is dry enough to allow introduction of the cement in one plug. The final step in implanting the glenoid component itself is then made. The glenoid component is tapped firmly into place using the ball impactor, and visible cement is carefully removed. No cement is intentionally placed between the articular surface of the component and that of the glenoid to prevent it from breaking out, leaving the prosthesis unsupported and leading to toggle motion and breakage of the stem of the glenoid component (see Fig. 3–98H). The component is held firmly in place and the wound is filled with antibiotics as the cement sets. When the cement is hard the component is tested to make sure there is no motion between it and the bone. If the glenoid component is loose, it is immediately removed; then, after removing the cement, the defect in the first implantation is corrected, and another component is cemented in its place.

Compensating for Bone-Deficient Glenoid

Glenoid deficiency may be caused by a number of processes, as listed in Table 3–2, including (1) uneven wear (osteoarthritis and arthritis of dislocation), (2) granulation erosion (rheumatoid arthritis), (3) skeletal underdevelopment (congenital hypoplasia, multiple epiphyseal dysplasia), (4) pressure erosion from longstanding dislocations (old trauma, Erb's palsy), (5) removal of bone (gunshot wound, surgical procedures), or (6) extreme glenohumeral instability causing Charcot-like erosion (cuff-tear arthropathy).

Although severe bone loss at the glenoid can prevent the use of a glenoid component, this problem can be overcome in many instances. Details of these techniques will be discussed separately with the descriptions of specific pathology according to diagnostic categories. An overall description of the techniques used is presented and illustrated in Figure 3–28. The technique depends on the severity of bone loss and the location of available bone.

Lowering the High Side. If the articular surface of the glenoid is worn unevenly on one side (as in osteoarthritis or arthritis of dislocations), support, front and back, for the articular surface of the glenoid component can be obtained in those with milder discrepancies by lowering the high side. However, larger discrepancies cannot be treated in this way for two reasons. First, lowering the high side to the level of an area of severe wear leaves an inadequate depth of bone for the keel of the glenoid component. Second, if the articular surface of the glenoid component is placed too far medially, increasing the distance from the articular surface of the glenoid to the greater tuberosity, the humeral component is rendered unstable and will tend to dislocate (see Fig. 3–27).

Avoid Cement Build-Up on the Low Side. Cement build-up on the low side to give support to the glenoid component when there is uneven wear of the articular surface is mentioned here only to condemn it and to emphasize that it should not be done. Bone support should be obtained on all sides behind the articular surface of the glenoid component. If there is cement build-up, the cement may break and fall out under the component, causing the articular surface to toggle until eventually breakage of the stem may occur (see Fig. 3–

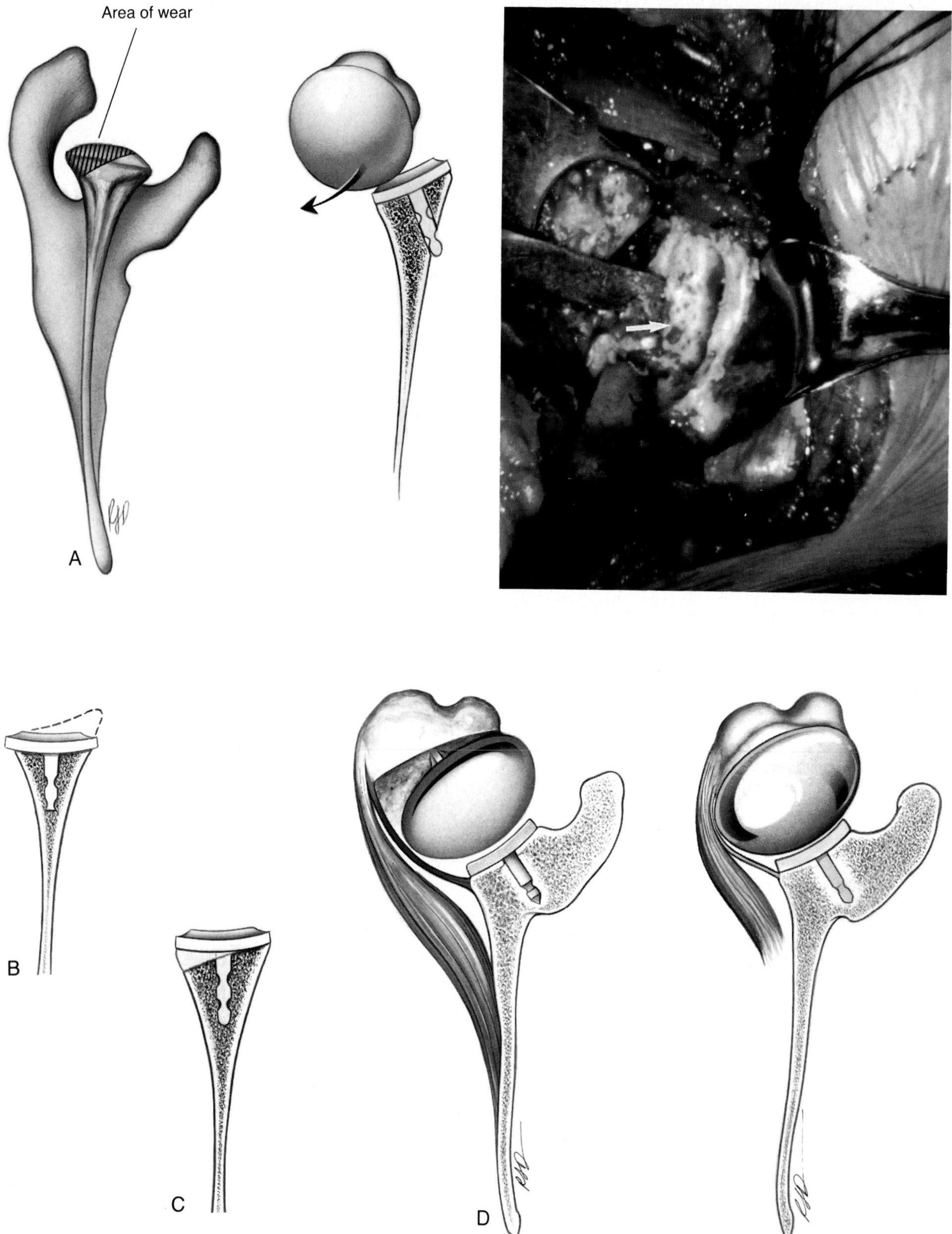

Figure 3–28 *See legend on opposite page*

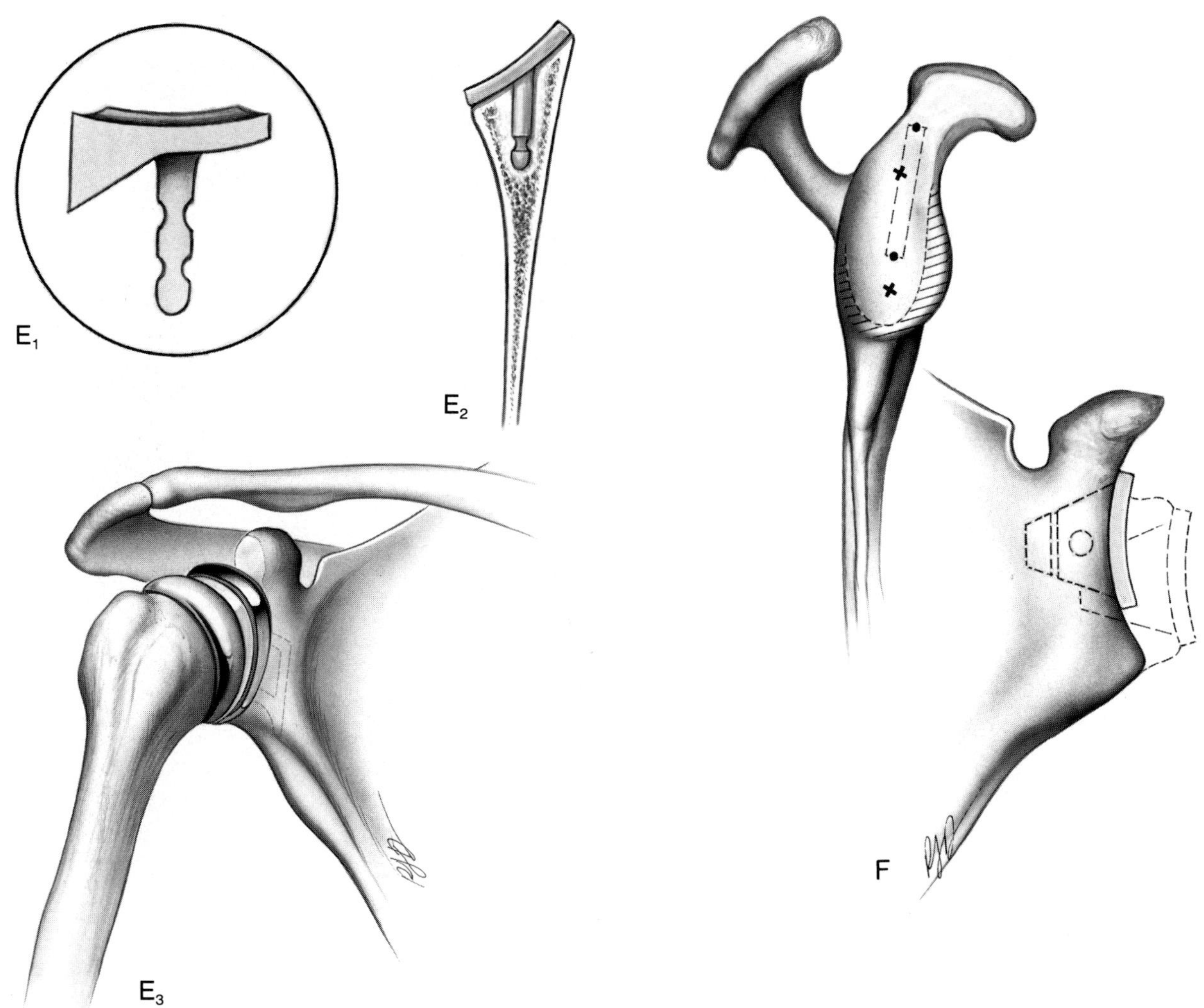

Figure 3–28. ***Technique of Total Shoulder Arthroplasty.*** Compensating for a bone deficient glenoid.

A, There are a number of processes that can cause bone deficiency at the glenoid that, unless compensated for, may make the components unstable. The photograph (right) illustrates posterior bone deficiency (arrow). Less often, the deficiency is anterior or superior. These glenoid bone deficiencies may be offset by one of the following techniques.

B, Lowering the high side.

C, Building up the low side with cement is to be avoided, as discussed in Figure 3–98G and H.

D, Altering the version of the glenoid component. This must be offset by altering the version of the humeral component in the opposite direction. The usual problem is loss of the posterior glenoid, causing the glenoid component to be implanted in retroversion and the humeral component in anteversion, as illustrated. The laxity or tightness of the posterior capsular pouch determines whether (1) the humeral component is implanted with space between the prosthesis and the greater tuberosity posteriorly to take up slack in the posterior capsule (left); or (2) because of short posterior capsule and short external rotators, the head is placed in the same position in which it presented (right). The first situation is seen in advanced osteoarthritis and in arthritis of recurrent dislocations and the latter in long-standing dislocations (see p. 208) and in arthritis occasionally seen after long-standing incomplete Erb's palsy (see Figs. 3–87 and 3–88).

E, Special glenoid components are used developmentally occasionally in less active patients with unusual bone loss from cuff-tear arthropathy, long-standing rheumatoid arthritis, or in a revision. Illustrated are (1) augmented side, (2) angulated stem, and (3) slightly oversized and thicker superiorly.

F, Coracoid (high) placement of the glenoid component utilizing the bone in the base of the coracoid can be helpful in cuff-tear arthropathy, advanced rheumatoid arthritis, and some congenital defects.

Illustration continued on following page

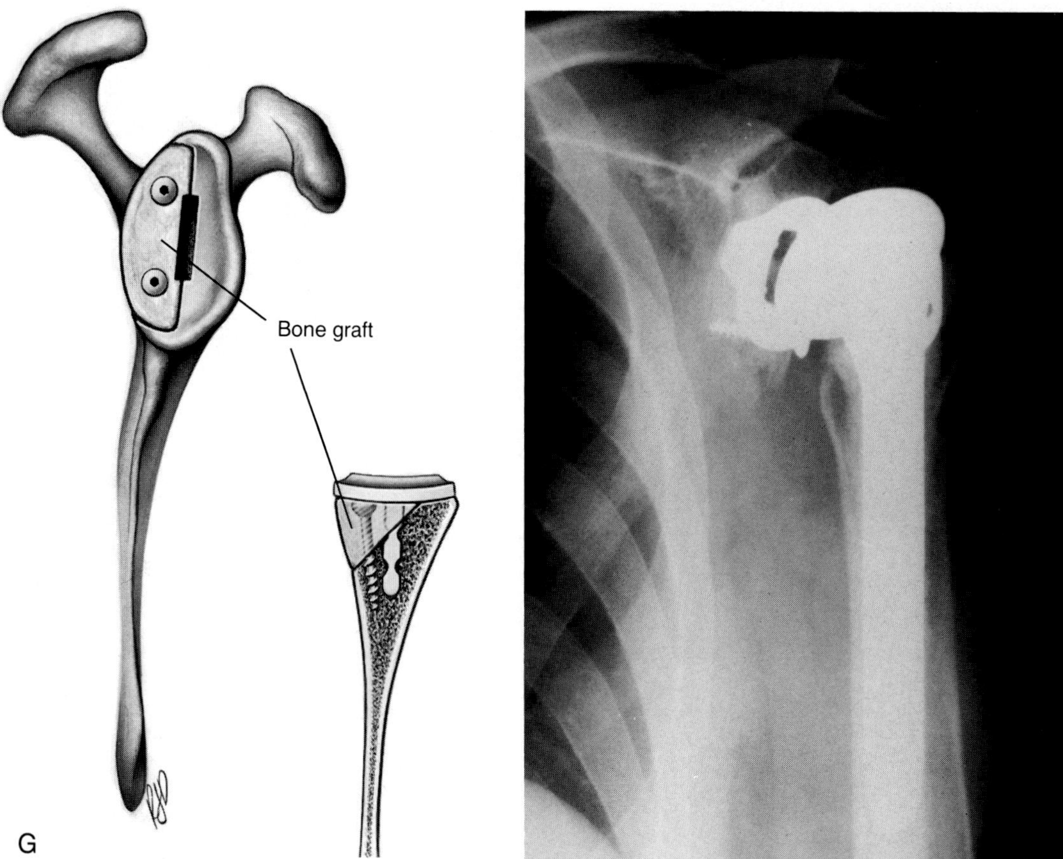

Figure 3–28 *Continued* G, Glenoid bone grafts. The technique is illustrated (left), and a 6-year follow-up appearance is shown (right). During recent years, I have tended to prefer altering the version rather than using glenoid grafts, but there have been exceptions.

Use of the humeral component alone is illustrated in Figure 3–49.

98G and H). This occurred in five patients in my series, and each required implantation of another glenoid component. At surgery, the tip of the keel remained firmly cemented in the bone, but the polyethylene stem had broken under the stress of toggling. Two steps have been taken to avoid this complication. The groove in the keel of the polyethylene glenoid component where the breakage always occurred has been removed, and second, cement build-up between the articular surface of the glenoid and the back of the component is avoided.

Alter the Version of the Glenoid Component. When there is excessive posterior wear the glenoid component can be placed in more retroversion (articular surface facing posteriorly), or, if there is more anterior wear, the glenoid component may be placed in more anteversion (articular surface facing anteriorly). If the version of the glenoid component is changed, the rotation of the humeral component must be changed in its relationship to the humerus so that the total combined retroversion of both the humeral and glenoid components does not exceed 40 degrees. Normally the glenoid component is near neutral (zero degrees), and the humeral component is in about 40 degrees of retroversion. Thus, if the glenoid component is placed in 30 degrees retroversion (because of posterior wear), the humeral component is placed at no more than 10 degrees retroversion (Fig. 3–28D). When this technique is used, care must be taken to have the glenoid component at the level of the base of the coracoid where the scapula is thickest (see Fig. 3–14); otherwise, the stem might protrude outside of the bone.

Special Glenoid Components. Although a bone-deficient glenoid may not support a special glenoid component, I have used one occasionally in an elderly or less active patient who puts less physical demands on the shoulders. Three designs are considered: (1) an augmented side front or back (Fig. 3–28E1), (2) an angulated stem for uneven anterior or posterior wear that allows the articular surface of the component to be in altered version but does not allow protrusion of the stem outside the bone (Fig. 3–28D2), and (3) a slightly oversized glenoid component that is thicker superiorly to compensate for superior wear (Fig. 3–28D3). In each case the back of the articular surface of the glenoid component is made to rest on bone.

Coracoid Placement. High placement of the glenoid component utilizing the base of the coracoid can be very useful when there is wear and loss of bone on the superior aspect of the glenoid, as seen in some patients with rheumatoid arthritis or cuff-tear arthropathy (Fig. 3–28F). Because much of the articular surface is gone, the eburnated surface of the base of the coracoid becomes continuous with the remains of the articular surface of the glenoid. The slot can be placed high, extending partly into the coracoid and using the coracoid for bone support. Bone is usually available at the inferior lateral margin of the scapula, and the loss of bone at the superior margin of the glenoid causes the articular surface of the glenoid to face upward, causing the humeral head to ascend.

Glenoid Bone Grafts. A piece of the head of the humerus may be used as a glenoid bone graft to fill large defects in the front or back of the scapula (Fig. 3–28G).[126] In addition, I have often used small amounts of cancellous or cortical bone from the head as bone grafts to build up weak spots in the scapula. Grafts taken from the inner table of the iliac crest are used when no head is available, as when doing a revision. Large grafts have been used in 30 of my shoulder arthroplasties; 20 of these were reported to the American Shoulder and Elbow Surgeons Open Meeting in 1986.[126] Although it is not possible to be sure all of the grafts are united by bone, none of the prosthetic components migrated, and the clinical results were satisfactory. The screws holding the grafts broke in two patients who subjected their shoulders to crutch-walking in the immediate post-operative period; however, the position of the screws and that of the component have remained stationary and without an enlarging line of lucency. The indications for the large, internally fixed glenoid bone grafts in this series were rheumatoid arthritis in seven, arthritis of dislocations (see Fig. 3–47) in five, osteoarthritis in two, old chronic dislocation in two, Erb's palsy deformity with arthritis in one, cuff-tear arthropathy in one, revision in one, and gunshot injury in one. A piece of the head was cut to the appropriate size to fit against a freshened surface of glenoid and was secured with two 4.0 mm. bone screws in 10 shoulders and with No. 2 nonabsorbable sutures and the cemented glenoid component in the other 10 shoulders. Good results of glenoid bone grafting can be seen in Figures 3–28G and 3–47C and D. The keel of the component is placed as far as possible inside the medullary canal of the scapula to prevent shear, while the wedge-shaped bone supporting one side is largely under compressive force, which may be one reason why the grafts have remained in place. In addition to the condition of the bone, the length of the available muscles is another factor in the decision as to whether a graft should be used. For example, I would no longer use a glenoid bone graft in Erb's palsy because positioning the components in their normal place leaves the external rotators too short to be re-attached (see Figs. 3–87 to 3–89).

Humeral Component Alone. A humeral component alone without a glenoid component is a valid choice when the glenoid is too frail and defective to support any type of fixation device. This is preferable to leaving the glenoid component unsupported by bone, as in long-standing rheumatoid arthritis (see Fig. 3–49B to D).

Anchoring the Humeral Component

Prior to permanent anchorage of the humeral component, anterior acromioplasty and cuff repairs are completed as indicated. The distal clavicle can be excised from below at this time without detaching deltoid origin. Large rotator cuff tears are more easily mobilized and repaired, in accordance with the principles outlined in Figs. 2–43 and 3–30, prior to implantation of the humeral component. The types of rotator cuff defects typical of impingement tears may be seen; in advanced rheumatoid arthritis (see Figs. 3–48 to 3–56), old trauma (Figs. 3–57 to 3–63), and cuff-tear arthropathy (see Figs. 3–72 to 3–82) the cuff defects may be much larger than those of impingement tears and require one of the transfers shown in Figure 3–30.

The humeral components of the Neer II System were designed for use with cement and are cemented except in younger patients with a good press-fit and in those occasional cases in which sepsis from previous surgery or injection is suspected (see p. 247 and Fig. 3–90). In my most recent 355 Neer II total arthroplasties, cement was used for the humeral component in all but 19. In an uncomplicated arthroplasty the humeral component is anchored in 30 to 40 degrees retroversion. Prior to cementing the component, a trial humeral component is inserted to determine the stability of the head in this position of rotation as well as the height of the head. The amount of retroversion can be judged by flexing the elbow and palpating the epicondyles to determine the rotation of the shaft. The head of the prosthesis should point toward the glenoid when the arm is held in neutral rotation (anatomical position). The head must extend slightly cephalad to the top of the greater tuberosity to prevent impingement of the tuberosity against the acromion. The head of the humerus must be thick enough to fill the space between the greater tuberosity and the glenoid component; otherwise the components may be unstable. The length of the humerus must be maintained with slight tension on the myofascial sleeve (see Fig. 3–26), as tested by applying downward traction on the arm. If there is loss of bone at the upper humerus, as from old trauma (see Figs. 3–57 to 3–63), or revisions (see Figs. 3–97 to 3–99), the gap between the tuberosities and the shaft is filled with bone grafts after cementing the humeral prosthesis proud. The height of the prosthesis is determined by placing traction on the arm with the prosthesis inserted in the medullary canal and lifting the head of the prosthesis upward until it is opposite the glenoid while traction is applied. Unless the length of the shaft is maintained with tension on the myofascial sleeve, the prosthesis will tend to subluxate or dislocate inferiorly, and the deltoid muscle will be too long to raise the arm. Either the humeral head or an iliac graft is used to fill the gap (see Figs. 3–26 and 3–29).

When the glenoid component has been implanted in retroversion or anteversion, the humeral component must be placed in the proper rotation, as discussed in Figure 3–28D.

If the prosthetic head is too long, it will make closure of the subscapularis or rotator cuff almost impossible, and, because the posterior capsule is intact, it will block internal rotation and cause the head to subluxate anteriorly. When there is "centralization" (medial displacement of the humerus due to medial erosion into the glenoid and coracoid, such as occurs with cuff-tear arthropathy and end-stage rheumatoid arthritis [see Figs. 3–48 to 3–56 and 3–72 to 3–82]), the long head (23 mm.) is usually used. In special cases a thicker glenoid component (see Fig. 3–28E) is considered. In shoulders with long-standing posterior dislocation or subluxation such as in old trauma, arthritis of dislocation, and advanced osteoarthritis, there is a pouch of capsule around the dislocated head, and the adjacent muscles become set in malalignment. The muscle forces and the pouch cause the humeral component to subluxate unless the glenoid–greater tuberosity distance is re-established by tightening the posterior capsule and eliminating the pouch. When the pouch is very redundant, it may be plicated through this anterior approach by placing double-looping, nonabsorbable suture from inside the joint. When there is a threat of subluxation, stressful internal rotation and flexion should be avoided during the early post-operative period.

In cementing the humeral component, after removing particles of loose bone, fat, and blood

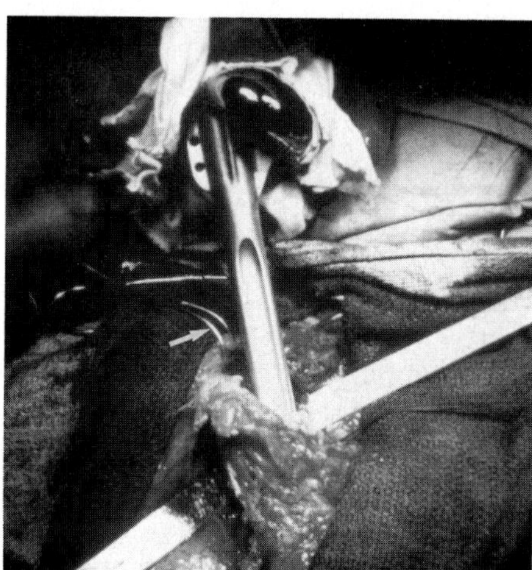

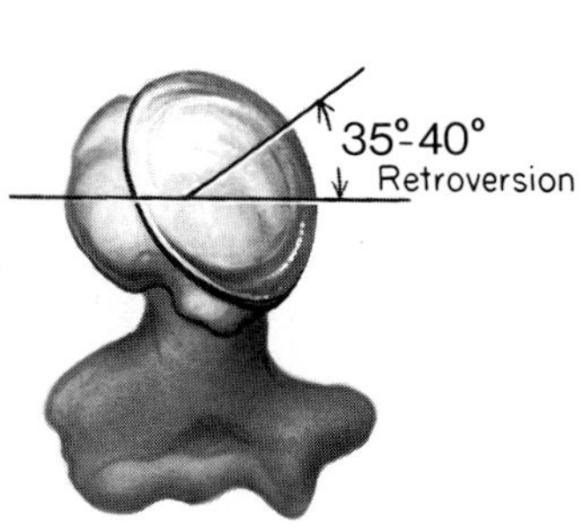

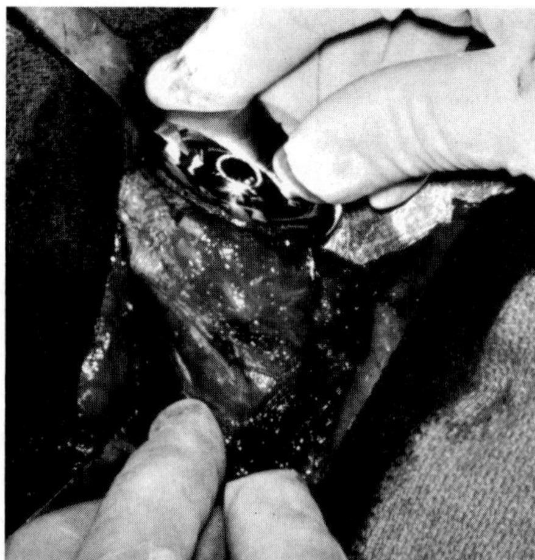

Figure 3–29. ***Technique of Shoulder Arthroplasty.*** Cementing the humeral component. A press fit is used only if there is a firm fit of the stem. Cement is inserted with vent tubes in place (arrow), which are withdrawn as the prosthesis is inserted (left). The length of the head, the height of the prosthesis above the greater tuberosity, and tension on the myofascial sleeve (with proper length of the shaft) are kept in mind as discussed in the text and in Figure 3–26.

Unless the glenoid is deformed, the humeral component is cemented in 40 degrees retroversion (middle); however, the final version of the humeral component is determined at this time (see Figs. 3–26 and 3–28D). All visible cement is removed from around the head of the prosthesis (right).

and irrigating with antibiotics, a tube to vent trapped air is inserted, and cement is injected from a syringe and compressed with finger pressure. A greater pressure on the cement, such as from a pressure syringe, is not tolerated by an osteopenic humerus. Several patients treated elsewhere with such pressure have had extrusion of the cement out of the shaft with involvement of the radial nerve.

When the cement is hard, the humeral component is relocated in the joint, and a final inspection is made for position and stability.

Restore Subscapularis Length

After the final seating of the humeral component, the subscapularis is re-attached in its normal anatomical position. It must first be mobilized by freeing it from the coracohumeral ligament and underlying capsule (Fig. 3–30). When normal length of the subscapularis tendon can be obtained, it is re-attached to its normal site on the humerus. If the subscapularis is short, it is lengthened by suturing it to the stump of the capsule, which remains attached to the humerus (Fig. 3–30). When the subscapularis tendon is more deficient, it can be rotated cephalically so that the upper part of its cut end is sutured to the supraspinatus tendon and the inferior margin of the subscapularis tendon is sutured to the soft tissue remaining on the humerus. In re-attaching the subscapularis, care should be taken to avoid injury to the biceps tendon, which is left free to run in its groove. Smaller tears of the rotator cuff should have been closed prior to re-attaching the subscapularis. Larger tears are mobilized prior to implanting the humeral component. Before cementing the humeral component, nonabsorbable sutures are placed through holes in the greater tuberosity in preparation for re-attaching the cuff. The joint capsule is left open except when it is used for lengthening the subscapularis.

Closing Large Cuff Defects

Some cuff defects encountered at the time of a glenohumeral arthroplasty are more extensive than those seen with impingement tears. In patients needing revisions and those with cuff-tear arthropathy the rotator cuff may have actually been excised at a previous surgery. If a patient has had a neoplasm requiring resection of the upper humerus, the entire rotator cuff would have been detached, and any part involved with tumor cells may have been excised. Severe trauma and long-standing rheumatoid arthritis are other sources of

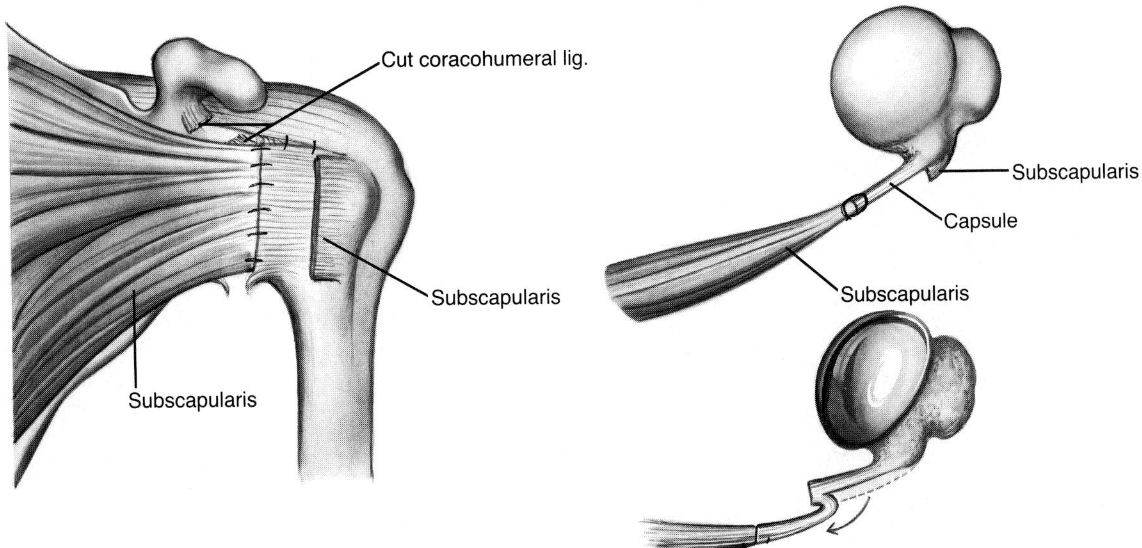

Figure 3–30. ***Technique of Shoulder Arthroplasty.*** Restoring subcapsularis length. As illustrated, and as shown in Figure 3–25, the usual way of gaining subscapularis length is by creating a flap of capsule attached to the humerus (right and left) during the approach. Note that the subscapularis tendon is made free to move by detaching all soft tissue connections between it and the coracoid process (including the coracohumeral ligament) (left) before sewing it to the capsular flap.

An alternative method, a Z-plasty of the subscapularis tendon, is shown in the inset, which may be used when the subscapularis is inadvertently divided too far medially.

extremely large tears. These large rotator cuff defects will be discussed in more detail under each diagnostic category; however, we can summarize the techniques used to close them at this time.

Capsular Flap. The capsular flap created by dividing the capsule more medially than the site of division of the subscapularis is helpful in closing large defects (Fig. 3–31A). If the rotator tendons have been well mobilized prior to implantation of the humeral component, the addition of this flap may be all that is needed to complete the closure.

Pectoralis Major (Sternal Head) Transfer. The sternal head of the pectoralis major with attached soft tissue can be used for the subscapularis (Fig. 3–31B).

Pectoralis Minor Transfer. Pectoralis minor transfer with a soft-tissue extension can be substituted for subscapularis (Fig. 3–31C).

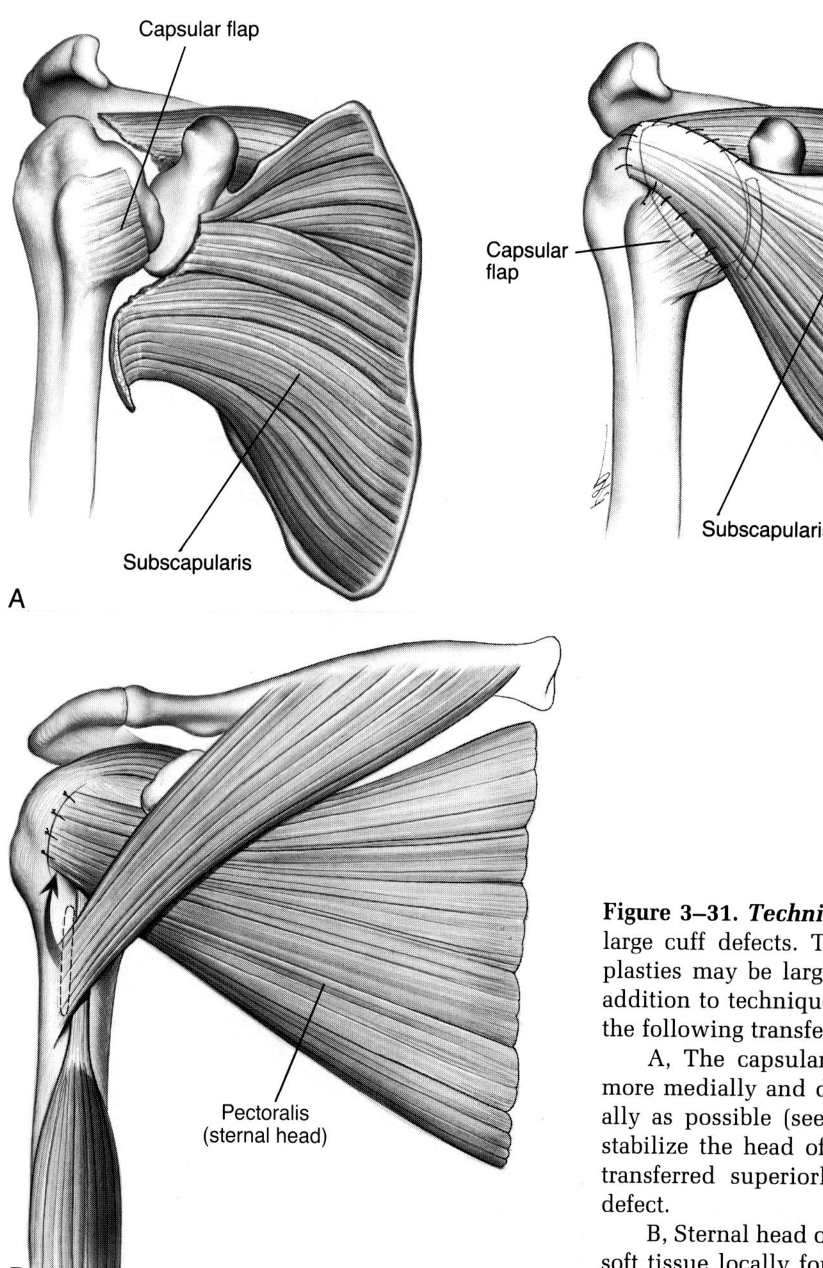

Figure 3–31. ***Technique of Shoulder Arthroplasty.*** Closing large cuff defects. The cuff defects encountered at arthroplasties may be larger than those of impingement tears. In addition to techniques discussed in Figure 2–43E through I, the following transfers have been helpful.

A, The capsular flap created by dividing the capsule more medially and detaching the subscapularis as far laterally as possible (see Figs. 3–25 and 3–30) can be used to stabilize the head of the prosthesis as the subscapularis is transferred superiorly to compensate for a supraspinatus defect.

B, Sternal head of the pectoralis major (with all available soft tissue locally for length) can be transferred upward for the subscapularis and, with a soft tissue extension, for loss of the supraspinatus.

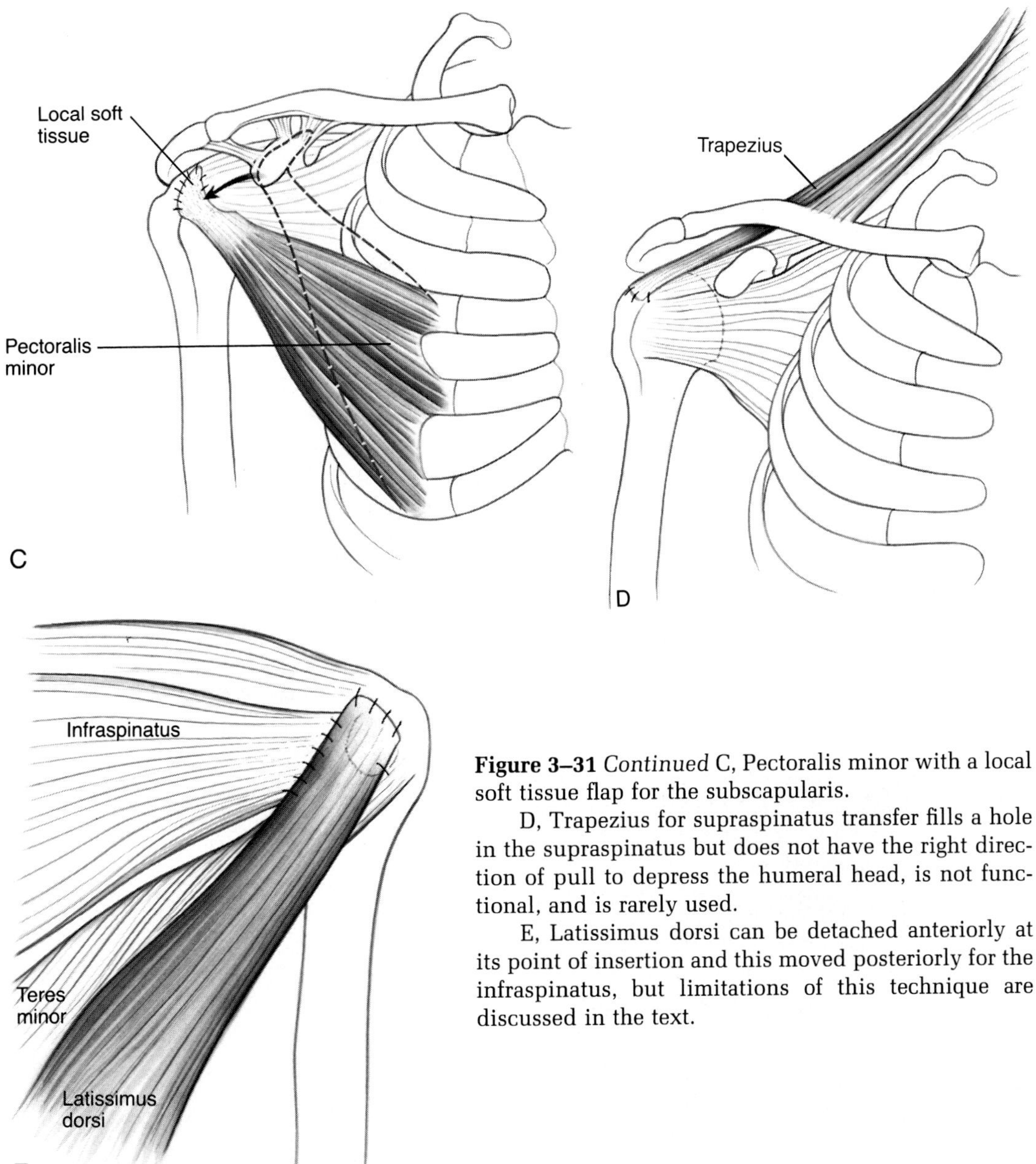

Figure 3–31 *Continued* C, Pectoralis minor with a local soft tissue flap for the subscapularis.

D, Trapezius for supraspinatus transfer fills a hole in the supraspinatus but does not have the right direction of pull to depress the humeral head, is not functional, and is rarely used.

E, Latissimus dorsi can be detached anteriorly at its point of insertion and this moved posteriorly for the infraspinatus, but limitations of this technique are discussed in the text.

Trapezius Transfer. Although it is tempting to use the trapezius for the supraspinatus, the trapezius fails to act as a head depressor and does not add very much. It might be substituted in a desperate case when there is no expectation of overhead function.

Latissimus Dorsi Transfer. The latissimus dorsi can be detached anteriorly and moved posteriorly high at the site of insertion of the infraspinatus to act as an external rotator and posterior head depressor (Fig. 3–31E). This procedure requires a posterior incision and care to avoid injury to the axillary nerve and also impair the function of the latissimus as a powerful extensor of the shoulder.

Closing the Deltopectoral Interval

The extended deltopectoral incision leaves the deltoid muscle intact except in situations in which a release of the anterior part of the deltoid insertion has been used (to avoid excessive retraction on the deltoid). If the anterior insertion has been released, it is re-attached to the pectoralis tendon with nonabsorbable 00 sutures. Suction drains are inserted between the deltoid muscle and the rotator cuff, and the deltopectoral interval is closed with interrupted 00 nonabsorbable sutures.

Deltoidplasties

When the deltoid muscle has been detached, denervated, or scarred by trauma or previous surgery, an effort must be made to restore function. As discussed in Chapter 1, p. 29, the anterior deltoid is of special importance. The middle deltoid may have been injured by a lateral acromionectomy, and reconstruction of the posterior deltoid occasionally becomes important in a complicated injury or paralytic problem.

Anterior Deltoid Repair. Methods used to repair the deltoid are illustrated in Figure 3–32. The most frequent problem is detachment or retraction injuries with denervation and scarring of the anterior part of the deltoid. This type of problem is usually treated by mobilization and approximation of the middle deltoid and pectoralis major. The ability to shift the clavicular head of the pectoralis laterally is limited by its nerve supply. Therefore, this type of deltoidplasty may be inadequate. If this proves to be the case, one can later consider shifting the middle and posterior deltoid anteriorly to fill the defect created by the loss of the anterior deltoid (Fig. 3–32A). This procedure stabilizes the shoulder but has not, in my experience, re-established overhead function. Augmenting the muscle with a transfer of the biceps to the clavicle also usually fails to restore overhead use of the arm. Another procedure we have considered to remedy loss of the anterior deltoid is transfer of the latissimus dorsi (Fig. 3–32D), as discussed below.

Middle Deltoid Repair. Surgical detachment of the middle deltoid, with or without lateral acromionectomy, causes a peculiar wasting of this part of the deltoid muscle and usually results in retraction of its origin. The retracted middle part of the deltoid adheres to the humerus and interferes with shoulder motion. When the muscle has been displaced down the arm, it is necessary to free it from the overlying skin as well as from the humerus and rotator cuff before it can be pulled upward onto the acromion. Rather than re-attaching the

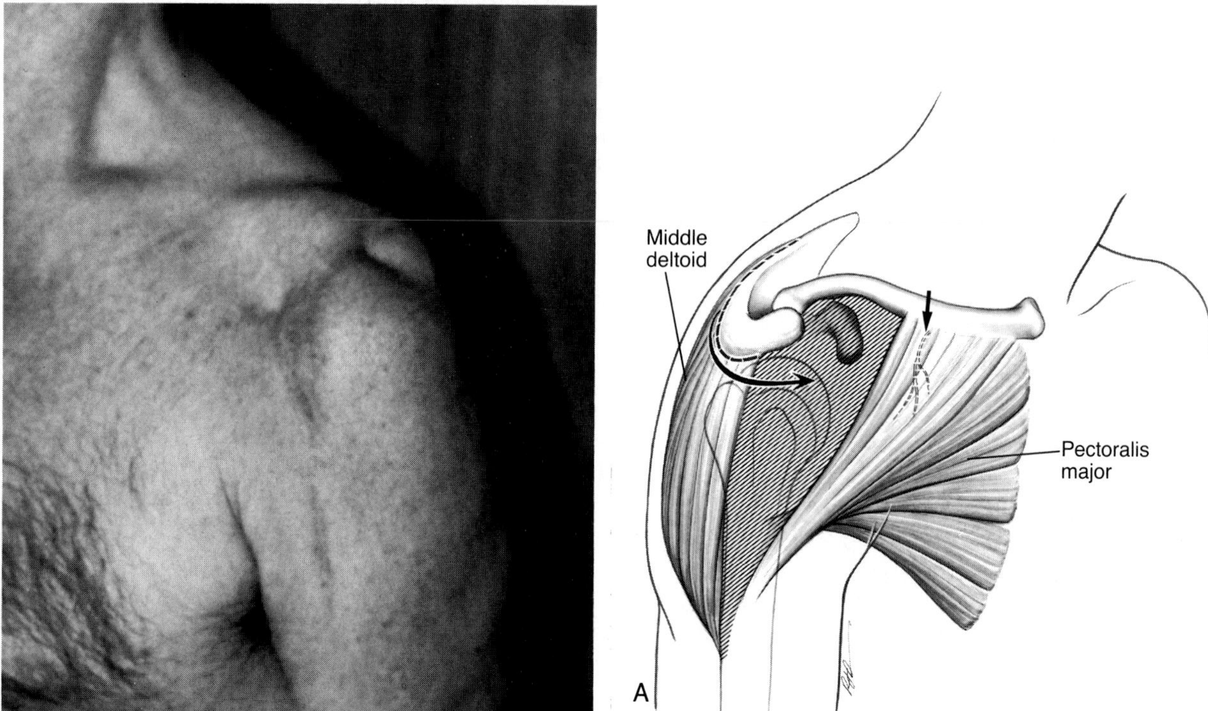

Figure 3–32. ***Technique of Shoulder Arthroplasty.*** Closing defects in the deltoid muscle (deltoidplasty). Typical problems following previous surgery are illustrated in the photograph here and in Figure 3–59. Methods of repair are the following.

A, Anterior deltoid defects of smaller size may be closed by mobilizing the edges of the middle deltoid and pectoralis major; however, this is limited by the nerves to the clavicular head of the pectoralis major (arrow), which cannot be mobilized very much. Larger defects require detaching the posterior deltoid and freeing it from the overlying skin (as illustrated). Alternatively, the latissimus dorsi can be transferred (see D) as discussed in the text.

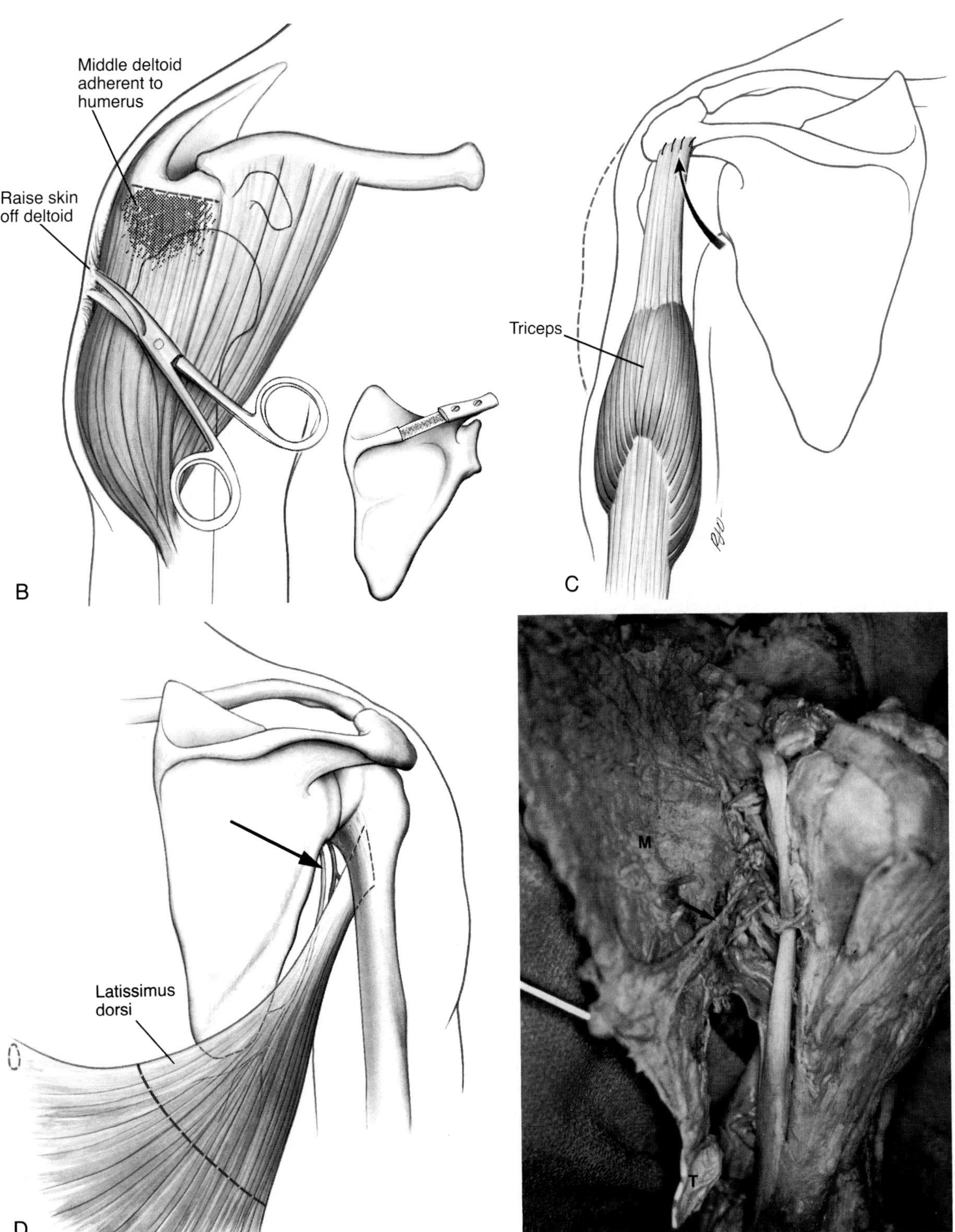

Figure 3–32 *Continued* B, Middle deltoid repairs are frequently required after surgical procedures that had detached this part of the deltoid and after acromionectomies (see Fig. 2–46). Overlying skin must be detached from the deltoid as well as freeing the deep surface of the deltoid, which is re-attached on top of the acromion and is protected with an abduction brace. A technique of sliding bone graft that can be considered for regaining acromial length is depicted in the inset.

C, Posterior deltoid can be effectively augmented by transferring the triceps to the acromion.

D, The latissimus dorsi has such a long neurovascular pedicle (arrow) that it can be rotated and used for any part of the deltoid. Limitations of this technique are discussed in the text. In this demonstration (right), the muscle (M) and tendon (T) have been detached and rotated to the front of the shoulder in the anatomy laboratory to show how the latissimus dorsi can fill the space of the anterior deltoid muscle without compromising its neurovascular bundle.

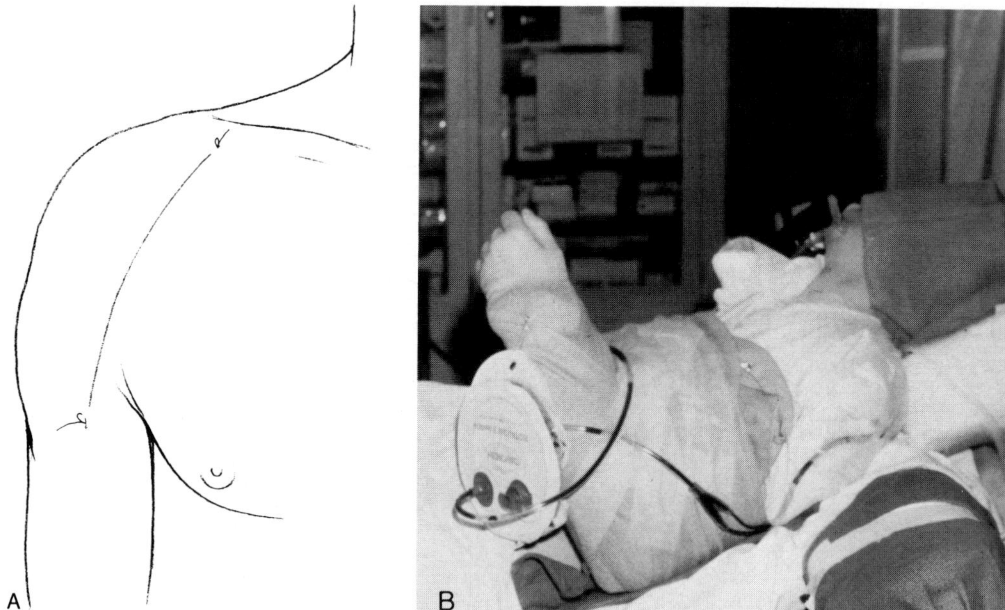

Figure 3–33. ***Technique of Shoulder Arthroplasty.*** Closure and dressing.

A, After placement of suction drains between the deltoid muscle and the rotator cuff, the deltopectoral interval is approximated with interrupted sutures with buried knots and the skin is closed with a removable subcuticular suture. Buried subcutaneous sutures are avoided.

B, Note that after applying the sling, the wrist is wrapped for 24 hours to prevent wrist flexion, which might compromise the median nerve in the carpal tunnel.

deltoid to the lateral edge of the acromion, I prefer to pull it up on top and suture it to the tendinous insertion of the trapezius muscle. A brace is then used for eight weeks to allow firm re-attachment of the deltoid before allowing use of the arm at the side. During this time, passive exercises maintain glenohumeral motion. When the middle deltoid is extremely atrophied and short, the clavicular and acromial insertions of the trapezius muscle can be detached and shifted over the top of the acromion to augment the function of the middle deltoid. Unfortunately, the trapezius usually adheres to the acromion and does not add very much function. A very important part of mobilizing and repairing the middle deltoid is freeing the humerus and rotator cuff to allow them to be moved. This alone can have a decidedly beneficial effect on the function of the shoulder, and if the middle deltoid is strong, further functional improvements are seen (Fig. 3–32B).

Posterior Deltoid Repairs. The latissimus dorsi usually compensates for loss of the posterior deltoid; however, there are special circumstances when the stability and strength afforded by the posterior deltoid become important. Transfer of the triceps from the glenoid to the posterior acromion (Fig. 3–32C) can be quite effective in restoring posterior stability.

Latissimus Dorsi Transfer for Deltoid. Because the latissimus dorsi has such a long neurovascular pedicle, it can be rotated and used for any part of the deltoid muscle (Fig. 3–32D). It is the largest of the broad muscles of the body, and its main vessels and nerves, arising from the subscapular artery and thoracodorsal nerve, enter this muscle in a similar plane at a point just superior and lateral to the inferior angle of the scapula. The diameter of the artery averages 1.2 mm., and the diameter of the nerve averages 1.3 mm. This muscle also receives blood from the transverse cervical artery, which descends along the vertebral border of the scapula. The relationships of the neurovascular bundle are so constant that it can be identified in the posterior part of the axillary fossa between the teres major and the latissimus dorsi. After dissecting out the neurovascular bundle, the amount of muscle tissue needed can be excised from the major part of the muscle and transferred through the axilla to present in the anterior incision. It is important to use dissecting loops and to avoid twisting the neurovascular bundle more than 50 degrees. Hemostasis with cautery is avoided. According to Lech,[141] it is possible to gain 10 cm. in length by ligating the circumflex branch (to the rhomboids) and the serratus anterior branch of the subscapular artery; however, the thoracodorsal artery must be left intact. Post-operatively, passive motion is started early, but active use of the deltoid is deferred for at least eight weeks. The latissimus may be rotated to any part of the deltoid. Although there has been considerable experience among plastic surgeons who use the latissimus transfer with overlying skin to fill cosmetic defects, there has been very limited experience using this muscle for deltoid power. Transfer of the latissimus dorsi for the deltoid has been used in patients with such severe muscle damage that it has been impossible to evaluate its full potential.

Pectoralis Major Transfer for Anterior Deltoid. It is logical to use the pectoralis major for the anterior deltoid because the two function in synchrony, and the pectoralis could be considered an extension of the anterior deltoid. Unfortunately, the clavicular head of the pectoralis major is tethered by its nerve supply, and although the neurovascular bundle for the sternal head of the pectoralis head is longer and it is possible to rotate the sternal head in position to act as an anterior deltoid, this failed in two attempts, and I do not expect to try it again.

None of these procedures have compensated for loss of the powerful deltoid, but those recommended for consideration have relieved fatigue ache and improved function. Axillary nerve palsy is discussed in Chapter 6, page 446; under unusual circumstances, it may require neurolysis.

Closure and Dressings

No buried subcutaneous sutures are used. They tend to migrate, probably because of the large excursion of motion in the exercise program post-operatively. A running, subcuticular, pull-out suture is used to close the skin (Fig. 3–33A), avoiding cross-marks caused by interrupted sutures or skin staples. A sling and swathe is applied (Fig. 3–33B) unless the repair of the rotator cuff or deltoid has been tenuous (requiring an abduction brace [see Fig. 7–15]) or if there is instability due to loss of bone or fixed malalignment of the soft tissue from an old dislocation (in which case a spica cast may be required to maintain the arm in external rotation). An x-ray of the shoulder is obtained prior to leaving the operating room if there has been any special problem; otherwise, it is obtained in the recovery room. Most patients are allowed a full fluid diet and are out of bed with assistance the first night, and are given a regular diet the following morning. The Hemovac is removed in 24 hours, and in an uncomplicated case early passive motion is begun on the second day (see Fig. 7–7).

Special Problems

The special problems encountered and their treatment are summarized in Table 3–3. The indications for special procedures will now be discussed according to the specific pathologic condition presented by each diagnostic category.

An "imprint" or frozen section analysis is indicated whenever suspicious tissue is encountered. If the histological sections suggest infection, the wound is closed and the arthroplasty is deferred until final culture results and further information can be obtained.

Bursectomy and synovectomy are indicated whenever thickening and scarring or proliferative changes are seen, as in patients with rheumatoid arthritis. Because tenderness and pain at the acromioclavicular joint are the most frequent indications for acromioclavicular joint resection, a determination about such a resection must be made preoperatively. Painful acromioclavicular arthritis is seen in some patients with rheumatoid arthritis and in a few with osteoarthritis. Resection of the acromioclavicular joint to provide more exposure of the supraspinatus is almost never indicated

Table 3–3. SPECIAL STEPS NEEDED DURING ARTHROPLASTIES (BY DIAGNOSIS)

1. Deficient deltoid (see Fig. 3–32)	Arthritis of recurrent dislocation, old trauma, acromionectomies, revision
2. Glenoid deficiency (see Fig. 3–28)	Long-standing rheumatoid arthritis, arthritis of recurrent dislocation, old dislocations, severe osteoarthritis, severe trauma, congenital dysplasia, Erb's, cuff-tear arthropathy
3. Rotator cuff deficiency (see Figs. 2—43, 3–30 and 3–31, 3–57 to 3–63, 3–72 to 3–82, and 3–83 to 3–86)	Long-standing rheumatoid arthritis, trauma, cuff-tear arthropathy
4. Deficient humeral shaft (see Figs. 3–26, 3–57 to 3–63, 3–94 to 3–95, and 3–97 to 3–99)	Trauma, neoplasms, revision
5. Short external rotators (see Figs. 3–57 to 3–63, 3–87 to 3–89)	Old retracted greater tuberosity, old posterior dislocation, Erb's palsy
6. "Imprint" for possible infection (see Figs. 3–90 to 3–93)	Previous surgery, contaminated injections
7. Bursectomy, synovectomy (see Figs. 3–48 to 3–56)	Rheumatoid
8. Acromioclavicular joint resection (see Fig. 2–14)	Osteoarthritis, rheumatoid arthritis (only if painful pre-operatively)
9. Anterior acromioplasty (see Fig. 2–41)	Impingement not relieved by the components

during shoulder arthroplasties because the rotator tendons can be mobilized more easily when the humeral head has been removed. Both acromioclavicular joint resection and anterior acromioplasty are performed if indicated prior to implanting the humeral component. However, it should be emphasized that proper positioning of the components usually eliminates the need for an anterior acromioplasty. Anterior acromioplasty is performed only in the occasional patient who has a bony prominence on the undersurface of the acromion or acromioclavicular joint that causes persistent impingement even after the components have been positioned correctly.

AVASCULAR NECROSIS OF THE HUMERAL HEAD

The humeral head is the second most frequent site of nontraumatic avascular necrosis, exceeded only by the femoral head. Yet although much attention has been given to the femoral head, little has been published about avascular necrosis of the humeral head except for an excellent article by Cruess[134] in 1976. Avascular necrosis resulting from fractures will be discussed with old trauma (Figs. 3–57 to 3–63). Idiopathic avascular necrosis of the femoral head is rather common; however, nontraumatic avascular necrosis of the humeral head can usually be traced to a cause.

The Anatomical Problem

Personal Series (1970–1980). A consecutive series of 37 shoulders with avascular necrosis of the humeral head in 26 patients treated by me during the ten-year period between 1970 and 1980 was reviewed with Dr. Kenji Takagishi in 1981.[135] The findings are summarized in Table 3–4. The etiological factor was systemic corticosteroid medications in 18, sickle cell anemia or trait in 4, Gaucher's disease in 2, alcoholism in 1, and idiopathic factors in only 1 patient.

Of the 18 who had received corticosteroid medications, prednisone or a similar substance had been given for or following spinal surgery in five, systemic lupus erythematosus in three, renal transplants in two, polymyositis in two, head injury in two, multiple sclerosis in one, reticulum cell sarcoma in one, Bell's palsy in one, and hyperparathyroidism in one. It was surprisingly difficult to determine the exact amount of steroids administered. The basis for the data seems inadequate to state with assurance the smallest amount of prednisone given prior to development of avascular necrosis. The duration between the beginning of steroid therapy and the onset of symptoms ranged from three months to nine years, and averaged three years and nine months. It is quite possible that some other etiological factor, such as systemic lupus erythematosus or another cause of shoulder pain, was responsible for the early onset of symptoms in those who became symptomatic within a few months after beginning steroid therapy. Seven of the 18 patients continued to take steroids for medical reasons after the diagnosis had been made. Total dosages were quite variable.

The age of the patients ranged from 21 years to 64 years and averaged 39 years. There were 12 males and 14 females. Bilateral lesions occurred in 11, of whom nine had corticosteroid therapy, one had sickle cell anemia, and one had sickle cell trait.

Avascular necrosis of the femoral head, often mild, could be detected radiographically at the time of diagnosis of avascular necrosis of the hu-

Table 3–4. ARTHROPLASTIES FOR AVASCULAR NECROSIS (1970–1980)

BACKGROUND MATERIAL	
Shoulders	37
Patients	26
Age	21–64 years (average 39 years)
Bilateral	11
Right	19
Left	18
Male	12
Female	14
ETIOLOGY OF AVASCULAR NECROSIS (26 PATIENTS)	
Steroid therapy	18
Sickle cell disease	4
Gaucher's disease	2
Alcohol	1
Idiopathic causes	1
REASON FOR STEROID THERAPY (18 PATIENTS)	
Spinal Injuries	5 (3 paraplegic)
Systemic lupus erythematosus	3
Renal transplant	2
Polymyositis	2
Head injury	2
Multiple sclerosis	1
Bell's palsy	1
Hyperthyroidism	1
Reticular cell sarcoma	1
TREATMENT (26 PATIENTS)	
Drilling and bone graft	2 (both failed)
Humeral head replacement	15
Total glenohumeral arthroplasty	9

Data from Takagishi, K., and Neer, C. S., II: Avascular necrosis of the humeral head. Presented to the Alumni Association, New York Orthopaedic Hospital, 1980; and at the Annual Meeting, Japanese Shoulder Society, 1982.

meral head in 16 of the 26 patients. Several of these had some avascular changes at the knee joint.

Interestingly, avascular necrosis of the elbow joint eventually developed in two patients who were paraplegic because of spinal injuries and used their arms for transfers from the wheelchair (see Fig. 3–37). Because no other patients developed this problem, one must assume that the weight-bearing pressure on the elbows precipitated the collapse of the subchondral bone in this joint. The effect of pressure explains why the humerus consistently first collapses at the point of maximum joint reaction force, as discussed below. The rotator cuff was intact in all shoulders except one 64 year old woman, who at the time of replacement arthroplasty was noted to have a tear of the supraspinatus tendon resembling an impingement tear. It was thought that the collapse of the head had caused the greater tuberosity to translocate upward against the acromion, leading to the impingement tear. There was an anterior acromial spur that was thought to have been caused by the impingement of the humerus against the acromion. These lesions were treated by an anterior acromioplasty and repair of the rotator cuff at the time of the replacement arthroplasty.

Treatment of these 26 patients consisted of a humeral head arthroplasty in 15, total glenohumeral arthroplasty in 9, and core decompression with a one-quarter inch drill and bone grafts surrounded by 3/32-inch drill holes into the involved part of the head in 2; the bone grafts were obtained from the upper shaft of the humerus. The results of those who received arthroplasties were generally satisfactory, as discussed later. Both shoulders treated by core decompression and bone grafts continued to deteriorate, and one was treated with a replacement arthroplasty two years later.

Classification

The pathologic changes that occur in the humeral head are similar to those occurring in the femoral head as described by Ficat[127] and Enneking[136] but with some differences. The differences are best explained by describing the point of maximum joint reaction force and the anatomical contour of the glenoid compared to that of the acetabulum. The glenoid is flat, and the point of maximum pressure on the head seems to occur when the arm has been raised about 90 degrees. At this point the scapula has rotated 30 degrees, so that the area of the head that is placed under maximum pressure is that contacting the glenoid when the humerus has been elevated 60 degrees. This area of contact is the site where the humeral head consistently collapses in avascular necrosis and where maximum wear and sclerosis occur in osteoarthritis.

Avascular changes with collapse of the articular surfaces in the elbows of two paraplegic patients, as mentioned above, confirm the importance of pressure and load in the configuration of avascular necrosis of the humeral head. In their discussions of the etiology of avascular necrosis, both Cruess and Enneking pointed out that the alterations in the femoral head did not match the anatomical configuration of the blood vessels in the femoral head nor the random site of infarction that might occur if the infarcts were due to "sludging." Since the location of the crescent sign (Fig. 3–34) and the later collapse at the head correspond to the point of maximum joint reaction force on the humeral head, I believe the consistent location of the wedge-shaped area of infarction is largely due to pressure.

To assist in describing the indications and treatment of this condition, I have adapted the excellent classifications of Ficat[137] and Enneking[136] to the shoulder, as illustrated in Figure 3–35.

Stage I. *Stage I* disease shows only subtle changes that are not always definitely diagnostic. Recent developments with magnetic resonance imaging (MRI) are helpful. The head retains its normal shape. There may be slight mottling of the trabecular pattern or an area of subchondral decalcification.[134] There may be no pain, but some patients do have pain. Patients with infarctional diseases (Gaucher's disease and sickle cell disease) have more very early pain. Unfortunately, at this time there is no infallible way to document the diagnosis.

Stage II. *Stage II* disease has an articular surface that is grossly round when inspected at surgery, and although the articular cartilage can be indented on pressure in an area where it has lost the support of the subchondral bone, it returns to its normal shape. This is the area where a "meniscus sign" can be seen (Fig. 3–35C). Tomograms and MRI are especially helpful in evaluating the extent of head involvement. Pain is usually present and may be severe. The severe pain probably corresponds to minute fractures and the sudden slight collapse of subchondral bone.

Stage III. *Stage III* disease is characterized by an area of wrinkled and loose articular cartilage (Fig. 3–35D). This corresponds to the wedge-shaped area of fracturing and collapse of subchondral bone. Eventually the edge of this detached cartilage may become torn, forming a flap. With each episode of collapse of the subchondral bone,

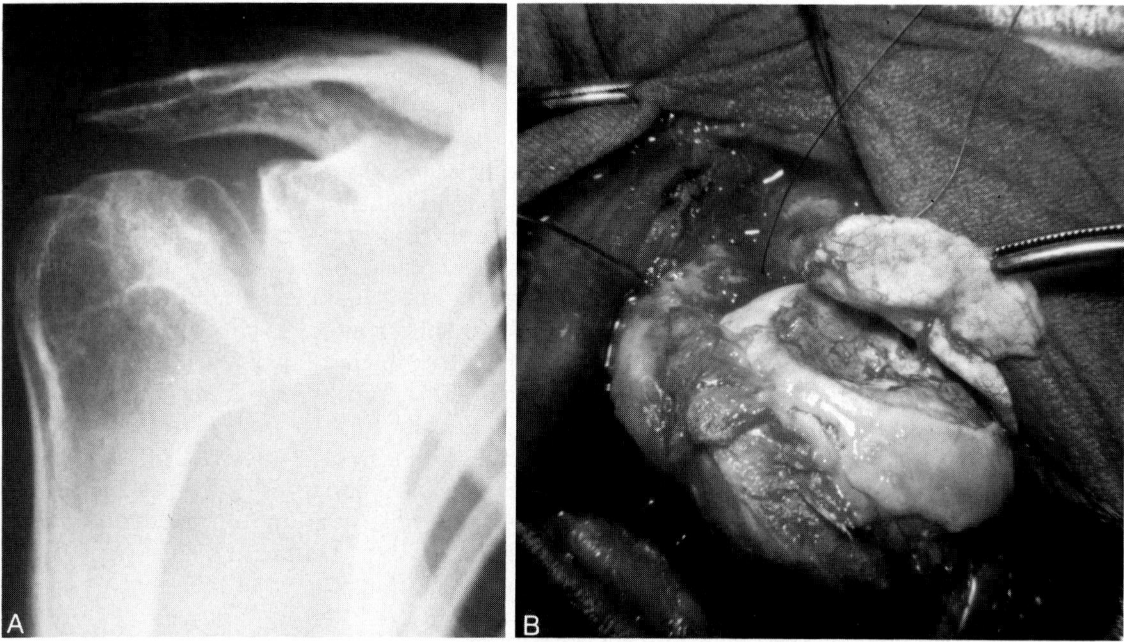

Figure 3–34A and B. ***Avascular Necrosis of the Humeral Head.*** Typical Stage III roentgen appearance (A) compared with appearance at surgery (B), showing the collapse of the subchondral bone beneath a loose flap of cartilage. There was no chance for a bone graft, core decompression, drilling, or a conservative regimen to result in healing. Humeral head arthroplasty prior to glenoid changes is preferred at this stage.

the pain is intensified. Eventually the x-ray film shows a "step-off" phenomenon, and the diagnosis is quite obvious. The articular surface of the glenoid remains intact.

Stage IV. *Stage IV* disease shows involvement of the articular surface of the glenoid due to the incongruity of the humeral head (Fig. 3–35E). As secondary arthritic changes occur, a ring of marginal excrescences develops around the head, particularly inferiorly, and the articular surface of the glenoid becomes worn unevenly, as in osteoarthritis (see p. 202). Because of the way the arms are used in everyday activities (see Fig. 2–3), the incongruous head presses more intensely on the posterior part of the glenoid, leading to uneven wear and eventually to a posterior subluxation. With the posterior subluxation, the posterior glenoid becomes rounded off and sclerotic, and an indentation develops in the head because of contact against the posterior edge of the glenoid. By this time, osteochondral bodies and a general synovitis of the joint are present.

The radiological changes seen in the infarctional diseases (sickle cell and Gaucher's) are similar to those described except that they show more mottling of the trabeculi as a result of patches of

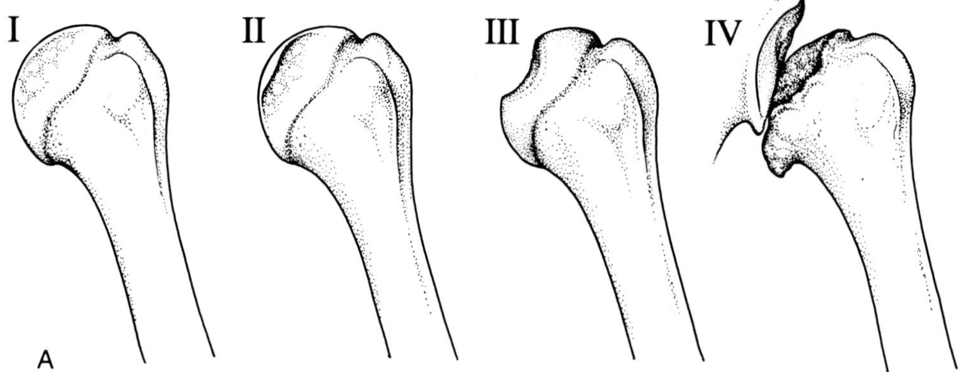

Figure 3–35. ***Avascular Necrosis of the Humeral Head.*** Author's classification.
A, Diagram of the classification.

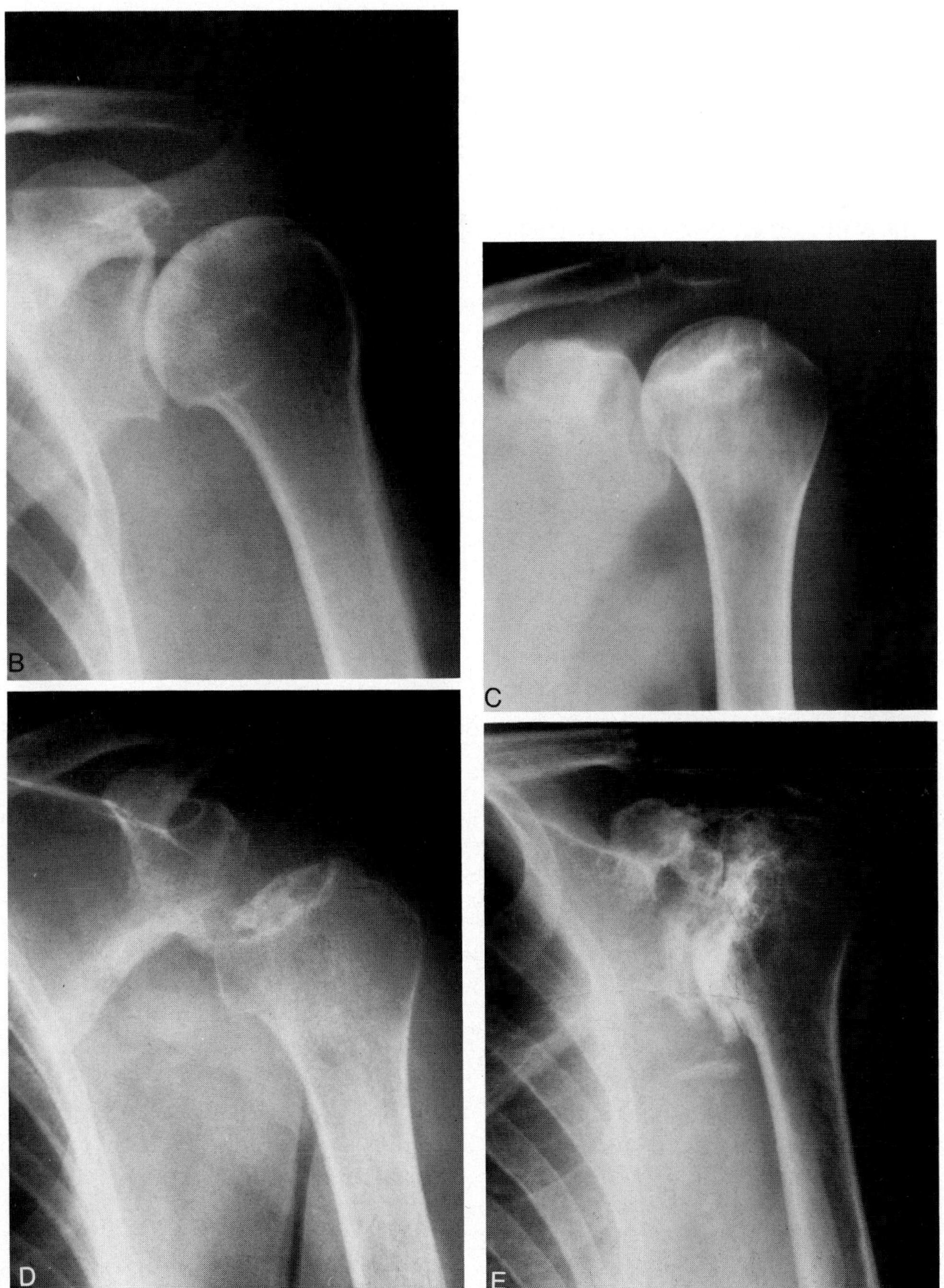

Figure 3–35 *Continued* B, Stage I. Only subtle changes are evident. There is no infallible way to diagnose this condition, but MRI holds promise.

C, Stage II. Meniscus sign ("crescent sign"). Diagnosis is definite. Conservative treatment is indicated.

D, Stage III. Subchondral bone collapse leaving a flap of cartilage. Humeral head arthroplasty is recommended.

E, Stage IV. Glenoid involvement and arthritis secondary to incongruity. Total shoulder arthroplasty is recommended if symptoms require it.

density mixed with areas of lucency. Otherwise, the alterations in the articular surfaces are similar. These conditions are discussed further on pages 199 and 201. Post-irradiation necrosis may be associated with even larger areas of sclerosis and mottling, as discussed on page 202.

Treatment of Avascular Necrosis of the Humeral Head

Tomograms in the anterior-posterior view, MRI, and CT scans are helpful in estimating the stage of involvement of the humeral head (Fig. 3–36A and B). The MRI is of greatest value in detecting early involvement. The CT scan and axillary views help to assess glenoid involvement.

Stage I and *Stage II* diseases are treated nonoperatively. In a limited experience, use of magnetic electric fields to induce re-vascularization, as well as drilling and bone grafting have in my experience been disappointing. Nonoperative treatment consists of reducing activity during periods when collapse and fracturing of the subchondral bone are threatening in the hope of preventing deformity of the subchondral plate or limiting it in hopes of avoiding an arthroplasty. Stretching exercises to prevent stiffness are performed, and nonaddicting pain medication is given as required. The course of involvement of the head is followed with the roentgen studies discussed above.

Stage III disease is treated with a humeral component without a glenoid component. Since most of the patients are young, the cortex of the humerus is usually thick and a good press-fit can be obtained; cement is usually unnecessary. This is considered a conservative procedure with known results for over 30 years and excellent durability (see Figs. 3–38, 3–103, and 3–104). The same preparations and procedures are carried out as have been described earlier (p. 168); but, because the rotator cuff and tuberosities are intact and it is unnecessary to implant a glenoid component, this is the most straightforward and simple type of arthroplasty. To date, it has been unnecessary to revise any of the shoulders treated in this way in our series. Examination of some unsatisfactory results from other hospitals has emphasized the importance of a firm fit of the stem of the humeral component to avoid loosening, proper height of the humeral head to avoid impingement, preservation of the length of the subscapularis to ensure external rotation and movement, and a meticulous exercise program to avoid a frozen shoulder. If

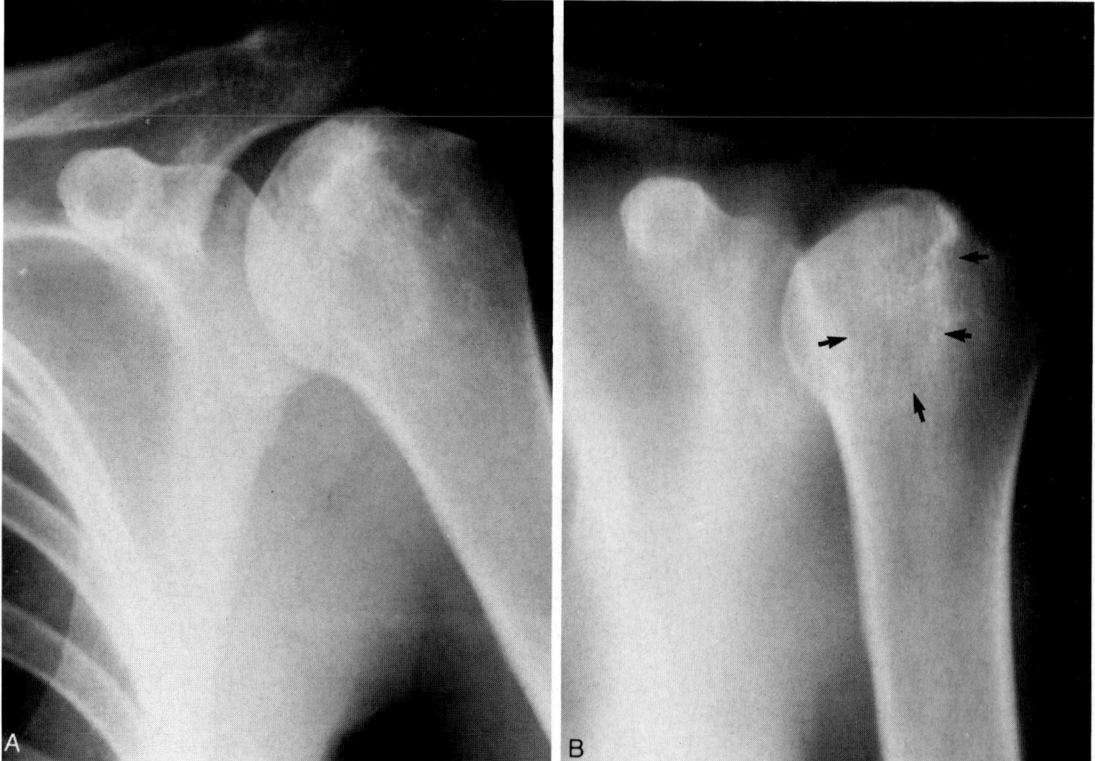

Figure 3–36. ***Avascular Necrosis of the Humeral Head.*** Tomograms, computerized tomograms, or MRI show extent of humeral head changes. A, Plain film. B, Tomogram. Arrows show the extent of bone loss much better than the plain film.

adhesions form and motion is restricted, the head of the prosthesis bears constantly on one area of the glenoid and erosion may occur. Early passive motion (EPM; see Fig. 7–7) can be started on the day after surgery. In patients with post-steroidal avascular necrosis, motion is rapidly regained and easily maintained; however, patients with sickle cell anemia and Gaucher's infarctional problems usually have more discomfort and difficulty with the rehabilitation program, as discussed below.

Stage IV disease may be obvious in plain x-ray films; however, the axillary view and CT scan may be needed to help assess the condition of the articular surface of the glenoid. Even then there are borderline cases in which the condition of the glenoid is determined only at surgery. A glenoid component is used if there is significant involvement of this articular surface. The technique is exactly as outlined on pages 168 to 193. Since the rotator cuff and tuberosities are normal and there is minimal glenoid deformity, no special difficulties should be encountered. In very advanced cases a number of osteochondral bodies are present and require removal.

Bilateral shoulder involvement is common in patients with avascular necrosis. When both shoulders are equally painful, the second arthroplasty is usually done about 10 to 14 days after the first.

The results of total shoulder arthroplasty, like those following humeral head replacement arthroplasty, have been very good, as would be expected when there is minimal bone deformity and the muscles are normal (see Fig. 3–101). One of the patients in the 1970–1980 series who had bilateral shoulder involvement and was paraplegic failed to follow advice to avoid using her arms for transfers during the early post-operative period. She may eventually require a repair of the rotator interval and subscapularis tendon, which was detached. Another patient in that series had an enlarging radiolucent line around the stem of the humeral component noted eight years following surgery. She had been ill and very inactive, and her humerus had become very osteopenic. She had very little shoulder discomfort and has never had a revision. The other 18 patients, who had either post-steroid, alcoholic, or idiopathic avascular necrosis, had results that were near normal, and there was no evidence of loosening.

I believe that when there is a painful deformity of the humeral head that threatens involvement of the glenoid, an uncemented humeral component is an extremely satisfactory and conservative operation. Very little bone is removed, the motion and function of the shoulder muscles are preserved, and full function is possible within a few weeks without waiting many months to learn the outcome of some of the other procedures that have a less certain prognosis. The results of humeral head replacement alone have been durable when the articular surface of the glenoid is in good condition (see Figs. 3–38, 3–101, and 3–103).

Avascular Necrosis of the Humeral Head in Paraplegics

Three patients in the 1970–1980 series and several others seen since then have had paraplegia following spinal injuries that had been treated with corticosteroids, subsequently developing avascular necrosis of the humeral heads.[95] Characteristically, both shoulders are involved, and the patients are between 20 and 30 years of age with a long life expectancy; they make extremely heavy use of their shoulders in all daily activities as well as in transferring their bodies to and from the wheelchair (Fig. 3–37).

I insist these patients agree pre-operatively to avoid shifting their body weight with their arms for at least six months following arthroplasty to allow the rotator interval and subscapularis tendon to become re-attached. Patients are taught the use of a wheelchair with a removable arm and a sliding board (see Fig. 7–16) pre-operatively and prior to discharge from the hospital.

The alternative treatments for this age group are less promising. Bilateral shoulder arthrodesis would prevent acceptable function. The results of core decompression, drilling, and bone grafts are uncertain and require a long period of time for revascularization, which seems unlikely to occur adequately. Therefore, an uncemented humeral head replacement prior to destruction of the articular surface of the glenoid seems to be the most satisfactory approach at this time.

Sickle Cell Disease

Osteonecrosis of the humeral head occurs with sickle cell anemia and sickle cell hemoglobin-C disease, and in those who have sickle cell thalassemia, or sickle cell trait. The life expectancy of those with sickle cell anemia is guarded; however, some do not die young. Patients with sickle cell anemia or sickle cell thalassemia are at considerable risk post-operatively. They have a greater risk for the development of wound infections, and it is very difficult to monitor this aspect because of the elevated sedimentation rate and fever, which may be due to the underlying sickle cell disease. Pain in the shoulder may also be due to a sickle cell

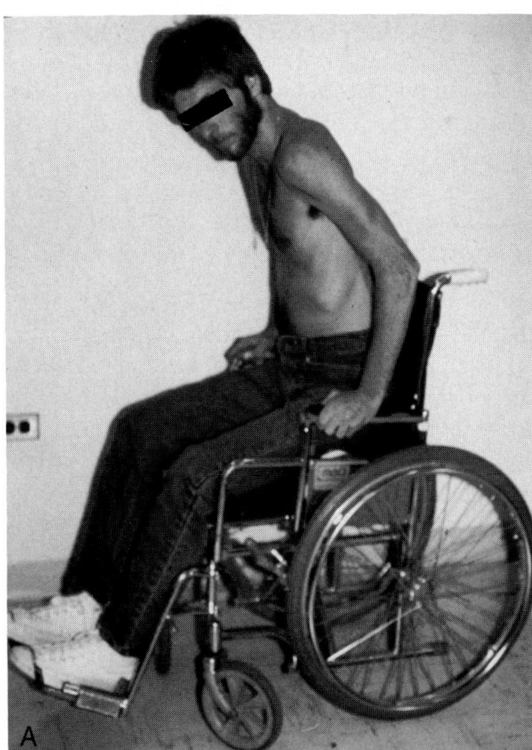

Figure 3–37. ***Avascular Necrosis of the Humeral Head.*** Bilateral avascular necrosis of the humeral heads in paraplegics after spinal injuries is not rare.

A, Paraplegic with bilateral uncemented humeral head replacements at the age of 25 years. This patient later developed avascular necrosis of the elbow.

B, X-ray with arm at side and arm overhead.

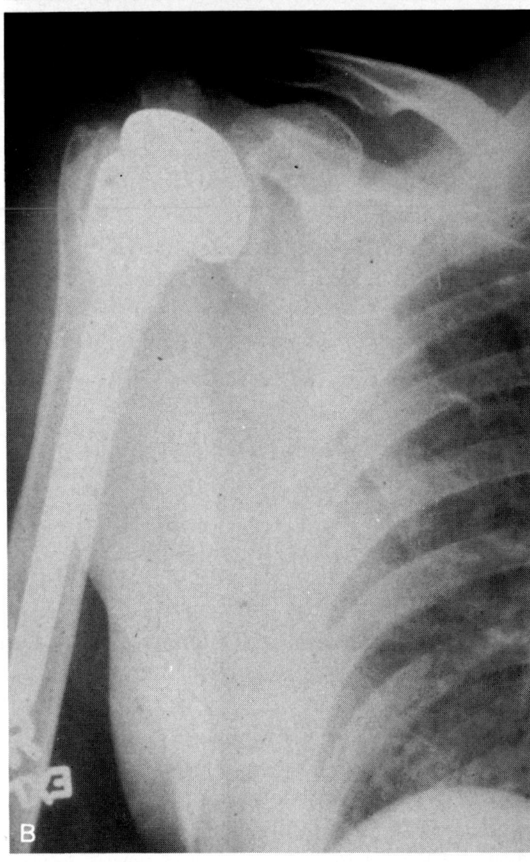

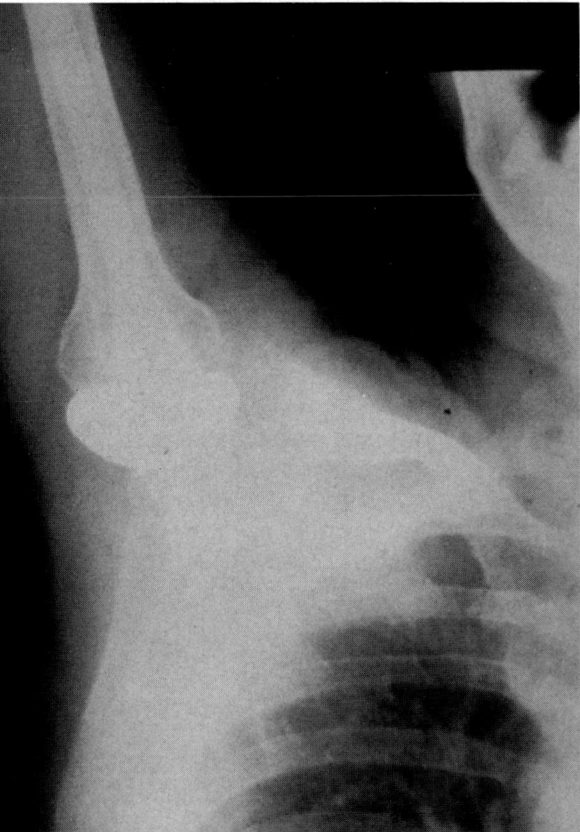

crisis. Beyond this, the patient may develop severe anemia and its complications. Pneumonia can also be a problem. For this reason, shoulder arthroplasty should be performed on patients with these conditions only as a last resort.

On the other hand, when collapse of the humeral heads has occurred and the pain is severe, these patients can be extremely grateful for the relief of pain and recovery of use of their arms. They will tolerate the procedure much better if they are given pre-operative transfusions and close medical supervision after surgery. Bilateral shoulder involvement is common, but the arthroplasty on the second shoulder is deferred at least two months until the patient has had time to recover from the first procedure. Those with sickle cell thalassemia and sickle cell trait are less apt to have such severe systemic reactions following this procedure.

Gaucher's Disease

Gaucher's cells may replace the bone marrow, causing an increased susceptibility to infection, fractures, and avascular necrosis of the femoral and humeral heads (Figs. 3–34 to 3–38). In the early stages there may be intense shoulder pain prior to evidence of upper humeral involvement. One patient in our series had had intolerable shoulder pain at night for two years prior to diagnosis, during which time she was being followed in one of our leading teaching institutions. The diagnosis of Gaucher's disease was made only after early evidence of avascular necrosis appeared in the humeral heads. An arthrodesis of the shoulder was performed in that institution without relief of pain. In time the patient developed similar humeral head changes in the other shoulder and was referred for a shoulder arthroplasty. I performed the arthroplasty on the other shoulder, but, although there was no evidence of infection or loosening of the components, the patient continued to have considerable discomfort in that shoulder as well.

The continuing pain in both shoulders despite a solid arthrodesis on one side and the apparently uncomplicated arthroplasty on the other had no apparent explanation other than the possibility of "infarctional pain" that continued after surgery. Since then, I have approached patients with this condition very cautiously, not only because of the risk of infection and possible risk of loosening of the implant in the abnormal bone, but also because of the possibility of ongoing "bone pain" even

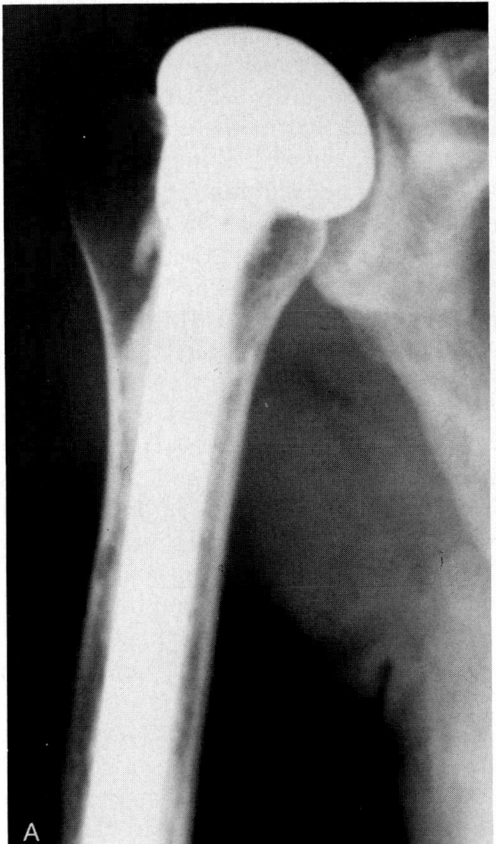

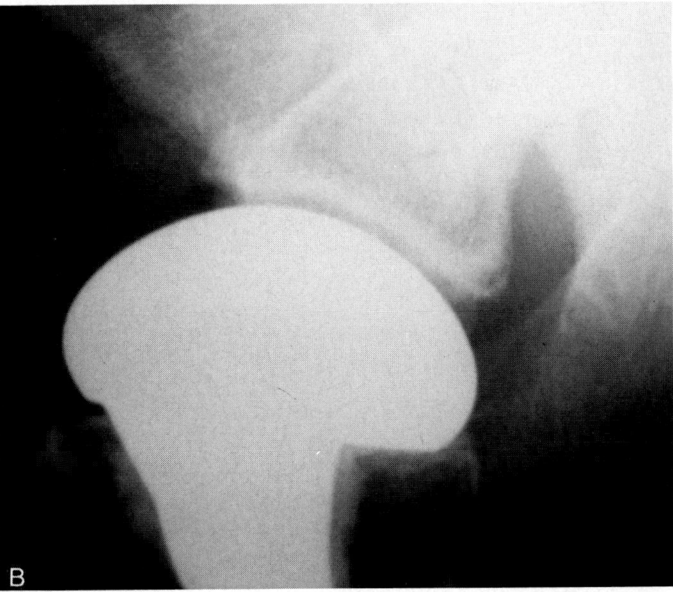

Figure 3–38. ***Avascular Necrosis of the Humeral Head.*** Roentgen results 11 years after humeral head replacement for a Stage III lesion in a 40 year old active tennis player.

A, Anterior-posterior view.

B, Axillary view without glenoid wear.

though an arthroplasty might be effective in alleviating the pain caused by incongruity of the articular surfaces.

Post-irradiation Necrosis of the Humeral Head

Roentgen therapy after radical breast surgery or for other neoplasms may cause bone infarction and secondary degenerative arthritis of the glenohumeral joint. These patients are usually worried about the possibility of metastasis. When a breast tumor requires an axillary node dissection, the pectoralis major has usually been removed, and lymphatic and venous return is often impaired by scarring, which has caused or threatens to cause elephantiasis. Scar may have been intensified by the radiotherapy. A shoulder arthroplasty can aggravate or precipitate an enlargement of the arm.

The first special step in treatment is to obtain appropriate studies and bone scans to relieve the patient's worry about metastasis. Second, the venous and lymphatic systems must be carefully appraised prior to reaching a decision about an arthroplasty. If an arthroplasty is being considered, I advise the patient of the risk of elephantiasis, the possibility of post-irradiation sarcoma, and the greater risk of post-operative wound infection, and more difficulty with the exercise program because of the scarring and loss of muscles. Considering all of these problems, I have usually advised against a shoulder arthroplasty (Fig. 3–39). However, in the few patients who have less post-irradiation scarring of the soft tissue and intense incongruity pain, very gratifying results can be obtained with an arthroplasty following these special steps:

1. Leave the cephalic vein intact.
2. Avoid retraction on the axillary vessels during the procedure.
3. Release the extensive adhesions around the rotator cuff and in the subacromial space.
4. Lengthen the subscapularis tendon (Fig. 3–30).
5. Because of the adhesions and scarred muscles, anticipate the need for establishing passive motion early and allowing a long time for recovery of maximum strength.

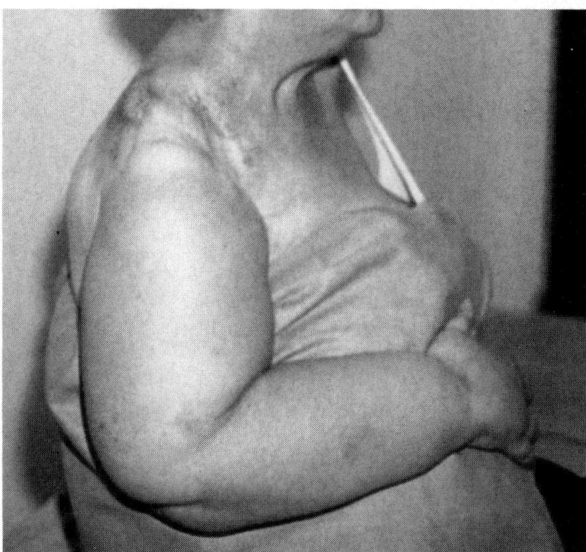

Figure 3–39. Postirradiation necrosis of the humeral head. Elephantiasis, muscle loss, and previous infection were thought to preclude an arthroplasty in this patient seen 20 years after radical mastectomy and radiation therapy.

GLENOHUMERAL OSTEOARTHRITIS

Systemic osteoarthritis of the glenohumeral joint is less common that that of the hip or knee, but it is not rare. No detailed description of a well-established lesion was made prior to 1974;[2] however, the term was used as early as 1961.[68] Since that time this condition has become familiar to American orthopaedic surgeons; it is less well-known to radiologists and is confused with rotator cuff tears in some parts of Europe, where the subacromial space is considered part of the glenohumeral joint and advanced cuff tears are referred to as "degenerative arthritis." It is important to recognize osteoarthritis of the glenohumeral joint as a distinct entity separate from tears of the rotator cuff characterized by (1) limitation of glenohumeral motion due to incongruity of the articular surfaces, (2) apparent enlargement of the head caused by marginal osteophytes (the reverse of the marginal erosion typical of rheumatoid arthritis), and (3) the rotator cuff and long head of the biceps are almost always intact. In contrast, in complete tears of the rotator cuff, glenohumeral motion is usually preserved, the articular surfaces are spared until the very end stages, and the long head of the biceps is often ruptured with the rupture of the cuff. Glenohumeral osteoarthritis produces constant and characteristic gross and roentgen appearances (Fig. 3–40A and B). Since the rotator cuff and long head of the biceps are almost always intact in osteoarthritis, this condition is ideal for nonconstrained arthroplasty.

Among the patients with primary glenohumeral osteoarthritis in the present series (Table 3–1), the age at the time of surgery ranges from 34 to 84 years and averages 60 years. In the original

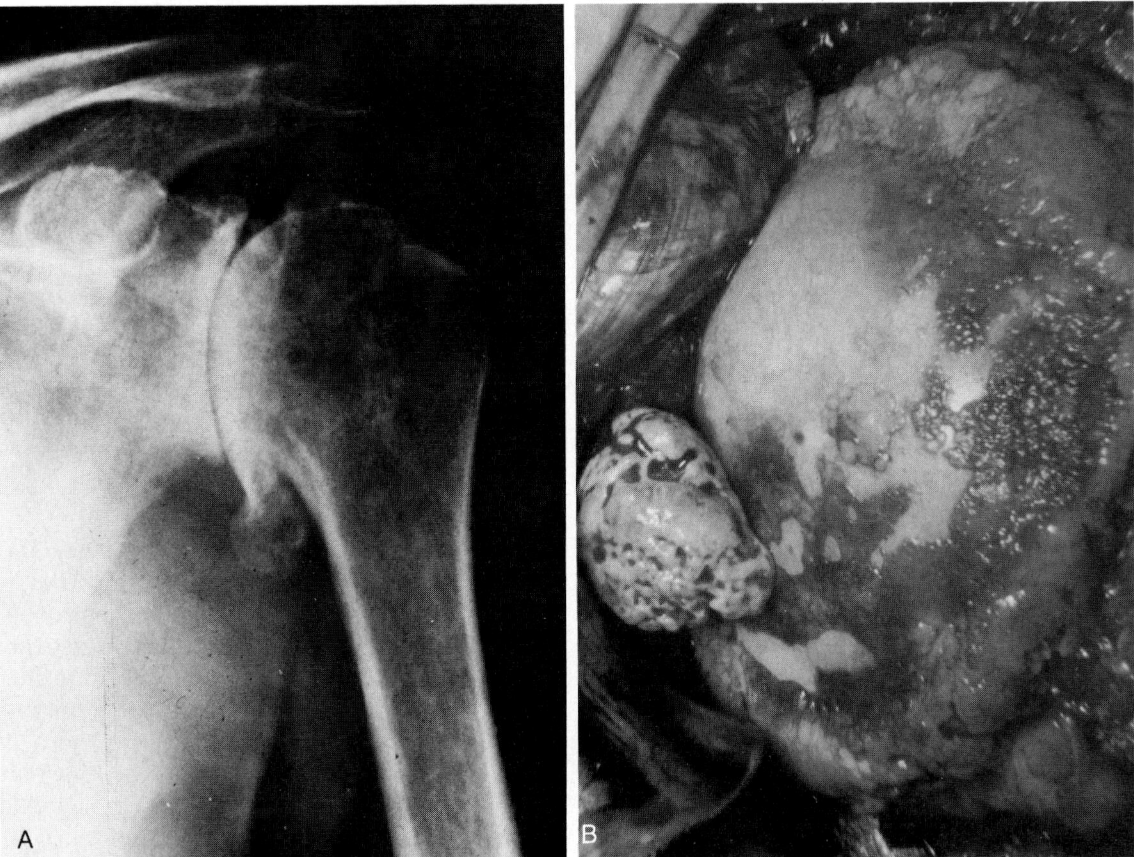

Figure 3–40. ***Glenohumeral Osteoarthritis.*** A and B, Typical appearance of moderately advanced glenohumeral osteoarthritis.

series of 48 shoulders,[2] the average age at the time of surgery was 55 years. Most of these patients are very active, in good general health, and in the prime of life. In the initial series 18 patients were men and 29 were women. In the present series, the 192 osteoarthritic shoulders occurred in women with equal frequency to men. These statistics contradict the impression that degenerative changes of the glenohumeral joint are limited to elderly men. The dominant shoulder was treated surgically twice as frequently as the other side.

The onset of symptoms is often gradual, becoming more intense. Pain is aggravated by activity and recumbency. Ultimately, the pain becomes almost constant and even light movements such as brushing the teeth or putting on a coat become impossible.

Anatomical Problem

I believe that the rotator cuff must be intact to develop the compressive forces required to produce primary osteoarthritis in shoulders subjected to ordinary activities (Fig. 3–41). Subsequent to the development of osteoarthritis, if the upper humerus displaces upward against the acromion because of wear on the joint surfaces, impingement may lead to degenerative lesions of the rotator cuff; however, this is extremely rare in osteoarthritis. The enlarged humeral head usually prevents significant upward displacement of the humerus and impingement tears after the development of osteoarthritis are very rare, whereas, as has been mentioned earlier, they do occur in patients with long-standing rheumatoid arthritis. I have seen a combination of osteoarthritis and cuff tears in paraplegics and circus performers who subject their shoulders to unusual activities. However, as a rule of thumb, the rotator cuff is almost invariably intact in patients who have the x-ray picture shown in Figure 3–40A.

Rupture of the long head of the biceps occasionally occurs with osteoarthritis but through a different mechanism than that producing biceps ruptures with impingement tears of the rotator cuff. In osteoarthritis, excrescences at the entrance to the bicipital groove can cause wear and eventual breakage of the long tendon, but this is surprisingly uncommon.

A similar pattern of hypertrophic spurs and wear may occur when the articular surfaces have been damaged by any one of many different processes (e.g., trauma, infection, gout, ochronosis, "low-grade" rheumatoid arthritis, and others). This is referred to as "secondary osteoarthritis." These lesions will be considered individually because of differences in clinical behavior.

When contemplating the cause of osteoarthritis, it is evident that shoulder problems due to gout and ochronosis, which are known metabolic lesions, can produce the exact same x-ray picture and gross configuration as primary osteoarthritis. Therefore, it seems only a matter of time before the metabolic disturbance leading to primary osteoarthritis will be understood.

The anatomical alterations seen at the end of the humerus, as shown in Figure 3–41, consist initially of thinning of the articular cartilage on that area of the humeral head that is in contact with the glenoid when the humerus is abducted between 60 and 90 degrees. This is the area of maximum joint reactive force (Fig. 3–41), and it becomes eburnated and sclerotic and eventually is worn away. Degenerative subchondral cysts often develop in this area just superior to the midportion of the articular surface, indicating the large amount of pressure exerted. Marginal osteophytes, which are more obvious in x-ray films inferiorly, enlarge to surround the head and obliterate the sulcus, blocking rotation, encroaching on the bicipital groove, and causing the head to appear much larger than normal. The largest osteophytes are located at the inferior margin of the joint, where they cover the calcar. At surgery, the marginal osteophytes are found to be larger than they appear in x-ray films because they have cartilage on the surface. The wear on the superior part of the articular surface and the large inferior excrescences often cause the surgeon to remove too much bone in preparing the upper humerus to receive the humeral component (Fig. 3–26).

At the glenoid, the articular cartilage is spared anteriorly at first because the wear is more intense posteriorly. Eventually, the articular surface of the glenoid becomes smooth and eburnated all the way across, but uneven wear causes more bone loss posteriorly than anteriorly. In long-standing cases, the loss of bone posteriorly necessitates special orientation of the glenoid component, and in extreme cases a glenoid bone graft is considered (see Fig. 3–26).

The capsule is distended by the enlarged head and contains an excess amount of synovial fluid. This distention of the joint can cause the synovial pouch to protrude inferiorly or between a cleft in the glenohumeral ligaments, which may be palpable and suggest a neoplasm. This problem caused needless biopsies elsewhere in two patients in the 1974 series[2] (see Fig. 3–44).

Osteochondral bodies, either loose or attached to the synovial lining, are usually present and may be so numerous that they suggest osteochondromatosis (Fig. 3–42). Large, loose osteochondral bodies are often trapped in the subcoracoid (subscapular) bursa, which normally communicates with the glenohumeral joint. Osteochondral bodies may increase in size and grow in the joint and radiographically may resemble a cartilaginous neoplasm (Fig. 3–42A). Free osteochondral bodies in the subcoracoid bursa may be easily overlooked; therefore, this bursa should be palpated during the arthroplasty to make sure there are no cartilaginous bodies entrapped there that do not appear on x-ray films.

The acromioclavicular joint may also be arthritic and should be examined carefully preoperatively to determine whether the outer clavicle should be excised at the time of shoulder arthroplasty. If so, this excision is done from below (without detaching the deltoid origin) prior to permanent implantation of the humeral component.

Treatment of Glenohumeral Osteoarthritis

Indications for Arthroplasty. As in osteoarthritis of other joints, exercises to maintain joint

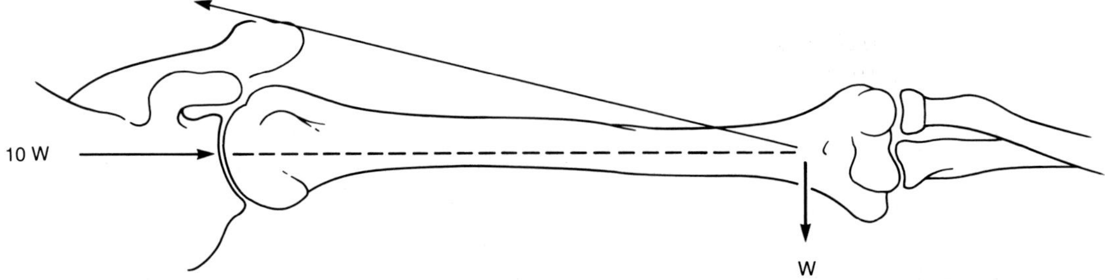

Figure 3–41. ***Glenohumeral Osteoarthritis.*** The maximum joint reaction force occurs at the point of greatest wear and erosion on the humeral head in patients with osteoarthritis. The rotator cuff must be intact to generate these forces. Wear on the glenoid is directed posteriorly because the arms are usually used in front of the body.

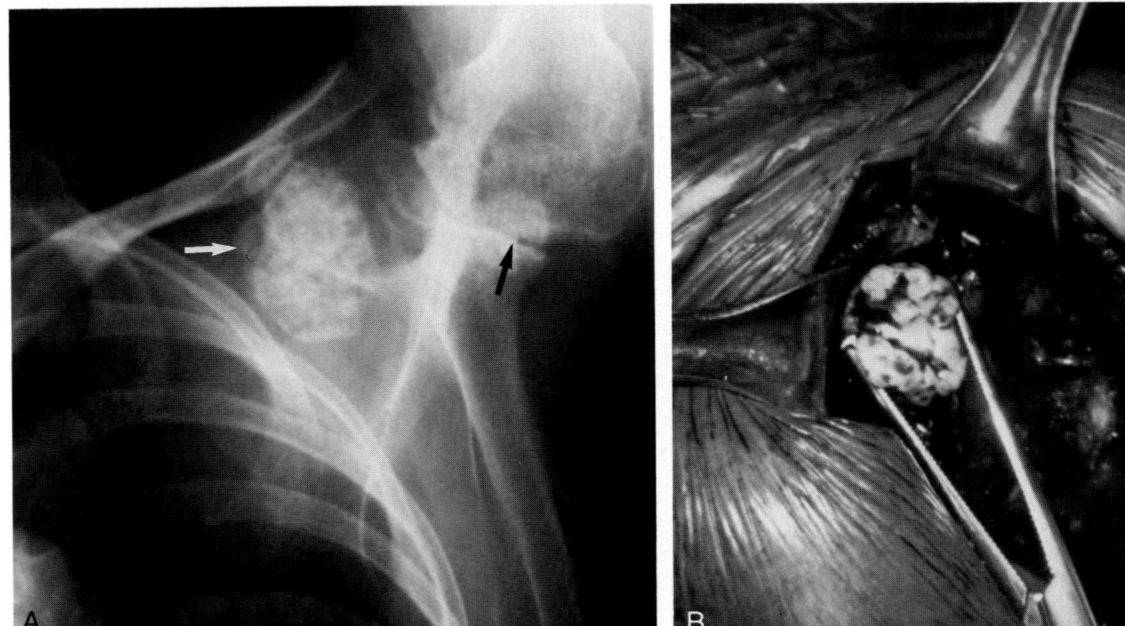

Figure 3–42. ***Glenohumeral Osteoarthritis.*** Osteochondral bodies in the subcoracoid bursa are easily overlooked.

A, Pre-operative x-ray shows a large osteochondral body anteriorly under the coracoid (white arrow), marked wear of the posterior glenoid (black arrow), and posterior subluxation of the humeral head, all of which are typical of glenohumeral osteoarthritis (see Fig. 3–21D).

B, With the glenohumeral joint open, the loose body could not be seen until the subcoracoid bursa was opened.

motion and strength, nonaddicting pain or anti-inflammatory medications, heat, and modifying activities should be given a trial. However, when pain becomes disabling and the axillary x-ray view shows loss of the joint space, uneven wear on the posterior glenoid, and posterior subluxation of the head (Fig. 3–42A), these measures are unlikely to be adequate. The alternatives, as discussed on page 161, include surgical or arthroscopic debridement (which has been, in my experience, unsatisfactory), arthrodesis (which is now unacceptable to most patients because they learn they have a good chance of retaining shoulder motion with another procedure), or nonconstrained glenohumeral arthroplasty.

Good results were obtained in many of our patients with glenohumeral osteoarthritis who were treated with humeral head replacement alone.[2] However, when the glenoid is worn unevenly or is enlarged and flattened, the speed and quality of rehabilitation have been improved when a glenoid component is used.

Special Steps in Arthroplasty for Glenohumeral Osteoarthritis. The procedure, as described in Figures 3–24 through 3–33 (pp. 170 to 192), illustrates all of the steps that might be encountered in a nonconstrained shoulder arthroplasty for osteoarthritis. The steps that are especially important to emphasize for this condition include the following:

1. *Pre-operative assessment of the acromioclavicular joint.* Concomitant painful arthritis of the acromioclavicular joint can spoil the result of a perfect arthroplasty. If this joint is tender and painful pre-operatively, the distal clavicle may have to be excised at the time of the arthroplasty, as shown in Figure 6–8, but performed through the arthroplasty incision. An injection of lidocaine (Xylocaine) into the acromioclavicular joint may be required to make this decision

2. *Lengthening the subscapularis.* The subscapularis muscle is often contracted and shortened, making external rotation impossible if it is re-attached to the humerus without lengthening, as shown in Figure 3–30.

3. *Removal of loose bodies.* A search for osteochondral loose bodies including palpation of the subcoracoid bursa (Fig. 3–42) is routine. A synovectomy is performed as required to remove subsynovial osteochondral bodies threatening to migrate into the joint.

4. *Compensation for uneven posterior wear.* Uneven wear on the posterior surface of the glenoid often makes it necessary to use one of the procedures shown in Figure 3–28 to compensate for the glenoid bone deficiency.

5. *Consideration of the long head of the biceps.* Occasionally the long head of the biceps is partially or completely ruptured by marginal osteophytes in the bicipital groove. If the biceps is frayed

and partially detached, it is tenodesed in the interval between the supraspinatus and the subscapularis or in its groove. Otherwise, it is left free to move in the groove rather than incorporating it during the re-attachment of the subscapularis tendon.

6. *Re-attachment of the subscapularis.* Double check during the re-attachment of the subscapularis tendon to make sure that adequate passive external rotation is maintained (see Fig. 3–30).

7. *Full exercise program.* Because the muscles are intact, the exercise program can be advanced as rapidly as tolerated. EPM (see Fig. 7–7) is begun by 48 hours after surgery and is advanced to the self-assistive program after five days. Active exercises are deferred until muscle soreness disappears, which is usually about three or four weeks after surgery.

Result to Be Expected. The functional results following replacement arthroplasty are determined by the strength of the muscles. Because the muscles are normal in patients with osteoarthritis, it is predictable that a near-normal shoulder should be obtained if nonconstrained arthroplasty is properly performed without complications and if the rehabilitation program is carefully directed. The only muscle disturbed in this procedure is the subscapularis, and there are many other internal rotators that can substitute for it until there is complete healing of the subscapularis in its lengthened position.

Glenohumeral Osteoarthritis in Paraplegics

As discussed on pages 120, 167, 199, 206, 492 and Figure 7–16, we have seen several patients with flail lower extremities due to poliomyelitis who have the roentgen picture of glenohumeral osteoarthritis but with an atypical tear of the rotator cuff. The immense stress and heavy use placed on the shoulders of these patients necessitates a radical change in their living pattern for many months if arthroplasty and cuff repair are to be attempted. If the rotator cuff tear is small, they might resume transfers after six months; however, they should be prepared to avoid using their arms for transfers for one year—the same time needed after cuff repairs in paraplegics without arthroplasty.

Osteoarthritis Treated with a Humeral Head Replacement Without a Glenoid Replacement

Of the 48 shoulders with osteoarthritis reported in 1974,[2] humeral head replacement without a glenoid component relieved the pain and gave excellent ratings with near-normal function in 43 per cent, and "satisfactory" ratings were achieved in 43 per cent. However, the speed of recovery of active motion and strength in patients with enlarged flat glenoids (Fig. 3–43) was thought to be slower than that achieved after the addition of glenoid components. The use of the extended deltopectoral approach since 1977, however, has been an important factor in improved strength and speed of recovery. Even now I see the occasional patient who fears a glenoid component because of conflicting articles in the literature on glenoid component loosening. Although I have not done an arthroplasty without a glenoid component for glenohumeral osteoarthritis in several years, this option does exist.

Osteoarthritis Associated with Acromegaly

Osteoarthritis of the glenohumeral joint may cause the primary disability and discomfort experienced in patients with acromegaly. The joint changes appear identical to those described above

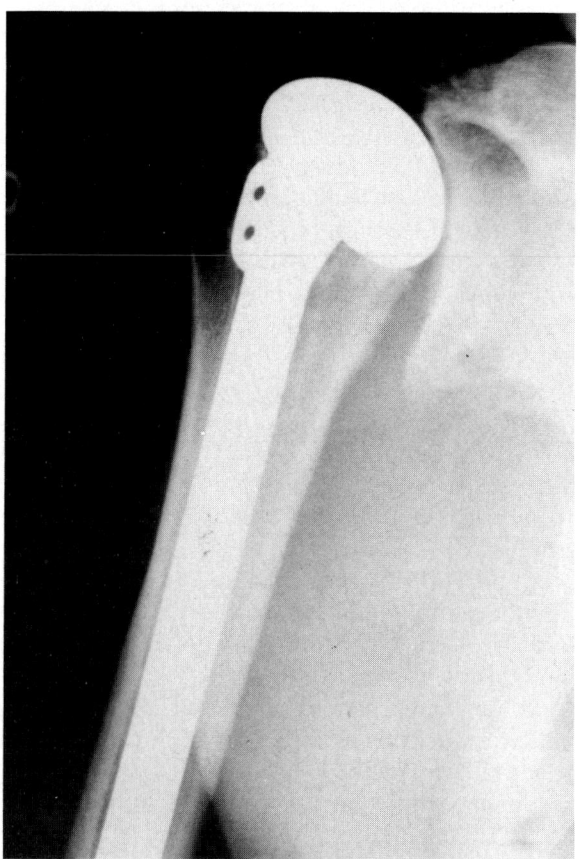

Figure 3–43. ***Glenohumeral Osteoarthritis.*** Enlargement, flattening, and posterior wear of the glenoid is typical of advanced osteoarthritis. This may retard the speed of recovery of active motion and strength when a humeral component alone is used.

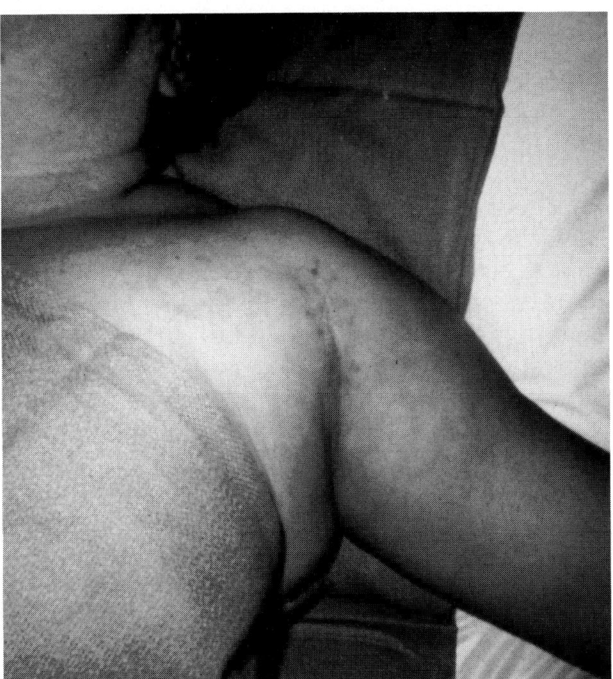

Figure 3–44. ***Glenohumeral Osteoarthritis.*** A biopsy had been performed elsewhere in error on this shoulder with osteoarthritis because of swelling. The swelling was due to osteophytes and fluid.

for primary osteoarthritis. The results following arthroplasty have been equally outstanding.

The major precaution to be taken in treating these patients is investigation for possible overgrowth of cartilage at the opening of the airway. This should be checked by a nose and throat specialist preoperatively. Also, the underlying cause of the acromegaly should, of course, be controlled.

Ochronosis

The roentgen appearance of shoulders with ochronosis is identical to that of primary osteoarthritis, although the cartilage is found to be discolored at surgery (Fig. 3–45). Interestingly, shoulder pain was the first symptom of this condition in two patients in my series. Both were younger than the average patient with osteoarthritis (in their late forties); both had dark cartilage in their ears, which made it possible to suspect the diagnosis preoperatively and confirm it with a simple urine test. One of these patients was treated with a humeral head replacement without a glenoid component and had an excellent result; he returned to a busy career as a taxi driver without shoulder difficulties. Unfortunately, he died from a heart attack ten years later. An autopsy showed no further wear of the glenoid[46] (see Fig. 3–103C).

Paget's Disease

Osteoarthritis of the shoulder may be symptomatic in patients with Paget's disease. Recommendations for surgery should be made cautiously as long as there is any possibility that the pain is due to a stress fracture or to Paget's sarcoma. In one instance in my series, a shoulder arthroplasty successfully stopped the pain and gave a very good functional result. Special care with drilling and reaming the bone is required, and excessive bleeding should be expected. Unfortunately, only a short follow-up was obtainable in my patient, and the long-term behavior at the bone-prosthesis interface is unknown.

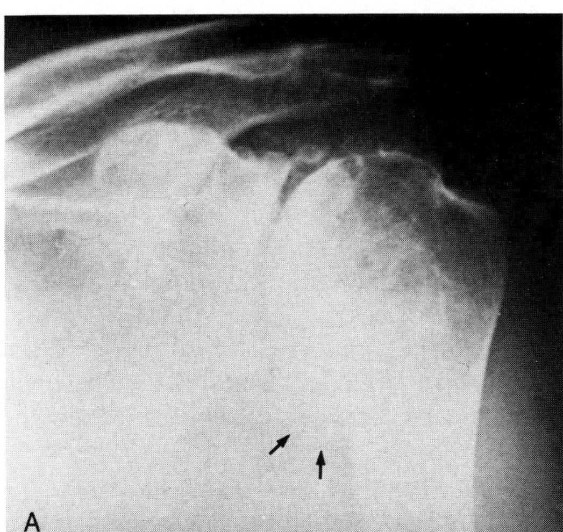

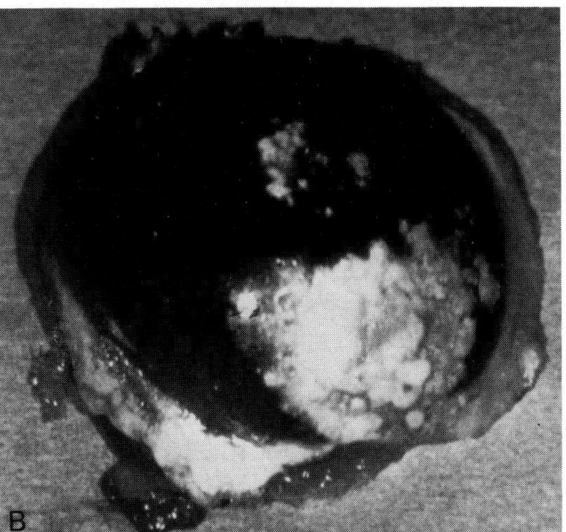

Figure 3–45. ***Glenohumeral Osteoarthritis.*** The gross appearance (B) and roentgen appearance (A) of ochronosis. The roentgen appearance of ochronosis is identical to that of glenohumeral osteoarthritis.

ARTHRITIS OF DISLOCATIONS

Arthritis of dislocations is an entity that has only recently been understood.[13, 22, 119] It is usually associated with multidirectional and inferior dislocations and subluxations of the glenohumeral joint and received almost no attention prior to our description in 1980.[13]

Anatomical Problem

Although degenerative arthritis of the glenohumeral joint can result from the trauma to the articular surfaces inflicted by many dislocations, this is uncommon. By far the most frequent etiological mechanism for the development of arthritis of recurrent dislocations is a "standard" operative procedure intended to remedy recurrent unidirectional dislocations that is unsuspectingly performed on a loose, multidirectional shoulder. Almost any of the standard operative procedures used for anterior or posterior dislocations can displace the head of the humerus, leading to these severe arthritic changes. The humeral head may be displaced in a multidirectional shoulder (one that is loose and dislocates or subluxes in all directions) by (1) tightening one side of the capsule, (2) transferring a muscle to reinforce one side of the capsule, (3) an osteotomy that tilts the articular surface of the glenoid, or (4) an anterior or posterior "bone block" (bone graft). All of these procedures can displace the humeral head in a loose shoulder away from the side of the repair, creating a fixed subluxation. The subluxed head wears unevenly on the glenoid, and arthritic changes can develop surprisingly fast.

Of the 61 shoulders with this condition in my current series (Table 3–1), surgery for recurrent dislocations had been performed elsewhere in all but eight. One patient had five operations, five had three operations, 15 had two operations, and 32 had one operation. Their shoulders were multidirectional prior to the initial procedure because of inherent generalized ligamentous laxity, acquired shoulder laxity due to repeated minor injuries (which had caused elongation of the ligaments and capsule), or a combination of the two, as discussed in Chapter 4, page 279.

Acquired laxity of the shoulder ligaments is an important new concept. It is the most frequent cause of multidirectional dislocations and, unfortunately, usually affects young patients who are athletic and muscular. It was a mistaken idea in the past to think of multidirectional dislocations as being limited to frail young women with loose joints. It is especially easy to miss multidirectional laxity of the shoulder in athletic persons with acquired laxity. Because almost any of the repairs used for unidirectional dislocations may cause malalignment of the humeral head and severe arthritis, it is important to know when to suspect and how to determine the presence of multidirectional dislocations (see Chapter 4, p. 288). The possible presence of multidirectional instability should be considered when an initial dislocation occurred without a significant injury and was spontaneously reduced, the patient has laxity of another joint, and a "sulcus sign" (see Fig. 4–17) is present in either shoulder (showing the presence of inferior instability).

The age of patients with arthritis of dislocations averaged only 38 years at the time of shoulder arthroplasty and ranged from 19 to 74 years. Thus, many are severely disabled when they are under 40 years of age. Although the majority are athletic young men, some are sedentary with generalized joint laxity. Bilateral shoulder laxity is common.

As indicated previously, the great majority (86 per cent) have had previous surgery. Because the procedure had usually been done on the anterior side, the humeral head was subluxated posteriorly (Figs. 3–46 and 3–47). On physical examination these shoulders resemble a traumatic posterior dislocation, with prominence of the coracoid, axis of the shaft of the humerus directed posteriorly, and restriction of external rotation. When a procedure had been done through a posterior approach, the head was subluxated anteriorly. Laxity of the opposite shoulder or other joints is a clue to suspect multidirectional instability as the underlying problem.

Treatment of Arthritis of Dislocation

Indications for Arthroplasty. Despite the young age of many of these patients, an arthroplasty is considered because of their intense pain and disability and the deformity of the joint surfaces. Although there has been some damage to the shoulder musculature in most cases, the prognosis for an excellent result after a nonconstrained arthroplasty is extremely good. A fusion is considered a last resort because it wastes good muscles and restricts motion and function. Debridement has been ineffective. Watchful waiting can lead to severe wear and further glenoid deficiency (Figs. 3–46 and 3–47).

On the other hand, some patients are referred who have pain and an unsatisfactory result following previous surgery, although the contours of the articular surfaces are maintained. These patients may have residual instability or a fixed subluxation

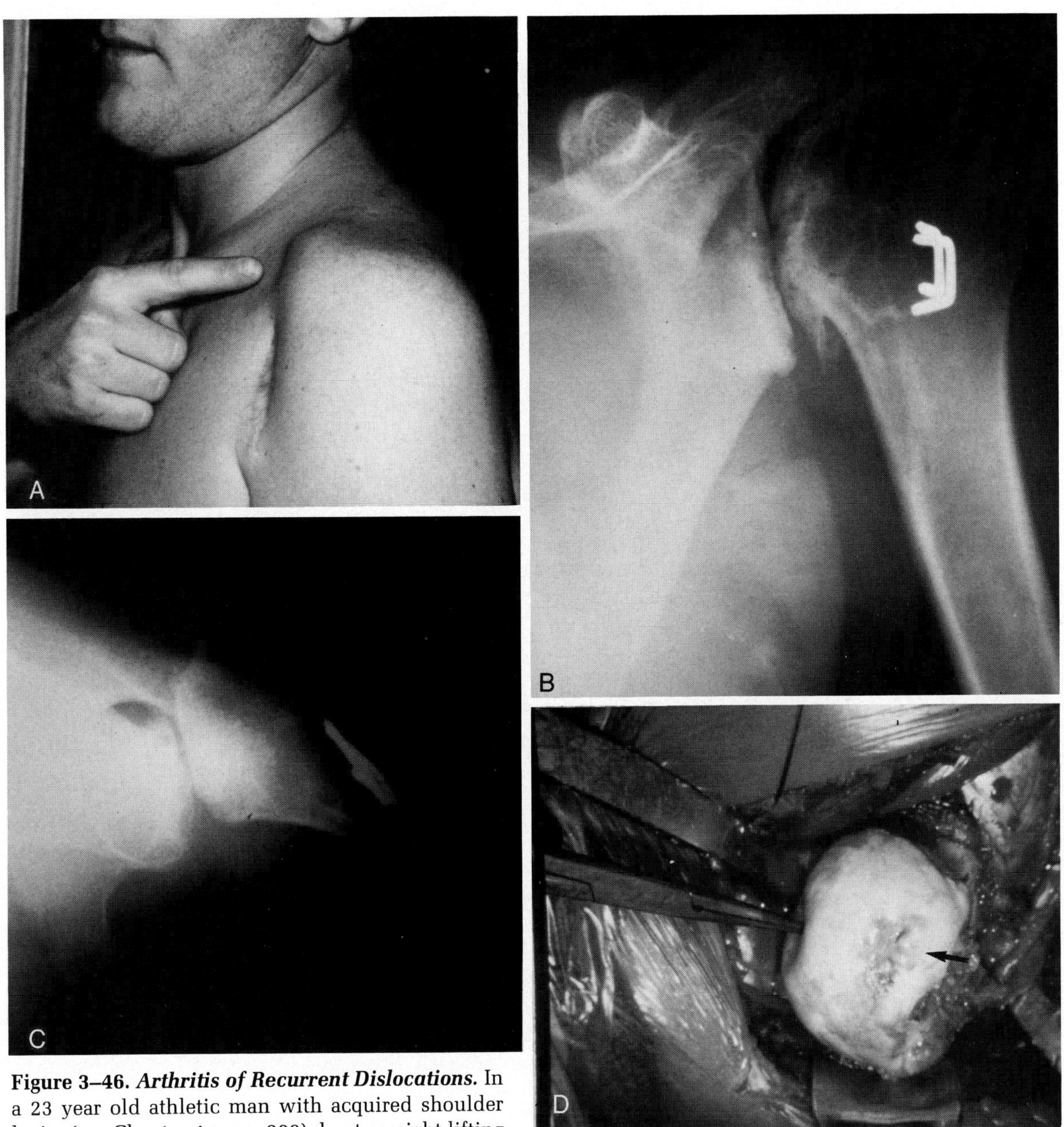

Figure 3–46. ***Arthritis of Recurrent Dislocations.*** In a 23 year old athletic man with acquired shoulder laxity (see Chapter 4, page 288) due to weight lifting the humeral head was subluxated posteriorly by a Magnusson-Stack procedure performed three years previously. He required a total shoulder arthroplasty.

A, The shoulder had the appearance of a locked, posterior dislocation with prominence of the coracoid anteriorly and of the head posteriorly.

B, Anterior-posterior view shows advanced arthritis and staples, which had been used in the previous surgery.

C, Axillary view reveals the posterior subluxation of the head with wear and sclerosis of the posterior glenoid.

D, At surgery, the humeral head was pushed out of the joint by the tight anterior capsule. The head was eburnated and sclerotic where it contacted the glenoid (arrow) but was soft and atrophic and could be indented with a clamp posteriorly (as shown).

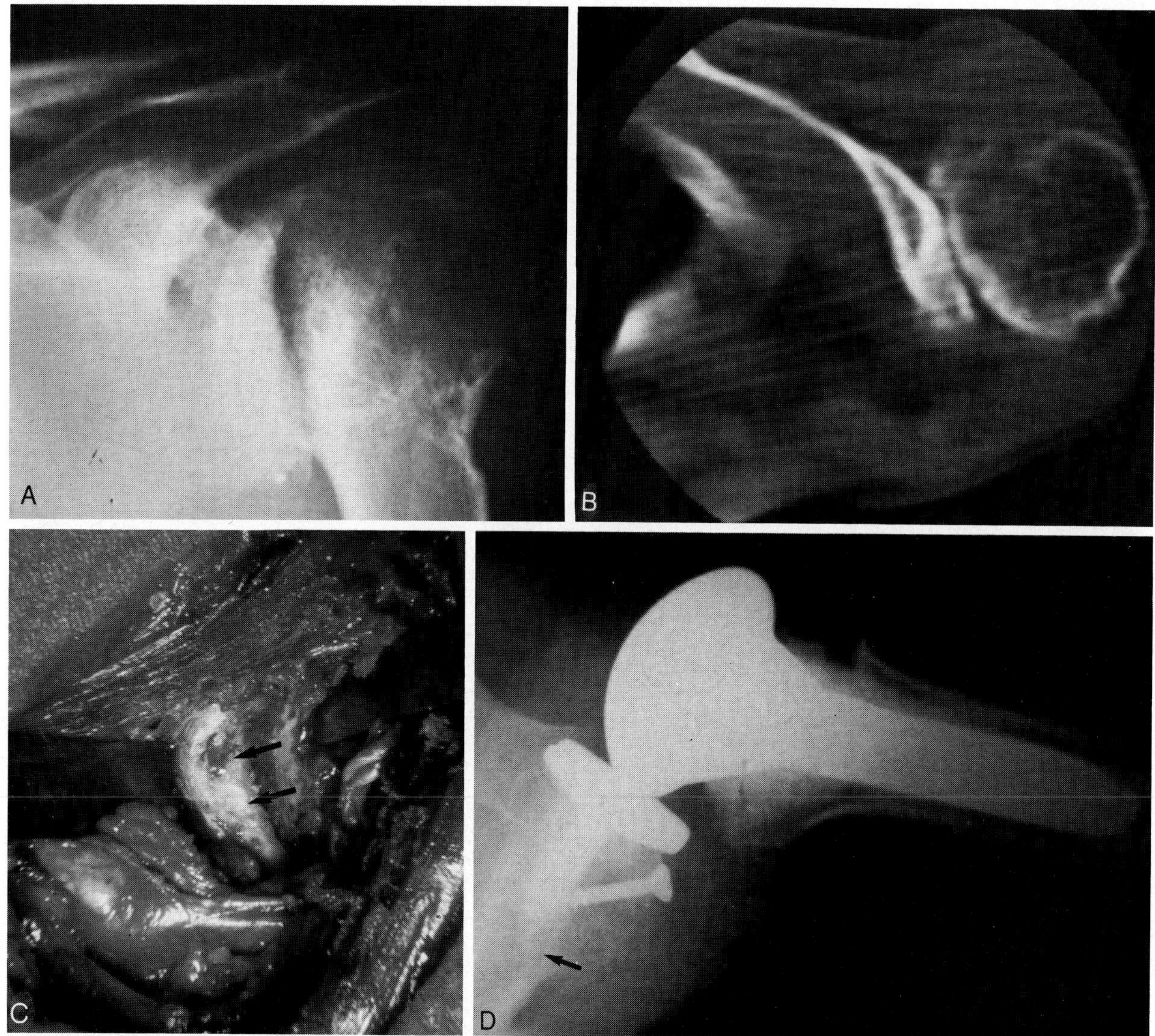

Figure 3–47. ***Arthritis of Recurrent Dislocations.*** A 34 year old man who had had a repair for recurrent anterior dislocation seven years previously required a total shoulder arthroplasty.

A, Anterior-posterior view shows posterior displacement of the head and severe arthritis.

B, Computerized tomography shows marked posterior dislocation of head, erosion of posterior glenoid and osteophytes, and sclerosis of the head.

C, Photograph at surgery shows complete erosion of the posterior half of the glenoid (arrows), which required a bone graft.

D, Axillary view of glenoid bone graft (a piece of humeral head held with a screw) shows it to be united to the scapula (arrow) and the components secure two years after surgery.

of the head. In this situation, the patient is warned that an arthroplasty may be required, the shoulder is explored, and the decision is made on the amount of instability or malalignment found and the condition of the articular surfaces. I am inclined to accept considerable loss of the articular cartilage provided that the shape of the surfaces remains sufficiently normal to allow releases and repairs of ligaments that maintain the head in proper alignment with stability. It is often necessary to release the soft tissues on the opposite side and eliminate an inferior capsular pouch with an inferior capsular shift,[13] as described in the discussion of re-operations for inadequate repairs of dislocation (see Chapter 4, p. 336). Arthroscopic examination of the articular surfaces may help to predict the likelihood of a replacement arthroplasty in borderline cases; however, the final decision is made on open inspection of the joint.

Glenoid involvement is almost always quite marked in arthritis of recurrent dislocation and precluded the use of a humeral component alone without a glenoid component in 52 of the 61 patients in the series outlined in Table 3–1.

Special Steps in Arthroplasty for Arthritis of Dislocations. Because the large majority of these patients have had previous surgery, the typical operation entails removing the previous scar, freeing the deltoid, lengthening the short muscles, dealing with a deficient glenoid, and coping with the special threat of instability of the components post-operatively.

1. *Incision.* Previous scars are excised and elongated or undermined as required rather than making new skin incisions.

2. *Possible deltoidplasty.* Previous surgery has usually made it difficult to locate the deltopectoral interval and has caused the anterior deltoid to be adherent to the coracoid and anterior humerus. Furthermore, the anterior deltoid may be scarred and weakened from retraction, necessitating a deltoidplasty (see Fig. 3–33), bringing the pectoralis and middle deltoid together when closing.

3. *Lengthening the subscapularis.* Previous anterior repairs have usually shortened the anterior capsule and subscapularis, limiting external rotation. These structures must be lengthened if overhead motion is to be restored. Because the subscapularis tendon and the capsule have usually been overlapped at previous surgery and made thicker than normal, it is easy to perform a "Z-plasty" in the coronal plane by raising all of the insertion of the subscapularis tendon off the humerus and thickened capsule (returning it to a normal appearance) and dividing the capsule transversely to create a thick flap of capsule that remains attached to the humerus and is later sewn to the end of the subscapularis tendon (Fig. 3–30).

4. *Glenoid bone deficiency.* Uneven wear of the articular surface of the glenoid may be more pronounced in arthritis of recurrent dislocations than in any other condition. Wear and loss of bone on one side of the glenoid can occur very rapidly when the humeral head is malaligned. It may be necessary to lower the high side (see Fig. 3–28B), alter the version of the components (see Fig. 3–28D), or use a glenoid bone graft (see Fig. 3–28G). In the most advanced stages of arthritis of dislocations, as illustrated in Figures 3–46 and 3–47, it may be preferable to compensate for glenoid bone loss by altering the version of the components rather than using a bone graft because the external rotators may have become retracted. Bringing the humeral head out to its normal position by using a glenoid bone graft may be incompatible with keeping the external rotators attached (see Figs. 3–28D, 3–88, and 3–89). To re-state this point, if the infraspinatus has been shortened by years of posterior dislocation, altering the version of the components is compatible with the short infraspinatus, but if a bone graft is used and the humerus is forced laterally, the contracted infraspinatus tendon may avulse an osteopenic greater tuberosity because it cannot reach that far (this happened in the case illustrated in Figure 3–47).

5. *Compensation for glenoid bone block, glenoid osteotomy, or coracoid transfer.* Surgical alterations of the glenoid must be corrected to permit implantation of the glenoid component with good bone support and proper version. If the subscapularis tendon is tethered by a coracoid process that has been transferred through it, the portion of subscapularis inferior to the transferred coracoid is divided so that the subscapularis can be dissected free to become an internal rotator again, allowing passive external rotation.

6. *Instability of the components.* The postoperative exercise program should take into consideration the possibility of instability of the components. Whenever there has been a long-standing subluxation or dislocation, the tissue becomes set around the upper humerus with shortening of the muscles and fascia on one side and a "pouch" or elongation of the capsule on the opposite side to accommodate the head. The tendency for instability is much greater if the glenoid–greater tuberosity distance has not been re-established (to eliminate the pouch—see Fig. 3–28D) or if the length and version of the head do not compensate for this defect. If the components tend to subluxate or dislocate posteriorly, supine elevation and forward flexion should be avoided in the early post-opera-

tive exercise program, during which the arm is raised in the scapular plane and the external rotators are strengthened for protection. If the humeral component tends to subluxate anteriorly, passive external rotation and abduction are restricted for several weeks while the internal rotators are strengthened. Active motion is deferred until healing of the soft tissue and protective muscles has occurred.

Results to Be Expected from Arthroplasty for Arthritis of Recurrent Dislocations

Although time is needed to establish stability of the components and deltoid strength, most late results have been quite good (see Table 3–7). Because the average age of the patients at the time of surgery was only 39 years and the patients were generally very athletic and active, the question arose as to what extent these activities should be restricted following arthroplasty. In general, I allow them to resume golf, tennis, and noncontact sports, but urge them to avoid lifting heavy weights overhead as an exercise (limiting the amount of weight to 50 pounds) and to avoid activities that entail hard falls (such as downhill skiing).

RHEUMATOID ARTHRITIS

Anatomical Problems

It is important to remember that rheumatoid arthritis is a systemic disease that involves the muscles, bursa, acromioclavicular joint, and, less frequently, the sternoclavicular joint.[21, 39] In the past, tears of the rotator cuff were considered an inherent and unavoidable part of rheumatoid shoulders, making them unsuited for an unconstrained arthroplasty.[104] Although I realized that tears of the rotator cuff were present in no more than 20 to 30 per cent of our patients who had shoulder arthroplasties for rheumatoid arthritis and Colfield's statistics agree,[103] I did not appreciate until recently the true mechanism of rotator cuff ruptures in patients with rheumatoid arthritis (Fig. 3–48A and B).

As discussed in Chapter 2 (Figs. 2–9A and 2–54), it is the loss of the articular surfaces that causes the head to translocate upward with impingement of the greater tuberosity under the acromion. This impingement, which is responsible for tears of the rotator cuff, can be prevented by a nonconstrained total arthroplasty in which the components are positioned to prevent ascent of the head.

Now the answer to an easier and more successful arthroplasty on a rheumatoid shoulder has become clear. The operation should be done prior to the development of severe bone loss from panus erosion and disuse osteopenia and prior to translocation of the humerus upward because of loss of the articular surfaces, which will eventually cause impingement erosion of the rotator cuff (Fig. 3–49E and F).

I once thought that an anterior acromioplasty should be a routine step in an arthroplasty on a rheumatoid shoulder, believing that the rotator cuff was weakened by rheumatoid disease and allowed the humerus to ascend, causing impingement.[21] Realizing that the components can be placed to act as a spacer against upward displacement of the humerus, I now very rarely do an anterior acromio-

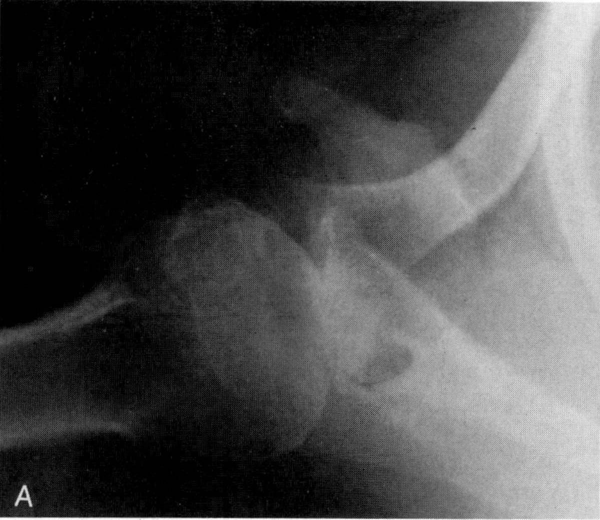

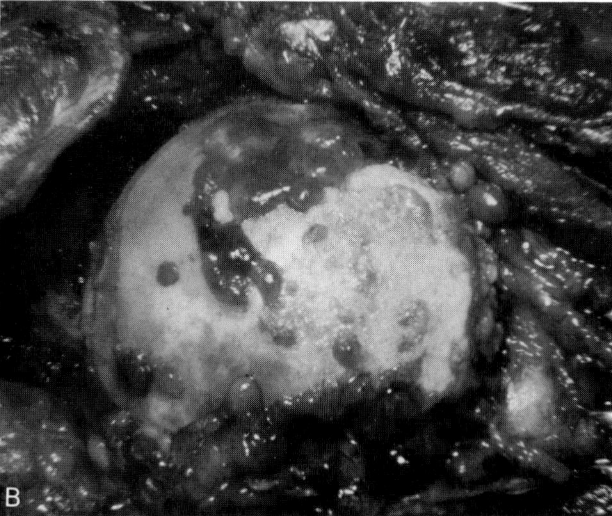

Figure 3–48. Axillary view (A) and photograph (B) in the operating room depicting the unpredictable nature of rheumatoid pannus erosion.

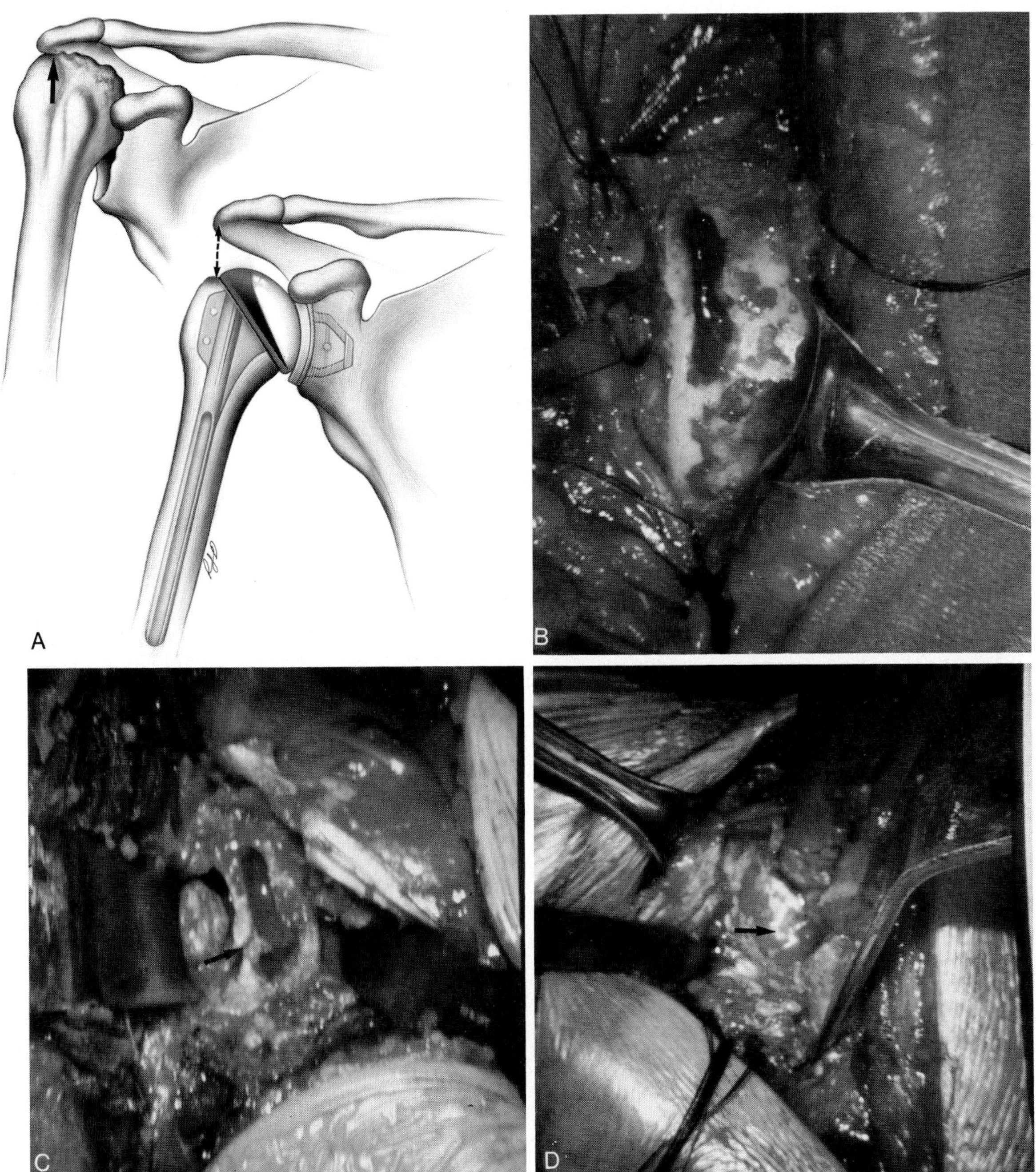

Figure 3–49. The secret of an easier and more successful arthroplasty in patients with rheumatoid arthritis is to perform it before there is severe loss of bone or rotator cuff.

A, Arthroplasty aims at eliminating upward translocation to stop cuff destruction caused by impingement.

B, Photographs taken in the operating room (B–D) show bone loss at the glenoid caused by delay. No wonder some have radiolucent lines! This figure shows perforation of the scapular wall and insufficient bone to permit making a slot large enough for the keel of the polyethylene glenoid.

C, Soft glenoid fractured (arrow) when inserting the guide.

D, The rheumatologist waited 11 years for the shoulder arthroplasty "to be perfected" and now there is no glenoid (arrow).

Illustration continued on following page

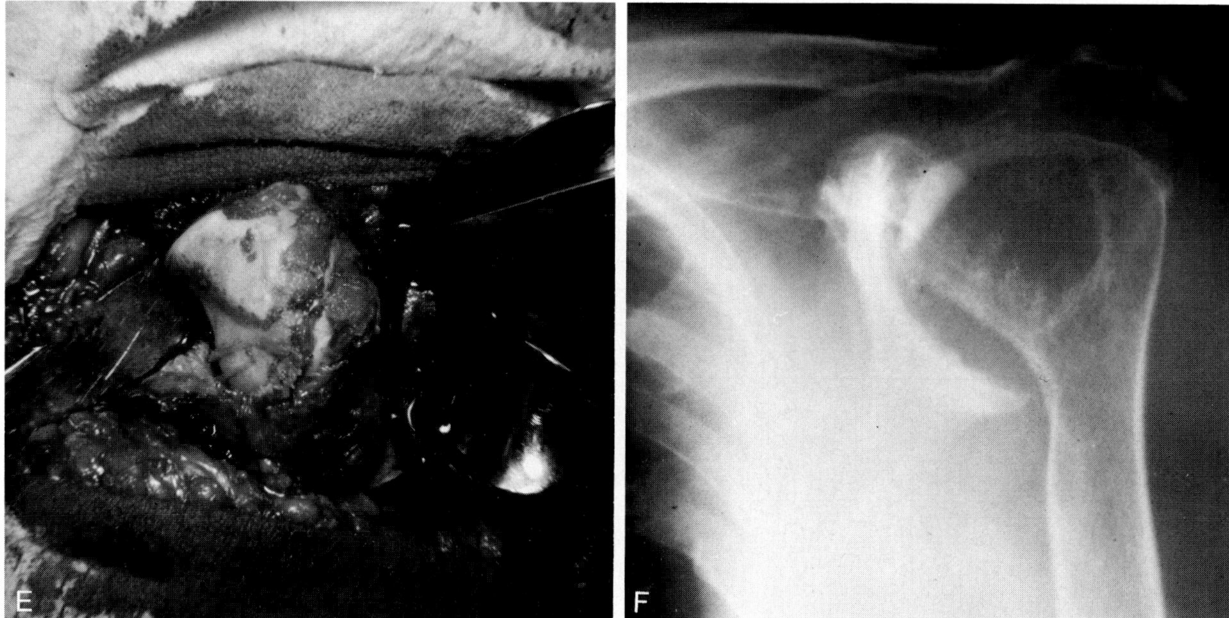

Figure 3–49 *Continued* E and F, End-stage loss of the rotator cuff. Severe, polyarthritic rheumatoid arthritis with long-standing loss of the rotator cuff. The irregular head has worn half-way through the coracoid, outer clavicle, and acromion, and there is no rotator cuff remaining on the humerus. Roentgen appearance resembles that of cuff-tear arthropathy. Nonconstrained arthroplasty and "limited goals" rehabilitation stopped the pain.

plasty during an arthroplasty for rheumatoid arthritis.[39] Painful rheumatoid arthritis of the acromioclavicular joint does occur and can spoil the rehabilitation program. Therefore, excision of the distal clavicle at the time of an arthroplasty on a rheumatoid patient may be required. This decision must be made pre-operatively and is based on pain and tenderness at the acromioclavicular joint rather than on the roentgen appearance. I have seen some acromioclavicular joints that were asymptomatic despite advanced roentgen changes, in which case the acromioclavicular joint is left undisturbed during the glenohumeral arthroplasty.

Personal Series

Of the 141 rheumatoid shoulders in Table 3–1, the average age of the patients was 59 years. Twenty-six patients had bilateral shoulder arthroplasties. There were eight patients with juvenile rheumatoid arthritis, all of whom were less than 29 years of age. The predominance of female patients was interesting; 105 procedures were performed in women and only 26 in men.

The incidence of right and left shoulder arthroplasties was about equal, unlike the situation in osteoarthritis, in which the dominant arm was affected more frequently and bilateral shoulder involvement was less common. Bilateral shoulder involvement was more frequent in rheumatoid arthritis than in other conditions.

A total elbow arthroplasty was performed in ten of the patients in this series. The elbow arthroplasty was performed prior to the shoulder arthroplasty in four patients who had predominantly more elbow symptoms than shoulder symptoms at the time of the elbow arthroplasty. The elbow arthroplasty was done after the shoulder arthroplasty in six patients. A number of patients who had both shoulder and elbow symptoms were relieved of both shoulder and elbow discomfort following a shoulder arthroplasty and were no longer interested in an elbow arthroplasty. It seemed two types of elbow pain, from strain placed on the elbow during everyday function when the shoulder is frozen and does not rotate and pain referred from the shoulder to the elbow, can be relieved by a shoulder arthroplasty. However, a shoulder arthroplasty has little effect on elbow pain caused by incongruity of the articular surfaces of the elbow joint.

Variations in Involvement and Pathology

Low-Grade, Intermediate, and Severe Involvement. There is a great deal about rheumatoid arthritis that is poorly understood. We do not know its cause or have a specific diagnostic test. In our present state of ignorance, it is helpful in making clinical decisions to classify the disease as low-grade, intermediate, or severe.

Post-operative rehabilitation is much easier in those with mild disease. Bone loss is apt to occur more slowly, and they may develop marginal os-

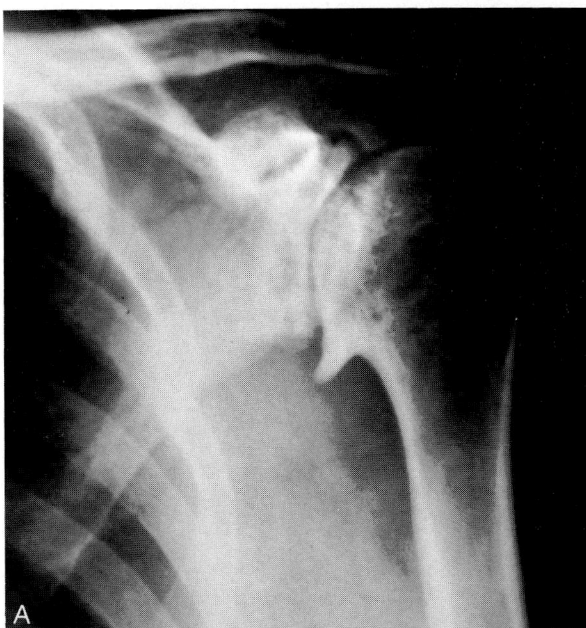

Figure 3–50. ***Variations in Involvement in Rheumatoid Arthritis.***

A, "Dry" form with stiffness, sclerosis, and marginal osteophytes similar to those seen in osteoarthritis.

B, "Wet" form with inflammation and abundant marginal erosion of the articular surfaces by the destructive granulation.

C, End-stage bone destruction with complete loss of glenoid and head after years of involvement.

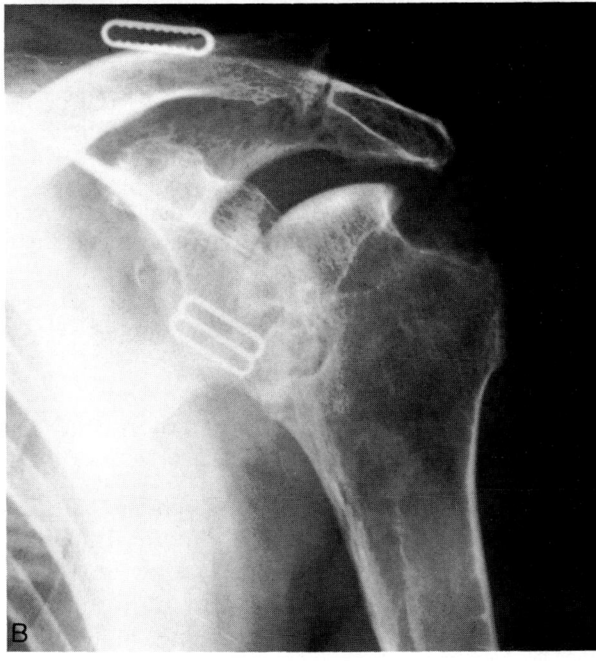

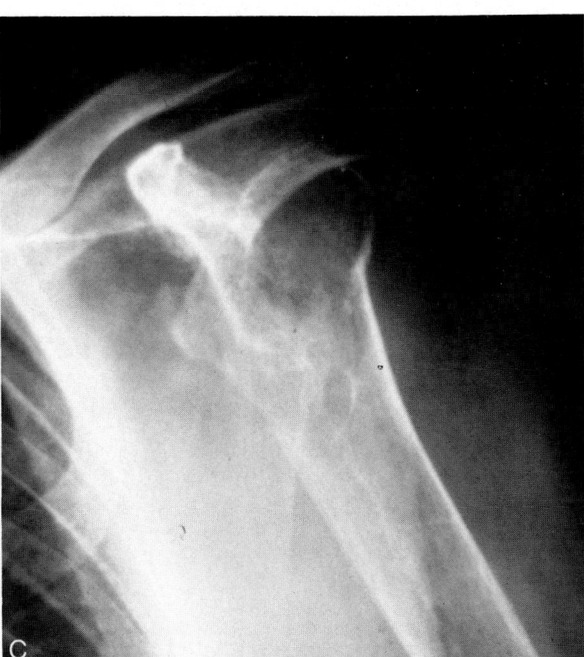

teophytes similar to those seen in osteoarthritis (Fig. 3–50A).

In the more severe form of rheumatoid arthritis, there may be rapid destruction of the joint surfaces with early ascent of the humerus and involvement of the rotator cuff. If shoulder arthroplasties are postponed unnecessarily, severe bone loss and rotator cuff damage can occur needlessly. In one major rheumatoid hospital in the United States, patients underwent an average of four other major arthroplasties (hips, knees, or elbows) prior to the first shoulder arthroplasty. The delays in performing shoulder arthroplasty undoubtedly contributed to their very high incidence of rotator cuff defects and severe glenoid bone loss.

Dry, Wet, and Resorptive. In addition to the variations in severity of the disease as discussed above, there are three clinical types of this condition, as illustrated in Figure 3–50A to C.

In the dry form there is sclerosis, subchondral cysts, and loss of joint space. Minimal margin erosion is seen, and marginal osteophytes may form similar to those characteristic of osteoarthritis. The joints tend to be stiffer than in the other types of this disease. Muscle wasting may be intense in patients with juvenile rheumatoid arthritis with this type of disease; however, muscles are usually in better condition in adults. When only a few joints are involved, many terms have been used, which probably apply to this condition: "inflammatory osteoarthritis," "low-grade rheumatoid arthritis," and "mixed arthritis."

In the wet form there are exuberant granulations with marginal erosion, which causes the ends of the bone to become pointed (Fig. 3–50). Severe destruction of the glenoid may occur not only because of granulation erosion and disuse osteopenia but also because the pointed end of the humerus causes pressure erosion of the glenoid.

There is a wet and resorptive form of rheumatoid arthritis associated with severe bone loss and central migration of the humerus that I have termed "centralization."

"Centralization"

Severe loss of bone is associated with loss of the contour of the shoulder. The point of the shoulder becomes flattened and resembles a Burgundy wine bottle without the shoulders of a Bordeaux bottle (Fig. 3–51), a finding that if looked for can easily be seen. This finding is significant in revealing marked bone loss and the probability of difficulty in implanting a glenoid component.

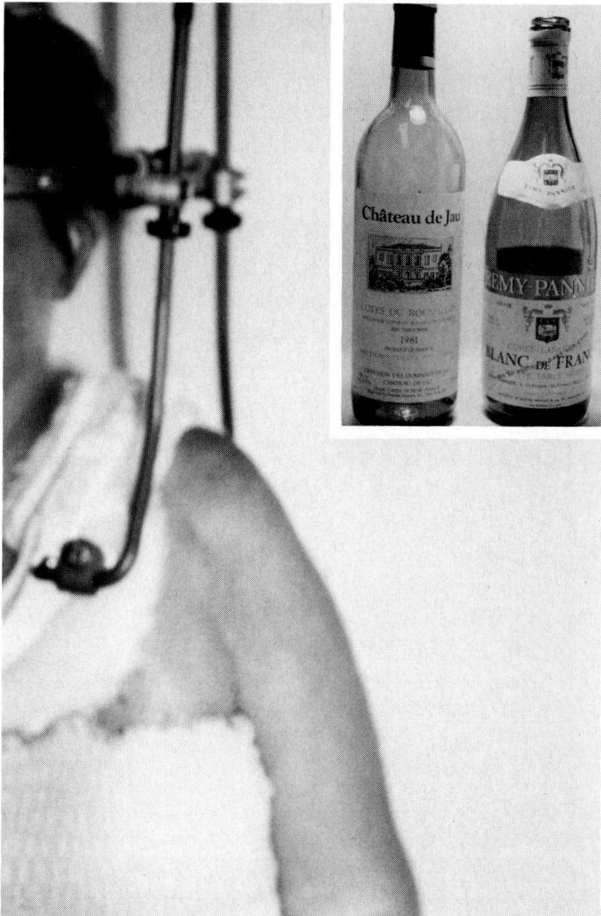

Figure 3–51. Preoperative assessment in patients with rheumatoid arthritis. Depicting the flat contour of a shoulder, which was due to "centralization" from bone loss. The centralized shoulder has the appearance of a burgundy wine bottle without the shoulders of a bordeaux (inset). Centralization is a warning that there is limited bone stock in the glenoid.

Special attention is given to the cervical spine in rheumatoid patients. This patient required a C1–C2 fusion and halo cast.

Unpredictable Granulation Erosion and Osteopenia

Unlike osteoarthritis, in which the pathological findings are constant and almost without variation other than that caused by slow erosion, the granulation erosion of rheumatoid arthritis is unpredictable and may involve any site on the glenoid or humerus. Because the glenoid has only a limited amount of bone, this type of destruction can interfere unexpectedly with secure anchorage of the glenoid component. The problem can be magnified by softening of the bone, which is due at least in part to the inactivity enforced by months of pain. Fractures of the greater tuberosity, the shaft of the humerus, and the glenoid may occur during this procedure unless the bone is handled with great respect. Because of the osteopenia with widening of the medullary canal in the shaft of the humerus, I routinely cement both the humeral and glenoid components in patients with rheumatoid arthritis.

Treatment

Indications for Arthroplasty. Nonoperative treatment can be continued as long as there is preservation of the humeral head, glenoid, and glenoid-tuberosity distance so that the greater tuberosity does not ride up against the acromion to threaten the rotator cuff. Once collapse of the articular surfaces occurs, there is no chance for success with medical treatment, and an arthroplasty is recommended to avoid loss of bone and damage to the rotator cuff.

The priorities for shoulder arthroplasty in rheumatoid patients are summarized in Table 3–2a. When only the upper extremity requires an operation, the primary goal is to relieve pain and preserve function. In the past, many hand surgeons insisted that all attention be directed initially to optimizing the function of the hand. To some of these surgeons, the only indication for a shoulder operation was so much stiffness of the shoulder that the arm could not be placed far enough out on an armboard for a hand operation. However, I believe most modern hand surgeons recognize that severe pain in the shoulder can be of much greater concern to the patient, the painful, stiff shoulder can have an adverse effect on the elbow and hand, and needless delay of shoulder arthroplasty is unwise because of the threat of destruction of the glenoid and rotator cuff. In my experience, patients who have primarily elbow pain without shoulder pain are relatively few. If the shoulder and elbow are equally painful, I advise doing the shoulder arthroplasty first because this should eliminate referred pain from the shoulder to the elbow, free the elbow from the strain placed on it by an immobile shoulder, and stop the progression of destruction at the rotator cuff and glenoid. A further point favoring performance of the shoulder arthroplasty first is the much higher incidence of serious complications, such as infection and instability, of elbow arthroplasties (Fig. 3–52).

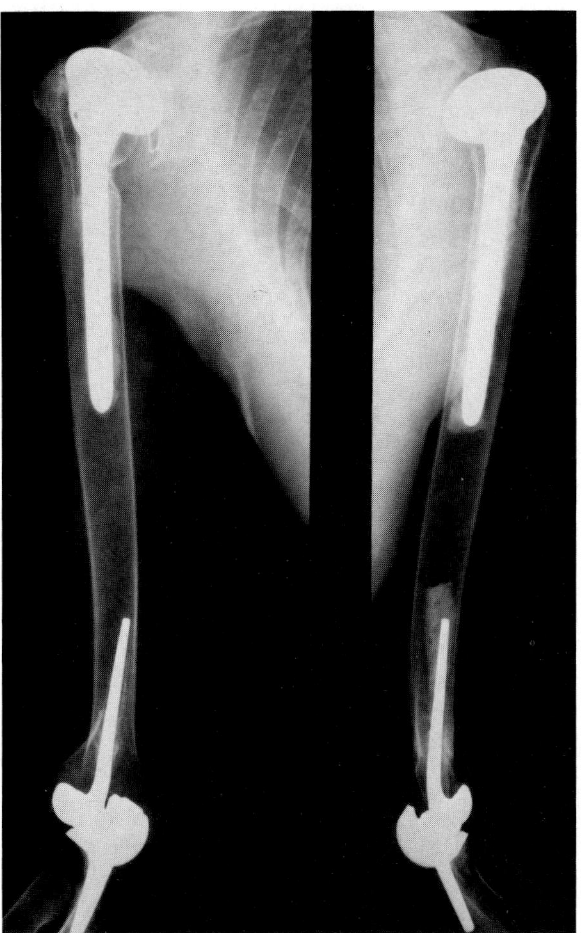

Figure 3–52. As was true of this rheumatoid patient who had all eight major joints replaced, shoulder arthroplasty takes a priority over elbow arthroplasty because of the threat of loosing the rotator cuff and for other reasons explained in the text.

When both the upper and lower extremities require an operation, the lower extremity generally has priority if the problem necessitates a wheelchair or constant walking aids. If the patient is ambulatory and shoulder pain is equally intense, the shoulder is given priority provided that the patient agrees to defer for at least six months lower extremity operations entailing walking aids that might stress the soft-tissue repair at the shoulder arthroplasty.

Nonoperative Treatment. Aside from safe and nonaddicting medications, conservative treatment is based on early detection of shoulder stiffness and eliminating it with exercises prior to the appearance of detrimental side effects. A flare-up of arthritis may cause the patient to clasp a painful shoulder against the side of the body to protect it from painful movements. After the arthritic process abates, however, stiffness of the shoulder may continue with pain at the extremes of movement because of contraction of the capsule and ligaments. This is "frozen shoulder" pain (see Chapter 6, p. 422), and a vicious cycle results with more stiffening of the shoulder as the arm is held rigidly against the side of the body. The immobility leads to stiffening of the elbow in a flexed position, stiffness and ulnar deviation of the wrist, and stiffening with ulnar drift of the fingers. The scapular musculature also becomes weak and short. Thus, the entire "upper extremity unit" (see p. 31) is affected. The nutrition of the articular cartilage is dependent on the joint fluid and pumping action of the joint. Inactivity and disuse impair the nutrition of the cartilage and may have an adverse effect on the joint surfaces beyond that of rheumatoid arthritis.

Low heat to relax the muscles and gentle passive external rotation and elevation of the arm are emphasized. A team approach is needed including the therapist, the internal medical consultant, and the surgeon. Physical therapy aims at restoring motion and strength. Medicine aims at controlling pain and inflammation. The orthopaedic surgeon evaluates the patient for nonoperative and operative treatment. A feeling of team play and mutual respect should prevail, with the common goal of controlling pain and re-establishing function by the safest and least harmful method available.

Passive exercises are the most important for regaining motion and are carried out with low heat and analgesia four or five times a day, as discussed in Chapter 7. Strengthening exercises are deferred until the pain subsides and then progress from isometric to assistive and eventually to resistive exercises. Braces may help to hold the shoulder out of the "protective position" and to allow air to reach an axilla that has been infested with fungus. Forceful manipulation has no role in rheumatoid shoulders and may fracture the osteopenic bone.

Alternative Procedures. Many procedures have been used in the past for rheumatoid shoulders, including glenohumeral arthrodesis, humeral head resection, and glenoidectomy, which are now rarely if ever used today and will not be discussed. The following operations deserve discussion.

Humeral Head Replacement Without a Glenoid Component. As described in 1971,[54] the results of shoulder arthroplasties using a humeral head component alone without a glenoid component were inferior to those now achieved with total shoulder arthroplasties.[21, 22] This is logical because both sides of the shoulder joint are involved in rheumatoid arthritis, and the muscles have often been weakened by the rheumatoid disease; however, when accounting for the improved results in recent years, one must appreciate that the extended deltopectoral approach (without detaching the deltoid origin) and the improved rehabilitation program (involving earlier passive motion) have been as important as the addition of the glenoid component.

When the articular surface of the glenoid has been destroyed by long-standing rheumatoid arthritis making it impossible to implant the glenoid component, or, if implanted, making it unlikely that the component can stay in place without loosening, the humeral component is used alone without a glenoid component. The methods used to compensate for a deficient glenoid (Fig. 3–28) are considered in borderline cases but should not be employed in patients with end-stage rheumatoid arthritis such as the shoulder illustrated in Figure 3–49.

Synovectomy and Joint Debridement. Synovectomy and joint debridement have been disappointing and are no longer used without concomitant replacement of the articular surfaces. The exception is the rare bursal type of rheumatoid shoulder, to be discussed.

Subacromial Spacer. An inert disc interposed between the greater tuberosity and the acromion was once used in a few rheumatoid patients with rotator cuff deficiencies by MacNab and also by Clayton.[140] This is of historic interest but is no longer used because it does not alleviate painful contact between the incongruous surfaces of the humeral head and the glenoid, nor does it provide stability against dislocations, which are apt to occur if the cuff tear is large enough.[112]

Bursal-Type of Rheumatoid Shoulder. I have seen two rheumatoid patients (three shoulders) with involvement of the subacromial bursa primarily without significant skeletal change at the glenohumeral joint.[21] The subacromial bursa was huge, but it is significant that no fluid could be aspirated from the bursa because it was filled with rice bodies (Fig. 3–53). There was some destruction of the acromioclavicular joint in each case. These shoulders were treated by bursectomy, excision of the distal clavicle, and inspection of the glenohumeral joint through the rotator interval. In each case there was moderate synovitis of the glenohumeral joint, and a synovectomy was performed by temporarily detaching the subscapularis tendon. The articular surfaces of the humeral head and glenoid were only minimally involved and were left intact. The results of these three shoulders have been satisfactory for more than ten years.

Special Steps in Arthroplasties for Rheumatoid Shoulders

Risk of Infection. Rheumatoid joints have a reputation for a higher rate of post-operative infection. There are several reasons for this. First, the soft tissue is involved in rheumatoid disease and has less ability to combat infection. Second, if corticosteroids have been administered, they have

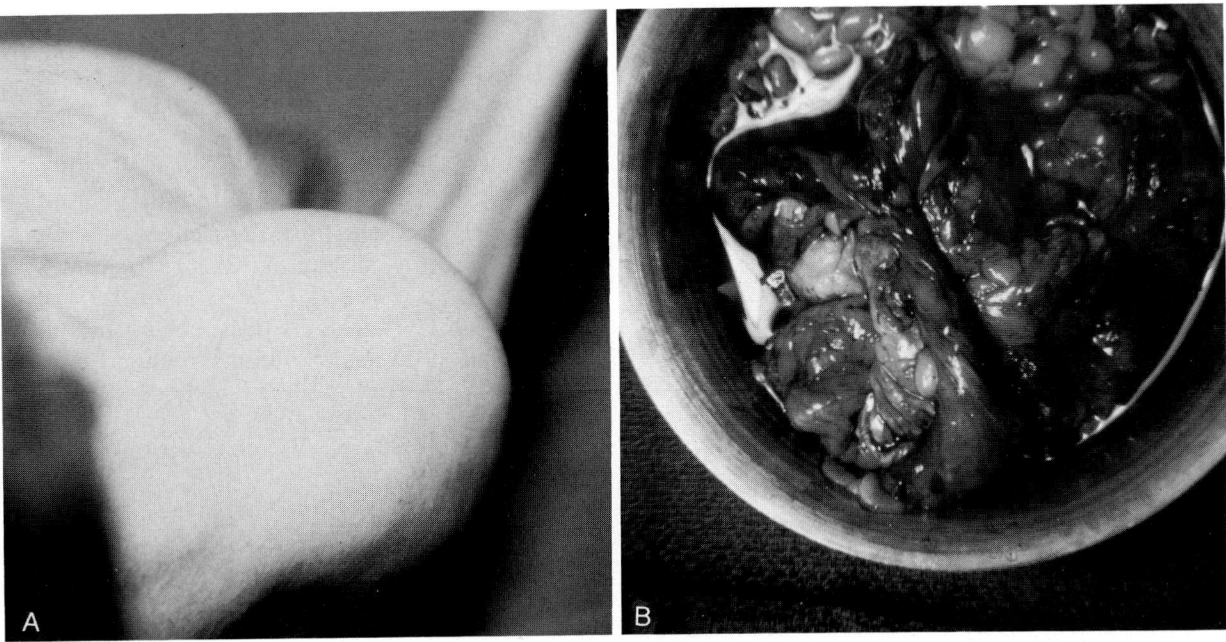

Figure 3–53A and B. Bursal type of rheumatoid shoulder treated by bursectomy, excision of the distal clavicle, and limited synovectomy. There was little glenohumeral joint involvement.

an adverse effect on healing. Third, injections have usually been given, and they may introduce microorganisms into the joint that may be present at the time of arthroplasty. Of the 776 shoulder arthroplasties described in Table 3–1, there were only two post-operative infections. One of these occurred in a rheumatoid patient whose culture at the time of the arthroplasty grew Staphylococcus aureus. The staphylococci in this case had been introduced by a prior injection, as discussed on page 262.

Antibiotics should be continued post-operatively until the final reports of the cultures taken at surgery have been received. Skin sutures are left in place until good healing of the skin edges has occurred, which may require three weeks in those who have been on corticosteroids.

Special General Precautions. Pre-operative cervical spine films are of special importance, with special attention to the C1–C2 relationships (Fig. 3–52). Juvenile rheumatoid arthritis patients and those with very long-standing disease often have small bones that require pre-operative study of the dimensions of the bones to make sure that the available components can be used. Plain x-ray films with a simple metallic marker of known length placed at the level of the bone show the diameter of the medullary canal. Many patients undergoing shoulder arthroplasties have been taking steroids and have suppression of the adrenal cortex. The usual supportive adrenal cortical extract is required as in other major surgical procedures.

Detachment of Subscapularis and Capsule Together. The glenohumeral ligaments and capsule in rheumatoid shoulder are usually frail and are inadequate to hold sutures. The subscapularis tendon is also thin and weak. When opening the joint, rather than separating the subscapularis tendon and capsule and dividing them at different levels, as is done in almost all other approaches (see Figs. 3–25 and 3–30), it is better to divide them together near the lesser tuberosity so that they will reinforce each other for holding sutures. Fortunately, these weakened anterior structures can easily be stretched out, and in most rheumatoid shoulders they are easily stretched out to obtain good external rotation and no lengthening of the subscapularis tendon is required.

Avoidance of Intraoperative Fractures. The osteopenic bones fracture easily. The shaft may be fractured during forced external rotation to expose the head. The greater tuberosity and upper humerus are often broken by the retractors holding the humerus posterior to the glenoid during implantation of the glenoid component. The glenoid wall is easily broken by levering retractors against it while implanting the glenoid component. If the greater tuberosity is broken and is displaced, just prior to cementing the humeral component, the greater tuberosity should be re-attached to the shaft with No. 2 nonabsorbable sutures and held in contact with the cement when the humeral component is in place. This, along with the closure of the rotator interval and subscapularis, secures the fractured tuberosity, allowing the normal post-operative exercise regimen without interruption.

Fractures of the shaft of the humerus are most apt to occur during the approach when the head is being dislocated anteriorly (see Fig. 3–25), and this complication can be avoided by levering the head forward with an elevator rather than by applying too much twisting force. The fracture is usually a spiral near the midshaft, and the periosteum is largely intact. This type of fracture may interfere with the post-operative exercise program and allow cement to leak out into the soft tissue, causing damage to the radial nerve. These potential problems can be avoided by introducing an intramedullary rod secured with cement at the time of implanting the humeral component (Fig. 3–54) or, if available, a long-stem humeral component to secure the fracture so that passive exercises can be given immediately after the arthroplasty. To avoid leakage of the cement into the soft tissue, it is important to expose the fracture, even if it requires lengthening the deltopectoral approach, and to hold the fracture firmly reduced while the intramedullary rod or long-stem component is being inserted. The fracture line is inspected, and any cement that has extruded is removed.

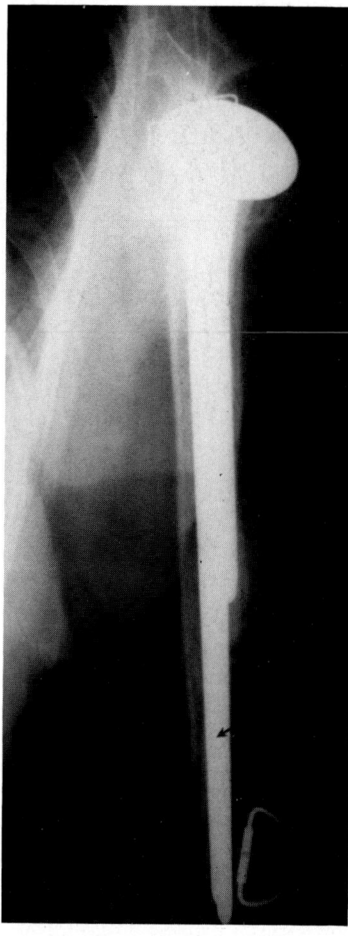

Figure 3–54. Intraoperative spiral fracture of the middle one-third of the shaft of the humerus was treated satisfactorily by incorporating two permanent intramedullary rods (arrow) secured with the cement of the humeral component.

Fractures and perforations of the glenoid are discussed below with glenoid deficiencies due to granulation erosion and are shown in Figure 3–49C.

Rotator Cuff Defects. Despite the reputation that has been created by long-standing, neglected rheumatoid shoulders, if the arthroplasty is done according to the indications discussed above, the rotator cuff is usually intact or can easily be repaired. Even long-standing rotator cuff lesions in rheumatoid shoulders can be repaired more easily than impingement tears because the articular surfaces have been destroyed and the humerus is centralized further medially under the rotator cuff because of the loss of bone.

Small tears are closed with nonabsorbable sutures when first seen, and the operation continues normally thereafter. Large tears (see Fig. 3–49E and F) are repaired after the humeral head has been excised and the glenoid component implanted but before final anchorage of the humeral component. The rotator cuff can easily be mobilized at this time, and holes can be made in the greater tuberosity nonabsorbable 0 sutures, which are inserted prior to cementing the humeral component (see Fig. 3–77). Anterior acromioplasty, such as is performed routinely for outlet impingement tears (see Chapter 2) is rarely done in rheumatoid arthritis because the components hold the greater tuberosity and rotator cuff away from the acromion, eliminating impingement. In rheumatoids, if a bony prominence on the acromion necessitates an acromioplasty, the coracoacromial ligament is reattached to the acromion (see p. 50).

Unpredictable Granulation Erosion. Erosion of the humerus and glenoid by panus and granulation tissue can occur. Surprisingly large areas of bone loss can occur that are not seen in plain x-ray films. Subchondral cysts and fibrous nodules are common. Marginal erosion may cause the proximal humerus to be pointed like a pencil. At other times, the head and glenoid are matched with areas of sclerosis mixed with areas of osteopenic bone, making it easy to produce a fracture when preparing the articular surfaces to receive the components. The cortices of the humerus as well as that of the glenoid are easily perforated. Perforations of the glenoid are very common, and when this happens, cancellous bone or a cement restricter is introduced into the holes prior to cementing the component. Some of the steps described for dealing with a deficient glenoid (see Fig. 3–28) may apply, but because the pattern of destruction in rheumatoid arthritis is unpredictable, no recipe applicable to all cases can be established, and when the bone loss is too great, it is more sensible to use a humeral component without a glenoid component.

Slow Recovery. Rheumatoid muscles are slow to gain strength but in most cases can be brought back to "excellent" function (see Table 3–7). A slower recovery should be anticipated, and during this time the surgeon should maintain good rapport with the internist and therapist and encourage the patient.

Earlier passive motion (see Fig. 7–7) has been a very significant advance for rheumatoid shoulders. An abduction brace is almost never necessary. A passive motion machine, which has the additional disadvantage of stressing the rheumatoid elbow, is avoided. A friend or member of the family can be taught how to perform the assistive exercises and can work with the patient after he or she goes home.

Patients with long-standing rheumatoid arthritis with loss of bone and loss of the rotator cuff may need "limited goals" post-operative rehabilitation, as discussed in Chapter 7, page 530.

If the patient's discomfort had been largely in the shoulder and pain is eliminated by the arthroplasty, it is often possible to stop corticosteroids, immunosuppressants, and other major drugs.

Result to Be Expected. Although progress may be slower, if the indications for arthroplasty outlined above are followed, the final results of most arthroplasties performed on rheumatoid shoulders are "excellent" (Fig. 3–55). Those with long-standing, advanced disease who require "limited goals rehabilitation" are grateful for the relief of pain and the ability to sufficiently rotate their shoulders internally and externally for self-care, sleep, and independent living.

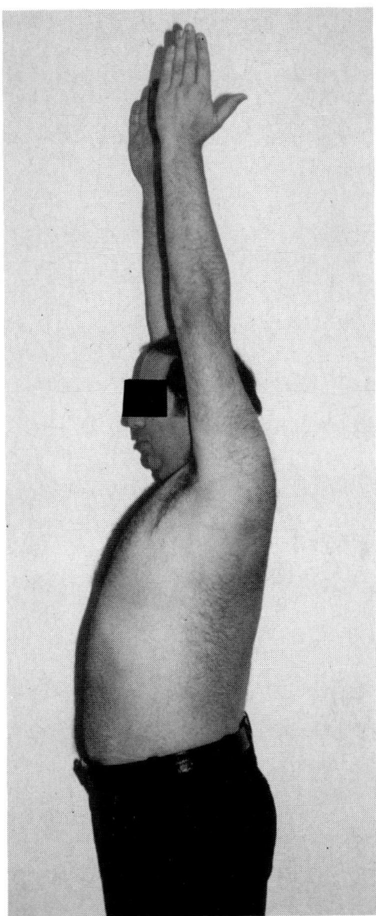

Figure 3–55. Following arthroplasty rheumatoid muscles are slow to gain strength, but most can be brought back to "excellent" function. Even years later, patients may have fleeting soft-tissue pain when their arthritis flares. They are advised to do occasional stretching exercises permanently to ensure keeping the range of motion, although they do not often lose motion once it is established.

A Rheumatoid Syndrome

A "syndrome" consisting of mild rheumatoid arthritis that is confined almost entirely to the shoulders, spares other joints, and is seen almost exclusively in women between 35 and 55 years of age, has been recognized.[21, 54] The diagnosis of rheumatoid arthritis was confirmed by a rheumatologist in all of my patients, and serologic test results were positive for the rheumatoid factor in each case. X-rays showed loss of the glenohumeral joint space, and both shoulders were usually involved with progressive cystic and sclerotic changes. Deterioration of the joint surfaces was usually observed to occur over a period of two or three years (Fig. 3–56).

The diagnosis can be difficult in the earlier stages but is confirmed by the positive serologic test results and eventual x-ray changes. As in the shoulders of patients with polyarthritis, mild shoulder involvement may occur that is responsive to nonoperative treatment and never requires an arthroplasty. However, seven of my patients with this syndrome of involvement confined to the shoulders had developed such extreme pain and disability that arthroplasties were indicated. They were ideal candidates for nonconstrained total shoulder arthroplasty and experienced results similar to those of patients with osteoarthritis.

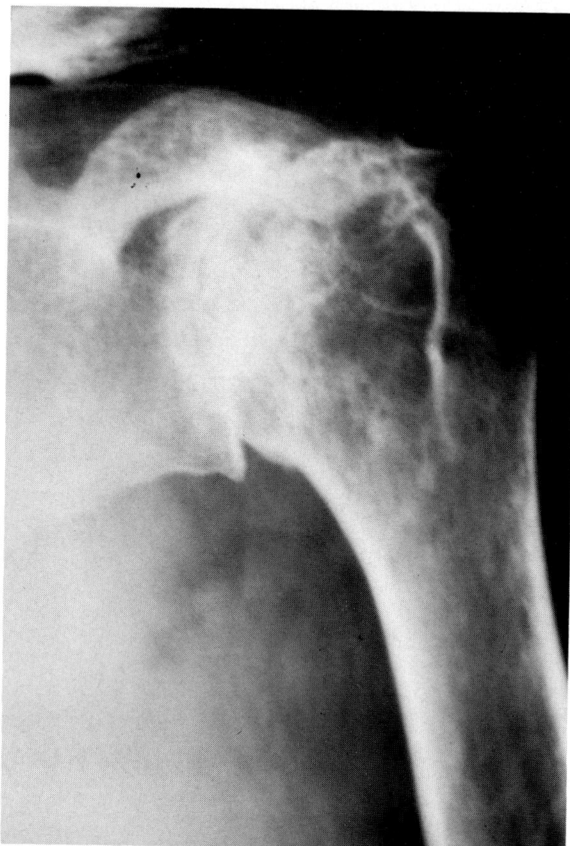

Figure 3–56. ***Rheumatoid Syndrome.*** There is a clinical syndrome of low-grade, atypical rheumatoid arthritis that occurs most often in women between 35 and 55 years of age, involves the shoulders almost exclusively, and spares other joints. Because of its slow progress, it is hard to diagnose in the early stages. Eventually, when roentgen changes occur and the serology is positive, the diagnosis can be made. The x-ray shown is of a 50 year old woman who developed these changes over a period of four years.

Related Conditions

"Psoriatic arthritis," "lupus arthritis," "inflammatory osteoarthritis," and "mixed arthritis" may or may not be related to low-grade rheumatoid arthritis. However, from a practical point of view, patients with these diagnoses usually have more trouble with the post-operative exercise program than those with straightforward osteoarthritis or steroid-induced avascular necrosis.

OLD TRAUMA

Anatomical Problem

Arthroplasties on old fractures and old fracture-dislocations are difficult because of retracted tuberosities, malunion and nonunion, loss of bone, shortening of the shaft (which weakens the deltoid muscle), and nerve injuries (Figs. 3–57 through 3–60). Further, these shoulders have often had previous surgery, which introduces the further problems of damage to the deltoid muscle and increased risk of infection.

Of the 157 shoulders in this category listed in Table 3–1, all had been initially treated in other hospitals and all had sustained the injuries more than six months prior to our shoulder arthroplasty. The interval from injury to operation ranged from seven months to 15 years and averaged two years. Recent fracture-dislocations are considered in Chapter 5.

The average age of the patients at the time of surgery was 56 years, ranging from 16 to 92 years. Pain and disability were characteristically intense. Some patients with seizure disorders had bilateral fracture-dislocations. Those with gunshot wounds had associated fractures of the acromion and deltoid muscle damage.

An axillary nerve palsy was present in 14 shoulders, and other infraclavicular plexus injuries existed in 20. Lateral or radical acromionectomy with severe damage to the deltoid muscle had been performed in six shoulders. The majority had had more than one previous surgical operation.

Nonunions of the surgical neck of the humerus with intact tuberosities and cuff were treated by bone grafting rather than replacement arthroplasty, and they will be considered separately (see Figs. 3–64 to 3–71). When this nonunion was associated with damage from the injury or softening and collapse from disuse and poor nutrition, a replacement arthroplasty was performed, as discussed further on page 232.

Treatment

Indications for Arthroplasty in Old Trauma. The decision to perform an arthroplasty in patients with old trauma cannot be made solely on the appearance of the x-rays. An attempt to ameliorate the discomfort with exercises and nonaddicting medications is routine. This also gives the surgeon an opportunity to evaluate the motivation and ability of the patient to cooperate with a post-operative exercise program. Some patients with old trauma have uncontrollable alcoholism, which in extreme cases can be a contraindication to an arthroplasty. If there have been severe muscle damage and loss of bone, the patient must accept a realistic goal but at the same time be willing to work for the best possible recovery. Indications for the arthroplasty are persistent pain and disability

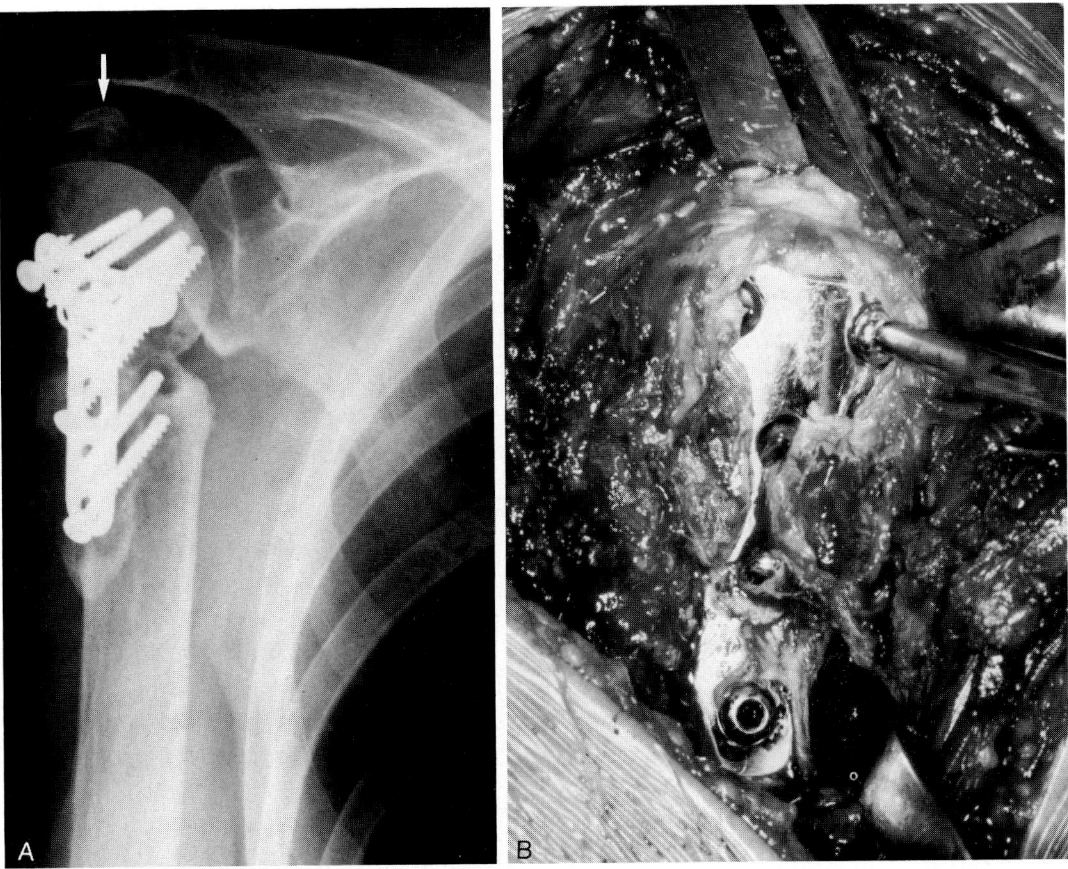

Figure 3–57A and B. ***Glenohumeral Arthroplasty for Old Trauma***
Arthroplasties on old fractures are difficult because of retracted tuberosities (arrow in A), malunion, nonunion, loss of bone, shortening, nerve injuries, and a greater risk of infection.

in a healthy, well-motivated patient who has not been helped by conservative treatment.

Special Steps in Arthroplasties for Old Trauma

Pre-operative Planning. If the history or the routine blood count and sedimentation rate suggest the possibility of an infection, the joint is aspirated and cultures are taken before an arthroplasty is recommended. One of the two infections in the series described in Table 3–1 occurred in a patient with old trauma who had had an aspiration and culture four days before the arthroplasty. The preliminary report of the laboratory on the morning of the arthroplasty showed negative culture results; however, two days later the report was changed to "a few *Staphylococcus aureus*." The cultures made during the arthroplasty grew *S. aureus*, and postoperatively an infection developed with this organism that required removal of the implant.

Prior to an arthroplasty on shoulders with old trauma and previous surgery, the pathologist is routinely alerted to the possible need for a frozen section. If an abscess or granulation tissue suggesting an infection is encountered during the arthroplasty, a frozen section analysis is obtained. The presence of many white cells and evidence of inflammation in the frozen section have been very reliable indexes to the need to discontinue the arthroplasty.

Roentgen studies should include the routine trauma series of anterior-posterior and lateral films in the scapular plane and the Velpeau axillary view (see Fig. 1–12B) to locate the four major segments of proximal humeral fractures. CT scans, when indicated, help to evaluate the articular surface of the glenoid.

The length of the arm should be measured and compared to that of the opposite side (see Fig. 3–58B). This measurement can be indicative of delayed recovery time for the deltoid muscle and may be an index to the likelihood of recovering overhead use (see Fig. 3–26D).

Draping for Access Posteriorly. Although the usual extended deltopectoral approach is generally

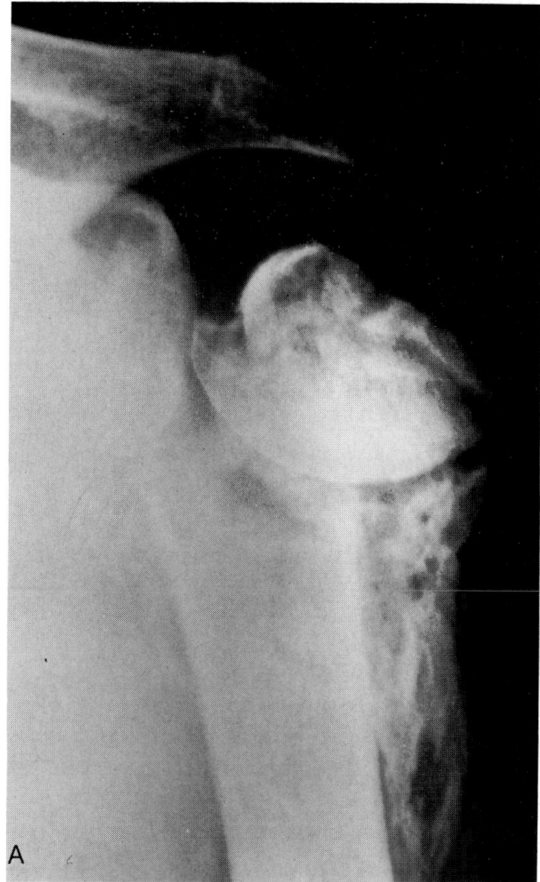

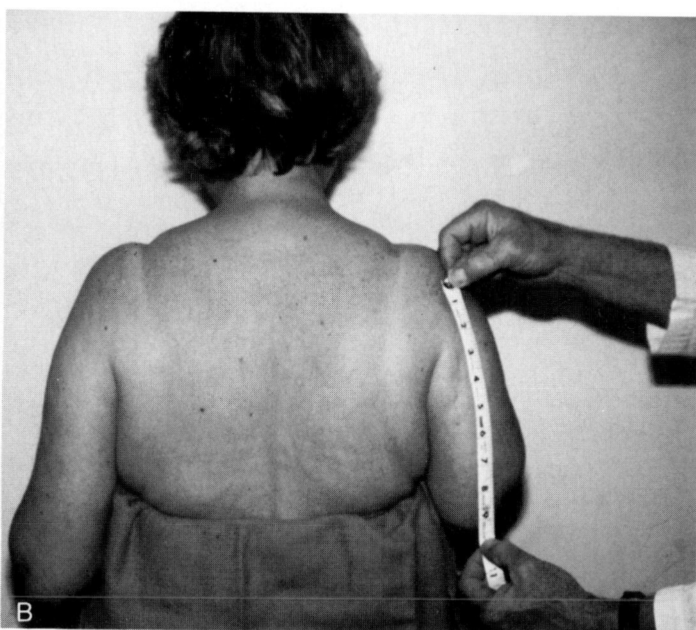

Figure 3–58A and B. ***Glenohumeral Arthroplasty for Old Trauma.*** Shortening makes the deltoid muscle too long to raise the arm and leads to dislocation of the implant (see Fig. 3–26). Tension on the myofascial sleeve must be regained by restoring length of the shaft as far as possible.

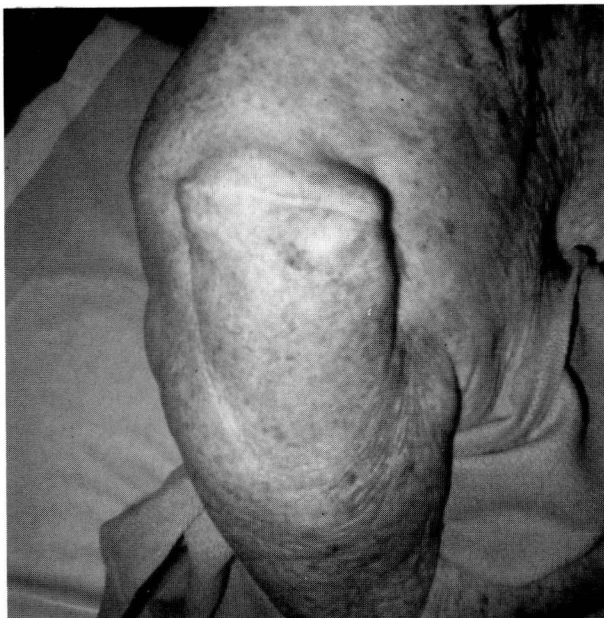

Figure 3–59. ***Glenohumeral Arthroplasty for Old Trauma.*** Damage to the deltoid muscle from injuries or prior surgery is a formidable problem. Function gained following deltoidplasties (see Fig. 3–33) has been disappointing.

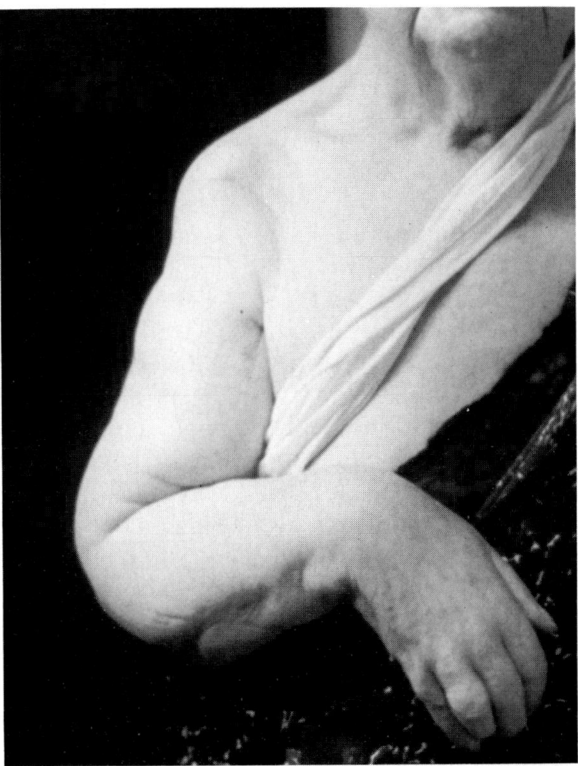

Figure 3–60. ***Glenohumeral Arthroplasty for Old Trauma.*** Old nerve injuries can be overwhelming, as shown in this patient who was seen two years after a failed open reduction of a four part fracture-dislocation. There is axillary and radial nerve palsy with stiffening of the fingers, wrist, elbow, and shoulder. It would have been of great help if the pliancy of the hand and elbow had been maintained with exercises.

adequate, if there is a retracted greater tuberosity, it may be impossible to mobilize it adequately from an anterior approach, and a second, posterior approach may be necessary to mobilize the infraspinatus tendon and the adherent tuberosity.

Use of Previous Skin Incision. Rather than making a new skin incision, excising and modifying a previous incision makes a better scar and usually can be accomplished without interfering with the exposure.

Early Detachment of Pectoralis Major in Anterior Approaches. The usual extended deltopectoral approach is made (see Fig. 3–25); however, it is helpful in patients with old trauma to detach the pectoralis major insertions on the humerus to mobilize the shaft. This is especially important if there is an old anterior or old posterior dislocation. The tendons are tagged with stay sutures and are re-attached during closure.

Osteopenia and Malunion of the Shaft. The upper part of the humerus may be malunited, interfering with introduction of the humeral component and requiring special drilling or reaming or the use of a short-stem component.

Osteopenia of the surgical neck and shaft may be severe, and twisting forces are avoided during the arthroplasty for fear of fractures.

Lesser Tuberosity Osteotomy. To enter the glenohumeral joint the lesser tuberosity is osteotomized and mobilized with the attached subscapularis tendon (Fig. 3–61, center). This facilitates mobilizing the subscapularis so that external rotation can be re-established. Later, when repairing the rotator tendons, the lesser tuberosity can be partially or completely excised to allow re-attachment of the subscapularis to the supraspinatus when it cannot be mobilized out to the proper length. Releasing the capsule beneath the subscapularis and dividing the coracohumeral ligament are important in mobilizing this structure.

Compensating for Malunion of the Greater Tuberosity. The greater tuberosity may have been displaced medially and posteriorly by the infraspinatus and teres minor, and when the supraspinatus remains attached, the greater tuberosity may also be displaced superiorly.[140] The displaced tuberosity often becomes adherent to the articular surface of the humerus, damaging the surface, blocking external rotation by impinging on the glenoid, and interfering with implantation of the humeral component in proper retroversion (Figs. 3–61 to 3–63). When the greater tuberosity is only moderately displaced, it should be possible to remove enough bone from the deep surface of the greater tuberosity to allow implantation of the humeral component and still maintain continuity of the tuberosity and rotator cuff to the shaft (Fig. 3–61). If so, the postoperative exercise program is greatly simplified and can be advanced rapidly.

With more severe displacement (Fig. 3–62), it is impossible to insert the humeral component in the medullary canal without osteotomizing and relocating the greater tuberosity. If the tuberosity is malunited, it must be osteotomized. If ununited it must be mobilized, which can be difficult. If mobilization is done, it is important to make the greater tuberosity fragment large enough so that firm fixation can be obtained with the shaft for bone union.

In some cases of borderline displacement, it is possible to place a small-stem humeral component with a short head in a varus position to avoid osteotomizing the greater tuberosity. This also eliminates the need to delay active exercises until the greater tuberosity unites.

Restoration of Length. In orienting the humeral component the length of the shaft of the humerus must be restored to create functional tension on the deltoid muscle and ensure stability of the components (see Fig. 3–26). This may entail a bone graft, as mentioned previously under Preoperative Planning.

Glenoid Component in Old Trauma. Because fractures and fracture-dislocations of the proximal humerus usually spare the articular surface of the glenoid, it may be possible to use a humeral component alone without a glenoid component if the articular surface of the glenoid is in good condition. A glenoid component is rarely used when the injury is less than six months old. The articular surface of the glenoid may remain adequate for a year or more.

Other factors in the decision are the condition of the deltoid and rotator cuff and the age of the patient. Theoretically, the slight constraint provided by the better conformity of the glenoid component offers a more stable fulcrum for the rehabilitation of weakened and damaged muscles. Therefore, a glenoid component may be selected in the hope of improving the function of damaged muscles. Regarding the age of the patient, because at this time the length of follow-up for glenoid components is limited to 15 years, there is a disinclination to use it in younger patients who have a reasonable glenoid and good muscles.

As shown in Table 3–1, a glenoid component was used in 118 of the 155 shoulders with old

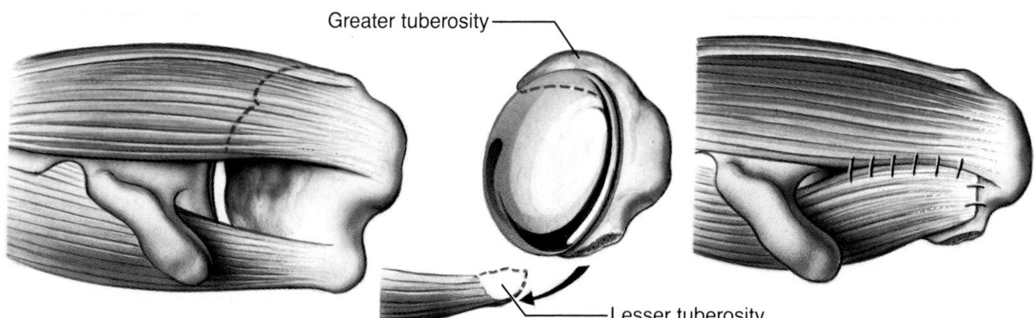

Figure 3–61. ***Glenohumeral Arthropolasty for Old Trauma.*** Sufficient retroversion for the humeral component must be regained when there is incongruity of the head and a moderately displaced malunion of the greater tuberosity.

Left, The malunion, with some retraction of the greater tuberosity, covers part of the head and blocks the insertion of the humeral component other than in anteversion. There is spreading of the rotator cuff near the rotator interval.

Center, In this approach the surgeon osteotomizes the lesser tuberosity to enter the joint. After removal of the head, a portion of the malunited greater tuberosity is excised from the inside the joint, leaving the insertion of the infraspinatus muscle intact as much as possible.

Right, If this permits implanting the humeral component in neutral version or slight retroversion it is possible to avoid osteotomizing the greater tuberosity and keep the infraspinatus intact. Most or all of the lesser tuberosity is excised, and the subscapularis and soft tissue anteriorly are freed to permit as much external rotation as possible (see Fig. 3–30), and if necessary the sternal head of the pectoralis major (which has been released) is used to supplement the shortened subscapularis to permit external rotation (see Fig. 3–32).

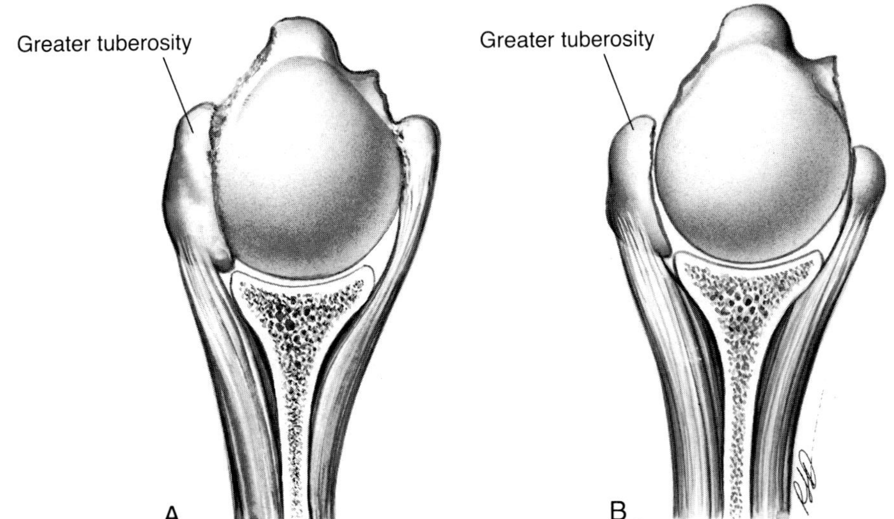

Figure 3–62. ***Glenohumeral Arthroplasty for Old Trauma.*** With marked retraction of the greater tuberosity, there is impingement on the glenoid (preventing external rotation) and on the acromion (preventing elevation), and the humeral component cannot be inserted until the tuberosity is mobilized (A) when there is a malunion, by osteotomy of the tuberosity, or (B) when there is a nonunion. In the latter case, the greater tuberosity must be mobilized and re-attached later in proper position (which can be very difficult).

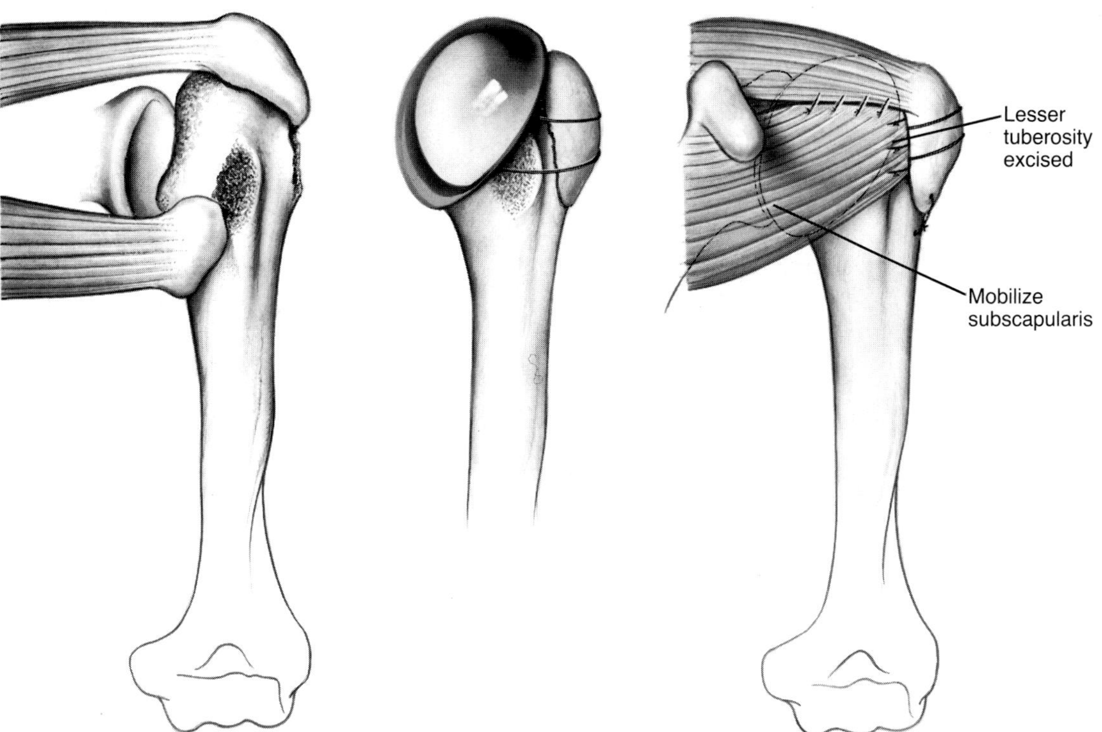

Figure 3–63. ***Glenohumeral Arthroplasty for Old Trauma.*** Re-attachment of a mobilized greater tuberosity with excision of the lesser tuberosity and mobilization of the subscapularis tendon (see Fig. 3–30), and, if necessary, transfer of the sternal head of the pectoralis major (see Fig. 3–30).

trauma (trauma of more than three months' duration) in that series. Of the 36 patients who were treated with a humeral component alone, the majority were under 40 years of age.

Freeing the Rotator Cuff and Tuberosities (Possible Anterior Acromioplasty). The surfaces of the rotator cuff and tuberosities are adherent to the acromion, acromioclavicular joint, and bursa, and the deep side of the tendons are attached to contracted joint capsule. The tuberosities must be mobilized for motion, and the rotator cuff must be mobilized for a "pull" for strength. Freeing the superficial surface of these structures may entail an anterior acromioplasty when the injury is old and the greater tuberosity has been in contact with the acromion for a long time. The coracoacromial ligament is excised to expose the superficial surface of the supraspinatus. The contracted coracohumeral ligament is divided, and adherent tissue is released from the base of the coracoid. After opening the joint the joint capsule is divided to gain length for the rotator tendons.

Closing the "Pouch" and Altering Version. When the humeral head has been dislocated for a long time, either anteriorly or posteriorly, the detached capsule forms a fibrous pouch around the head. If the head is reduced, the pouch remains as an empty space into which a new dislocation can easily occur. When the dislocation has been present for a long time, the muscles re-align themselves around the humerus in the position of dislocation and tend to cause re-dislocation. These problems can be corrected by a prosthetic head placed in the reduced and properly aligned position and careful post-operative rehabilitation.

Regarding the orientation of the humeral prosthesis, a length of head should be selected that produces tension on the pouch. If the trial component tends to re-dislocate, it is possible to eliminate some of the redundancy of the pouch by sewing a freshened surface against the edge of the glenoid with nonabsorbable sutures. This can be done from inside the joint prior to the final insertion of the humeral component; however, this is rarely necessary.

In addition to selection of the proper length of head to place tension on the pouch, the version of the humeral component can be altered to offset the tendency to dislocate. If the long-standing dislocation has been anterior, the humeral component is placed in more retroversion than normal. If the dislocation has been posterior, the humeral component is placed in less retroversion.

One must also remember the importance of maintaining tension on the myofascial sleeve and the length of the arm in stabilizing the components. If the humeral component is set too low and this tension is lost, the prosthesis will tend to dislocate regardless of the version.

If instability persists after carrying out these steps, a spica cast may be required during the immediate post-operative period.

Deltoidplasty. The injury and previous surgery have often inflicted muscle loss and nerve injury to the deltoid muscle. It may be possible to compensate for these injuries by one of the steps outlined in Figure 3–32.

Individualizing the Exercise Program. Following an arthroplasty for old trauma, the scar tissue that has been released can quickly become re-attached, and adhesions blocking motion may form within a few days. Furthermore, the muscles have been weakened by injury and disuse. Early passive motion (EPM) (see Fig. 7–7) has been especially helpful in maintaining motion in this group. The arm is raised by the surgeon and therapist by the second day after surgery provided that stability of the components permits.

Recovery from nerve injuries is followed with electromyograms. I have a distinct impression that electrical stimulation is beneficial in regaining function when the deltoid muscle has been paralyzed.

Precautions should be discussed with the therapist in positioning the shoulder during exercises following arthroplasties on old trauma, especially when there has been an old dislocation. If the shoulder had been dislocated posteriorly, forward flexion and horizontal adduction are avoided during the first six weeks to allow repaired tissue to obliterate the pouch. The arm may be elevated in the scapular plane, but care is taken to avoid stressing the posterior capsule. If there has been an anterior dislocation, external rotation beyond 40 degrees and abduction are avoided during the first six weeks. Again, the arm may be raised in the scapular plane, taking care to avoid stress on the anterior capsule.

Patients with old injuries may make gains in motion and strength for many months after the arthroplasty. It is very advantageous to have discussed this point with the patient pre-operatively so that he or she will anticipate the slow speed of recovery. Patients who are forewarned are able to go further without discouragement.

For those who have too much loss of bone and loss of muscles, the "limited goals" rehabilitation program is followed (see Chapter 7, p. 530).

Result to Be Expected. Functional results vary from excellent to "limited goals," depending on the quality of the muscles. The overall results of patients with old trauma are definitely inferior to the results currently being obtained in patients with recent four-part fractures and fracture-dislocations who are treated initially with humeral head replacement and reconstruction of the tuberosities and cuff (see Chapter 5, p. 396 and Fig. 5–25).

Nonunion of the Surgical Neck

Nonunion of the surgical neck rapidly becomes a true pseudarthrosis rather than a fibrous union with a cavity that communicates to the glenohumeral joint. The tuberosities remain attached to the head, giving it a blood supply (Figs. 3–64 and 3–65).

Textbooks on fractures have implied that healing always occurs in proximal humeral fractures because these fractures occur through cancellous bone. However, in fractures at the surgical neck level, the distal fragment is cortical bone. Nonunions at this level are not rare. I reported 50 examples and described the pathology to the American Orthopaedic Association in 1983.[114] I briefly discussed treatment in Rockwood and Green's *Textbook on Fractures*.[71, 73]

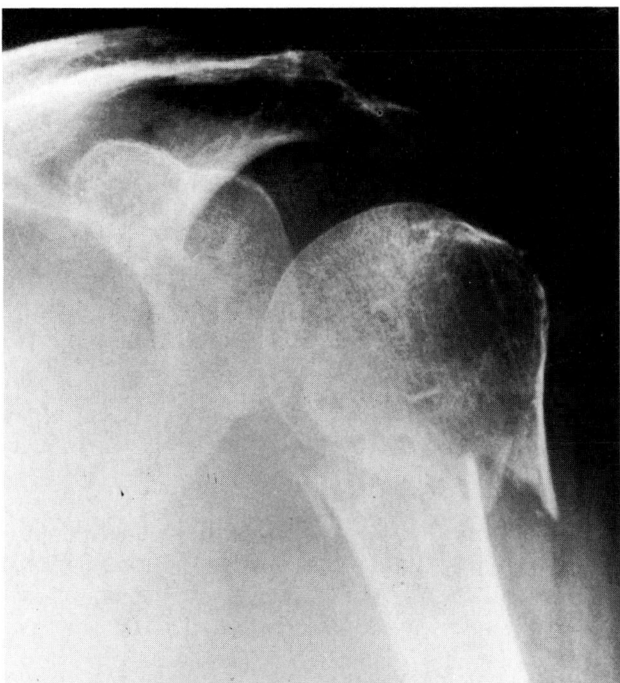

Figure 3–64. ***Nonunion of the Surgical Neck.*** Pathology. The original fracture usually looks harmless. Distraction or inadequate immobilization can lead to a nonunion that can be very disabling and difficult to treat.

This lesion is important clinically not only because it can occur unexpectedly but also because treatment is unexpectedly difficult.

Etiological Factors

This type of nonunion may occur when a patient is started on simple pendulum exercises before there has been enough impaction of the fragments or healing for the head and shaft to move in unison. Other factors include interposition of the deltoid muscle or long head of the biceps, and distraction caused by overhead traction or a hanging cast. Inadequate immobilization is important in the etiology, as exemplified by alcoholic patients and those with multiple injuries.

Anatomical Factors Making Treatment Difficult

1. *Muscle forces.* In addition to the distraction caused by gravity, forces acting against bone union include the pull of the powerful pectoralis major, which displaces the shaft anteriorly and medially while the rotator cuff rotates the proximal fragment (Fig. 3–65). The proximal fragment is rotated by the rotator cuff, but the shaft does not move with it (Fig. 3–66).

2. *Softening of the head.* Because of the vascularity of the shoulder, softening of the proximal fragment occurs unusually rapidly. This precludes the use of screws and pins for fixation.

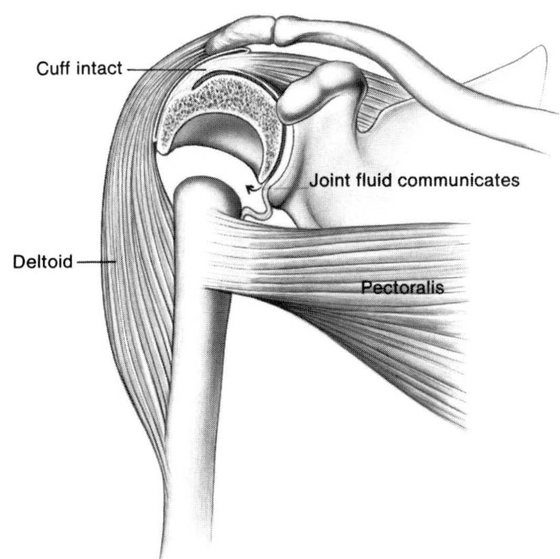

Figure 3–65. ***Nonunion of the Surgical Neck.*** The pathology is shown with the muscle forces. Joint fluid communicates with the nonunion, and the distraction of gravity and muscle pulls interferes with healing.

3. *"Cavitation" of the head.* Resorption of bone at the nonunion site reduces the size of the proximal fragment. The impact of the shaft against the head often leads to a hollowing-out or cavitation of the head (Figs. 3–65 and 3–67A). Further loss of the head due to resorption adds to the difficulties of internal fixation with standard methods.

4. *Shortening of the shaft.* Resorption of the shaft of the humerus may weaken the deltoid muscle by rendering it too long (Fig. 3–66) and may cause the head of the humerus to subluxate inferiorly; the head may eventually become fixed in an inferiorly subluxed position. Shortening of the shaft complicates an arthroplasty because there is a tendency to implant the humeral component too low, resulting in inferior subluxation and deltoid weakness.

5. *Pseudarthrosis communicating with the joint.* Characteristically, a fibrous union is soon converted to a space with an enlarging cavity lined by synovial membrane and fibrocartilage with fluid communicating to the glenohumeral joint. The joint fluid acts as a deterrent to bone union.

Thus, the adverse mechanical forces of gravity, the pectoralis major, and the rotator cuff muscles; the difficulty of achieving internal fixation because of the small, soft proximal fragment; and the glenohumeral instability and weakening of the deltoid muscle, which may be caused by shortening of the shaft, all contribute to the difficulty of treatment.

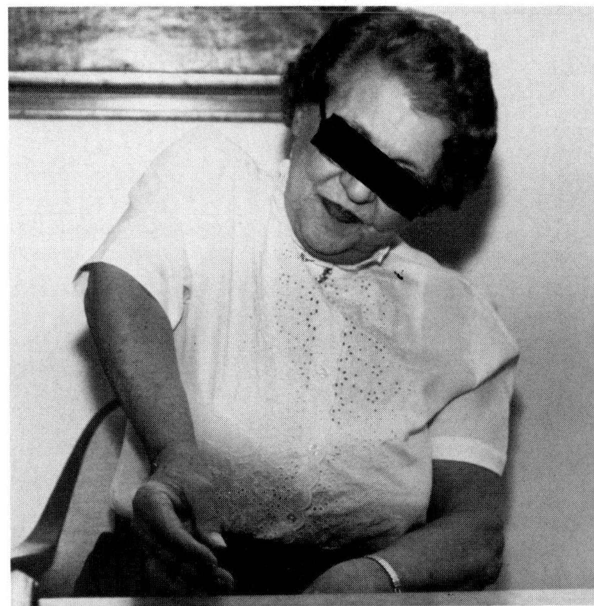

Figure 3–66. ***Nonunion of the Surgical Neck.*** When a true pseudarthrosis tends to form, the shoulder is rendered flail because there are no effective external rotators. The patient usually has pain, a "dropping sign," and inability to raise the arm.

Treatment of Nonunion of the Surgical Neck

The difficulty of repairing these lesions is illustrated by the fact that there were 35 failed attempts at repair in the 50 nonunions of the 1983 series. Anyone attempting to repair this lesion should double the precautions taken and "wear both belt and suspenders."

Conservative treatment has been ineffective. Electrical stimulation had been tried in several of my patients prior to surgery without success, as would have been predicted by the proponents of this method because of the gaping pseudarthrosis and the difficulty of obtaining adequate immobilization against the forces of gravity and the opposing muscles.

In operative treatment, occasionally the bone in the proximal fragment is hard, and one can use an AO T-plate for internal fixation. However, the bone in the proximal fragment is usually too soft, and it is necessary to use some type of cerclage fixation in the form of a "compression band." I use an intramedullary nail and nonabsorbable sutures. Aside from the method of internal fixation, an autogenous iliac bone graft is used, and a spica cast is applied for external support until bridging callus appears. In patients with long-standing nonunions and after failed surgery, the articular surface of the head may have partially resorbed or become soft and collapsed due to atrophy and osteopenia. When this has occurred, especially in older patients, a replacement arthroplasty is performed taking special care to regain the length of the shaft of the humerus and obtain union between the greater tuberosity and the shaft, as discussed below.

Compression Band and Bone Graft. The technique of bone grafting and a "compression band" to prevent distraction and immobilize the bone is illustrated in Figure 3–68. Only four shoulders in the 1983 series had bone hard enough to hold an AO T-plate and screw fixation. The compression band was used in 13 shoulders, of which 12 united by bone.

Pre-operatively, I ask the patient to think of this as a two-operation procedure. The long period of immobilization required to ensure bone union usually results in adhesions and stiffening of the shoulder, which requires a release operation and removal of the internal fixation device as a second procedure. The iliac donor site is also explained to the patient and prepared for the procedure in case it is needed.

The nonunion site is prepared for the bone graft by removing the fibrocartilage and freshening

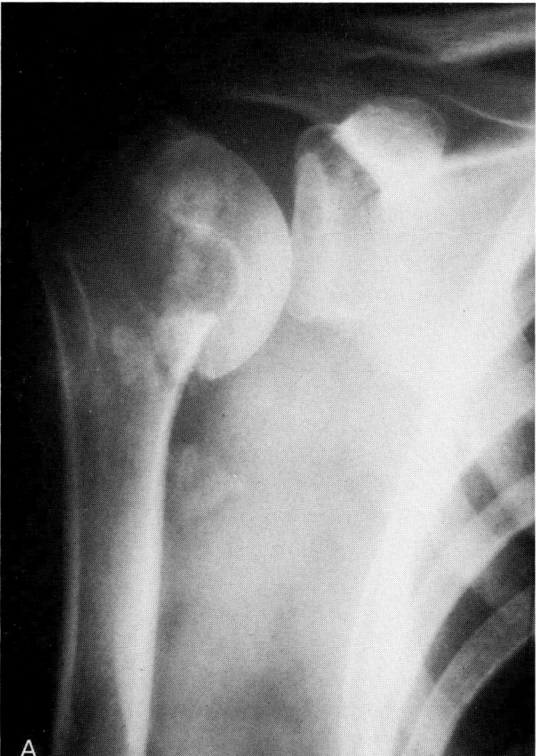

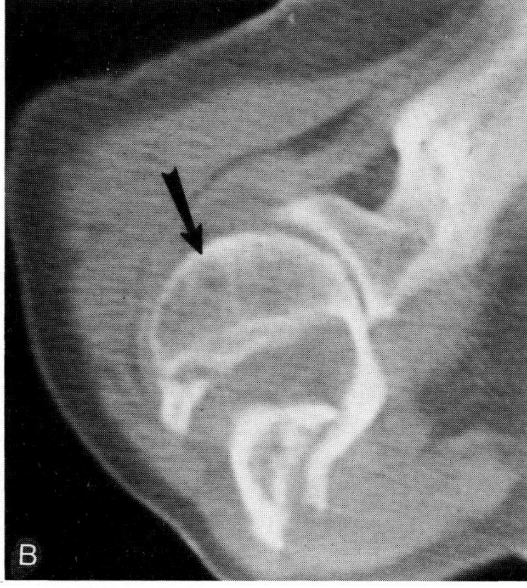

Figure 3–67A and B. ***Nonunion of the Surgical Neck.*** Typical nonunion of the surgical neck following closed treatment with an intact head (arrow). It was treated successfully with compression band and bone grafts and a spica (see Fig. 3–68).

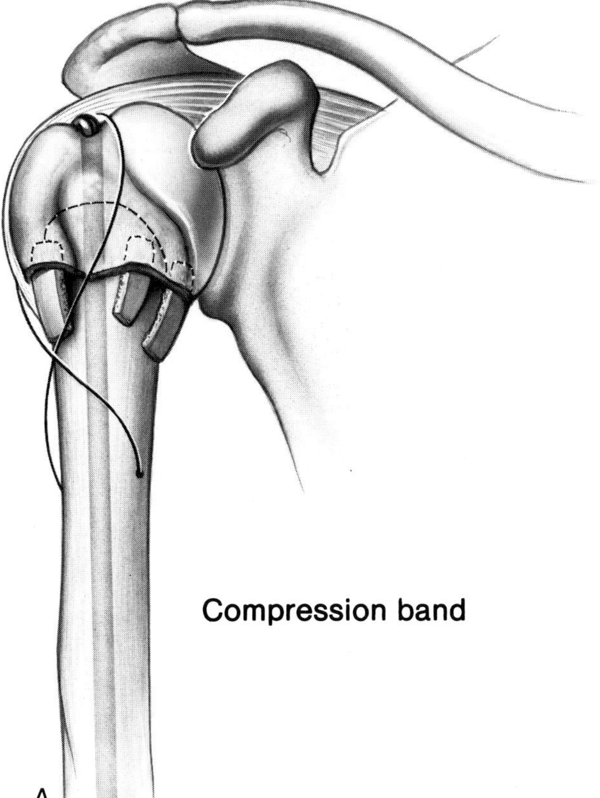

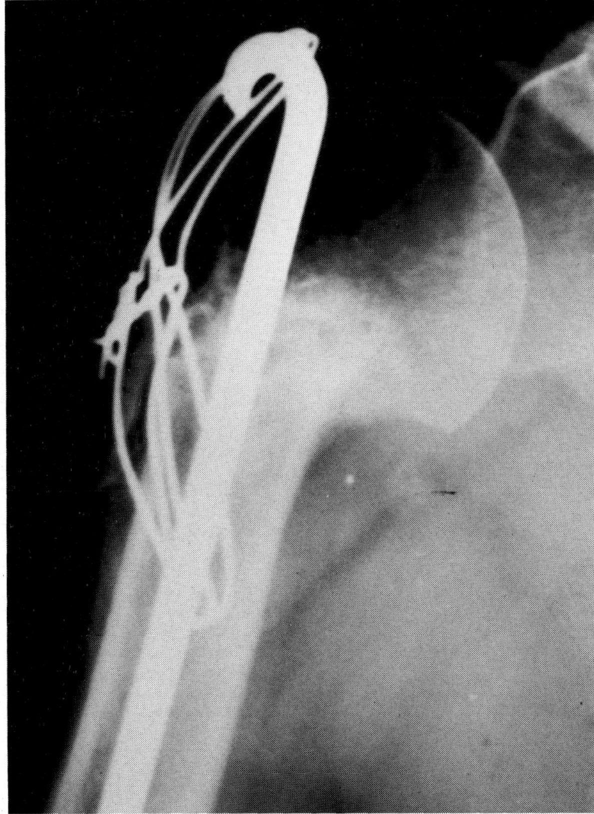

Figure 3–68A and B. ***Nonunion of the Surgical Neck.*** Compression band technique with iliac grafts and a spica cast. The x-ray film shows good healing with this method. The wire in B depicts the technique; however, nonabsorbable sutures are now preferred.

the ends of the fragments, maintaining firm contact between the shaft and the head with the compression band (or AO T-plate), packing cancellous iliac bone adjacent to the ends of the fragments, and applying a spica cast with the arm near the side in neutral rotation. A new, light plastic spica cast is applied prior to discharge from the hospital and is used until x-rays show that union has occurred (usually 14 weeks). After removal of the spica cast, a sling may be worn prior to beginning exercises depending on the firmness of union. Some patients develop enough motion that they do not wish to have a release or the internal fixation device removed. However, if there is marked stiffness or prominence of the intramedullary rod, the upper 10 cm. of the previous site of incision is excised, and after removing the internal fixation device, adhesions are divided around the upper humerus to re-establish passive motion. Because the rotator cuff and bone are intact, early passive motion can be started in two days, and the patient can progress to a self-assistive program very soon.

Replacement Arthroplasty and Nonunion of the Surgical Neck. In cases of long-standing nonunion when the head has resorbed or collapsed, a replacement arthroplasty is considered (Figs. 3–69, 3–70, and 3–71). If this procedure can be accomplished with sufficient fixation of the greater tuberosity to the prosthesis and shaft to permit bone union, early passive motion can be given to avoid adhesions. However, it is more important to establish bone union of the greater tuberosity to the shaft than to preserve motion. If the greater tuberosity fragment is precarious, the arm should be immobilized until union occurs, even though a subsequent release of adhesions may be required to re-establish motion.

The soft and deformed head is removed by performing an osteotomy between the lesser and greater tuberosities. If the long head of the biceps is intact, it is dissected free and retained to be incorporated later in the rotator cuff repair. The attachments of the subscapularis on the lesser tuberosity are retained, as are the attachments of the supraspinatus and external rotators on the greater tuberosity. It is important to keep the fragment of greater tuberosity large so that it will not resorb and will offer as much surface as possible for the bone grafts between it and the shaft. The fragments of head are removed from the tuberosities with a rongeur and are retained for bone grafts. The articular surface of the glenoid is protected in the hope that it will be adequate and a glenoid component will be unnecessary.

The humeral component is cemented in 35 to 40 degrees retroversion with the head opposite the articular surface of the glenoid when traction is applied to the arm. At this level, the humeral component will retain the proper tension on the deltoid and myofascial sleeve (see Fig. 3–26). Al-

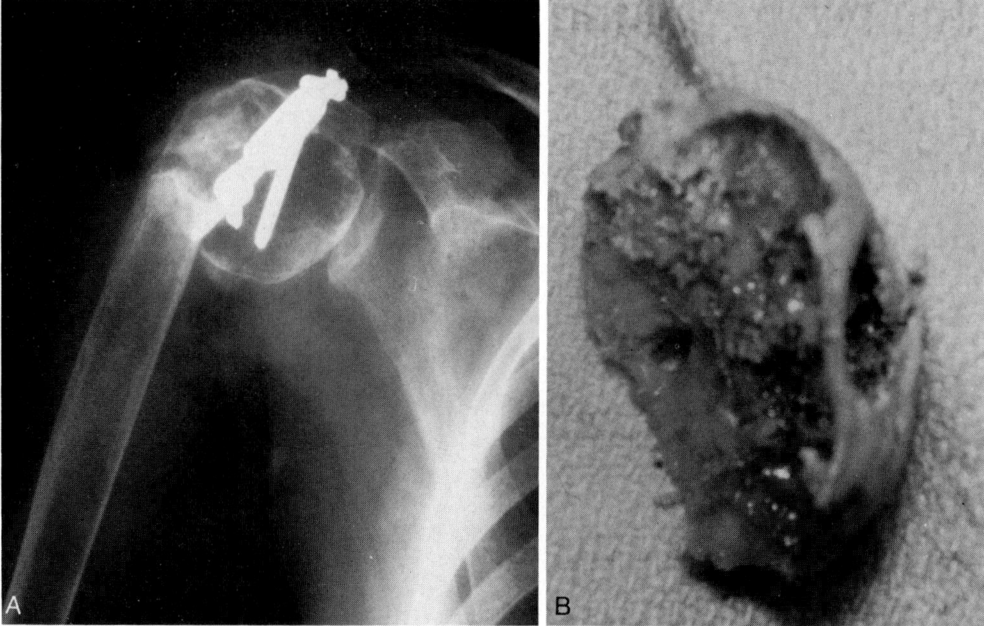

Figure 3–69. ***Nonunion of the Surgical Neck.*** A preoperative film (A) and the head removed (B) of a 55 year old woman who had six failed repairs over an eight-year period. The head was extremely soft. She was treated with a prosthesis and tuberosity-to-shaft graft, as illustrated in Figure 3–70.

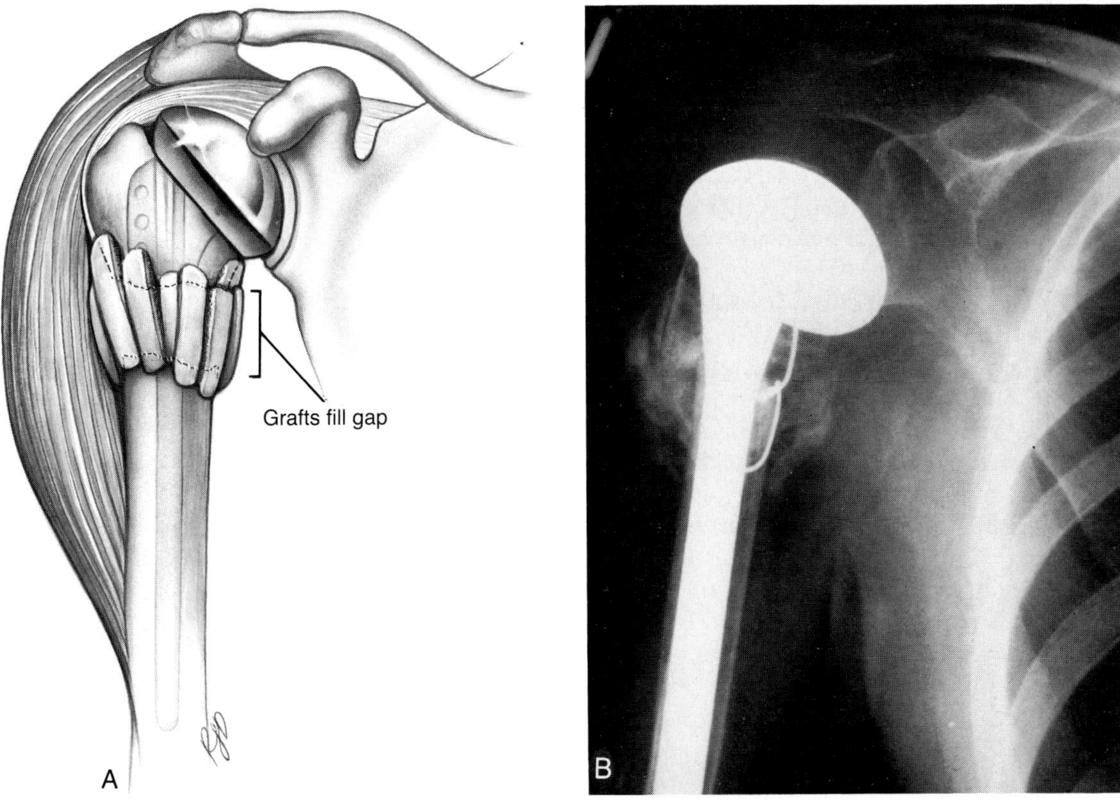

Figure 3–70A and B. ***Nonunion of the Surgical Neck.*** Technique and a successful result of arthroplasty to replace the head and prosthesis-to-tuberosity bone graft. It is important to regain as much length of humerus as possible (Fig. 3–26).

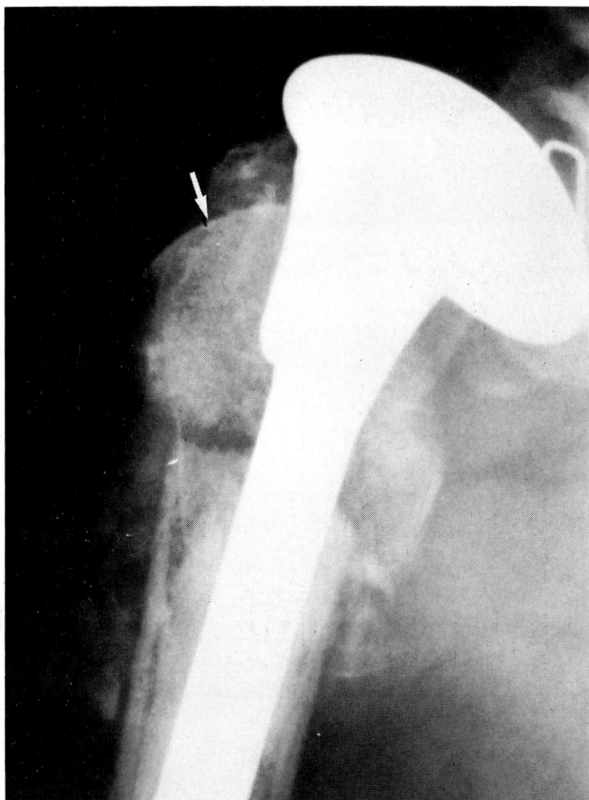

Figure 3–71. ***Nonunion of the Surgical Neck.*** In some cases the humeral head (arrow) may be used as a bone graft to maintain length, especially when the tuberosities have united on the head in three-part or four-part fractures with a nonunion.

though it is important to achieve firm fixation between the greater tuberosity fragment and the prosthesis and to keep that fragment as large as possible, the lesser tuberosity can be excised when necessary to attain adequate length for external rotation. If the lesser tuberosity is excised, it is important to re-attach the subscapularis to the supraspinatus and to make a soft-tissue repair anteriorly for stability.

In regard to bone grafts, the humeral head is often soft and can be indented like a ping pong ball, indicating the loss of subchondral bone and poor quality for bone grafting. However, in some patients who have a large greater tuberosity fragment that is in reasonably good contact with the shaft, the head fragment may be sufficient for the bone grafts with no need to supplement with iliac grafts.

It is important not only to achieve firm fixation between the greater tuberosity and the prosthesis but also to have a freshened bone surface between the greater tuberosity and the shaft if it can be obtained. The rotator tendons must be dissected free prior to re-attaching the tuberosities.

If the articular surface of the glenoid has deteriorated, a glenoid component may be used. This decision is made at surgery.

If secure fixation of the greater tuberosity fragment has been obtained and the grafts are secure, early passive motion can be started, and passive motion can be continued during the four months while union between the tuberosity and shaft is being established. However, if there is any doubt about the quality of the fixation or if the patient is having persistent and unusual pain, I prefer to restrict motion until union of the greater tuberosity and shaft has occurred, even though this may entail a subsequent release of adhesions.

Result to Be Expected. The compression band technique evolved during the course of the 1983 study and was successful in obtaining union in 90 per cent of the patients in whom it was used. However, it should be emphasized that six patients with histories of uncontrollable alcoholism were judged unsuitable for this type of surgery. The patients were carefully selected. Those with the most severe anatomical problems were treated with a prosthesis. Subsequent removal of the internal fixation device and release of adhesions were almost routine in the later cases, and when patients were given early passive motion and an intensive exercise program, their functional results were very good.

Those treated with a prosthesis often had had previous surgery, and the deltoid muscle was weakened not only by shortening of the humerus but also by surgical incisions. Those with a combination of impairment of both the rotator cuff and the deltoid muscles rarely achieved overhead motion. However, characteristically they were satisfied with the relief of pain and function with the arm at the side. Patients with good deltoid and rotator cuff muscles (about 40 per cent) achieved excellent functional ratings.

CUFF-TEAR ARTHROPATHY

The pathology and etiological mechanism of this condition are discussed in detail in Chapter 2, page 124, and Figures 2–47 to 2–52. Its treatment is considered in this section.

Anatomical Problem

The combination of painful incongruity of the articular surfaces and a massive rotator cuff tear is very difficult to treat (Figs. 3–72 to 3–76). The end-stage cuff tear would seem to preclude a nonconstrained shoulder arthroplasty, and yet the alternatives also present problems. One hesitates to perform a fusion because the typical patient is older and is not young enough to tolerate the period of immobilization required and because the opposite shoulder is almost always involved. A con-

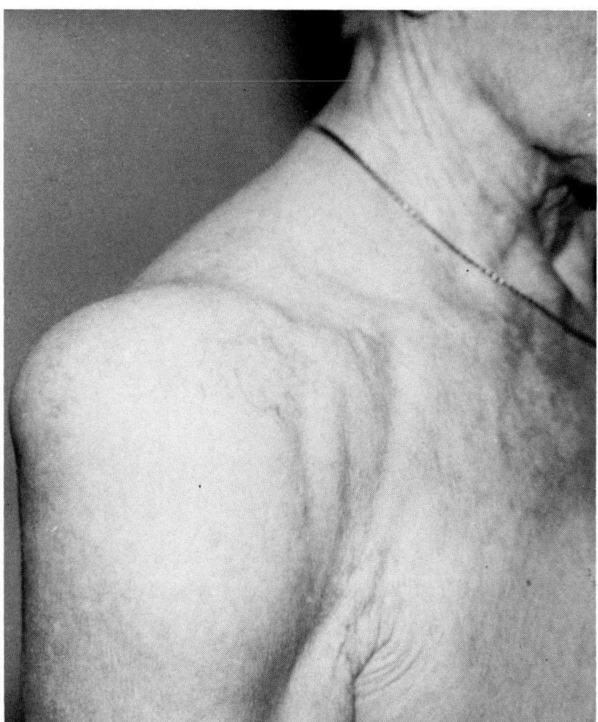

Figure 3–72. ***Treatment of Cuff-Tear.*** A 69 year old woman with the typical fluid and instability of cuff-tear arthropathy. Special care must be taken to make sure there is no infection.

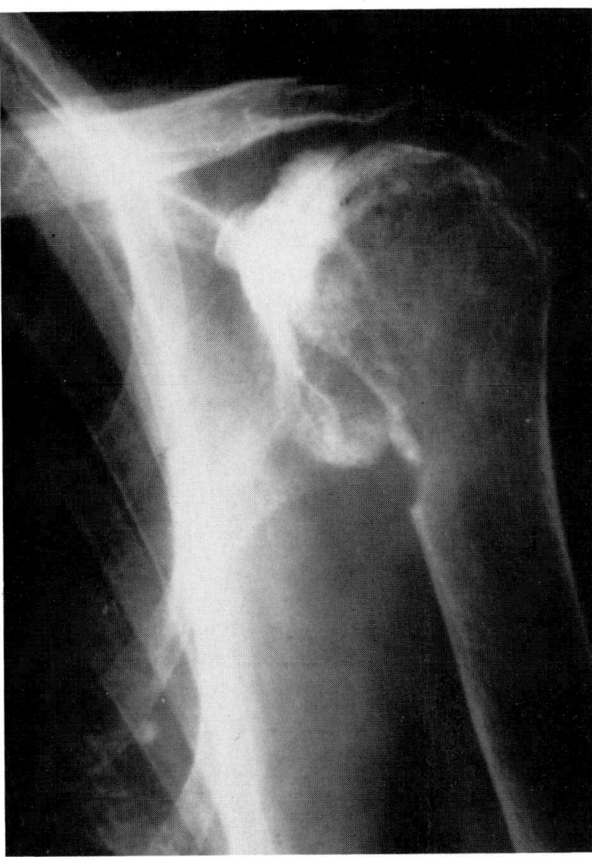

Figure 3–73. ***Nonconstrained Total Arthroplasty for Cuff-Tear Arthropathy.*** Preoperative anterior-posterior x-ray.

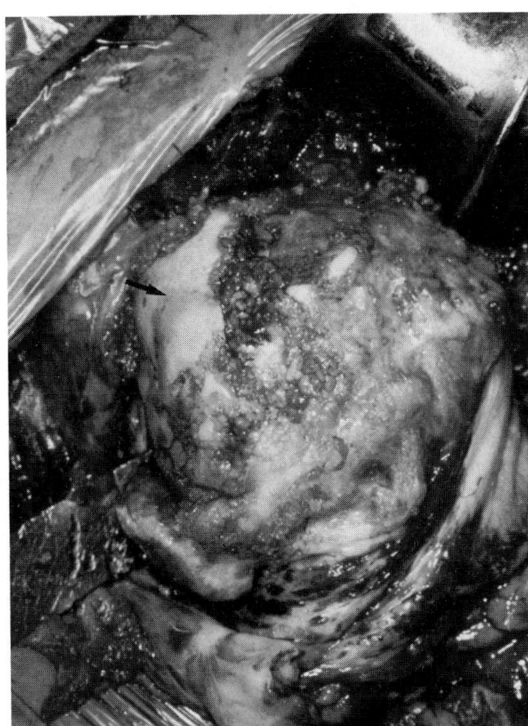

Figure 3–74. ***Nonconstrained Total Arthroplasty for Cuff-Tear Arthropathy.*** Appearance of the head (arrow). All of the supraspinatus and infraspinatus and half of the subscapularis have been detached.

strained, fixed-fulcrum shoulder arthroplasty is likely to result in loss of scapular fixation because of the erosion, fragmentation, and softening of the glenoid. A "subacromial spacer," as discussed (p. 158), when used with a humeral head component is apt to fail because a large tear of the rotator cuff left unrepaired will allow the humeral component to dislocate. A humeral head replacement used alone without a glenoid component is more apt to dislocate even when the rotator cuff is repaired because of loss of bone at the glenoid; however, when the glenoid is too destroyed to permit implantation of a nonconstrained glenoid component without the likelihood that it will loosen, a humeral component alone may be the best choice.

Although an arthrodesis can be considered in some special cases, I prefer to use a nonconstrained shoulder arthroplasty with limited goals rehabilitation (see Chapter 7, p. 530) in virtually all of these patients who are in good general health and have uncontrollable pain. The series of 26 patients treated this way and reported in 1983[24] were operated on between the years 1975 and 1983. During

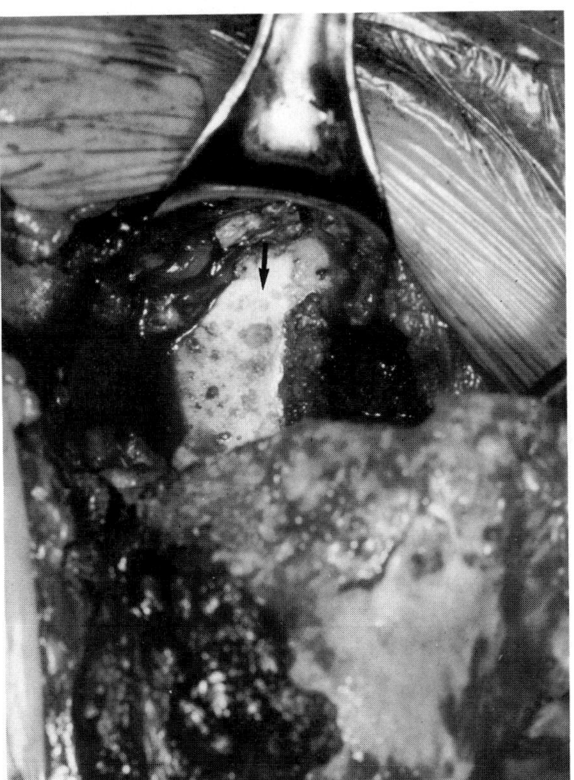

Figure 3–75. ***Nonconstrained Total Arthroplasty for Cuff-Tear Arthropathy.*** Appearance of the glenoid, which was very deeply eroded up to the base of the coracoid (arrow).

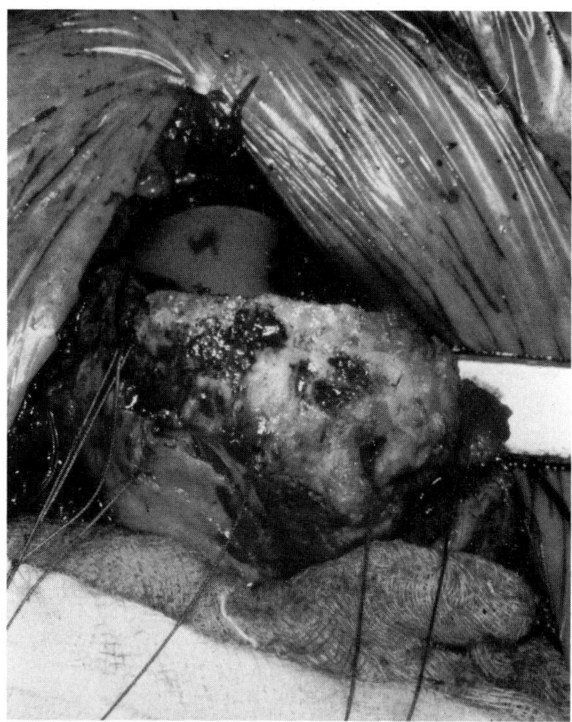

Figure 3–76. ***Nonconstrained Total Arthroplasty for Cuff-Tear Arthropathy.*** Standard metal-backed glenoid component in place, and awl holes with nonabsorbable sutures are visible in the bald greater tuberosity prior to implanting the humeral component.

the same period of time an equal number of shoulders with cuff-tear arthropathy were not treated operatively either because of the poor general health of the patient or because the patient was tolerating the pain or feared surgery. My patients averaged 69 years of age at the time of nonconstrained arthroplasty, and their ages ranged from 50 to 87 years. All had severe pain and the physical signs and disability of a large tear of the rotator cuff superimposed on painful glenohumeral incongruity.

Special Steps in Arthroplasty for Cuff-Tear Arthropathy

This operation aims to eliminate painful glenohumeral incongruity while at the same time repairing the massive cuff tear and decompressing it from impingement. The likelihood of a limited functional result and limited goals rehabilitation is carefully explained to the patient.

1. Explanation of Limited Goals. Make sure that the patient and the family understand the expected results and the likelihood that the muscles are inadequate for overhead function.

2. Mobilization of the Rotator Cuff. The repair of the rotator cuff must be kept in mind throughout the operation. The usual extended deltopectoral approach is made, but, when clearing the subacromial space, the edges of the rotator tendons are tagged with stay sutures. The superficial surfaces of the tendons are cleared of scar tissue prior to dividing the subscapularis tendon. The subscapularis tendon is divided near the lesser tuberosity, and the capsule is divided near the glenoid, as shown in Figure 3–77. This flap of capsule can be invaluable in the subsequent closure of the rotator cuff, which usually entails transferring the subscapularis tendon upward to compensate for the loss of the supraspinatus tendon.

3. Decompression of Subacromial Impingement. Three of the twenty-six patients in this series had unfused anterior acromial epiphyses that were treated by internal fixation and bone grafting because the epiphyseal fragment was too large to be excised (see Figs. 2–55 through 2–57). Four other patients had such long-standing impingement that the acromion had worn through and had fractured. The paper-thin fragment of acromion rested on the humerus and had to be excised prior to re-attaching the deltoid. Five patients in this series had undergone a radical acromionectomy elsewhere prior to the arthroplasty; this procedure had increased the disability, had not relieved the pain, and had weakened the deltoid beyond repair (see Fig. 2–46). However, when residual narrowing of the supraspinatus outlet was found, an anterior acromioplasty was performed, but care was taken to maintain the superficial surfaces of the acromion and clavicle intact, preserving the attachment of the origin of the deltoid muscle (see Fig. 2–41). It is important to remember, however, that it is impossible to eliminate impingement by enlarging the supraspinatus outlet unless the prosthetic components are stabilized against riding upward (by repair of the rotator cuff and careful placement of the components).

4. Glenoid Component Selection and Placement. In an effort to prevent the humerus from riding upward, oversized glenoid components were used developmentally in 12 shoulders in this series—ten 200 per cent larger and two 600 per cent larger (see Figs. 3–11 and 3–12). In cuff-tear arthropathy wear usually occurs on the superior aspect of the glenoid and into the coracoid (see Fig. 3–75). This causes the articular surface of the glenoid to face upward. A glenoid component with an overhanging superior rim seems logical; however, it adds little support because whenever an effort is made to raise the arm, the scapula rotates upward, causing the glenoid to face upward and rendering the overhang ineffective. In the final analysis, the rotator cuff repair must be strong enough to stabilize the head of the humerus against

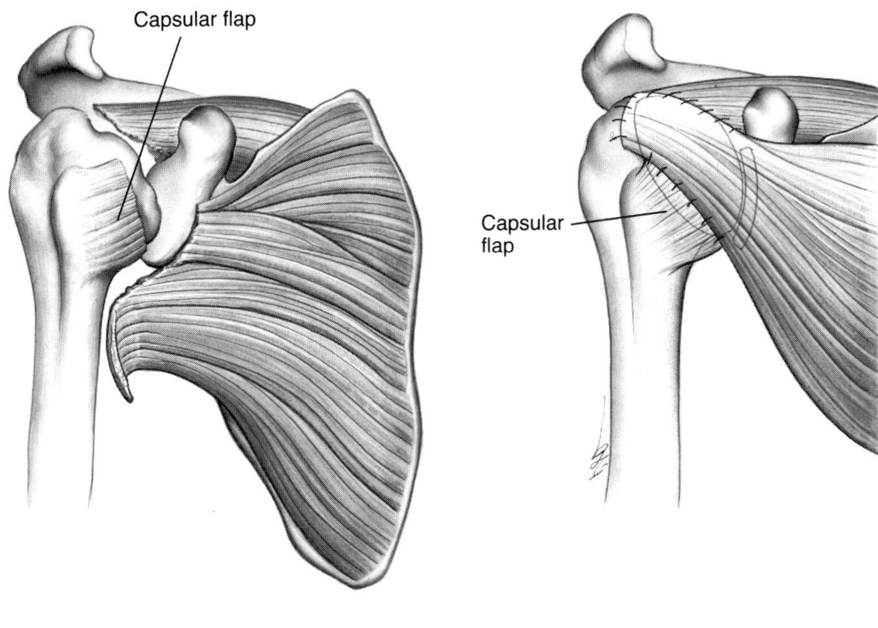

Figure 3–77. ***Nonconstrained Total Arthroplasty for Cuff-Tear Arthropathy.*** Method usually used for closing the cuff. The subscapularis tendon is separated from the capsule, and a flap of capsule is left attached to the humerus (left). After implanting a short head humeral component, the subscapularis is transferred cephalically to be sutured to the stump of the supraspinatus and infraspinatus. The capsule, which has been left attached to the humerus, is sutured to the subscapularis tendon to stabilize anteriorly (right). (*Note* that centralization of the head places it further under the rotator cuff, which is an advantage for closing the tendons.)

ascent. The larger (600 per cent) glenoid component precluded closing the rotator cuff and did not improve the functional results. Although to date I have removed only one of the 200 per cent glenoid components because of loosening, I believe the radiolucent lines around these components are more prevalent and there is a greater likelihood of loosening because of the increased mechanical forces caused by the constraint. Therefore, I have come to prefer a standard-sized glenoid component in treating cuff-tear arthropathy (Fig. 3–78), as in other conditions, and only very rarely use a 200 per cent glenoid component when the scapula is large and there is adequate bone inferiorly to support the component but severe bone loss superiorly. In any case, the quality of the cuff repair is considered more important in stabilizing the humeral head.

Loss of bone at the glenoid can make it impossible to insert even a standard polyethylene glenoid component without shortening and trimming the keel. In one patient, the scapula fractured during implantation of the glenoid component, and no glenoid component could be used. Large bone grafts were used in four patients in this series to support the glenoid component (see Fig. 3–28G), and high placement of the glenoid component (see Fig. 3–28F) was frequently necessary.

5. Selection of the Humeral Component. After mobilizing the rotator cuff tendons, a careful trial to determine the appropriate length of head is very important. Although a long head component affords better leverage, it may preclude repairing the cuff. On the other hand, in some patients who have very deep wear and loss of glenoid bone, the long head prosthesis is more stable. A short head humeral component facilitates closure of the cuff and may be preferable.

6. Closing the Cuff. Having mobilized the rotator cuff from beneath the acromion and acromioclavicular joint as well as anteriorly and posteriorly, and having divided the subscapularis tendons as far laterally as possible while preserving an anterior capsular flap on the humerus (Fig. 3–77[left]), the rotator cuff is pretty well prepared for closure. However, prior to the final implantation of the humeral component, the glenohumeral joint capsule is freed posteriorly so that it does not tether the infraspinatus and teres tendons. Also, before cementing the humeral component, awl holes with nonabsorbable sutures are placed in the greater tuberosity to be used for re-attaching the cuff after the humeral component has been cemented (see Figs. 3–76 and 3–77).

7. Implantation of the Humeral Component. A final check for the proper length of the humeral head is made by pulling the mobilized rotator tendons around the head of a trial prosthesis prior to cementing the humeral component. After the cement has set, the rotator cuff is closed with whatever transfer of the subscapularis tendon is required. The flap of capsule is retained to stabilize the head against dislocating anteriorly (see Fig. 3–77).

8. Limited Goals Exercise Program. As outlined in Chapter 7 (Fig. 7–14, p. 530), the limited goals exercise program is aimed at the stability of the shoulder and use of the arm at the side. No abduction brace is used, and no overhead exercises are given. The arm is protected in a sling, and pendulum exercises are performed several times a day during the first three months. Starting at about three or four months isometric exercises are begun, and the patient progresses to the "instability exercises" (see Fig. 7–13) as tolerated. The strength of the rubber used for resistance is gradually increased. Carrying more than 15 pounds of weight is forbidden for at least nine months.

Results To Be Expected After Nonconstrained Arthroplasty for Cuff-Tear Arthropathy

The "limited goals" exercise program trades range of motion for stability. It is intended to allow the patient to have about 110 degrees of passive elevation and 20 degrees of passive external rotation at the time isometric exercises are begun. Of the 26 patients in the reported series, 25 were very pleased with the relief of pain and improved function they enjoyed (Figs. 3–79 through 3–82). One patient, who had received a 200 per cent glenoid component, re-tore the rotator cuff when lifting a very heavy machine seven years after the arthroplasty. The rotator cuff was re-repaired, and the glenoid component was inspected and found to be firm and not loose. Another patient who had received a 200 per cent glenoid component did well for nine years, at which time the glenoid component suddenly became loose and painful and was removed. At the time of removal of this glenoid component, the rotator cuff was found to be remarkably restored, as shown in Figure 3–82.

CONGENITAL DEFECTS OF THE GLENOHUMERAL JOINT

In the series shown in Table 3–1, six shoulders had developmental defects requiring total shoulder

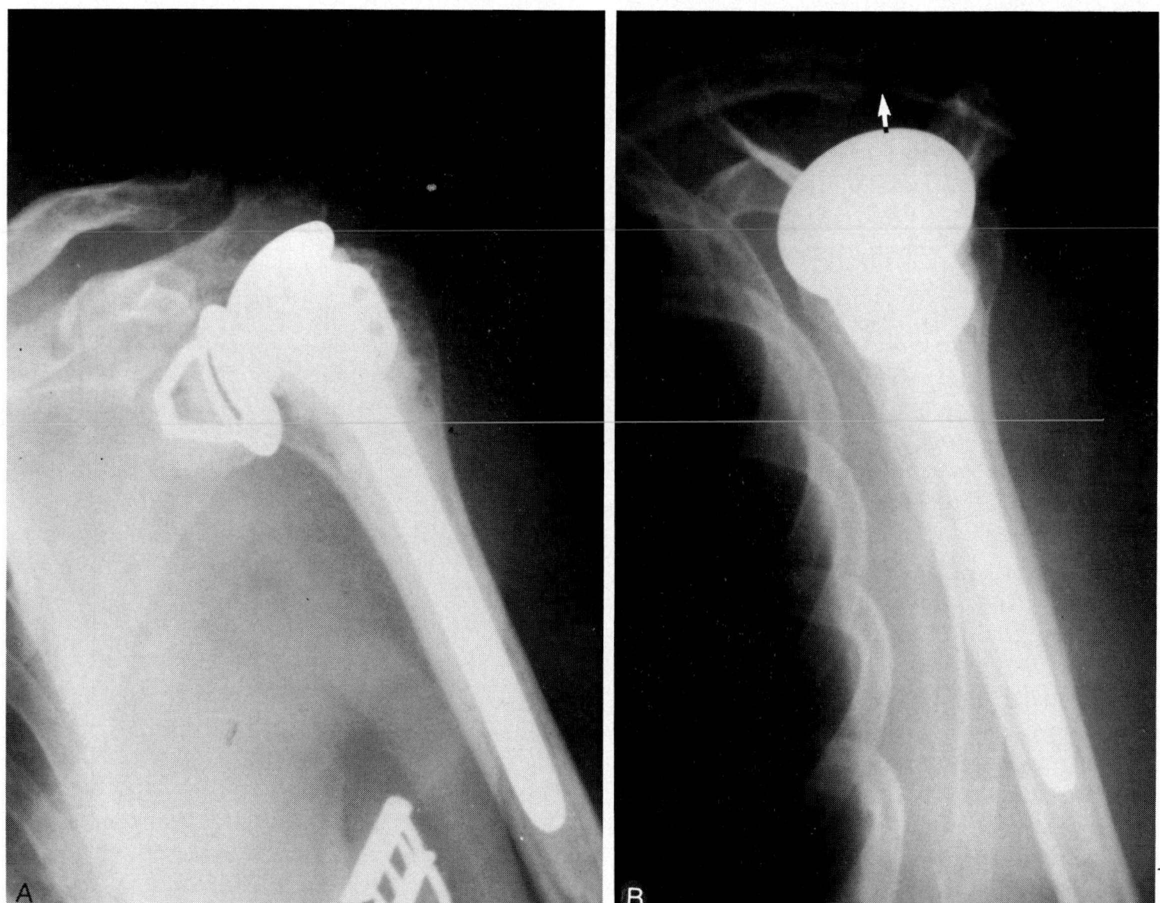

Figure 3–78A and B. ***Nonconstrained Total Arthroplasty for Cuff-Tear Arthropathy.*** Follow-up x-rays. Limited goals rehabilitation was given (Chapter 7, p. 530). The components became stabilized. Note the preservation of the acromial distance in the outlet view (arrow in B).

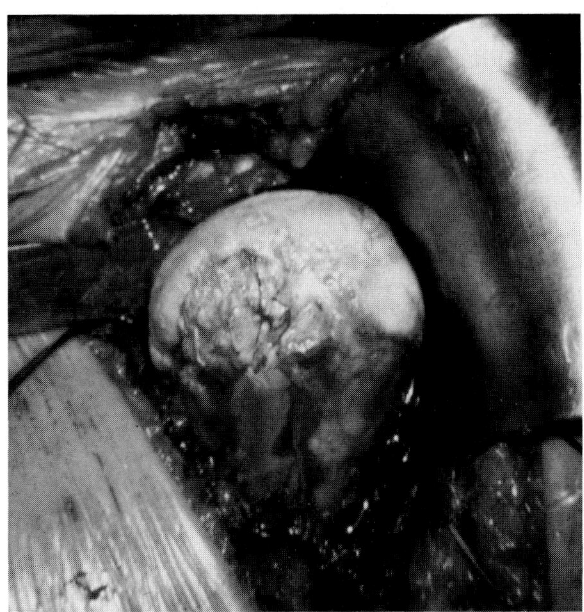

Figure 3–79. ***Cuff-Tear Arthropathy.*** Figures 3–79 through 3–82 show an 11 year follow-up of a cuff repair that demonstrates remarkably strong healing of the tendon. This figure shows the massive cuff tear at arthroplasty in 1977.

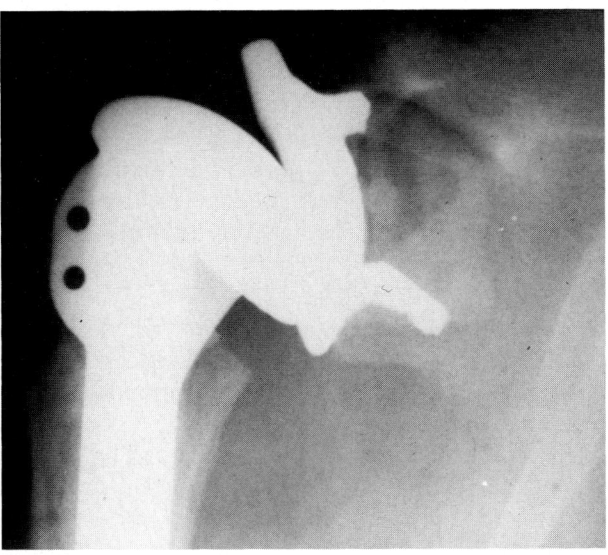

Figure 3–81. ***Cuff-Tear Arthropathy.*** The shoulder functioned well for nine years, when the glenoid component loosened.

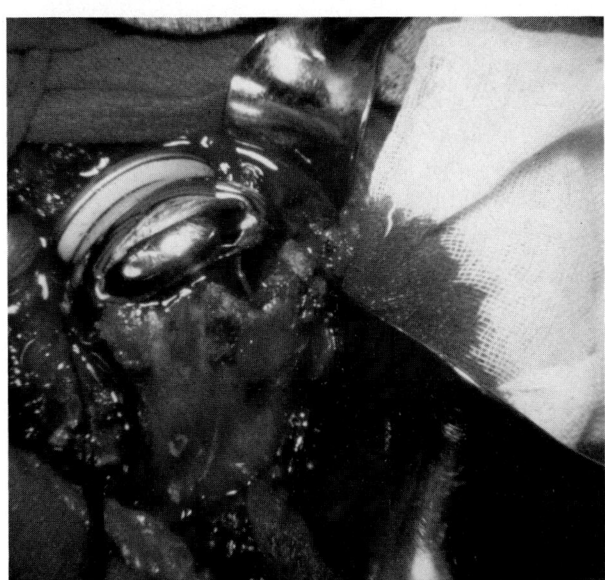

Figure 3–80. ***Cuff-Tear Arthropathy.*** A 200 per cent developmental glenoid component was used. Note the bald greater tuberosity. The cuff was closed in a manner similar to that shown in Figure 3–77.

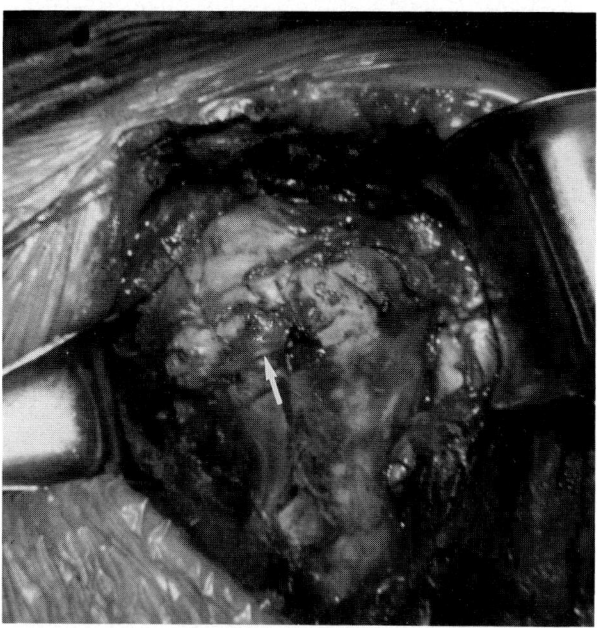

Figure 3–82. ***Cuff-Tear Arthropathy.*** This photograph of the cuff was made at removal of the loose glenoid component in 1988, showing a surprisingly good tendon and the nonabsorbable sutures in place (arrow).

arthroplasties. Severe pain and limitation of motion was the indication for surgery in each case.

Multiple Epiphyseal Dysplasia

Nonconstrained total shoulder arthroplasty was performed in three shoulders with this condition (Fig. 3–83). The age of the patients at the time of surgery ranged from 23 to 35 years, averaging 29 years. Pain had gradually increased over a number of years and had become intolerable. The anatomical findings were similar in each case. The humeral heads were underdeveloped, deformed, and subluxated. The glenoid was also deformed and sloping. The articular surfaces were eburnated at the point of contact between the head and the glenoid, and this area of eburnation was surrounded by marginal osteophytes. The bone was soft where no contact had occurred. The deltoid and rotator cuff muscles were intact; however, the rotator cuff muscles and tendons were very thin and small. The rotator cuff tendons looked as if they had never been used. The bones were small.

The underdeveloped rotator cuff tendons and the small, deformed bones demanded special consideration during the arthroplasty. The thin subscapularis tendon was carefully tagged with stay sutures and mobilized. The sternal head of the pectoralis major was advanced upward during closure to compensate for the deficient subscapularis in one patient. The small humerus required a short-head humeral component with a 6.3 mm. stem diameter in each of the three shoulders. The glenoid component was difficult to implant. It was necessary to re-shape the scapula so it would have a bearing surface to support the glenoid component and an adequate slot to receive the stem. A power burr was the key instrument in the preparation of the glenoid. Because of the small amount of bone available, a polyethylene glenoid component was used in each case. Good bone support was eventually obtained by seating the glenoid components in some anteversion. This was compensated for by cementing the humeral components in more than the usual 40 degrees of retroversion.

The post-operative course was slow because of weak muscles. One male patient eventually obtained an "excellent" rating. The other two had good pain relief and were pleased with the result, but their functional ratings were marked down to "satisfactory" because of their weak muscles. There have been no complications to date with follow-up ranging from 6 to 11 years (Fig. 3–84).

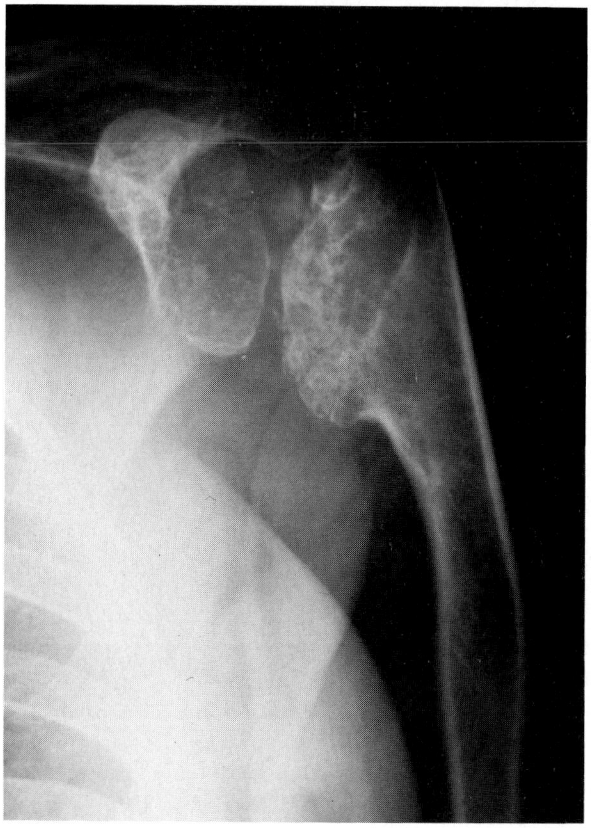

Figure 3–83. ***Arthroplasty for Congenital Defects.*** Anterior-posterior view of multiple epiphyseal dysplasia.

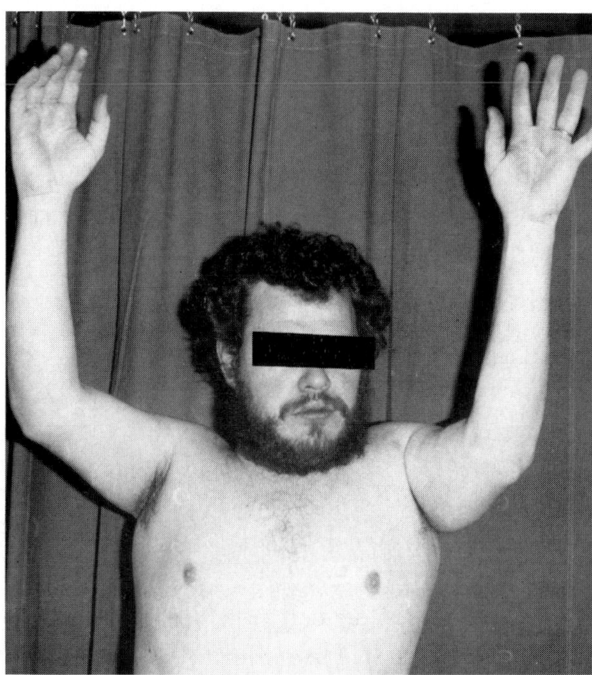

Figure 3–84. ***Arthroplasty for Congenital Defects.*** An 11 year follow-up of a total arthroplasty for painful multiple epiphyseal dysplasia of the right shoulder. Patient had little or no pain, was active, and had the active range of motion demonstrated.

Glenoid Hypoplasia[194]

Bilateral shoulder arthroplasties for this condition were performed in a 44 year old man who had progressive shoulder pain over 15 years. The arthroplasties were performed two weeks apart. This patient had become addicted to a number of medications and was helpless because of severe pain with movement of either arm. He could not sleep, eat, dress himself, or perform any of the functions of self-care.

Similar anatomical findings were present in both shoulders (Fig. 3–85C and D). The glenoids were very small and sclerotic and had pointed ridges articulating with the humeral heads. Deep grooves had been worn into the humeral heads at their points of articulation with the glenoid ridges. The scapula and arm musculature of this patient had become markedly atrophied from disuse (because of pain). The muscle atrophy was so striking that it suggested the possibility of a disorder of the muscles.

The main special step in these arthroplasties was the preparation of the glenoids. The ridges of bone on the glenoid were excised; then, after leveling the surface to support the back of the glenoid

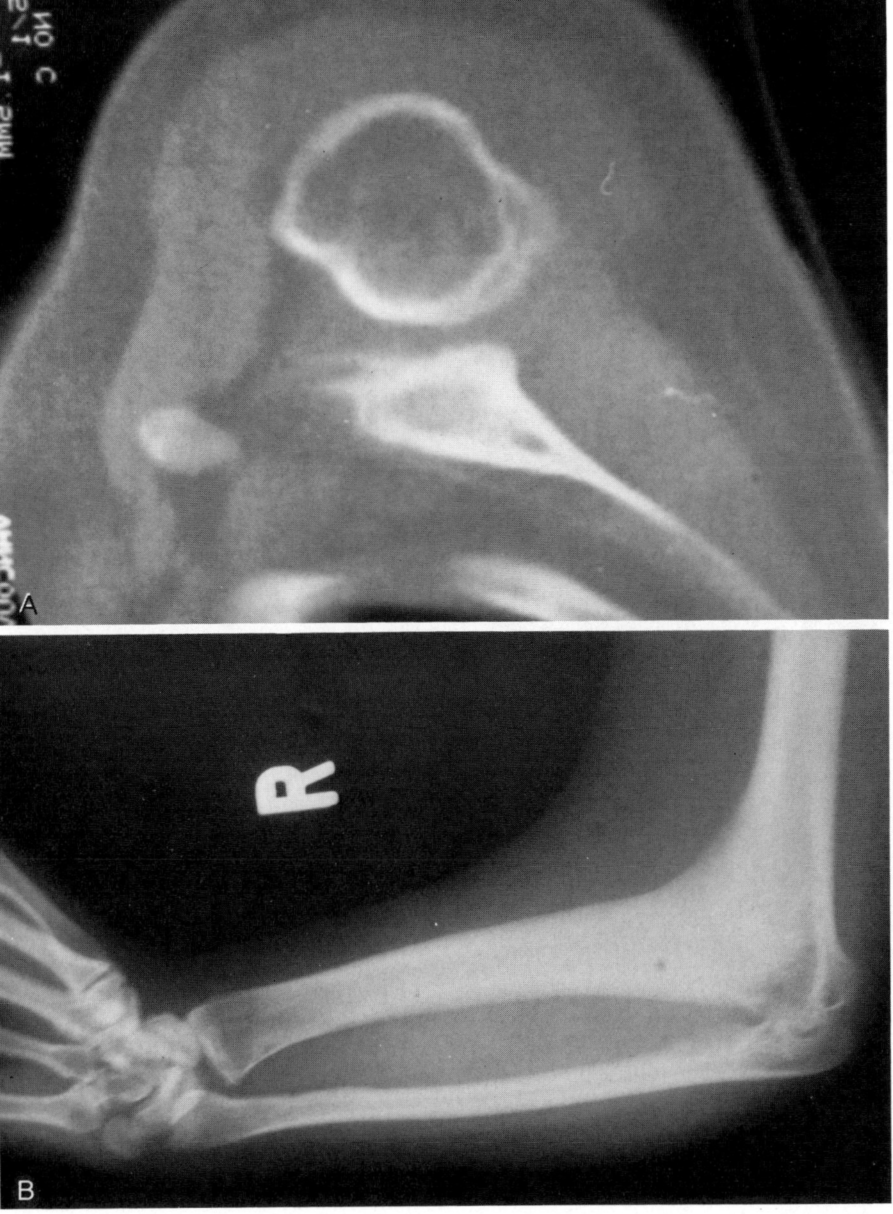

Figure 3–85. ***Arthroplasty for Congenital Defects.*** Computerized tomography of the right shoulder (A) and lateral x-ray of the right elbow (B) in a patient who had severe glenoid hypoplasia.

Illustration continued on following page

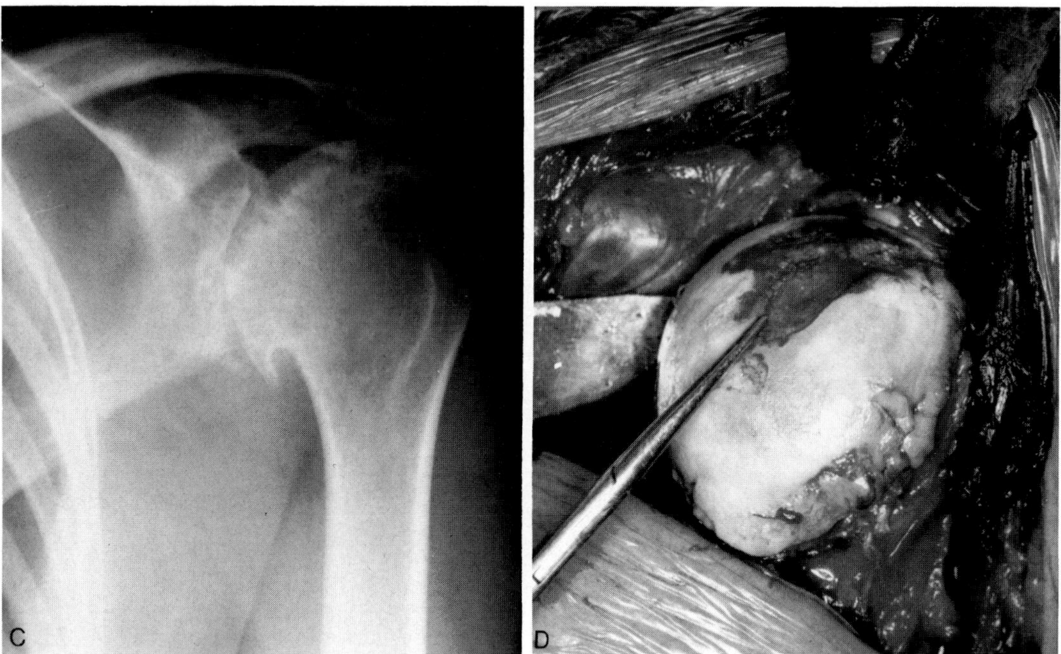

Figure 3–85 *Continued* C and D, Anterior-posterior x-ray view and photograph at arthroplasty of another patient (a 44 year old man), who had extremely painful arthritis of both shoulders as a result of glenoid hypoplasia.

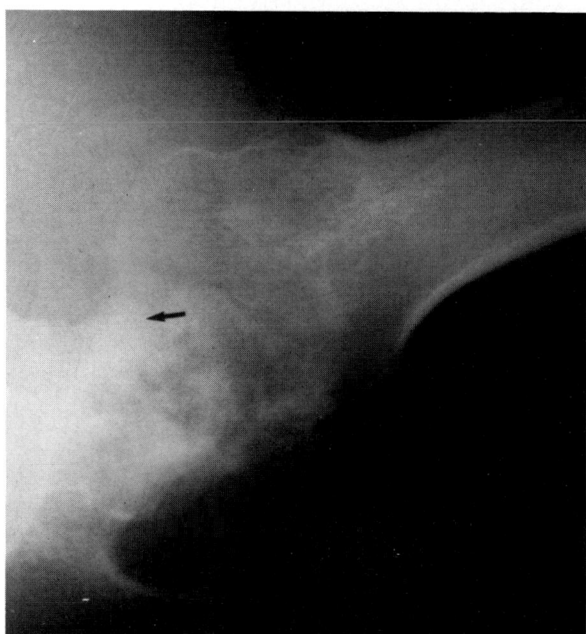

Figure 3–86. ***Arthroplasty for Congenital Defects.*** Axillary view showing dysplasia epiphysealis hemimelica of the posterior glenoid, which is displacing the humeral head anteriorly, causing changes in the humeral head secondary to disuse anteriorly and to pressure posteriorly. The anteror rim of the glenoid (arrow) was almost normal.

component, slots of sufficient size could be developed to contain the keels of standard metal-backed glenoid components.

These arthroplasties were performed only one and one-half years prior to this writing. The early results have been very good. Since being freed from the pain in the shoulders, the patient's muscles have regained strength, and he is handling the addiction problem.

Dysplasia Epiphysealis Hemimelica of the Glenoid[198]

We reported the first case of dysplasia epiphysealis hemimelica in the scapula in the English literature[94] and have not seen another. The patient's parents could recall that he seemed to have some limitation of shoulder motion all his life and at age 14 began to experience progressive swelling, pain, and more restriction of movement. X-rays of his shoulder were first made at the age of 18, and the patient was referred to me for a biopsy and treatment with a diagnosis of chondrosarcoma of the scapula.

Because the axillary x-ray showed a lesion in the posterior glenoid that spared the anterior half of the articular surface of the glenoid and had displaced the humeral head forward long enough to have produced secondary arthritic changes (Fig. 3–86), it was thought that the process must have been long standing. I made a tentative diagnosis of dysplasia epiphysealis hemimelica of the glenoid, which was substantiated at surgery by Dr. May Parisien and Dr. Austin Johnston, who later made further histological studies of the tumor mass, which was subsequently excised.

Following excision of the mass, the shoulder was observed for two years without recurrence of the tumor; however, shoulder pain continued because of the arthritic changes. A total shoulder arthroplasty was done when the patient was 20 years of age, and further specimens were sent to the pathologist. The diagnosis was further substantiated. The total shoulder arthroplasty stopped the patient's pain and allowed satisfactory but imperfect motion. There has been no complication or recurrence of the tumor at seven years of follow-up.

ARTHRITIS OF ERB'S PALSY

Anatomical Problems

The soft-tissue aspects of Erb's palsy are discussed in Chapter 6, page 452.

The intensity of muscular and skeletal involvement in patients with birth palsies is quite variable. In my experience the specific muscles involved in Erb's palsy do not always conform to the textbook picture of weak external rotators, strong subscapularis, and weak deltoid. However, some of these muscles are usually involved. The skeletal structures in shoulders with mild birth palsies may be relatively normal. Those with more severe muscle involvement develop an overhanging acromion, retroversion and posterior subluxation of the humeral head, underdevelopment of the posterior glenoid, and a prominent coracoid process, which may impinge on the humerus (Fig. 3–87). In those with skeletal deformities, secondary arthritic changes may develop in later life between the retroverted and deformed humeral head and the deficient glenoid. The combination of muscle deficits, painful glenohumeral arthritis, and skeletal abnormalities is a very challenging problem that has interested me for a long time. I believe we have recently evolved a very satisfactory nonconstrained arthroplasty technique for this condition.

Surprisingly, some patients with this condition go through early life without a diagnosis, and the lesion is overlooked until shoulder pain begins. At that time the residual paralysis is incomplete,

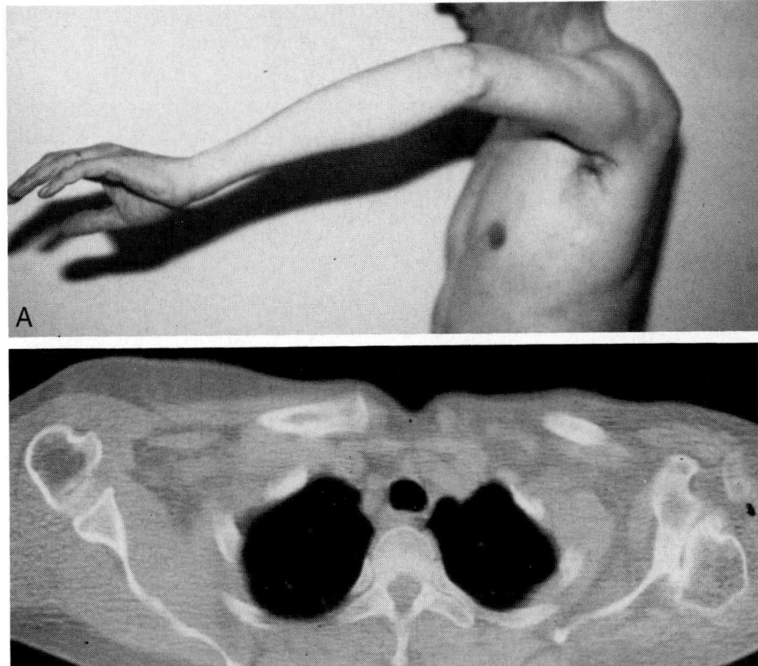

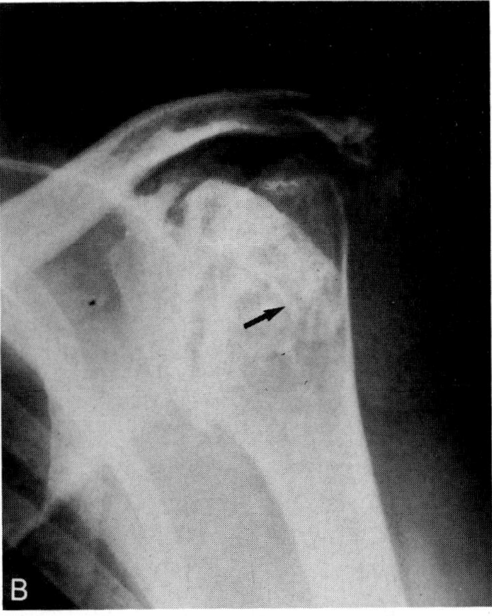

Figure 3–87. ***Arthritis of Erb's Palsy Deformity.*** A, The skeletal defects in a 62 year old man with Erb's palsy since birth. B, The glenoid is underdeveloped and in marked retroversion. The humeral head is posteriorly dislocated. The coracoid is elongated and protrudes anteriorly (arrow). The acromion is overhanging and impinges. There has been variable recovery of the muscles. C, The CT scan is especially helpful in demonstrating the pathology and treating this condition.

but the diagnosis can be made by means of electromyograms. The skeletal abnormalities can be evaluated with axillary and lateral x-ray views supplemented with CT scans (Fig. 3–87C). The age of patients at the time of onset of arthritic symptoms has ranged from 18 to 35 years. The ages of the three patients with this condition noted in Table 3–1 at the time of shoulder arthroplasty ranged from 50 to 65 years; however, since then two other younger patients (in their twenties) had sufficient pain to require arthroplasties.

The key anatomical lesion in an arthroplasty for this condition is the shortened infraspinatus and teres minor muscles (Fig. 3–88). Although some motor power has returned to these muscles, the humerus has been dislocated all the patient's life, and the posterior capsule and external rotators are short. Using bone grafts for the glenoid component and positioning the humerus in its normal location laterally fails because the short external rotators pull away or fracture the soft greater tuberosity and cannot be re-attached. This loss of the external rotators spoils the functional result. About two years ago I first began to leave the posterior capsule and the external rotators attached to the posterior humerus without attempting to displace the humerus laterally; the glenoid component was then implanted in marked retroversion while the humeral component was implanted in anteversion (Fig. 3–89). Because the internal rotators are usually short, the subscapularis and pectoralis major are detached early during the procedure and lengthened.

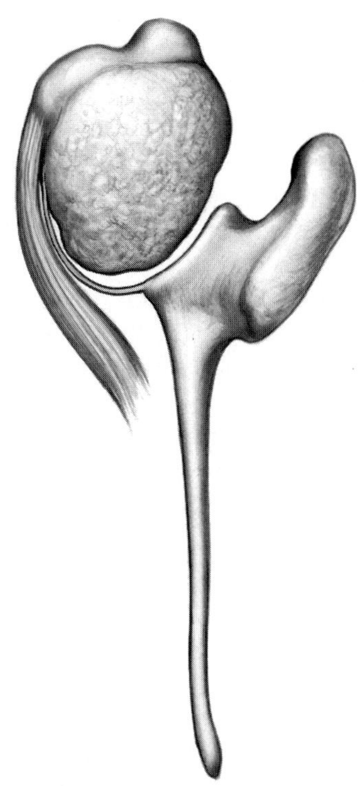

Figure 3–88. Arthritis of Erb's palsy deformity. Illustrating the skeletal and soft-tissue deformity. The external rotators and posterior capsule are shortened. The same problem is encountered in arthroplasties for long-standing posterior dislocations.

Treatment

Indication for Arthroplasty in Erb's Palsy. The objective of this procedure is to relieve pain and increase the range of external rotation. Although one cannot hope to substantially increase strength, if the internal rotation contracture is eliminated and the humerus can be externally rotated, the use of the hand and elbow is greatly improved. Muscle deficits should be carefully documented and discussed with the patient prior to surgery. Patients who have incapacitating pain and have a clear understanding of these objectives and their irreparable muscle deficits are very grateful for the results achieved.

Special Steps in the Arthroplasty for Erb's Palsy. As mentioned previously, the infraspinatus and teres minor have been short throughout the life of the patient, and they cannot be lengthened or transposed to reach the humerus if the humerus is placed in its normal location on the scapula. Any attempts to lengthen or slide these muscles would weaken them, and they are stronger if left in situ. Therefore, the posterior capsule is left intact, the internal rotators are lengthened, and the version of the components is made to comply with the deformed glenoid. This condition illustrates a principle applicable to all old posterior dislocations with fixed shortening of the external rotators, as in old trauma (p. 222) and extreme displacements in arthritis of dislocations (p. 208).

1. *Pre-operative assessment.* The shoulder musculature is carefully assessed pre-operatively, and the prognosis and limitations imposed by these muscles are discussed with the patient.

2. *Partial paralysis of the deltoid.* Because the deltoid muscle is often partially denervated, it is important to handle it with care and to avoid traumatizing the axillary nerve. Early detachment of the pectoralis major makes it possible to achieve the exposure of the posterior scapula required without forceful retraction on the deltoid.

3. *Early detachment of the pectoralis major insertion.* The usual deltopectoral approach is made except that the insertions of both the sternal and clavicular heads of the pectoralis major are detached and tagged early. This, with the detachment of the subscapularis, overcomes the internal

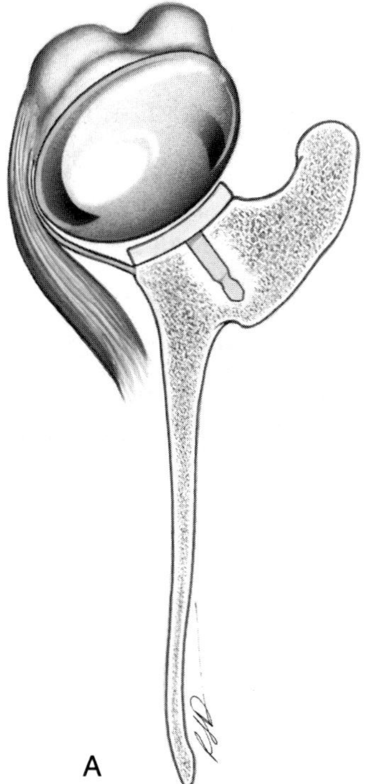

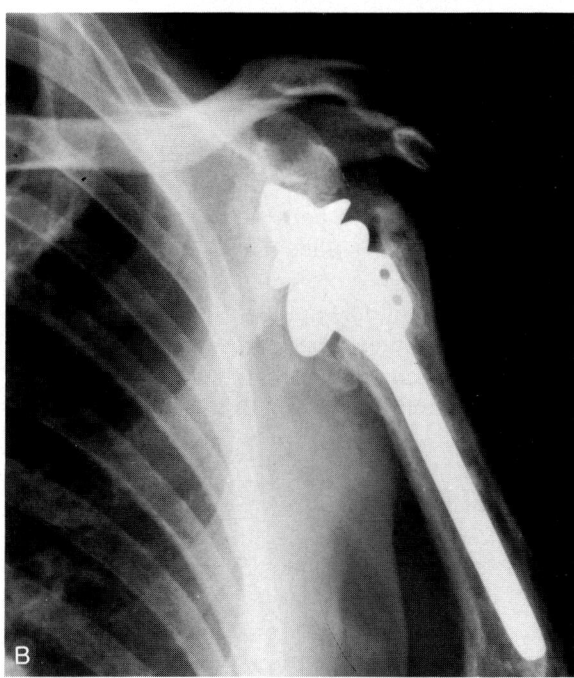

Figure 3–89. ***Arthritis of Erb's Palsy Deformity.*** The recommended repair leaves the posterior capsule and external rotators in place.

A, The positioning of the components.

B, Post-operative appearance in the anterior-posterior view.

C, Because of the short external rotators and short posterior capsule, positioning the glenoid component in a normal location is avoided.

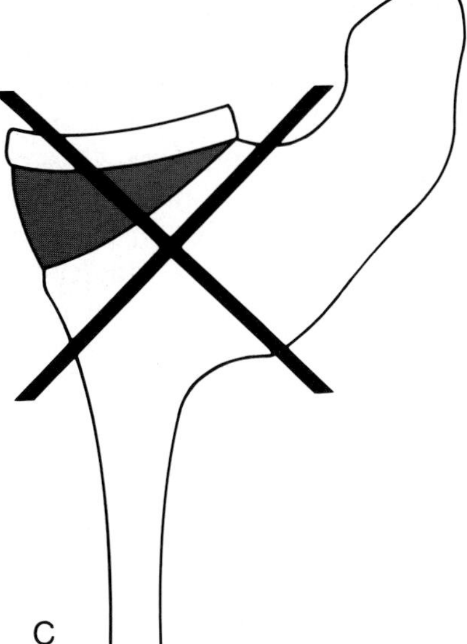

The pectoralis major and subscapularis tendons are released early. The glenoid component is placed on the existing glenoid and the humeral component is anteverted to point toward the glenoid in the same alignment as it presented. Bone is trimmed from the undersurface of the acromion, leaving the deltoid origin intact. The coracoid is trimmed. Because it is usually impossible to lengthen the subscapularis, after it is released the sternal head of the pectoralis is transferred upward to augment it and still allow external rotation.

This principle also holds for some old posterior dislocations. The glenoid component with an angulated stem may have a place, as here, when the posterior capsule is short, but it would be very unstable if the posterior capsule and external rotators were redundant (see Figure 3–28).

rotation contracture and allows the humerus to be retracted posteriorly.

4. *Lengthening of the subscapularis.*

5. The subscapularis was underdeveloped in all of my patients and required augmentation with pectoralis major after being released (Fig. 3–31).

6. *Glenoid component placed in retroversion.* Place the back of the articular surface of the glenoid component on the site of the existing articular surface of the glenoid. The existing articular surface faces posteriorly, and the stem of the glenoid component may have to point toward the front of the scapula. There is adequate bone to permit this when the stem is pointed toward the base of the coracoid (Figs. 3–28D and 3–89).

7. *Version of the humeral component.* The humeral component is oriented so that it points toward the glenoid component when the arm is held in neutral rotation. This may place the humeral component in 20 or 30 degrees anteversion rather than the usual 40 degrees retroversion. A short-head humeral component is usually necessary because of the underdevelopment of the soft tissue.

8. *Minimum 20 degrees of external rotation established.* At least 20 degrees of external rotation must be established as the soft tissue is closed anteriorly. As noted in No. 4 above, the subscapularis may be too short to be re-attached and must be supplemented with the sternal head of the pectoralis major. The clavicular head of the pectoralis major is re-attached to the deltoid insertion.

9. *Correction of acromial and coracoid deformities.* To correct the overhanging, drooping acromion, bone is excised from the undersurface of the acromion to make room for the humeral component rather than osteotomizing the acromion. Some of the attachment of the origin of the deltoid on the deep edge of the acromion is detached; however, the superficial layers of the deltoid origin are left intact. If the coracoid impinges on the humerus, the lateral half of the coracoid can be excised with a rongeur without detaching the short head of the biceps or coracobrachialis.

10. *Sling in neutral rotation and extension.* The sling to be worn post-operatively is applied with the arm in slight extension and neutral rotation to relieve tension on the external rotators. The sling can soon be discarded and the regular exercise program advanced. Because of the unusual version of the components, overhead elevation is expected to be limited to about 140 degrees. After the initial soreness has subsided, active exercises that emphasize strengthening the external rotator and deltoid muscle are added.

Result to Be Expected. In addition to passive motion being limited by the version of the components, active motion is limited to the capabilities of the deltoid and rotator cuff. Residual nerve deficits to the deltoid and rotator cuff have generally limited active external rotation to 20 degrees and total elevation in the scapular plane to 90 degrees. However, with this amount of motion, the patient can perform most everyday activities. The last man with Erb's palsy who had an arthroplasty of this type was mowing his lawn six months after the operation and was very pleased with the freedom from pain.

SHOULDER ARTHROPLASTY AFTER INFECTION

Infection of the Glenohumeral Joint

Incongruity of the articular surfaces of the humeral head and glenoid caused by injections or soft-tissue procedures that do not invade the bone (such as infections after repair for recurrent dislocations or cuff repairs) may, after the infection has disappeared and there is no evidence of infection systemically or in the shoulder, be treated selectively by an uncemented humeral head replacement without a glenoid component (Fig. 3–90). This procedure was performed in six patients in the series reported in Table 3–1. The likelihood of causing the infection to flare, resulting in failure, depends on the strength of the organism, the quality of the tissue, and the presence or absence of bone involvement. In my patients the infection must have been limited to the joint, with no bone involvement or osteomyelitis below the joint surfaces, and it must have been inactive for a minimum of one year. Old infected fractures are treated by joint debridement and possible subsequent arthrodesis (see Chapter 6, p. 442). A prosthesis is no longer used in old fractures after infection (because the recurrence of clinical infection was too high), and these lesions are treated according to the principles of debridement and possible subsequent arthrodesis as discussed in Chapter 6, page 438. The patient's erythrocyte sedimentation rate must be normal, and there must be no clinical suggestion of activity of the infection. The patient is warned that if a focus of residual infection is encountered, the operation will be discontinued.

The initial part of this procedure is considered an exploration with antibiotic irrigation, cultures, and a frozen section analysis ("imprint") of any abnormal tissue encountered during surgery. The articular surface of the humerus is cleanly excised with an osteotome, and the bone remaining must be free of involvement. The articular surface of the

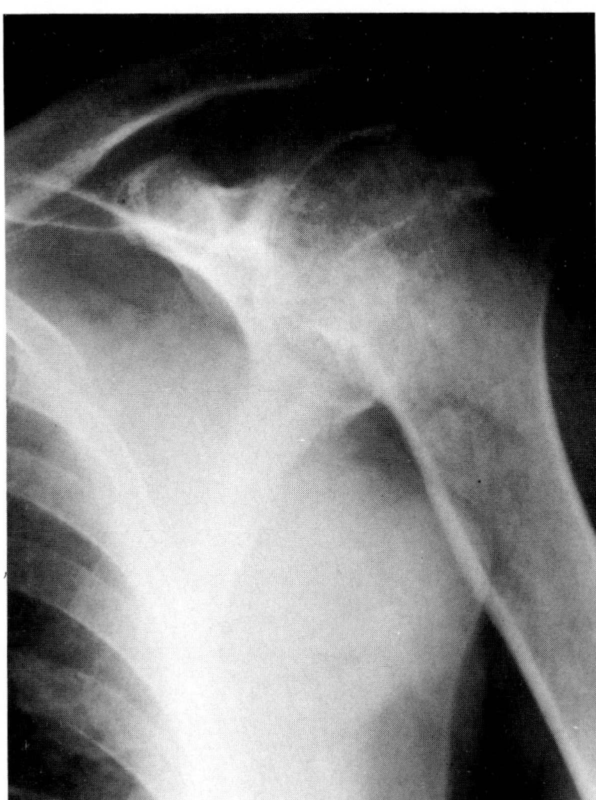

Figure 3–90. ***Shoulder Arthroplasty After Infection.*** Degenerative arthritis occurred four years following a *Staphylococcus aureus* infection in a repair for recurrent dislocations. There was no definite bone involvement, and the infection had been quiescent since a few weeks after onset. Several highly selected patients of this type without bone involvement have been treated successfully with an uncemented humeral component.

glenoid is inspected, and scar tissue is removed. The articular surface of the glenoid is left undisturbed, however, and no glenoid component is used even when there has been some damage to the articular cartilage of the glenoid. The humeral component is press-fit without cement. The subscapularis and deltopectoral closures are performed in the usual way. Intravenous antibiotics are given paraoperatively, and oral antibiotics are continued for three months. The standard postoperative exercise regimen is followed, with early passive motion started on the second day, progressing to the self-assistive regimen by the fifth day.

This technique was used in six patients in the series listed in Table III–1 who had previously had infection due to surgery for recurrent dislocations in three, injections in two, and a previously infected cuff repair in one. These patients have been followed for from 2 to 20 years, and results have been excellent to satisfactory in five and gradually increasing discomfort in one patient who has had insufficient pain to desire further surgery.

Infantile Suppurative Glenohumeral Arthritis

A successful total glenohumeral arthroplasty was done in a 40 year old woman who had had suppurative arthritis of the glenohumeral joint during infancy. Her shoulder had been drained when she was only a few months old. The proximal humeral epiphyseal plate must have been damaged, and the humerus became shortened and deformed, as illustrated in Figure 3–91. The incongruity between the upper humerus and the glenoid eventually led to disabling pain. There had been no evidence of active infection since infancy.

The rotator cuff muscles were found to be very thin and underdeveloped, similar to those seen in patients who have congenital defects, and the bones were small. The smallest (15 mm. head and 6.3 mm. diameter stem) humeral component and a standard polyethylene glenoid component were implanted 14 years ago without complications. Considering the underdeveloped musculature, the result has been very good. The patient has had complete relief of pain and the strength and size of the deltoid muscle have improved with time.

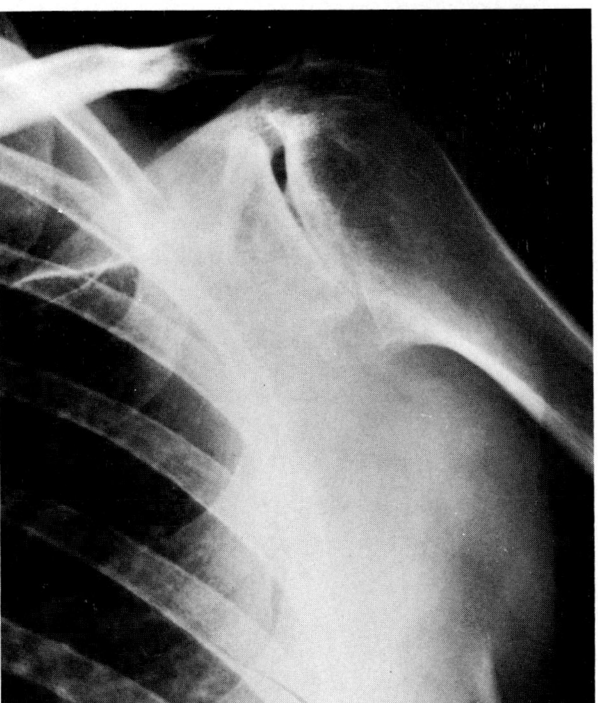

Figure 3–91. ***Shoulder Arthroplasty After Infection.*** A 40 year old woman with a painful glenohumeral arthritis following infantile suppurative arthritis of the glenohumeral joint was treated with total shoulder arthroplasty; a 14-year follow-up showed no recurrence of infection. Although the muscles were very atrophic and underdeveloped, good function was obtained.

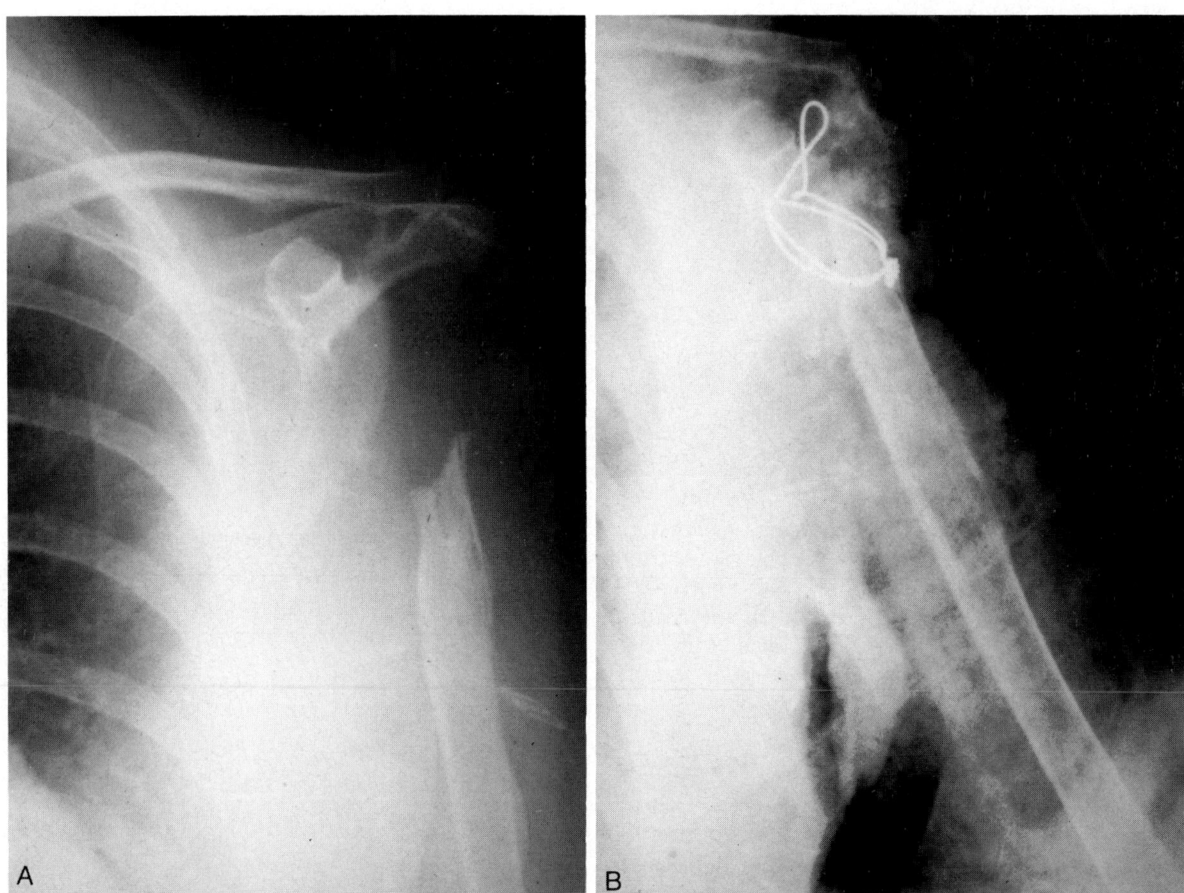

Figure 3–92. ***Shoulder Arthroplasty After Infection.*** An infected prosthesis was treated with two cleanouts, but because of ongoing pain one year after control of infection, an arthrodesis was performed.

A, Appearance after two debridements and one year of quiescence. Note the thinness of the cortical bone of the humerus.

B, Despite the adversity of bone loss, the distraction of gravity, and the normal uncontrollable movements of the scapula, a fusion was accomplished with iliac grafts, wire sutures to prevent distraction, and a spica cast for six months.

This woman has continued in her regular job as a bank teller.

A similar patient presented recently who is considering this procedure.

Treatment of Infected Shoulder Prostheses

The treatment of infected prostheses is discussed with revision arthroplasty (p. 255) and with resection and fusions (Chapter 6, p. 442, and here, in Figs. 3–90 through 3–93). I am very reluctant to use another prosthesis in a shoulder that has previously had an infected prosthesis. In active patients with one shoulder involved I would prefer to do debridement and resection with possible subsequent arthrodesis. There have been a few exceptions to this rule; however, I almost never advise another prosthesis when there has been a previously infected prosthesis.

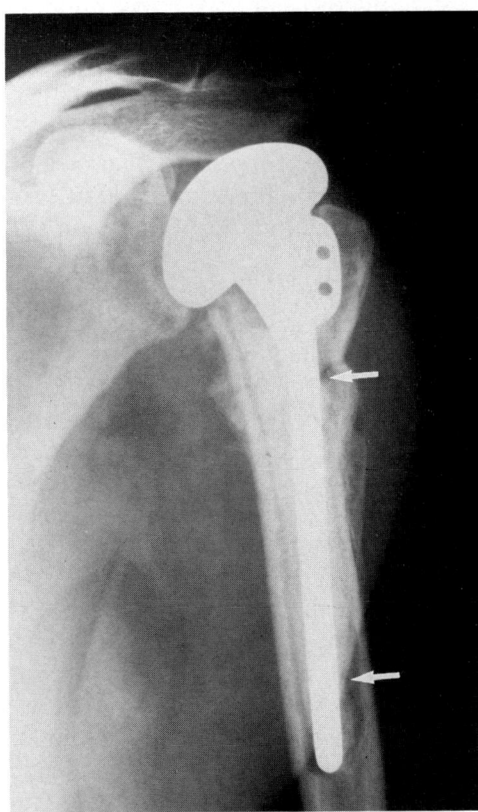

Figure 3–93. ***Shoulder Arthroplasty After Infection.*** Anterior-posterior view of an infected prosthesis showing bone involvement (arrows). I do not use another prosthesis in this situation but do a "cleanout," administer appropriate antibiotics, and prescribe sling immobilization for three or four months. An arthrodesis later is rarely required.

RECONSTRUCTION AFTER PROXIMAL HUMERAL NEOPLASMS

The proximal humerus is one of the sites of predilection for low-grade malignant tumors requiring en bloc resections such as fibrosarcomas, chondrosarcomas, and giant cell tumors, as discussed in detail in Chapter 6, p. 458. En bloc resection usually involves removal of the articular surface, the tuberosities, and varying lengths of the diaphysis of the proximal humerus.[93, 142] Rarely, as in two shoulders I have treated with "recurrent" chondroblastoma, it is possible to excise the tumor, leaving at least a portion of the greater tuberosity with some of the insertions of the supraspinatus and external rotators. On these rare occasions it is possible to do a simple head replacement with rotator cuff reconstruction.

These two possibilities will be considered separately. A key to preserving the muscles essential for active motion following arthroplasties for neoplasms is a carefully planned and carefully executed biopsy;[116] the technique of biopsy will also be discussed.

Greater Tuberosity Spared

Neoplasms requiring humeral head replacement alone are rare. The requirements are a benign tumor with destruction and collapse of the articular surface that spares most of the greater tuberosity (see Chapter 6, p. 465 and Fig. 6–27). The only condition I have seen meeting these requirements is a very large chondroblastoma. Perforations of the articular surface, as occur when treating smaller lesions, are treated by filling the defect with an iliac bone graft rather than a prosthesis.

In either case, previous scars are excised, and a deltopectoral approach is used. I prefer to detach the subscapularis and make a window in the lesser tuberosity for the removal of the tumor. Gouges and osteotomes are used rather than a curette to excise the lesion cleanly without spreading tumor cells in the wound. Complete excision of the tumor is the first objective. Following this, the humeral component can be implanted in the usual way. The full standard exercise program can be given, and near normal function can be expected.

Reconstruction After Proximal Humeral Resection

This procedure is performed after resection of the proximal humerus for a fibrosarcoma, giant cell tumor, or chondrosarcoma, but to date has not been performed for a metastatic tumor or a high-grade primary neoplasm. Possibly in the future if pharmaceutical and roentgen control of these latter lesions is improved, en bloc resection of them may also be indicated.

Removal of the proximal humerus detaches all of the rotator cuff muscles as well as the pectoralis major, teres minor, and latissimus dorsi. The deltoid insertion is usually spared. The long head of the biceps remains intact and acts to stabilize the head when it can be saved.

Although such an extensive loss of bone and soft tissue would seem to preclude an unconstrained glenohumeral arthroplasty, stability can be regained if two essentials are achieved. First, the length of the humerus should be maintained to exert tension on the myofascial sleeve, as shown in Figures 3–26D, 3–94, and 3–95. Second, the rotator cuff should be re-attached at least in back (and if at all possible in front) to prevent anterior and posterior dislocation. If the subscapularis is lost, the pectoralis major can be used as a substitute. Of course, if the rotator cuff tendons are available, all are carefully re-attached to the fibular graft. Ideally, one day a material capable of allowing ingrowth and re-attachment of tendons will be developed; however, it is useless to sew tendons to present materials, and bone grafts must be used for re-attachment of the soft tissues. Retaining active overhead elevation of the shoulder depends on preserving the deltoid muscle. This structure must be kept in mind during the biopsy, during the approach, and, as far as possible, during the extraction of the tumor. A posterior approach might seem logical to preserve the anterior deltoid intact, and this approach is more feasible after an en bloc resection because, unlike the situation in standard glenohumeral arthroplasties in which the importance of retaining the external rotators intact is recognized, removal of the upper humerus detaches the external rotators anyway. Therefore, a posterior approach might be valid as far as preserving the deltoid muscle is concerned. Of course, the axillary and radial nerves are more in the way and must be respected if a posterior approach is selected. In all of my patients there have been previous surgical scars anteriorly that required excision at the time of the en bloc resection, and therefore an anterior approach was used.

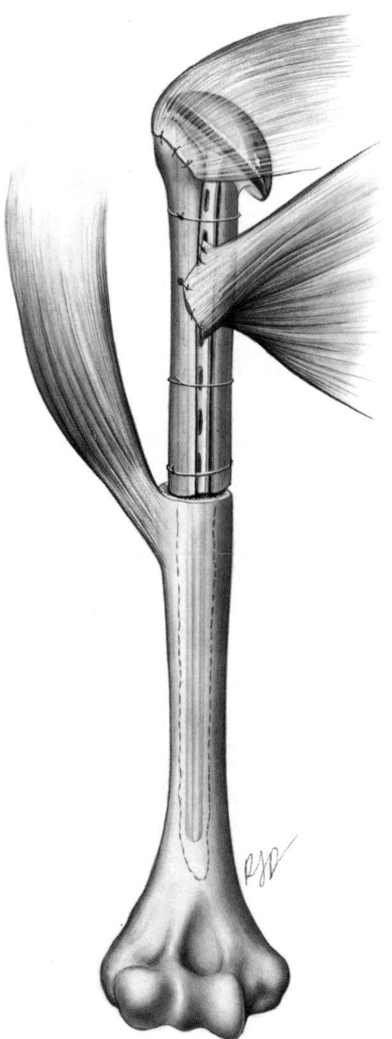

Figure 3–94. ***Arthroplasty After En Bloc Resection of Proximal Humeral Neoplasms.*** Objective of the procedure. The cemented long-stem humeral component maintains the normal length of the arm, placing tension on the neurovascular sleeve, which, along with the re-attachment of the muscles, gives stability. The autogenous fibular grafts are protected against fractures by the prosthesis as they become re-vascularized. My personal series is described on page 251.

Substitutes for the loss of the rotator cuff muscles are illustrated in Figure 3–31. If the infraspinatus and teres minor have been excised, the latissimus dorsi can be re-attached posteriorly to give some external rotating power and to act as a humeral head depressor; however, it is a less effective stabilizer of the head. The sternal head of the pectoralis major can be re-attached at a higher level in an effort to replace the subscapularis.

If resection of the humerus must be done below the deltoid insertion, the deltoid is re-attached to the bone graft at the normal distance from the acromion to preserve its length.

A long-stemmed humeral prosthesis is used, and the stem must be cut at the proper length preoperatively. An x-ray is made of the good humerus with a metal ruler or marker to determine the proper length of stem. Prior to cementing the humeral component, a biopsy is made of the stump of the humerus. The humeral component is then cemented in the remaining shaft of the humerus to give it the necessary stability for healing of the bone graft.

A glenoid component is used if the tumor involves the joint mandating resection of the articular surface of the glenoid, if the articular surface of the glenoid is atrophied and imperfect due to previous surgery or delays, or if the rotator cuff is defective and in the surgeon's judgment a glenoid component might improve the stability of the head.

After resecting the upper tumor, the length of the fibular graft is determined by measuring from the glenoid to the stump of the humerus and adding 2.0 cm. for overlap. The grafts are allowed to overlap at their junction with the shaft for better healing. The fibula is split with a hand drill and osteotome (rather than a power tool, which heats the bone). When the humeral component has been cemented at the proper length, the fibular grafts are anchored to the stem of the prosthesis with No. 5 or No. 2 nonabsorbable sutures. Extra bone fragments are distributed about the junction of the grafts and the humeral stump. Drill holes are made at the top of the graft for nonabsorbable sutures that are used to re-attach the rotator cuff. All other tendons that have been detached are re-attached to the bone graft at their approximate normal site of insertion using nonabsorbable sutures.

It is especially important for the surgeon to set goals for a realistic exercise program and to eliminate confusion between the patient and therapist In addition, he can reassure the patient, who constantly worries about recurrence of the neoplasm. The patient needs cheer and confidence to have peace of mind.

The arm is maintained in a sling for five months to allow the tendons to become re-attached to the grafts before the limited goals exercise program is started (Chapter 7, p. 530). A few patients have enough muscles remaining to be advanced to overhead exercises.

Among the seven patients who had been followed for two years, in the series shown in Table 3–1, one case of radial nerve palsy and one case of perineal nerve palsy cleared spontaneously without residuum. One nonunion between the graft and the humerus occurred in an early case in which no cement was used to anchor the stem of the prosthesis. This required cementing the stem and bone grafting. There were no other significant complications and no recurrences of the tumor. One patient whose deltoid muscle had been preserved by a well-planned biopsy and resection was able to achieve essentially a full range of active motion. The others had too much loss of muscle tissue; however, they were pleased with good function of the arm at the side with stability, freedom from pain, and the ability to perform everyday activities.

None of the patients in this series was under

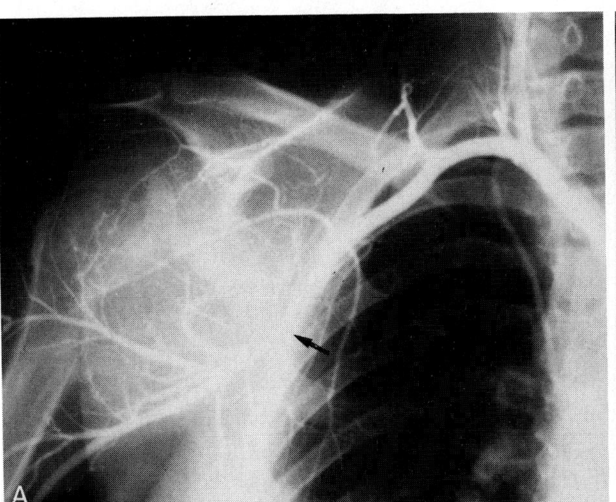

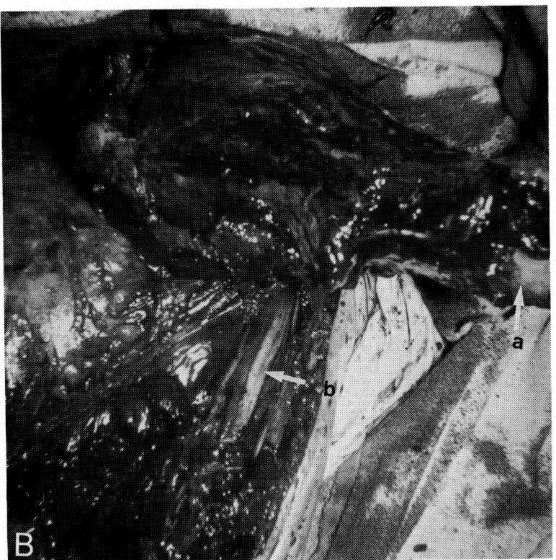

Figure 3–95. ***Arthroplasty After En Bloc Resection of Proximal Humeral Neoplasms.*** An example of this method is shown in parts A through F.

A, Arteriogram in a 19 year old patient who had had two recurrences of a chondroblastoma. The large tumor displaced the neurovascular bundle (arrow), protruded toward the infraclavicular region, and involved the glenohumeral joint. Nevertheless, re-biopsy revealed the histology of typical chondroblastoma. En bloc resection without entering the tumor was advised.

B, All previous operative scars and the part of anterior deltoid exposed were removed with the specimen, as was the glenohumeral joint including the articular surface of the glenoid and the intact joint capsule. This photograph was made after the humerus had been divided just proximal to the insertion of the deltoid muscle. The humeral shaft is at (a) and the neurovascular bundle is at (b). The axillary nerve is intact, as are the posterior and medial parts of the deltoid muscle. Frozen section biopsy of the distal stump of humerus showed no tumor cells.

Illustration continued on following page

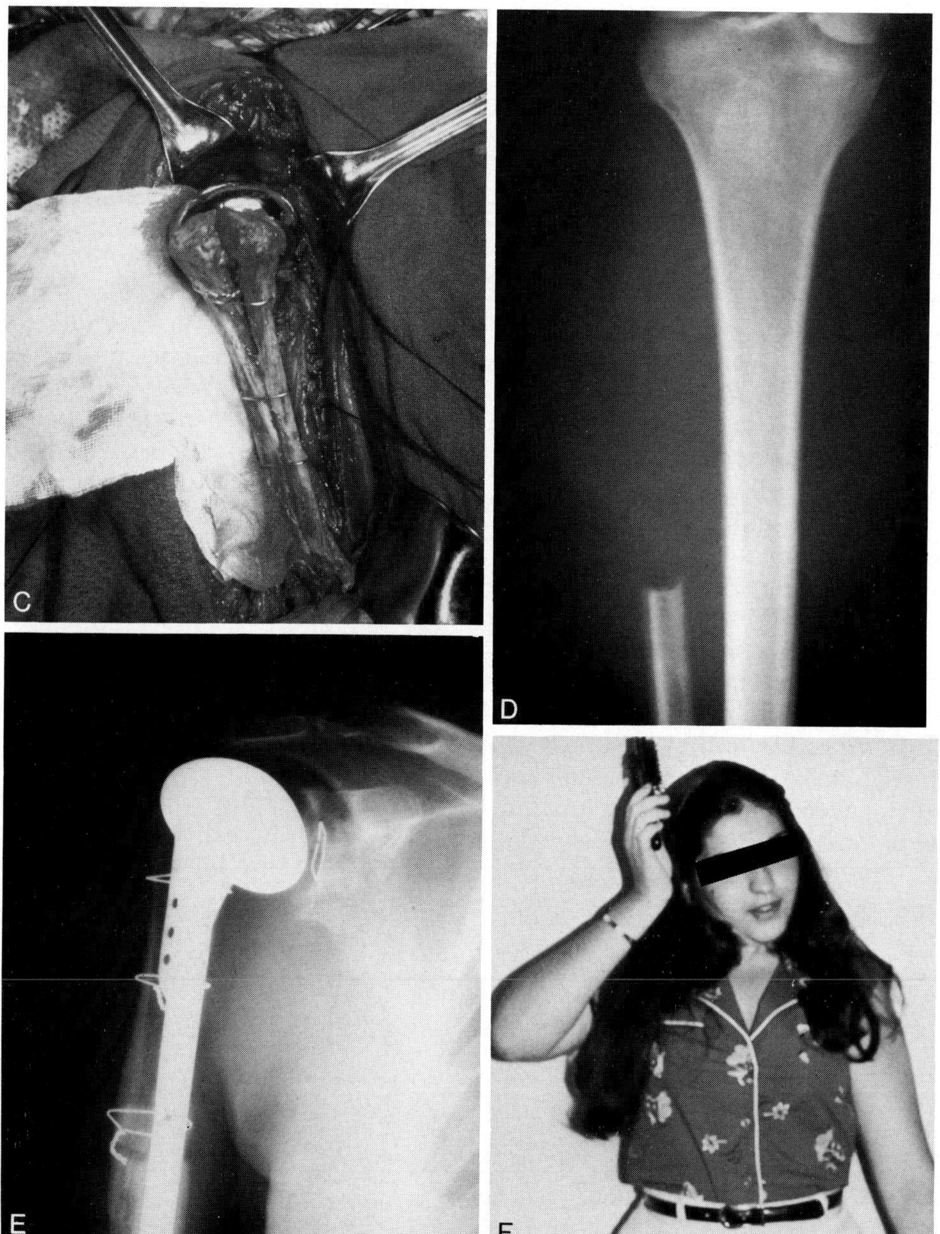

Figure 3–95 *Continued* C, Pre-operative scanogram for length on the humerus had been made, and the stem of the prosthesis had been cut at the proper length pre-operatively. After cementing a standard polyethylene glenoid component into the re-contoured stump of the glenoid, the humeral prosthesis was cemented in place while light traction was applied to the arm. The head of the humeral prosthesis was maintained in 40 degrees retroversion and opposite the glenoid component for proper length. After measuring the length of fibula required (to re-form a greater tuberosity and overlap the humeral shaft by 2.0 cm.), a fibular graft was obtained. The fibular graft was split in half lengthwise and secured to the prosthesis with circlage wires (nonabsorbable sutures are now used instead of wire). All of the muscles were then attached to the grafts. The arm was protected with a sling for six months, and a limited goals rehabilitation program followed.

D, The fibular donor site.

E and F, Follow-up four years later. The grafts had united with the shaft. Function was limited only by the loss of the anterior deltoid (F). Patient has now been followed eight years without recurrence of tumor or other complications.

At late follow-up there was stress-shielding osteopenia at the proximal end of the graft in all of the patients in this series, but the muscles remained attached, and the prostheses remained stable.

17 years of age; however, I have seen two other patients operated on elsewhere who had growing epiphyses at the time of removal of the proximal humerus. Although the proximal humeral epiphysis supplies 80 per cent of the length of the arm, continuing growth eventually made the humeral prostheses that were used in these patients too short. A humeral component with an expandable stem should be considered if a prosthesis is used when the bone is still growing.

Technique of Biopsy of Proximal Humeral Neoplasms

The objective of a biopsy is to obtain adequate samplings of tissue for formal histological sections and cultures without spilling tumor cells outside of the humerus. A cannulated trocar is preferred when possible, but adequate tissue may not be obtained with it. I prefer to have the pathologist in the operating room to perform frozen sections to determine whether the specimen is adequate. If an open biopsy is required, it can be done as described below.

When a cannula is used, it is inserted in the deltopectoral interval so that the track can later be easily excised with little loss of deltoid muscle.

If it is necessary to do an open biopsy, the smallest possible incision is made with minimal stripping of the humerus. The tissue is covered with packs and plastic drapes to prevent contact with the tumor cells. A 2.5 cm. incision and a 1.0 cm. window in the bone should be adequate to obtain tissue from several parts of the lesion. An angulated curette is used for this purpose. When adequate tissue has been removed, the window in the bone is sealed with acrylic cement to prevent spillage of tumor cells outside of bone.[116] The skin is closed in hairline fashion with a single running subcuticular suture for direct and rapid healing.

As mentioned above, after division of the shaft of the humerus, a biopsy is made of the stump, and a frozen section is made to be sure there is no "skip area" of tumor cells, which is especially likely to occur in chondrosarcoma (see Chapter 6, Fig. 6–31).

ARTHROPLASTY AFTER GLENOHUMERAL FUSION

Anatomical Problem

Following glenohumeral fusion, shoulder motion is limited to scapular movements as discussed in Chapter 6, page 438. Elevation is limited to about 60 degrees, and rotation of the humerus, which is the most important function of the glenohumeral joint, is lost. At best, a fusion creates difficulty in reaching the top of the head, the opposite axilla, or the anal region for self-care. It usually precludes sleeping on the involved side.

The technique of arthroplasty after glenohumeral fusion (Fig. 3–96) involves exacting osteotomies. To preserve the glenoid and acromion, it is better to err on the side of removing too much humerus. An anterior acromioplasty makes room for the trapezius or whatever muscle is to be used for the supraspinatus. The trapezius is most available but is not ideal because it does not depress the humeral head but instead tends to displace it upward. The "calcar sling" (Fig. 3–96C) is helpful

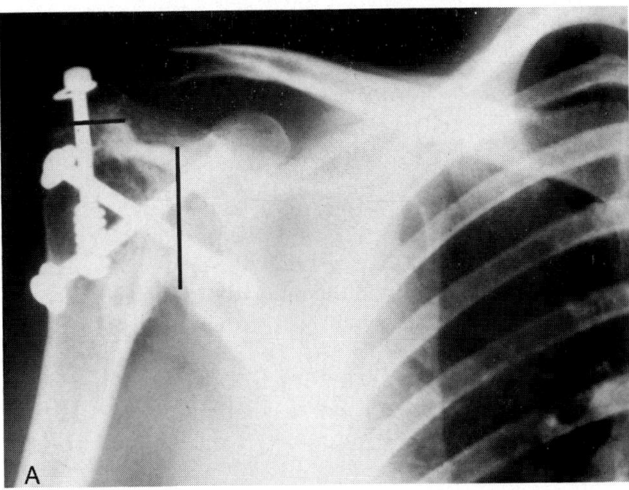

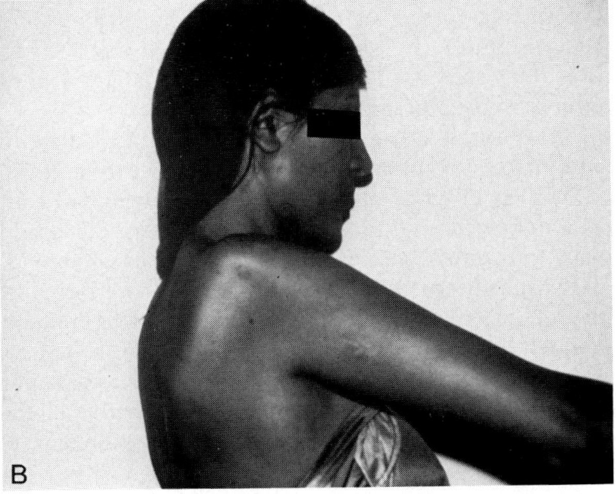

Figure 3–96. ***Arthroplasty After Glenohumeral Fusion.***
A and B, Preoperative appearance. Film is marked at the sites for osteotomies. Anterior acromioplasty is planned. Finding the correct levels for the osteotomy cuts is made easier at surgery by seeing the remains of the capsule and ligaments.

Illustration continued on following page

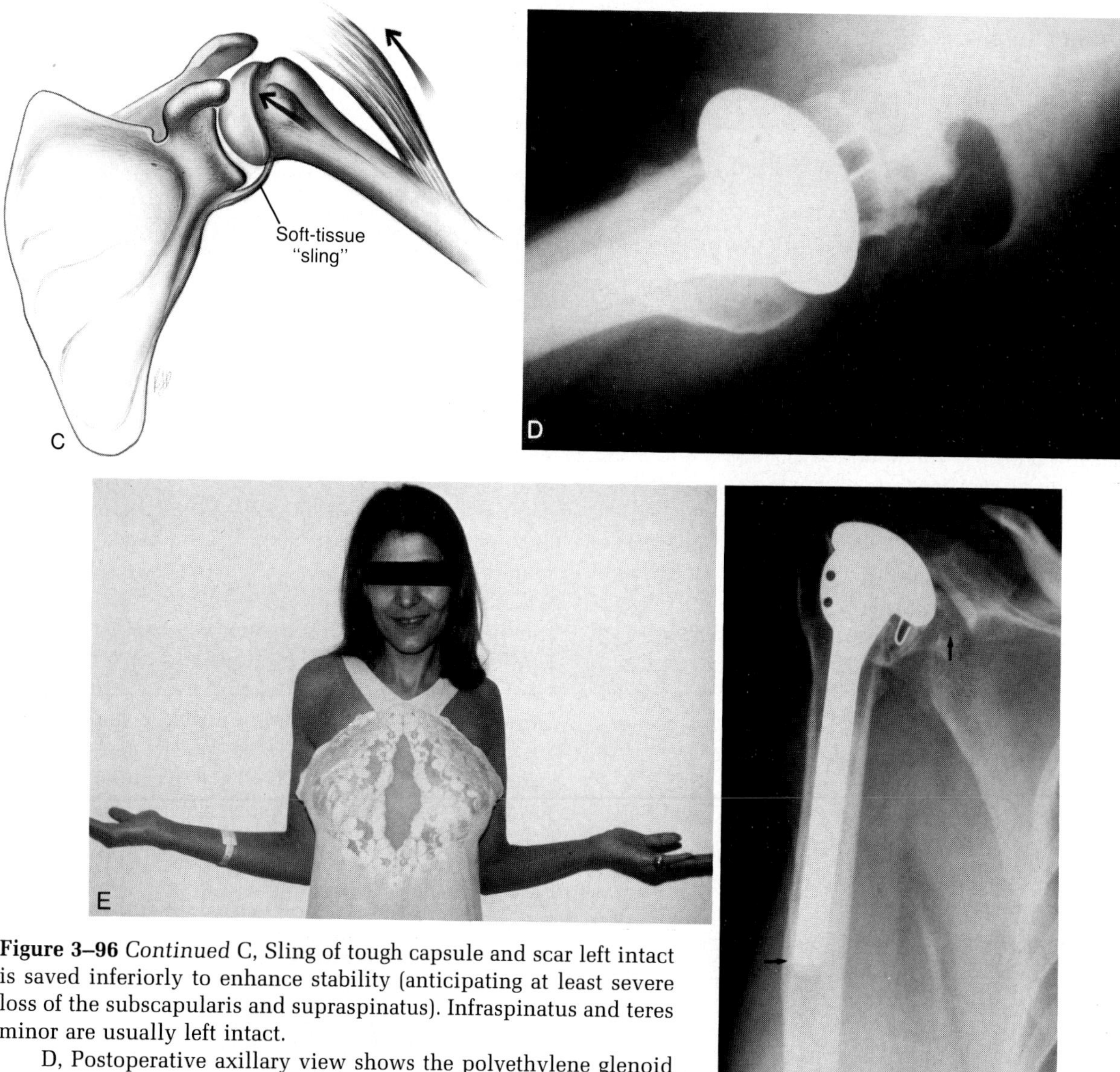

Figure 3–96 *Continued* C, Sling of tough capsule and scar left intact is saved inferiorly to enhance stability (anticipating at least severe loss of the subscapularis and supraspinatus). Infraspinatus and teres minor are usually left intact.

D, Postoperative axillary view shows the polyethylene glenoid and humeral component implanted at the correct level.

E, An 11 year follow-up of a patient who had had this procedure (with a strong calcar sling capsule) as well as a deltoidplasty (transferring the posterior and middle deltoid anteriorly; see Fig. 3–33), and a transfer of the pectoralis minor with extension for the subscapularis and of the trapezius for the supraspinatus. A revision of the deltoidplasty was done nine years after the arthroplasty, at which time the components were inspected through the rotator interval and found to be intact without much wear. The patient had no pain, felt strong, went swimming frequently, and was pleased with the result.

F, Radiographic follow-up at 11 years showing dense bone at the tip of the stem of the uncemented humeral component (lower arrow), which was indicative of good active use of the arm. There was no radiolucent line at the bone-cement interface of the glenoid component (upper arrow).

in obtaining stability immediately, and because the muscles are usually inadequate for more than limited goals function to be expected (see p. 530), it is not important that it might restrict overhead motion.

It is hoped that, with a clearer definition of the indications for fusion and its limitations, the procedure of converting a fusion to an arthroplasty will not be required in the future.

REVISION ARTHROPLASTY

Anatomical Problem

Bone loss, muscle loss, scar, the threat of fractures, and the greater risk of infection make this category the most difficult for arthroplasty. The problem differs from that in the hip or knee because of the great importance of the rotator cuff and other muscles in regaining function. The procedure aims to achieve not only a painless, stable fulcrum but also reconstruction of the rotator cuff while leaving the deltoid undisturbed or, if detached, in a functional state.

It is important to analyze the cause of the failure as much as possible pre-operatively. The factors needing investigation are listed in Table 3–5 with the means of investigation to be considered. Analysis of specific anatomical problems requires a good understanding of the principles discussed in Figures 3–24 through 3–33 and illustrated in Figures 3–97 to 3–99.

Table 3–5. PRE-REVISION INVESTIGATION FOR CAUSES OF FAILURE

GENERAL	
Psychological	Lack of motivation, alcoholism
Nerve injury or cervical root defect	Electromyograms, etc.
Arthritis	Acromioclavicular or sternoclavicular joints
Scapulothoracic mechanism	Weakness or deformity
LOCAL	
Infection	Aspiration and cultures, scans, frozen section during surgery
Instability	Dislocations
Heterotopic bone	Delay revision if active
Deltoid defects	Detached, retracted, scarred
Cuff defects	Contractures, adhesions, detached
Bone defects	Bone loss, bony prominence, nonunion, impingement, retracted tuberosity, retained head, too long, loss of length, glenoid slope, "centralization," pannus erosion
Contractures and adhesions	Always present
IMPLANT	
Humeral component	Version, height, head length, stability, stem size, loosening, breakage, cement
Glenoid component	Version, face upward, height, loosening, breakage, wear, cement

Personal Series

In 1982, Kirby and I published a report on a series of 40 revision arthroplasties I had performed between 1973 and 1981. During the past six years there have been 22 additional revisions, making a total of 67 in the present series. The most frequent causes of failure in fixed-fulcrum implants have been loss of the external rotators and mechanical failure. The safest fixed-fulcrum implant is one buried in scar tissue for support.

The most common causes of failure of unconstrained implants include deltoid scars and detachment, tight subscapularis tendon with loss of external rotation, prominent or retracted greater tuberosity, loss of humeral length, inadequate glenoid, and an inadequate exercise program causing adhesions, as illustrated in Figure 3–97A.

Contraindications to revision arthroplasty are (1) infection, or (2) paralysis or loss of both the rotator cuff and the deltoid muscles.

The results of 40 revisions were analyzed[22, 110] and were not as good as results in the other diagnostic categories because, as illustrated in Figure 3–97, many difficult lesions were accepted for reconstruction. Nevertheless, satisfactory pain relief and function for daily activities were obtained in all but five patients using a nonconstrained prosthesis and reconstructing the tissue as discussed. The full rehabilitation program was followed in 23 patients with an "excellent" rating in only ten patients. Seventeen patients required a limited goals program, and the remaining had marginal results, usually because of muscle deficits rather than pain (see Fig. 3–100).

Special Steps in Revision Arthroplasty

Rather than making more general statements, it seems necessary to illustrate some specific problems that show the primary defects and the treatment employed (see Figs. 3–98 to 3–99). All of the principles of unconstrained arthroplasty are used in these procedures (see Figs. 3–24 through 3–33).

Text continued on page 262

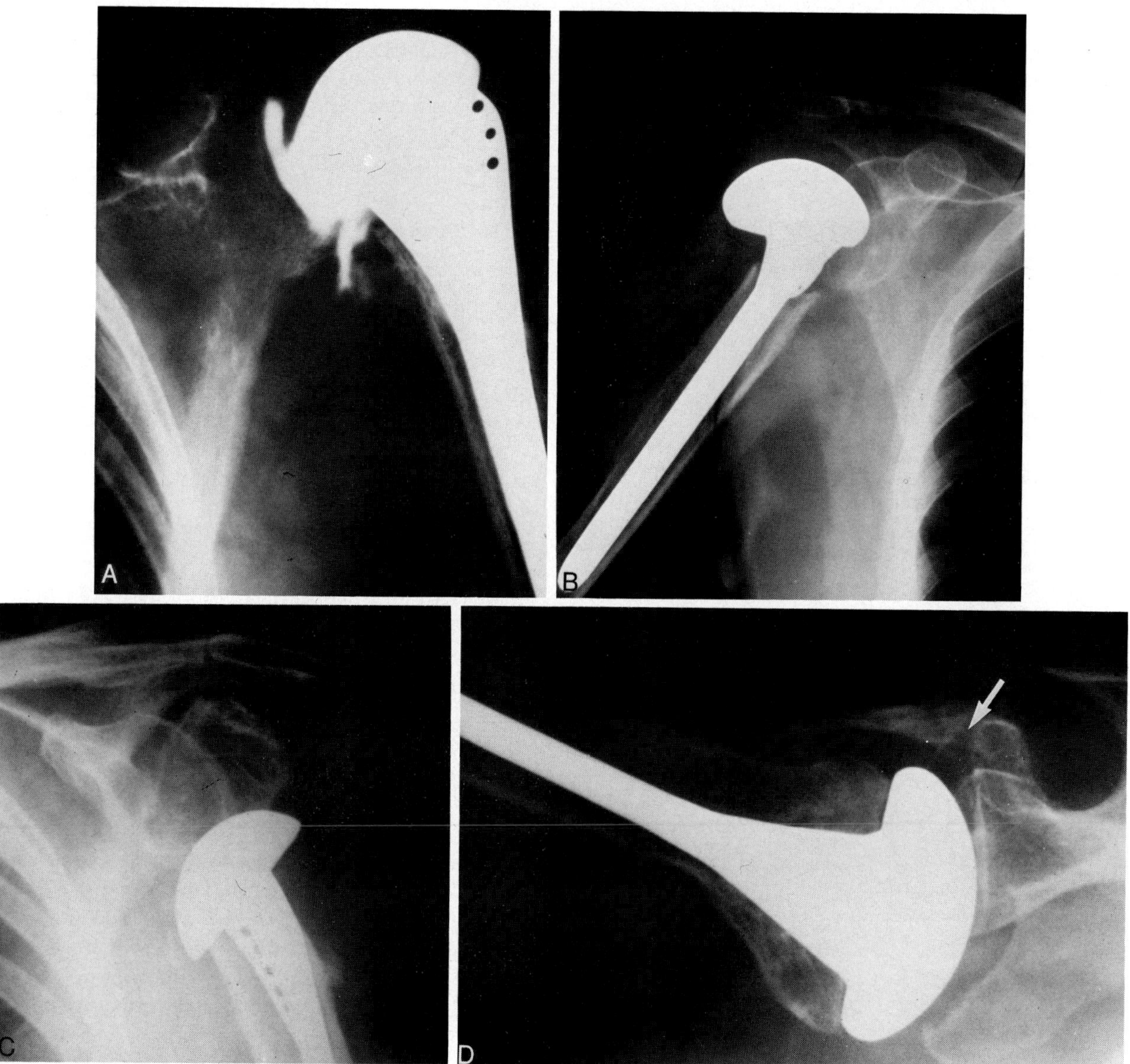

Figure 3–97. Some causes of failure encountered at revision surgery after replacement of the humeral head for fractures.

A, The most common cause of failure is inadequate aftercare. Arthrogram shows almost complete obliteration of the joint space due to scar tissue, indicating a "frozen shoulder." All "failed prostheses" are surrounded by scar. Extensive releases and early motion are required.

B, Tuberosities had been excised. The stem of the prosthesis is loose and spins in the humerus. This situation is treated by cementing the humeral component, inserting an iliac bone graft for the tuberosity, and reconstructing the rotator cuff.

C, Fractured tuberosities were not connected. The prosthesis was seated too low and has dislocated because of loss of length.

D, Axillary view shows a greater tuberosity (arrow) that has united to the scapula with a retracted, short infraspinatus. This required a second approach posteriorly.

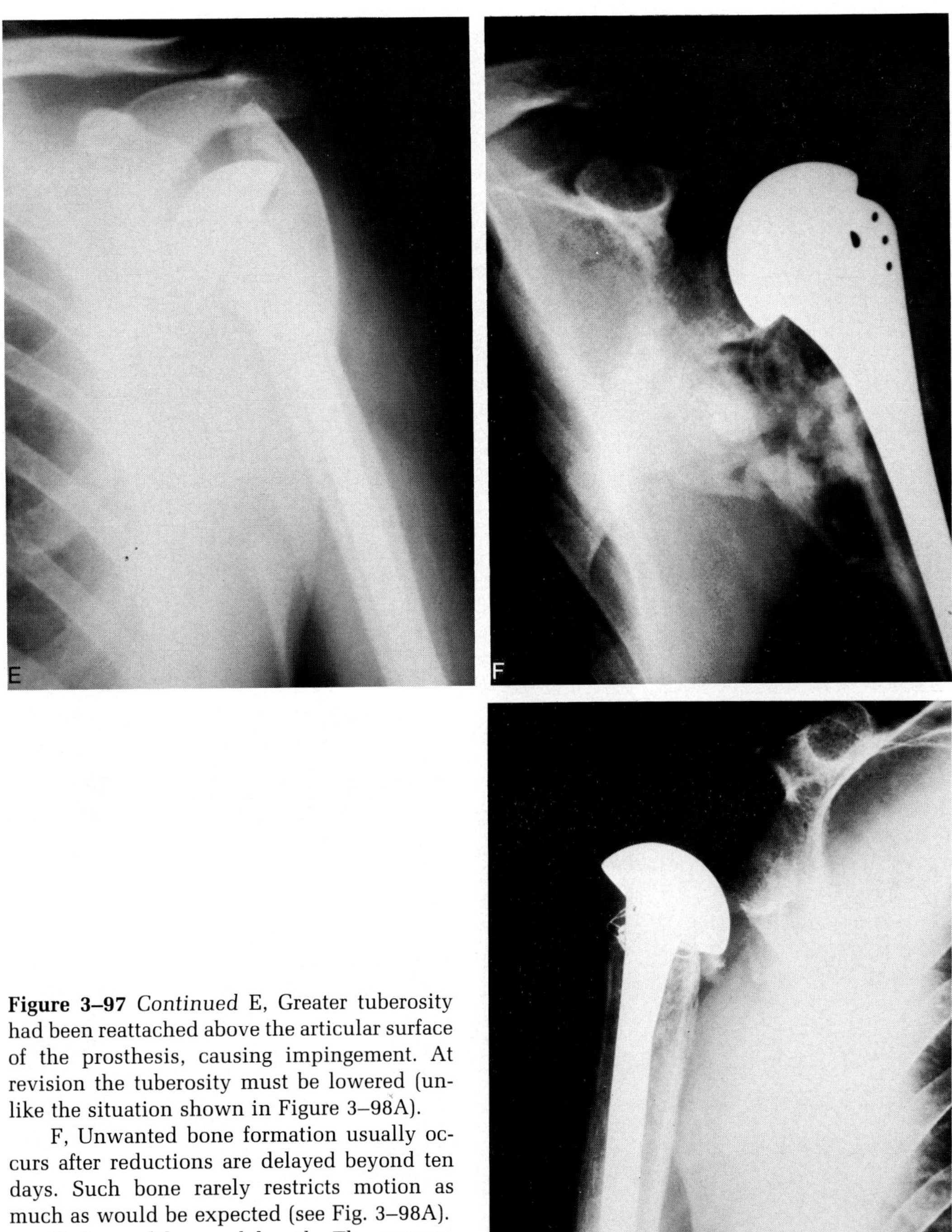

Figure 3–97 *Continued* E, Greater tuberosity had been reattached above the articular surface of the prosthesis, causing impingement. At revision the tuberosity must be lowered (unlike the situation shown in Figure 3–98A).

F, Unwanted bone formation usually occurs after reductions are delayed beyond ten days. Such bone rarely restricts motion as much as would be expected (see Fig. 3–98A).

G, Loss of humeral length. The surgeon failed to put tension on the myofascial sleeve, the prosthesis dislocated, and the deltoid muscle could not raise the arm. The rotator cuff alone does not keep the head in the socket. This situation required bone grafts to regain humeral length and reconstruction of the tuberosity and cuff.

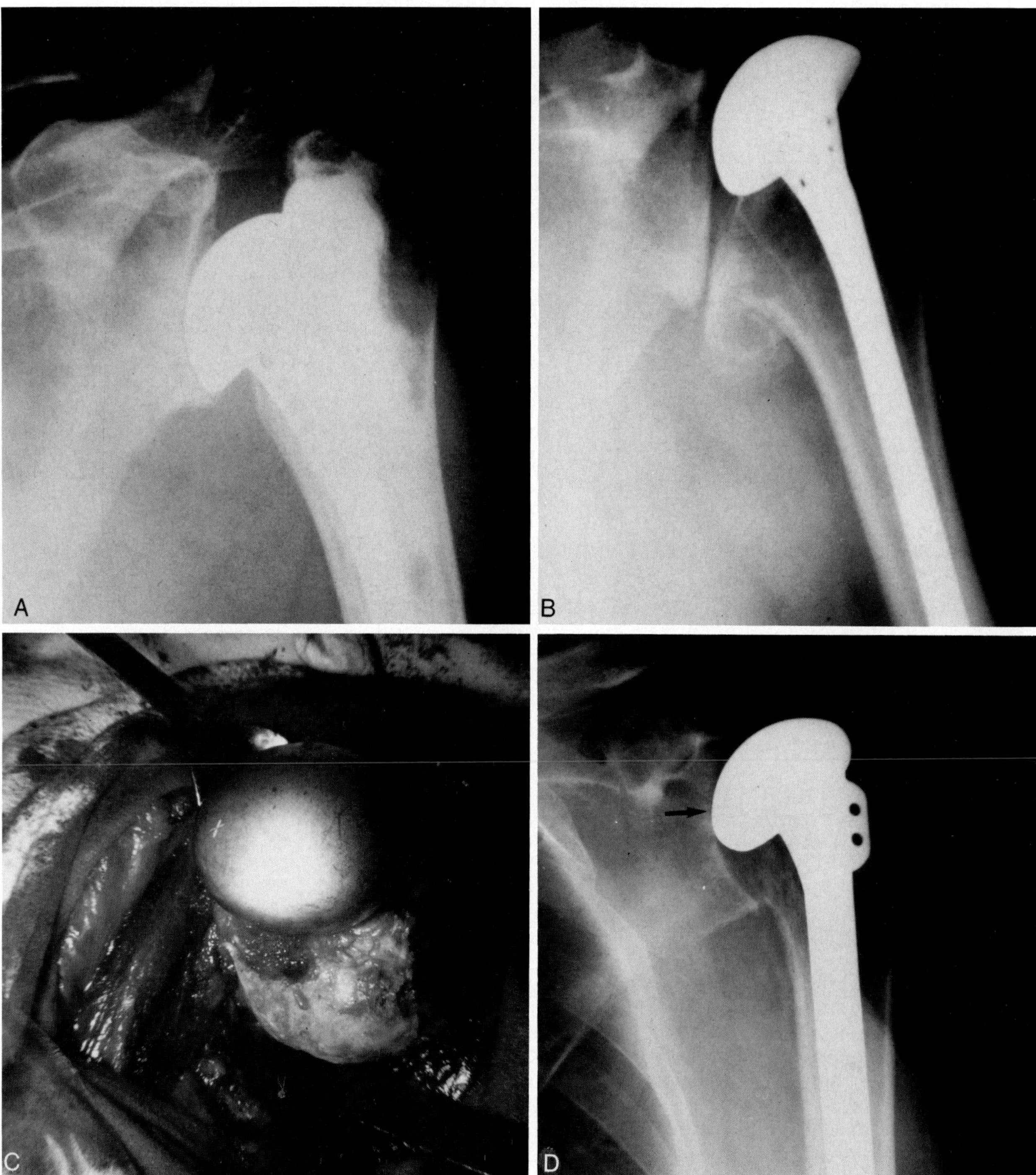

Figure 3–98. Some causes of failure encountered at revision arthroplasty are shown in this figure.

A, Low placement of prosthesis causing a prominent greater tuberosity with impingement. At revision the new prosthesis must be set higher, unlike the situation shown in Figure 3–97E.

B and C, Retained humeral head.

D, Stiff shoulder causing erosion of the glenoid (arrow) by the prosthesis.

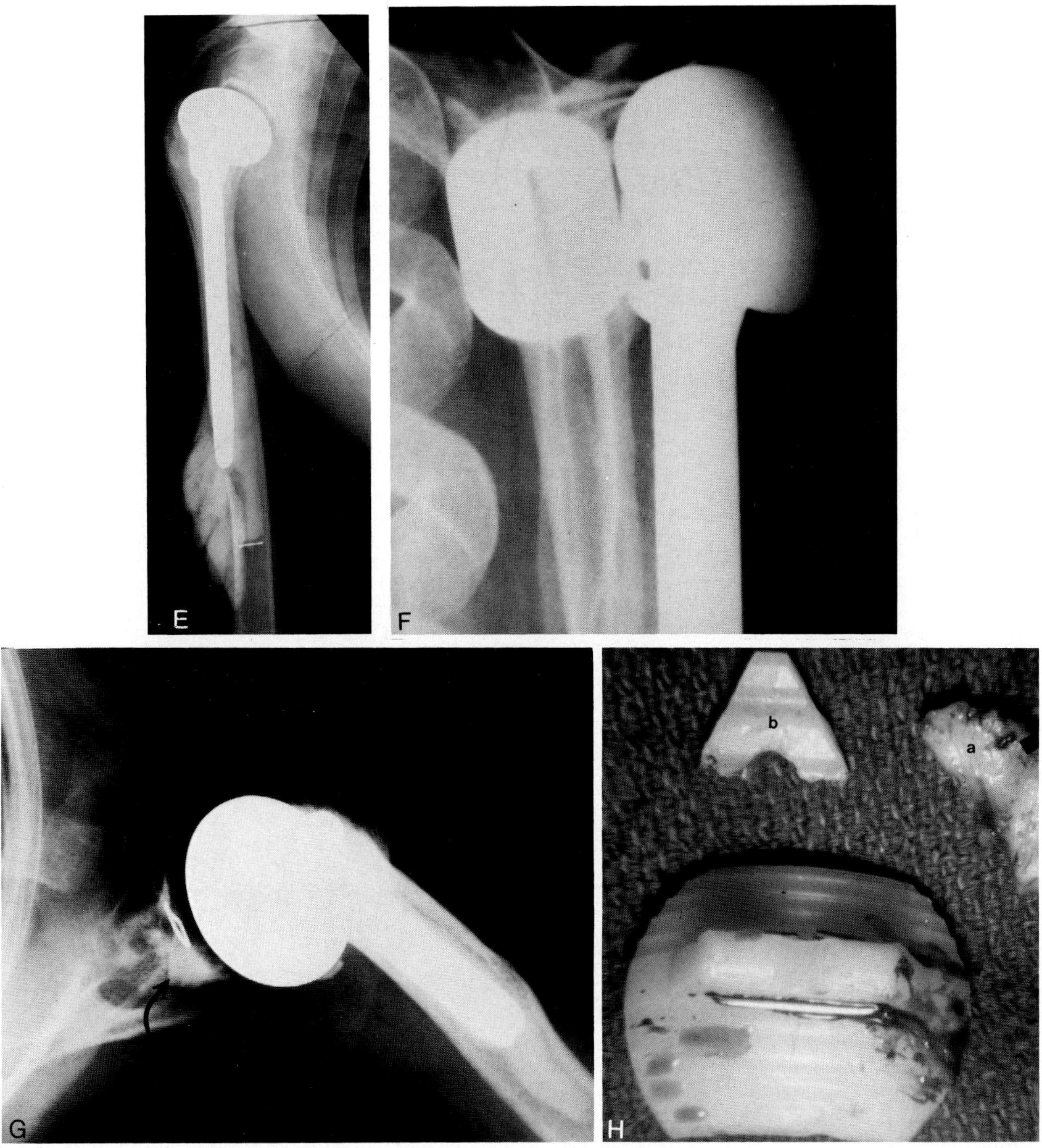

Figure 3–98 *Continued* E, The humeral shaft can be very soft, especially in patients with rheumatoid arthritis. Cement-gun pressure has been seen to cause extrusion of cement with radial nerve palsy in two patients.

F, Loose placement of the glenoid component at surgery caused the components to dislocate at the end of the operation.

G and H, The error was made of building up cement under the prosthesis (arrow) to compensate for uneven glenoid erosion (axillary view). H, The cement (a) broke out from under the prosthesis, causing a toggling motion of the glenoid, which finally broke the stem of the polyethylene glenoid at the proximal groove. The tip of the stem (b) was firmly imbedded in the bone and cement and was not loose (see I and J). To remedy this problem, the groove in the polyethylene component was removed and a new metal-backed glenoid component was cemented, making sure it was supported by bone on all sides.

Illustration continued on following page

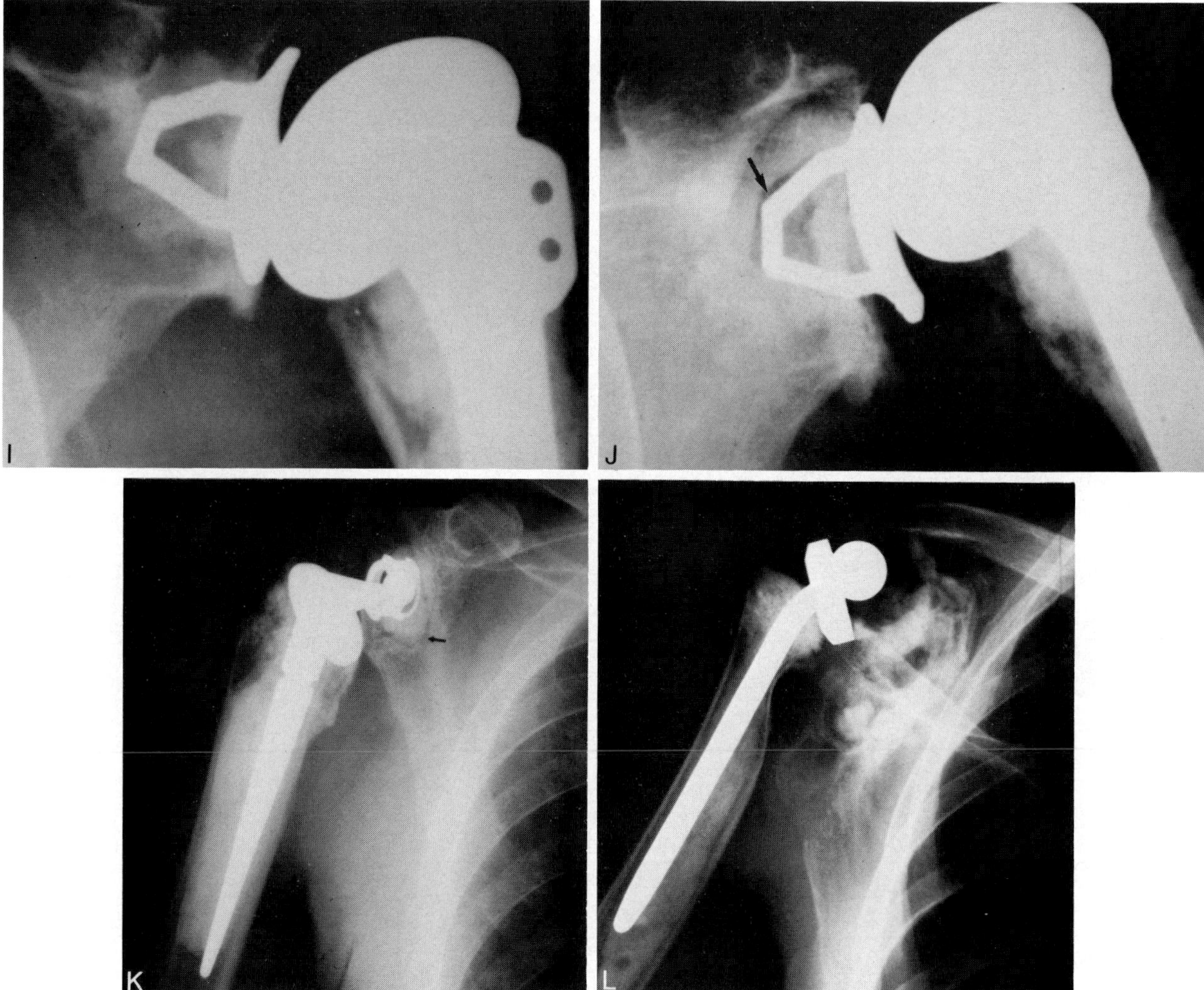

Figure 3–98 *Continued* I and J, Error of shallow seating of the glenoid component placing tilting (rocking) stress on the component is shown in I. This mistake caused the component to break out of the cement (arrow) about three months after surgery (J). (Note that the bone-cement interface remained solid.)

K, Error of detachment of the rotator cuff and partial detachment of the deltoid. The shoulder was stiff and painful, but despite the lucent line (arrow) at the bone-cement interface, the prosthesis was firmly anchored in the scapula.

L, Depicting the errors of a fixed fulcrum broken out of the glenoid, a radical acromionectomy, and excising the tuberosity and cuff.

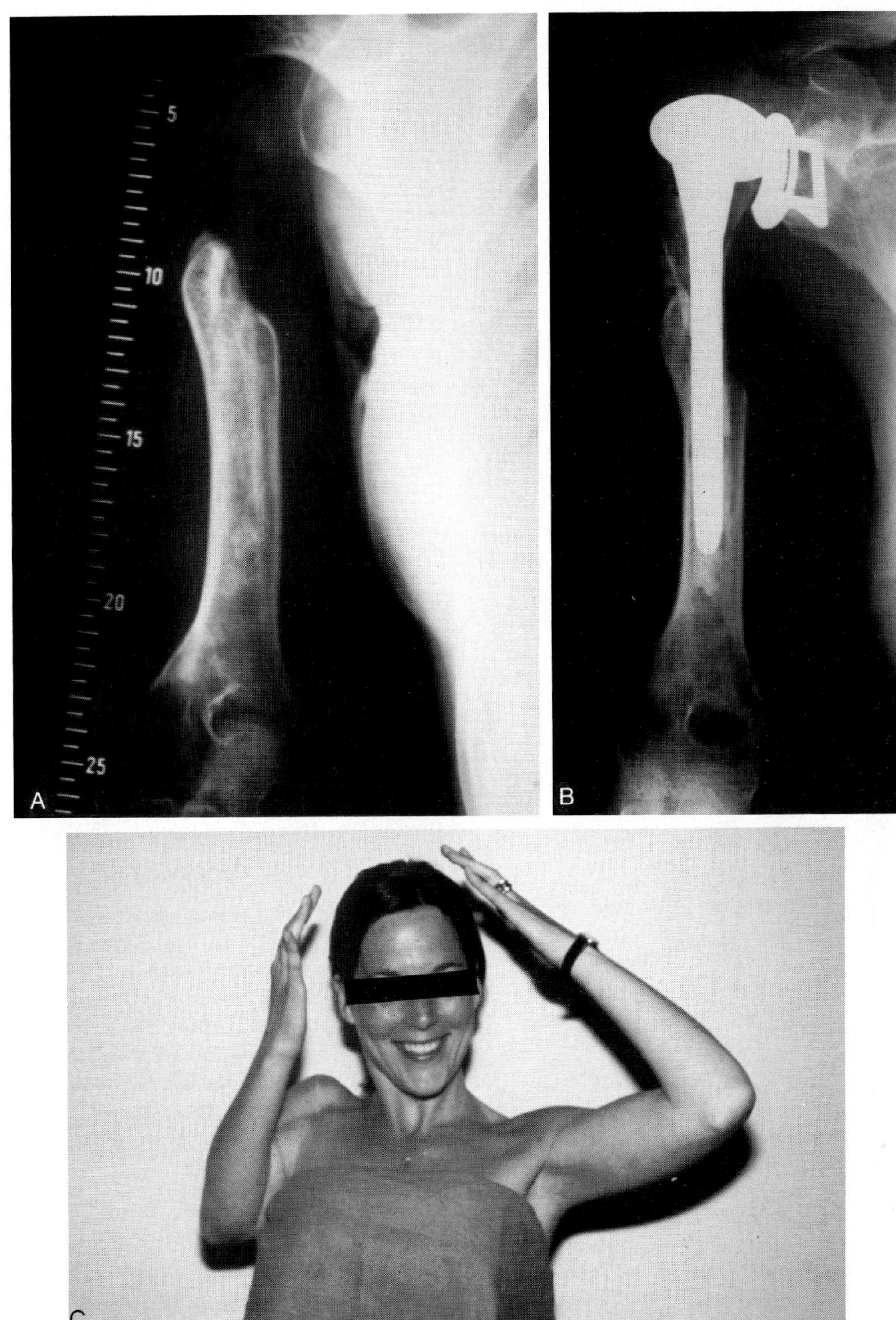

Figure 3–99. A, Proximal humeral prosthesis implanted at the age of 12 because of a tumor became too short, dislocated, and had been removed ten years previously.

B, Autogenous fibular grafts, humeral and glenoid components (as in Fig. 3–95), and re-attachment of available muscles stabilized the shoulder.

C, Four years later there was good function at the side, the shoulder was stable, and rotation was possible despite deltoid muscle deficits.

RESULTS OF NONCONSTRAINED SHOULDER ARTHROPLASTY

The results to be expected have been considered under each specific diagnostic category. In this section, we briefly summarize the overall results and complications in my personal series and then briefly review the results in the literature. The results of humeral head replacement alone have been comparable (see Figs. 3–101 and 3–103).

Recent Personal Series

Overall Functional Results

The overall functional results of my recent series of 615 total shoulder arthroplasties in all diagnostic categories are shown in Figure 3–100 and Table 3–7 (see also Table 3–2). As of June 1988, the functional results in 408 shoulders in this series have been reviewed by examination for more than two years after total arthroplasty.[22, 269]

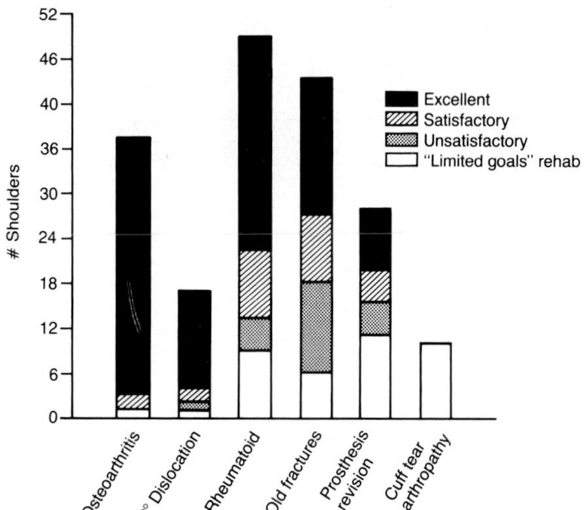

Figure 3–100. ***Results of Nonconstrained Shoulder Arthroplasty: Functional Results.*** Overall functional results of the 615 total shoulder arthroplasties (see Tables 3–1 and 3–7) are depicted. An excellent rating was achieved in the great majority of those with good muscles (patients with osteoarthritis or arthritis of dislocations). Many patients with low-grade rheumatoid arthritis have excellent ratings, but their recovery is slower, and some have bouts of muscle soreness when their arthritis flares. Some patients with long-standing rheumatoid arthritis have large rotator cuff defects and bone destruction requiring limited goals rehabilitation; this was true also of patients with old fractures and prosthetic revision. All of those with cuff-tear arthropathy had limited goals rehabilitation (but a few of those on the limited goals program were later advanced to the full program).

Forty-one shoulders were given limited goals rehabilitation and are considered separately.

Full Exercise Program

The criteria for rating the results of patients on the full exercise program are shown in Figures 3–101 and 3–102. The average gain in active total elevation in our 1982 series[22] was 77 degrees in patients with osteoarthritis, 57 degrees in patients with rheumatoid arthritis, 33 degrees in patients with old trauma, and 39 degrees in patients with revisions. The average gain in external rotation was 51 degrees in patients with osteoarthritis, 66 degrees in patients with arthritis of dislocations, 60 degrees in patients with rheumatoid arthritis, 58 degrees in patients with old trauma, and 44 degrees in patients with revisions. The functional results have improved during recent years because of the extended deltopectoral approach with an intact deltoid origin and improvements in earlier passive motion and exercise.

One of the patients (not in the above series) with a Neer I humeral head replacement and more than 30 years of follow-up who was last seen three years ago is illustrated (see Fig. 3–104). She is now 92 years of age. It is remarkable that none of the Neer I prostheses has required removal except in one patient—a clean case with a fracture, who had an early post-operative Staphylococcus aureus infection—and in six others who had their prostheses implanted after old infected fractures.

"Limited Goals" Rehabilitation

Those on the limited goals rehabilitation program were rated "satisfactory" if they had no significant pain, were pleased with the procedure, and were able to live normally with independent self-care. Otherwise, they were rated unsatisfactory. Of the 41 rated, 40 were satisfactory and one man was rated unsatisfactory. He is an illustration of how essential it is to stress pre-operatively that there is no chance of use of the arm overhead.

Complications

The complications in the 776 nonconstrained shoulder arthroplasties in the current series are listed in Table 3–6. Both of the infections occurred in patients who had positive culture results for Staphylococcus aureus in the shoulders at the time of the arthroplasty: one in an old fracture with internal fixation and the other in a patient with long-standing rheumatoid arthritis who had been treated with injections prior to surgery.

The broken polyethylene glenoid stems (see Fig. 3–98G and H) occurred because cement broke

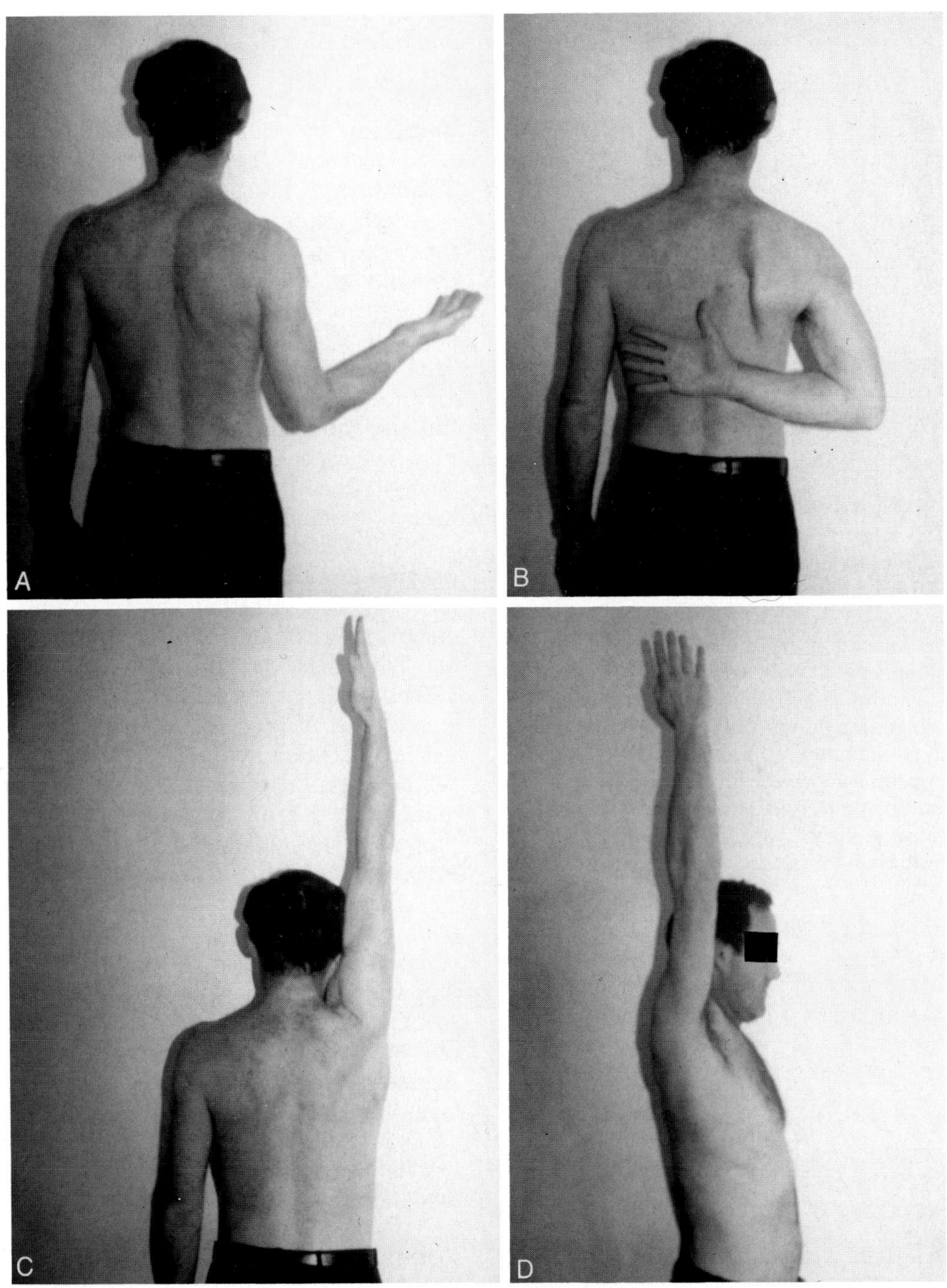

Figure 3–101A–D. ***Criteria for an "Excellent" Functional Result of Nonconstrained Shoulder Arthroplasty.*** Criteria for an "excellent" functional result for those on the full exercise program were as follows: The patient needed to demonstrate enthusiasm about the procedure, no significant pain, full use of the shoulder (except as advised against impact loads and heavy weight lifting exercise), muscle strength approaching normal, and active elevation to within 35 degrees and 90 percent of the rotation of the normal side. These patients did normal work (except heavy overhead steamfitting) and engaged in sports such as bowling, tennis, golf, and swimming. This patient, who had an "excellent" rating, illustrates his range of motion 11 years after arthroplasty: A, external rotation; B, internal rotation; C and D, elevation.

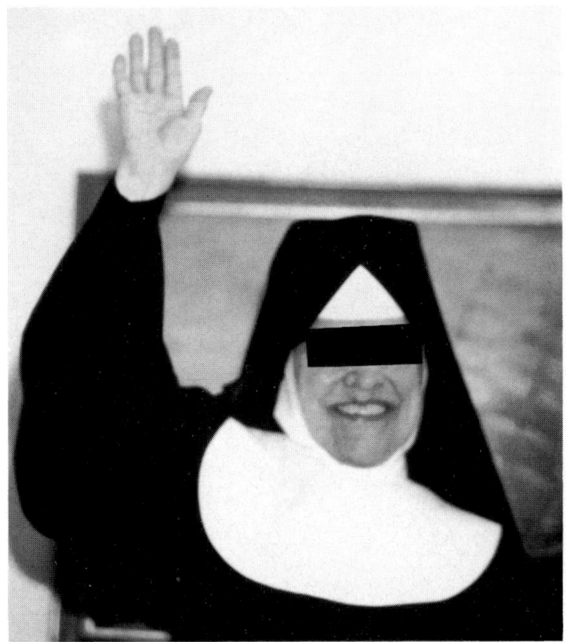

Figure 3–102. ***Criteria for a "Satisfactory" Functional Result of Nonconstrained Shoulder Arthroplasty:*** Criteria for "satisfactory" functional rating for those on the full exercise program were as follows: Patient was satisfied with the operation; had no more than occasional pain or weather-ache; at least good use of the arm for daily functions from the top of the head (to groom the hair) down, including crutch walking; and a minimum of 30 percent strength, 90 to 135 degrees elevation, and 50 percent rotation compared with the expected normal. This rheumatoid patient (who also had arthritic knees) exemplifies a satisfactory result. In an "unsatisfactory" result these criteria were not met.

out from under the component, and with loss of support, toggling motion occurred, eventually fatiguing the stem until it broke at the proximal groove. This emphasized the importance of ensuring bone support for the glenoid component and avoiding cement build-up. Also, the proximal groove was taken out of the polyethylene component. This complication has not recurred since the problem was recognized. It should be noted that the tip of the stem of the prosthesis was firmly embedded in bone and cement and was not loose. All five of these patients had been very active in sports and work and had had "excellent" functional results prior to this complication, and all have recovered completely after re-implantation of glenoid components.

Table 3–6. COMPLICATIONS REQUIRING FURTHER SURGERY IN CURRENT PERSONAL SERIES (776 NONCONSTRAINED ARTHROPLASTIES)

	NO. PATIENTS
Infection	2
Fracture out of bone	2
Re-repair of cuff	3
Late breakage of tuberosity wire	2
Excess anteversion	2
Nonunion of greater tuberosity	2
Broken stem of glenoid component	5
Loosening of glenoid component	2
Unexplained pain	2
	22*

*No alteration of components in seven. Alteration of components required in 1.9 percent, average follow-up six years.

Both of the glenoid component loosenings in this series have been treated surgically and have been illustrated. Shallow implantation of the component caused rocking stress and loosening of the component in the cement (see Fig. 3–98I and J). This loosening occurred in a recent case, and another glenoid component was re-implanted in this patient within a year from the original insertion. The second glenoid loosening involved a 200 percent glenoid component ten years after it had been implanted for cuff-tear arthropathy (see Fig. 3–96). The quality of bone in this glenoid had been poor originally, and the loose component was removed without further effort to implant another glenoid component. This stopped the patient's pain and had little effect on his function. I know of a patient with severe rheumatoid arthritis who had extremely bad glenoid bone at surgery and now has a definitely loose glenoid component with some migration of position; however, he has so many polyarthritic problems that the shoulder problem does not trouble him enough at this time to have the glenoid component removed.

The significance of radiolucent lines at the bone-cement interface without migration of the component is unclear, as illustrated in Figure 3–98K and discussed further in the next section on roentgenographic results. However, it is fair to say that the incidence of clinical loosening (with shifting in position of the component) in this series has been low. Of the 176 shoulders with glenoid components that have had more than ten years follow-up, 46 have had recent roentgen evaluation without evidence of clinical loosening.

Roentgenographic Results

There have been two reviews of the x-ray films in this series. Watson (1982)[22] studied the films of 174 shoulders with from 24 to 99 months roentgen follow-ups, averaging 37 months, and Satterlee (1988) studied an additional 214 with minimum 24 months follow-up, bringing the review up to date (Figs. 3–103 to 3–107 and Tables 3–8 and 3–9).

It was surprising that the overall incidence of some type of radiolucent line at the bone-cement

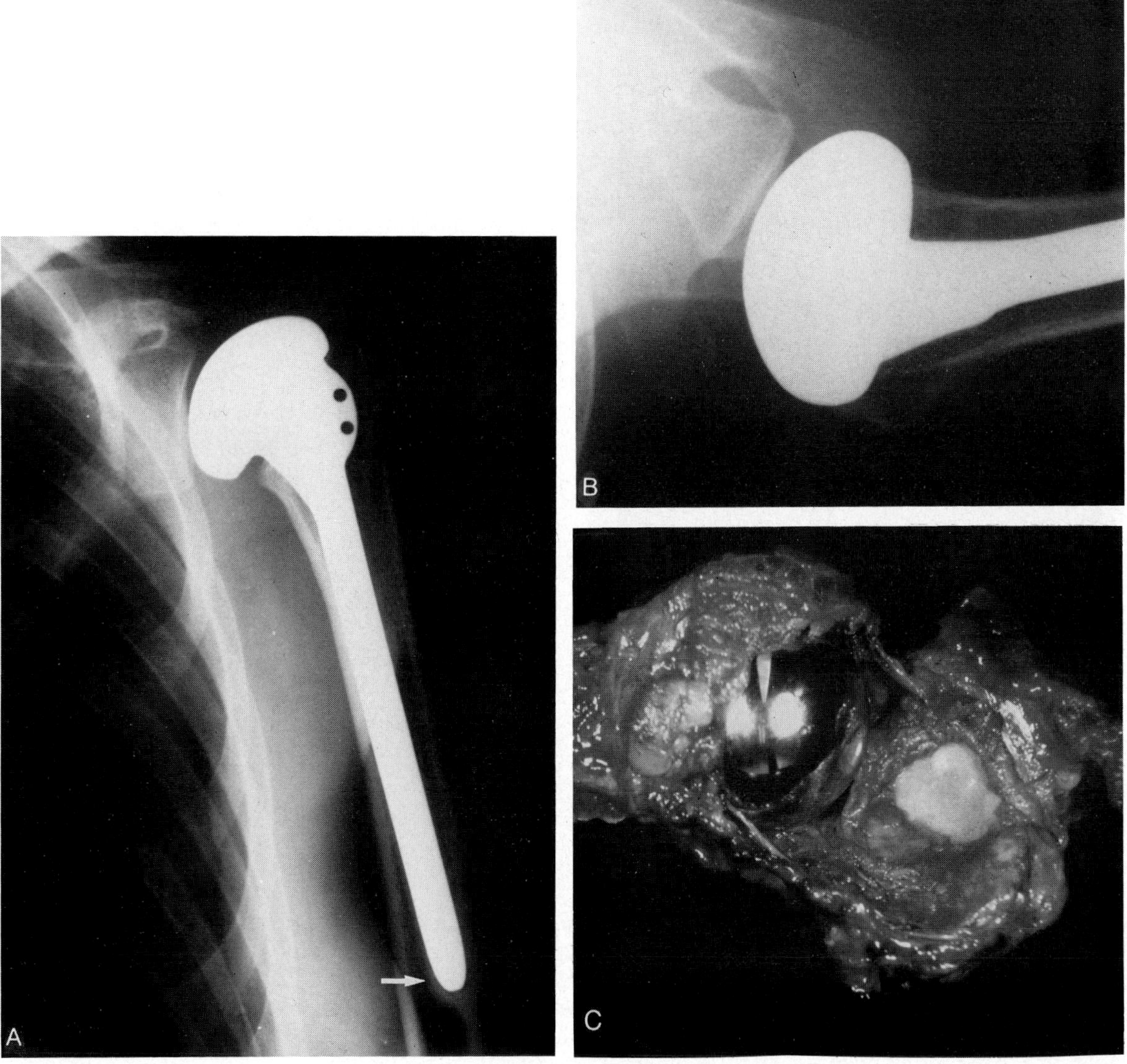

Figure 3–103. ***Results of Humeral Head Replacement Shoulder Arthroplasty:*** Roentgen findings 11 years after humeral head replacement without a glenoid component for Stage III avascular necrosis. A, Anterior-posterior view showing sclerotic bone at the tip of the uncemented stem (arrow) indicates good use of the arm. B, Axillary view shows freedom of glenoid erosion. C, Autopsy specimen of the glenohumeral joint 10 years after a humeral head replacement for ochronosis (illustrated in Fig. 3–45). Patient had an excellent functional result and died suddenly of an unrelated cause. There was no deformation of the glenoid, although it had little articular cartilage at the time of the arthroplasty.

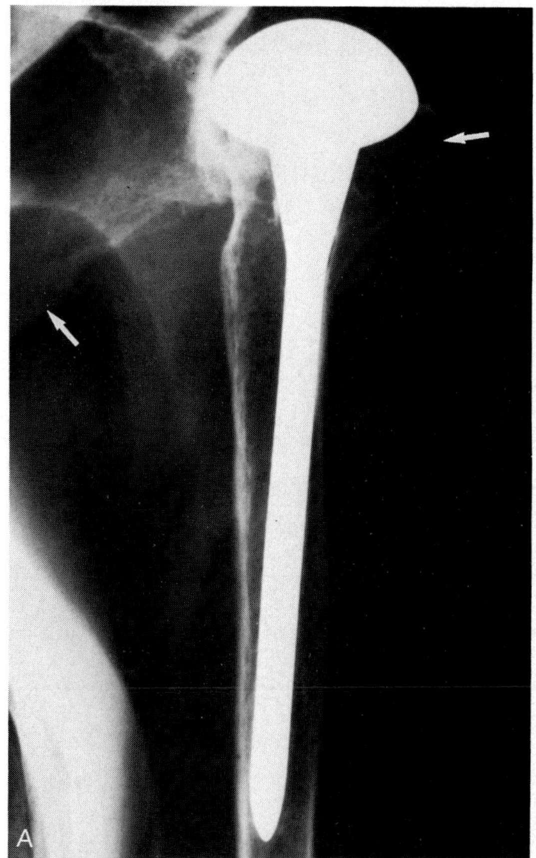

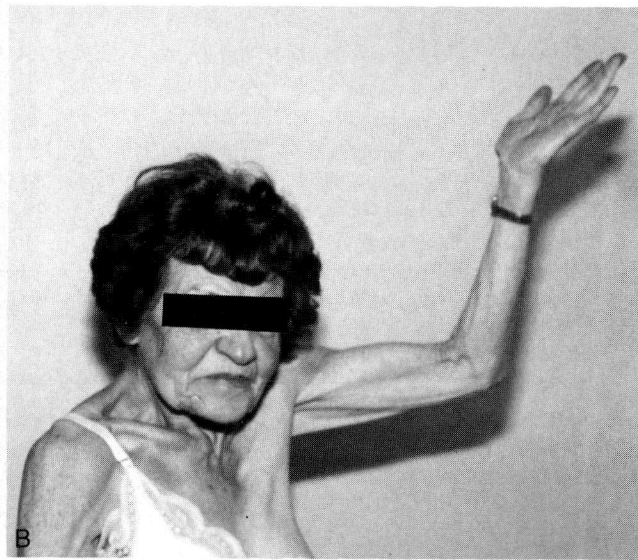

Figure 3–104A and B. ***Long Term Result of Humeral Head Replacement Arthroplasty.*** A 32-year follow-up of a 92 year old woman who had glenohumeral arthritis due to avascular necrosis after a fracture of the humeral head. She had always had some limitation of abduction because (1) a partial scapulectomy had been performed prior to the fracture (left arrow), which restricted scapular motions, and (2) a prominent malunited greater tuberosity had resulted from the fracture (right arrow). Range of motion had changed little from her initial result other than a slight loss of elevation due to the rounding of the dorsal spine from osteoporotic spine fractures.

Roentgenographically, the glenoid had changed very little (it had been abnormal before the prosthesis because of wear from the deformed head), and the sclerotic bone at the tip of the stem indicated good active use. She had no shoulder pain and used the arm normally.

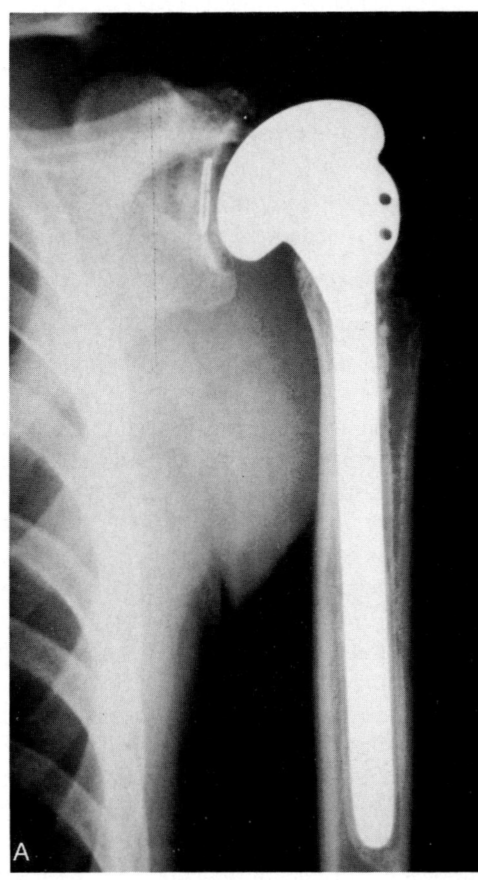

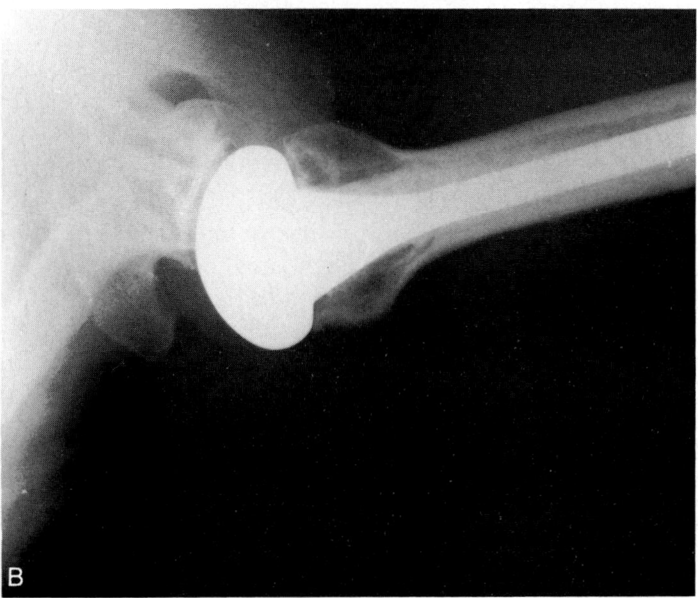

Figure 3–105. ***Results of Nonconstrained Total Shoulder Arthroplasty.*** Roentgen findings ten years after total shoulder arthroplasty showed no radiolucent lines at the bone-cement interface. A, Anterior-posterior view (both components cemented). B, Axillary view.

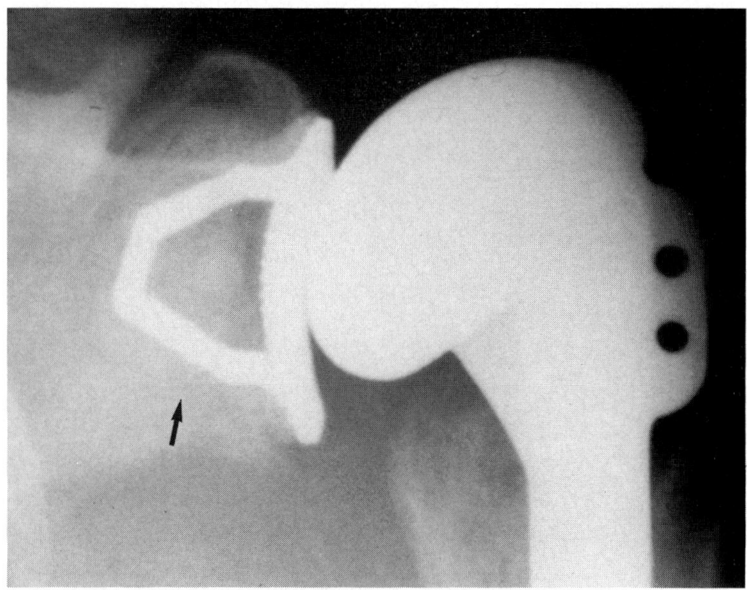

Figure 3–106. Anterior-posterior film showing a faint, incomplete radiolucent line inferiorly (arrow) at the bone-cement interface, which had been seen in the initial postoperative films and was essentially unchanged 1 year later. This type of line was thought to be caused by faulty cementing technique rather than by mechanical forces with loosening.

interface of the glenoid component, considering all diagnostic categories together, was nearly the same in the two studies (e.g., 33 percent in the 1982 study and 31 percent in the 1988 study). However, the incidence of complete lines was much lower in the later study. Of 59 patients with "glenoid lines" in the 1982 study, 23 had complete lines. Of 68 with lines in the later study, only 5 had complete lines. This result suggests improved cement technique and bone of poor quality can be expected to result in a higher incidence of lucent lines.

In both studies the incidence of radiolucent lines at the bone-cement interface of the glenoid component was higher in patients with rheumatoid arthritis and cuff-tear arthropathy. In the later study some type of line was present in 27 percent of patients with osteoarthritis, 12 percent of those with arthritis of dislocations, 48 percent of those with rheumatoid arthritis, 26 percent of those with old trauma, 47 percent of those with cuff-tear arthropathy, and 67 percent of those in the miscellaneous category, which includes congenital hypoplastic glenoids, tumors with excision of the glenoid, and several other unusual glenoid problems.

Humeral Component

The humeral component has always been almost trouble-free provided it has been seated firmly and there is no low-grade infection, severe osteopenia from disease, or some other circumstance. In the first series, methylmethacrylate had been used to anchor the humeral component in 144 shoulders and was not used in 50 shoulders. A 4.0 mm. lucent line was present in one patient, and a 3.0 mm. lucent zone was seen in another. One of these patients had had prior internal fixation of a fracture. Differential gallium scans and special cultures were negative for infection. Although these findings suggested clinical loosening, neither patient had significant symptoms that would justify revision surgery. Both have been followed for more than ten years since the arthroplasty and continue status-quo.

In the 1988 series methylmethacrylate was used at the humeral component in 195 shoulders

Table 3–7. FUNCTIONAL RESULTS*

		FULL EXERCISE PROGRAM			"LIMITED GOALS"	
SHOULDERS	INDICATION	Excellent	Satisfactory	Unsatisfactory	Satisfactory	Unsatisfactory
118	Osteoarthritis	105	7	5	1	
35	Arthritis dislocations	26	3	5	1	
106	Rheumatoid arthritis	65	21	9	11	
69	Old trauma	30	14	18	7	
43	Revision	12	9	9	13	
26	Cuff-tear arthropathy				25	1
11	Miscellaneous	4		3	4	

*408 total shoulder arthroplasties with two years minimum follow-up.

Table 3–8. ROENTGEN RESULTS OF THE GLENOID COMPONENTS*

	WATSON AND NEER[22] (1973–1980)	SATTERLEE AND NEER[281] (1980–1986)
Overall (number of shoulders)		
Number studied	174	214
Incomplete radiolucent lines	36	63
Complete radiolucent lines	23	5
Percentage with lines (incomplete and complete combined)		
Overall	33%	31%

*388 total shoulder arthroplasties with 24 to 171 months follow-up; 46 followed for more than 10 years.

and a press-fit in 19 shoulders. There were no complete radiolucent lines other than those expected with uncemented components (e.g., lines reflecting a thin fibrous interface and of no significance).

COMMENTARY ON THE LITERATURE AND ON RADIOLUCENT LINES

The literature on nonconstrained shoulder arthroplasty by other authors has described consistent pain relief, function according to the capability of the muscles, and few humeral component complications. A few authors have expressed great concern about the high incidence of radiolucent cement lines at the glenoid component in their series and equate lucent lines with loosening of the component.

I cannot agree with the few authors who infer from their incidence of radiolucent lines that there has been frequent glenoid component loosening due to the design of the component or some inherent biomechanical shear force on the scapula (Figs. 3–107 and 3–108). In the first place, the reported incidence of re-operation for loosening of the prosthesis has been low (Table 3–9). As of 1987, only ten cases had been reported for revision of the glenoid component. Second, the meaning of the radiolucent lines seen at the bone-cement interface of the glenoid component is unclear. Of course they could mean loosening, but beyond this consider the following:

1. These lines vary with the roentgen projection and exposure. The films should be made with consistent radiologic technique in the same projections.

2. The study must include films from the time of surgery compared with repeated studies at yearly intervals to make the assumption there has been loosening rather than that the component had never been firmly secured. (A high proportion of incomplete lines in our study were present in the immediate post-operative films, implying imperfect technique; however, these components have not yet progressed to clinical loosening with enlarging lines and migration of the component.) In Brems' study,[279] as in ours, there was a higher incidence of complete cement lines in the earlier cases in the series performed during the learning period.

3. The great variability in density and strength of bone has been described in the discussions of the various diagnostic categories. The fact that lucent lines are more prevalent in shoulders with rheumatoid arthritis and those with cuff-tear arthropathy must undoubtedly be related to the qual-

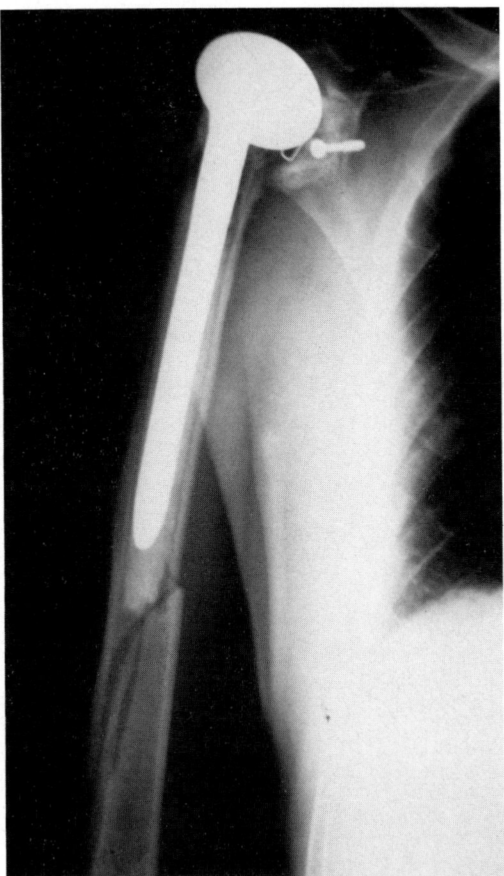

Figure 3–107. ***Results of Nonconstrained Shoulder Arthroplasty: Roentgen Results.*** The durability of nonconstrained shoulder arthroplasty and the unknown significance of radiolucent lines in one-third of our patients are demonstrated by this patient. He required a glenoid bone graft during his arthroplasty and had always had an asymptomatic 0.5-mm. radiolucent line at the bone-cement interface. Seven years after surgery he fell down some stairs, fracturing the humerus without dislodging the prosthesis and showing no subsequent roentgen changes.

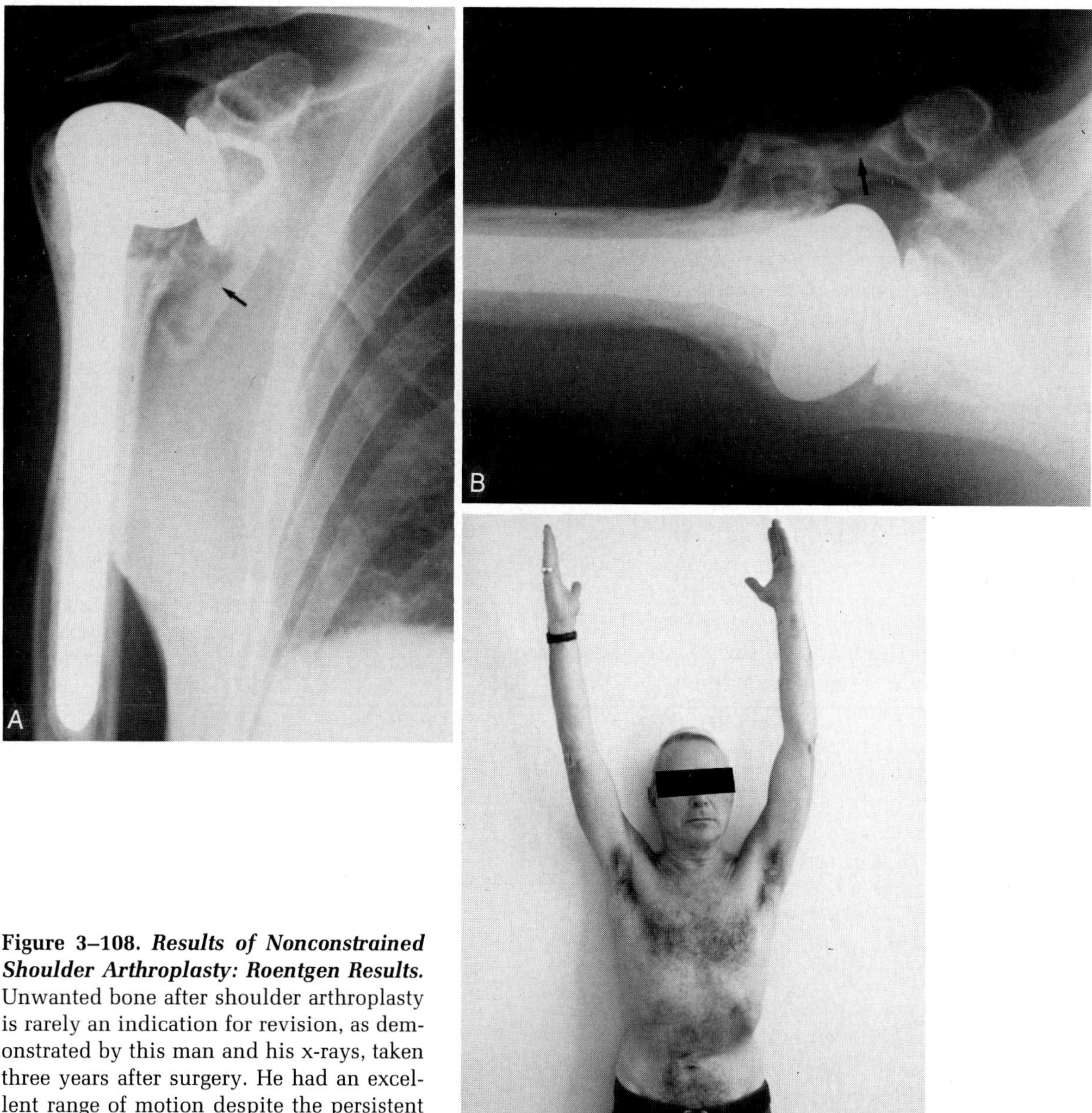

Figure 3–108. ***Results of Nonconstrained Shoulder Arthroplasty: Roentgen Results.*** Unwanted bone after shoulder arthroplasty is rarely an indication for revision, as demonstrated by this man and his x-rays, taken three years after surgery. He had an excellent range of motion despite the persistent bone in his follow-up films.

Table 3–9. REVISIONS REPORTED IN THE LITERATURE FOR GLENOID LOOSENING OF THE NEER II SYSTEM ARE UNDER 1.0 PERCENT.

INVESTIGATOR	LOCATION	REVISIONS/SERIES (TOTAL ARTHROPLASTIES)
Adams (1986)[273]	Toronto	0/33
Bade (1984)[274]	Hospital of Special Surgery	0/27
Barrett (1987)[104]	University of Washington	4/50
Clayton (1986)[275]	Denver	0/15
Cofield (1986)[276]	Mayo Clinic	3/73
Hawkins (1986)[277]	Ontario	3/70
Thornhill (1983)[278]	Boston	0/146
Brems (1986)[279]	Cleveland	0/69
Neer (1988)[280]	New York	2/615

ity of bone. Rheumatoid granulations and unpredictable pannus erosion have destroyed some glenoids to the point where the decision must be made between bone grafts or no implant at all (and the latter may be the wiser choice in these situations in which the disease has gone on too long).

4. Stress shielding by the glenoid component may cause adjacent osteoporosis. Watson[280] thought this was the probable cause of the incomplete lines often seen at the inferior aspect of the glenoid component in symptomless patients.

5. Disuse osteoporosis is a possibility. Rheumatoid arthritis and cuff-tear arthropathy patients are certainly less active. The more active patients have a better quality of bone. Overuse could be a problem but to date has not appeared to be a clinical problem.

6. Other types of osteopenia, as in patients with a systemic osteoporosis from several causes, have been noted to cause a generalized thinning of the cortex of the humerus with widening of the bone–implant space of press-fit humeral components. Some type of systemic osteopenia could be a factor in some patients with rheumatoid arthritis.

7. Unrecognized low-grade infection could be a factor in selected cases, as proved to be true in a patient with mysterious loosening of a humeral component in one of our earlier series who later developed identifiable infection.

8. Biomechanical factors have been proposed by some, and, of course, if enough pressure and stress is placed on any type of foreign body it will loosen inside a living bone. One has only to consider the way dentists straighten teeth. However, as discussed earlier (p. 154), the shoulder enjoys favorable biomechanical forces, mostly compressive and with a socket that rotates as the humerus rotates and has "give" on impact.

9. We have seen lucent lines and expected to find a loose glenoid component at the time of revision in a number of patients referred from other hospitals with failed arthroplasties but instead found no demonstrable loosening of the component at surgery (Fig. 3–98K).

Obviously, it is easy to implant a glenoid component incorrectly, resulting in rocking and loosening. Also, it should be obvious that some bone is inadequate to hold a component. It is desirable to have a holding device for the glenoid component that has as large an area as possible for diffusion of force at the bone–prosthesis interface so that there will be less tendency for resorption of bone. However, the stem must be implantable without excessive removal of bone. As discussed earlier (p. 158), surface ingrowth requires good contact between the bone and the prosthesis, and this is hard to obtain in the glenoid in actual practice, especially in soft glenoids. Therefore, I believe there will always be a use for some type of grouting for many glenoid components; and although experimentation with cementless glenoid components is justified by a limited number of surgeons, one must keep in mind that the complications with cemented glenoid components have been very few—significantly fewer than with prosthetic replacement at other joints.

Improvement in the future should concentrate more on materials than on design. The normal anatomical design should give the best function and be the most lasting design. A material with the modulus of elasticity of bone that could be attached with a holding device that becomes incorporated in the bone would be an improvement. However, until real improvements in materials are made, let us make changes slowly and keep the implant simple because complications have been very few.

4

DISLOCATIONS

GLENOHUMERAL INSTABILITY

Historical Background

Because dislocations occur at the glenohumeral joint more frequently than at any other joint, and the deformity and impairment of function that occur with a shoulder dislocation are usually obvious, it is not surprising that these lesions were among the earliest recognized surgical conditions. Murals in Egyptian tombs depicted glenohumeral dislocations as early as 3000 B.C. Undoubtedly, prehistoric cave men also recognized these lesions.

In the late fifth century B.C., the remarkable Hippocrates described dislocations resulting from injuries and other dislocations that loose-jointed individuals could produce at will. Thus he made the first classification of dislocations, "traumatic" and "atraumatic," and he recognized voluntary dislocations. He also recognized the importance in glenohumeral stability of muscle tone, which is the basis for conservative treatment today. The translation by Withington[143] of the writing of Hippocrates on dislocations is as follows:

> One should bear in mind that there are great natural diversities as to the ease of reductions of dislocations. There may be some difference in the sockets, one having a rim easy to cross, the other one less so; but the greatest diversity is in the attachment of the ligaments, which in some cases is yielding, in others constricted. For the humidity in individuals as regards the joints comes from the disposition of the ligaments which may be slack by nature and easily lend themselves to extensions. In fact one may see a person of so humid a temperment that when they choose they can dislocate or reduce their joints without pain. The state of the body makes a further difference, for in those who are muscular and have the limb in good condition dislocation is rarer and reduction more difficult, but when they are thinner and less muscular than usual, dislocation is more frequent and reduction is easier.

Hippocrates also recognized the greater likelihood of recurrent dislocations when no inflammation of the surrounding parts occurred after reduction of a dislocation. In addition, he described a method of repair for recurrent dislocations by cauterizing the axillary soft tissues with white-hot irons followed by immobilization of the shoulder in adduction and internal rotation. He also described his famous heel or fist in the axilla method of closed reduction of acute dislocations. He recognized that chronic (long-standing) dislocations could not be reduced by closed methods. It is of interest that he thought the shoulder always dislocated inferiorly rather than anteriorly or posteriorly. I came to recognize the importance of inferior instability[13, 158–160] as a major cause of failure of the "standard repairs" that have been devised for recurrent anterior and recurrent posterior dislocations (see Figs. 4–3, 4–22, and 4–23 and Table 4–2).

During the eighteenth century, prior to roentgenography, anatomists described lesions found at autopsy dissection. The late H. F. Moseley made an outstanding description of their findings in his excellent monograph, "Recurrent Dislocation of the Shoulder."[144] After Lister's work on aseptic technique published in 1867, various surgical procedures began to be introduced. Language barriers among the English, French, and German anatomists must have been responsible for many re-discoveries of previously established information. It is impossible to know everything that each contributor observed, and most of them appreciated more than one aspect; thus, it is difficult to construct an accurate chronology of events.

Perhaps the first description of a posterior head defect was written by Malgaigne[161] (French, 1855). Many others followed. The roentgen appearance of this lesion was brought to the attention of radiologists and clinicians by Hill and Sachs[162] in the United States in 1940. Detachment of the anterior labrum was probably recognized by many. The first clear descriptions were by Caird (Scottish, 1887) and Broca and Hartman (French, 1890).[163] Perthes (German, 1906)[164] was the first to describe re-attachment of the anterior labrum both with sutures and with staples. He also described repair of the rotator cuff if a cuff defect was present with a dislocation. Bankart (English, 1923)[16] popularized labral re-attachment in the English-speaking world. Jossel (German, 1880)[165] was probably the first to describe the relationship of rotator cuff tears with shoulder instability ("posterior mechanism," p. 68). The treatment of instability with glenoid bone defects was suggested by Eden (German, 1918)[166] and Hybbinette (Swedish, 1918).[167] A variety of capsular and fascial repairs were discussed in an important symposium in the British volume of the Journal of Bone and Joint Surgery in 1948, which had an impact on the surgical procedures done in recent years (e.g., the Bankart[16, 168] repair [suture re-attachment of the anterior labrum to the glenoid rim], the Putti-Platt[169] repair ["double-breasting" the anterior capsule with the subscapularis tendon], and the Galli-Lemesurier[170] repair [fascial repair modified by Bateman[75]]).

Since then, bone operations such as the Webber[174] (rotational osteotomy of the humerus), Trillat[182, 183] (osteotomy of the coracoid), and Eden-Hybbinette (bone blocks) have been used more in central Europe than elsewhere. Latarjet[184] in France described transfer of the coracoid through the subscapularis to the anterior glenoid in 1954. This procedure is very much like the Helfet[177a] (1958) modification of the Bristow operation (in which the osteotomized coracoid is transferred to the glenoid and attached with a screw). This operation has been modified by May[177] and is widely used by sports medicine surgeons in the United States. Tullos[178] and others have modified the technique of coracoid transfer by placing the subscapularis tendon superficial to the coracoid to gain more external rotation. A very excellent monograph on coracoid transfer has been written by Hovelius[181] (Swedish, 1982).

In America the Magnuson-Stack[175] procedure (part of the subscapularis tendon is transferred laterally) became more popular than the Nicola[176] procedure (the long tendon of the biceps is transferred through a hole in the humeral head). The Magnuson-Stack procedure was preferred by many because it was less difficult and avoided the Bankart bone sutures. The Putti-Platt[169] procedure was also commonly used for the same reasons. Rowe[145, 169, 171–173] has made many contributions to the surgery of shoulder instability, perfecting the technique of the Broca-Perthes-Bankart repair of a detached anterior labrum and offering a method of capsulorrhaphy when no detachment of the labrum is present. He has emphasized the importance of avoiding surgery on improperly motivated voluntary dislocators.[172] Hippocrates recognized the existence of this group of patients, but it is important to re-emphasize the point that those with poor motivation should not be operated on. Rowe described a method of approaching the glenohumeral joint posteriorly.[172a] He believes that recurrent anterior subluxation is an important surgical entity.[173] Jobe,[179] a leader in sports medicine, has developed a technique for the repair of anterior instability in the throwing arm of athletes. He splits the subscapularis tendon longitudinally to keep it intact.

During recent years, arthroscopy has been used in the evaluation and treatment of instability. Leaders in this field in the United States include Johnson,[283] Andrews,[284] Richardson, Caspari,[285] and Lombardi.[286] To date, the results of arthroscopic repairs for recurrent glenohumeral dislocations have been distinctly inferior to those of surgical repairs. The consensus at present favors the use of arthroscopy for diagnosis at the time of examination under anesthesia in selected patients, but arthroscopic repairs for dislocations are considered developmental at this time. The arthroscope also has potential value for research.

My contributions to the treatment of the unstable glenohumeral joint have been as follows:

1. To urge surgeons to correct the pathology actually present when performing surgical repairs for all types of instability, striving to return the joint to as near the normal anatomical condition as possible, rather than performing one standard procedure for all and distorting the anatomy. It is my belief that this is the key to restoring normal function, which should be the goal, in addition to the elimination of redislocation.[19, 158–160, 190, 197]

2. In the classification of dislocations and subluxation, to add to the two categories of Hippocrates (traumatic and atraumatic) a third category, "acquired laxity." This condition is caused by repeated minor injuries, rather than by either major trauma or congenital joint laxity (Table 4–1),[13, 158–160, 192] although there may (or may not) be elements of generalized laxity of varying degrees.

3. To point out that this third etiological mechanism leads to enlargement of the joint volume (see Fig. 4–2). Laxity of the inferior capsule and of both sides of the joint precludes correction with a standard procedure devised for unidirectional dislocations. I recognized it as an important cause of failure of standard repairs (as Rockwood[186] and others have since verified).

4. To describe a method of treatment for multidirectional dislocators by reducing the joint volume on all sides by "inferior capsular shift."[13]

5. To describe the etiology, pathology, and treatment of "arthritis of recurrent dislocations."[13, 20, 22, 119, 158]

Terminology of Glenohumeral Instability

In traveling around the United States and the world, I have heard similar terms used with different meanings. For example "voluntary" indicates

Table 4–1. CLASSIFICATION OF RECURRENT DISLOCATIONS

	ETIOLOGY	PATHOLOGY	CLINICAL	TREATMENT
Atraumatic	Congenital laxity (*no* injury)	Generalized joint laxity Labrum intact; no bone changes X-rays negative (except for evidence of laxity)	No injury; patient always had been "loose jointed," first dislocation ill defined No labral tear or bone changes Self-reduced Often asymptomatic	Treatment of initial dislocation: Immobilization does not affect outcome Recurrences: Exercises
Traumatic	One major injury (hard fall, wrestling)	No joint laxity Labrum detached or middle glenohumeral ligament torn X-rays—usually a traumatic humeral head defect and glenoid rim fragment	No prior shoulder symptoms Definite injury (e.g., hard fall, wrestling); swelling and pain from injury; possible nerve injury Requires help to reduce Unidirectional	Treatment of initial dislocation: Immobilization five weeks Often effective Recurrences: Surgery (unidirectional)
Acquired	Repeated minor injuries (swimming, gymnastics, weight lifting, overhead work)	Possible finger laxity Increased glenohumeral joint volume (other joints spared) Labrum often intact, later may be detached May develop a humeral head defect X-rays—negative early, bone changes later	Minimal trauma at first dislocation (e.g., swinging a bat, lifting weight overhead, etc.) Less soreness Usually self-reduced Threat of multidirectional instability	Treatment of initial dislocation: Immobilization unlikely to be effective Recurrences: Surgery (possible inferior capsular shift or modification)

to me that the shoulder can be dislocated at will but does not imply that the patient always has a psychological problem. "Habitual" in some places implies a psychological problem such as a nervous tic, but for me this term can be used in the same way as "recurrent." It seems important to clarify terminology before proceeding further.

Instability: A subluxation or dislocation
Traumatic: Caused by one major injury
Atraumatic: No injury
Repetitive microtrauma: Many small injuries
Voluntary: At will or intentional
Involuntary: Against one's will or unintentional
Habitual: Same as *Recurrent*
Chronic: Longstanding; same as *Perpetual* or *Old*
Unidirectional: One way (e.g., *anterior* or *posterior*)
Multidirectional: Inferior, anterior, posterior, and, potentially, superior.

Etiology and Proposed Classification of Recurrent Dislocations

The great majority of recurrent dislocations are due to an abnormality of the ligaments rather than to bone defects or muscle imbalance. The latter categories will be dealt with separately.

Hippocrates classified recurrent dislocations as "traumatic" and "atraumatic." He recognized that dislocation could be instituted at will ("voluntary") or against one's will, and he noted that muscle tone had an important bearing on the stability of the glenohumeral joint. The validity of these observations has stood the test of time for more than 2000 years.

I suggest no alteration of Hippocrates' classification except for the addition of a large and important category that comprises patients who have had neither a significant injury nor generalized joint laxity (Table 4–1). In this group, repetitive activities have led to loosening of the shoulders. The other joints are usually normal, but in some cases some degree of generalized ligamentous laxity, such as a mild varient of Ehlers-Danlos syndrome (Fig. 4–1), may be demonstrated by laxity of the fingers, elbows, knees, and perhaps other joints.

As discussed in our article in 1980,[13] in our patients with recurrent dislocations we see combinations of three etiologies in varying proportions: (1) inherent congenital laxity of the glenohumeral capsule, (2) trauma (a major injury), and (3) activities that repeatedly stress the joint capsule such as swimming, weight lifting, and gymnastics. Therefore, my classification of recurrent dislocations is as follows:

I. Atraumatic: No injury
II. Traumatic: One major injury
III. Acquired: Repeated minor injuries

I. Atraumatic Dislocations

At one end of the scale, as in Figure 4–1A, a person with extremely hypermobile shoulders may have experienced subluxations and dislocations all his or her life. These may become symptomatic without unusual stress merely from everyday activities. This patient is in the "atraumatic" category. There has been no tearing of ligaments nor detachment of the labrum.

There is no point in immobilizing the shoulder at the "initial" episode in hopes of eliminating the problem. In the first place, this "initial episode" is characteristically ill defined. The only treatment indicated is "rest" until the soreness disappears and exercises to improve muscle tone (Table 4–1). In rare cases the person may have enough persistent pain with activities to eventually consider an inferior capsular shift (see p. 316).

II. Traumatic Dislocations

At the other end of the scale is the person who has no joint laxity but sustains the initial dislocation from a rather violent injury (Fig. 4–1B). Detachment of the labrum from the glenoid rim occurs in the majority of these cases, and there may be tearing of the capsule, especially attenuation of the middle glenohumeral ligaments.

Initial treatment in this group consists of immobilization (at the time of the first dislocation), with a good chance that healing of the ligaments will occur and a very low incidence of recurrent dislocations.[186, 187] If recurrent dislocations do occur, conservative treatment based on exercises has little chance of success, and I recommend considering surgical repair. The labrum is often detached from the scapula. It should be repaired because the anterior labrum is the attachment of the important inferior glenohumeral ligament to the scapula (see Fig. 1–18). Occasionally the middle glenohumeral ligament has failed, and the labrum remains intact. Therefore, I routinely reinforce the middle glenohumeral ligament when repairing recurrent anterior dislocations (see Fig. 4–31). I attempt to restore intact ligaments of sufficient length to allow an excursion of motion that is normal for the average

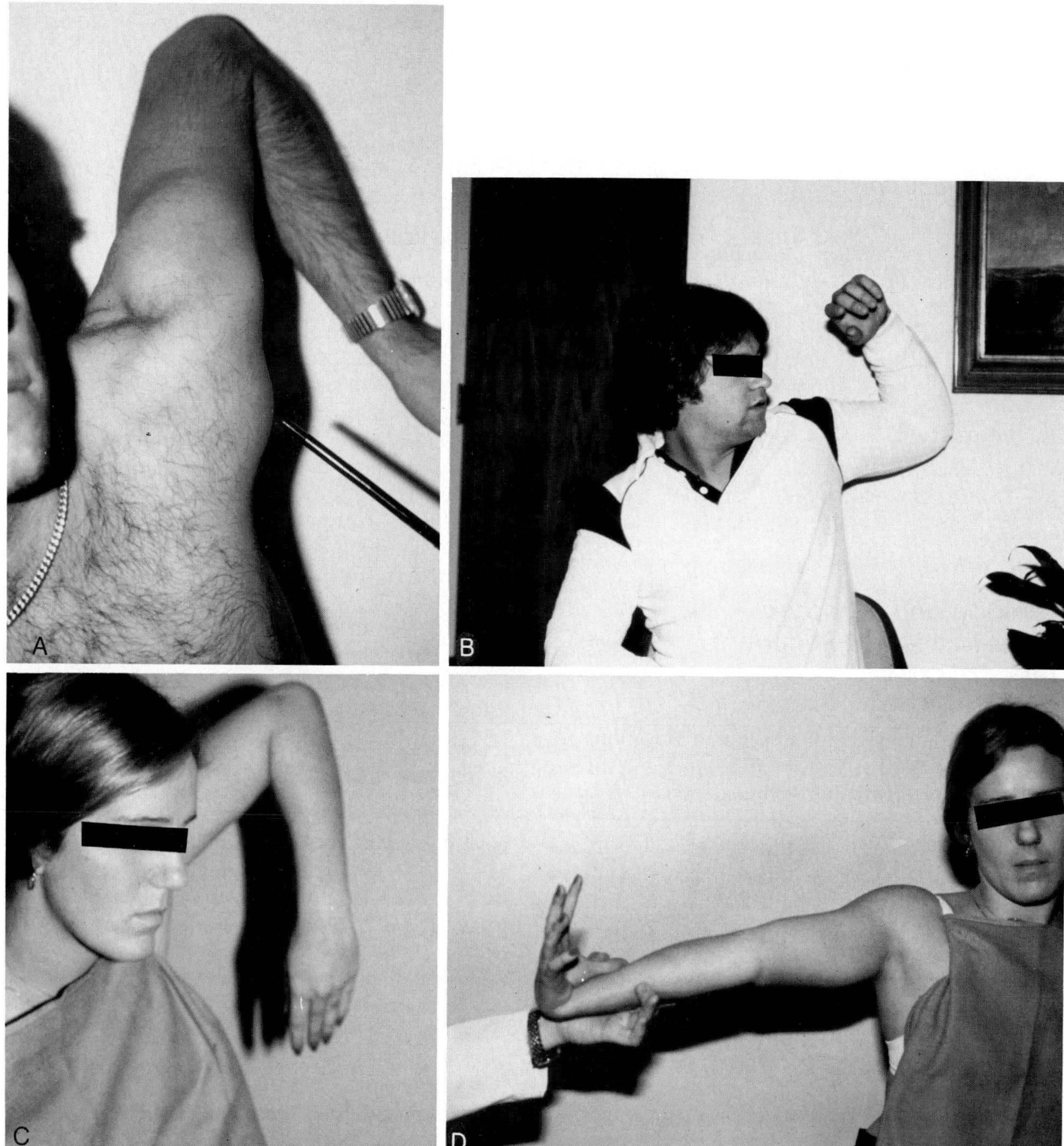

Figure 4–1. ***Classification of Recurrent Dislocations.***

A, The "atraumatic" category at one end of the scale is congenital laxity, as in this patient with Ehlers-Danlos syndrome, who has dislocated his shoulders all his life.

B, "Traumatic" dislocation belongs at the other end of the scale and comprises those who have no joint laxity but sustained the initial dislocation from a single, violent injury.

C and D, Persons with "acquired" dislocations develop laxity because of repeated minor injuries such as butterfly swimming, weight lifting, and gymnastics, as in this Olympic swimmer (C). The patient never had a single injury sufficient to cause dislocation but may or may not have some element of congenital laxity, as shown by the hypermobile thumb and hyperextended elbow (D). Both unidirectional and multidirectional dislocations may originate in this manner.

patient (not necessarily equal to that of the opposite shoulder of the patient concerned because the opposite shoulder may be hypermobile).

III. Acquired Dislocations

In my series, this third category is the largest. The incidence of one major injury at the time of the initial dislocation was 49 percent in our series of recurrent anterior dislocations.[185] The incidence of a significant injury in those with posterior dislocations and multidirectional instability has been much lower. As discussed above and outlined in Table 4–1, these patients have engaged in repeated minor trauma such as swimming (butterfly and backstroke), weight lifting, gymnastics, or working with the arms overhead. Their injuries are less severe than those in the traumatic group. They often have some inherent joint laxity, but this is less than in the atraumatic group (Fig. 4–1C and D). The basic lesion is acquired enlargement of the glenohumeral joint volume (their other joints are usually normal). Initially, the anterior labrum is intact, but in some patients splitting and partial detachment develop. After the shoulder has dislocated many times, detachment of the labrum may occur, and a posterior head defect may develop similar to that seen in the traumatic group but differing in that there is laxity of the glenohumeral joint capsule.

Laxity inferiorly and on the opposite side may cause a standard operation for traumatic unidirectional dislocations to fail and at times produces the most serious complication, arthritis of dislocations (Figs. 4–3C to F, 4–56, and 4–57). The enlargement of the joint volume and the extent of inferior laxity vary. Therefore, I routinely test all directions of instability three times during *all* repairs for recurrent dislocations, either anterior or posterior, to be sure I am not overlooking another direction of instability that would cause trouble after the repair. The aim is to restore normal anatomy, as shown in Figure 4–31. In performing repairs from either the anterior or posterior approach, inferior laxity, if present, is corrected by a partial or complete inferior capsular shift, as required, to eliminate instability in all directions.

Importance of Recognizing the "Acquired" Category

The importance of adding the acquired category to the classification of dislocations:

1. The group with acquired laxity is larger than either the purely traumatic or the atraumatic group. A careful history of the mechanism of injury at the time of the first dislocation will convince the clinician of the validity of this statement. The majority of dislocations occur the first time either

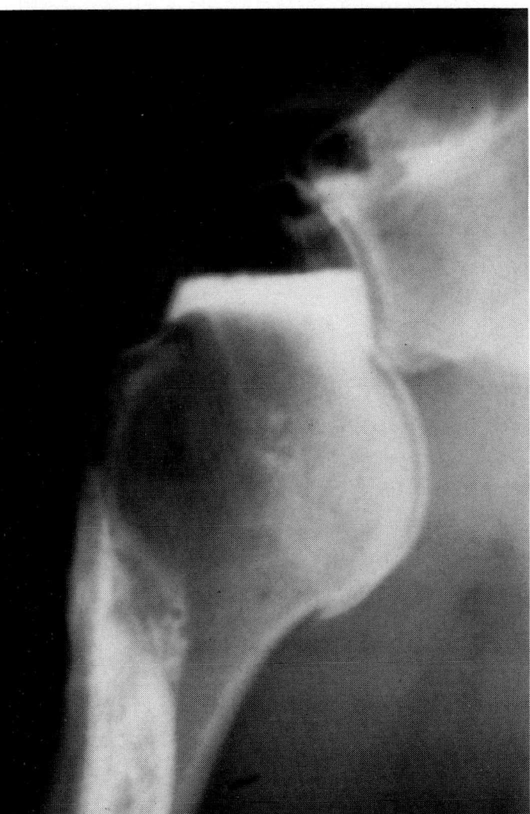

Figure 4–2. ***Why Multidirectional Dislocations Are Important.*** The basic lesion in multidirectional dislocations is increased joint volume, as shown in this arthrogram. Multidirectional instability is the most frequent cause of failed standard repairs for recurrent dislocations (see Figs. 4–8, 4–38 to 4–42, and Table 4–3). It is a diagnostic pitfall because it usually occurs in the category of acquired dislocations, which affect all types of strong, athletic people, both men and women, often those who would not be expected to have hyperlaxity of a joint.

Table 4–2. CAUSES OF FAILURE IN "STANDARD" REPAIRS FOR RECURRENT ANTERIOR DISLOCATIONS

120 re-repairs (1976–1983)[197]	
Residual instability	
Missed multidirectional instability	23
Missed anterior labrum detachment (Broca, Perthes, Bankart)	19
Arthritis of dislocations	30
Too tight	7
Voluntary dislocations	9
Error in diagnosis	7
Infection	9
Seizures	5
Metal complications	11
	120

without injury or with injuries that would not dislocate a normal shoulder.

2. The shoulders in the acquired group have the potential of developing an enlarged joint volume inferiorly and on the opposite side as well as on the side of the greatest instability. Failure to consider the possibility of more than one direction of instability has been the most common cause of failure in repairs for anterior dislocations, as shown in Table 4–2 and in Figures 4–3, 4–56, and 4–57. In a shoulder with multidirectional instability, not only may a standard procedure fail to prevent redislocations (because of failure to control inferior instability), but a standard procedure may also displace the humeral head, leading to a more serious complication, the arthritis of recurrent dislocations.

3. Examination under anesthesia at the time of all surgical repairs for recurrent dislocations is important to avoid these complications.

OVERALL ASSESSMENT OF INSTABILITY

Unreduced Dislocations

The diagnosis can be easy in a straightforward, unreduced, traumatic *anterior dislocation*. The typical findings (see Fig. 4–51A) are loss of the rounded contour of the point of the shoulder, long

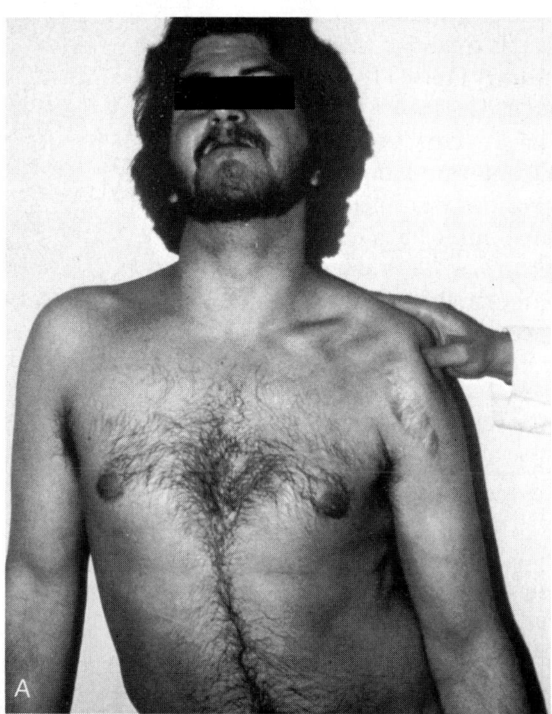

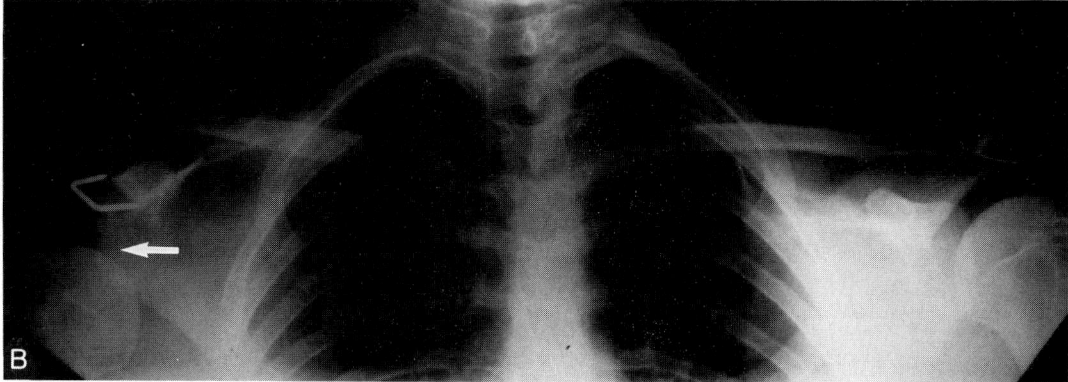

Figure 4–3. ***Why Multidirectional Dislocations Are Important.*** A and B, An example of multiple failed repairs for recurrent dislocations caused by multidirectional instability. A Putti-Platt repair anteriorly and a Boyd-Sisk repair posteriorly failed because standard repairs for unidirectional dislocations do not control inferior instability, as shown by the "sulcus sign" (B) and descent of the humeral head (arrow) when the patient holds a weight (C).

axis of the shaft of the humerus pointing toward the cervical region rather than toward the acromion, prominence of the head anteriorly, and inability to touch the elbow against the side of the body. Rarely, one sees a *dislocation erecta*, in which the arm remains elevated overhead and the prominence of the head can be palpated inferiorly to the glenoid (see Fig. 4–14). A posterior dislocation rarely remains unreduced long enough to be seen by a physician unless there is an impression

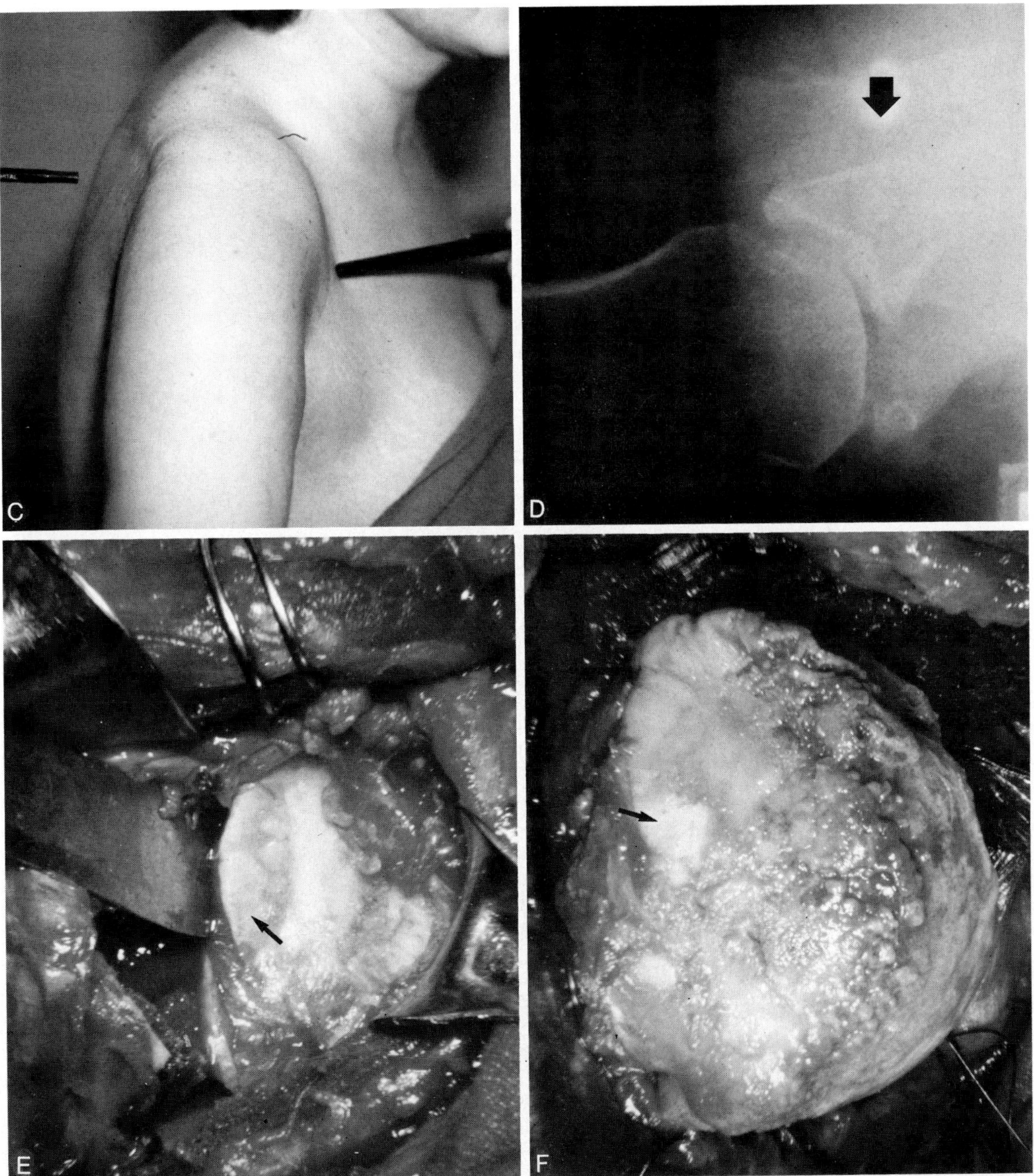

Figure 4–3 *Continued* C to F, Arthritis of recurrent dislocations after six failed operations for recurrent dislocations, three anteriorly and three posteriorly, in a multidirectionally unstable shoulder. One operation had been a posterior glenoid osteotomy, as seen in the axillary view (D). The arrow points to the osteotomy site, and the deformity of the glenoid articular surface it produced is shown. The osteotomy displaced the head out of the front of the joint, leading to destruction of the joint and necessitating a total shoulder arthroplasty when the patient was only 27 years of age. E, Appearance of the glenoid, showing sclerosis (arrow) where the glenoid was prominent prosteriorly. F, Appearance of the head, which was sclerotic (arrow) where it had contacted the glenoid. The head was soft and atrophied anteriorly. This case illustrates an important principle: an osteotomy to alter the version of either the humerus or the glenoid, performed in an effort to control recurrent dislocations when the true anatomical problem is a loose joint capsule, is a very dangerous thing to do because it may sublux the head and cause this type of arthritis (see p. 333).

fracture of the humeral head (see Fig. 4–15). There have been extensive lectures and publications on the error of missing locked posterior dislocations, yet more than 50 percent are still missed by the initial examiner. The physical and roentgen findings and treatment are discussed in Chapter 5, pages 393 and 394. As indicated in Table 4–1, many dislocations occur initially without significant trauma and are self-reduced, making the diagnosis and identification of the directions of instability more difficult.

Difficulty of Evaluation of Self-Reduced Dislocations

A few years ago the military services, as well as training programs in orthopaedic surgery, required documentation by x-rays of a dislocation before surgery could be performed. Our military and naval hospitals created new x-ray views to show bone defects in shoulders with self-reduced dislocations (e.g., the Stryker notch view for a

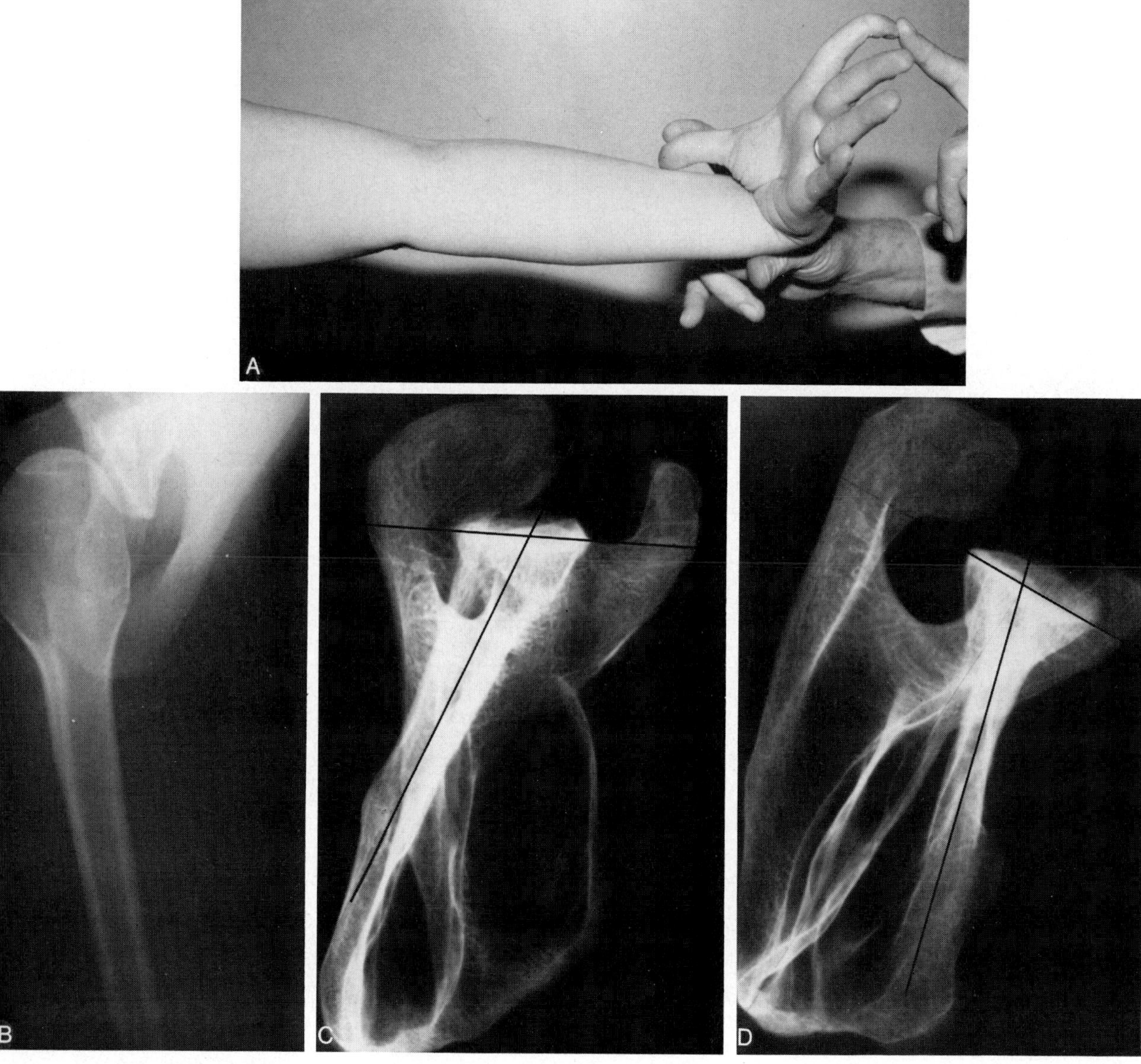

Figure 4–4. ***Overall Assessment of Instability.***

A, During the initial assessment, the thumb, fingers, elbow, and opposite shoulder should be tested for hypermobility in every patient with glenohumeral instability.

B to D, Do not trust a plain film to show retroversion (retrotorsion) or anteversion of the articular surface of the glenoid. In an axillary view of a normal shoulder (B), 20 degrees of anteversion is suggested. Axillary views (C and D) of a dried bone rotated 30 degrees between the two exposures show that its articular surface appears to grow from 20 degrees retroversion to 8 degrees anteversion.[270]

posterior head defect, and the West Point view for an anterior glenoid rim "fragment"). These roentgen techniques have been of great help in the diagnosis of these self-reduced lesions. Nevertheless, in some cases, clear roentgen evidence is lacking. Avoid the error of overreading plain films (Fig. 4–4B to D).

In recent years, surgery for subluxations (incomplete dislocations) has become accepted, introducing a much greater possibility of diagnostic error. Roentgen documentation of a dislocation is no longer required for surgery. The three errors to avoid in evaluating self-reduced dislocators are as follows:

1. *Avoid an error in diagnosis.* Make sure that the pain and disability are due to instability rather than some other diagnostic category. Not all loose shoulders are painful! There may be another diagnosis such as systemic arthritis, neurological pain from the neck, hemorrhagic subacromial bursitis, or impingement (see Fig. 4–5). The laboratory routines (see Figs 1–4 and 4–22) and a careful examination are important.

2. *Avoid a motivation problem.* This is a most difficult step. However, it is necessary to evaluate the motivation of the patient and exclude voluntary dislocators from surgery (see Fig. 4–20). Such patients want to attract attention or gain something by dislocating the shoulder. They can make the surgery fail despite the best efforts of the surgeon.

3. *Determine all directions of instability.* Avoid a standard operation designed for unidirectional dislocations in a patient who has multidirectional instability, as discussed previously (see Fig. 4–3). Because pain causes muscle guarding, it is often difficult to detect the full extent of instability without an examination under anesthesia (to be described later) (see Fig. 4–24). Apprehension tests (see Figs. 4–9 and 4–16) in all directions should be made repeatedly pre-operatively. Preoperative examination of the fingers, thumb, and elbow for hyperlaxity should be routine (Fig. 4–4A).

History

Details of the initial dislocation should be obtained including mechanism of injury (Fig. 4–5), position of the arm, method of reduction, neurological symptoms, and aftercare. This helps identify the direction and classification of the instability (Table 4–1 and Fig. 4–5).

If there have been subsequent dislocations, the mechanism of injury and position of the arm during injury also help to identify whether the dislocation has been anterior or posterior. The arm is almost always above the horizontal plane when an anterior dislocation occurs and below shoulder level when a posterior dislocation occurs.

The classic mechanism for the initial dislocation, in the case of a traumatic anterior dislocation, is a fall on the outstretched hand, causing continuing abduction of the arm without rotation. A classic history for a traumatic posterior dislocation is a seizure (Fig. 4–6), electrical shock, or hard fall with the arm in front holding a football against the chest. As indicated in Table 4–1, in atraumatic dislocators there has been no trauma, and the onset is vague. In the acquired group, there is a history of repeated minor injuries rather than a single major injury, and the initial dislocation occurs with little or no trauma, such as swinging a bat or making a turn while swimming.

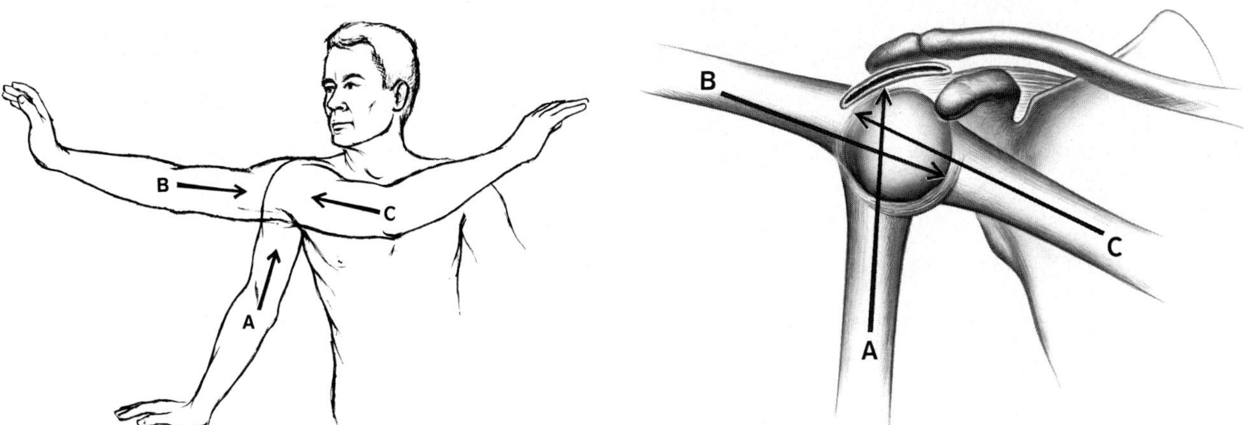

Figure 4–5. History of the mechanism of injury at the initial examination. A, A fall with the hands down at the side may produce an acute subacromial hemorrhagic bursitis (see Chapter 2, p. 81), which can mimic a dislocation. B, Continuing abduction without rotation of the arm can produce an anterior dislocation. C, A fall forward with the bent elbow in front may cause a posterior dislocation.

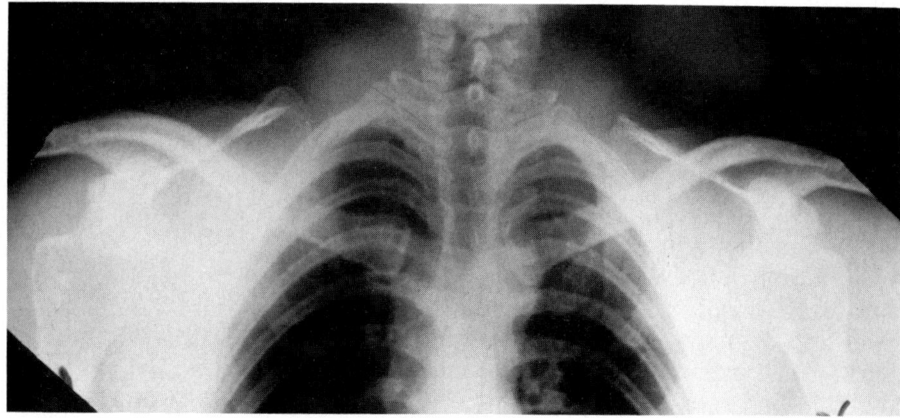

Figure 4–6. Unreduced bilateral anterior dislocations after a seizure. The history must include a statement about seizures before treatment is started.

Physical Signs and Roentgen Diagnosis of Instability

Anterior Instability

Traumatic Dislocations

Unreduced, anterior dislocations should be easily diagnosed by the physical findings shown in Figure 4–7. Most traumatic anterior dislocations require reduction at the time of the initial injury. Nerve injuries, especially injury to the axillary nerve, are not rare and should be diagnosed prior to reduction.

Signs of Self-Reduced Anterior Instability

The anterior instability test and the anterior apprehension sign are demonstrated in Figures 4–8 and 4–9.

An undescribed sign that I have found helpful in detecting anterior instability is forced external rotation with the arm at the side and the elbow bent 90 degrees. This sign I call the *anterior instability test* (Fig. 4–8). It helps in the differential diagnosis between Stage I and Stage II impingement and anterior subluxation. Although forced external rotation does cause the humerus to ascend a bit, it usually does not cause pain when there is an impingement problem but does cause pain if there is symptomatic anterior instability. The impingement injection test (see Fig. 2–30) is also a most helpful test.

Shoulders with anterior instability that are not too acutely tender may have a large excursion of external rotation when the arm is held at the side compared with the opposite side. Baseball pitchers develop acquired laxity of the anterior capsule that

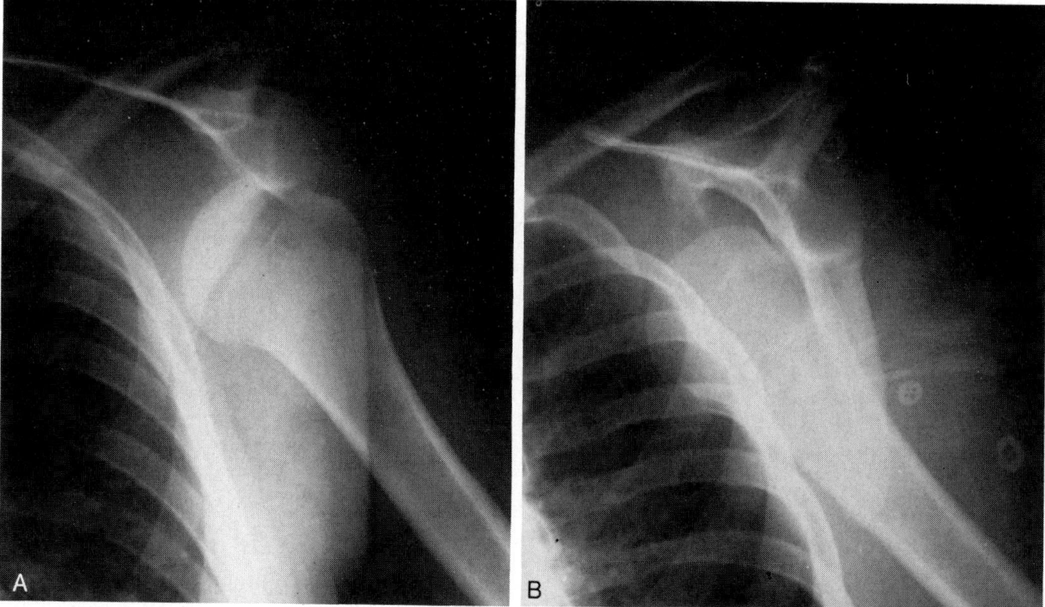

Figure 4–7. ***Roentgen Findings in Unreduced Anterior Dislocations.*** Trauma series (see Fig. 1–12) and computerized tomography of unreduced anterior dislocations. A, Anterior-posterior view. B, Lateral view.

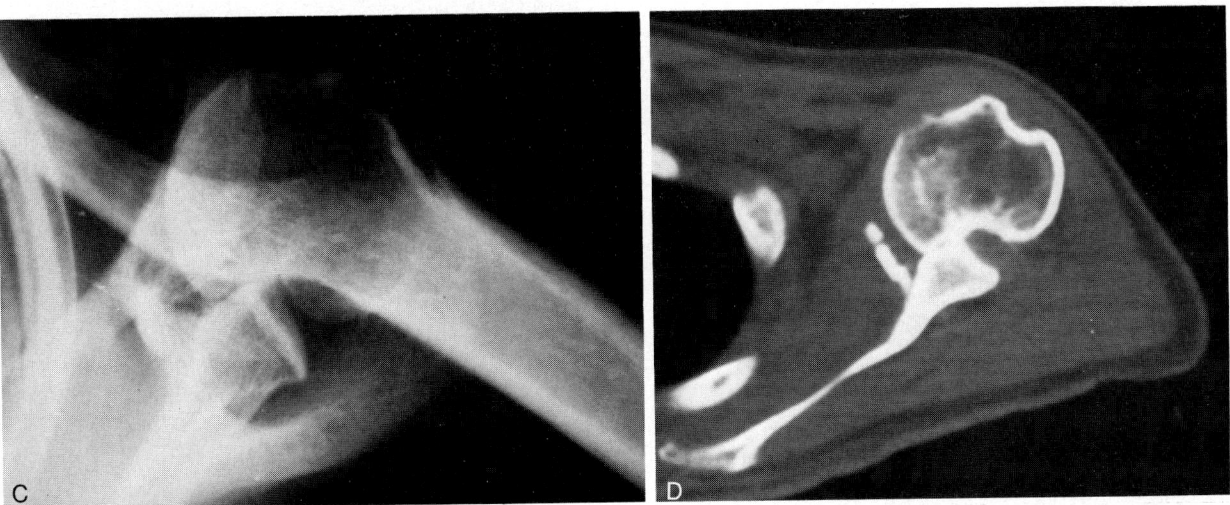

Figure 4–7 *Continued* C, Axillary view of another patient shows a small anterior glenoid rim fragment, which was confirmed with computerized tomography (D).

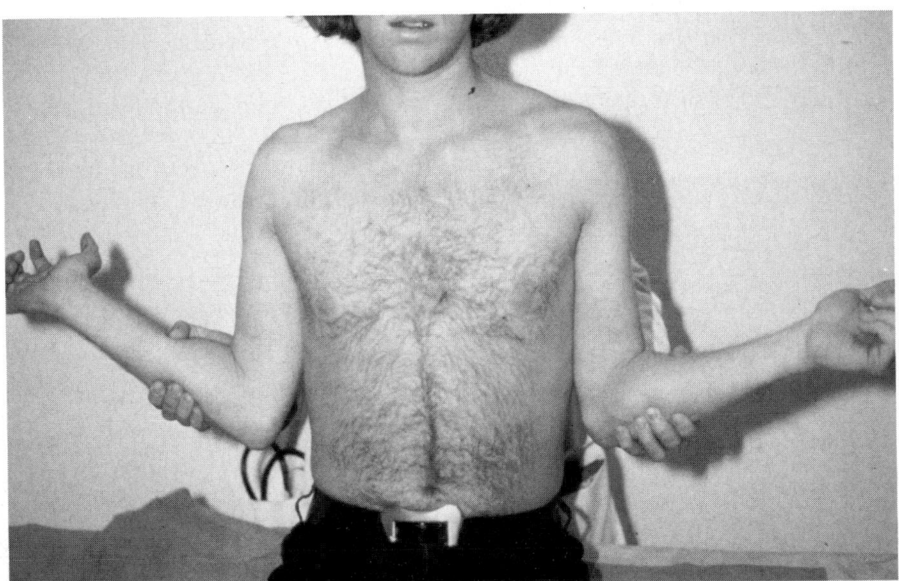

Figure 4–8. ***Anterior Instability Test.*** This unpublished sign is helpful in distinguishing anterior instability from impingement. External rotation with the arm held at the side causes pain in most patients if there is anterior instability. There may be more external rotation on the involved side, as is the case on this patient's right side. Unfortunately, acutely painful impingement lesions also hurt when the arm is externally rotated; therefore, it may also be necessary to perform the impingement injection test (see Fig. 2–30) just prior to this test to make the differential diagnosis.

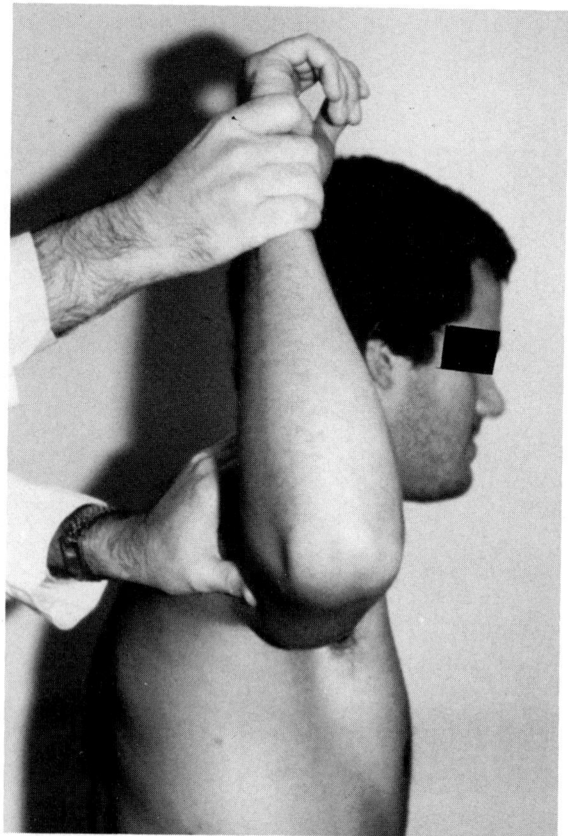

Figure 4–9. Anterior apprehension sign. Pressure is applied on the humerus as the arm is extended and externally rotated.

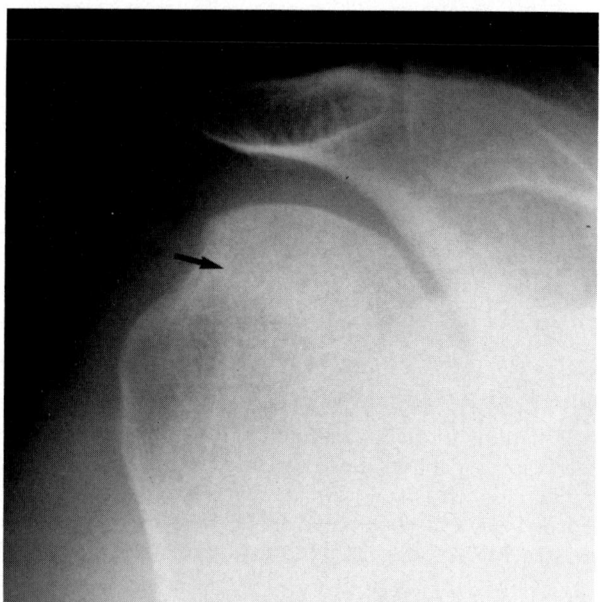

Figure 4–10. Roentgen findings in recurrent, traumatic anterior dislocations (see also Figs. 4–11 through 4–13). Anterior-posterior view with the arm in internal rotation shows an average posterior head defect (arrow—Hill-Sachs defect).

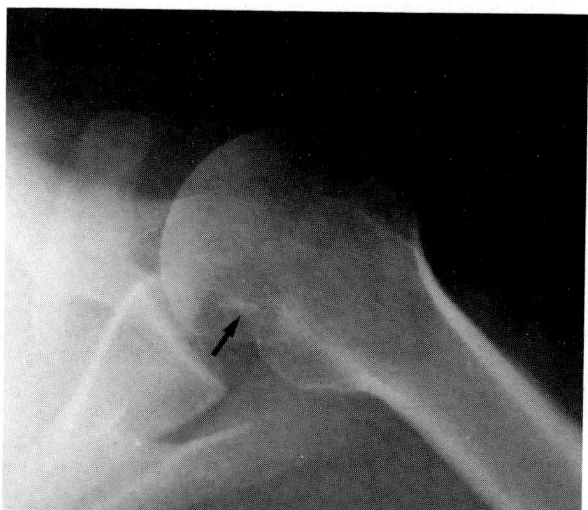

Figure 4–11. Axillary view of a more recent posterior head defect (arrow).

is an extreme example of this; however, others may also exhibit this finding. Throwing arms, as in baseball pitchers with acquired anterior laxity, demonstrate even more external rotation when the arm is tested in 90 degrees of abduction (see Figs. 1–7 and 4–43).

The x-ray findings seen in recurrent traumatic anterior dislocations are the posterior head defect and the anterior glenoid rim reaction (Figs. 4–10 through 4–13). Patients with acquired anterior laxity may have minimal x-ray findings but eventually develop similar bone changes.

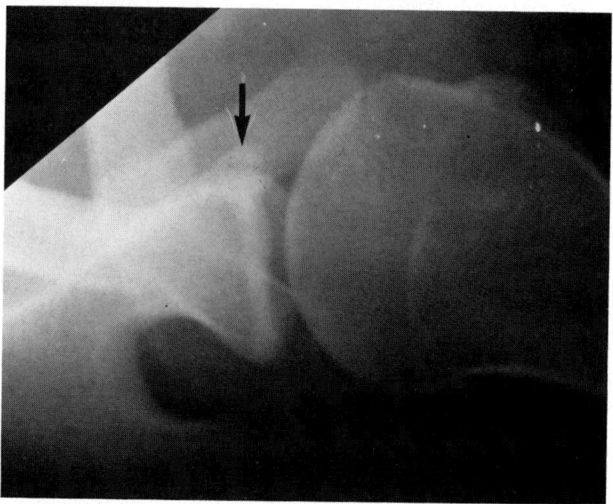

Figure 4–12. Supine axillary view with the arm held in external rotation and 10 degrees cephalic tilt of the tube (see Fig. 1–12) shows the reactive bone at the anterior rim of the glenoid (arrow) that is pathognomonic of anterior instability.

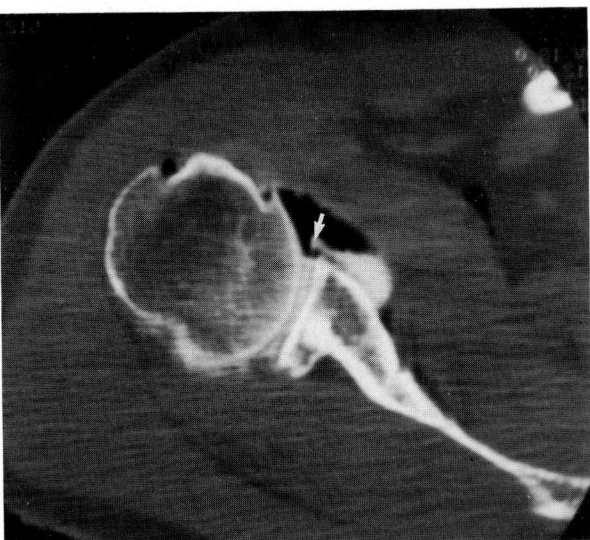

Figure 4–13. Computerized tomography of an arthrogram was read as showing an avulsion of the anterior glenoid labrum (arrow); however, minimal labrum defect was found at surgery. In problem cases, this test has not been as dependable as examination under anesthesia.

Diagnosis of Dislocation Erecta

The diagnosis of dislocation erecta should be easy (Fig. 4–14). The incidence of axillary nerve injuries is greater with this injury than with other types of dislocations. X-rays may reveal a superior head defect (see Fig. 4–45). Treatment is discussed on pages 300 and 309.

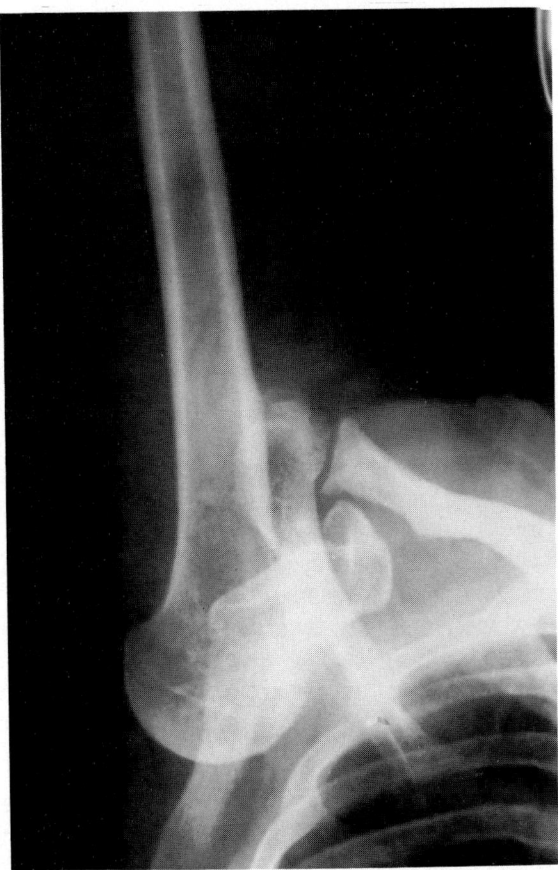

Figure 4–14. Dislocation erecta. An antero-inferior dislocation that occurred with the arm fully elevated.

Diagnosis of Unreduced Posterior Dislocations

Very few pure posterior dislocations (dislocations without a fracture) remain dislocated long enough to be examined by a physician or to have an x-ray made (Fig. 4–15). One of the few I have seen is illustrated in Figure 4–2A. Dislocations with anterior impression fractures often "lock" in the dislocated position; they are discussed in Chapter 5 with proximal humeral fractures (pp. 392 to 395).

The appearance of a patient with a locked posterior dislocation is illustrated in Figure 5–32. The two most helpful signs are loss of external rotation and extension and, as illustrated, an altered axis of the shaft of the humerus so that the arm points behind the acromion rather than toward the anterior acromion. In slender patients it may be possible to detect a prominence of the coracoid and of the head posteriorly, but these signs are of little value in obese and muscular patients.

The most useful x-ray study for the diagnosis of a posterior dislocation is the axillary view. The

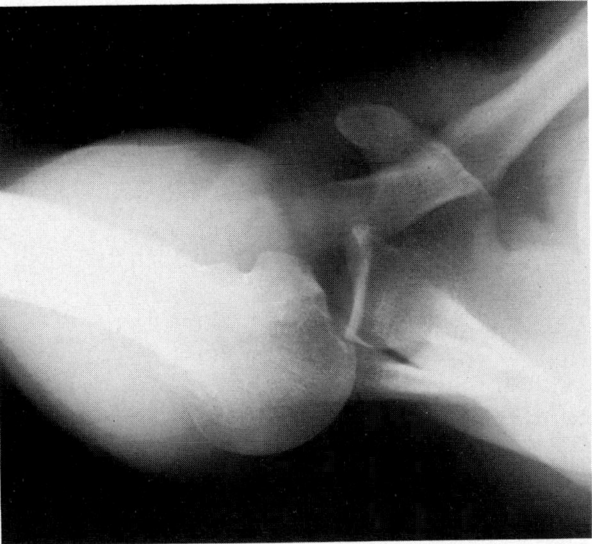

Figure 4–15. Roentgen appearance of unreduced posterior dislocation. Axillary view of a posterior dislocation in a patient with acquired dislocations. It is very rare to see this type of dislocation unreduced unless there is an impression fracture of the humeral head.

extent of bone damage can be estimated with a CT scan (see Fig. 4–13).

Signs of Self-Reduced Posterior Instability

The posterior apprehension signs and other signs of posterior instability are illustrated in Figure 4–16. Most patients with posterior instability are young women who have self-reducing subluxations that require extremely careful clinical judgement and conservative treatment before considering a surgical repair. Most of these patients have some elements of inferior instability. Male patients with injuries occasionally have self-reduced traumatic posterior dislocations that often go undiagnosed or are misdiagnosed, and they usually require surgery. The acquired type of posterior laxity should also be treated conservatively initially but may, because of persistent disability, require surgery as discussed in Figure 4–34.

X-ray signs may include an anterior head defect and rounding off or bone reaction at the posterior rim of the glenoid in the more long-standing cases. Abnormal retroversion of the glenoid is very rarely present, although imperfect axillary views made with oblique projections give the false appearance of abnormal version.[270]

Recognition of Multidirectional Instability

The *sulcus sign* and multiple apprehension signs are illustrated in Figures 4–17 and 4–18. Inferior instability is a requirement for multidirectional instability. The recognition of multidirectional instability depends on the following factors:

1. Dislocation occurred without significant injury and was self-reduced.
2. Some generalized laxity (as evidenced by hypermobility of the fingers and elbow) may be present or none.
3. Patient is often athletic (swimmer, weight lifter, gymnast). Male and female patients are affected with about equal frequency.
4. Pain is brought out by carrying loads at the side or lifting overhead.
5. Sulcus sign is present.
6. Multiple apprehension signs (e.g., inferior,

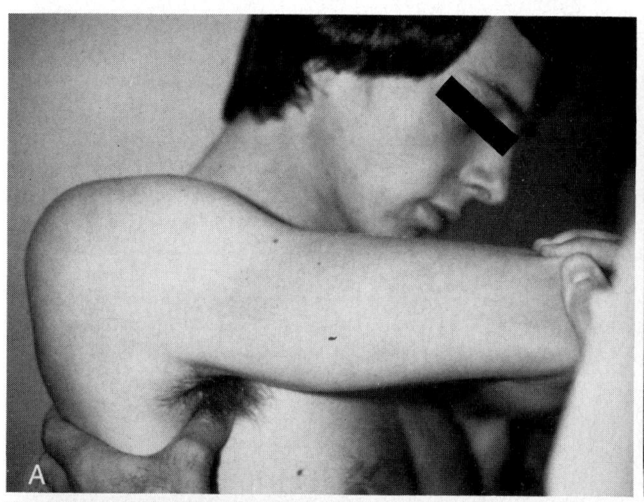

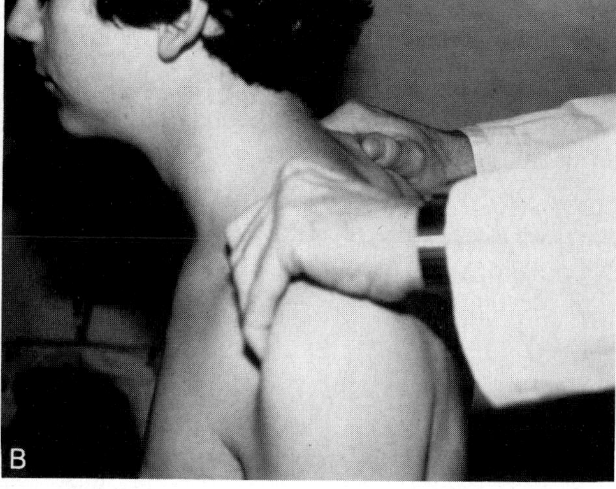

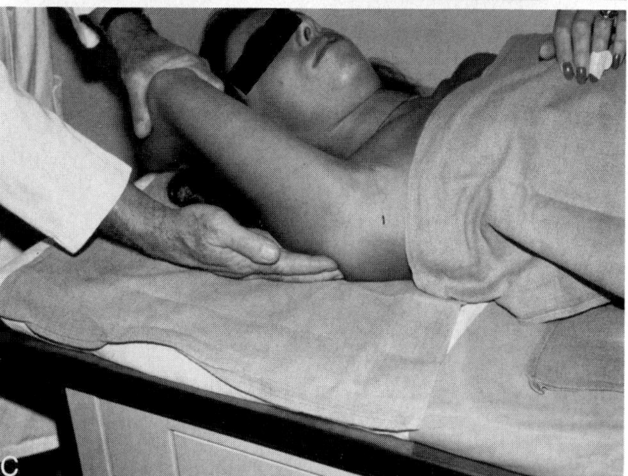

Figure 4–16. Physical signs of posterior instability.

A, Posterior apprehension sign. Pressure is applied to the scapula and at the elbow as the arm is flexed, adducted, and rotated in various angles to cause pain or a subluxation of the head.

B, Posterior translocation of the head ("Fukuda test") is done on both shoulders at once to compare the two sides.

C, Posterior subluxation can also be elicited with the patient supine. The humeral head jumps back as it is allowed to reduce. This is a very useful sign, especially during examination under anesthesia.

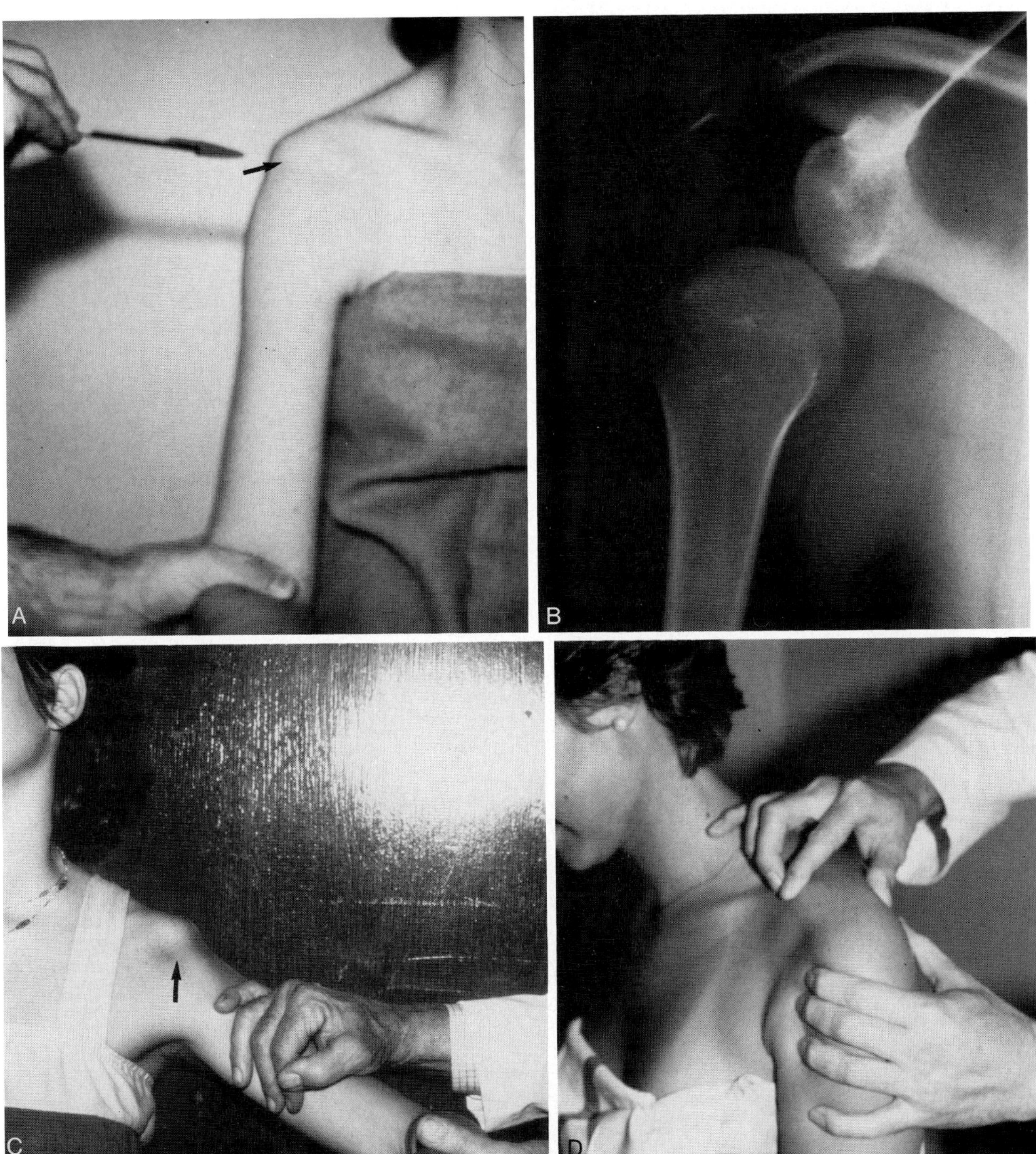

Figure 4–17. Physical signs of multidirectional instability.

A and B, Sulcus sign shows inferior instability. An indentation below the acromion (arrow in A) appears on downward traction (patient must relax the deltoid muscle). Roentgen appearance (B) with downward traction.

C, Inferior subluxation can be demonstrated with the arm in abduction, again showing the sulcus sign (arrow).

D, Translocation of the head both anteriorly and posteriorly (as well as inferior instability) is shown, as can be elicited if the patient can relax the muscles.

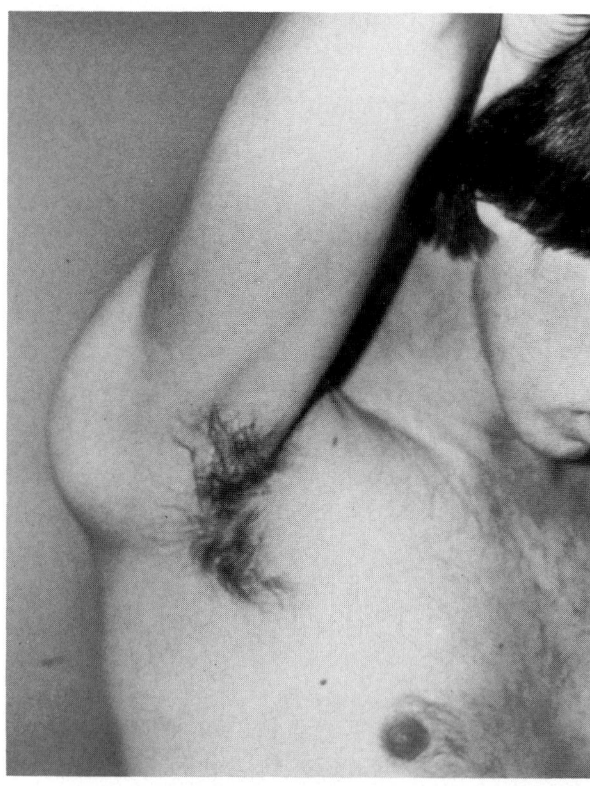

Figure 4–18. Patients with multidirectional instability can often subluxate their shoulder both forward and backward and have all three apprehension signs—anterior, posterior, and inferior—as in this swimmer, who has acquired multidirectional instability and is subluxating his shoulder posteriorly.

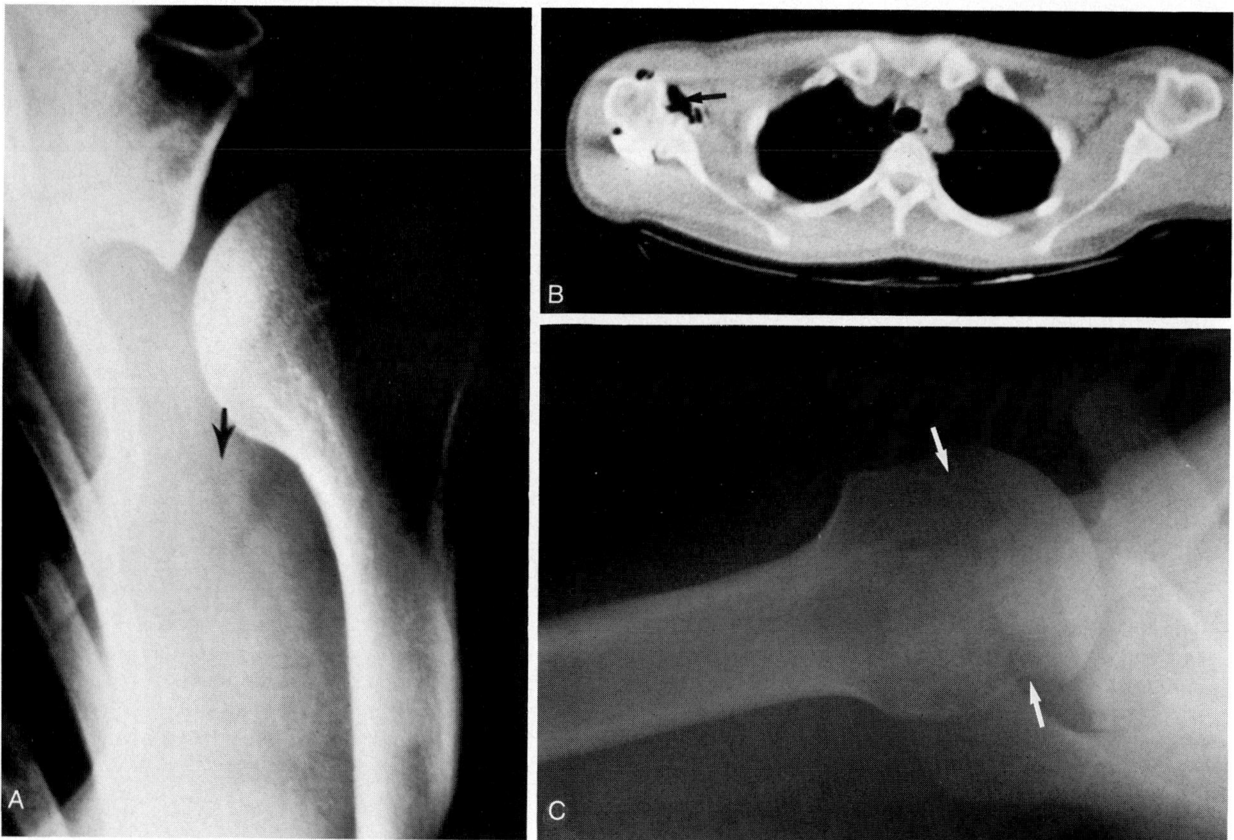

Figure 4–19 *See legend on opposite page*

anterior, and posterior [Figs. 4–17 and 4–18]) are present.

7. Special x-rays (25-pound weights [Figs. 1–12 and 4–19A], stress x-rays, and fluoroscopy) may be necessary.

Recognition of Motivational Problems

"Voluntary" dislocators are rarely psychiatric patients but may be motivated to dislocate their shoulders to attract attention or to avoid some unpleasant task. I used the term "involuntary"[13] dislocators in 1980 to refer to patients who had shoulders so unstable that they dislocated against their will, unexpectedly, and with real disability.

The distinction between the two types of patient can be very difficult. Most psychiatrists who are consulted return a report indicating that "no psychosis is present and patient is satisfactory for surgery;" however, the surgeon needs to have some information about the maturity and motivation of the patient.

The age of patients with maturity and motivational problems is usually between 14 and 20 years (Fig. 4–20), but some are older. To the delight of the patient, the parents are usually very concerned. During the initial interview, the patient usually smiles and shows far less concern than the parents.

The most valuable sign in my examination occurs during an attempt to reduce the shoulder while palpating the resistance of the patient's muscles. These patients make an effort to hold the humerus out of the joint. This is called the "resistance to reduction" sign.

I re-examine voluntary dislocators repeatedly at intervals of from three to six months and advise daily home "instability exercises" (Fig. 7–13) between examinations. This prevents the patient from having an undesirable surgical procedure and allows some time for maturity. I assure the parents and the families there is no harm if an episode of dislocation occurs. The more disinterested the parents become, the faster the cure. Identification of those with motivational problems who have had previous failed surgery is more difficult.

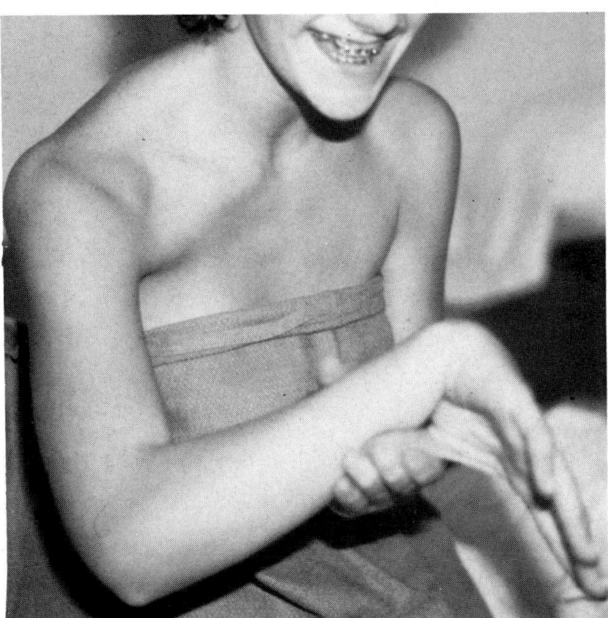

Figure 4–20. *Voluntary Dislocator.* A 16 year old girl demonstrating her "posterior dislocation" and thumb hypermobility. This upsets her parents, but she is smiling without genuine concern. Surgery is contraindicated.

Superior Dislocations

A violent injury may cause this lesion (Fig. 4–21).

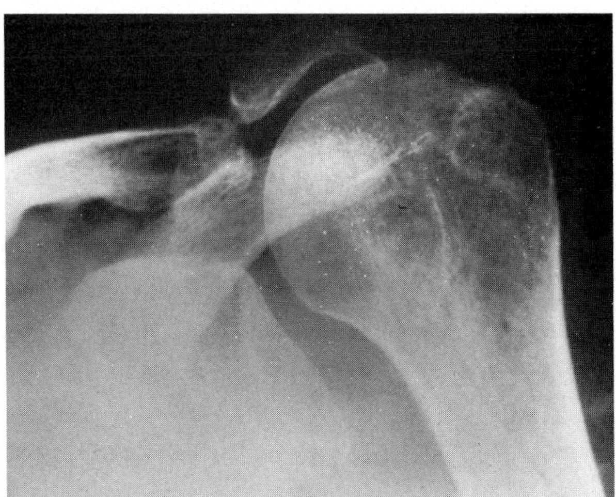

Figure 4–21. *"Superior Dislocation."* Violent trauma has driven the humerus upward, fracturing the acromion and avulsing the rotator cuff. This is a diagnostic pitfall. An arthrogram is indicated, and treatment is given as discussed in Chapter 5, page 416.

Figure 4–19. Roentgen findings in multidirectional instability.

A, Inferior instability (arrow) shown with the 25-pound weight films in a patient who had had two failed standard procedures for recurrent dislocations, one anteriorly and one posteriorly.

B, Arthrogram–computerized tomogram showing the enlarged joint space (arrow), which is the basic lesion in multidirectional instability.

C, There are usually no humeral head defects in multidirectional instability, but in this case of long-standing instability there were small defects both anteriorly and posteriorly (axillary view).

Differential Diagnosis

As mentioned earlier, the presence of a loose shoulder does not finalize the diagnosis. Not all loose shoulders are painful; the pain may be due to some other condition. In the course of my practice I have performed total shoulder arthroplasties on five patients with rheumatoid arthritis who had been treated elsewhere initially with some standard procedure for unidirectional instability.

Impingement and instability can be confusing and, as shown in Figure 4–22, can occur together. A multidirectionally unstable shoulder that is unstable anteriorly, posteriorly, and inferiorly may also be unstable superiorly, causing impingement with the clinical picture of a Stage I or Stage II impingement lesion (see Chapter 2). Because subacromial impingement is often associated with symptoms at the long head of the biceps, this type of pain may be present as well. The impingement injection test (see Fig. 2–30) does not completely relieve the pain from this type of inpingement and the remedy is stabilization of the shoulder with an inferior capsular shift (see Figs. 4–38 to 4–42), avoiding the error of a biceps tenodesis or an anterior acromioplasty (Fig. 4–22).

A large Stage III impingement cuff tear (as seen in some patients over 40 years of age) can cause instability by the posterior mechanism, which is treated by repair of the rotator cuff rather than a capsulorrhaphy. A few patients have combined Bankart lesions and cuff tears. The technique for treating them is described in Chapter 2.

In patients under 40 years of age, more violent and repeated microtrauma (as in a javelin thrower) can cause acquired glenohumeral dislocations, which, like most multidirectional dislocations, are associated with an enlargement of the cleft between the superior and middle glenohumeral ligaments.[13] Eventually, this enlargement spreads further and is associated with a defect at the rotator interval between the supraspinatus and subscapularis tendons. At first this defect may be seen in an arthrogram as a bulging of the synovial lining, but later it breaks through (see Fig. 2–21) as a complete thickness tear in the rotator interval, and arthrogram dye leaks into the subacromial bursa. This type of tear is treated by stabilization of the unstable shoulder with an inferior capsular shift (or variant of it) as well as closure of the tear at the rotator interval.

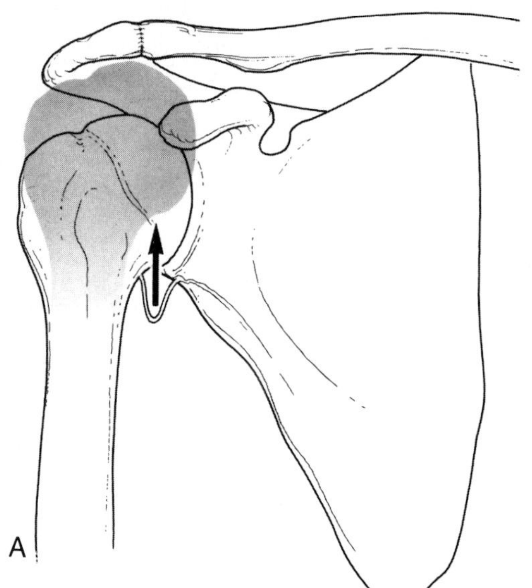

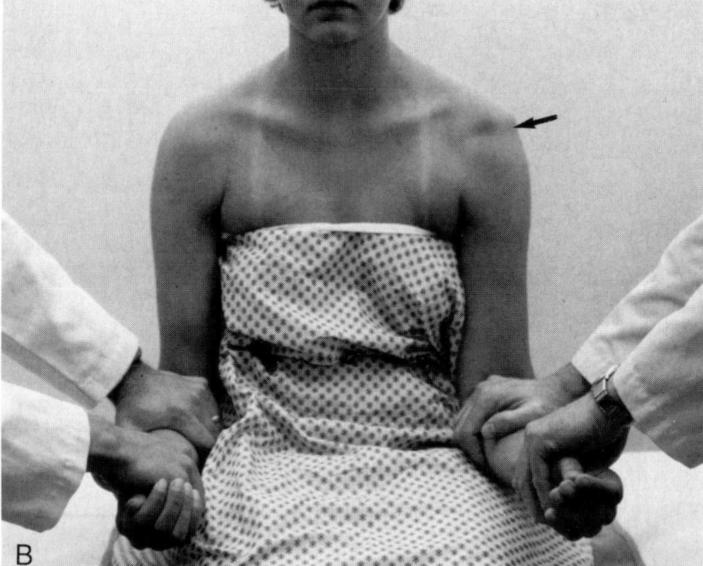

Figure 4–22. ***Differential Diagnosis.*** The differential diagnosis between pain due to impingement and pain due to glenohumeral instability is important.

A, Multidirectional instability can cause impingement.

B, A failed left anterior acromioplasty (arrow) in a 24 year old patient demonstrating a sulcus (arrow). She had undiagnosed multidirectional instability. The pain was eliminated with an inferior capsular shift (see Figs. 4–38 to 4–42) to control the instability. The impingement injection test (see Fig. 2–30) is most helpful for making the distinction to ensure appropriate treatment.

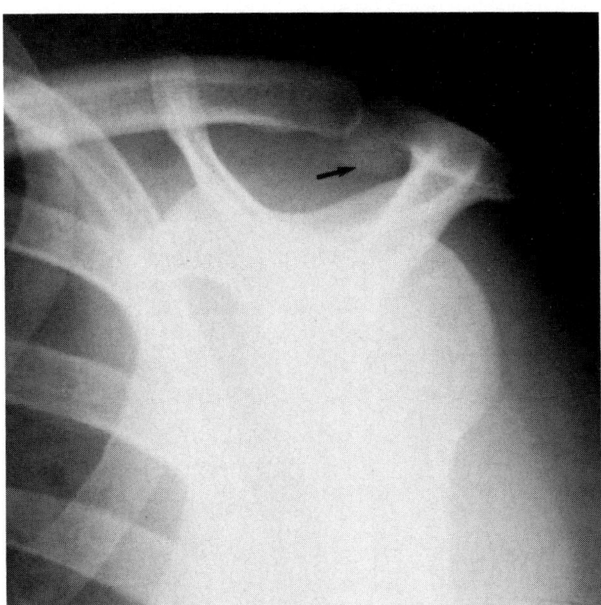

Figure 4–23. ***Differential Diagnosis.*** An extremely rare cause of persistent pain after a repair for recurrent anterior dislocations in a 24 year old man. This true bony deformity (arrow) of the acromion was causing impingement, and although the patient was younger than the usual acceptable age for an anterior acromioplasty, this procedure was successfully performed with relief of pain.

Evaluation During Surgery

Examination Under Anesthesia

Muscle guarding can preclude an accurate estimate of the extent of instability. The amount of laxity present can be judged better after relaxation of the muscles with anesthesia. On the other hand, a patient who is awake during the examination can communicate which directions are associated with pain (apprehension tests). Therefore, both types of examination are valuable and should be used to complement each other.

In a patient with a possible multidirectional problem, I repeat the apprehension tests at each office visit and again on admission to the hospital. These tests usually give a good idea of which directions bother the patient most, but muscle guarding can conceal areas where pain would otherwise have been encountered.

Examination under anesthesia is conducted prior to the skin preparation for either arthroscopy or surgery; at surgery it is performed after the deltoid has been retracted out of the way prior to detaching the rotator cuff and again when the joint is open. Stress x-rays or fluoroscopic studies may be made prior to making the skin incision during this examination under anesthesia (Fig. 4–24).

Technique of Examination Under Anesthesia

This procedure has a learning curve before it is satisfactory, but with experience it is quite accurate. It requires placing the humerus in a number of positions and patience.

The surgeon and assistant wear sterile gloves and avoid scratching the skin. After the muscles are relaxed, folded towels are placed beneath the scapula, and additional stabilization of the scapula is given by the assistant, who grasps the scapula and places the index finger of his or her other hand on the coracoid process with the thumb on the posterior corner of the acromion so that he or she can tell the surgeon whether the humeral head is being dislocated anteriorly or posteriorly or is remaining in place in the joint. Anterior instability can be elicited by abduction and external rotation in some cases but is usually better elicited by translocation of the head with direct pressure (Fig. 4–24). Posterior instability can also be brought out by translocation or by flexion, elevation, and internal rotation, (which causes the head to subluxate backward and downward into the pouch) followed by lowering the arm and external rotation to cause the head to reduce. Inferior instability can be brought out by traction such as that producing the sulcus sign (see Fig. 4–17A). It may take repeated testing to determine whether the head has left the joint and is dislocated or whether the head has been reduced and remains in the joint.

Some surgeons claim that normal shoulders show instability when tested in this way, making this examination of little value. This is not so in my experience. One has merely to examine a number of shoulders of patients who are under anesthesia for some other procedure to realize that not all shoulders are unstable and to appreciate the amount of instability that is within normal limits. Of course, as has already been emphasized, instability when present is not always painful and must be interpreted in light of the apprehension signs and injection tests performed when the patient is awake.

Arthroscopic Examination of Instability

Hawkins and I became interested in arthroscopic examination of instability in 1977, and in selected diagnostic and litigation problems it has a place in diagnosis. As I have become better at

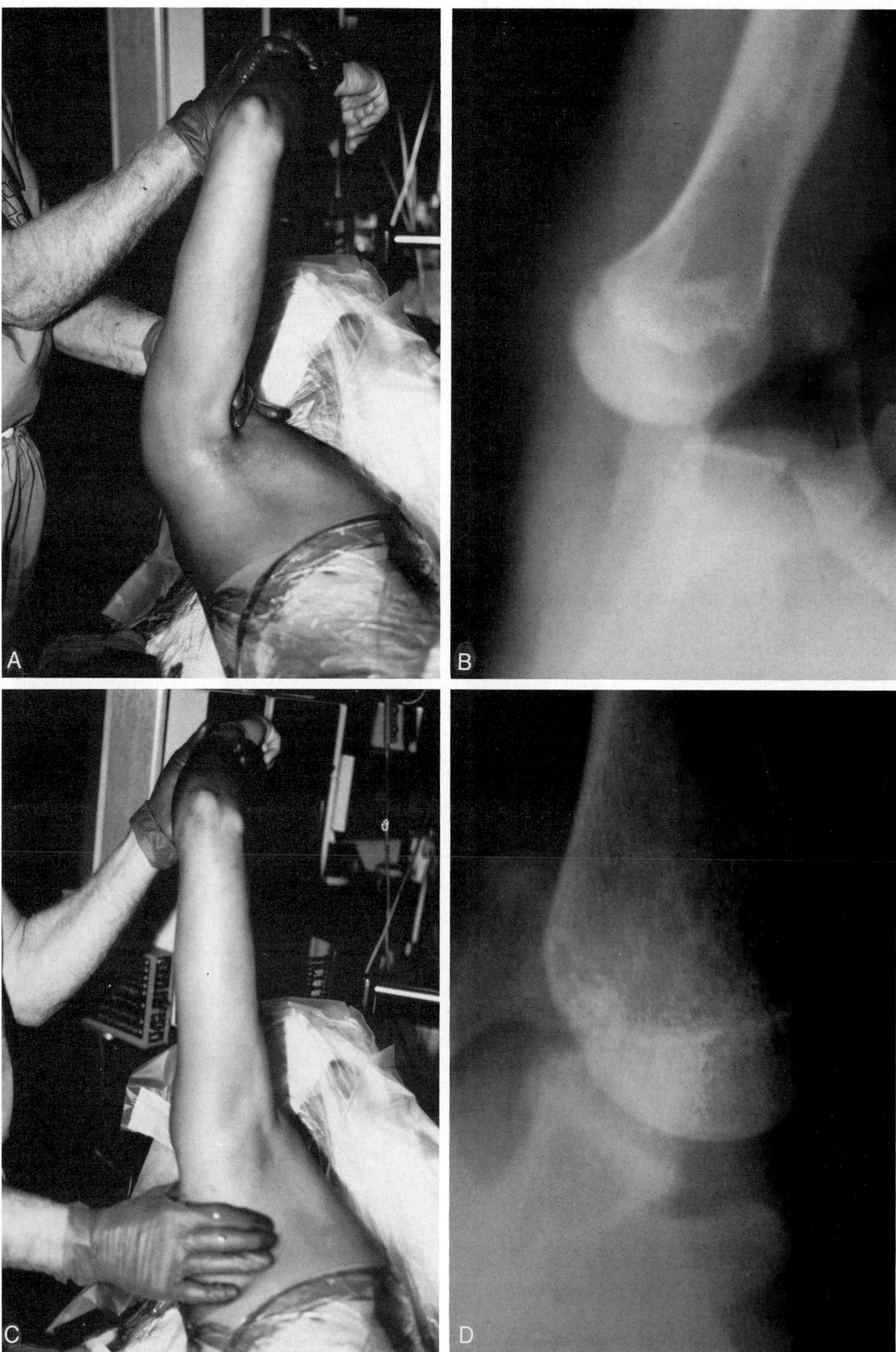

Figure 4–24. Examination under anesthesia of a posterior dislocator without anterior instability. A and B, The head can be displaced backward. C and D, It cannot be displaced forward. Inferior instability is judged by placing traction on the arm and the sulcus sign.

examination under anesthesia, however, I have found myself rarely using arthroscopy to evaluate instability.

Arthroscopic repairs for minor instability problems can be challenged unless adequate time and exercise therapy (see Fig. 7–13) have been given to make sure that the symptoms would not have been controlled by conservative treatment. Arthroscopic repairs for straightforward, two- or three-time recurrent traumatic dislocations that are unidirectional are of interest, but to date the results have been definitely inferior to those achieved by surgical repair. Although continuing developmental use of the procedure by those most expert in the field is justified, it seems impossible to achieve the same quality of capsular repair with an arthroscope as can be accomplished surgically, especially in a long-term dislocator or one with capsular laxity.

Therefore, since surgical repairs have been superior, I almost always prefer examination under anesthesia at the time of surgical repair and find myself using the arthroscope only occasionally in patients with negative or confusing examinations under anesthesia who have had a long history of unexplained shoulder disability. In doubtful cases, the operating room is set up for arthroscopy so that it can be used diagnostically if desired, but this is very rarely necessary if one is familiar with the technique of examination under anesthesia.

Operative Findings

As discussed in the preceding paragraphs, I rely on examination under anesthesia and the findings at surgery to direct the procedure. The operation should correct the pathology actually present in that particular shoulder. Since in many cases one does not always know prior to anesthesia whether the shoulder instability is unidirectional or multidirectional or whether it is primarily anterior or posterior, it is better to consider the operative findings of all types of shoulder instability together, just as one must be prepared to do at surgery. At surgery, a shoulder with the major instability in either an anterior or posterior direction should again be stressed in all directions and examined because it may have some pathology inferiorly or even prove to have multidirectional instability. Operative findings are illustrated in Figures 4–25 through 4–29.

Evidence of Anterior Instability

The findings listed below are frequently present in those in the Traumatic category, may de-

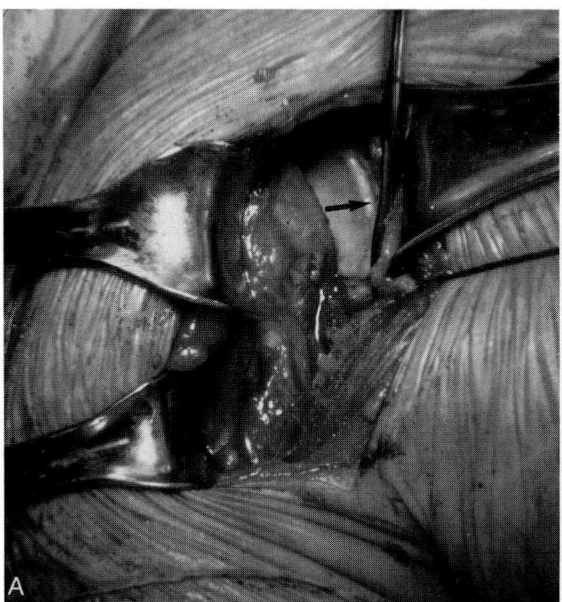

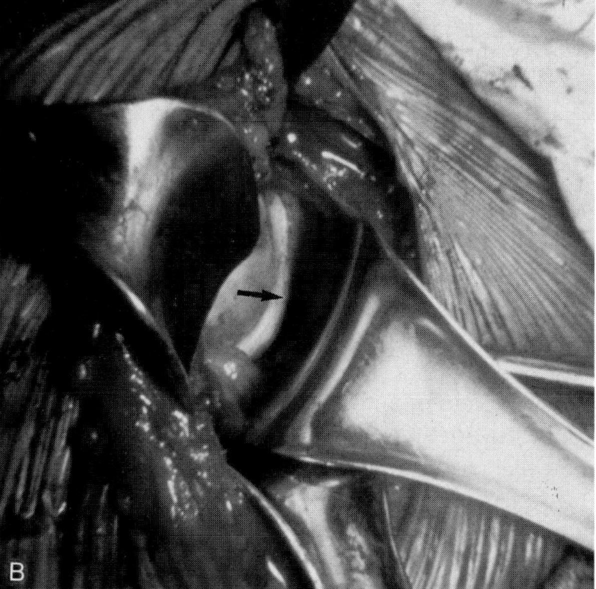

Figure 4–25. ***Operative Findings in Recurrent Anterior Dislocations.*** Detachments of the anterior glenoid labrum (Bankart, Broca; arrows) are frequently seen in those with traumatic dislocations, eventually appear in acquired dislocations of long standing, but are rarely seen in those with atraumatic dislocations. Detachment of the labrum should be treated by re-attachment because the labrum is the scapular attachment of the important inferior glenohumeral ligament.

A, An anterior detachment.

B, A larger anterior and inferior detachment.

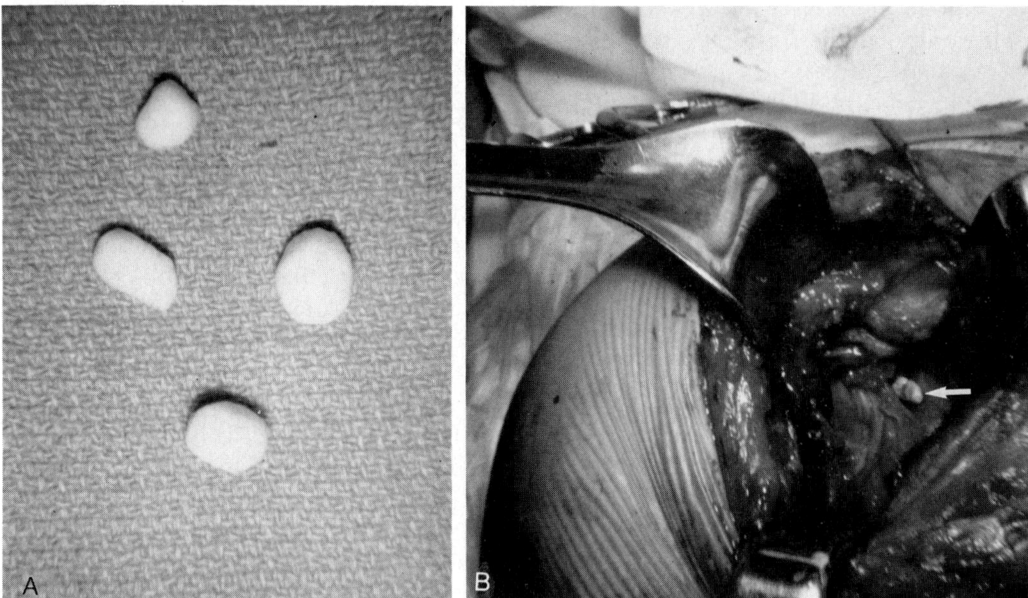

Figure 4–26A and B. ***Operative Findings in Recurrent Anterior Dislocations.*** Osteochondral bodies tend to migrate to the recess at the insertion of the long head of the biceps, the posterior-inferior pouch of the glenohumeral joint, and, as illustrated in B, in the subscapularis bursa (beneath the coracoid). Unless removed they can spoil the result of a repair.

velop with time (but are not present initially) in those in the Acquired category, and are rarely seen in patients in the Atraumatic group (see Table 4–1). Hypermobility and enlarged capsular recesses are more notable in those in the Acquired and Atraumatic categories. Gross evidence of *anterior instability* includes:

1. Fraying, splitting, or detachment of the anterior labrum (Fig. 4–25A and B).
2. Attenuation or splitting of the middle glenohumeral ligament.
3. Cartilage wear or eburnation at the anterior rim of the glenoid.
4. Loose osteochondral bodies (which usually result from a posterior head defect—Fig. 2–26A and B). The head defect is not seen at surgery unless it is located more superiorly because of inferior dislocations.
5. Enlargement of the cleft between the middle and superior glenohumeral ligaments or a rotator interval tear of the rotator cuff (see Figs. 2–21 and 2–22). Impingement tears may also be associated with anterior instability (Fig. 2–19), as may massive tears tht occur occasionally with unusually violent injuries (see Fig. 2–24).

Evidence of Posterior Instability

1. The posterior labrum serves as the attachment for the long head of the biceps and is not an important structure in stability. However, it may be frayed or split, as shown in Figure 4–28A. I do not recall seeing it detached from the scapula except in violent trauma, and it is not to be compared with the anterior labrum in importance in stability problems.
2. A posterior "pouch" forms in which the posterior-inferior capsule is distended to hold the

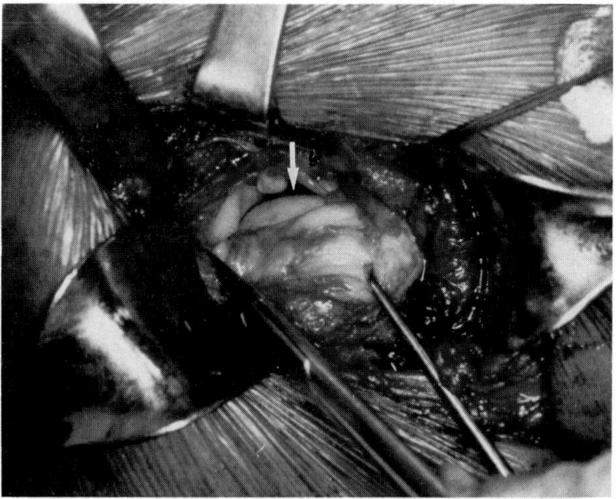

Figure 4–27. ***Operative Findings in Recurrent Anterior Dislocations.*** This traumatic anterior dislocation occurred in a 56 year old woman who fell. It was easily reduced but was unstable. An arthrogram showed a tear of the rotator cuff. At surgery four months later, this rotator interval tear (arrow) was found and repaired through an anterior acromioplasty approach, as seen. The anterior glenoid labrum was found to be intact, but if it had been detached, it could have been re-attached through this approach if the arm were held in forward flexion.

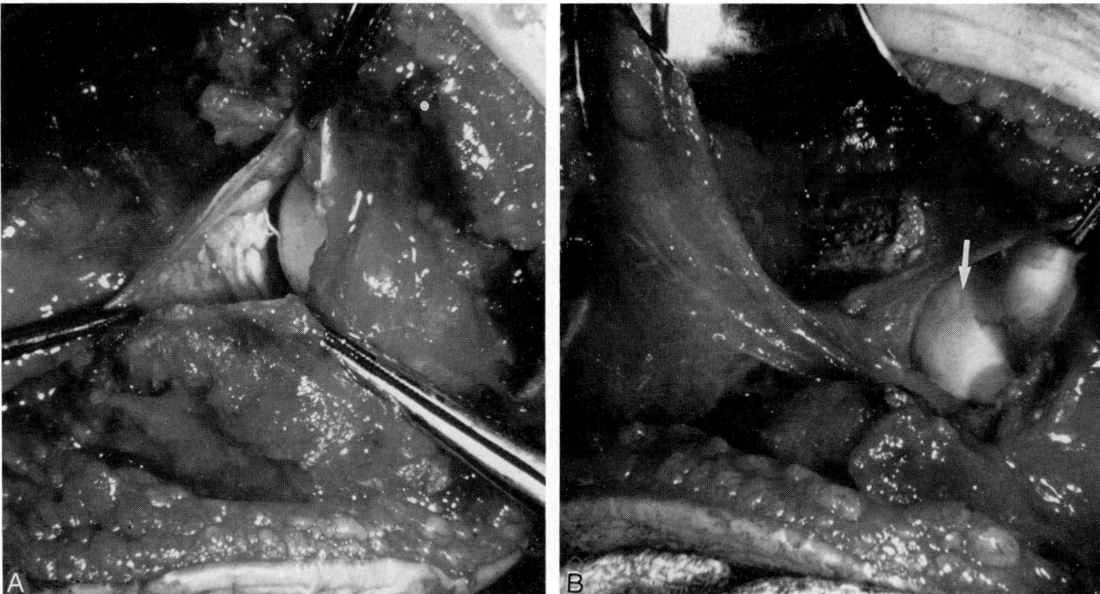

Figure 4–28. Posterior view of a shoulder with recurrent posterior dislocations.

A, A large posterior capsular "pouch" and fraying of the posterior glenoid labrum, seen with the head reduced.

B, The humeral head (arrow) is dislocated posteriorly into the pouch.

humeral head when it is dislocated (Fig. 4–28A and B).

3. An anterior counterpart of the Malgaigne-Hill-Sachs posterior head defect that is seen with anterior dislocations may be present, as illustrated in Figure 4–19C, but it is smaller unless there has been an impression fracture of the articular surface, such as occurs with a seizure (see Figs. 4–45 and 4–46).

4. With long-standing recurrent posterior in-

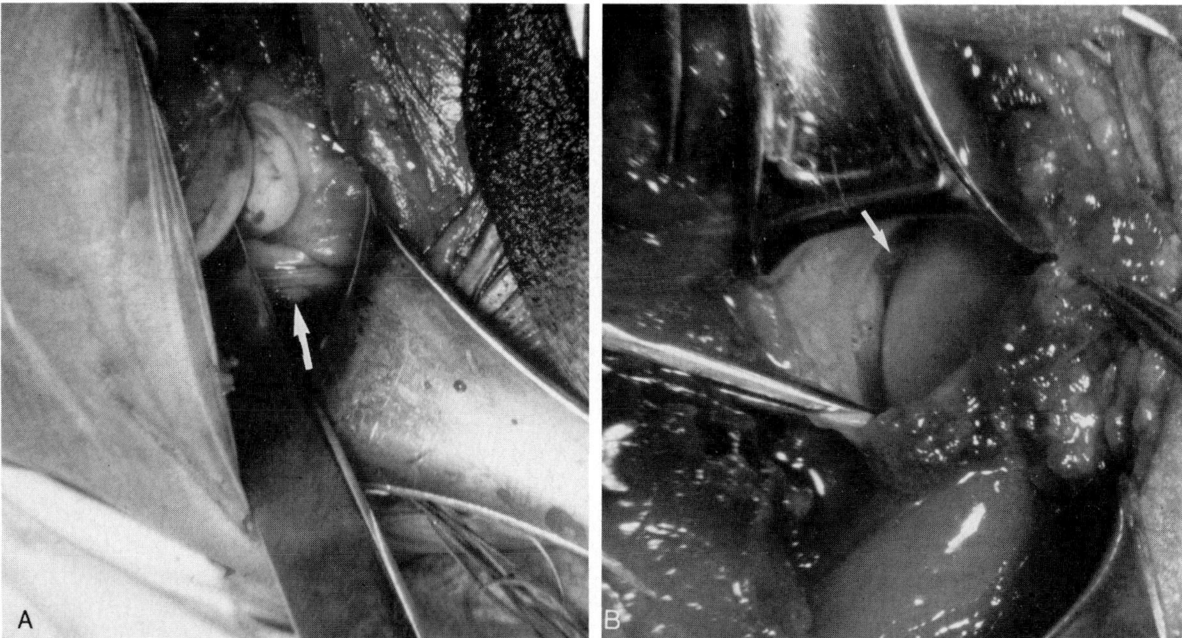

Figure 4–29. ***Operative Findings in Multidirectional Dislocations.***

A, Anterior view of a shoulder with multidirectional dislocations showing the large inferior capsular pouch (arrow) after it has been partially released from the humerus.

B, Posterior view of a multidirectional unstable shoulder joint showing a large posterior capsular pouch; the humeral head is retracted anteriorly and laterally to show a detachment of the anterior glenoid labrum (arrow). A second approach was made in front (of this one) to re-attach the labrum before the inferior capsular shift (see Figs. 4–39 to 4–42) from the posterior side was completed.

stability, there may be loss of articular cartilage and rounding off of the posterior glenoid rim. This, along with an inadequate posterior capsule, as is seen at times in patients undergoing surgery for posterior repairs, is my indication to consider a posterior bone block (see Fig. 4–34G).

Evidence of Inferior Instability

1. Traumatic inferior dislocation can occur in injuries in which the arm is abducted overhead, which produces a "dislocation erecta" (see Fig. 4–14). The humeral head is driven downward and may have an impression fracture superiorly (see Fig. 4–46), which is visible from an anterior approach. The inferior labrum between 5 and 7 o'clock is detached. If the arm is lowered, the head is locked tightly onto the glenoid and cannot be closed reduced. The arm must be fully elevated overhead with traction upward to reduce this type of dislocation (see Fig. 4–30).

2. Acquired and atraumatic inferior instability is associated with an inferior capsular pouch large enough to hold the head below the glenoid (Fig. 4–29A). The labrum is intact early but eventually begins to fray and eventually becomes detached and may require re-attachment to the rim of the glenoid at the time of an inferior capsular shift (Fig. 4–29B).

Evidence of Multidirectional Instability

1. Detachment of the anterior glenoid labrum is less likely to be present but may be present (Fig. 4–29B), apparently as a result (not the cause) of repeated dislocations. In our series published in 1980,[13] we excluded patients with multidirectional instability with detachment of the anterior labrum because we thought that they would confuse the analysis of inferior capsular shift (because they would need the additional procedure of re-attachment of the labrum). This led to the erroneous statement by some surgeons that we thought detachment of the anterior labrum never occurred with multidirectional instability. Detachment of the anterior labrum is less common but certainly does occur, and fraying of the inferior and posterior glenoid labrum is usually present in multidirectionally unstable shoulders.

2. The constant finding is a redundant capsule inferiorly, posteriorly, and anteriorly in varying proportions (Fig. 4–29A).

3. Enlargement of the cleft between the superior and middle glenohumeral ligaments is characteristically present (see Fig. 4–31E).

4. By applying traction, the head can be dislocated inferiorly, and with direct pressure it can be subluxated or dislocated anteriorly and posteriorly before opening the capsule and with the joint open.

TREATMENT OF INITIAL DISLOCATIONS

Treatment of Initial Anterior Dislocation

As indicated in Table 4–1, an initial anterior dislocation that results from a significant injury (e.g., a traumatic anterior dislocation) usually remains dislocated until a closed reduction is performed. After a trauma series of x-rays (see Fig. 1–12) to exclude a fracture and a neurological appraisal, especially for an axillary nerve injury (sensory loss over the middle deltoid and inability to set the deltoid muscle), the dislocation is reduced by closed manipulation.

The method of closed reduction that I consider least traumatic is continuous traction on the arm as the arm is gradually elevated while an assistant holds a sheet wrapped around the patient's chest for countertraction (Fig. 4–30). From time to time the surgeon applies pressure on the humeral head, pushing it backward into place with gentle rotation of the arm when necessary to disengage the head. Elevation of the arm relaxes the rotator cuff and usually allows the head to reduce without force with analgesia provided by Demerol and Valium. Another method that is tried when this fails is the Stimson[271] method, in which the patient lies prone with the arm off the side of the table with weights attached to the wrist to attempt to overcome muscle spasm as the surgeon from time to time pushes the humeral head toward the glenoid. If these methods fail, I prefer to use general anesthesia to relax the muscles. Once reduction is obtained, the arm is placed in internal rotation and flexion in a sling and swathe.

There has been considerable dispute about whether the shoulder should be immobilized after the initial dislocation in the hope that the tissue will heal to avoid recurrent dislocations. I feel very strongly that this confusion has resulted from failure to distinguish those with pure traumatic dislocations from the large group with acquired glenohumeral laxity. Thus, the importance of the proposed classification in Table 4–1 is emphasized again.

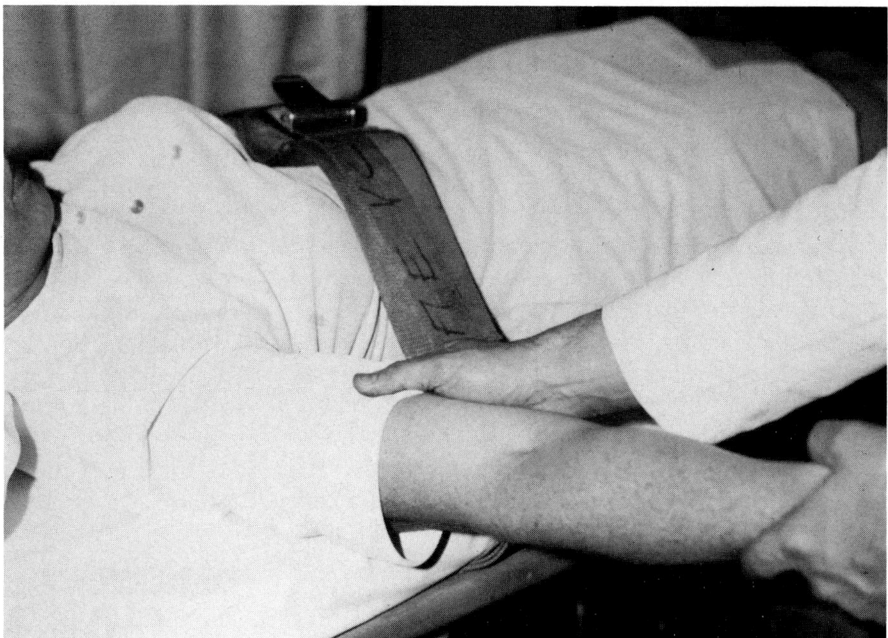

Figure 4–30. A method of closed reduction of an anterior dislocation that is atraumatic. The assistant holds a sheet wrapped around the chest, and continuous traction is applied to the arm as the arm is gradually abducted. Pressure is intermittently applied on the humerus to relocate the head. At times slight gentle rotation is necessary to disengage the head.

In my experience, patients with traumatic dislocations have an excellent chance of healing and avoiding recurrences if the shoulder is "immobilized" five to six weeks to allow torn soft tissue to heal and rehabilitation exercises are performed afterward to strengthen the subscapularis. The subscapularis is the most important active defender against recurrent anterior dislocations. My experience[185] is similar to that of McIntosh,[187] who found a very low rate of recurrence after anterior shoulder dislocations in athletes at the University of Toronto when they were treated initially with immobilization. Cofield[189] also favors immobilization after the initial dislocation.

The better prognosis of those with traumatic anterior dislocations treated with immobilization after the initial dislocation compared with those with acquired laxity has never been recognized. I believe that this is the key to settling the time-worn controversy about whether immobilization after the initial dislocation is of any value. It is another reason for recognizing the group with acquired laxity in our classification (Table 4–1).

Should a patient with acquired laxity who has an initial self-reduced anterior dislocation be "immobilized" and treated in the same way as a person with a traumatic dislocation? I believe this is optional. I explain the poor prognosis to the patient regardless of whether the arm is immobilized or not. Most patients want to have the benefit of any doubt and request immobilization.

The method I use for immobilization after the initial dislocation is similar to that used after repair for recurrent anterior dislocations. A sling and swathe is worn for a few days until the initial soreness abates. At that time a removable sling is provided (see Fig. 7–2A), which can be easily unsnapped to use the arm at the side; however, the patient is instructed not to carry more than five pounds of weight or to move the arm into more than 20 degrees of external rotation or to raise the hand higher than the top of the head. After two weeks, the sling is discarded during the day (with the same restrictions on the use of the arm); however, a sling (with a strap around the body to prevent abduction and external rotation) is worn at night for five or six weeks. After five weeks, light use of the arm is allowed as desired. The "instability exercises" (see Fig. 7–13) are begun at three months. Heavy lifting and contact sports are avoided for at least nine months.

Using this regimen for patients with traumatic anterior dislocation, the recurrence rate in those with traumatic dislocation has been under 20 percent. Those with acquired laxity (no significant injury) have a high rate of recurrence.

In the past, emphasis has been placed on the difference in prognosis after a first dislocation between patients in the young age group (20 years old) and those in the older age group (50 years old). Older patients are found to have a much lower rate of recurrence. My experience agrees with that of Cofield.[189] The recurrence rate in the younger age group with traumatic dislocations who were treated with restricted motion and did not return to heavy activities too soon (before healing and rehabilitation were complete) was no higher than that in the older age group.

Treatment of Initial Posterior Dislocation

A discussion of treatment of acute posterior dislocations must include failure to diagnose a locked posterior dislocation. This is an ever-threatening diagnostic pitfall.[192] It has received much attention in the literature, and yet it continues to be a common error in patients with fractures, as described in Chapter 5, pages 392 to 395. Almost all posterior dislocations without fractures are self-reduced. It is very rare to see one that is unreduced; however, an x-ray of such a case is shown in Figure 4–15, and that shoulder reduced spontaneously shortly after the x-ray was made. Thus, when we hear talk about a "missed posterior dislocation," for all practical purposes the speaker is actually talking about a missed fracture-dislocation.

The initial treatment of an early recognized, locked posterior dislocation with an impression fracture of less than 40 percent is a trial of closed reduction. The closed reduction is performed with the patient supine. The shoulder is flexed 90 degrees and adducted (to displace the head lateral to the posterior glenoid so it will clear the posterior rim when traction in a forward direction is applied [see Fig. 4–33]), and countertraction is applied on the scapula. It is helpful during this maneuver to apply pressure directly on the humeral head, pushing it forward. Ideally, three people are involved in the reduction: one stabilizing the scapula, one applying forward traction on the flexed and adducted arm, and the third applying pressure on the head to move it forward. When the head slips forward, the humerus is externally rotated and lowered to the side. It is immobilized in external rotation and moderate extension. I prefer a light plastic spica cast (see Fig. 4–34) to maintain this position for approximately five or six weeks. Later, after the shoulder has regained a reasonable range of motion, the patient is given the instability series of strengthening exercises (see Fig. 7–13). Larger humeral head defects are discussed in Chapter 5, page 395.

I have never had an opportunity to perform such a reduction on a pure posterior dislocation without a fracture. Self-reduced posterior dislocations may be diagnosed by a small anterior head defect ("reverse Hill-Sachs defect"), posterior apprehension signs, and examination under anesthesia. If symptoms of instability persist after conservative treatment, surgical repair is indicated.

Treatment of Initial Dislocation Erecta

The closed reduction of a dislocation erecta (see Fig. 4–14) is best achieved by traction cephalically with countertraction, similar to that just described for an unreduced anterior dislocation. When the head is opposite the glenoid, the arm is lowered to the side. Immobilization is similar to that described for an initial unreduced anterior dislocation. The arm is used at the side for five or six weeks without heavy lifting and is immobilized with a sling at night. After three months, strengthening exercises (see Figs. 7–10 and 7–11) are given. Heavy use of the arm is avoided for at least nine months.

SURGICAL REPAIR FOR RECURRENT ANTERIOR DISLOCATIONS

Indications

More than one complete anterior dislocation is justification for considering surgical repair because:

1. Patients with this problem are usually unable to participate in overhead activities and are handicapped in other ways.
2. Each complete dislocation inflicts some articular surface damage, although there is no urgency to perform the repair.
3. Conservative treatment is not effective in preventing continuing instability (although exercises to help control instability are advised if surgical repair is delayed).

I use a modification of an inferior capsular shift, termed the reinforced capsular cruciate repair,[19] for all recurrent anterior dislocation procedures when there is anterior instability, possibly with inferior instability but no posterior instability.

Reinforced Capsular Cruciate Repair for Recurrent Anterior Dislocations (Modified Inferior Capsular Shift)

I have preferred this method since 1978.[19] The technique differs from an inferior capsular shift from the front (see Figs. 4–38 to 4–42) only in that there is no detachment of the capsule from the posterior neck of the humerus and no spica cast is used post-operatively. Two prospective studies have been made and reported,[19, 190] as described later.

The principles and advantages of this technique are as follows:

1. The middle glenohumeral ligament is reinforced with half the thickness of the subscapularis tendon and with the tissue formed by creating two anterior capsular flaps, which are closed in a cruciate manner to double the thickness of the anterior capsule. Reinforcement of the middle glenohumeral ligament is routine because this ligament has been shown to be deficient in more than 20 percent of cadaver shoulders and in an even higher percentage, in my experience, of those with recurrent anterior dislocations.

2. Good exposure for repairing the intra-articular pathology is provided (the detached anterior labrum is re-attached, loose osteochondral bodies are removed, and in the rare case when there is a bone deficiency at the glenoid, a coracoid transfer to the scapula or other skeletal procedure can be done).

3. A sufficient length of reinforced anterior capsule is provided for flexibility in adjusting the tension at the time of closure to preserve shoulder motion. (Some standard procedures for recurrent anterior dislocations create a fixed length of capsule and tendon, which at closure may be too short for proper external rotation.)

4. This technique offers the possibility of doing an inferior capsular shift to eliminate posterior and inferior instability exactly as in Figures 4–38 to 4–42. If multidirectional instability is unexpectedly found, all directions of instability are checked during the procedure.

5. I have found that this technique is well suited for re-operations on failed repairs because the glenohumeral ligaments, which are often attenuated, can be reinforced, good exposure is provided for correcting anatomical defects inside the joint, and, if multidirectional instability is encountered, an inferior capsular shift can be performed.

It is recommended that the patient use an antiseptic soap with the daily shower beginning a few days prior to the operation. Acne and skin blemishes in the area of the incision should be cleared.

The patient is positioned in the beach chair position with a short arm board under the elbow to prevent the arm from falling backward in hyperextension from the side of the table (Fig. 4–31). Folded towels are placed under the scapula to hold it forward. Our anesthesiologists prefer general endotracheal anesthesia. Prophylactic antibiotics are given during surgery and post-operatively.

Prior to the skin preparation the shoulder is examined (with the patient under anesthesia) to determine all directions of instability (see Fig. 4–39). After skin preparation and prior to applying the adherent plastic drapes, the site of the skin incision is located in the skin creases (as seen when the arm is held at the side) and marked with a marking pencil. The incision, 6.0 cm. long, is made starting at the anterior margin of the axilla and extending upward toward the coracoid in the axillary skin folds. I use this approach of Leslie and Ryan[191] for all anterior procedures for instability (Fig. 4–31B). The area over the deltopectoral interval is undermined, and the deltopectoral interval is opened. The cephalic vein is retracted laterally (because there is less bleeding and the amount of exposure required at the upper end is less than that needed for total shoulder arthroplasties and some larger procedures). After opening the full length of the deltopectoral interval, a Darrach retractor is placed between the deltoid and the humeral shaft to retract the deltoid and cephalic vein laterally, and after dividing the clavipectoral fascia, a second Darrach elevator is placed between the acromion and the humeral head. The coracoid and its attached muscles are left intact to protect the neurovascular bundle from a retractor (Fig. 4–31C).

With flexion and external rotation of the arm, the subscapularis tendon and the circumflex artery and vein can be seen. The axillary nerve is located on the front of the subscapularis by palpation and is displaced away from the inferior capsule. The anterior circumflex vessels are then cauterized and divided.

Next, the subscapularis tendon is divided transversely halfway through, near the lesser tuberosity. Using sharp dissection the anterior half of the subscapularis tendon is raised, tagged with stay sutures, and freed so that it remains with the subscapularis muscle. The posterior half of the subscapularis is left in continuity with the middle glenohumeral ligament to reinforce it (Fig. 4–31D).

The cleft between the middle and superior glenohumeral ligaments (see Chapter 1, p. 25, Fig. 1–18 and Fig. 4–31E) can be identified and is closed with interrupted nonabsorbable sutures. The lateral vertical limb of the "T" opening is made over the sulcus (to avoid lacerating the articular cartilage of the humeral head), and the horizontal limb of the "T" is made through the reinforced capsule at the level of the center of the head of the humerus (Fig. 4–31F). The corners of the reinforced capsular flaps thus created are tagged with stay sutures. The "T-ing" of the capsule should give ample exposure for inspecting the interior of the joint. If the shoulder is unstable

Text continued on page 307

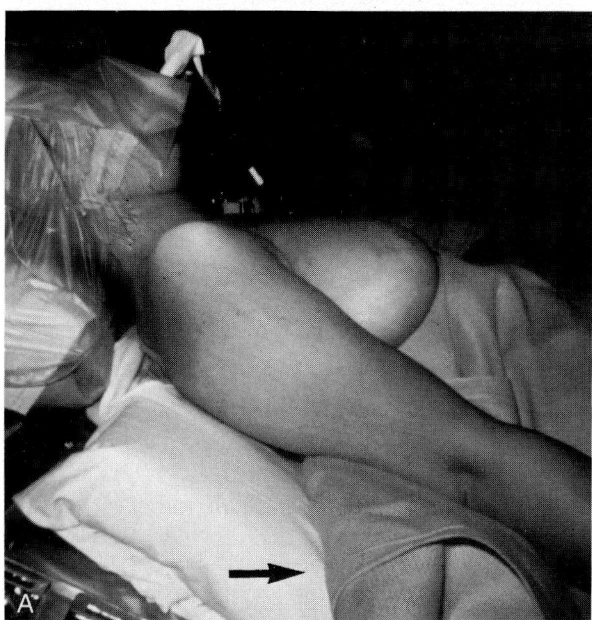

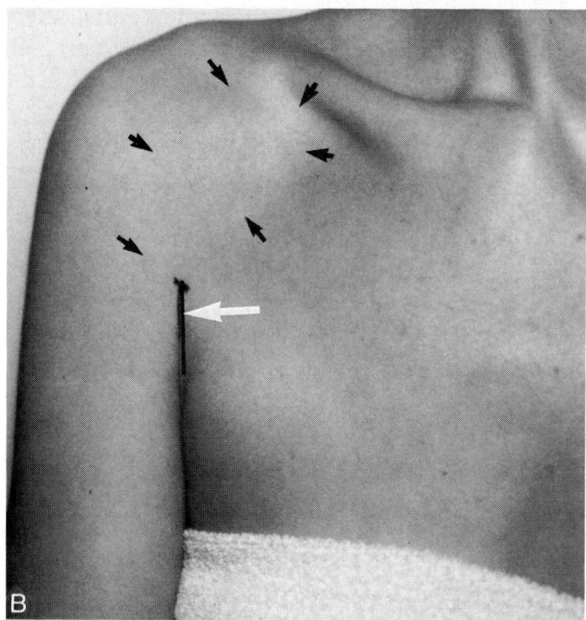

Figure 4–31. ***Reinforced Capsular Cruciate Repair for Recurrent Anterior Dislocation.*** The technique is the same as for inferior capsular shift through the anterior approach (see Fig. 4–40), except the capsule is not detached posteriorly and, although inferior redundancy is eliminated as desired, a true shift with obliteration of the posterior pouch is not performed.

A, Position. The patient is supine in the 35 degree beachchair position with folded towels under the scapula to hold it forward and a well-padded armboard or table (arrow) on which a bolster can be placed after the joint is open to prevent the arm from falling backwards in hyperextension (which interferes with exposure of the interior of the joint). Examination under anesthesia (see Fig. 4–39) is performed prior to the skin preparation and again as needed during the procedure to determine all directions of instability.

B, Incision. After the skin preparation and prior to applying adherent plastic drapes, the anterior axillary crease is marked for a 6.0 cm. incision (white arrow). This incision is undermined over the deltopectoral interval up to the clavicle (as indicated with black arrows) (see Figs. 1–25 and 1–26).

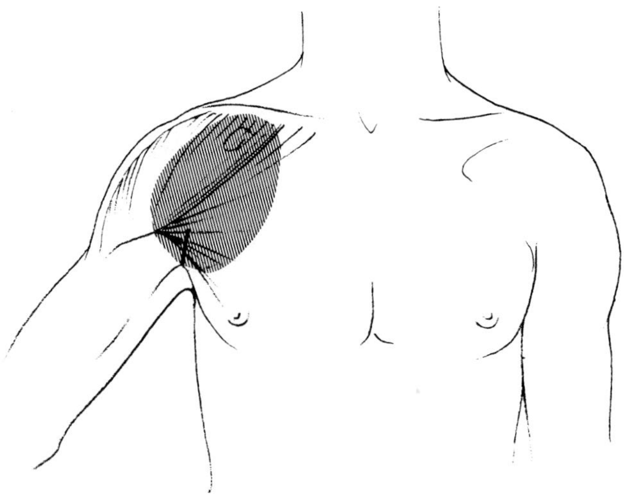

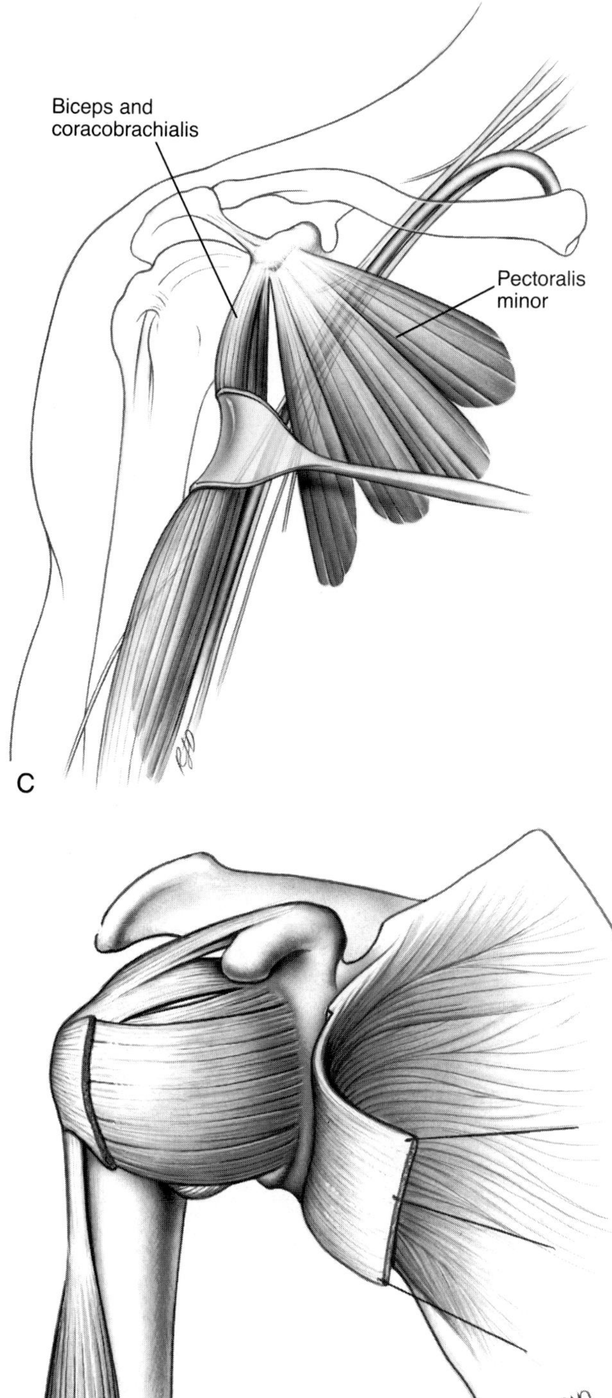

Figure 4–31 *Continued* C, The cephalic vein is retracted laterally with the deltoid muscle. The coracoid muscles are left intact to protect the neurovascular bundle from retractors (see text for details and Fig. 1–30).

D, Reinforcement of the glenohumeral ligaments. The posterior half of the subscapularis tendon is left attached to the capsule, and the "cleft" between the middle and superior glenohumeral ligaments is closed with interrupted sutures.

E, The "cleft" that is closed is illustrated (arrow).

Illustration continued on following page

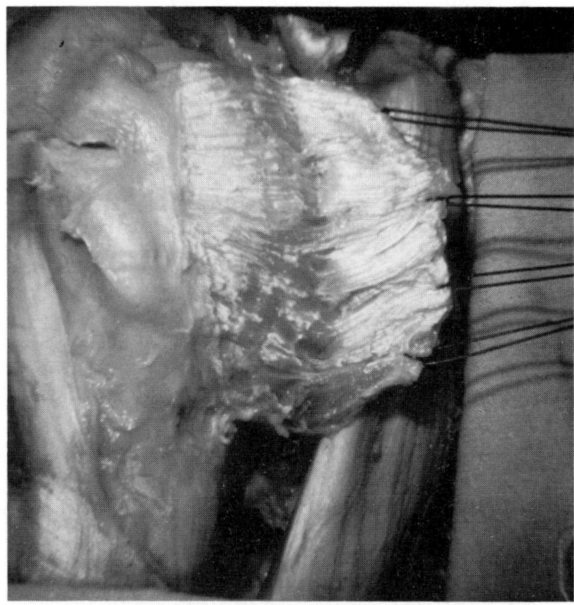

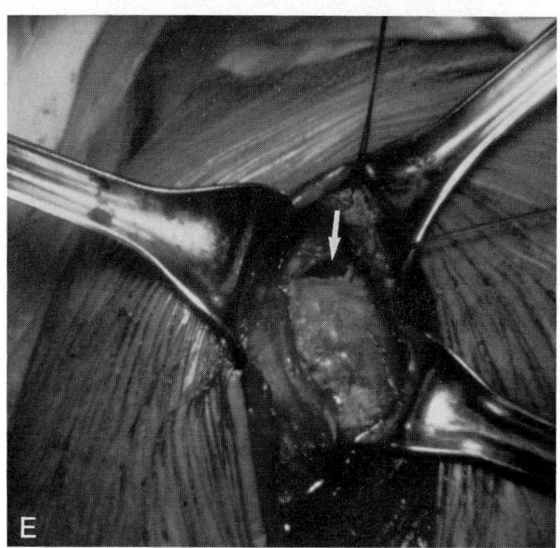

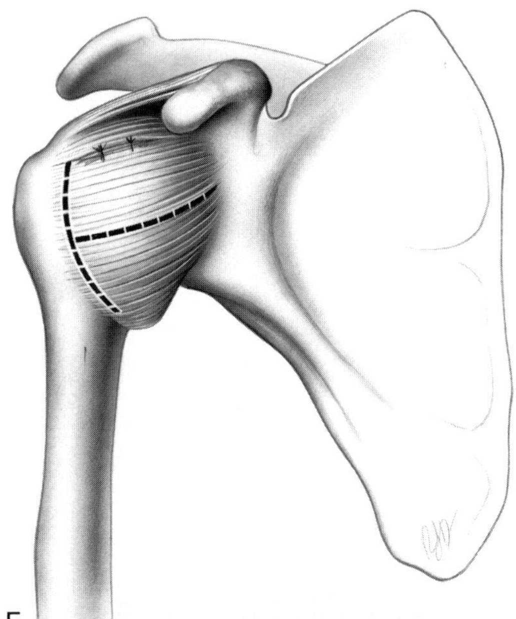

Figure 4–31 *Continued* F, After closing the cleft as shown, a T-opening in the reinforced capsule gives an optimum view of the interior of the joint and permits an inferior capsular shift (see Fig. 4–40) if required.

G, Interior of the joint is inspected, and anatomical defects are corrected. 1. If the anterior labrum is detached (right), it is re-attached (left) as described in the text.

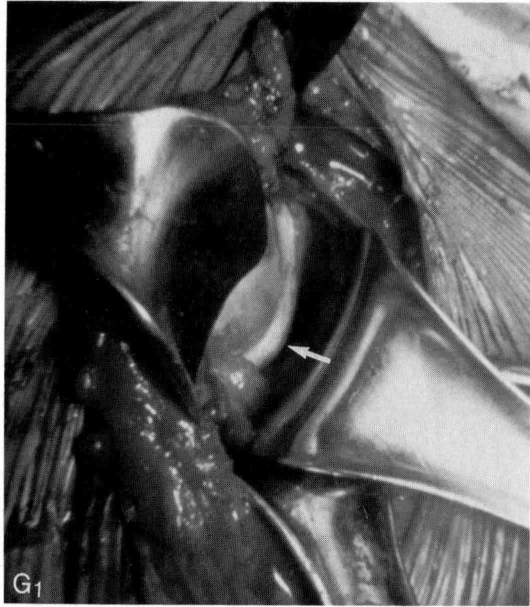

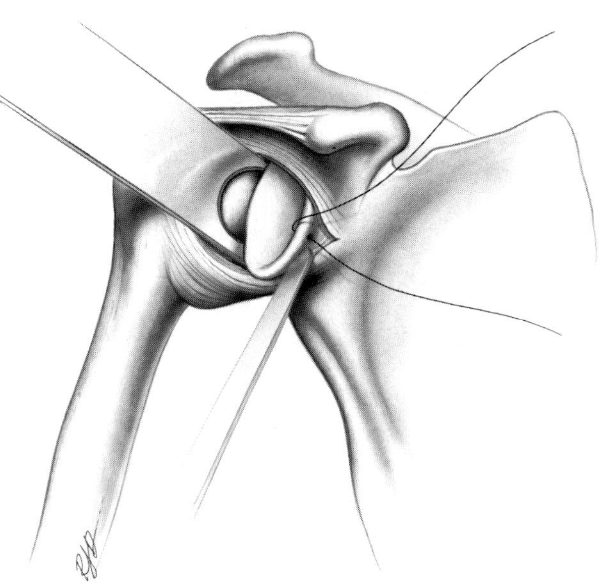

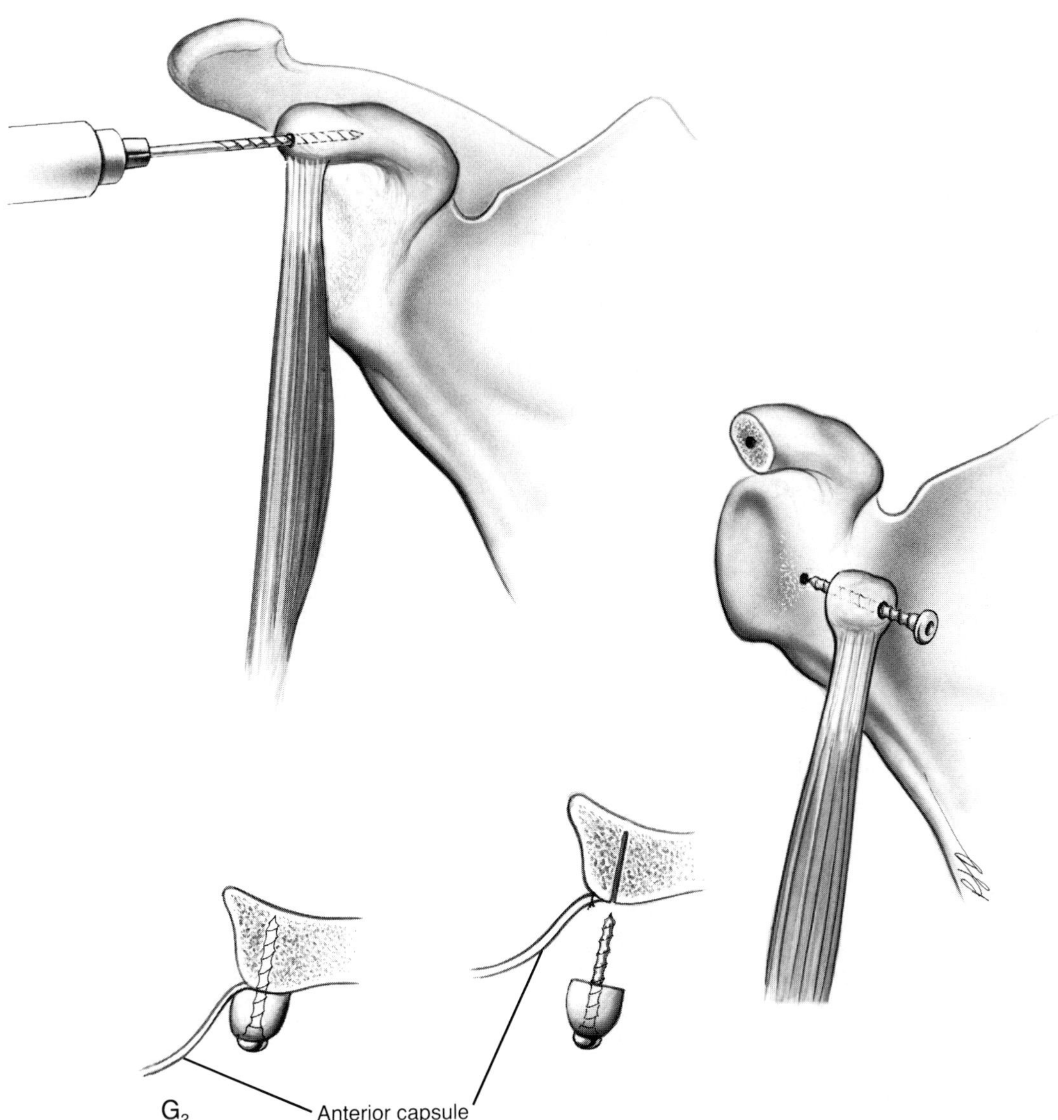

Figure 4–31 *Continued* G, 2. In the rare instance when the anterior glenoid is worn and sloping, a coracoid transfer is performed by pre-drilling the coracoid before cutting a 1.5 cm. length of it to be transferred with the attached muscles outside of the anterior capsule and beneath the subscapularis tendon. I delay complete closure of the capsule until the screw is in place to make sure it does not enter the joint. Loose bodies are removed.

Illustration continued on following page

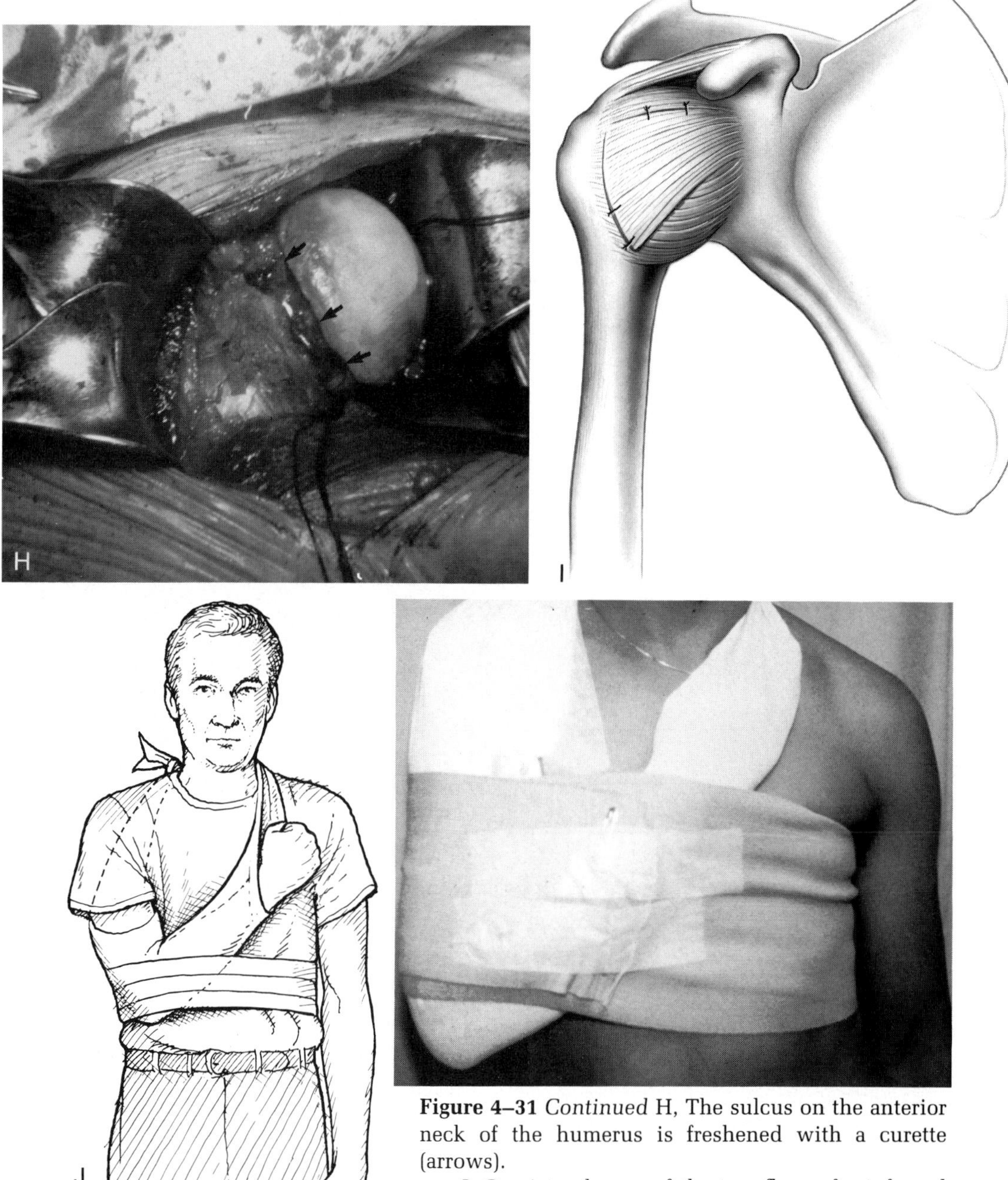

Figure 4–31 *Continued* H, The sulcus on the anterior neck of the humerus is freshened with a curette (arrows).

I, Cruciate closure of the two flaps of reinforced capsule with the arm at neutral flexion-extension and 10 degrees external rotation. Note the "cleft" had been closed at step E. The subscapularis tendon is re-attached in its normal anatomical location.

J, Stockinette Velpeau to hold the shoulder in moderate flexion and internal rotation at least until the anesthesia has worn off.

inferiorly as well as anteriorly, the capsule is detached from the neck of the humerus inferiorly so that it can later be pulled up to eliminate inferior instability as required (see Fig. 4–40).

A Fukuda-Ogawa[127] ring retractor is inserted in the joint to hold the humeral head back to allow inspection of the anterior rim of the glenoid and anterior labrum (Fig. 4–31G1) and to look for loose bodies (which are more apt to lie in the recess near the origin of the long head of the biceps or near the neck of the humerus in the inferior capsular pouch).

If a Bankart-Broca detachment of the anterior labrum is present, it is re-attached to the freshened scapula with one or two nonabsorbable sutures through drill holes placed in the rim of the scapula. This can be a very tedious task or not, depending on the preparation of the drill hole and the needle used. An osteotome is used to freshen the cortical surface of the anterior glenoid and to cut a small trough into the cortical surface at the point where the suture is to emerge below the glenoid rim. A Darrach elevator is then placed in front of the scapula for retraction. Using a drill and a small angulated curette, this hole is enlarged as much as desired without harm. Using a hand drill or power drill, a small hole is made through the articular cartilage and subchondral bone near the rim of the glenoid to meet with the anterior hole. Using the angulated curette inserted into the anterior opening (outside of the joint), the canal can be enlarged as much as desired and the two holes connected without damage to the articular cartilage. A nonabsorbable suture on a No. 4 bone-cutting needle is then passed from inside the joint out through the larger opening anteriorly. When properly done, the larger opening in the anterior cortex allows the needle to be passed without resistance. After changing the Darrach elevator to a position outside the capsule and beneath the subscapularis, the bone-cutting needle is then passed through the labrum to emerge in front of the capsule. Using a cutting needle on the other end, the bone suture is again passed through the labrum and out the front of the capsule, where, after removing retractors that might impede good approximation of the labrum to bone, the bone suture is tied securely with the knot outside the joint (see Fig. 4–31G1).

In the rare instance when the anterior glenoid is worn and sloping, a coracoid transfer (beneath the subscapularis tendon and outside of the joint capsule) is performed, as shown in Figure 4–31G2.

Next, the bone at the sulcus at the anterior neck of the humerus (adjacent to the anterior articular surface) is freshened with a curette or gouge to encourage healing of the ligaments and capsule to bone (see Fig. 4–31H). If inferior instability is present, the inferior neck of the humerus is also freshened with a curette and more of the inferior flap is mobilized and pulled upward to eliminate slack in the inferior capsule. The lower flap of the reinforced capsule is closed first.

With the patient's elbow resting on a bolster on the arm board to maintain slight flexion and with the elbow flexed 90 degrees, the shoulder externally rotated 10 degrees, and the patient's forearm resting on the surgeon's chest (to maintain neutral flexion and extension), the lower flap is pulled up and laterally as desired and sutured to the soft tissue just lateral to the trough to hold the capsule and ligaments against the trough. A 0 or 00 nonabsorbable suture is passed through the central portion of the lower flap and into the middle of the upper flap to approximate them. The upper flap is sutured downward and laterally as a further aid in preventing anterior and inferior instability (see Fig. 4–31H).

The subscapularis tendon is pulled up into position and sutured in its normal anatomical location with 0 or 00 nonabsorbable sutures. The deltopectoral interval is closed with two 00 nonabsorbable double-looping sutures passed through the subcutaneous layer to eliminate the dead space created when the skin was undermined during the approach. The skin is approximated with a continuous subcuticular pull-out suture, avoiding unsightly cross marks and staple holes.

The arm is placed in a "stockinette Velpeau" (see Fig. 4–31J) in internal rotation and flexion to prevent dislocation while the patient recovers from the anesthesia. This stockinette is changed to a removable sling within 48 hours. I continue antibiotic coverage for about five days and discharge the patient when he or she is comfortable with the arm in a removable sling that permits use of the arm at the side during the day.

Although the aftercare program varies according to the stiffness of the shoulder as determined by examination about every two weeks, in general the sling is discarded within two weeks after surgery during the day but is re-applied at night. External rotation of the arm beyond 20 degrees or elevation of the hand above the top of the head is usually prohibited for five or six weeks, at which time the sling is also discarded at night. Patients who are noted to be very stiff and apprehensive are advised to discard the sling altogether after about three weeks. Full light use of the arm is then permitted. Three months after surgery strengthening exercises (see Fig. 7–13) are begun. Lifting weights of more than 20 pounds and contact sports are not advised for about 10 to 12 months. For example, I usually allow ground strokes in tennis at six months and overhead strokes after nine months; the short game of golf at six months and the long game at nine months; and swimming without formal strokes at three months and butterfly and backstroke after 12 months.

Results of Reinforced Capsular Cruciate Repair (Modified Inferior Capsular Shift) for Recurrent Anterior Dislocations

Two prospective studies have been made[185, 190] of this procedure, the "reinforced capsular cruciate repair," for primary repair of recurrent anterior dislocations. Another study of the use of this procedure for failed repairs is discussed on page 336.

In my personal series[19] of repairs of primary anterior dislocations done between 1978 and 1982 with two years' minimum follow-up (follow-up ranged from two to five years and averaged three years) there were no recurrences and no complications, and all patients returned to regular activities (Fig. 4–32); however, one patient was afraid to resume wind surfing and another said he could not throw as well as previously. A significant injury had occurred at the time of the initial dislocation in 49 percent, and no significant injury occurred in 51 percent. Detachment of the anterior glenoid labrum was found in 57 percent. A coracoid transfer to the scapula was performed in only one shoulder. During this same period of time I used this technique in an equal number of shoulders with failed repairs that had been performed elsewhere and performed an inferior capsular shift in an equal number of patients who had been referred with multidirectional instability.

Mendoza,[190] using essentially the same technique in patients with primary anterior dislocations and allowing the same period of immobilization and inactivity postoperatively in 29 shoulders in patients followed a minimum of two years, had similar good results. He noted also that a history of a significant injury at the initial dislocation was less frequent than no significant injury. A detached labrum was present in 15 shoulders

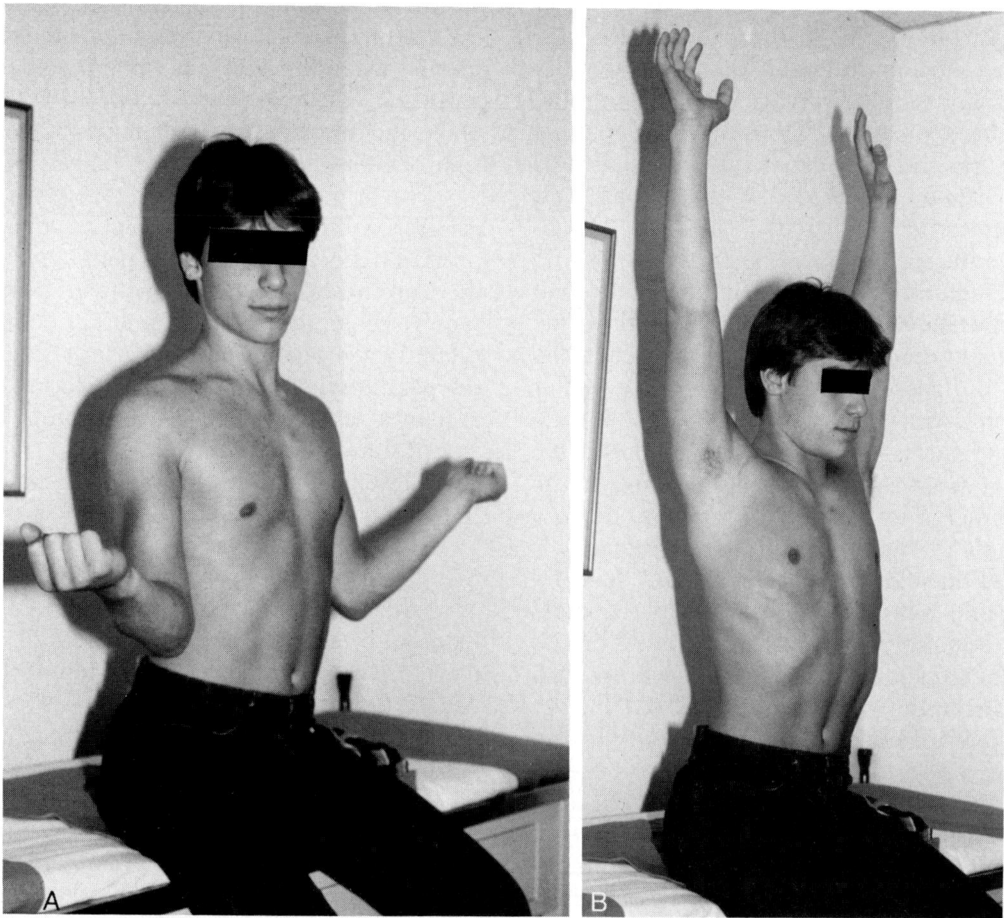

Figure 4–32A and B. The repair for recurrent anterior dislocation should strive for slightly less motion than that in the opposite shoulder (which is often hypermobile), no recurrences of instability, and recovery of function.

(51 percent). Glenoid bone deficiency requiring a coracoid transfer to the scapula was present in only one shoulder. Osteochondral loose bodies were removed from four shoulders. The results were no re-dislocations and strong shoulders without significant loss of external rotation or elevation in 28 shoulders (97 percent). A superficial infection occurred in one shoulder. Mendoza concluded that the repair had provided physiological restoration of anatomy and successful recovery of function in almost all patients.

Welsh,[188] in his study in Toronto of 120 functional results after various standard procedures for recurrent glenohumeral instability (Putti-Platt, Bankart, duToit staple capsulorrhaphy, and anterior glenoid osteotomy), found a re-dislocation rate of 8 percent, significant loss of motion in 30 percent, and "weakness" in 16 percent (which interfered with overhead activities). He very correctly emphasized the importance of considering not only the dislocation recurrence rate but also the quality of function.

I heartily concur with Welsh's opinion and believe we should strive for more normal and physiological recovery of function in repairs for recurrent dislocation. This is the aim of the procedure described previously.

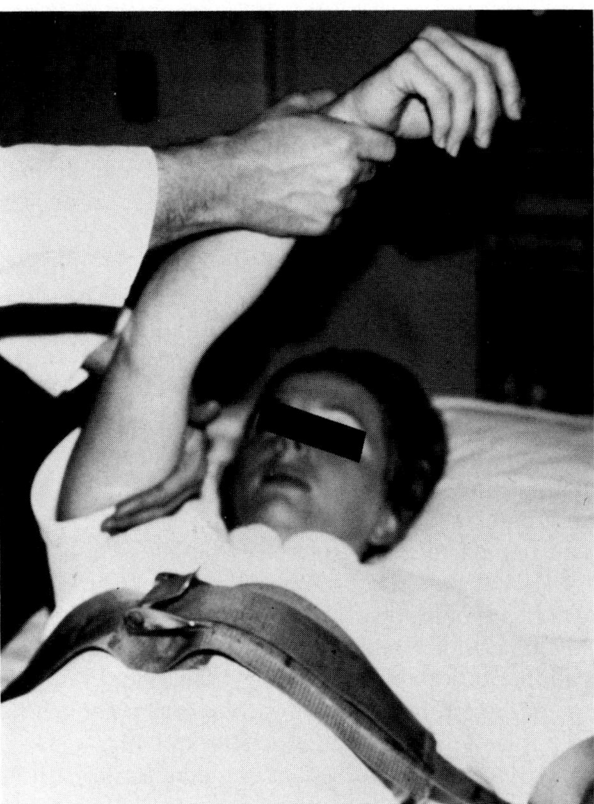

Figure 4–33. Method of closed reduction of a "locked" posterior dislocation. In my experience, this condition is almost always associated with an impression fracture (see Chapter 5 p. 394); otherwise, posterior dislocations self-reduce. An exception is shown in Figure 4–15. The assistant places countertraction on the scapula as traction forward is applied to the arm in the direction shown. A third person applies direction pressure on the head of the humerus to push it forward. The arm is then adducted, levering the shaft on the glenoid to displace the head laterally. After the head slips forward opposite the glenoid, the arm is externally rotated and lowered to the side. The arm is immobilized in external rotation and extension (see Fig. 4–34H).

SURGICAL REPAIR FOR RECURRENT POSTERIOR INSTABILITY

Indications

Recurrent posterior dislocations, like recurrent anterior dislocations, may be traumatic, atraumatic, or acquired through repeated minor trauma (Table 4–1). They are almost always self-reduced. An unreduced posterior dislocation is very rarely seen without an impression fracture. The key to avoid missing an unreduced posterior dislocation is to obtain an axillary view radiograph. This is done without moving the patient's arm and without pain (see Fig. 1–12).

The treatment of locked posterior dislocations with impression fractures is discussed in Chapter 5, pages 394 to 396. Other posterior fracture-dislocations are also considered in Chapter 5.

The rare unreduced posterior dislocation occurring without a fracture is reduced by the closed maneuver shown in Figure 4–33 and described under treatment of initial dislocations (see p. 300); as described, initial traumatic posterior dislocations are immobilized in external rotation with an extension spica cast for six weeks. Traumatic posterior dislocations with more than one recurrence are considered for surgical repair.

Acquired (by repeated minor injuries) recurrent dislocations and atraumatic recurrent posterior dislocations are more common than the literature of the past would indicate. They are usually posterior-inferior dislocations; multidirectional instability must be excluded at the time of surgical repair when surgery is undertaken. I have little hesitation in recommending repair for those with acquired posterior dislocations when discomfort and instability with recurrent dislocations persist despite conservative treatment. (Conservative treatment emphasizes strengthening the infraspinatus muscle [see Chapter 7].)

Prior to a surgical repair for recurrent posterior dislocations or subluxations, the patient is warned about the wide scar, post-operative spica cast, and one-year period of reduced activities following the repair and also about the possibility that a posterior bone block and screw to reinforce it may be necessary if the capsule or posterior glenoid proves to be deficient.

My repair is a reinforced posterior capsular cruciate repair (modified posterior inferior capsular shift omitting detaching and tightening the anterior capsule). When this repair is performed, if the capsule is found to be deficient or—as can occur in traumatic lesions—torn, a posterior bone block is added to reinforce the repair. The posterior bone block is rarely used in primary repairs but is added in about half of the re-operations for failed posterior repairs referred from elsewhere (see p. 313).

An osteotomy of the posterior glenoid has been used as an accepted and not infrequent procedure in the United States for recurrent posterior dislocations; however, I do not perform glenoid osteotomies except in a rare effort to correct a congenital hypoplastic glenoid (see p. 330 and Fig. 4–47). I agree with Randelli[180] that skeletal abnormalities of version are very rarely a cause of recurrent dislocations. To perform a glenoid osteotomy on a normal glenoid is a distortion of anatomy that can result in disaster (see Figs. 4–3 and 4–52A). Hawkins[193] has shown it has had a poor record in the treatment of recurrent posterior instability. I cannot believe that an operation on the glenoid should be done unless there is a skeletal defect of the glenoid. Even then, if there is only rounding off and wear of the posterior rim of the glenoid, as occasionally seen in persons with long-standing instability and often associated with an attenuated posterior capsule, I prefer to do a bone block (Fig. 4–34G) capsule rather than a glenoid osteotomy.

The usual basis for posterior instability is a pouch of capsule, which, when the bone is normal, is treated with a reinforced capsular cruciate repair and spica cast (with or without reinforcement with the infraspinatus tendon), depending on the condition of the posterior capsule bone block. A bone block is less frequently performed in primary repairs.

Reinforced Capsular Cruciate Repair for Recurrent Posterior Dislocation

An antiseptic soap is used by the patient prior to entering the hospital, and careful skin preparation is given as described under repair of an anterior dislocation. Antibiotics are used.

The technique is illustrated in Figure 4–34. The patient is positioned in a high tilt position, almost all the way over on the opposite side (Fig. 4–34A). A pad is placed between the chest and the table to prevent pressure on the opposite shoulder. The head is supported on a padded head rest, taking care to avoid pressure or irritating solutions on the face. Adherent plastic drapes are applied, exposing the front of the shoulder and the midline posteriorly.

Prior to skin preparation and with the patient under anesthesia, the shoulder is manipulated to determine all directions of instability (see Fig. 4–24). Directions of instability are tested again later after detaching the deltoid (before spreading the interval between the infraspinatus and the teres minor) and after the joint is open.

The skin incision is 12.0 cm. long and may be horizontal or vertical (see Fig. 4–31). I have a preference for the vertical incision. The skin is undermined, and a self-retaining (Gelpi) retractor is placed to expose the lateral three-quarters of the spine of the scapula and posterior acromion. The origin of the deltoid muscle is detached from 1.0 cm. anterior to the posterior prominence of the acromion to 3.0 cm. lateral to the medial border of the scapula. In this step, care is taken in elevating the deltoid from the spinous process to avoid injury to the suprascapular nerve as it winds around the base of the acromion. Care should be taken to find the superficial surface of the infraspinatus muscle before detaching the deltoid origin, which lies superficial to the axillary nerve. The interval between the lateral and posterior parts of the deltoid muscle is separated 5.0 cm., and a stay suture is implanted in the deltoid muscle at the distal end of the split to avoid splitting it further. The bursa is removed to expose the superficial surface of the infraspinatus and teres minor muscles.

At the point of insertion of the teres minor on the humerus, there is a distinct prominence, which is a help in identifying the teres minor to separate it from the infraspinatus. This interval can be developed without fear of damaging either the suprascapular nerve or the axillary nerve (see Figs. 4–33 and 4–34). The infraspinatus is retracted upward, exposing the posterior capsule. The superficial surface of the posterior capsule is further exposed with an elevator, taking care to avoid injury to either the suprascapular or the axillary nerve.

The posterior capsular pouch is then opened along its full length horizontally at the level of the

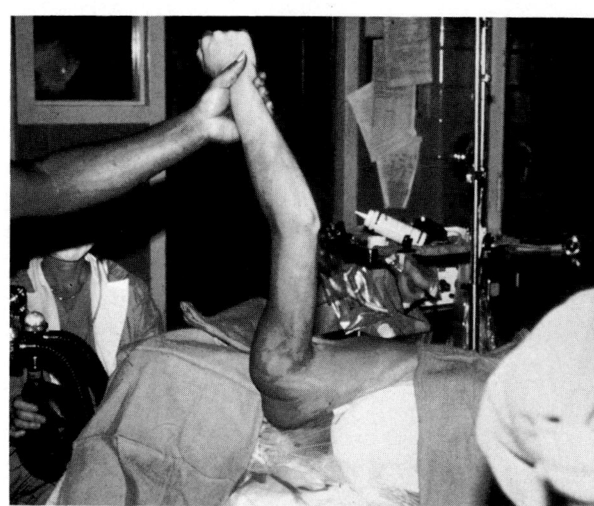

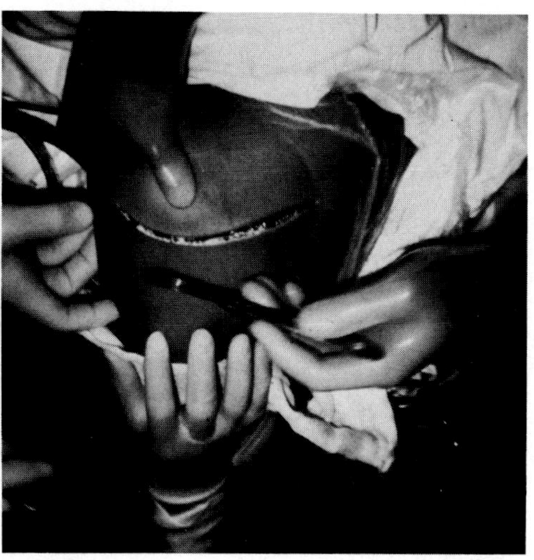

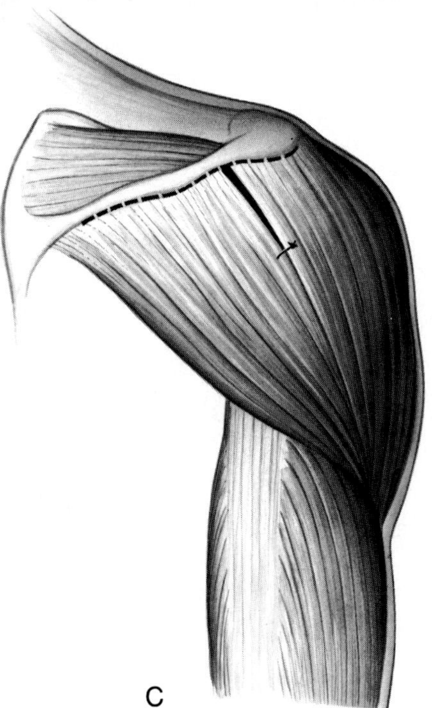

Figure 4–34. *Reinforced Capsular Cruciate Repair for Recurrent Posterior Instability.*

A, Position the patient almost all of the way on the uninvolved side as described in the text. The shoulder is manipulated under anesthesia prior to the skin preparation to make sure of the direction of instability and to exclude multidirectional instability (as in Fig. 4–39).

B, A vertical incision 20.0 cm. long is preferred (see Figs. 1–25, 1–26, and 4–36).

C, The origin of the deltoid is detached, and the deltoid is split 5.0 cm. at the posterior corner of the acromion as shown. A stay suture is placed to avoid splitting further.

Illustration continued on following page

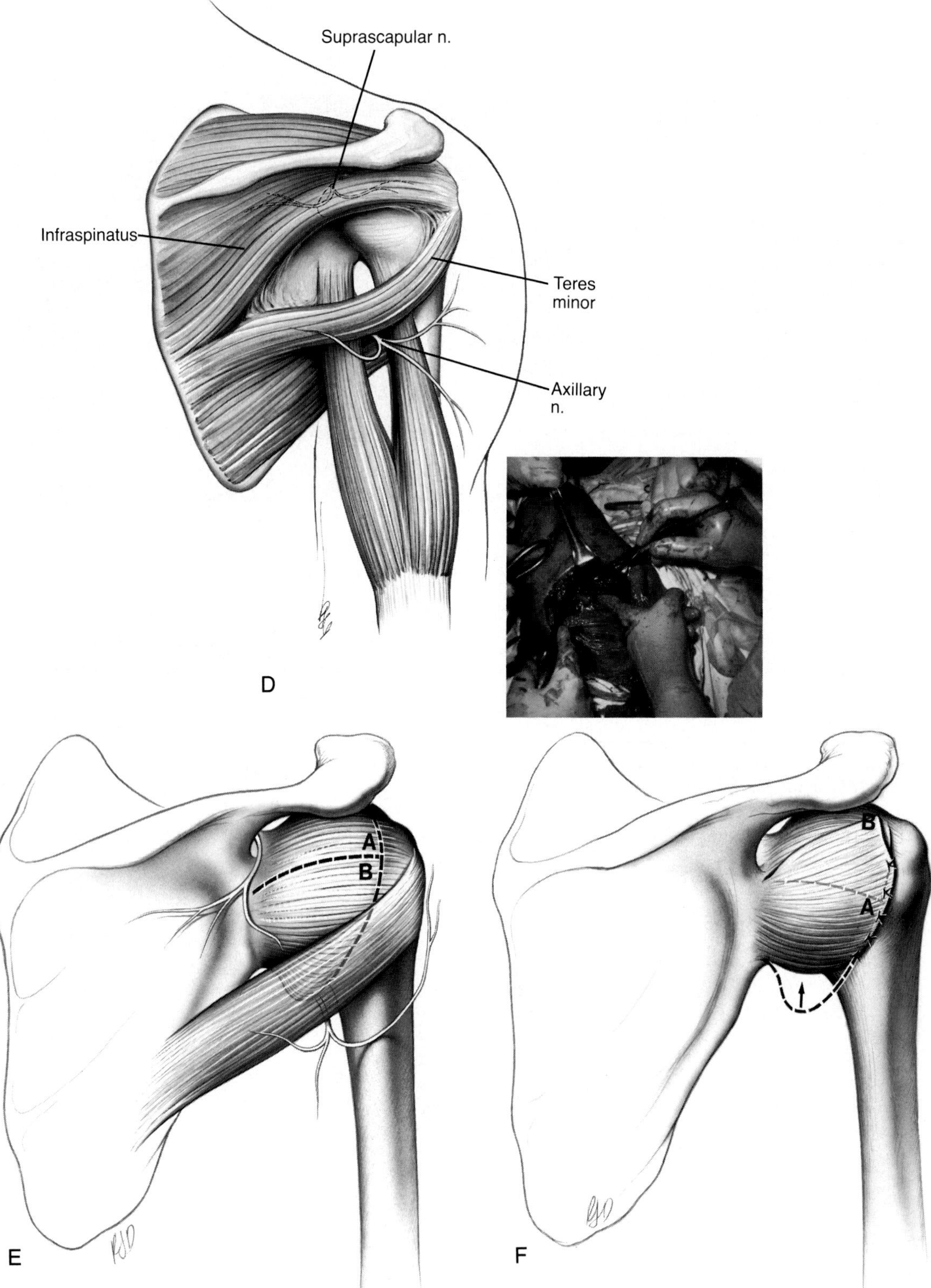

Figure 4–34 *See legend on opposite page*

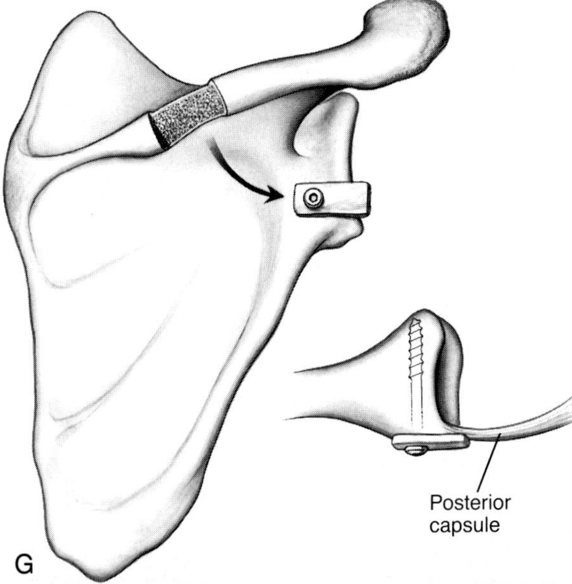

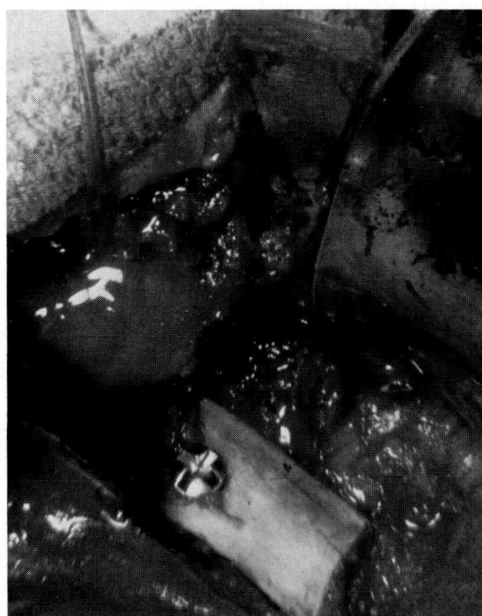

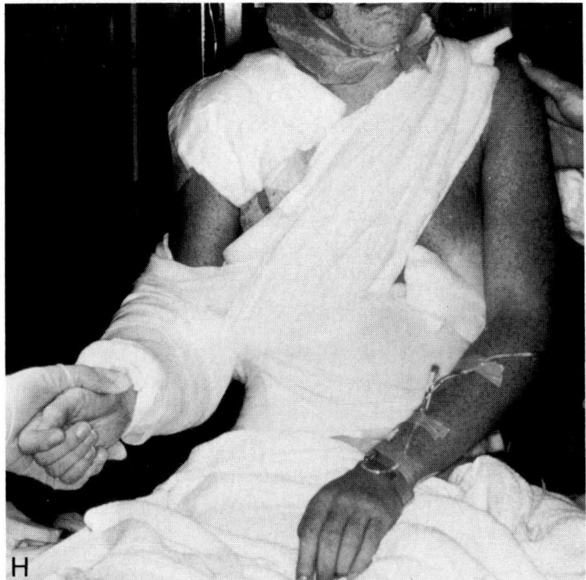

Figure 4–34 *Continued* D, After separating the deltoid off of the infraspinatus muscle (with care to avoid injury to the suprascapular nerve), the interval between the infraspinatus and teres minor is spread. Note that the suprascapular nerve is above and axillary nerve is below this line of approach. I palpate the base of the acromion to locate the suprascapular nerve at this time (inset).

E, "T-ing" the posterior capsular pouch. Unlike in the inferior capsular shift, the capsule is not detached from the front of the neck; however, since the direction of instability is usually posterior-inferior, some inferior capsule is often detached from the neck of the humerus. Note the proximity of the horizontal opening to the suprascapular nerve.

F, Cruciate closure usually closes a posterior-inferior pouch. In most situations, it is easier to suture the upper flap first (after freshening the posterior neck with a curette). The lower flap overlaps, creating a double thickness of capsule and eliminating the pouch. If the capsule is thin, a portion of the deep surface of the inferior part of the infraspinatus tendon is used to reinforce the capsule.

G, If the glenoid rim is rounded and sloping (or in re-operations if the posterior capsule is defective), a 2.5 cm. graft is taken from the spine of the scapula to deepen the socket. The graft protrudes no more than 5.0 mm. beyond the posterior rim of the glenoid, is outside of the capsule, and is held with a screw. I delay complete closure of the capsule until the screw is in place to make sure it does not enter the joint, as described in the text.

H, The arm is held in slight extension and 40 degrees external rotation as the wound is closed. The patient is allowed to wake up by the end of the subcuticular skin closure so that he or she can be sat up for the plastic cast.

center of the humeral head and vertically for a distance of 2.5 cm. After "T-ing" the capsule, the interior of the joint is inspected and loose bodies are removed. The anterior labrum is visualized, and the final stressing of the joint is made (to be sure that there is no anterior instability). The posterior rim of the glenoid is inspected for eburnation and wear, and if no significant amount of either is present, the capsule is closed as follows to eliminate the posterior pouch and reinforce the posterior capsule. If the posterior capsule is unusually thin, making the repair weak, a portion of the infraspinatus tendon is detached to reinforce it, as shown in Figure 4–34. If the posterior rim of the glenoid is rounded and worn, consideration is given to adding a posterior bone block (outside the capsule—Fig. 4–34).

If reinforcement of the posterior capsule with a portion of the infraspinatus tendon is desired, the tendon is detached from the deep surface of the infraspinatus tendon, leaving the superficial part of the tendon intact, as shown in Figures 4–34F and 4–41.

If reinforcement of the posterior capsule by deepening the glenoid is indicated, the bone graft is taken from the spine of the scapula, pre-drilled, threaded, and fitted with a 4.0 mm. screw, usually 20 to 28 mm. long depending on the size of the scapula as later determined with a depth gauge (Fig. 4–34G). The drill hole is made in the scapula to receive the screw, the adjacent bone is decorticated, and a trial placement of the graft is made prior to closing the capsule to make sure that the screw will not enter the joint and the graft will extend only 4.0 or 5.0 mm. beyond the posterior rim of the glenoid.

While the arm is held in 40 degrees external rotation with the elbow at the side, the capsule is closed by overlapping the two flaps to make a double thickness of capsule. Just prior to this, an area of sulcus is decorticated with a curette to obtain capsule-to-bone healing on the neck of the humerus (Fig. 4–34E and F). If there is a significant element of inferior instability, the lower flap is mobilized further on the humeral neck and pulled up first to close the redundancy inferiorly and posteriorly. The superior flap is approximated to it with a central stitch and closed over it (Fig. 4–34F).

When the posterior bone block is added, it is placed in position temporarily, and the scapula is drilled, tapped, and decorticated to receive the graft prior to closure of the capsule. After capsular closure, the graft is anchored in place with the screw. The screw should hold the graft firmly, but because no early motion of the shoulder is allowed, it need not engage the anterior cortex. Local bone fragments are placed around the area of contact between the graft and the scapula to expedite healing.

While the arm is held in 40 degrees external rotation, the interval between the infraspinatus and the teres minor is closed, and the deltoid origin is re-attached with interrupted 00 nonabsorbable sutures. The skin is closed with a subcuticular pull-out suture.

The patient is allowed to wake up, and a lightweight plastic cast is applied with the patient sitting up (Fig. 4–34H). The cast holds the arm in slight extension and 40 degrees of external rotation.

When the suture is removed, adherent plastic strips are re-applied to prevent early spreading of the skin incision. The cast, which is worn for six weeks, is changed before the patient leaves the hospital if it is uncomfortable or loose. An x-ray of the shoulder is made with the patient standing prior to discharge to make sure the cast is not distracting and displacing the humerus inferiorly.

Following removal of the cast, a sling is worn (with the arm held in near-neutral rotation) between exercises for two weeks; if a bone block was used, x-rays, including an axillary view, are then made to follow healing of the graft. Light activities are advised.

At three months following surgery isometric and progressive strengthening exercises with the arm held below the horizontal plane are begun. Whereas exercises after surgery for anterior instability are aimed at strengthening the subscapularis muscles, strengthening exercises after posterior repairs are aimed primarily at the infraspinatus and deltoid muscles, because they are the most important muscles for protecting this repair (see Fig. 7–13). Impact loads and heavy use of the shoulder are avoided for one year.

Results of Repairs for Recurrent Posterior Dislocation

Since 1977 I have used a reinforced capsular cruciate repair in 23 recurrent posterior dislocations. I am unaware of a single instance of a recurrence, and the patients returned to regular activities (Figs. 4–35 to 4–37). The results have been much better than those generally reported for soft-tissue repairs of posterior dislocations.

One of the patients, who probably had a congenital hypoplastic glenoid and whose son definitely has a hypoplastic glenoid (see Fig. 4–47), developed degenerative arthritis and had a total shoulder arthroplasty eight years later. Whether a

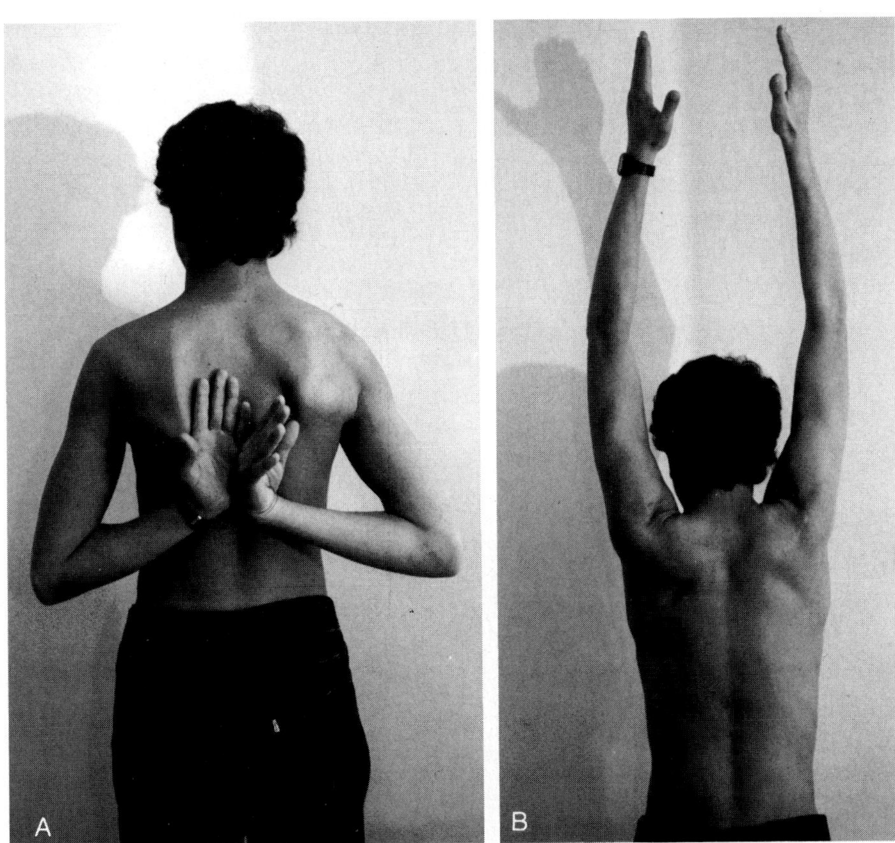

Figure 4–35. ***Results of Reinforced Capsular Cruciate Repairs for Recurrent Posterior Dislocations Have Been Good.*** A and B, Ten-year result of a right posterior capsular cruciate repair (modified inferior capsular shift) for recurrent posterior dislocations. Posterior repairs tend to lose a little internal rotation rather than external rotation. The indications for adding a posterior bone graft are discussed in the text.

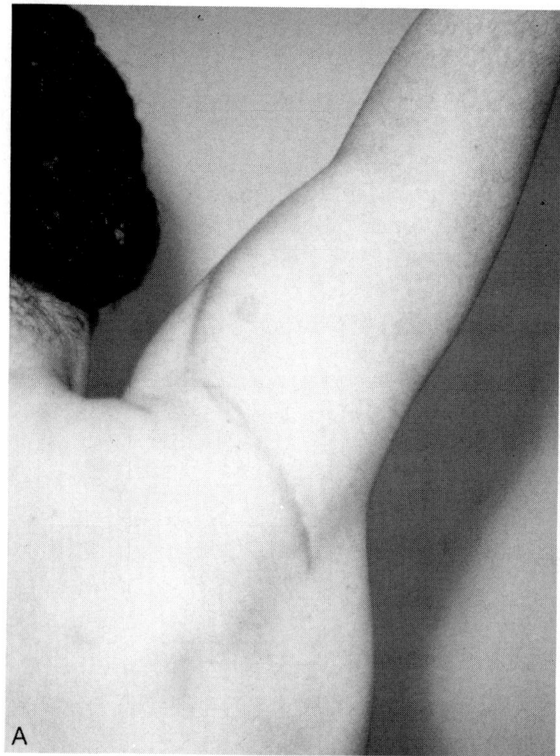

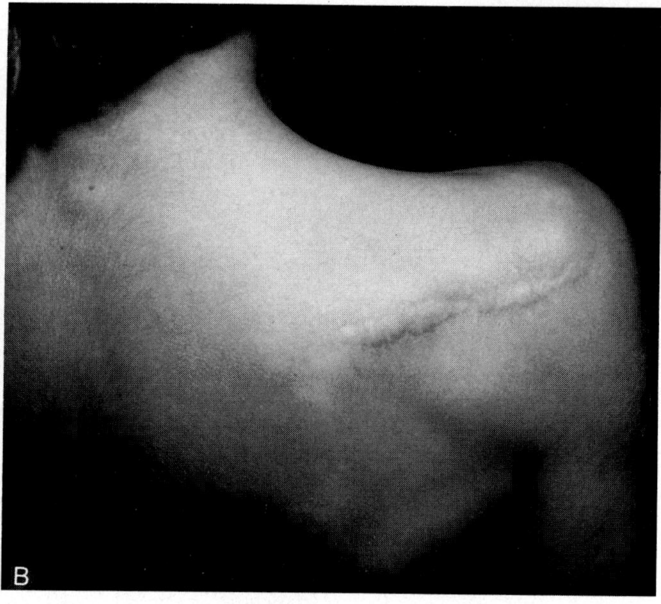

Figure 4–36. Choice of scars for posterior repairs. Both widen. My patients prefer the vertical scar (A) to the horizontal (B).

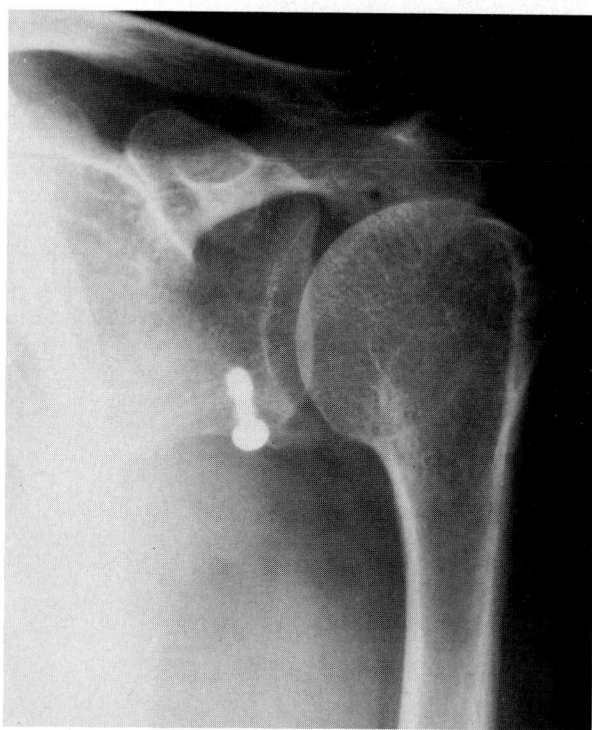

Figure 4–37. A 45 degree angle view (see Fig. 1–12F) made 11 years after a posterior bone block. Union of the graft is present, and there is room for the attachment of the capsule between it and the head. The graft protrudes just enough to deepen the socket. Some of the tip of the graft has been remodeled according to use.

posterior bone block or glenoid osteotomy would have improved this result, I do not know. Several patients have returned for surgery on the other shoulder. During the same period I used a posterior bone block (outside of a capsular repair) in 10 shoulders. One of these patients, who had early degenerative arthritis initially, developed further arthritis with symptoms at 11 years following the bone block; however, the symptoms were insufficient to consider an arthroplasty.

INFERIOR CAPSULAR SHIFT FOR INFERIOR AND MULTIDIRECTIONAL INSTABILITY[13]

Indications

As has been discussed earlier (p. 280), the evaluation of shoulder instability can be extremely difficult. Not all loose shoulders are painful, and not all require surgery. Some patients with loose shoulders may have pain because of another condition such as acromioclavicular arthritis, neoplasm, and so on. Not all patients are motivated for successful surgery, and there are some "voluntary dislocators" who are dedicated to making sure the operation will fail. Finally, all directions of instability must be evaluated. Standard procedures to correct unidirectional dislocations often fail if inferior and multidirectional instability is present. Multidirectional instability is not rare, and it can be easily overlooked if we become too routine in evaluating patients presenting with recurrent dislocations. All directions of instability must be tested by repeated examinations preoperatively, with the aid of anesthesia, and again during surgery.[13]

In view of the above factors, in patients who have not had previous surgery, I require that symptoms be present for a minimum of one year despite conservative treatment (based on the exercises as described in Chapter 7, Fig. 7–13). This gives an opportunity to see whether the shoulder soreness might disappear spontaneously or with the aid of "rest" and carefully progressive strengthening exercises to improve muscle tone to protect the capsule and ligaments. It also gives the clinician an opportunity to evaluate the motivation of the patient and to observe the stress of the environment on the patient.

In the final analysis, the surgeon can better judge the motivation of the patient by attempting to reduce a subluxated shoulder against the patient's will and palpating the muscle spasm (the "hold-out sign") and judging the sincerity of the patient. "Involuntary" multidirectional dislocators usually show the normal fear of surgery and yet at the same time display a desire to be rid of a truly painful disability. They speak of their inability to engage in sports or perform work they would like to do and ask how soon they might be able to resume activities after surgery. In contrast, there is usually an aura of panic and excitement around a voluntary dislocator that does not ring true. But the difference can be very subtle.

Patients with multidirectional instability who are having persistent pain after previous surgery elsewhere are even more difficult to evaluate. Of course, they would have been observed for some time by a physician, and the one-year pre-operative observation rule is often modified. If a gross anatomical defect is present, such as instability in the opposite direction from that of the side of the previous operation, a sulcus sign showing inferior instability, or fixed subluxation, I see little alternative in attempting to repair it unless the patient has obvious psychological problems. However, although we have made very few mistakes in judging the motivation of those who have never had surgery, we have made several in operating on patients with failed surgery.

Anatomical evidence of laxity on the inferior part of the capsule and both sides of the joint is determined in part by pre-operative examinations and special x-rays (scapular plane, axillary, stress, weights [Fig. 4–38], fluoroscopy, and cineradiography). Arthrograms (regular or with CT scans) may document the enlarged joint volume but do not give me other useful information. With experience in examining under anesthesia, arthroscopy is rarely, if ever, needed to determine the major direction of instability (see Fig. 4–39).

To summarize, my indications for an inferior capsular shift are:

1. Presence of inferior and multidirectional instability that has caused true pain and disability despite conservative treatment for a minimum of one year.

2. Failed surgery with definite anatomical evidence of residuals of multidirectional instability and no apparent emotional problem.

Technique of Inferior Capsular Shift

The objective of this procedure is to reduce the volume of the glenohumeral joint on all three

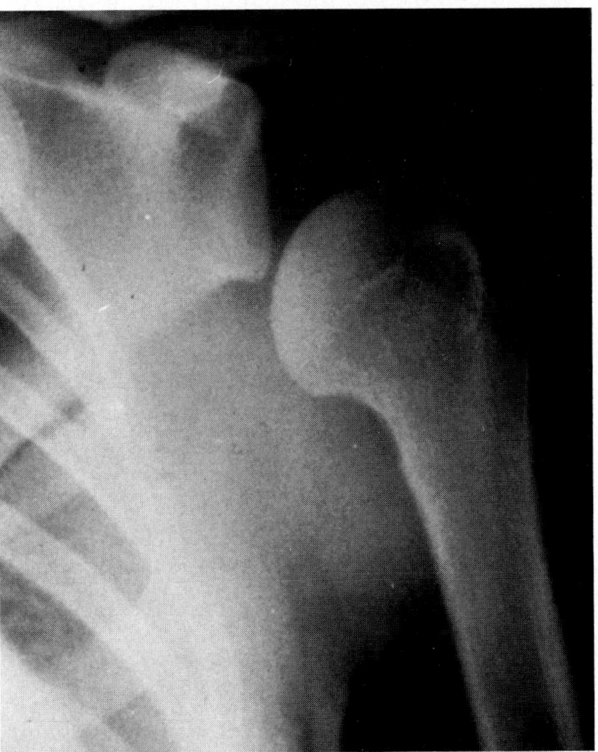

Figure 4–38. ***Objective of Inferior Capsular Shift.*** This film, made with the patient under anesthesia while downward traction is being applied to the arm, demonstrates the inferior instability that denotes multidirectional instability. The basic lesion in this condition is an increase in the joint volume due to a loose capsule. The objective of inferior capsular shift is to reduce the joint on all three sides, usually through one approach.

sides (inferiorly, anteriorly, and posteriorly), placing the humeral head in balance and equalizing tightness and laxity on all sides, usually through one approach. The approach is made on the side of greatest instability as determined preoperatively and under anesthesia just prior to the skin preparation for surgery (Fig. 4–39). As experience with examination for instability under anesthesia has improved, arthroscopy has been used less frequently (see Fig. 4–24).

The patient is informed pre-operatively of the following: (1) The incision might be made in front or in back, and occasionally both; (2) a special risk to the axillary nerve exists; (3) a spica cast is to be expected; and (4) heavy activities are restricted for 18 months following surgery. Patients are advised to clean the axilla daily with bactericidal soap for several days prior to admission. Prophylactic antibiotics are used.

After determining the side of the approach by examination under anesthesia (which is more accurate than an examination with the patient awake and guarding with the muscles), the skin is prepared and the arm draped free with access to both the front and back of the shoulder (Fig. 4–31).

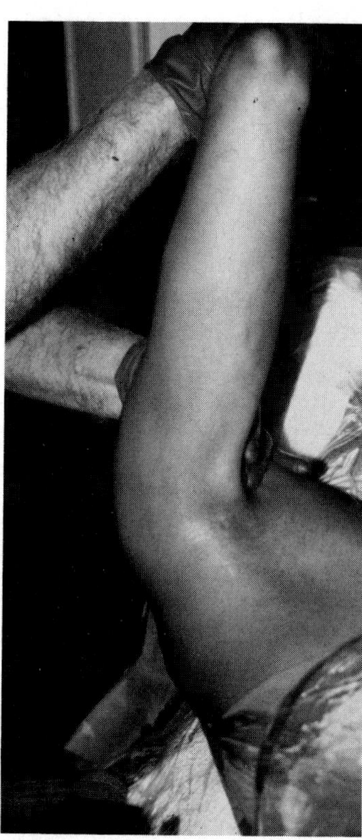

Figure 4–39. ***Inferior Capsular Shift for Multidirectional Instability. Examination Under Anesthesia and Position.***

Prior to final positioning and before the skin preparation, the shoulder is examined under anesthesia for all directions of instability, judged by palpating the posterior acromion and coracoid as the humeral head is dislocated. It is often possible to feel three stops. The first is when the head is dislocated to the side of greatest instability. The second is when the head is opposite the glenoid. The third is when the head is subluxated or dislocated toward the opposite side. If the greatest instability is anterior, the patient is positioned as in Figure 4–31A. If the greatest instability is posterior, the patient is positioned as in Figure 4–34A. In the latter position, the patient can be tilted backward for a second anterior approach if desired as the operation progresses. In either case, the shoulder is draped so that both anterior and posterior incisions can be utilized in the unexpected event that a second approach might be required, as discussed on page 325. Examinations for instability are repeated during surgery, after spreading the deltoid muscle and again after opening the joint.

Anterior Approach

When the anterior approach is used (Fig. 4–40A), the skin creases are marked after the skin preparation and just prior to applying adherent plastic drapes. A short arm board is attached to the side of the table at the level of the patient's elbow to prevent extension of the arm off the side of the table. A 6.0 cm. incision is made in the skin creases from the anterior axillary border of the axilla toward the coracoid process. The subcutaneous tissue is mobilized from the clavicle and on each side of the deltopectoral interval to expose the deltopectoral interval and cephalic vein.[191] The deltopectoral interval is developed medial to the cephalic vein, and the deltoid is retracted laterally. The clavipectoral fascia is divided, and the muscles attached to the coracoid are retracted medially. The subdeltoid bursa is excised to expose the subscapularis tendon and anterior circumflex vessels. The anterior vessels are cauterized after making sure the axillary nerve is safe medially on the subscapularis and inferiorly beneath the capsule.

Prior to detaching the subscapularis, the stability of the joint is again tested. An effort is made to dislocate the humeral head posteriorly and anteriorly as well as inferiorly while the surgeon palpates the anterior glenoid to make sure of the pattern of instability.

With the arm in slight flexion and external rotation and supported by a bolster on the arm board, the superficial half of the thickness of the subscapularis tendon (Fig. 4–40B) is divided transversely 1.0 cm. medial to the biceps groove, leaving a short stump of soft tissue on the lesser tuberosity to be used in the repair. The deep half of the subscapularis tendon is left attached to reinforce the anterior aspect of the capsule (see Fig. 4–38). The superficial half of the tendon is tagged with

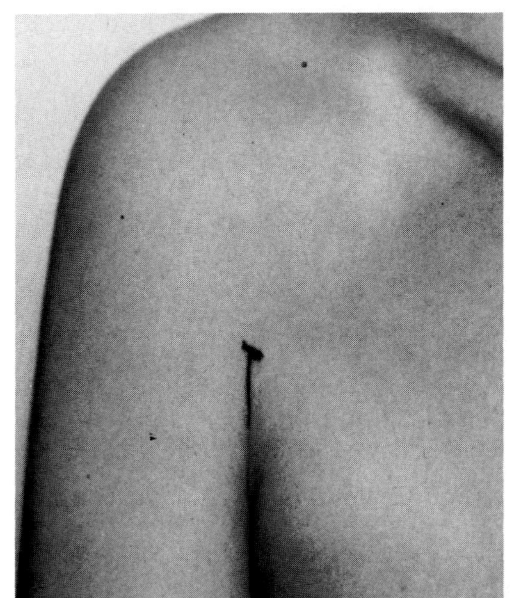

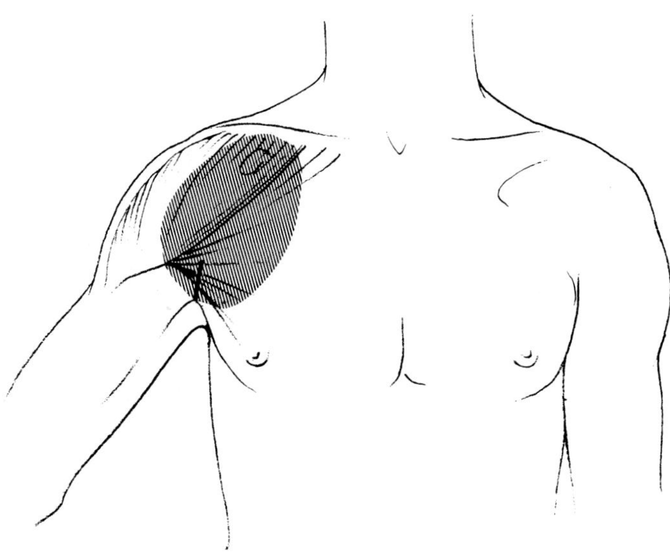

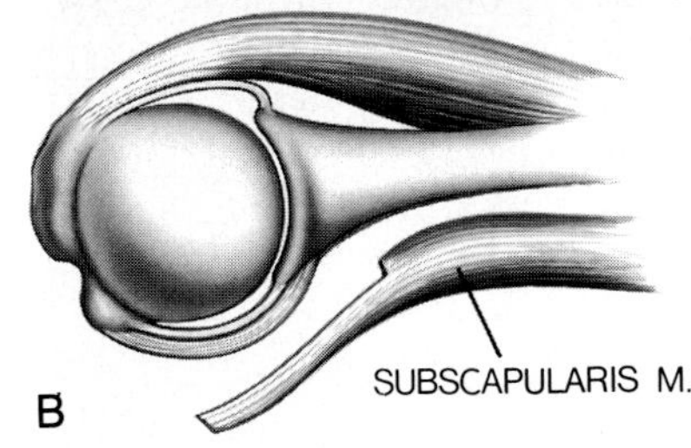

Figure 4–40. ***Inferior Capsular Shift Through the Anterior Approach.*** This procedure is the same as the reinforced capsular cruciate repair for recurrent anterior dislocation (see Fig. 4–31) except the lower flap of reinforced capsule is detached from the inferior and posterior aspects of the neck of the humerus, the surface of the neck is freshened on all three sides, and when the inferior flap is pulled upward it closes the posterior pouch as well as eliminating inferior redundancy and stabilizing anteriorly. Great care is necessary to avoid injury to the axillary nerve (D). The arm is immobilized in a plastic spica with care to avoid inferior subluxation of the humeral head in the cast. The text should be read for details.

A, The skin incision and position are as in Figure 4–31A and B.

B, One-half of the subscapularis tendon is left attached to the anterior capsule to reinforce the glenohumeral ligaments.

Illustration continued on following page

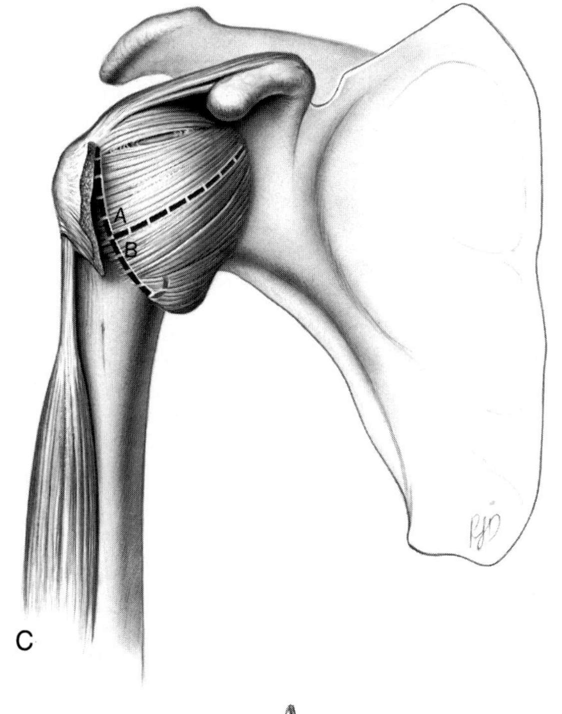

Figure 4–40 *Continued* C, After closing the cleft between the middle and superior glenohumeral ligaments, the reinforced capsule is "T-ed" as illustrated and the edges tagged with traction sutures. The inferior and posterior attachments of the lower flap are detached with great care, as shown in the next illustrations.

D, The axillary nerve is identified by palpation with the index finger (left) or is visualized (right), and the arm is externally rotated (arrow) to bring the posterior side of the neck of the humerus into view before attempting to detach the capsule posteriorly.

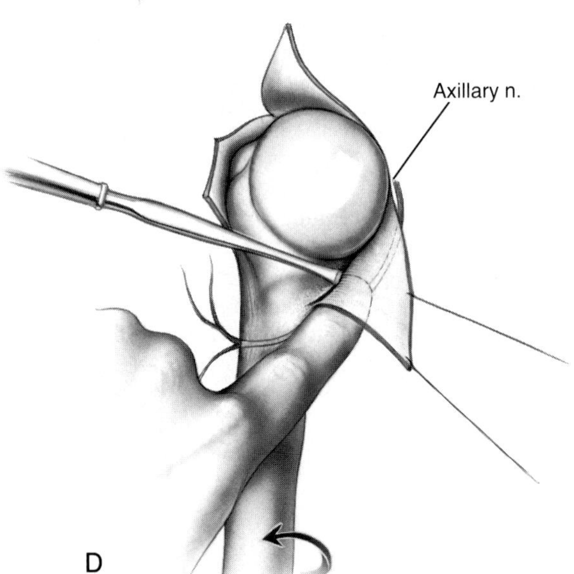

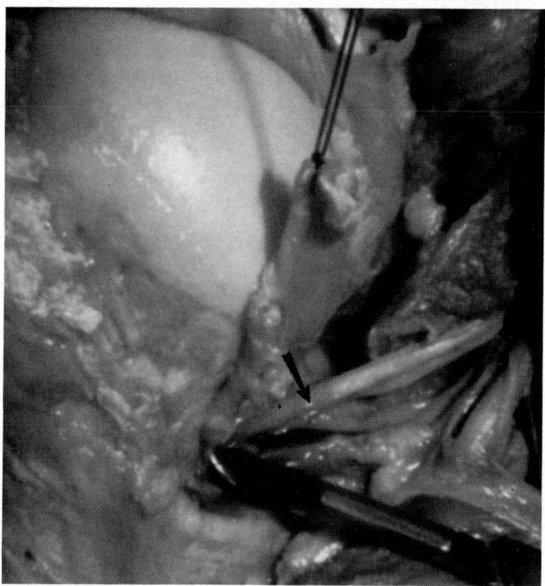

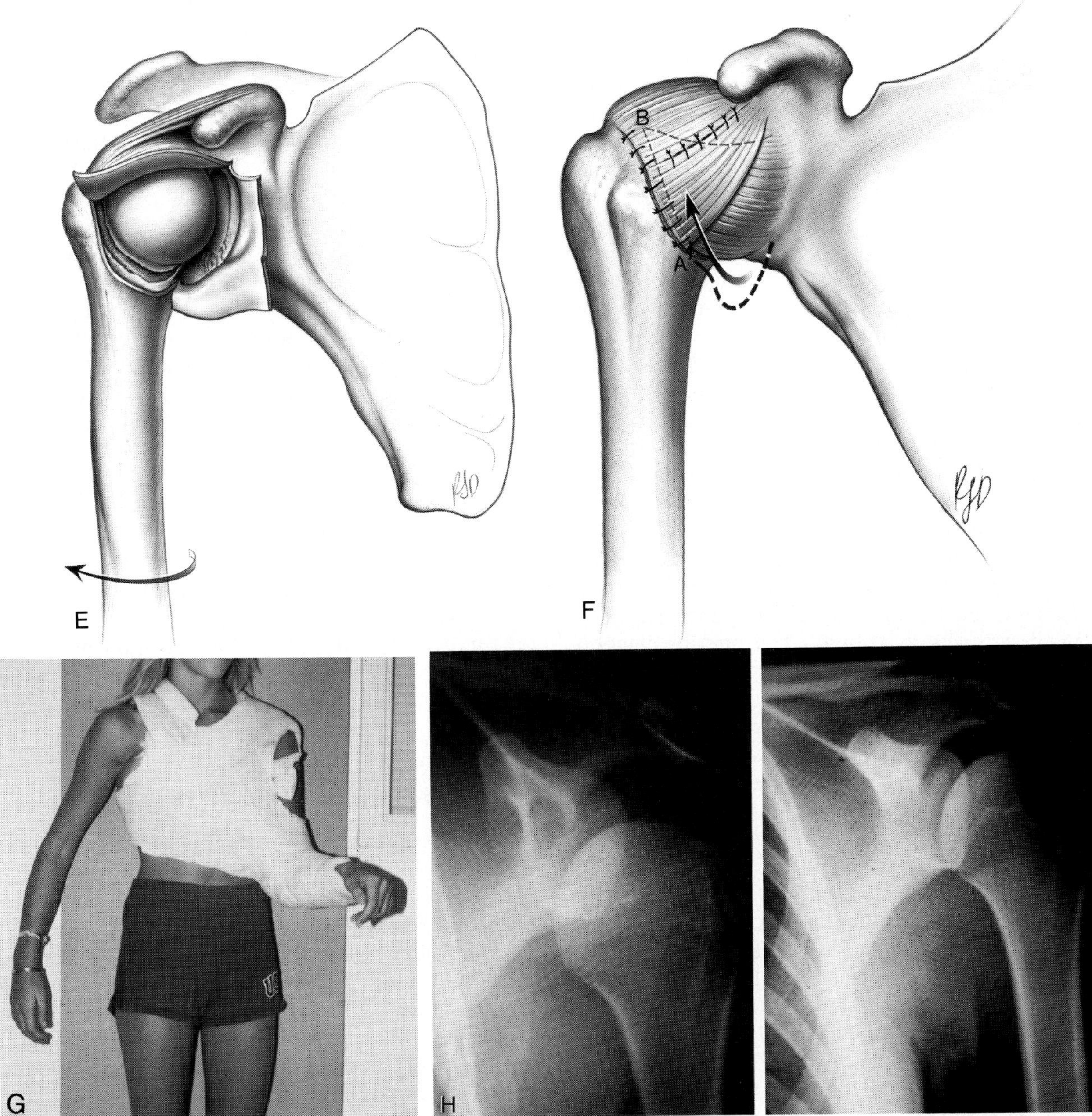

Figure 4–40 *Continued.* E, With the arm in external rotation for exposure, a shallow trough is made with a curette or gouge on the posteror, inferior, and anterior sides of the humeral neck.

F, Cruciate closure shifts the lower flap forward and upward, laterally reducing the joint volume and eliminating redundancy on all three sides. The upper flap is sutured over the lower one to reinforce it further and to prevent inferior instability. The subscapularis is re-attached anatomically.

G, A lightweight plastic spica cast with at least one shoulder strap to prevent downward displacement of the head is applied with the patient awake enough to be sat up with the arm in neutral flexion-extension and 10 degrees external rotation. In female patients, the final cast rests on the iliac crest, at least on the side of the repair.

H, Unless post-operative x-rays made with the patient standing show the head opposite the glenoid (right) without inferior subluxation (left), the cast must be changed before discharge of the patient from the hospital.

stay sutures and retracted medially. It is considered important that this superficial half of the tendon be free so that the action of the subscapularis muscle is not tethered (Fig. 4–40B).

Originally, the cleft between the superior and middle glenohumeral ligaments was used as the horizontal limb of the opening into the joint, and the reinforced capsule was detached from the neck of the humerus inferior to this point. However, this caused the creation of an excessively long inferior flap of capsule, which made it difficult to use the inferior glenohumeral ligament efficiently. Therefore, the cruciate repair was designed to create two flaps, an upper and a lower flap, which could be overlapped with double the thickness of the anterior capsule (Fig. 4–40F). Thus, in the next step the cleft between the superior and middle glenohumeral ligaments is closed with one or two interrupted 0 or 00 nonabsorbable sutures, and a T-opening (Fig. 4–40C) is made in the reinforced capsule. The upper and lower flaps of reinforced capsule are tagged with stay sutures.

The interior of the joint is inspected, and any osteochondral loose bodies or fragments of labrum are removed. The stability of the humerus is again tested with the joint open. The inferior glenohumeral ligament and capsule are then detached from the inferior and posterior aspects of the neck of the humerus with a sharp, small periosteal elevator and curette while the arm is progressively rotated externally until the posterior aspect of the neck can be clearly visualized by the surgeon. During this step, the index finger of the free hand is held on the axillary nerve to protect it from injury (Fig. 4–40). Additional stay sutures are added to the inferior flap to pull it forward as the arm is rotated externally. A finger can be placed in the posterior pouch and tension placed on the inferior flap to make sure this pouch will be eliminated at the time of closure. If the axillary nerve cannot be definitely located by palpation, it is dissected free and exposed prior to this step (Fig. 4–40D). Soft tissue is removed from the posterior, inferior, and anterior surfaces of the neck of the humerus with a curette and freshened to bleeding bone (for healing of the shifted capsule to bone); this is shown in Figure 4–40E. At this time, if the anterior labrum is detached or split and is partially detached sufficiently to make a step-off into which a posterior head defect might catch, the labrum is re-attached to the scapula as described earlier in the section on repair of recurrent anterior dislocations (Fig. 4–31G).

The capsular flaps are then closed with the arm supported by the bolster in slight flexion and held in 10 degrees external rotation. The inferior flap is pulled upward and forward first to eliminate the posterior pouch, inferior redundancy, and anterior redundancy. It is re-attached to the soft tissue on the lesser tuberosity with two 00 nonabsorbable sutures so that the capsular flap is held against the shallow slot of raw bone. A suture is placed through the middle of the upper edge of the inferior flap to secure it to the base of the upper flap. The upper flap is then pulled down and sutured to the soft tissue on the humerus and to the underlying lower flap to reinforce anteriorly to prevent descent of the head (Fig. 4–40F).

The subscapularis tendon is then brought over the capsule and sutured in its normal position with 00 nonabsorbable sutures. It is expected to adhere to the capsular repair to reinforce it further and also eventually to act normally as an internal rotator. After closure of the deltopectoral interval with two interrupted sutures, the skin is closed with a removable continuous subcuticular suture. The patient is allowed to wake up for application of the cast. The arm is maintained at the side in neutral flexion-extension and about 0 to 10 degrees external rotation in a light plastic spica cast, which includes a shoulder strap over the opposite shoulder to prevent inferior subluxation of the humeral head (Fig. 4–40G and H).

Posterior Approach

The preparation, positioning, testing of instability, and approach used in the posterior approach are the same as those described for the reinforced capsular cruciate repair for recurrent posterior and postero-inferior dislocations (see Fig. 4–34) except that the inferior capsular flap is detached from the front of the neck of the humerus in the inferior capsular shift for multidirectional instability, and some infraspinatus tendon is routinely obtained to reinforce the capsular repair (Fig. 4–41).

A 10.0 cm. vertical skin incision is preferred (see Figs. 4–34B, 4–36, 4–41B, and 1–25). The deltoid origin is carefully detached to avoid injuring the suprascapular nerve and split 5.0 cm. as described in Figure 4–41. The infraspinatus tendon is divided obliquely from medial to lateral, as described in the original article,[13] or from lateral to medial; alternatively, a flap of infraspinatus tendon can be taken from the inferior margins of the tendon after the interval between the teres minor and infraspinatus has been developed. I usually prefer to detach and re-attach it as described in the original article (Fig. 4–41B).

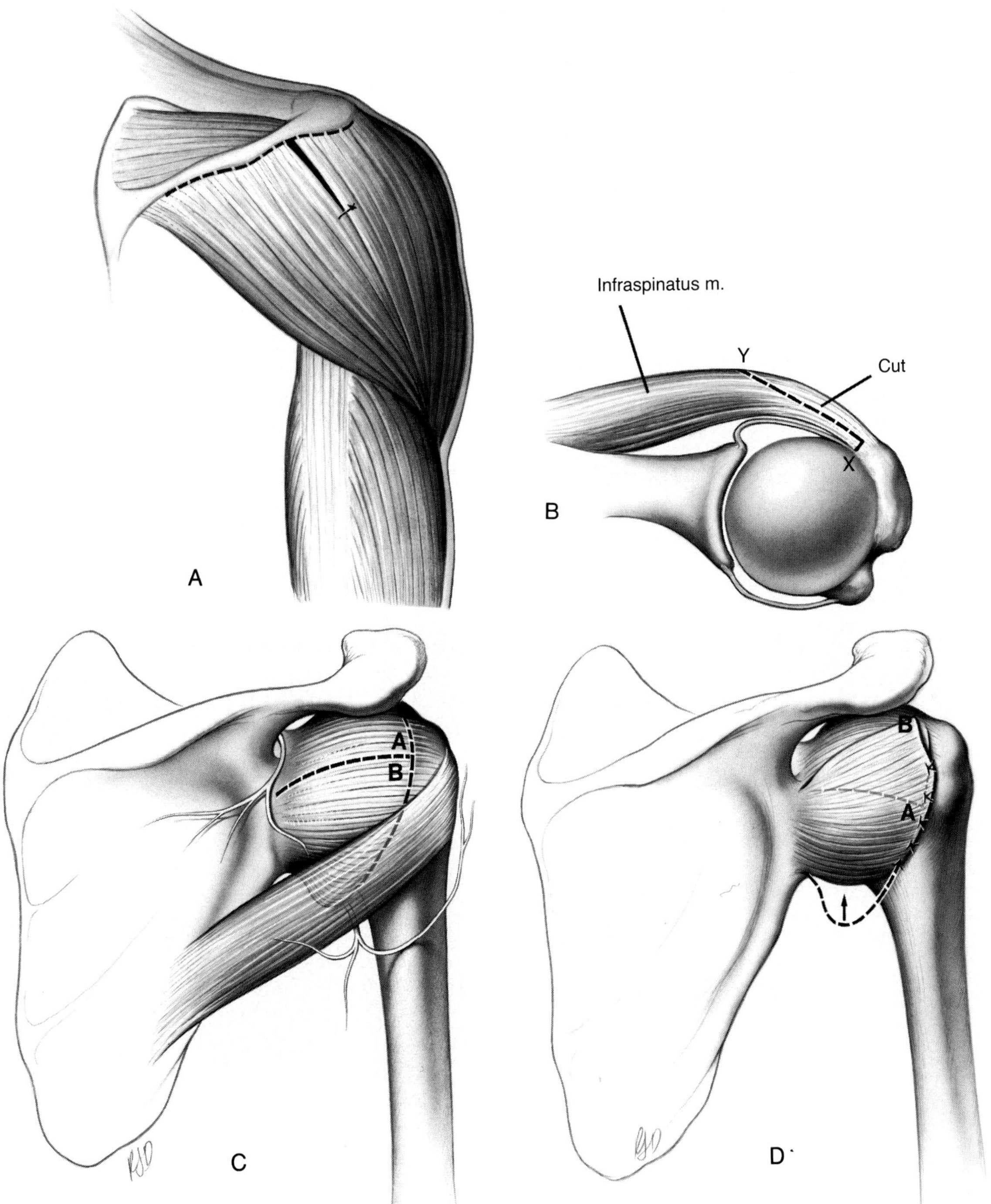

Figure 4–41. ***Inferior Capsular Shift Through a Posterior Approach.***

A, A vertical skin incision 20.0 cm. long is made, and the deltoid muscle is detached as shown (see Figs. 1–25, 1–26, and 4–34).

B, Either the superficial or the deep surface of the infraspinatus tendon may be used for later reinforcement of the capsule. I usually prefer the superficial part and divide the infraspinatus tendon as shown in F.

C, "T-ing" the capsule forms upper and lower flaps. The teres minor is left intact to lend some protection for the axillary nerve. The capsule is detached from the inferior and anterior sides of the humeral neck only after an index finger has located the nerve and protects it. The arm is internally rotated to expose the anterior side of the neck.

D, After inspecting the anterior labrum to make sure it is attached and after re-attaching the upper flap, the lower flap is pulled upward against the curetted anterior, inferior, and posterior neck to eliminate redundancy on all three sides.

Illustration continued on following page

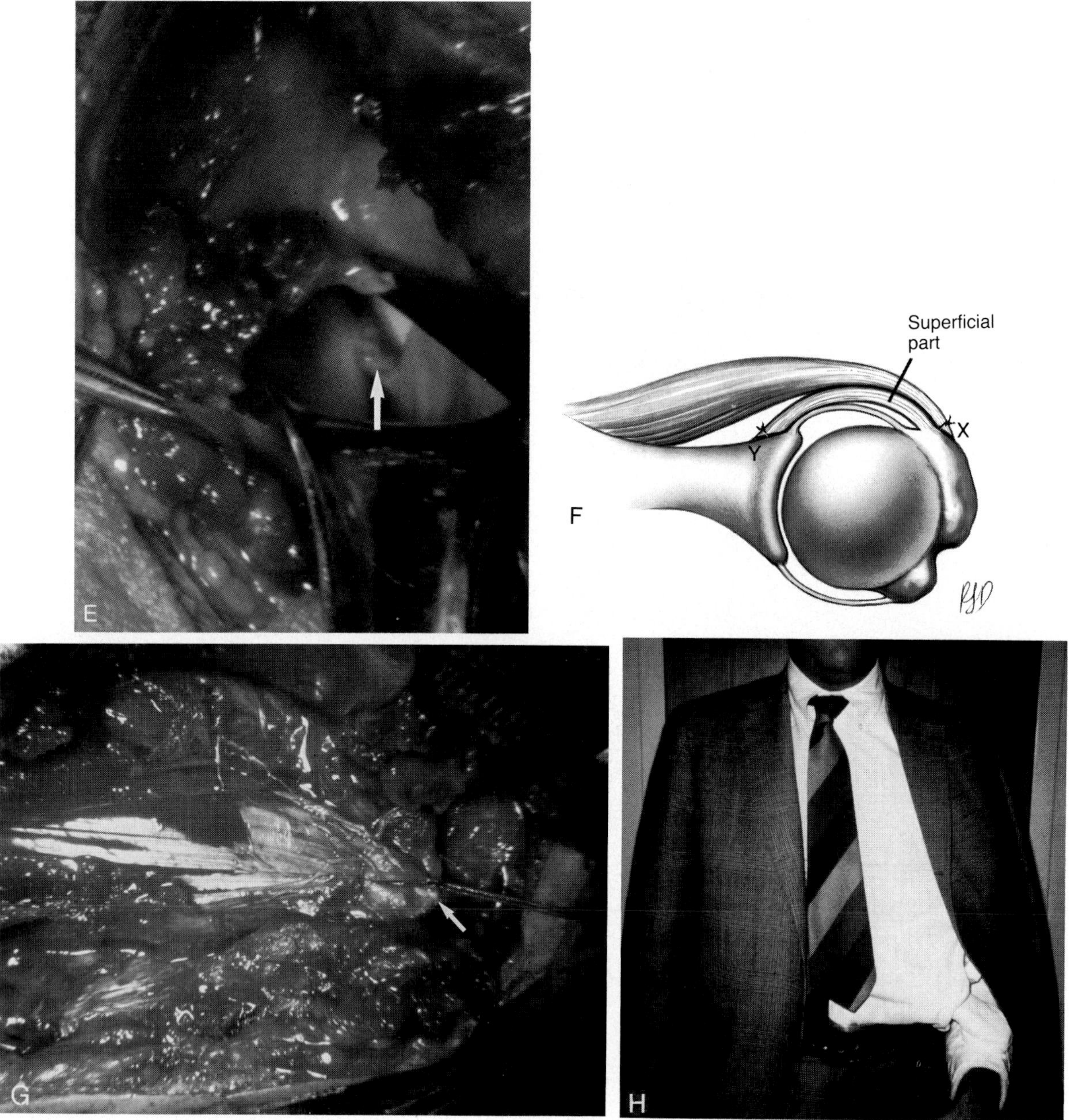

Figure 4–41 *Continued* E, If on inspection of the anterior glenoid labrum it is found detached as illustrated (arrow) (the articular surface of the humeral head is white), a second approach is made anteriorly to re-attach the labrum before proceeding with step D.

F, The superficial layer of the infraspinatus tendon is sutured to the scapula to reinforce the capsule.

G, The infraspinatus (arrow) is re-attached in anatomical position with interrupted sutures.

H, A lightweight plastic spica is applied, as shown in Figure 4–40, with the arm in neutral flexion-extension and 10 degrees external rotation. Standing x-rays are made to confirm the absence of inferior subluxation of the head (see Fig. 4–40) prior to discharging the patient from the hospital.

Detaching the capsule from the anterior surface at the neck of the humerus is done with an index finger palpating and protecting the axillary nerve and with progressive internal rotation of the arm to expose the anterior surface of the neck of the humerus. The inferior flap is pulled up against the curetted neck of the humerus to eliminate anterior, inferior, and posterior redundancy (Fig. 4–41D). The superior flap may be re-attached first, depending on which seems easier at the time. The infraspinatus tendon is re-attached as illustrated to reinforce the repair (Fig. 4–41G).

After re-attaching the deltoid origin with 00 nonabsorbable sutures and closing the skin with a removeable subcuticular suture, the patient is allowed to wake up and sit up as the light plastic spica cast is applied with the arm held in about 10 to 20 degrees external rotation and protected against inferior subluxation as in Figures 4–34I and 4–41H.

Inferior Capsular Shift with Two Approaches

Although the inferior capsular shift is usually performed through one approach, I do not hesitate to add a second approach if

1. When performing the operation through a posterior approach a significant detachment of the anterior glenoid labrum is found.
2. I am in doubt during the surgery about having adequately stabilized the opposite side of the joint.
3. At re-operations a release is required on the short side before proceeding with the shift on the other side.

Posterior Approach Adding Anterior Approach to Re-Attach the Anterior Labrum

As pointed out in our discussion of operative findings, anterior labrum detachment can develop in shoulders with multidirectional instability. Detachment of the anterior labrum is, as described in Chapter 1, pages 25 and 26, and Figure 1–18, actually a detachment of the medial portion of the inferior glenohumeral ligament, and it is important to re-attach this structure to the scapula when repairing an unstable shoulder. This is especially true in a patient with multidirectional instability because without this attachment of the important inferior glenohumeral ligament, the capsular shift would have no anchorage medially to prevent inferior and anterior instability.

Therefore, when doing an inferior capsular shift through a posterior approach, if detachment of the anterior labrum is present (Fig. 4–42B), I make a second incision anteriorly and repair the

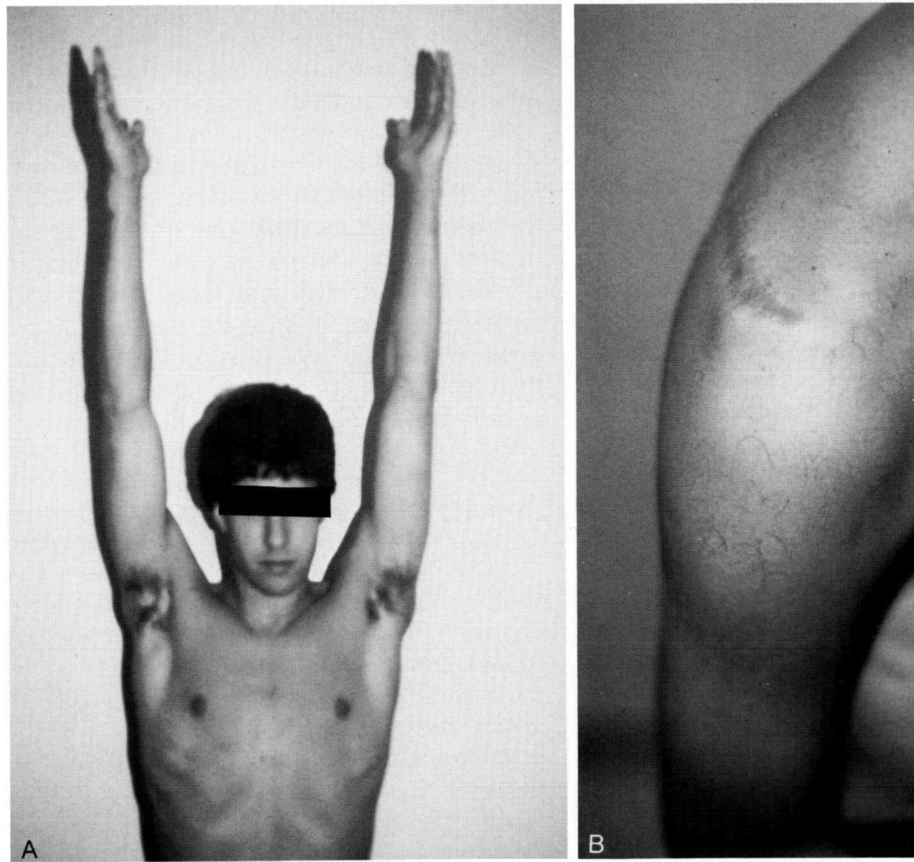

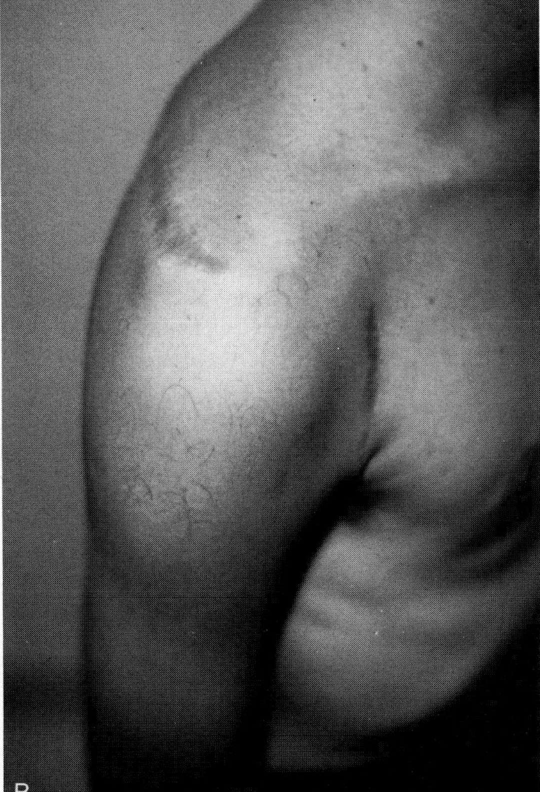

Figure 4–42. ***Results of Inferior Capsular Shift.***

A, Illustrating an excellent result eight years after bilateral inferior capsular shifts. The patient had returned to two years of college level swimming and continues to be active and free of pain.

B, Another patient with an excellent result who had a second anterior approach made to re-attach the anterior glenoid labrum at the time of an inferior capsular shift through the posterior approach. Ten years after this procedure, he continues to play weekend basketball and perform normal activities. We now prefer a lower anterior incision and a vertical posterior incision.

detached labrum to bone, as shown in Figure 4–31G, before proceeding with the shift from the posterior approach.

In our original article on multidirectional instability in 1980,[13] we excluded shoulders that had both a Bankart repair (re-attachment of the anterior labrum) and an inferior capsular shift from the anterior approach because we thought these two procedures together would confuse the analysis of the results of inferior capsular shift. However, five shoulders that were more unstable posteriorly than anteriorly and had had inferior capsular shifts performed from the posterior approach were included even though a second approach had been made anteriorly to re-attach the anterior labrum to make the shift effective. It was thought, since the major direction of dislocation was posterior, re-attaching the anterior labrum would not detract from the analysis of results.

It is important to emphasize that, although not typical, detachment of the anterior labrum may be present in patients with multidirectional instability; if so, re-attachment is thought to be important. This is true regardless of whether the approach is made from the front or the back. This special explanation seems necessary to clarify the significance of a Bankart lesion in multidirectionally unstable shoulders and to explain why two incisions are used when this lesion is found during an operation through the posterior approach.

Second Approach When in Doubt

Earlier in my experience I sometimes made an approach on the opposite side (usually in back after doing a shift from the front) to make sure that the shift had stabilized the opposite side. With increased confidence in the operation, I have not done this in recent years. However, when in doubt, a small approach can be made on the opposite side so that a finger can be inserted near the joint line to check the effectiveness of the shift; and, of course, if stabilization in that direction is inadequate, the second approach can be enlarged to augment the repair with local tissue.

Second Approach in Re-Operations to Release the Opposite Side

In re-operations after failed anterior repairs in which tightening of the anterior capsule caused a posterior subluxation of the humeral head, the anterior side may be released first to re-establish passive external rotation prior to performing the shift from the posterior side (see Figs. 4–52 to 4–57). It is much less common to perform a release of the posterior side first before tightening the anterior side after failed posterior repairs, but the problem does arise.

In the majority of re-operations on patients with multidirectional instability in my series, release and shift from one side have been done without using a second approach.

Aftercare Following Inferior Capsular Shift

Aftercare following an inferior capsular shift is extremely important and aims to allow mature healing to occur before stressing the repair. Prior to discharge, an x-ray of the shoulder is obtained with the patient standing to make sure that the cast is preventing downward subluxation of the humeral head. The cast is usually changed to ensure a good fit.

The cast is removed after six weeks, and a sling is worn with the arm placed in near-neutral rotation for three additional weeks. Gentle isometric exercises are begun at about three months that are gradually progressed as illustrated in Figure 7–13 to avoid stress on the repair. Other strengthening exercises and lifting more than 20 pounds are deferred for one year. I advise against performing strengthening exercises above the shoulder level and heavy weight lifting permanently. Full use of the shoulder—backstroke and butterfly swimming, impact sports, and so on—are prohibited for 18 months to allow mature healing of the capsule and recovery of muscle strength and tone. The ideal range of motion is, in my opinion, slightly less than that of the opposite side because the opposite shoulder is usually hypermobile.

Results of Inferior Capsular Shift

Our grading of results after inferior capsular shift for inferior and multidirectional dislocations is simply "satisfactory" or "unsatisfactory." Prospective grading of these results has been ongoing during the past 14 years. A "satisfactory" result meant that there was no recurrence of dislocation or subluxation, no significant pain, participation in a full range of activities, normal strength on manual testing compared with the contralateral shoulder, and full elevation within 10 degrees and rotation within 20 degrees compared with the contralateral shoulder. The contralateral shoulder is often hypermobile, and about 20 degrees less rotation is considered ideal for the repaired shoulder. In an "unsatisfactory" result these criteria were not met.

In the overall results of the initial series of 40

shoulders in 36 patients treated between 1974 and 1975,[13] 32 had been followed for a minimum of one year and 17 for more than two years. Only one shoulder was graded "unsatisfactory." That shoulder subluxated anteriorly seven months following an inferior capsular shift performed from the posterior approach. At re-operation from the front a detachment of the anterior glenoid labrum was found and repaired. It was thought that this lesion had been overlooked at the initial operation. One other patient had experienced two bouts of pain two years apart that had abated at the time of this preliminary report in 1980.

These patients have continued to remain asymptomatic except for the patient who had the bouts of unexplained pain. She subsequently became quite depressed and was considered to have a serious psychological problem. With time and observation her symptoms have regressed. No redislocations have occurred other than the one described above, and some of these patients have been followed for more than ten years.

Since the report of 1980, more than 100 additional inferior capsular shifts have been done with similar satisfactory results.

In the initial series, neurapraxia of the axillary nerve occurred in three patients. Fortunately, all recovered spontaneously. This is a stern warning of the threat of injury to this nerve.

Although the inferior capsular shift is more difficult than most standard repairs for unidirectional dislocations and requires a great deal of time for mature healing before stressing the capsule, it offers the advantage of stabilizing this type of shoulder, usually through one approach. Because the capsule and ligaments form the only inelastic barrier against dislocation and because excessive joint volume appears to be the cause of this problem, it is logical to use a direct repair with reinforcement of these structures rather than some less anatomical method.

I believe that the lasting results are due to reduction of the joint volume rather than simple reinforcement of the ligaments and capsule. Hyperelasticity of the capsule has not been a cause of late recurrent dislocations in this series, although I can see that it might be in some patients with extreme congenital laxity.

SPECIAL INSTABILITY PROBLEMS

Anterior Subluxation

Pitfalls in Diagnosis

During recent years, repair of incomplete anterior dislocations has been accepted as a surgical entity. This has opened a gate for many errors in diagnosis. A few years ago in my city, the most unsatisfactory and yet commonly used procedure was a biceps tenodesis. Now this is less frequently performed, and anterior subluxation surgery has taken its place.

The signs are the same as those characteristic of recurrent anterior dislocation (e.g., the anterior apprehension sign and the anterior instability test [see Figs. 4–2 and 4–3]). The impingement injection test (see Fig. 2–30) does not relieve the pain when the shoulder is stressed. Unfortunately, the same clinical picture can be produced by a slightly frozen, stiff shoulder, which can result from many causes, such as low-grade rheumatoid or other type of arthritis or an injury that has led to stiffness and scarring. Of great assistance in this dilemma was the work of Rokous, Feagin, and Abbott,[179a] who made a real contribution in showing reactive bone at the anterior rim of the glenoid, often seen in an axillary view, is concrete evidence for this diagnosis (Figs. 1–12C and 4–12). I have become unwilling to diagnose subluxation without this roentgen finding or a history of previous dislocation. Many patients with real pain prove to be recurrent anterior dislocators rather than subluxators.

The arthroscopic finding of fraying of the labrum is not a reliable indication that instability is present and causing pain. I have performed anterior repairs on several patients with long-standing diagnostic problems on the basis of arthroscopic evidence of fraying with frequent failure to relieve the symptoms. Of course, if a detachment of the anterior glenoid rim was seen arthroscopically, it would be proof of the presence of recurrent anterior dislocations; however, labrum detachment is not expected to be present in subluxating shoulders.

Other points important in the differential diagnosis of anterior dislocations and subluxations are illustrated in Figures 4–22 and 4–23 and in Table 4–1.

Indications for Repair of Recurrent Anterior Subluxation; Baseball Pitcher's Shoulder

Activities that cause pain are discontinued, and a trial of exercises to strengthen the muscles stabilizing the humeral head is given. Exercises are continued as long as improvement is occurring (see Fig. 7–13). The exercises are done without causing discomfort, are kept below the horizontal plane, and are gentle at first, adding progressive resistance to strengthen the internal rotators. Oral anti-inflammatory medications may help to eliminate the soreness. Isokinetic (Cybex) exercises may be helpful later. After the pain has disappeared and the arm has been strengthened, occupations or sports that place abnormal demands on the anterior capsule are studied for ways in which the arm could be spared before allowing the patient to resume these activities. The problem of a baseball pitcher's shoulder is shown in Figure 4–43.

Without objective roentgen signs to support the diagnosis, surgery is considered only if these conservative measures have failed and a true disability has been present for at least one year.

Technique and Results of Repair for Recurrent Anterior Subluxation

The approach, closure, and aftercare are the same as those used for recurrent anterior dislocations. As shown in Figure 4–44, the subscapularis tendon is maintained intact except for a slight release superiorly and is split longitudinally to expose the capsule. The anterior-inferior capsule is then plicated with double looping sutures as illustrated in Figure 4–44. Activities may be progressed to easy throwing after 12 months, but hard throwing is prohibited for 18 months.

This procedure is done only occasionally and then in carefully selected patients who place unusual demands on the shoulder. In my series, two high-level tennis players have benefited from the operation, and these repairs have endured for over 10 years. There have been other successes but also failures. A policeman and an industrial worker who had been referred as diagnostic problems were

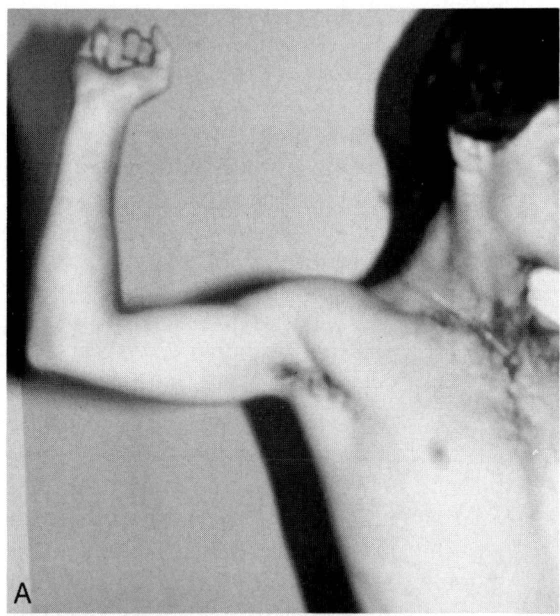

Figure 4–43A and B. The problem of a baseball pitcher's shoulder. The axillary view demonstrates anterior subluxation with reactive bone at the anterior glenoid rim (arrow) and an indentation in the back of the humeral head (arrow); the left shoulder is shown for comparison. This laxity, the extreme positions of the arm in throwing, and the force of throwing all cause impingement and stress the anterior capsule. Tightening the anterior capsule would solve all of these problems; however, the patient would then be unable to pitch. Anterior acromioplasty would make more room for the abnormal excursion of the arm and might relieve the impingement caused by a relaxed capsule, but could it be adequate and lasting?

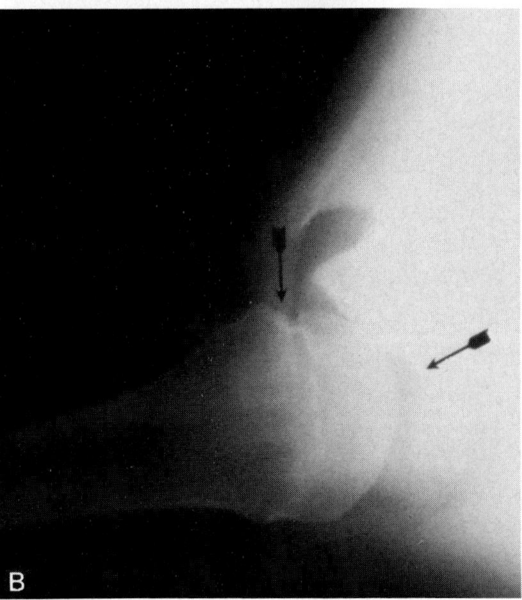

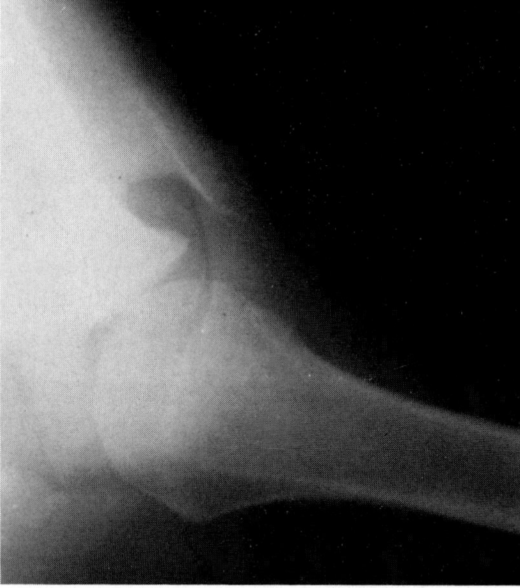

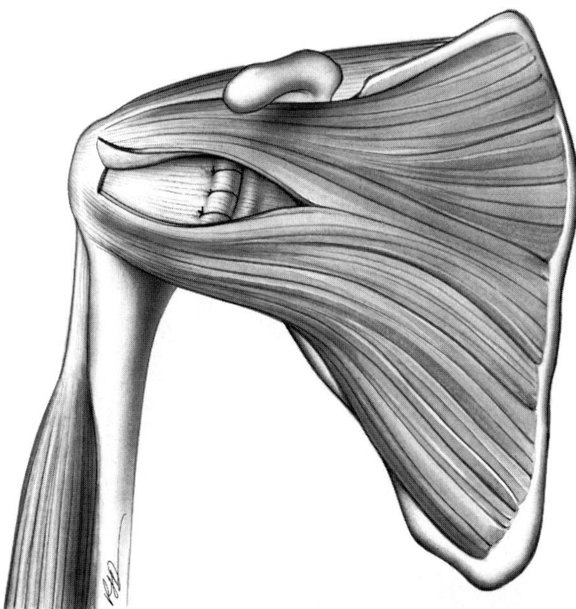

Figure 4–44. Repair for recurrent anterior subluxation.

operated on without improvement after fraying of the labrum and some laxity anteriorly were noted arthroscopically. Patient selection for this procedure is especially difficult. In addition, it is difficult to separate patients with true anterior dislocations who require a better stabilization procedure, as in Figure 4–31, from those with subluxation unless a careful examination under anesthesia is performed. Jobe[179] has devised an operation for throwers who have stretched out the anterior capsule using a similar technique of splitting the subscapularis tendon longitudinally and making a short T-opening in the capsule with the top of the "T" at the level of the glenoid rim. This offers exposure to allow inspection of the interior of the joint and perhaps a more controlled capsular closure such as a modified shift. The problem of patient selection and careful analysis of the degree of instability remains difficult in treating patients in a general population, compared with an athletic team in which all of the patients are young, healthy, and highly motivated and there is a greater incidence of traumatic dislocations (see Table 4–1).

Large Posterior Head Defect (Hill-Sachs Lesion)

As described in Figures 4–10 and 4–11, in patients with traumatic dislocations and longstanding acquired dislocations, wear and traumatic changes occur in the posterior part of the humeral head. The large groove in the back of the head may become hung up on the anterior glenoid rim when the arm is externally rotated (Fig. 4–45). A large anterior head defect may hang up when the arm is internally rotated.

Surprisingly, one very rarely sees hanging up of the head defect to be the cause of failure following repairs for recurrent anterior dislocations. Rather than doing one of the bone grafting procedures or osteotomies that have been described to fill the head defect, I perform the anterior repair (see Fig. 4–31) but shorten the capsule slightly more than usual to partially restrict external rotation. To date, following this policy, I have had no difficulty.

Impression Fractures

Indentation of the articular surface of the humeral head occurs more often with posterior dis-

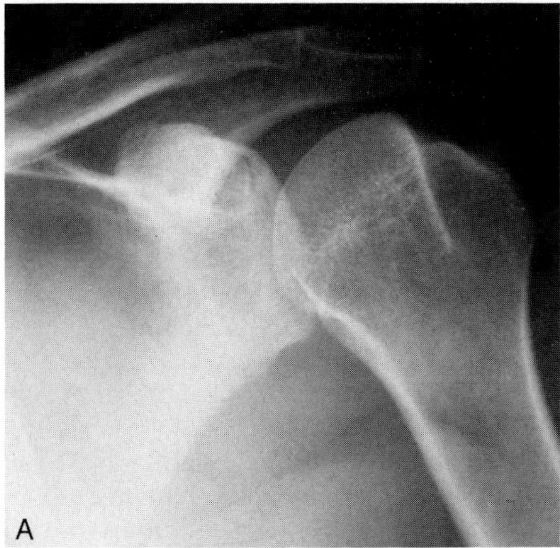

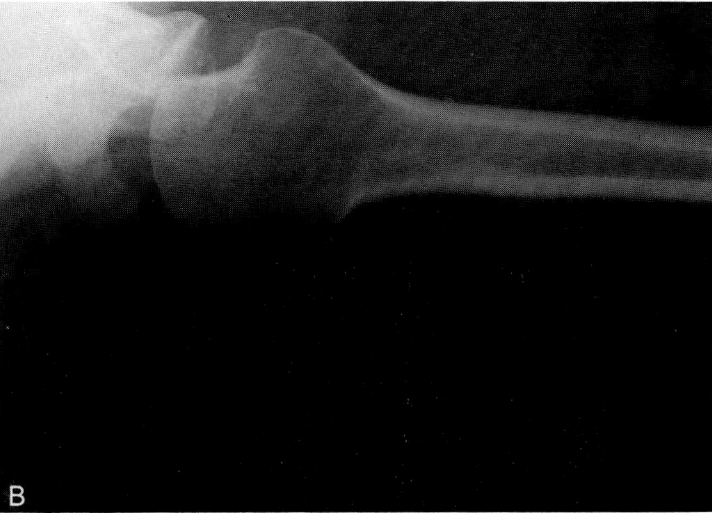

Figure 4–45A and B. Recurrent anterior dislocations with a large posterior head defect (Hill-Sachs defect) in the anterior-posterior and axillary views. The usual repair was done but with a little more shortening of the anterior capsule than usual.

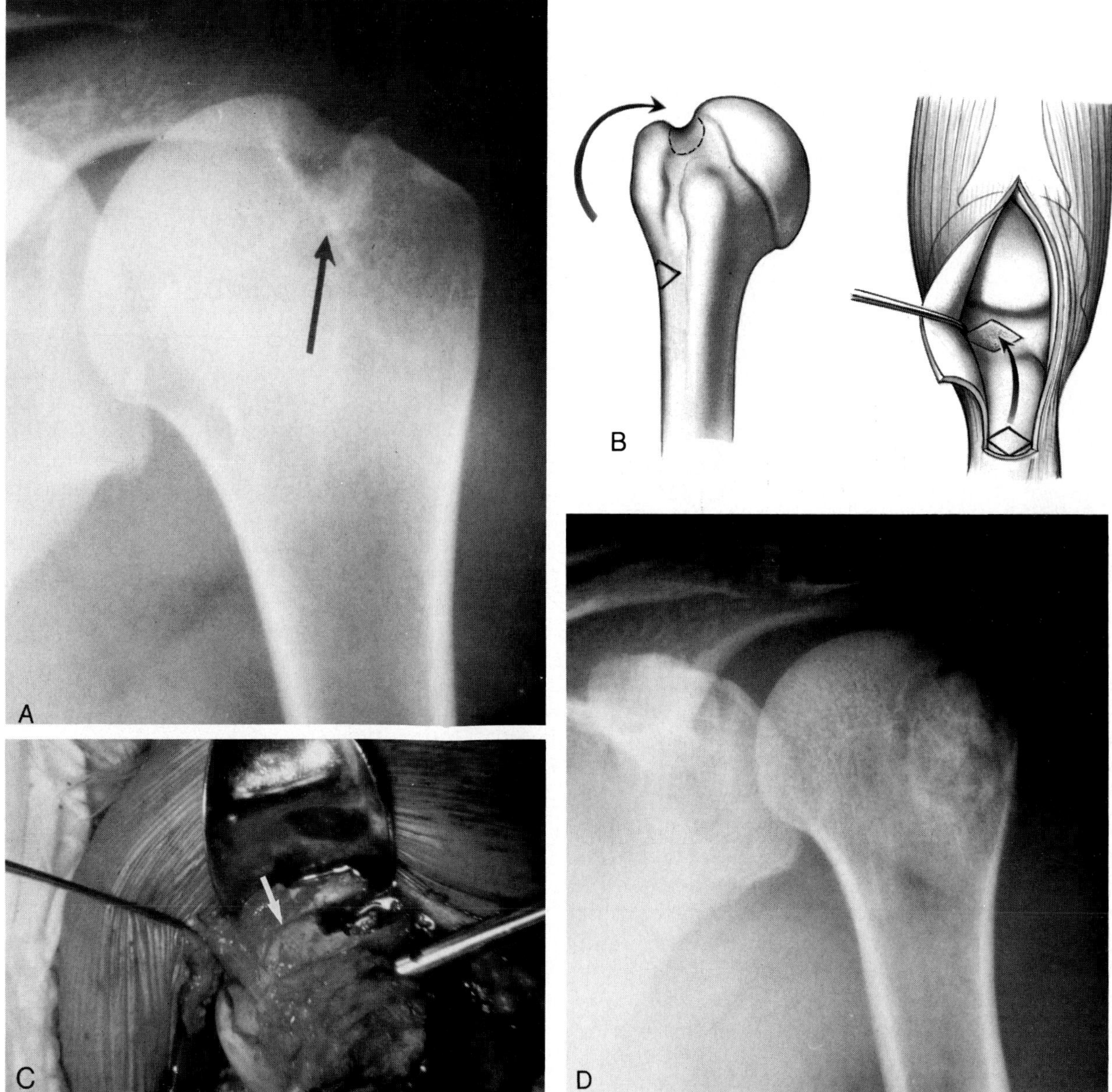

Figure 4–46A to D. Traumatic inferior dislocations can cause a high head defect (A, black arrow), which may require a bone graft (C, white arrow). The graft is taken from the surgical neck of the humerus. Roentgen appearance two years later is shown in D, at which time the shoulder was functioning normally.

locations than with anterior dislocations. Occasionally it occurs with an inferior dislocation requiring a bone graft (Fig. 4–46). An anterior approach is used (see Fig. 4–31), and the diamond-shaped graft is taken from the surgical neck region of the humerus.

Hypoplastic Glenoid

Congenital underdevelopment of the glenoid (Fig. 4–47) is not common but is seen about once a year in my experience, sometimes in several members of a family. It differs from multiple epiphyseal dysplasia in that the latter involves the humeral head and other joints are involved. Both of these conditions can lead to degenerative arthritis and require a shoulder arthroplasty (see Chapter 3, p. 208, and Figs. 3–46 and 3–47).

This condition can occur as an incidental finding without symptoms. It may cause symptoms of instability or, in the late stages, symptoms of degenerative arthritis. With symptoms of instability this condition is one of the few entities that requires consideration of a glenoid osteotomy.

Glenoid osteotomy for this deformity is undertaken only after careful roentgen analysis, including CT scans to determine whether the approach should be made from the front or the back. A bone

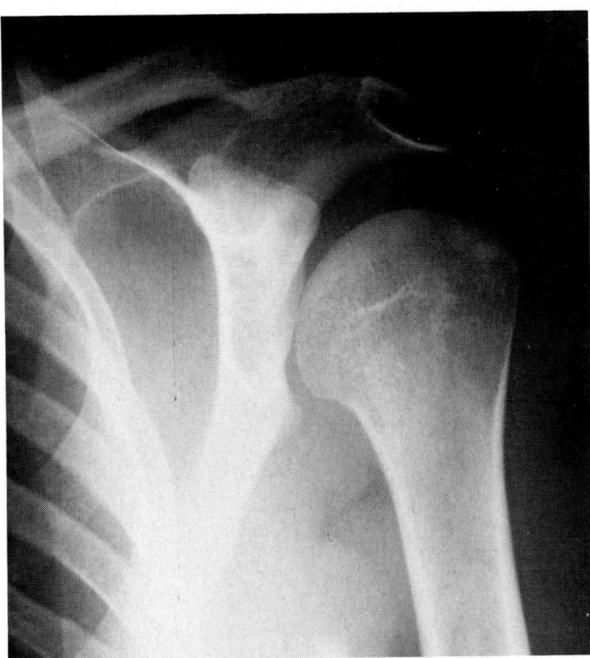

Figure 4–47. Congenital glenoid hypoplasia. This can be associated with instability requiring an osteotomy but is often seen as an incidental finding without symptoms. Rarely, as discussed in Chapter 3, it can lead to degenerative arthritis.

graft from the inner table of the iliac crest or spine of the scapula (if a posterior approach is used) is wedged into the osteotomy site after carefully cutting across the neck of the scapula at least 1.0 cm. from the articular surface with an osteotome, taking care to guard the axillary nerve with an elevator placed just inferior and anterior (or posterior if operating from the front) to the capsule of the glenohumeral joint. A screw is used to maintain position if needed. A spica cast is worn for eight weeks.

It is logical to perform an osteotomy of the glenoid when bone deficiency of the glenoid is the basis for symptomatic instability. However, I do not have adequate statistics on the results of osteotomy repair of this condition. Dysplasia epiphysealis multiplex with deformity on both sides of the joint seems less amenable to correction by osteotomy. A glenoid osteotomy, as illustrated in Figure 4–3, is wrong when the problem is a redundant glenohumeral capsule and the skeletal structures are normal.

Instability After Proximal Humeral Epiphyseal Fractures

I have seen a group of patients with complicated problems and failed surgery because of recurrent dislocations and subluxations after healing of fractures of the proximal humeral epiphysis. I am not referring to the transitory inferior subluxations often seen after humeral fractures and that disappear as the deltoid and rotator cuff muscles regain tone. These are patients with persistent recurrent multidirectional dislocations who were referred to me several years after fractures.

Hansen[196] and I reviewed these patients in 1984 and were unable to find a report of this complication of proximal humeral fractures. Yet the six patients in this series, two males and four females ranging in age from 5 to 21 years (average 13 years), all sustained significant proximal humeral epiphyseal fractures and, without prior shoulder disability, developed symptomatic instability that was treated elsewhere surgically without success, in my judgement, because of multidirectional instability.

Of the six epiphyseal fractures, all were Salter-Harris Type II fractures; five were treated closed with simple immobilization, and one older patient had been treated with closed reduction, percutaneous pinning, and three weeks of cast immobilization. All healed uneventfully, and there were no nerve injuries. Following fracture healing, normal shoulder function was reported from 1 to 11 years, after which a slow onset of shoulder symptoms developed when the patient lifted heavy objects and used the arm overhead, and there were episodes of slipping and catching during activities. None of the patients had further significant injuries.

Operative repairs had been performed elsewhere in three patients—two had had one procedure, and one had had three failed procedures (Fig. 4–48). None were suspected of having multidirectional dislocations prior to these procedures. The three other patients were referred because multidirectional instability was recognized.

At the time of our examination, all six had clinical evidence of multidirectional instability, as discussed in Figures 4–17, 4–18, and 4–19. Our initial treatment was conservative and consisted of exercises and altering activities, without success. Following this treatment, I performed an inferior capsular shift repair in each case. Of the three re-operations, a release of the anterior capsule and a shift repair made through the posterior approach was performed in two patients, and a posterior bone block was added because of a deficient posterior capsule after repeated failed operations in one case, as discussed under re-operations for failed instability surgery on page 313, Figure 4–34G.

I believe it is important to recognize this group of patients who, following proximal humeral epi-

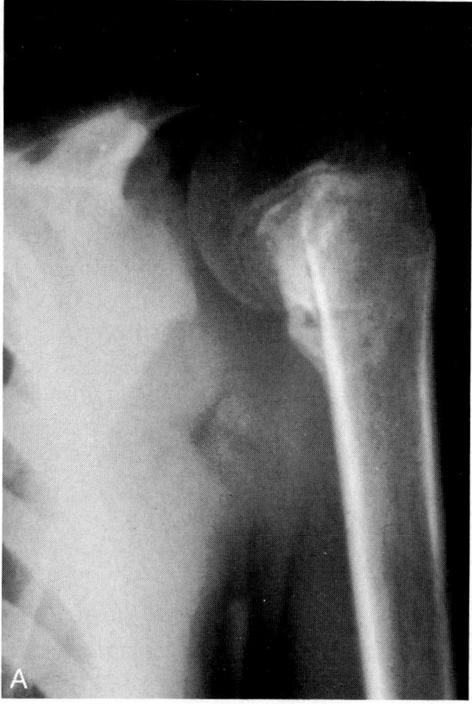

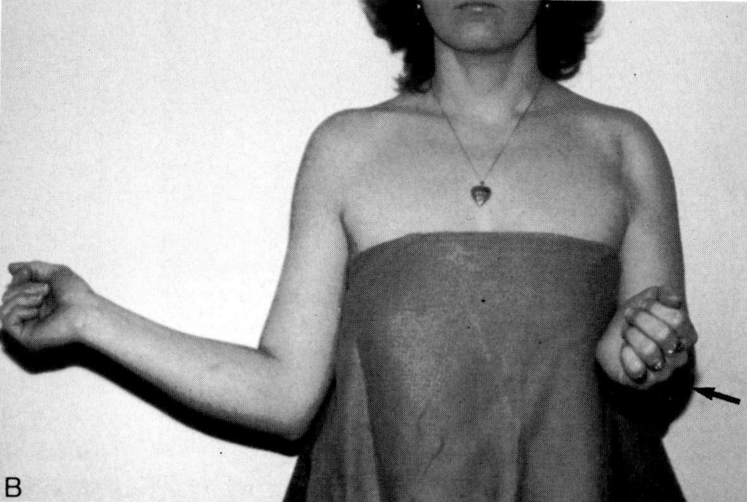

Figure 4–48A and B. One of a group of patients with complicated multidirectional dislocations after proximal humeral epiphyseal fractures. This patient had three failed repairs (scars front and back) and 5.0 cm. shortening of the humerus (arrow). The epiphyseal fracture had been sustained ten years previously.

physeal fractures, develop capsular laxity, probably because of pre-existing laxity in some cases (all were in the young age group) and also because of the effects of the injury on the capsule. Another factor to consider is altered version (torsion) of the humeral head. These patients should be carefully evaluated for unusual capsular laxity and, less importantly, altered humeral version prior to undertaking a surgical repair.

Glenoid Rim "Fragments" and Fractures

Small "fragments," which are more often reactive bone at the rim of the glenoid rather than true fractures, are common after traumatic dislocations and may develop with acquired dislocations. These lesions are best seen in axillary view roentgenograms or CT scans. When a bone fragment is present it is important to make sure during the repair to eliminate a step-off at the anterior glenoid rim that might catch on a posterior head defect and predispose to continuing instability. Otherwise, re-attachment of the labrum proceeds essentially as usual except for prying the "fragment" of bone up to the level of the articular surface of the glenoid prior to the bone suture. This is done with a thin, flat osteotome, and holes are made through the fragment to secure it to the glenoid with a nonabsorbable suture (Fig. 4–49).

Larger fragments of the glenoid articular surface can make the joint unstable and may create a fixed subluxation of the head (see p. 414), leading to severe post-traumatic arthritis. Optimum treatment entails repositioning of the fragment and internal fixation. Screw fixation is easier and is preferable when feasible. In my experience, in the majority of these fractures the piece of glenoid is too fragmented or too soft to hold a screw. Com-

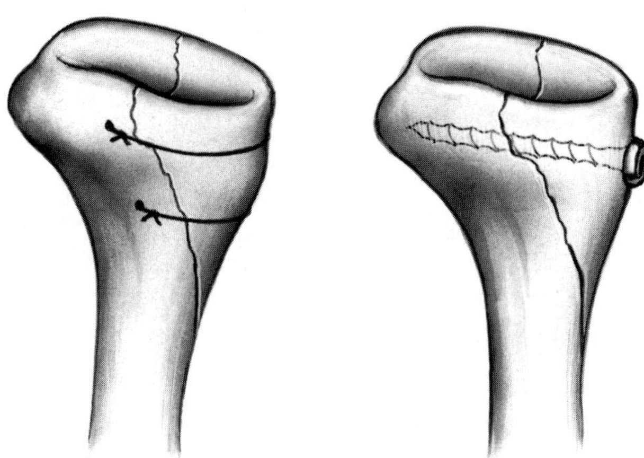

Figure 4–49. Large glenoid rim fragments require internal fixation. If the bone does not hold a screw (right), nonmetallic sutures (left) can be used effectively.

minuted fragments are anchored to the scapula with nonabsorbable sutures (see Fig. 4–49). Comminuted fragments usually require protection with a sling or cast for from four to six weeks.

Osteotomies for Recurrent Dislocations. Version (Torsion of the Upper Humerus or Glenoid) Rarely Indicated

I agree with Randelli[180] that abnormal torsion of the upper humerus or abnormal version of the articular surface of the glenoid is almost never a significant factor in everyday, recurrent glenohumeral dislocations. Rarely, in congenital defects (p. 330) it is a consideration in some patients but not in others. The major problems are the capsule and the ligaments.

In Europe, derotational osteotomy of the humerus has been a common operation for correcting recurrent anterior dislocations. In the United States, osteotomy of the glenoid has been used for correction of recurrent posterior dislocations. This requires a comment. I have not performed an osteotomy of the glenoid or humerus in repairs for recurrent dislocations (except in patients with extremely rare congenital defects with obvious bone abnormalities (see Fig. 4–47) for the following reasons:

1. An osteotomy done to alter a normal bone in the presence of instability that is due to a loose or detached capsule distorts anatomy and can cause subluxation of the humeral head, leading to the arthritis of dislocations (see Fig. 4–3C to F).

2. When a loose capsule is at fault an osteotomy alone will fail to control the instability.

3. An osteotomy on a normal bone reduces the range of motion or at least causes abnormal stress on the articular surfaces. For example, the combination of an osteotomy and capsulorrhaphy, as performed by some surgeons, may succeed in controlling the dislocations (provided that the capsulorrhaphy is adequate), but the alteration in the contour of the articular surfaces restricts the range of motion and reduces the functional result.

4. An osteotomy makes the procedure more difficult and adds the risks of possible complications in bone healing and, in the case of glenoid osteotomies, possible damage to the articular surface (e.g., fracturing through the articular surface).

Instability with Muscle Imbalance

Because the glenohumeral ligaments and capsule are normally loose enough to allow them to twist when the arm is raised, imbalance of the surrounding muscles can cause subluxation or dislocation of the humeral head. This may occur when the muscles on one side of the joint are flaccid, in which case the normal muscles on the other side displace the head, or it may occur when the muscles are spastic with uneven overactivity. Secondary features are alterations in the capsule and overlying muscles, which may become contracted or, on the side that has fewer muscles for protection, elongated. Neurotrophic joints are discussed in Chapter 6.

Shoulders with Flaccid Paralysis (Poliomyelitis)

In poliomyelitis the deltoid muscle is more frequently involved than the other muscles of the shoulder; however, the severity of involvement and number of muscles affected vary.

If the rotator cuff is spared and the deltoid muscle is paralyzed, inferior subluxation often occurs. If the inferior subluxation is causing pain, an inferior capsular shift to correct it (Figs. 4–38 to 4–42), is helpful. Otherwise, no surgical procedure is performed.

Deltoid paralysis was once treated in the United States almost routinely with a glenohumeral arthrodesis. Now, many surgeons recognize the functional advantages of preserving rotation of this joint rather than performing a fusion when the rotator cuff is functioning. It is preferable for most patients to keep rotation of the humerus to allow positioning the elbow, so that the elbow, by flexion and extension, can place the hand where it is needed. A fusion is stronger if the scapular muscles are intact, but rotation is lost.

If there is paralysis of both the deltoid muscle and the rotator cuff, a fusion is considered unless both shoulders are involved. Bilateral shoulder fusions are not performed because of the functional loss that would result (e.g., inability to reach in back or reach the top of the head). Therefore, if both shoulders are paralyzed, an inferior capsular shift to stabilize the joint and muscle transfers are done when there is some residual rotator cuff power. Transfer of the pectoralis minor, subscapularis, or the latissimus dorsi for the infraspinatus, as shown in Figure 3–31, can be considered.

Shoulders with Spastic Paralysis (Strokes)

Because the muscles controlling internal rotation are much stronger than those controlling external rotation, an internal rotation and adduction contracture (as in "frozen shoulders," p. 422) may

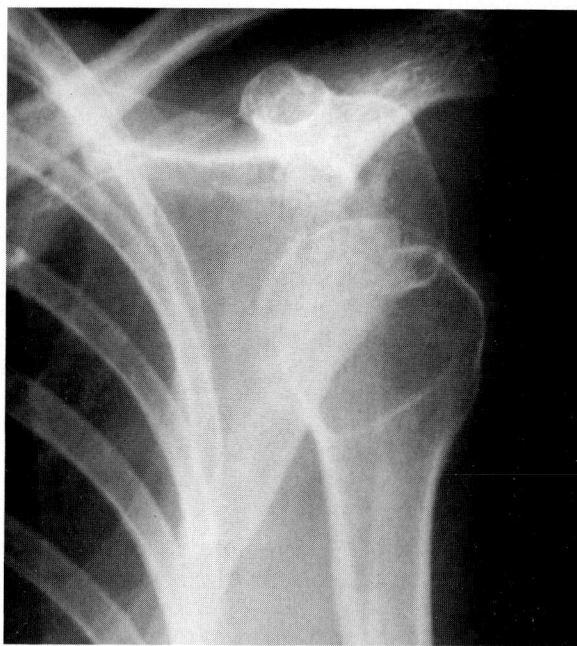

Figure 4–50. Paralytic "stroke" shoulder with subluxation.

occur in patients who have had "strokes" (cerebrovascular accidents). The internally rotated humeral head may subluxate if the deltoid and rotator cuff are sufficiently weakened (Fig. 4–50).

Conservative treatment, consisting of heat and passive and assistive exercises to overcome stiffness, almost always relieves pain and is all that is required. Intermittent use of a sling or strap to prevent subluxation may be helpful. Release and lengthening of the subscapularis tendon, or tenotomy of the pectoralis major have been described; however, I have never encountered a patient whose symptoms could not be controlled adequately with heat and stretching exercises. Nor have I, to date, performed an inferior capsular shift for this condition. Home helpers or members of the family are taught how to raise and externally rotate the arm after the application of low heat to relax the muscles.

Initial Dislocation After Age 40

Those who experience a first dislocation after the age of 40 may, unlike younger individuals, have concomitant tears of the rotator cuff. This and the "posterior mechanism" of anterior dislocation are discussed in Chapter 2, page 68. However, it is important to reiterate that the majority of this older age group have pathology similar to that of younger patients and are treated in essentially the same way. Some older patients have a greater tendency to develop stiffer shoulders after surgery or immobilization, but this is not always the case. Some younger patients also have a tendency to become stiff, so patients in both age groups require re-examination and individualized post-operative exercise programs.

The treatment of those with a combination of a tear of the rotator cuff and detachment of the anterior labrum is discussed with Figure 4–27.

Chronic Dislocations

Old dislocations without fractures are considered in this section. Old fracture-dislocations are discussed in Chapters 3 and 5.

Old Anterior Dislocations

The physical and roentgen findings of old dislocations are similar to those of acute dislocations, discussed earlier in this chapter and illustrated in Figure 4–51. A chronic anterior dislocation is easier to recognize clinically than a missed posterior dislocation or posterior fracture-dislocation.

Treatment should not be undertaken without careful consideration of the neurovascular status, condition of the articular surfaces, softening of the bone, and psychological attitude of the patient. Alcoholic and noncompliant patients are especially prone to this problem and may not give reliable histories or be capable of cooperating with the aftercare program. Softening of the bone may pose a threat of fracturing the humeral shaft and preclude efforts at closed reduction. Destruction of the articular surfaces from fractures or wear may demand replacement arthroplasties. CT scans and good quality axillary view x-ray films are essential in planning treatment.

No Reduction

If the patient is cooperative and nonalcoholic and has no undue risk for anesthesia, reduction is advised except in the occasional patient who has minimal pain and prefers disability to treatment.

Reduction Under Six Weeks After Anterior Dislocation

If there is severe osteopenia, open reduction is preferred; otherwise, closed reduction is attempted with the understanding and permission of the patient to proceed to open reduction if closed reduction is unsuccessful. Contractures of the soft tissue have, in my experience, prohibited closed reduction after six weeks, and usually after three weeks.

Closed reduction is performed with the patient under general anesthesia. Traction, countertrac-

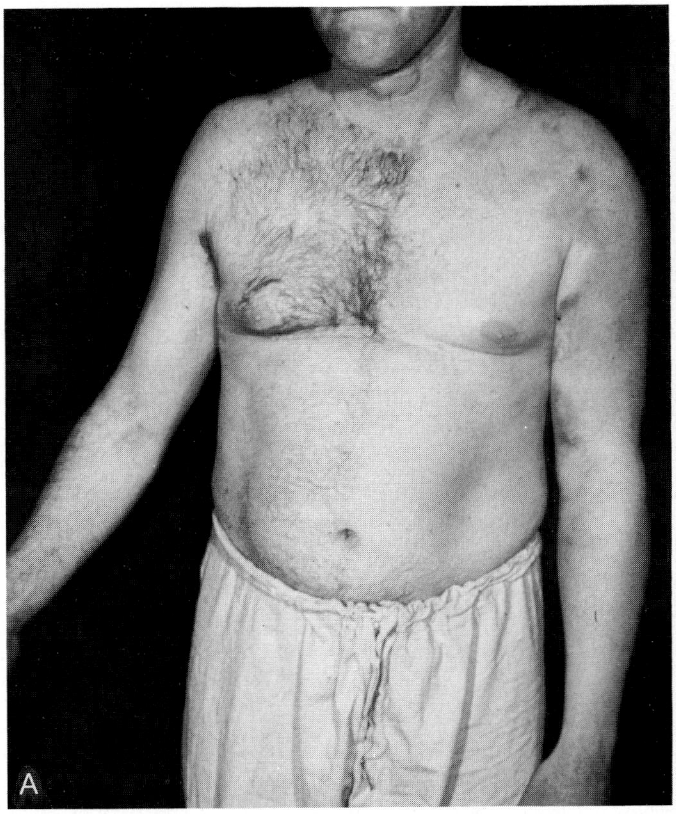

A

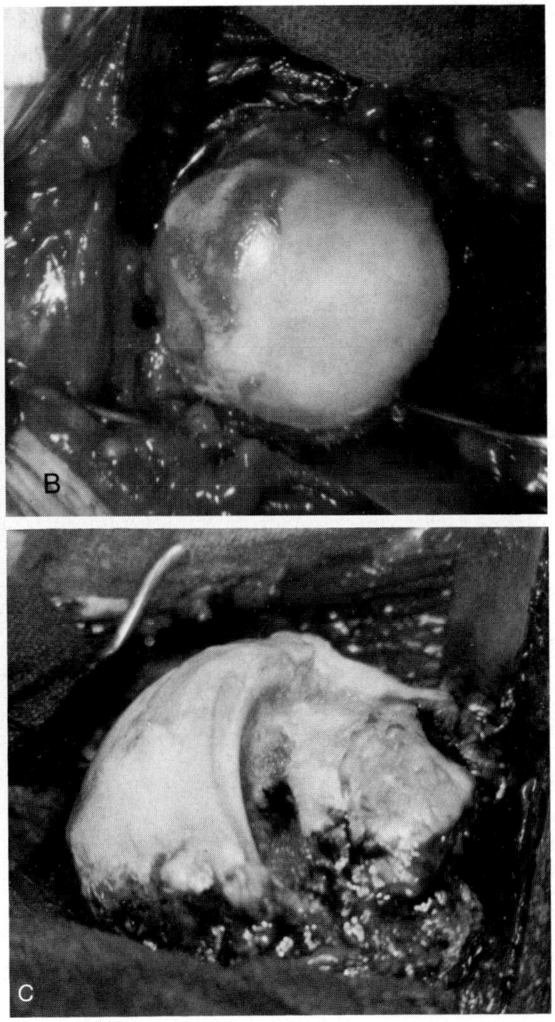

B

C

Figure 4–51A to C. Chronic dislocations. A missed anterior dislocation of the right shoulder and a missed posterior dislocation of the left shoulder seen nine months after electroshock treatment. The right shoulder (A) was treated with open reduction, and the left shoulder (B) was treated with a prosthesis.

tion, and gentle rotation, flexion, and extension are used to free the humeral head from repair tissue as the arm is gradually abducted. Attempts are made to re-locate the head by direct pressure on it at various levels of abduction (see Fig. 4–30). If these maneuvers are unsuccessful, the shoulder is prepared for surgery, and an open reduction is performed.

The same approach as for repairing a recurrent anterior dislocation is used. The subscapularis tendon is detached, and an anterior capsular repair is made. The labrum usually requires re-attachment, as shown in Figure 4–31.

Reduction Six Weeks to Nine Months After Dislocation

During the first six to nine months after dislocation, the humeral head is usually preserved, and open reduction is performed. The same approach used for repairing recurrent anterior dislocations (Fig. 4–31) is used, except that the insertion of the pectoralis major is detached early to free the proximal humerus so that it can be re-aligned. The subscapularis tendon is detached, and a T-opening is made in the anterior capsule. After freeing the glenoid of scar tissue, the head should be reduced without great force or effort. The detached labrum is re-attached to the scapula with a suture placed through a drill hole (Fig. 4–31G), the capsule is closed, and the subscapularis tendon is re-attached in its normal location.

Post-operatively, the arm is immobilized in internal rotation and slight flexion for approximately three to four weeks. No transfixing pin is required. External rotation is prohibited for at least six to eight weeks. Pulley and pendulum exercises (forward) can be allowed six to eight weeks after surgery, and the shoulder is then allowed to regain motion slowly at its own speed.

If the articular surfaces have been maintained and the subchondral bone is not too soft, these patients can be expected to obtain a result similar to patients having repairs for recurrent anterior dislocation.

Treatment After One Year Following Anterior Dislocation

The head is almost always too soft and the articular cartilage too atrophied to permit a trial of closed reduction (Fig. 4–51). Replacement of the head is usually preferable. This is done through the extended deltopectoral approach (see Fig. 3–25). The pectoralis major and subscapularis tendons are detached early. The scar tissue is then released to mobilize the upper humerus and clear the glenoid. Erosion of the glenoid may demand use of a glenoid component, which, in the case of long-standing dislocations, may become very difficult because of loss of bone (Figs. 3–24 through 3–33 and 3–57 through 3–65).

Chronic Posterior Dislocations

These are discussed with fractures (Chapter 5, p. 393), because they are always, in our experience, associated with impression fractures.[118, 192]

RE-OPERATION FOR FAILED REPAIRS

Causes of Failure in Repairs for Recurrent Dislocation

The causes of failure in 120 consecutive shoulders referred to me because of unsatisfactory repairs for recurrent dislocations between 1978 and 1983[197] are listed in Table 4–2. I performed further repairs for residual instability in 50, releases for stiffness in 7, and arthroplasties in 30 with severe arthritis; some of these are illustrated in Figures 4–52 to 4–57.

There is undoubtedly a higher proportion of patients with advanced arthritis of recurrent dislocations in this series than is found in the general surgical experience because of my special interest in shoulder arthroplasty. Almost all of these shoulders with arthritis had had standard unidirectional dislocation repairs performed when there was unrecognized multidirectional instability. Patients with multidirectional disability with residual instability formed the second largest group. Thus, unrecognized multidirectional instability was the most common cause of failure in these repairs done for recurrent anterior instability. This has been discussed previously (pp. 280 and 281). It is the reason I use an approach in which, if needed, I can do an inferior capsular shift. This makes it possible to correct unexpected inferior laxity or laxity on the opposite side of the capsule at the time of an anterior or posterior repair.

The second most important cause of failure was overlooking a detachment of the anterior labrum. This lesion renders the inferior glenohumeral ligament ineffective and results in persistent anterior instability.

Next in frequency was the complications caused by metal. Late loosening or migration of metal and damage to the articular surfaces are especially common in the shoulder because of the large excursion of motion of the glenohumeral joint. My use of metal in procedures for repairing recurrent dislocations is limited to a few excep-

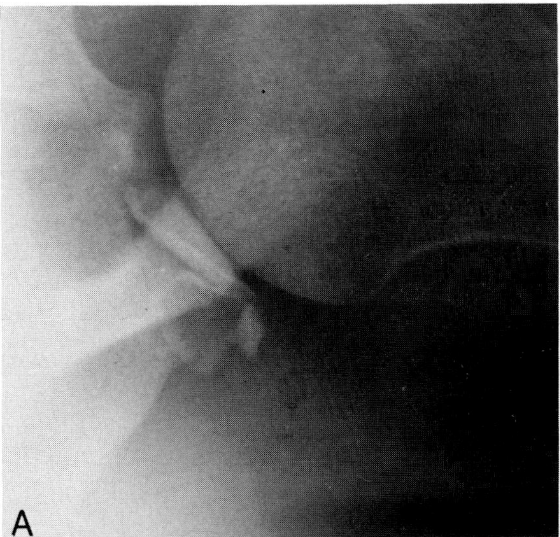

Figure 4–52. ***Complications and Failed Repairs for Recurrent Dislocations.*** A, Nonunion of a posterior glenoid osteotomy with early arthritis. B, Stiffness after an anterior repair. C, Paralysis of the arm. D, Staples in the joint.

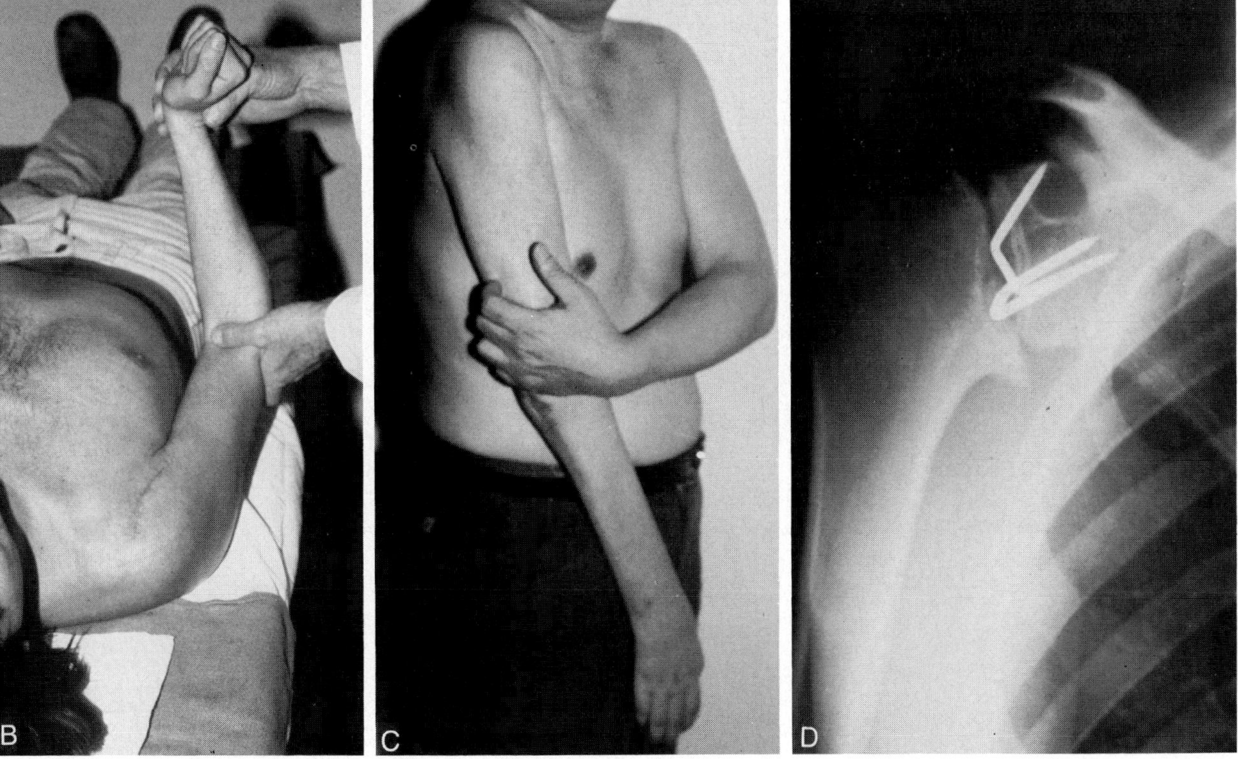

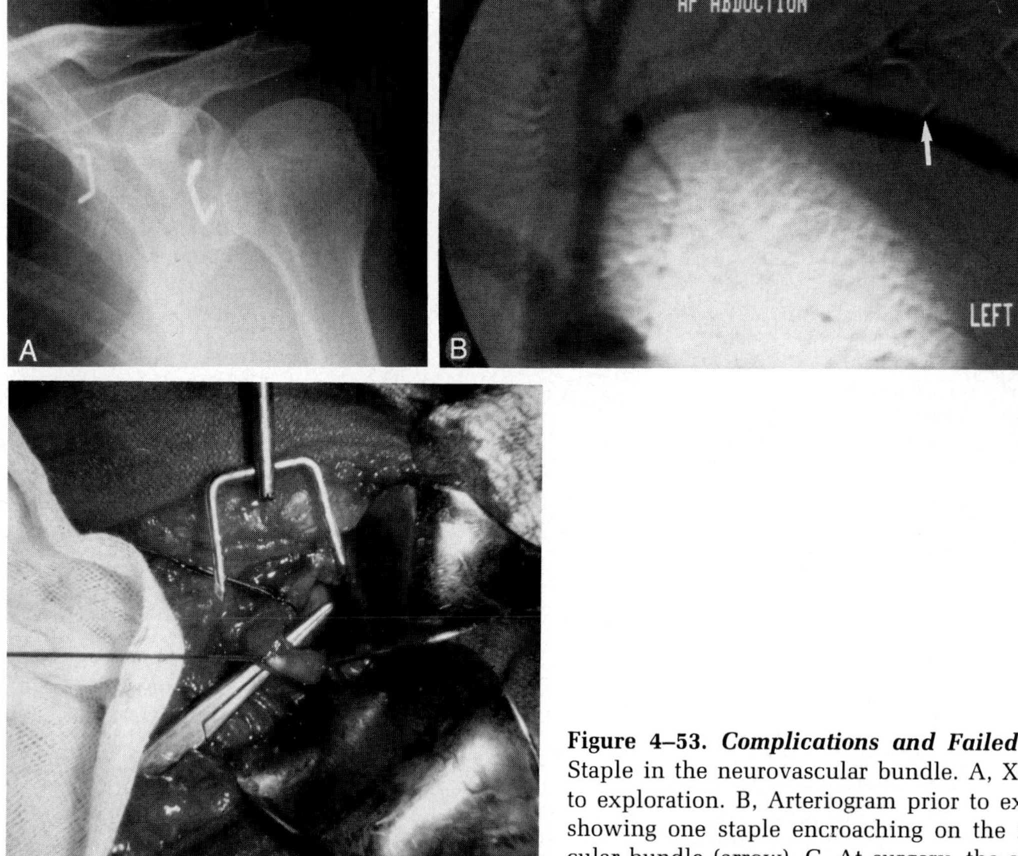

Figure 4–53. ***Complications and Failed Repairs.*** Staple in the neurovascular bundle. A, X-ray prior to exploration. B, Arteriogram prior to exploration showing one staple encroaching on the neurovascular bundle (arrow). C, At surgery, the staple was found to be through the brachial plexus.

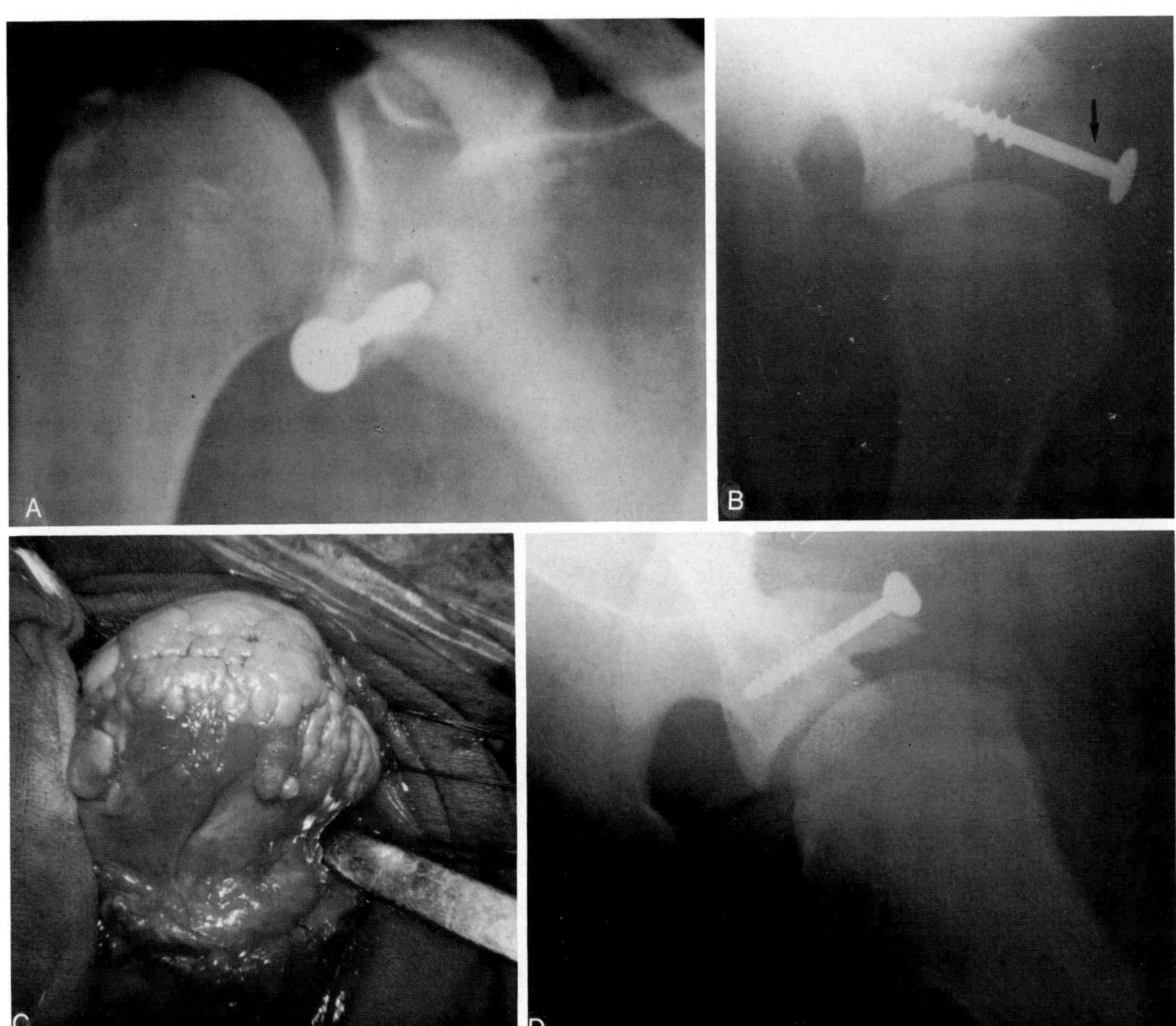

Figure 4–54. ***Complications and Failed Repairs. Ununited Coracoid Transfer Inside the Joint.***

A, Ununited coracoid transfer.

B, Axillary view showing the subluxated head against the coracoid (arrow points to the coracoid).

C, Erosion of the front of the head because the coracoid is inside the joint.

D, Axillary view one year after rebuilding the anterior capsule with a cruciate repair, re-attaching the glenoid labrum, and bone-grafting the coracoid process (outside the capsular repair and outside the joint).

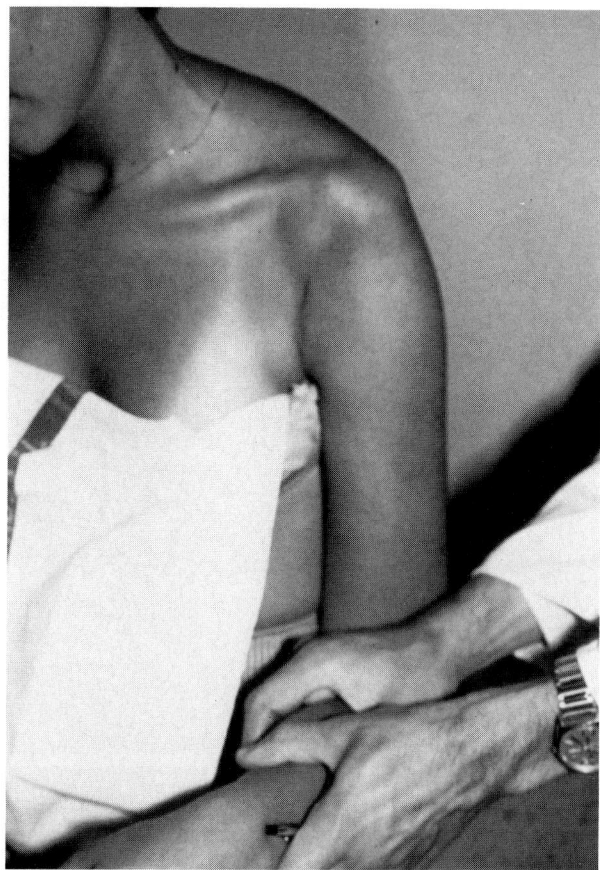

Figure 4–55. ***Complications and Failed Repairs.*** Patient with a failed Bankart repair because of multidirectional instability. There was a sulcus sign and residual inferior and posterior instability.

tional cases—for example, in the rare case of a coracoid transplant (see Fig. 4–31G), posterior bone block (see Fig. 4–34G), and selected glenoid rim fractures (see Fig. 4–49).

Voluntary (intentional) dislocators were the cause of failure after nine procedures. They were considered inoperable, and no further surgery was advised.

Infection was found to be more common after surgery for recurrent anterior dislocation than is generally recognized. If infection is treated early and adequately, the joint may be saved. Later, débridement of the damaged articular surfaces and drainage may be inadequate, and eventually further reconstruction or a fusion may be required, as discussed in Chapter 3 and shown in Figure 3–92.

Stiffness of the shoulder with pain and inadequate motion is a common cause of dissatisfaction. Some patients accept it, but others have sufficient pain and disability to want further surgery. At surgery, the tight structures are released but integrity of the anterior capsule is re-established by using an inferior capsular shift approach with cruciate repair to reinforce the lengthened capsule against re-dislocation.

Errors in diagnosis included surgery for recurrent anterior instability in five shoulders with rheumatoid arthritis and one with acromioclavicular arthritis and one with impingement (see Fig. 4–23).

Uncontrolled seizures were the cause of failure in five patients who did not take their medication regularly. No further surgery was done on these patients unless they became compliant.

Technique of Re-repair for Failed Repairs

The objective of surgery is to restore as near-normal anatomy as possible. This includes elimi-

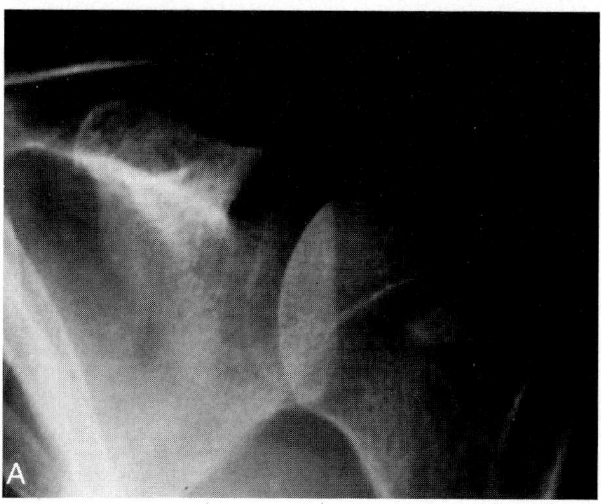

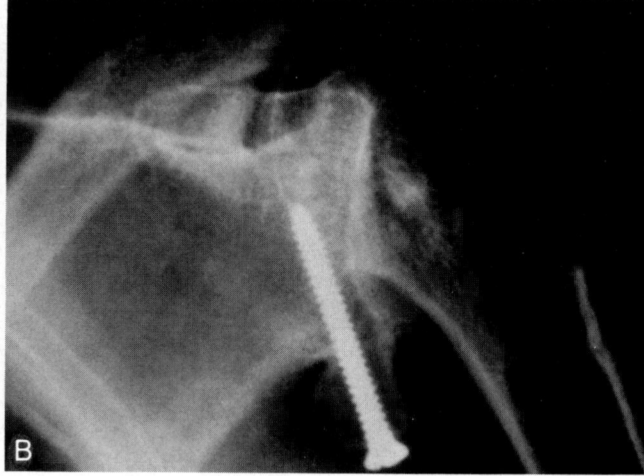

Figure 4–56. ***Complications and Failed Repairs.*** A coracoid transfer (modified Bristow repair) in a 54 year old woman pushed the humeral head out of the back of the joint, leading to severe arthritis of recurrent dislocations.

A, Prior to the Bristow repair, the joint appeared normal.

B, After the Bristow repair, the posterior dislocation of the head is visible. There was complete destruction of the articular surface of the head, requiring a total glenohumeral arthroplasty.

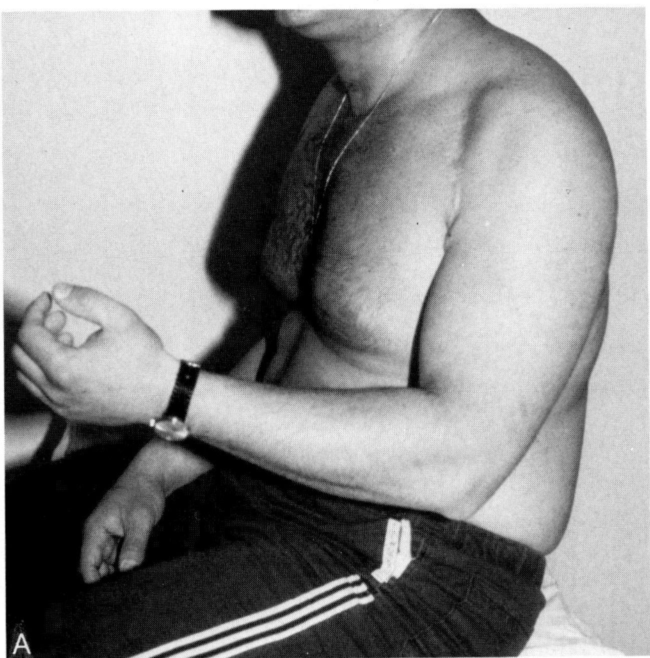

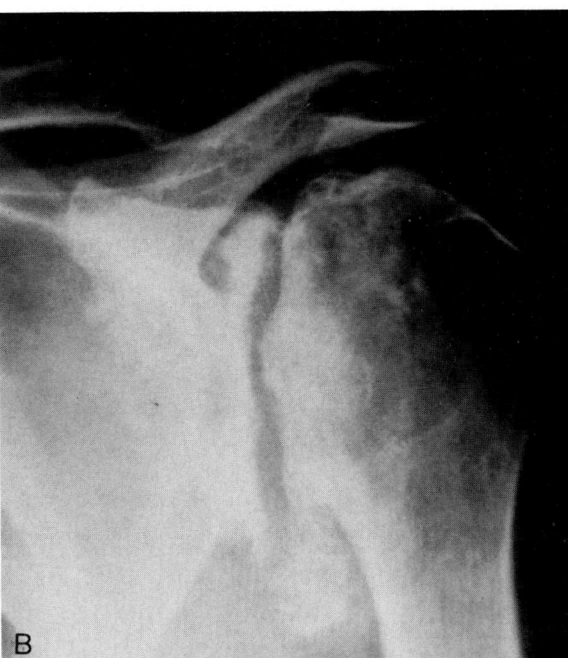

Figure 4–57. ***Complications and Failed Repairs.*** A Putti-Platt anterior capsular repair had pushed the humeral head out of the back of the joint because of multidirectional dislocations in this 28 year old weightlifter. This required a total glenohumeral arthroplasty. Note in A the axis of the humeral shaft is directed posterior to the acromion and in B there is marked joint deterioration with the posterior dislocation.

nating any defects causing instability or stiffness and removing foreign bodies as necessary. The various problems encountered are discussed above and in Figures 4–52 through 4–57.

The preparation and approach are the same as those used for an inferior capsular shift (see Figs. 4–38 to 4–42). The direction of greatest instability determines whether the approach will be in the front or the back, but often it is necessary to make a second approach on the opposite side to release tight structures prior to repairing the loose structures.

In re-operations varying degrees of scarring of the deltoid muscle are encountered. This muscle is carefully elevated off the underlying structures to preserve its strength. In loosening a tight side the capsule is often found to be thicker than normal, and creating the superior and inferior capsular flaps is not very difficult. In contrast, difficulty can be encountered in creating these flaps on the loose side, where the capsule may be attenuated and thin. Osteochondral fragments and metallic foreign bodies are removed. If the labrum is detached, it is sutured to the glenoid (see Figs. 4–30 to 4–32). If there is inferior laxity, it is corrected with a capsular shift. If there is deficiency of the articular surfaces of the glenoid or capsular deficiency, a bone block (coracoid transfer in front [see Fig. 4–31] or spine of the scapula posteriorly [see Fig. 4–34]) is considered. The capsule is closed as in the capsular shift by overlapping the flaps and suturing them as shown in Figures 4–38 to 4–42.

ACROMIOCLAVICULAR JOINT

Acute Acromioclavicular Separations

Hippocrates recognized acromioclavicular dislocations, emphasized the importance of distinguishing them from glenohumeral dislocations, devised a sling for treating them, and thought they were rarely disabling. With the advent of aseptic technique many methods of surgical repair were devised in the hope of improving the anatomical results and eliminating the confining slings. Some of these operative techniques were not anatomical and were poorly tolerated. Resection of the distal clavicle in the presence of torn coracoclavicular and acromioclavicular ligaments allowed the scapula to drop further and the clavicle to appear even higher. Metal that crosses joints tends to break or migrate if joint motion occurs. Dynamic muscle transfers were inadequate to replace the strong ligaments normally present at this joint. Thus, a controversy developed between proponents of operative repair, users of supporting casts or slings, and advocates of "skillful neglect."

The confusion caused by this controversy among surgeons on operative versus nonoperative treatment continues today. Obviously, the treatment logically selected to repair acromioclavicular dislocations depends on the activities, health, and life expectancy of the patient as well as on the precise anatomical problem. In this section, I attempt to describe the logic of my approach, which is based on observations of a number of long-term results of both operative and nonoperative treatment. I have also included an analysis of the cause of pain and treatment of long-standing acromioclavicular dislocations with persistent disability. Because some patients with long-standing acromioclavicular dislocations have little pain or handicap, it is impossible to be dogmatic.

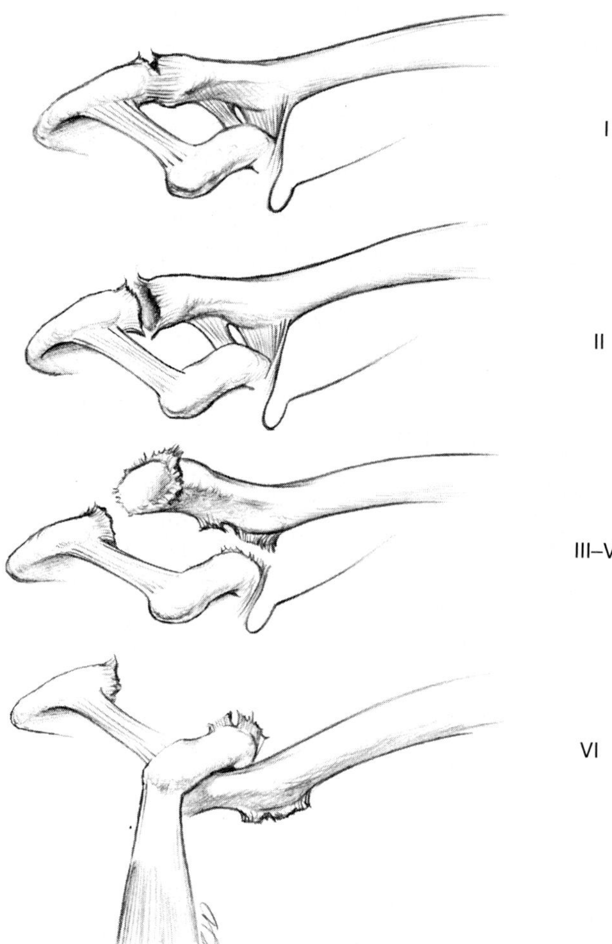

Figure 4–58. Acute *Acromioclavicular Dislocations.* Classification of acute acromioclavicular separations (viewed from top to bottom).

Type I, Incomplete tear of acromioclavicular joint capsule.

Type II, Complete tear of acromioclavicular joint capsule.

Types III, IV, V, Complete disruption of the acromioclavicular joint capsule and the coracoclavicular ligaments.

Type VI, Clavicle displaced beneath the coracoid.

Classification and Pathology

The patients are usually young, active adults, but they may be any age. The lesions are most frequently caused by a blow on the posterior aspect of the acromion and spine of the scapula (Fig. 4–59). Allman[99] classified these lesions into three grades: Grade I—partial tear of the acromioclavicular joint capsule; Grade II—complete tear of the acromioclavicular joint capsule; and Grade III—complete tear of the acromioclavicular joint capsule and of the coracoclavicular ligaments. Rockwood[199] uses six "types" in his classification and during recent years this classification has become widely used in the United States. I have modified Rockwood's classification, as shown in Figure 4–58, by combining Types III, IV, and V into one group.

Type I. There is a sprain or incomplete tear of the acromioclavicular joint capsule. There is no major break in continuity, and the lesion is treated like a sprain of any other joint (cold initially followed by exercise and use as pain allows). Despite some recent reports of disability resulting from this injury, I have never seen persistent trouble unless an occult fracture of the articular surface of the clavicle (see Chapter 5) was overlooked initially, leading to late acromioclavicular arthritis.

Type II. There is a complete tear of the acromioclavicular joint capsule. The coracoclavicular ligaments are intact. Clinically, it is impossible for me to separate these lesions from those of Type I. They are treated the same way and have the same good prognosis provided that no fracture is present. These first two categories are the same as Allman's Grade I and Grade II.

Type III, Type IV, and Type V. There is a complete disruption of the acromioclavicular joint capsule and the coracoclavicular ligaments. Type III corresponds to Allman's Grade III separation, in which there is less severe or extreme displacement. Rockwood identifies lesions with more posterior displacement of the scapula as Type IV and those with more downward displacement of the scapula as Type V. Because I advise operative repair for all Type III or higher-

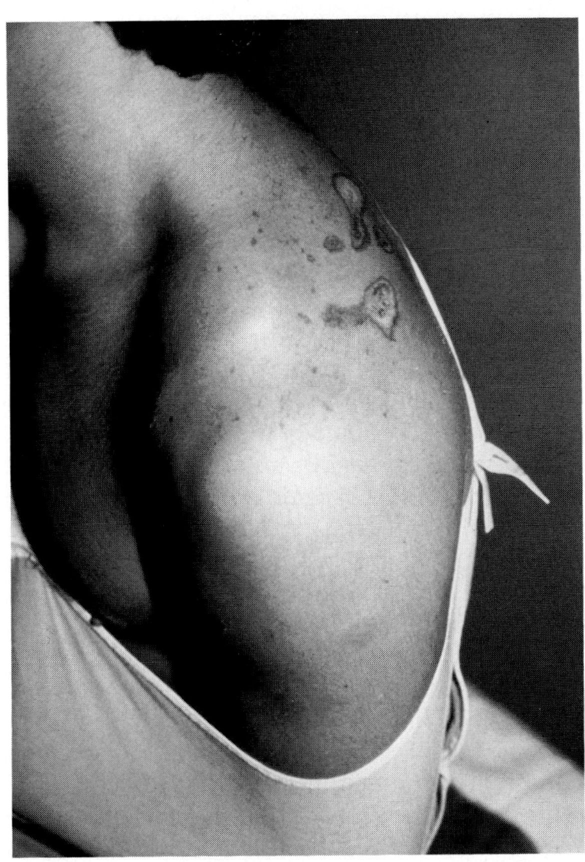

Figure 4–59. ***Acute Acromioclavicular Dislocations.*** Abrasions often are present to show that the mechanism of injury is usually a blow on the posterior acromion or the spine of the scapula.

grade lesions in active patients, the amount of displacement seems less critical. Some anterior displacement of the scapula is present in most of these lesions, making it hard to state the precise amount of displacement. In addition, the trapezius muscle tends to displace the clavicle posteriorly in many. As shown in Table 4–3, which summarizes the evaluation and treatment of old acromioclavicular dislocations, I find it helpful to recognize a subgroup with less displacement than the diameter of the clavicle and which tends to heal with stability but may cause late pain due to impingement or incongruity. I have referred to them as "Type II½." In these lesions there may be some parts of the coracoclavicular ligaments that remained intact sufficiently to allow healing with stability, and yet they cause persistent impingement.

Type VI. There is displacement of the clavicle beneath the coracoid, and of course, both the acromioclavicular joint capsule and the coracoclavicular ligaments are torn. I have never seen this lesion in my patients; however, it has been reported by more than one surgeon,[201] and I have seen the radiographs of two of Dr. Rockwood's patients. Operative repair is usually indicated.

Treatment of Acute Acromioclavicular Separations

Anatomical Rationale of Treatment

The functions of the acromioclavicular joint and its associated ligaments are shown in Figure 4–60 and are summarized as follows:

1. The coracoclavicular ligaments and acromioclavicular ligaments suspend the scapula from the clavicle and support the weight of the upper extremity.

2. The clavicle maintains the width of the shoulder, providing anchorage and leverage to guide scapular rotation. Scapular rotation moves the acromion out of the way, preventing impingement with the greater tuberosity when the arm is raised.

3. The "suspensory" (coracoclavicular) ligaments protect the infraclavicular part of the brachial plexus.

Table 4–3. EVALUATION AND TREATMENT OF OLD ACROMIOCLAVICULAR DISLOCATIONS WITH PAIN

	GRADES I AND II	GRADE II½	GRADE III OR HIGHER
Pathology	Suspensory ligament is intact	Partial dislocation with stability	Complete dislocation with stability
Possible source of pain	Occult fractures with osteolysis or arthritis	Subacromial impingement	Muscle fatigue Acromioclavicular joint incongruity Neurological signs (coracoid displaced) Impingement (faulty scapular rotation)
Clinical assessment	Xylocaine injection acromioclavicular joint	Impingement injection test Arthrogram Acromioclavicular injection test	Weight duration test (Fig. 4–63C) Horizontal adduction test (Fig. 4–63D) Electromyogram Impingement injection test Arthrogram
Operative treatment (if indicated)	Excise distal clavicle (see Chapter 6)	Anterior acromioplasty with or without cuff repair	Reconstruction of the coracoclavicular ligament with excision of the distal clavicle and anterior acromioplasty

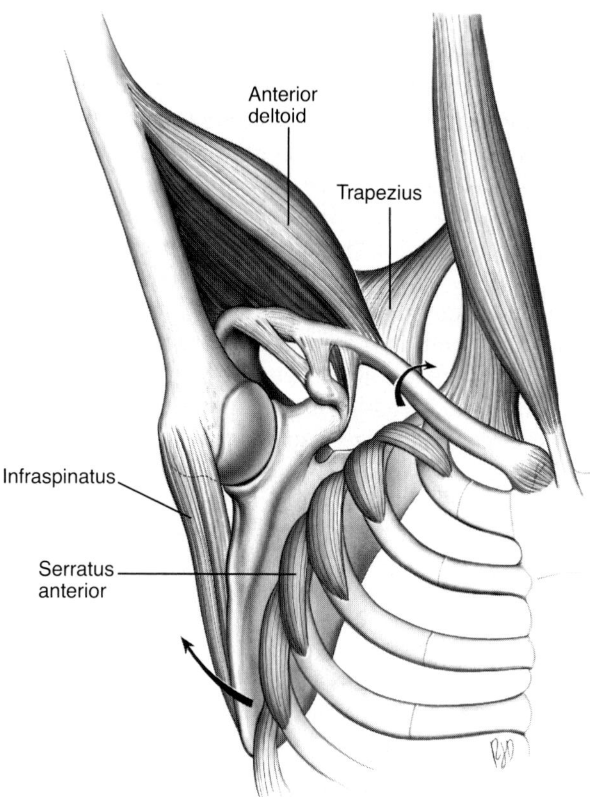

Figure 4–60. ***Acromioclavicular Dislocations.*** Functions of the acromioclavicular joint and its associated ligaments are (1) to suspend the scapula and weight of the upper extremity; (2) to transmit the action of the clavicle in guiding scapular rotation (which moves the acromion out of the way (preventing impingement) as the arm is raised (arrows), and (3) to protect the brachial plexus from downward displacement of the coracoid process.

As summarized in Table 4–3 and depicted in Figure 4–63C, some patients with long-standing complete acromioclavicular dislocations of Types III, IV, or V have pain because of muscle fatigue through loss of the suspensory ligament, because of incongruity of contact between the clavicle and the acromion, or because of impingement through faulty scapular rotation as well as encroachment of the acromion on the supraspinatus outlet (see Chapter 1, Figs. 1–13 and 1–14; and Chapter 2, Fig. 2–10B). Occasionally, the downward displacement of the coracoid causes neurological symptoms because of traction on the brachial plexus. Therefore, it is logical to attempt to restore the continuity of the coracoclavicular ligaments; because the acromioclavicular joint capsule contributes to anterior and posterior stability, [9] it is logical to restore it as well. Treatment by "skillful neglect" is reserved for those with health problems and those who desire to accept the risk of these impairments.

Immobilization with slings, strapping, or casts is unsuccessful in maintaining reduction of complete (Types III, IV, and V) dislocations because pressure on the bone prominence cannot be tolerated for the long period required to heal the ligaments and because of the shifting forces acting on the clavicle and scapula during recumbency and sleeping. Skin breakdown is not uncommon (Fig. 4–61).

Resection of the distal clavicle when the coracoclavicular ligaments are torn can result in further downward displacement of the scapula (giving the appearance of a further prominence of the clavicle). I have seen several patients who have

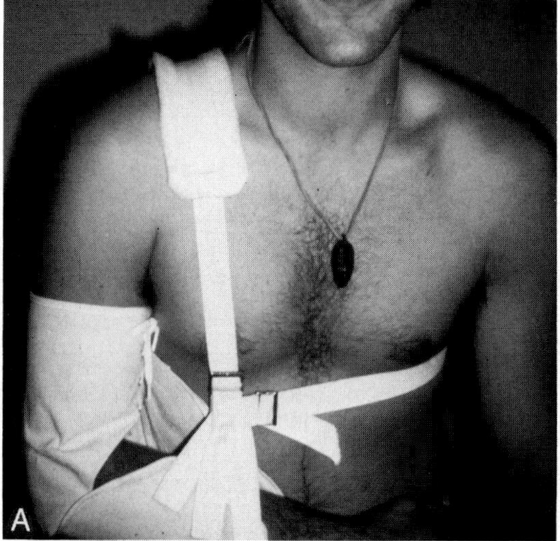

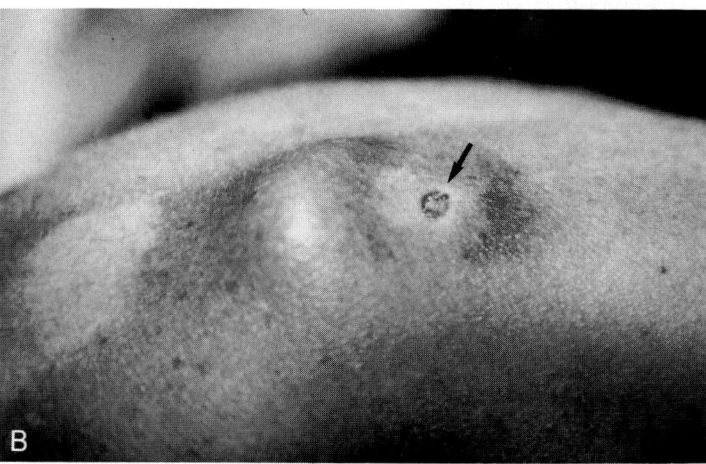

Figure 4–61A and B. ***Acute Acromioclavicular Dislocations.*** Slings fail to maintain reduction of acromioclavicular dislocations and often cause skin breakdown (arrow).

had multiple resections of the distal clavicle. Each resection resulted in greater prominence of the clavicle. Finally, almost all of the clavicle had been excised without relief of symptoms.

Surgical repair, of course, introduces the possibility of complications from metal (breakage or migration), wound infection, scars, and the possible inconvenience of more than one in-hospital procedure. However, the same is true of most surgical procedures, and because it offers the best chance of restoring normal anatomy, I inform my patients that its advantages usually outweigh these disadvantages.

Indications for Surgical Repair

Type I and Type II injuries are treated nonoperatively with a sling and progressive activities as pain subsides.

Many of my patients with Type III, IV, or V injuries have seen more than one physician and have received conflicting opinions prior to seeing me. I show them a photograph of a shoulder with a persistent prominence of the outer clavicle to illustrate the expected appearance if no repair is done. At the same time I explain that some patients go through life with this condition without significant pain or disability while others do not, and some of these patients later request surgical repair. With this explanation, the majority desire surgical treatment despite the risks and inconvenience. A few do not, and they are treated with a simple sling and progressive use of the arm as the pain subsides.

If abrasions are present, as illustrated in Figure 4–59, the operation is either done immediately without allowing time for growth of bacteria and with careful draping of the abrasions with adherent plastic drapes, or the abrasions are allowed to heal before repair is attempted.

If a patient is likely to be uncooperative during the recovery period, such as an alcoholic or a drug addict, a simple sling is recommended.

The chronological age of the patient is of less importance than his or her physical demands, activities, and general health. I have seen active patients in their sixties and seventies who did not want to "accept the deformity;" however, many of them prefer to accept it.

Some young, athletic patients will not stay away from their sport long enough to allow the shoulder to be repaired. This is understandable in the case of highly paid, professional athletes who might lose their position on the team if they are away long enough for the ligaments to heal. They may never again have an opportunity to receive such a large income. A trial of nonoperative treatment may well be justified because of the economic pressure; however, this does not alter the anatomical problem. Results in such patients are too often judged solely on the basis of how soon they returned to the sport, and their early functional recovery (without consideration for the effect on the shoulder in later life). What may be best for a professional athlete may not be best for the overwhelming majority of patients. Most patients have no such economic pressures and usually want what is best for their shoulder. It is surprising that serious traction injuries to the infraclavicular plexus have not occurred more often in athletes who return to contact sports without the protection rendered by the coracoclavicular ligaments against downward displacement of the coracoid process.

If the interval between the injury and surgery exceeds three months, transfer of the coracoacromial ligament to reinforce the coracoclavicular ligaments is advisable, as discussed on page 346.

Technique of Surgical Repair

There are several good methods for repairing complete (Types III, IV, V, and VI) acute acromioclavicular dislocations. They fall into three general categories: (1) transacromial fixation, (2) "coracoid screws," and (3) subcoracoid sutures.

Transacromial Fixation. Pins,[206] Kirschner wires, or screws across the acromioclavicular joint have the advantage of good alignment of the clavicle in relation to the acromion with a minimal incision. This method violates the articular surfaces of the acromioclavicular joint, but surprisingly, in a large series from our hospital reviewed by Wilson,[203] late arthritis of the acromioclavicular joint was found to be extremely rare. This method is preferred when the acromioclavicular dislocation occurs with a fracture of the coracoid process. Tilting motion occurs at the acromioclavicular joint when the arm is raised; therefore, overhead activities should be avoided until the pin or screw has been removed. The major disadvantage of this method is breakage or migration of the metal.

Coracoid Screw. A general surgeon, B. M. Bosworth, whose brother David is well known to orthopaedic surgeons, described the method of the coracoid screw in 1941.[204] It later became popular with sports medicine surgeons in the United States. Rockwood[199] has improved the technique. Although this is referred to as the "coracoid screw," the screw actually is inserted into the scapula posterior to the coracoid, where, if properly inserted, it holds the clavicle in normal relationship to the scapula, does not harm the articular surfaces of the acromioclavicular joint, and has distinct advantages. Removal of the screw after healing of the ligaments is a simple matter. The only problem I have seen is loss of fixation when the screw has been improperly inserted or the patient has been too active.

Subcoracoid Fixation. Alldredge[205] described using a wire loop beneath the coracoid and around the clavicle. This is a very effective method, but it has two disadvantages: breakage of the wire and anterior displacement of the clavicle by the wire, because the coracoid process is anterior to the normal location of the clavicle. Therefore, I modified this technique by using strong, nonabsorbable sutures rather than wire, which are passed through a drill hole in the clavicle to reduce the anterior displacement of the clavicle that occurs when the sutures are placed around the clavicle. This technique also has the advantage of avoiding cutting through the entire thickness of the clavicle, as can occur when wire, plastic sutures, or grafts are placed around the clavicle. The technique is illustrated in Figure 4–62.

Technique of Subcoracoid Suture Repair

The skin incision is made from the coracoid process to the acromioclavicular joint (Fig. 4–62A). After elevating the subcutaneous fat from the remains of the acromioclavicular joint capsule, the meniscus is removed if it is detached (Fig. 4–62C). The deltoid with the attached periosteum and capsule is elevated off the anterior edge of the distal 2.0 cm. of the clavicle and is split in the direction of its fibers until the coracoid process is exposed. Using sharp dissection, the posterior part of the pectoralis minor tendon is divided where it inserts on the coracoid. A curved clamp is passed through this opening, staying very close to the coracoid process until it emerges on the other side. It is important to pass this clamp as far posteriorly as the contour of the coracoid process allows to minimize pulling the clavicle forward. A long piece of No. 5 nonabsorbable suture is then doubled and grasped with the clamp so that two strands are drawn under the coracoid. At this time, if the interval between injury and surgery exceeds three weeks, the coracoclavicular ligaments are inspected, and, if indicated, a suture is placed in them to ensure their accurate approximation. This suture is tied later after the subcoracoid sutures have been secured. In cases of longer standing, the coracoacromial ligament is used to reinforce the repair, as shown in Figure 4–67. A $^{3}/_{32}$-inch drill hole is made in the middle of the clavicle at a point directly above the coracoid process (as seen in Fig. 4–62D). The two strands of No. 5 nonabsorbable suture are passed through this hole. After the distal clavicle has been reduced and held against the acromion with a towel clip, the subcoracoid sutures are tied, as illustrated in Figure 4–62. The deltoid muscle is sutured to the trapezius muscle to cover the clavicle. The acromioclavicular capsule is repaired anatomically with interrupted sutures, and the skin is closed with a removable subcuticular suture. A sling and swathe are applied. Post-operatively, light use of the arm at the side is allowed, but heavier use is avoided for at least 12 weeks. A sling is worn at night during this period. After 12 weeks, gradual resumption of normal activities is allowed, but contact sports and impact loads are avoided for nine months.

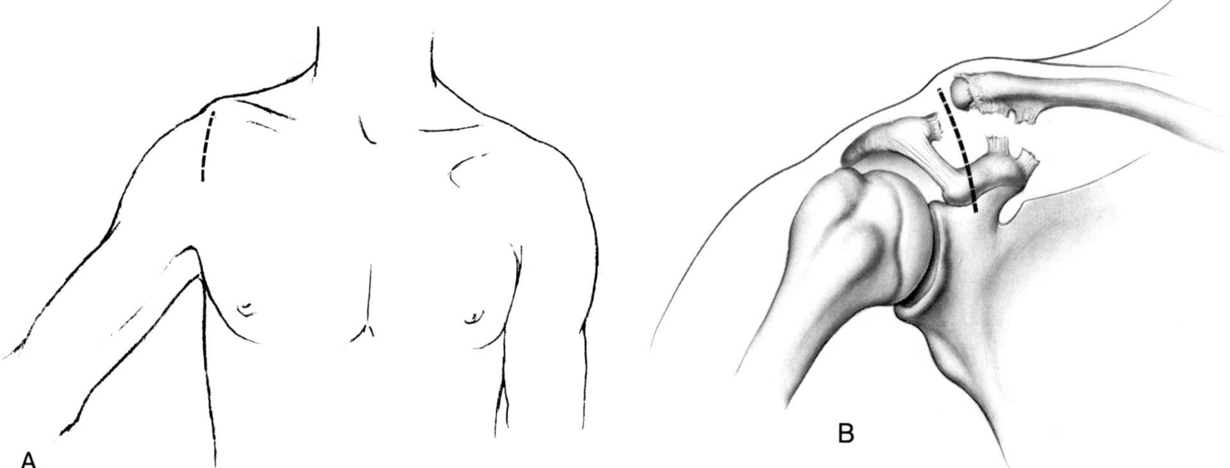

Figure 4–62. ***Acute Acromioclavicular Dislocation.*** Surgical repair of *acute* acromioclavicular dislocations.
A, Incision.
B, Subcoracoid, nonabsorbable sutures (No. 5) through a drill hole in the clavicle.

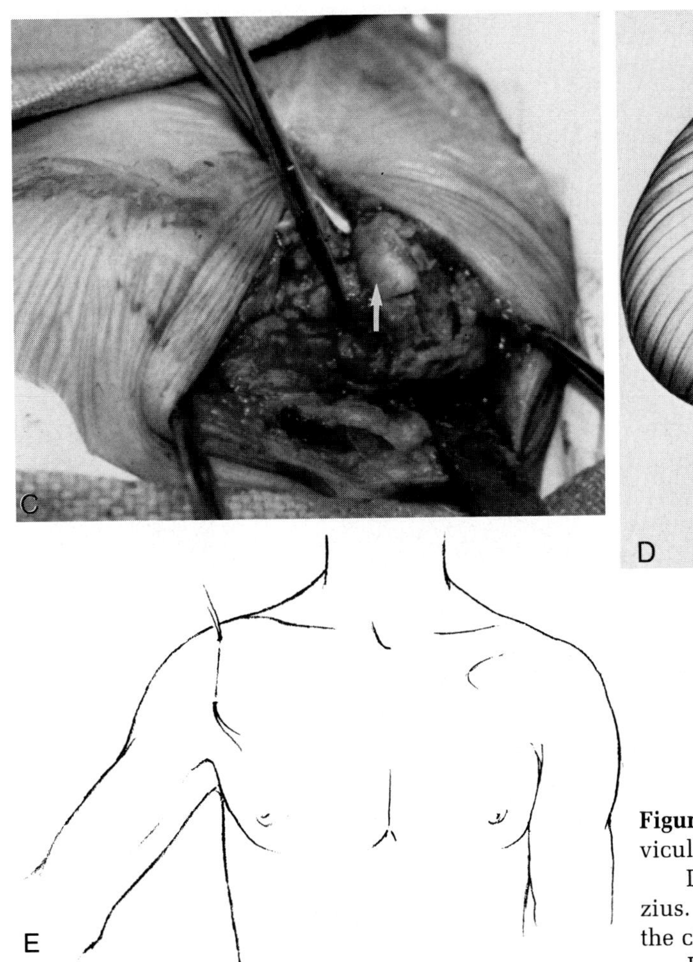

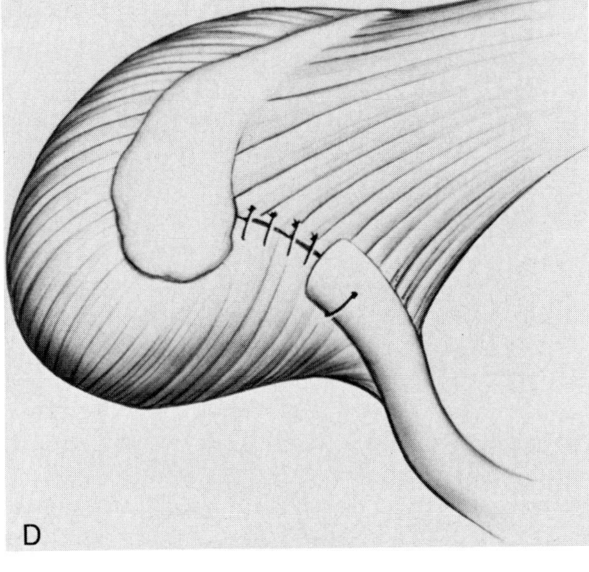

Figure 4–62 *Continued* C, Repair of the acromioclavicular joint capsule (arrow).

D, Closure approximating the deltoid and trapezius. The No. 5 sutures are seen in the drill hole in the clavicle.

E, Subcuticular closure.

In a series of eight such procedures, the results were good. There were no complications. Since the glenohumeral joint is spared in acromioclavicular injuries, glenohumeral motion remains good regardless of the treatment. It has always seemed inappropriate to cite the good range of shoulder motion obtained as a point in favor of either an operative or a nonoperative method of treatment of acute acromioclavicular dislocations because glenohumeral motion is preserved in either case. The real issue is whether the shoulder has as good a chance to remain symptom free with years of use (see Table 4–3).

Acromioclavicular Dislocations with Fractures of the Coracoid or Avulsion of the Undersurface of the Clavicle

In these lesions, the acromioclavicular joint capsule is disrupted but the coracoclavicular ligaments remain intact. If repair is done early, the fragments may fall into good position as the dislocation is reduced. Any of the methods of internal fixation discussed above (transacromial, "coracoid screw," or subcoracoid sutures) may be used if indicated when there is a clavicular avulsion. Transacromial fixation is used when indicated for acromioclavicular dislocations with coracoid fractures.

Old Acromioclavicular Dislocations

Some long-standing lesions are asymptomatic, and in others the symptoms are too mild to warrant treatment. Patients with pain and disability require a cautious approach with consideration of all possible causes of pain. The results of resection of the distal clavicle have generally been inadequate except in old Type I and Type II injuries in patients with acromioclavicular arthritis who have intact coracoclavicular ligaments (see pp. 433 to 436). Resection of the distal clavicle in unstable Type III acromioclavicular dislocations may make the instability worse, leading to more prominence of the distal clavicle and more pain due to muscle fatigue or impingement (Fig. 4–63A).

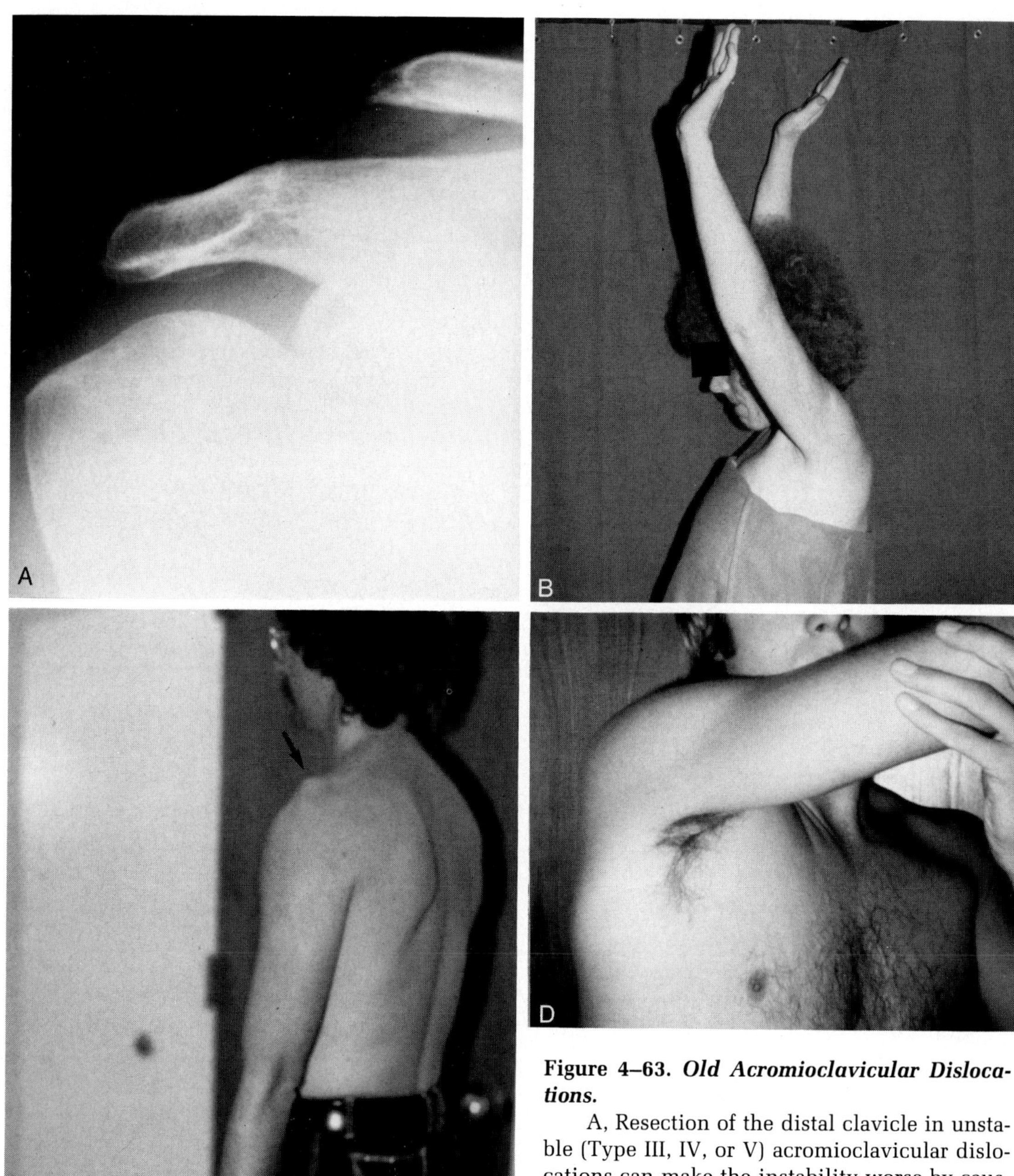

Figure 4–63. ***Old Acromioclavicular Dislocations.***

A, Resection of the distal clavicle in unstable (Type III, IV, or V) acromioclavicular dislocations can make the instability worse by causing more scapular drop and more clavicular prominence. Reconstruction of the coracoclavicular ligament is indicated.

B, Resection of the distal clavicle, which had been done three times, failed to relieve pain due to improper scapular rotation (causing impingement) and to muscle fatigue (from loss of the suspensory ligament). Reconstruction of this ligament was indicated.

C, Weight endurance test. This old acromioclavicular dislocation (arrow) caused pain due to fatigue. When it was not responsive to exercises to strengthen the muscles, a reconstruction of the coracoclavicular ligaments was performed.

D, Horizontal adduction test for incongruity. If lidocaine (Xylocaine) injection into the acromioclavicular joint relieves the pain caused by this maneuver, excision of the distal clavicle and reconstruction of the coracoclavicular ligament are considered (see Chapter 6).

Four Types of Pain

It is helpful to consider four types of pain in patients with disability from long-standing acromioclavicular dislocations, as summarized in Table 4–3.[202]

Weight Endurance Test (Muscle Fatigue)

The coracoclavicular ligaments are of great importance in the mechanism for suspending the upper extremity (Chapter 1, Fig. 1–13). Fatigue pain in the trapezius muscle is not rare in patients with old acromioclavicular dislocations. This type of pain can be brought on by having the patient hold a chair for several minutes, as in Figure 4–63C. If this causes the appearance or exacerbation of the pain, symptoms may be helped by exercises to strengthen the scapular muscles, but more often, repair of the disrupted coracoclavicular ligaments will be required.

Horizontal Adduction Test (Incongruity)

Forceful adduction of the arm across the front of the body (Fig. 4–63D) impacts the scapula against the distal clavicle. This brings out pain due to incongruity between the scapula and the distal clavicle. If this pain is relieved by lidocaine (Xylocaine) injected at the distal end and posterior aspect of the clavicle, this type of incongruity is the source of pain. Excision of the distal clavicle (see Fig. 6–8) is usually indicated. If arthritis has developed at the acromioclavicular joint after a Type I or Type II acromioclavicular injury with intact coracoclavicular ligaments, simple excision (see Fig. 4–64) should be adequate. If there has been a true acromioclavicular dislocation with torn coracoclavicular ligaments, repair of these ligaments is required at the time of excision of the distal clavicle (Fig. 4–63B and C).

Neurological Studies (Infraclavicular Plexus)

As Bateman[75] has described, pressure may develop on the neurovascular bundle due to a chronic rupture of the suspensory ligament. If tingling, numbness, or weakness of the hand is present, an electromyogram is obtained. These signs may be an indication to repair the coracoclavicular ligaments (see Fig. 4–67). This repair relieves the downward pressure of the coracoid. Paresthesias of this type have been present in several patients in whom I repaired old acromioclavicular dislocations, and in each case the symptoms disappeared after the repair.

Impingement Tests (Subacromial Impingement)

Acromioclavicular dislocations can cause subacromial impingement in two ways: (1) by distortion of the supraspinatus outlet (Fig. 4–64B and C),

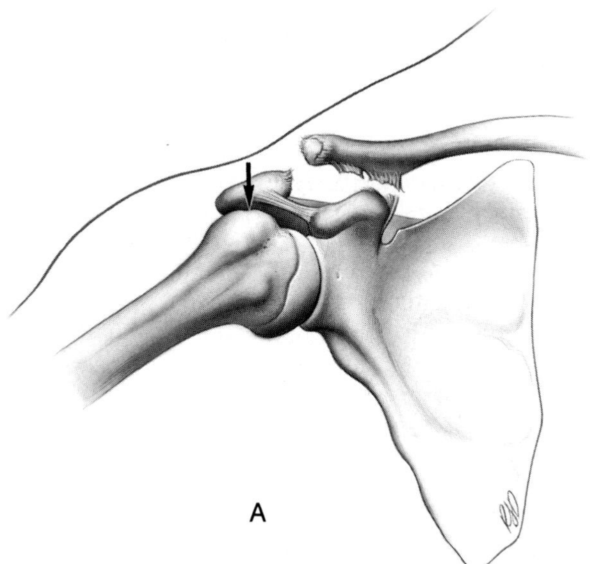

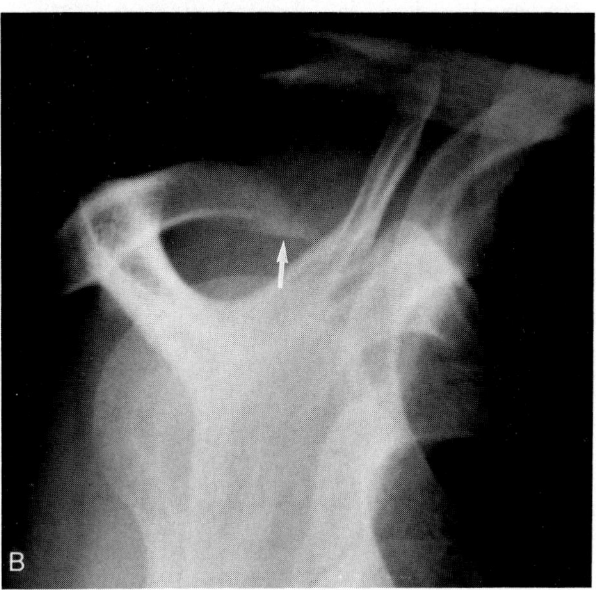

Figure 4–64. Impingement caused by old, unstable acromioclavicular dislocations is logically treated by reconstruction of the coracoclavicular ligaments.

A, Loss of the ligaments causes improper scapular rotation when the arm is raised and may cause impingement (see Fig. 2–10B).

B, Outlet view (lateral view of the scapula) of a 20 year old patient with a type III acromioclavicular dislocation showing downward projection of the anterior acromion (arrow) with reactive bone caused by impingement.

Illustration continued on following page

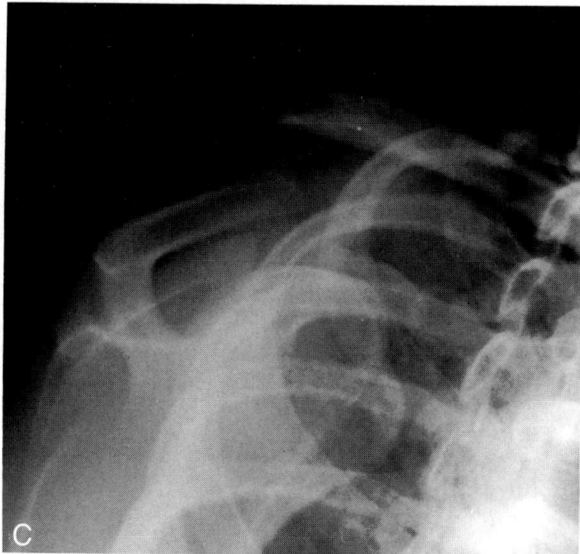

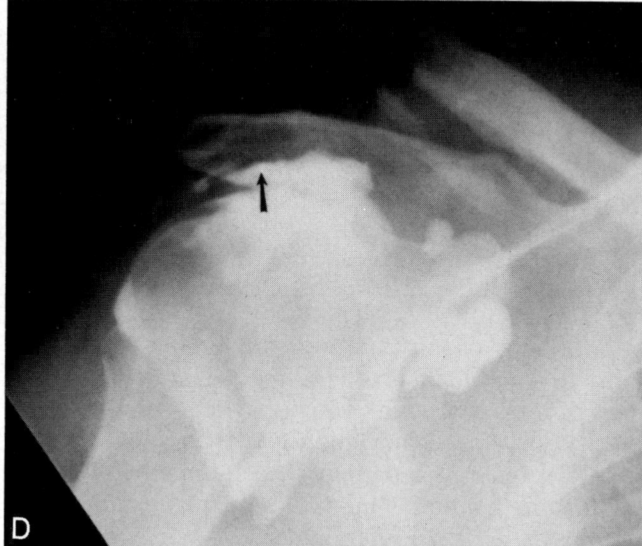

Figure 4–64 *Continued* C, Outlet view of an earlier Type III lesion also shows distortion of the space for the supraspinatus tendon.

D, A positive arthrogram showing a cuff tear (arrow) in another patient with an old acromioclavicular dislocation following an unsuccessful resection of the clavicle.

and (2) if the coracoclavicular ligaments are torn and the acromioclavicular dislocation is unstable, by faulty rotation of the scapula. The presence of impingement as the cause of pain can be demonstrated by the impingement injection test (see Fig. 2–30), and, in long-standing cases when a complete cuff tear has developed, by an arthrogram. Impingement due to a stable, moderate "Type II½ displacement" can be relieved by an anterior acromioplasty (Figs. 4–65 and 4–66). The main problem is the narrowing of the supraspinatus outlet. Unstable acromioclavicular dislocations with impingement cannot be relieved by acromioplasty alone, but in addition require reconstruction of the coracoclavicular ligaments (Fig. 4–67) to correct the downward displacement and abnormal rotation of the scapula.

Treatment of Old Acromioclavicular Separations

Nonoperative Treatment

If the only type of pain present is trapezius muscle fatigue, as evidenced by the weight endurance test (other tests being negative), a change in the use of the arm and scapular muscle strengthening exercises should be given a thorough trial before surgery is considered.

Excision of the Distal Clavicle (Ligaments Intact)

Excision of the distal clavicle without ligament reconstruction (see Fig. 6–8) is indicated when the primary cause of pain is the incongruity of the acromioclavicular joint, as shown by relief of pain when Xylocaine is injected into the acromioclavicular joint and the coracoclavicular ligaments are intact. The arthritis of the acromioclavicular joint that occurs after a Type I or Type II acromioclavicular separation may have resulted from an unrecognized articular surface fracture or cartilage injury.

The technique is the same as that used for repair of "weightlifter's clavicle" and other types of arthritis of the acromioclavicular joint (see Chapter 6, p. 433).

Anterior Acromioplasty for Stable, Old Acromioclavicular Dislocations

Anterior acromioplasty alone, as shown in Figures 2–41 and 4–66, is indicated when pain is primarily due to subacromial impingement, as evidenced by relief of pain with the impingement injection test and, at times, abnormal results of a glenohumeral arthrogram, provided that the acromioclavicular dislocation has become stabilized with repair tissue. If a tear of the rotator cuff is present, it is repaired during the same procedure. The acromioclavicular dislocation is usually a Type II½ dislocation in which a portion of the clavicle still articulates with the acromion, as shown in Figure 4–65A.

If the clavicle is found to be hypermobile and unstable, the procedure described below of reconstructing the coracoclavicular ligaments is performed because anterior acromioplasty alone will be inadequate. On the other hand, if the clavicle is firmly connected to the acromion and coracoid by repair tissue, acromioplasty alone greatly simplifies aftercare, especially when there is a tear of the rotator cuff.

In my series[202] of 11 patients with Type II½ dislocations and increasing symptoms in later life, the average interval from injury to anterior acromioplasty was 20 years. Arthrograms showed complete tears of the rotator cuff in ten patients and an incomplete tear in one patient. The average age of the patients was 51 years, and all were men.

The technique is the same as described in Figure 2–41, except that care is taken to preserve the soft tissue on the superficial surface of the acromioclavicular joint intact (Fig. 4–66). Of course, the repair tissue between the coracoid and clavicle is left undisturbed. A skin incision as shown in Figure 4–67 is used if there is doubt about the stability of the acromioclavicular joint and it is thought that a transfer of the coracoacro-

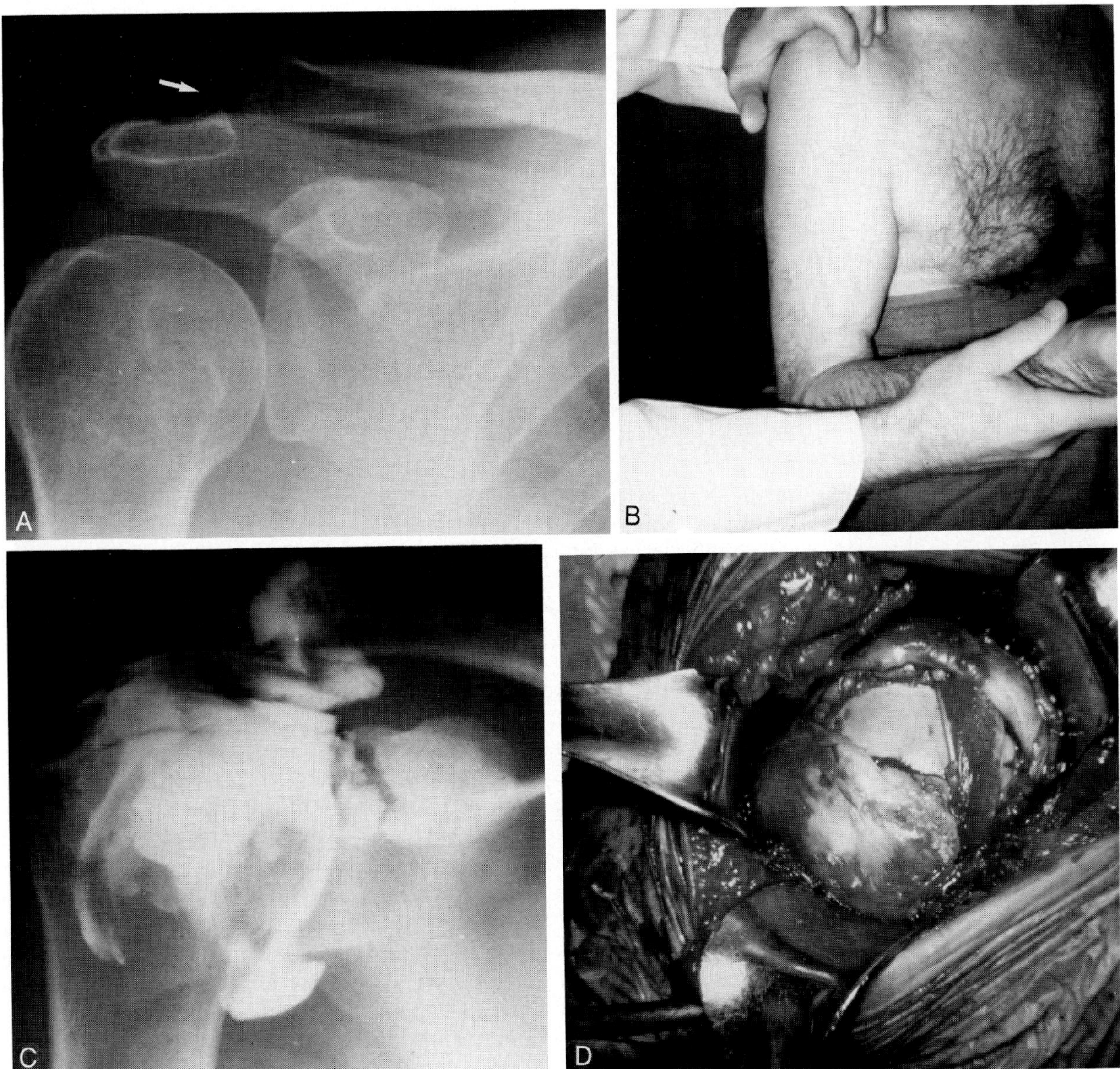

Figure 4–65. Impingement caused by old, stable acromioclavicular dislocation is treated by anterior acromioplasty.
A, Type II½ acromioclavicular dislocation (arrow) of 18 years duration.
B, Crepitus and weakness of external rotation.
C, An arthrogram showed a tear of the rotator cuff, which was repaired after an anterior acromioplasty.
D, Cuff tear found at surgery in C (see Fig. 4–66).

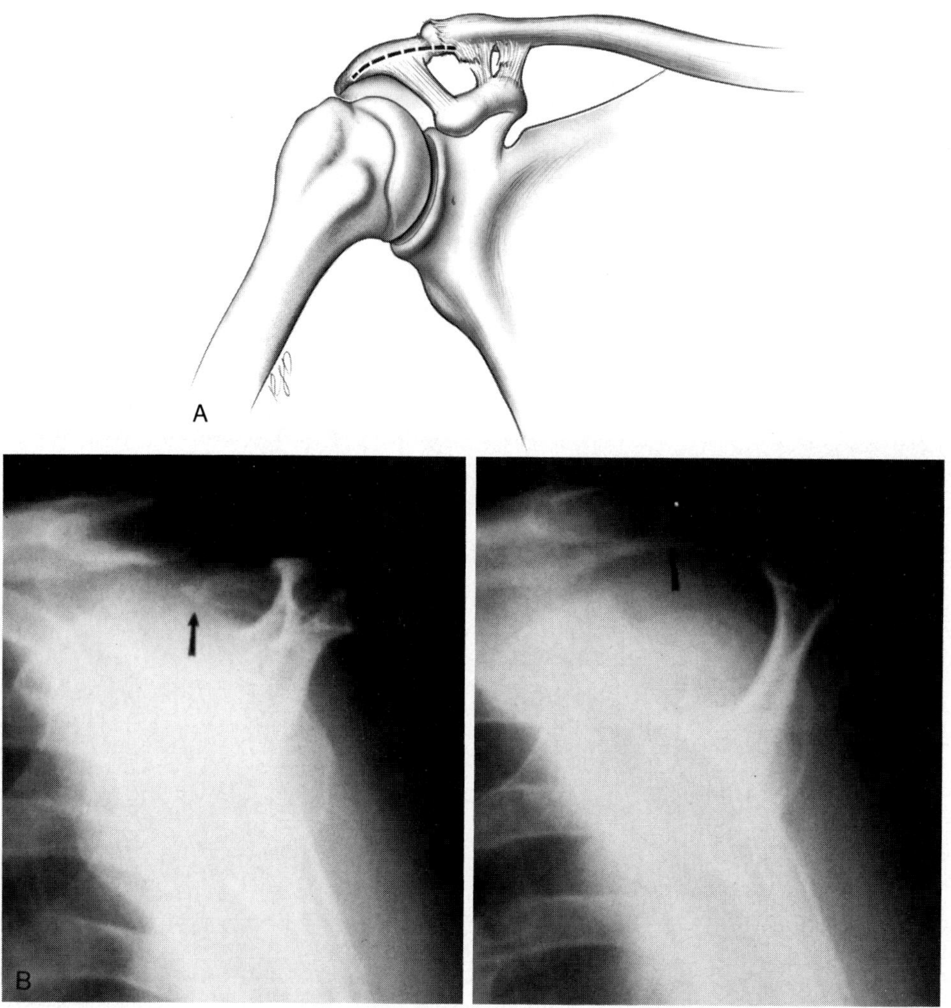

Figure 4–66. A, Repair for old, stable acromioclavicular dislocations is accomplished by anterior acromioplasty and repair of the rotator cuff if it is torn.

B, Outlet views of a 20 year old, stable acromioclavicular dislocation in a 57 year old man seen pre-operatively (left) and after this procedure (right). The rotator cuff had been torn and was repaired with a good result. Arrows point to the undersurface of the anterior acromion.

mial ligament to the clavicle, as in Figure 4–67C, might be required. As illustrated in Figure 4–66, in the acromioplasty more bone is removed from the undersurface of the acromion than from the clavicle, and a tunnel for the supraspinatus tendon is created. This makes the remaining anterior acromion thin, but complete excision of the anterior acromion is avoided. Rather than excising the distal clavicle, some contact is left between the acromion and the clavicle to enhance stability of the clavicle.

The results of repairs in the 11 patients with long-standing acromioclavicular dislocations and cuff tears treated in this way have been quite good, in contrast to results in three other patients with tears of the rotator cuff and unstable acromioclavicular dislocations who required reconstruction of the coracoclavicular ligaments, as shown in Figure 4–64E, at the time of cuff repair. Passive exercises could be started early and the usual rehabilitation program advanced as for tears of the rotator cuff (see Chapter 7, p. 491), when the anterior acromioplasty and cuff repair alone were done. The rehabilitation program was difficult when coracoclavicular reconstruction was required at the same time as the cuff repair. Therefore, it seems important to consider anterior acromioplasty alone without reconstruction of the coracoclavicular ligaments in this special group with cuff tears whenever there is stability between the clavicle and the scapula.

Coracoclavicular Ligament Reconstruction for Unstable, Old Acromioclavicular Dislocations

Coracoclavicular ligament reconstruction is considered when the acromioclavicular dislocation is unstable. Evidence of instability of long-standing acromioclavicular dislocations includes hypermobility of the clavicle on clinical examination preoperatively, hypermobility of the clavicle at surgery, and at times, traction x-rays with measurements of the coracoclavicular distance. Patients with neurological symptoms should be strongly considered for reconstruction of the coracoclavicular ligaments. Young athletic patients who have persistent disability after Type III, IV, or V dislocations are advised to consider ligamentous reconstruction, and because the injury is more than 12 months old when they are referred for surgery, excision of the distal clavicle, as described in Figure 4–67, is performed at the time of the repair as in older patients with long-standing lesions.

As mentioned previously, if at the time of repairing an acute dislocation the interval between injury and surgery is more than three weeks, a suture is added to the coracoclavicular ligament to ensure its accurate approximation. Transfer of the coracoacromial ligament to reinforce the coracoclavicular ligament and subcoracoid suture fixation is performed if the lesion is more than three months and less than one year old. After one year, reconstruction of the ligament as described below is performed with excision of the distal 1.5 to 2.0 cm. of the clavicle and an acromioplasty.

The technique is a modification of the method of Weaver and Dunn[10] and is illustrated in Figure 4–67. The patient is positioned in a beach chair position, and the arm is draped free as in Figure 2–41. The skin incision extends from the anterior margin of the acromioclavicular joint to the coracoid. The deltoid and trapezius muscles are elevated off the distal 2.0 cm. of the clavicle by subperiosteal dissection. The distal 1.5 to 2.0 cm. of clavicle is cut off with a rib cutter, removing more bone anteriorly than posteriorly and more superiorly than inferiorly. Irregular edges are trimmed with a rongeur. The deltoid muscle is split in the direction of its fibers from the stump of the clavicle to the top of the coracoid, and stay sutures are placed to mark the corners of the split in the deltoid muscle and to mark the trapezius muscle to facilitate accurate approximation of these structures at closure. The posterior part of the insertion of the pectoralis minor on the coracoid is divided. A curved clamp is passed under the coracoid through this opening, staying very close to bone and as far posteriorly as the contour of the coracoid will permit. The point of the curved clamp is made to present lateral to the coracoid to grasp two strands of No. 5 nonabsorbable suture. The two strands of suture are pulled under the coracoid and temporarily secured while the acromioplasty is performed. The coracoacromial ligament is dissected free of soft tissue and detached from the undersurface of the acromion, preserving as much length as possible. It is tagged with a stay suture. Using a 22 mm. beveled osteotome, an anterior acromioplasty is performed to remove the overhanging edges of the anterior acromion, as in Figure 2–41. A $\frac{3}{32}$-inch drill hole is made through the midpoint of the stump of the clavicle as shown in Figure 4–64B, and the two No. 5 nonabsorbable sutures are threaded through this hole and tied individually quite firmly as the clavicle is held close to the coracoid in anatomical alignment. A fine drill hole is then made through the superficial cortex of the clavicle nearer the end of the clavicle for a 00 suture to hold the transferred coracoacromial ligament. The acromial end of the coracoacromial ligament is then inserted inside the clavicle and secured with the bone suture at proper tension. The split in the deltoid muscle is closed, and the deltoid and trapezius muscles are approximated to cover the stump of the clavicle and fill the dead space. The skin is closed with a continuous removable subcuticular stitch. A sling and swathe are applied.

A sling is worn at night for 12 weeks, during which time only light use of the shoulder with the arm at the side is permitted. Activities are gradually increased after this, but heavy lifting and impact loads are avoided for at least nine months.

The results of this procedure have been good (Fig. 4–68), with the exception of three older patients who had tears of the rotator cuff. They were mentioned earlier on page 352. The protection and relative immobilization required for healing of the coracoclavicular ligament reconstruction is counter to the early passive motion required to prevent adhesions at the cuff repair. Of the three poor results, one lost fixation of the clavicle and had a recurrence of the deformity, one developed adhe-

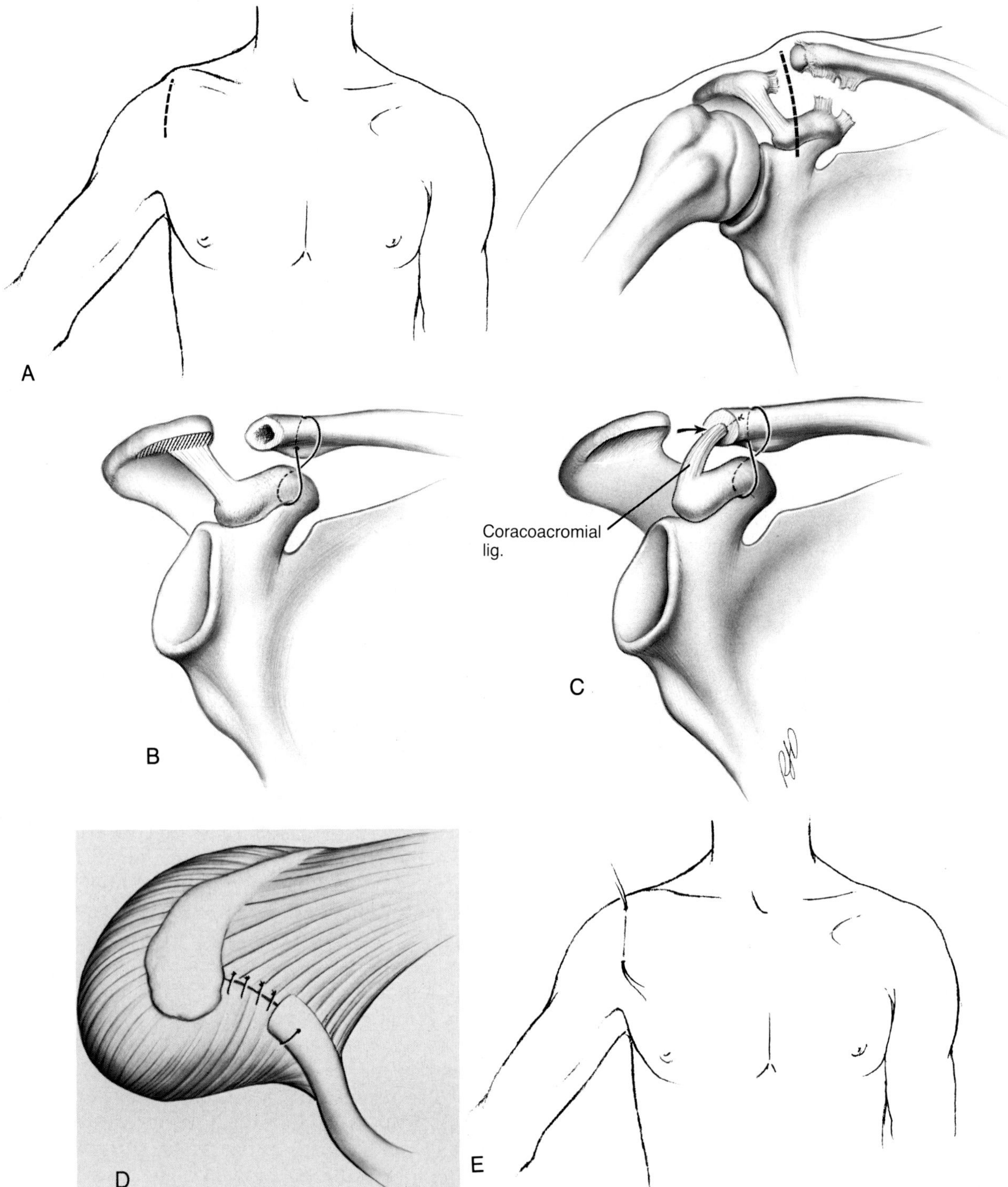

Figure 4–67. ***Repair of Old, Unstable Acromioclavicular Dislocations.***

A, Incision and pathology.

B, Excision of distal clavicle and drill hole in clavicle and subcoracoid fixation.

C, Transfer of coracoacromial ligament from acromion.

D, Closure with deltoid and trapezius muscles.

E, Skin closure.

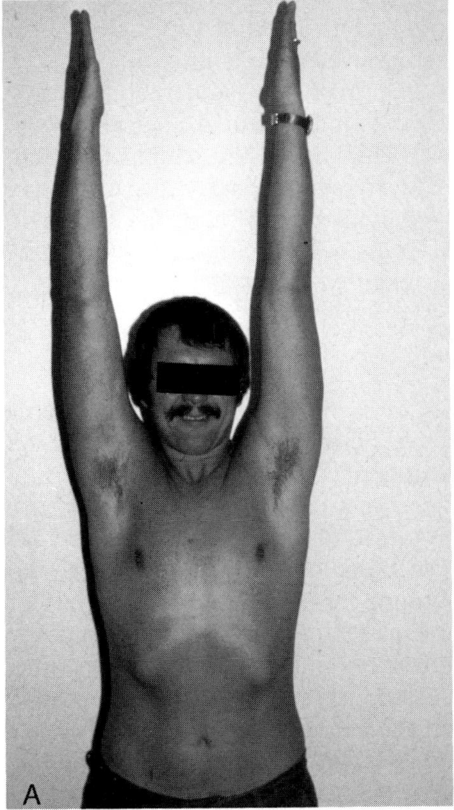

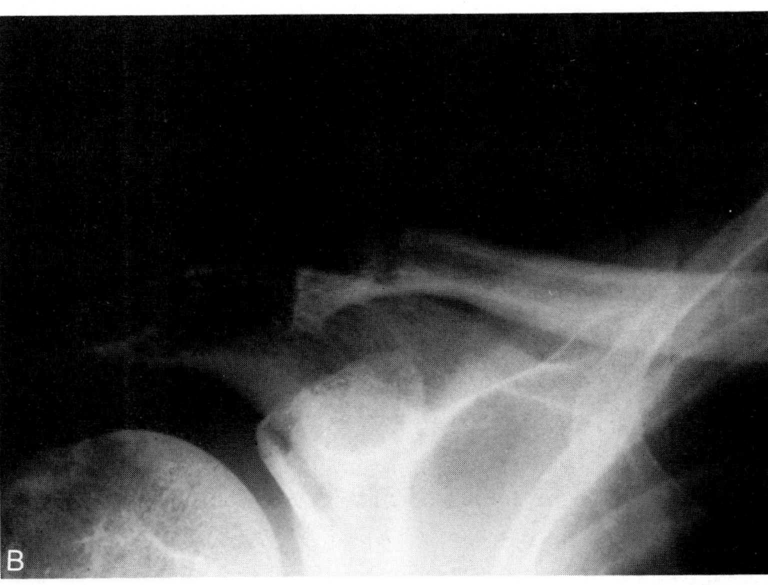

Figure 4–68. Results of the repair for old, unstable acromioclavicular dislocations.

A, Regaining glenohumeral motion is easy after acromioclavicular injuries (provided that there is no rotator cuff involvement).

B, Follow-up x-ray two years later shows the excised clavicle, drill hole in the clavicle, and proper coracoclavicular distance maintained.

sions and a re-tear of the rotator cuff, and the other was impaired by adhesions. In the others, glenohumeral motion was quickly recovered and rehabilitation was easy.

STERNOCLAVICULAR JOINT

The sternoclavicular joint is subjected to considerable stress, and as the only joint connecting the upper extremity to the body, moves with nearly all movements of the arm. The clavicle rotates more than 40 degrees in its long axis and can be moved in all directions at this joint. Yet the sternoclavicular joint is much less frequently dislocated than the acromioclavicular joint. Anterior-superior sternoclavicular dislocations are much more common than posterior sternoclavicular dislocations; however, the latter are more dramatic and have been recorded more consistently, causing inaccuracies in incidence reports.

Classification of Sternoclavicular Dislocations

It is of interest that of 14 sternoclavicular dislocations studied by Salvatore[207] in our institution, athletic injuries accounted for five, automobile accidents for three, and, of the remaining six patients, four had only trivial injuries such as reaching or lifting. Two experienced spontaneous onset of sternoclavicular instability with no known cause. Of these 14 sternoclavicular dislocations, 12 were anterior and 2 were posterior. Both of the posterior sternoclavicular dislocations resulted from direct trauma to the clavicle in athletics.

Sternoclavicular dislocations can be classified into the following categories:

I. Traumatic
   A. Anterior-superior
   B. Posterior (retrosternal)

II. Atraumatic
   A. Voluntary
   B. Involuntary

Traumatic Sternoclavicular Dislocations

Mechanism of Injury

The mechanism of injury producing a sternoclavicular dislocation may be either a direct blow on the clavicle or a transmitted force. Displacement of the inner clavicle occurs much more frequently anteriorly than posteriorly. Anterior dislocation is usually produced by an indirect force. Posterior displacement is almost always caused by a direct force and is more significant because of the proximity of important mediastinal structures. In patients under 17 years of age, epiphyseal fractures of the inner clavicle almost always occur rather than sternoclavicular dislocations (Fig. 4–69).

Acute Traumatic Sternoclavicular Dislocations

Clinical and Roentgen Assessment

Strong ligaments (the costoclavicular, sternoclavicular, and interclavicular ligaments) provide the strength of this joint. There is very little skeletal support. Traumatic displacement of the inner clavicle occurs with varying degrees of disruption of these ligaments. In my experience, anterior sternoclavicular subluxations or dislocations are usually unstable after reduction. (In contrast, the two posterior dislocations I have reduced were both stable after closed reduction, apparently because the anterior capsule remained intact.)

On physical examination the inner clavicle is prominent and tender after anterior dislocation (Fig. 4–69). In contrast, the prominence of the inner clavicle is lost and the alignment of the whole clavicle is altered compared with the opposite side after posterior dislocation. However, local swelling occurs and usually obscures these findings. Therefore, careful roentgenographic evaluation is important.

A standard anterior-posterior view is hard to interpret. The 45 degree angle view of the clavicles (Fig. 1–12), comparing the two sides, is helpful. A lateral view of the sternum often shows the displacement when there is a posterior dislocation. CT scans are not always available and are confusing when the patient is positioned with the shoulders at unequal levels, as shown in Figure 4–69A. Anterior-posterior laminograms of both sternoclavicular joints can be of great value, especially when a fracture of the inner clavicle is present.

Physical examination should include assessment of the circulation and neurological status of the injured arm. The life of the patient illustrated in Figure 4–70 was saved by early recognition and repair of this tear in the intima of the subclavian artery before traumatic attempts were made to reduce the dislocation.

Treatment of Acute Traumatic Sternoclavicular Dislocations

Treatment of Acute Anterior Sternoclavicular Dislocations. Closed reduction is usually obtained easily by placing traction on the arm and direct pressure on the inner clavicle. Unfortunately, it is usually hard to maintain reduction with closed methods. A plastic spica cast is applied with flexion and adduction of the glenohumeral joint to compress the inner clavicle against the posterior capsule. The cast should include a strap over the opposite shoulder to prevent the spica from dropping down. In the few anterior dislocations I have seen treated with closed reduction, the prominence of the inner clavicle usually returned to some degree. However, because closed reduction can be obtained easily, usually without anesthesia, I believe it should be tried and a cast applied as described above. If this fails, I am inclined to accept the prominence of the inner clavicle rather than proceed with an open reduction and internal fixation. If there is unusual displacement or for some other reason an open reduction seems warranted, it is done through a 7.0 cm. incision made in line with a necklace inferior to the prominence of the inner clavicle. The clavicle is fixed to the sternum with a drill hole and No. 2 or No. 5 nonmetallic sutures. The anterior sternoclavicular capsule is repaired. A spica cast is applied after open reduction with the arm in flexion and adduction, and support for the weight of the cast is provided by including the top of the opposite shoulder.

Because of the large amount of motion at the sternoclavicular joint and the proximity of vital structures (pleura, pericardium, and great vessels), metallic fixation across this joint is especially prone to migration with serious consequences (Fig. 4–71). I know of a fatality that occurred in a nearby hospital from a broken wire that migrated into the heart.

Treatment of Acute Posterior (Retrosternal) Sternoclavicular Dislocations. As discussed above, the first step in treatment of a posterior sternoclavicular dislocation is careful assessment of the

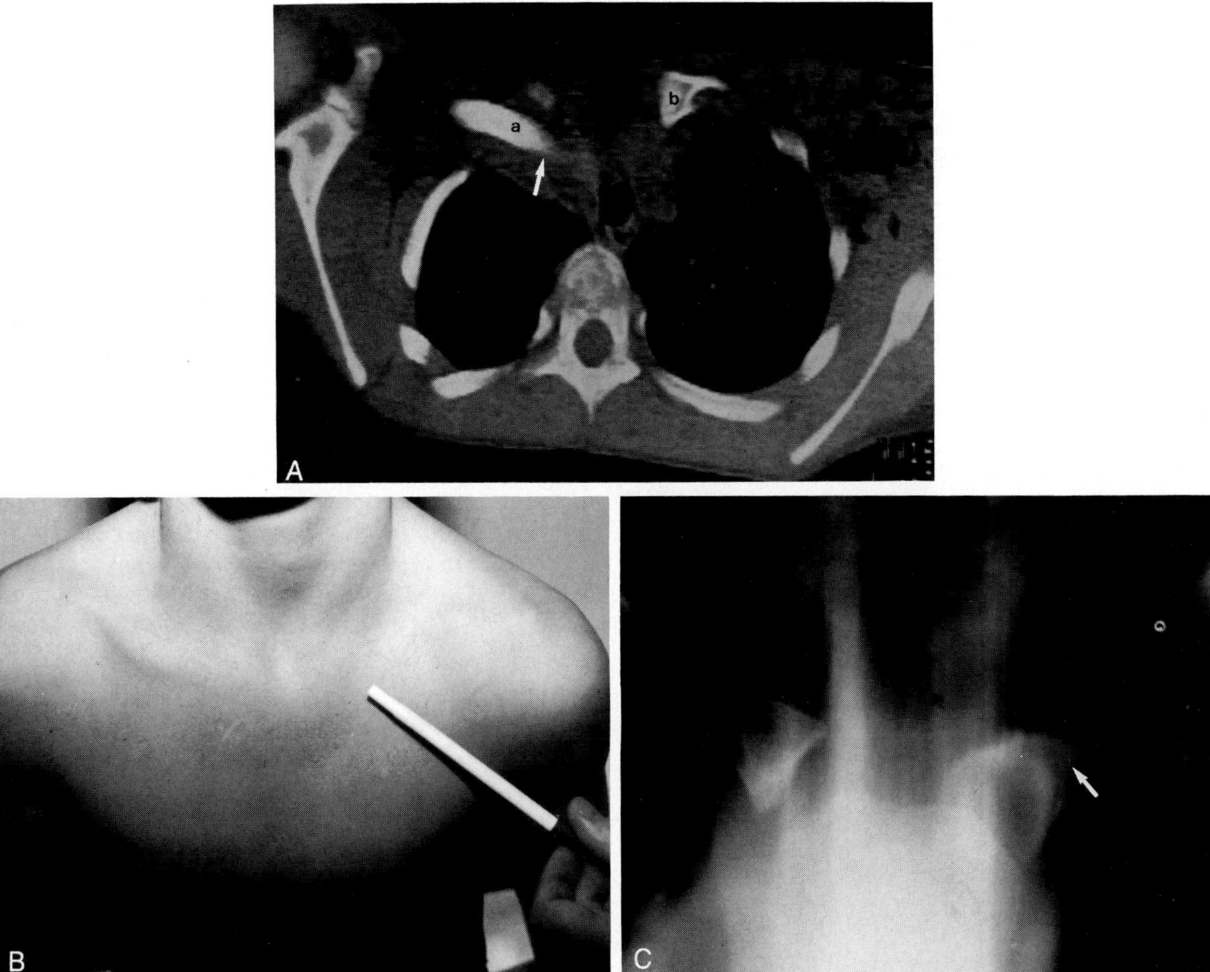

Figure 4–69. ***Sternoclavicular Dislocations.*** Epiphyseal fractures of the medial end of the clavicle in a 14 year old boy who was referred for emergency surgery with the erroneous diagnosis of a markedly displaced sternoclavicular dislocation.

A, Computerized tomogram showed that the left clavicle (a) was posterior to the right clavicle (b), suggesting the need for surgery.

B, On examination the medial end of the clavicle was found to be palpable, although the shaft of the clavicle was displaced backward. The patient lacked the systemic signs or tenderness of a recent fracture, and further history revealed that other injuries had occurred in the past. The tentative diagnosis of an old epiphyseal fracture was made, and observation was advised.

C, A tomogram of the sternoclavicular joints made nine months later showed new bone connecting the shaft to the epiphysis (arrow), confirming the diagnosis of epiphyseal fracture. The patient had no symptoms. His clavicle now has a near-normal roentgen appearance.

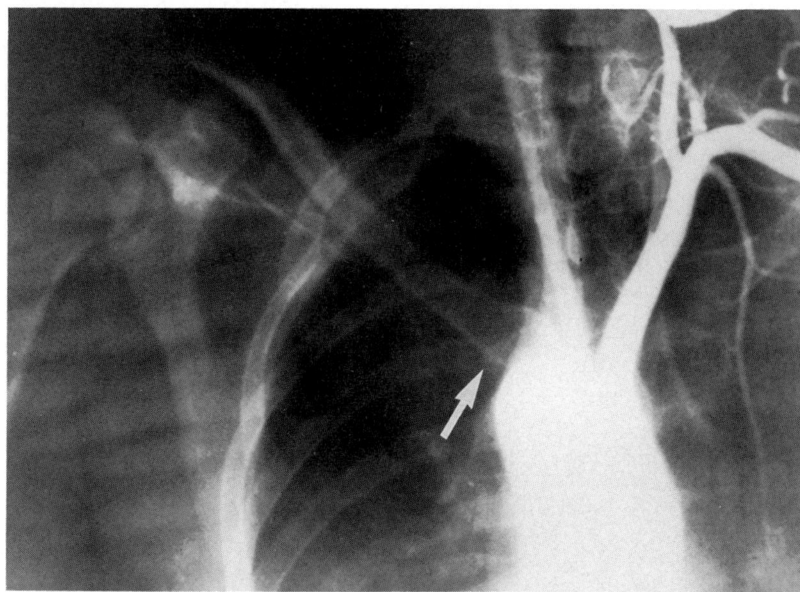

Figure 4–70. Arteriogram of a patient with acute posterior sternoclavicular dislocation shows occlusion of the artery (arrow) due to a large intimal tear of the artery adjacent to the inner end of the clavicle.

neurovascular status of the upper extremity. The signs and symptoms may vary from mild tenderness to hoarseness, dyspnea, paralysis or ischemia of the upper extremity, or cardiovascular collapse. The subclavian vein, cardiac vessels, trachea, esophagus, brachial plexus, and pleura have all had reported injuries.

Closed reduction is usually successful. Relaxing anesthesia is given, and with the patient supine and with folded towels between the scapulae, lateral traction is applied with the arm abducted off the side of the table in slight hyperextension. If this fails, after proper skin preparation, a sterile towel clip placed on the clavicle gives more leverage. If closed reduction is unsuccessful, open reduction is indicated because of the encroachment of the clavicle on the mediastinal structures.

Open reduction is performed through a 7.0 cm. incision placed inferior to the bone prominence in line with a necklace. The skin is undermined, preserving the anterior capsule intact as much as possible. The inner clavicle is exposed from above downward with extreme caution. The subclavian vein is directly in back of the clavicle and is easily torn. The pleura is also easily entered. The clavicle is grasped with a towel clip, reduced, and secured

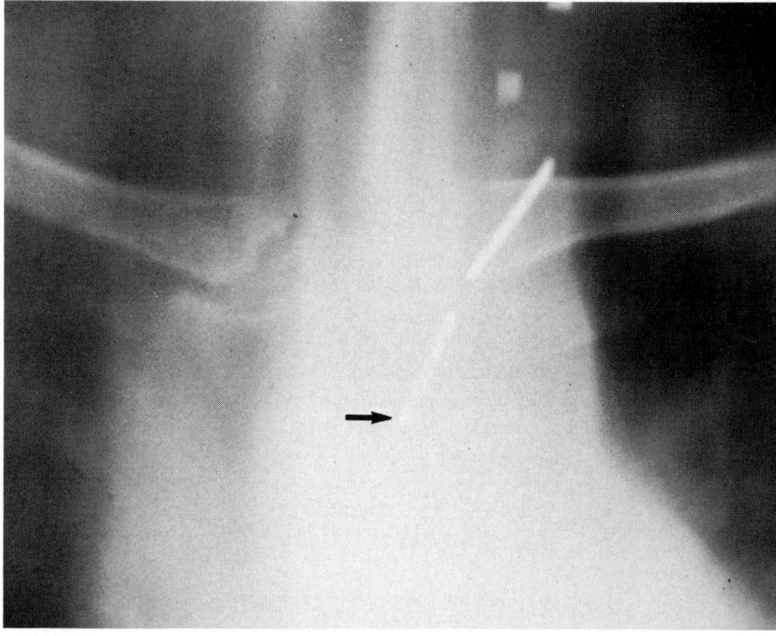

Figure 4–71. A broken pin (arrow) in the sternoclavicular joint migrated into the pericardium.

with a drill hole and No. 2 or No. 5 nonmetallic sutures to the sternum. The cervical fascia is closed and the skin approximated with a continuous subcuticular suture.

Following either closed or open reduction, the shoulders are immobilized with a plastic spica cast, which incorporates a carefully padded plastic "figure-of-eight" to prevent the shoulders from slumping forward and to protect the clavicle during sleep (see Fig. 5–38C). The cast is used for approximately eight weeks and is followed by a sling and gradual resumption of activities. Heavy lifting and impact loads are prohibited for at least nine months.

As mentioned above, the two acute, unreduced posterior sternoclavicular dislocations I have treated were both stable after closed reduction and were treated successfully with figure-of-eight dressings. However, I now advise a spica cast that holds the shoulders back like a figure of 8 but provides better protection when the patient is recumbent and sleeping.

Epiphyseal Fractures of the Inner Clavicle

The ossification center at the inner end of the clavicle appears late, usually after age 17 years. Prior to that time it cannot be visualized on x-ray films. As illustrated in Figure 4–69, displaced fractures at this epiphysis in patients under 17 years of age appear in x-ray films to be sternoclavicular dislocations. The prognosis and treatment differ in that the epiphyseal fracture can unite inside a periosteal sleeve, and remodel to near-normal appearance. Rockwood[200] reviewed the literature on this injury and rightfully emphasized its clinical significance. As long as the patient is free of mediastinal symptoms, these epiphyseal fractures can be treated nonoperatively with so much probability of a satisfactory end result that operative intervention is withheld.

Old Traumatic Sternoclavicular Dislocations

Old anterior sternoclavicular dislocations are usually asymptomatic and require no treatment. Old dislocations occasionally become painful. When pain and disability persist, surgery may be indicated as described below.

If the inner clavicle is stable, the proximal 0.5 to 1.0 cm. of clavicle is resected and the dead space filled with the clavicular head of the sternocleidomastoid muscle, as shown in Figure 6–11. This is the same treatment as the procedure used for arthritis of the sternoclavicular joint.

If the inner clavicle is unstable and slips about, the costoclavicular ligament is reconstructed at the time of resection of the inner clavicle. Several methods have been described for doing this. The method I have evolved that seems to carry the least risk and inconvenience to the patient is shown in Figures 4–72 and 4–73. A 7.0 cm. incision is made in the necklace line below the bone prominence. The soft tissue is carefully elevated, staying very close to the clavicle. Darrach elevators are placed behind the clavicle to protect the subclavian vein. The superior surface of the first rib is cleared of soft tissue, and two drill holes are made through the outer cortex 1.5 cm. apart. An angulated curette is used to connect these holes and enlarge them sufficiently so that the tendon graft can be passed through them; a bridge of cortex of at least 1.25 cm. is left. The inferior (deep) surface of the rib is left intact. I have used both palmaris and plantaris tendon grafts but prefer the palmaris tendon from the side of the sternoclavicular repair if it is available because it leaves the other upper extremity and both legs free of surgical incisions. The graft should be about 6.0 cm. long and is placed along with two strands of No. 2 nonabsorbable suture in the tunnel under the outer cortex of first rib. Next, the inner clavicle is trimmed with a rongeur, removing 0.5 cm. inferiorly and 1.0 cm. superiorly (Fig. 4–72). A drill hole is then made through the center of the stump of clavicle to receive the graft and nonabsorbable sutures. The clavicular head of the sternocleidomastoid muscle is detached (which has the beneficial effect of eliminating its pull on the clavicular repair) and is sutured into the dead space between the stump of the clavicle and the sternum. The cervical fascia and platysma muscle are approximated. The skin is closed with a continuous subcuticular suture. A spica cast is applied and is used for 10 to 12 weeks; this is followed by a sling and gradual resumption of activities.

My results in three patients with this procedure were very satisfactory. There were no complications, and the stabilization of the clavicle has held. The cosmetic result is illustrated in Figure 4–73. The patients have been satisfied with the appearance and pleased with the functional improvement.

Atraumatic Sternoclavicular Dislocations

Sternoclavicular instability is seen in hypermobile individuals with generalized joint laxity. In addition, as discussed below, sternoclavicular dis-

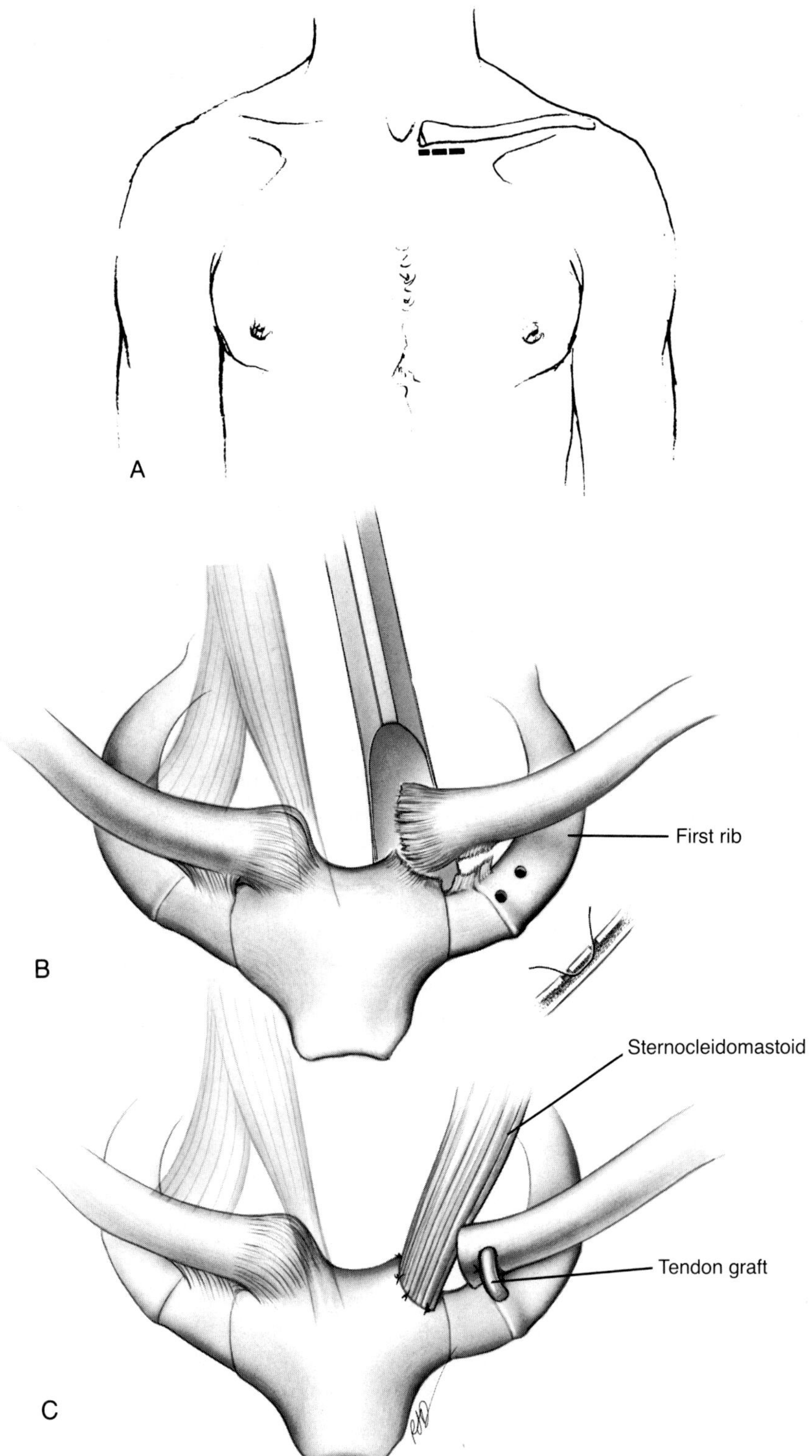

Figure 4–72. ***Repair of Old, Unstable Sternoclavicular Dislocations (Palmaris Graft).***

A, Incision.

B, Detachment of clavicular head of sternocleidomastoid. Holes in first rib and clavicle.

C, Excision of inner clavicles, palmaris graft in place, transfer of clavicular head of pectoralis major to fill the dead space.

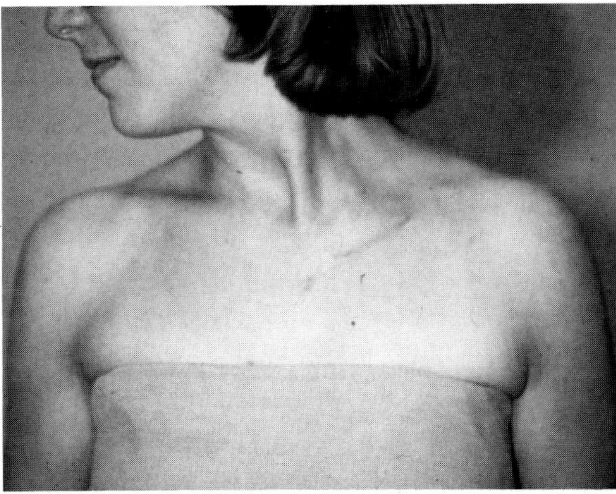

Figure 4–73. Results after excision of inner clavicle and palmaris graft, as in Figure 4–72, for an unstable old sternoclavicular dislocation. In this example, the stump of the clavicle has remained in place, and the patient can perform a full range of activities without pain and is pleased. She is tensing the sternocleidomastoid showing how the clavicular head has been transferred medially.

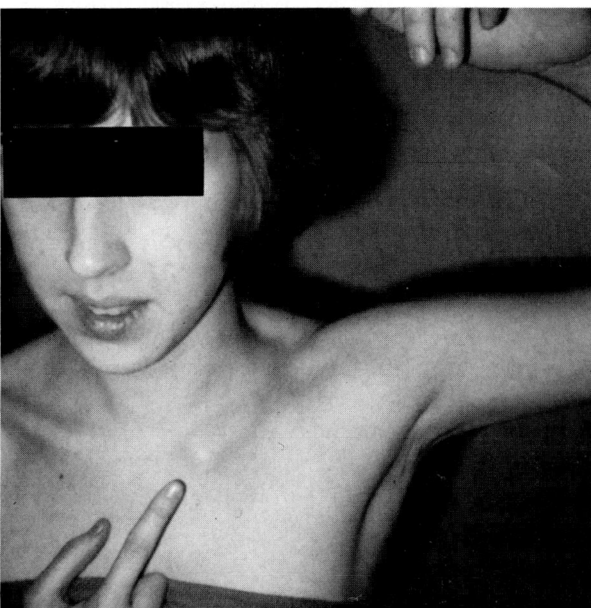

Figure 4–74. Voluntary sternoclavicular dislocation.

locations may be noted for the first time by young adults who have had no significant or only trivial trauma. The literature contains a number of reports of this and in the early series from our institution,[207] 6 of the 14 sternoclavicular dislocations occurred without major trauma. "Spontaneous" dislocations may occur unintentionally and unexpectedly or intentionally (voluntarily).

The literature on atraumatic dislocations sometimes includes a discussion of degenerative changes, as will be considered in Chapter 6, page 436 (sternoclavicular osteoarthritis in older patients).

Voluntary Sternoclavicular Dislocations

Patients who subluxate the sternoclavicular joints intentionally to attract attention are usually immature individuals between 9 and 20 years of age (Fig. 4–74). Hypermobility is usually demonstrable at other joints. Because of the motivation and immaturity of these patients, surgical repair is contraindicated just as in persons with voluntary glenohumeral dislocations.

This condition is painless, and no treatment is indicated. It is important, however, to reassure the patient and the parents that no harm is being done and that the prognosis is excellent for recovery.

I operated on a nurse who at age 28 years had painful degenerative changes at the sternoclavicular joint. She probably had been a voluntary sternoclavicular dislocator in her adolescence. If so, she is the only voluntary sternoclavicular dislocator I have seen who required surgery in later life. The operation described in Figure 4–72 was performed in this patient with a good result.

Involuntary, Spontaneous Sternoclavicular "Dislocations"

These very rare lesions are only occasionally seen in young adults. The displacement is usually incomplete, and there is little if any pain.

A 30 year old male patient I have seen with this condition first noticed it a year and a half ago when playing tennis. On examination, the inner clavicle can be subluxated both anteriorly and posteriorly without pain. He develops moderate pain, however, if he attempts athletic activities that involve overhead use of the arm, such as serves and overhead strokes in tennis or throwing a ball. He also develops discomfort after raking leaves. He does not have enough pain, however, to desire reconstruction of the costoclavicular ligaments. Conservative treatment consists of avoiding the activities that cause soreness and reassurance that there is no indication to perform surgery to avoid further trouble. I have never operated on a patient with this condition, but if symptoms truly demanded it and the pain brought out by exercises prior to the office visit could be relieved with a lidocaine injection into the sternoclavicular joint, the operation depicted in Figure 4–72 might be considered. I have seen this problem on only two or three occasions and have never seen it with sufficient disability to warrant surgery.

DISLOCATION OF THE CLAVICLE

Concomitant dislocations of both the sternoclavicular and acromioclavicular joints have been referred to as "floating clavicle" or dislocation of the clavicle (Fig. 4–75). I have seen it on several occasions but never without an articular surface fracture of either the inner or outer clavicle, and all have had associated rib fractures.

The mechanism of injury is a compression between strong forces. For example, one patient was lying on his side under a car when the jack fell, causing the weight of the car to compress one shoulder against the other shoulder, which was lying on the cement floor.

I performed a reconstruction of the coracoclavicular ligaments and resection of the distal clavicle, as shown in Figure 4–66, in one patient two years after injury, with relief of pain at the acromioclavicular joint, which was his main complaint. Otherwise, I have not performed surgery for this type of injury. In two other patients seen two or three years after injury, it was difficult to localize the exact source of symptoms, and no surgical repair was attempted.

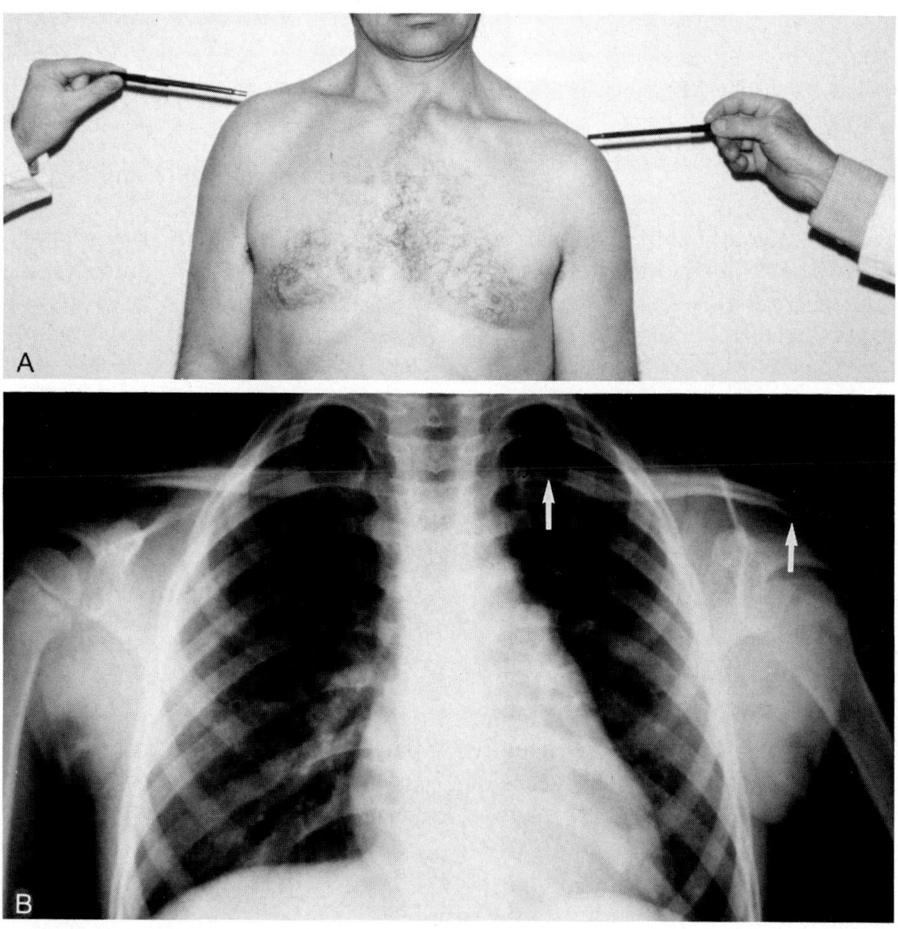

Figure 4–75. ***Dislocation of the Clavicle.***

A, Note the dropped scapula and the prominent inner end of the clavicle on the left side (arrows).

B, Anterior-posterior view. The inner clavicle is dislocated anteriorly (arrow), and there is a Type III dislocation of the acromioclavicular joint (arrow).

5

FRACTURES

FRACTURES OF THE UPPER HUMERUS

Proximal humeral fractures are frequent. They account for about 4 to 5 per cent of all fractures. They occur more often in older patients, after the cancellous bone of the humeral neck has become weakened by senility, but they are seen in patients of all ages and merge with epiphyseal separations. In older patients, the fracture often results from a minor fall and is usually minimally displaced. The more serious fractures and fracture-dislocations are usually seen in active, middle-aged patients (averaging 55 years of age in my series). Some of these lesions can be extremely disabling, and their management demands experienced surgical skill and judgement.

Previous classifications according to the level of the fracture or mechanism of injury were inadequate to identify accurately the more difficult displaced lesions and have caused confusion in the literature.[214] In this discussion, the four-segment classification[8, 71, 73, 77, 150] is used. This system simply insists on the accurate identification of the location and relationship of each of the four major groups of fragments by good initial x-ray studies. Nothing has to be memorized, but a knowledge of the anatomy and insertions of the tendons of the rotator cuff is essential.

In 80 per cent of upper humeral fractures, none of the four major segments is significantly displaced and the fragments are held together by the attachments of the tendons of the rotator cuff, joint capsule, and intact periosteum. These lesions are amenable to simple treatment by early functional exercises and can all, regardless of the number of fracture lines, be considered together as minimal displacement because of similarity in treatment and prognosis.

In 15 to 20 per cent of upper humeral fractures, one or more of the major segments are displaced. These displaced fractures are associated with characteristic soft-tissue injuries. They are often unstable, may not be reducible by closed methods, and can be associated with distortion of the rotator mechanism or even loss of circulation to the head (articular segment). The pathology and treatment of each displaced lesion are considered individually in the four-segment classification.

Anatomy of Upper Humeral Fractures

Muscle Forces

The muscle forces acting on the four major segments are shown in Figure 5–1. For example,

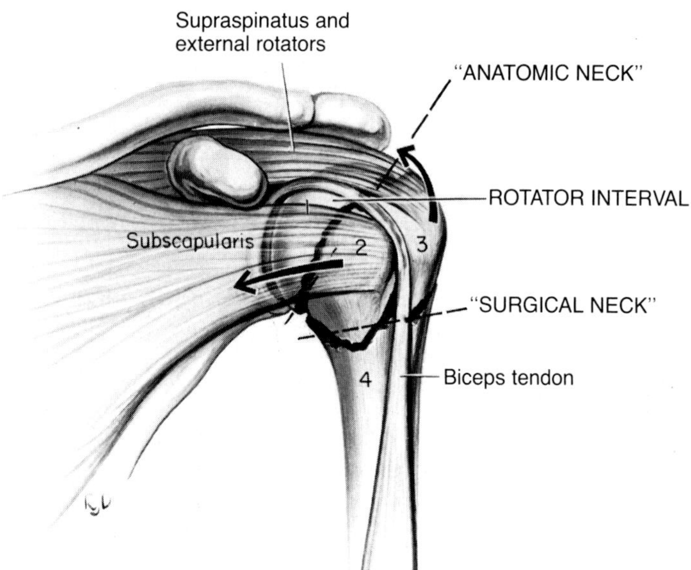

Figure 5–1. Muscle forces acting on the four major segments of proximal humeral fractures: (1) the head, (2) the lesser tuberosity, (3) the greater tuberosity, and (4) the shaft. Displacements of the tuberosities tear the rotator interval and involve both the surgical neck and the anatomical neck levels. (From Neer, C. S., II: Displaced proximal humeral fractures: I. Classification and evaluation. J. Bone Joint Surg. *52A*:1077, 1970.)

the greater tuberosity may be retracted by the supraspinatus and external rotators, and the lesser tuberosity may be retracted by the subscapularis. The shaft tends to be displaced medially and anteriorly by the pectoralis major. These active forces and the status of the rotator cuff must be considered when reduction is being contemplated. Displaced fractures at the anatomical neck level separate the head from its blood supply and result in a high incidence of aseptic necrosis.

Blood Supply

The blood supply to the humeral head is derived from both the anterior and the posterior circumflex vessels, which give branches entering the tuberosities and biceps groove. Laing[147] indicated that the most consistent and important source of circulation to the head appeared to be from the ascending branch of the anterior circumflex humeral artery, which enters the bone in the vicinity of the bicipital groove. It is important in performing open reductions of proximal humeral fractures to avoid further injury to the circulation, being especially careful to avoid injury to the soft tissue in the vicinity of the bicipital groove (Fig. 5–2). In four-part displacements (in which both tuberosities are displaced), the circulation to the head has been so severely damaged by the injury that the incidence of avascular necrosis with late collapse of the head has, in my opinion, been quite high.

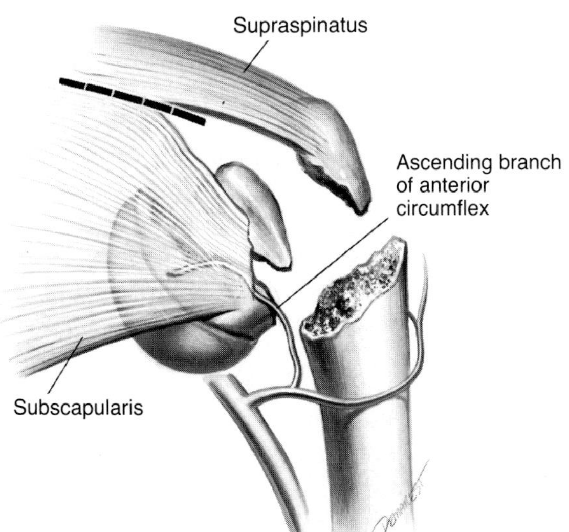

Figure 5–2. Relationship of proximal humeral fractures to the blood supply of the humeral head. Arterial branches enter both the greater and the lesser tuberosities and the biceps groove. When the greater tuberosity remains attached to the head, the blood supply is adequate. When the greater tuberosity is separated, the main remaining source of blood supply to the head is from the ascending branch of the anterior circumflex artery, which enters at the lesser tuberosity and bicipital groove.

Nerve Injuries

The neurovascular bundle is anteromedial, and the axillary nerve is just inferior to the glenohumeral joint. They are in greatest peril in anterior fracture-dislocations and displacements at the surgical neck level (Fig. 5–3).

Mechanism of Injury

A fall on the outstretched arm is the classic mechanism of injury. Continuing abduction may exceed the check-point of the ligaments. In younger patients, in whom the breaking strength of the bone may be greater than the tensile strengths of the ligaments, a dislocation usually occurs. When the bone is weaker than the ligaments, as in older patients, a fracture of the humeral neck occurs. As

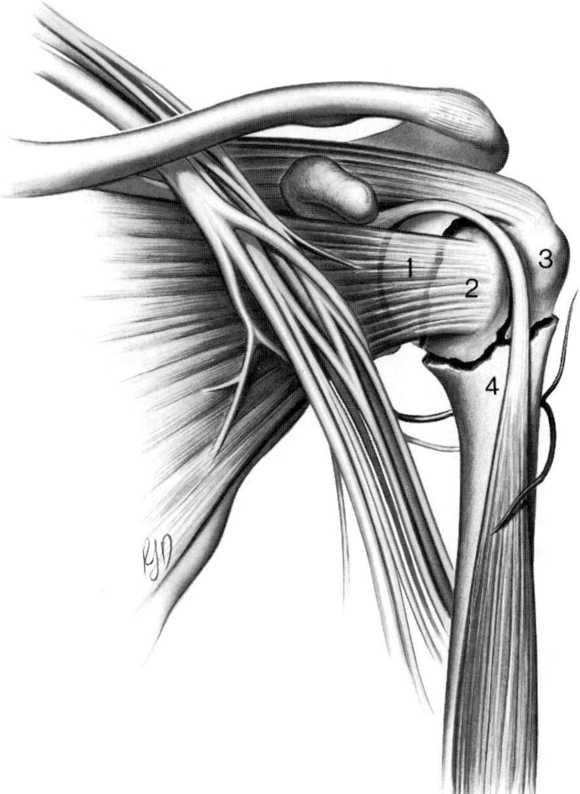

Figure 5–3. The nerves are in greatest peril in anterior fracture-dislocations (from the displaced head) and surgical neck fractures (from a displaced spike of medial calcar, as is almost always present on the stump of the shaft). The four segments will be marked with numbers throughout this part of the book as follows: (1) the head, (2) the lesser tuberosity, (3) the greater tuberosity, and (4) the shaft.

might be expected, the most severe combination of injuries—fracture-dislocation—usually results from hard falls in middle-aged patients.

Upper humeral fractures can also result from a blow on the lateral side of the arm. Most patients are unable to recall the details of the injury, but the fact is that some of them fall while carrying an object in their arms, such as a bag of groceries, and are still holding the object after the fracture has occurred. In these cases, the injury must have been a blow on the lateral side of the arm rather than one on the outstretched hand.

Four-Segment Classification

The original four-segment classification described in 1970[8] was simplified and modified in 1975 by deleting the Roman numerals.[77, 150] The key to understanding this four-segment system is to recognize it as a concept rather than as a numerical classification. Again, there is nothing to memorize, but accurate initial radiographic evaluation is essential.

It has been observed that upper humeral fractures occur among one or all of four major segments: (1) the articular segment or "anatomical neck" level; (2) the greater tuberosity, which often has been broken into a number of fragments; (3) the lesser tuberosity; and (4) the shaft or "surgical neck" level (see Fig. 5–1). Any segment may have multiple fracture lines or fragments. The location of each of these four major segments must be carefully identified in the initial x-rays. It is impossible to state in precise numbers the amount of displacement requiring manipulation or surgery, but in an effort to be specific, it was arbitrarily stated that if any of the four segments is displaced over 1.0 cm. or angulated more than 45 degrees, the fracture is considered to be displaced. These figures are intended as a guide to the surgeon but need not be considered exact. Less displacement is categorized as minimal displacement, regardless of the number and level of the fracture lines.

For clarity, a fracture with "minimal displacement" could be called a "one-part fracture." A "two-part fracture" is one in which only one segment is displaced in relationship to the three that remain undisplaced. A "three-part fracture" is one in which two segments are displaced in relation to other segments that are in apposition; however, to meet the criteria for this classification, there must be an unimpacted surgical neck component and rotatory displacement. In a "four-part fracture," all four major segments are displaced. Thus, there are four major categories of fractures, based on the number of displaced segments rather than on the number of fracture lines: "minimal displacement," "two-part displacement," "three-part displacement," and "four-part displacement." The thera-

Table 5–1. TREATMENT ACCORDING TO FOUR-SEGMENT CLASSIFICATION*

	INCIDENCE† (%)	PROBLEM	AUTHOR'S TREATMENT
Minimal displacement	80	Adhesions	Passive exercises progressing to active exercises as continuity permits
Two-part	10	Usually amenable to closed reduction	Closed treatment, except for greater tuberosity and some shaft displacements
Three-part	3	Rotary forces of muscles prevent accurate closed reduction	Open reduction, internal fixation, and cuff repair, except prosthesis is now preferred in older patients and greater tuberosity three-part displacement with frail head attachments
Four-part	4	High incidence of avascular necrosis or post-traumatic arthritis	Prosthesis to replace the head with accurate fixation of the tuberosities and cuff repair
Articular surface fractures	3		
"Impression"			
Under 20%		Stable	Closed reduction, immobilization in external rotation
20% to 40%		Often unstable after closed reduction	Transplant lesser tuberosity if unstable
Over 50%		Re-displace into head defect	Prosthesis
"Head-splitting"		Articular surface crushed	Prosthesis

*These generalizations apply only to active patients who are good operative risks and have good motivation and reasonable life expectancy.

†Expressed as percentage of all upper humeral fractures and fracture-dislocations.

Modified from Neer, C. S., II: Fractures about the shoulder. *In* Rockwood, C. A., Jr., and Green, D. P. (eds.): Fractures in Adults, 2nd ed. Philadelphia, J. B. Lippincott, 1984.

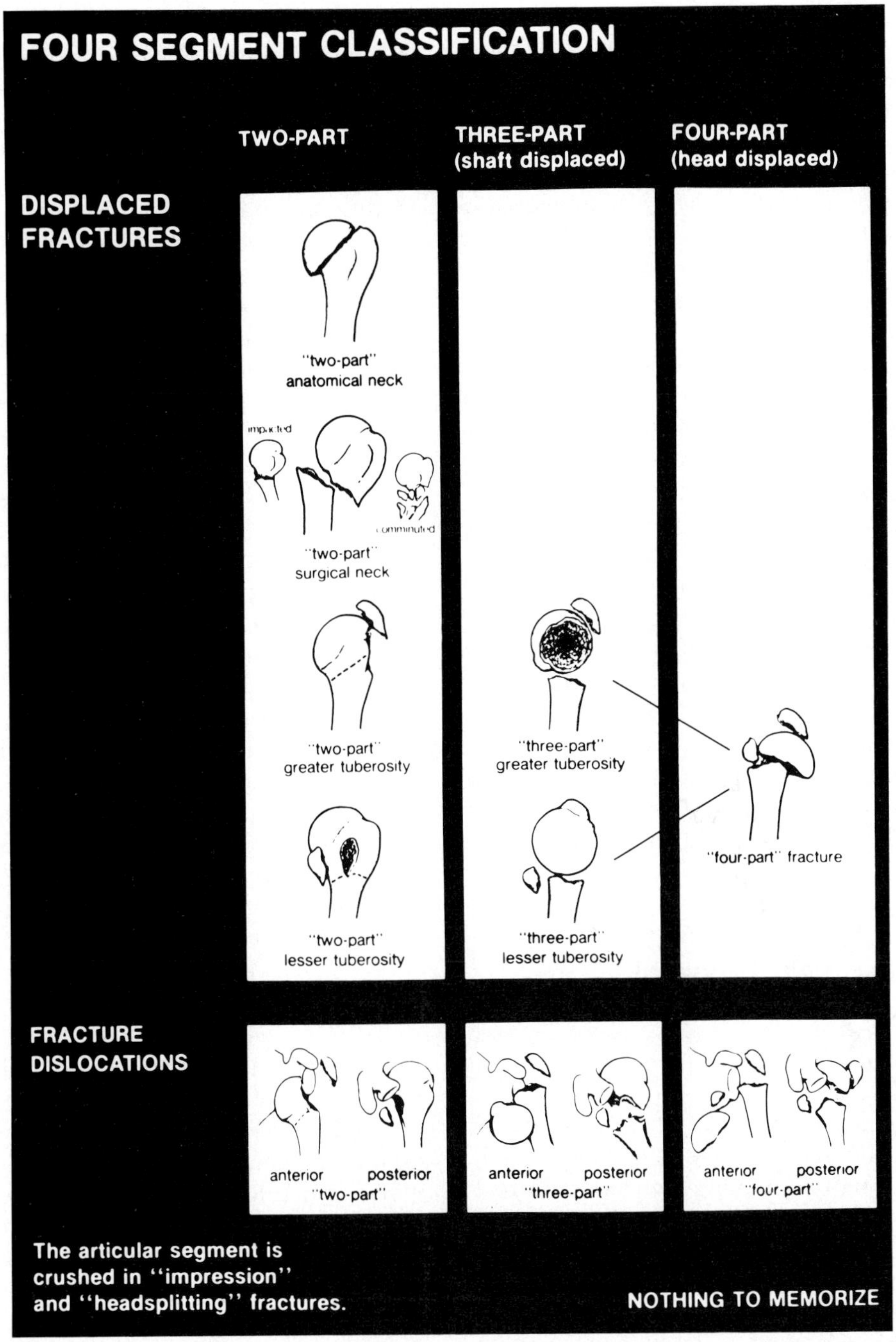

Figure 5–4. ***Modification of the Original Four-Segment Classification of Displaced Proximal Humeral Fractures.*** As stated in the illustration, there is nothing to memorize, but good x-rays (the "trauma series"—see Fig. 1–12C) are essential. Nondisplaced fractures (defined for general purposes as less than 1.0 cm. or angulated less than 45 degrees) are not considered in this classification, although for clarity they might well be termed "one-part." "Two-part displacements" include isolated displacements of the head (anatomic neck), shaft (surgical neck), greater tuberosity, and lesser tuberosity. "Three-part displacements" are associated with an impacted surgical neck component that allows the head to be rotated by either the external rotators or the subscapularis, depending upon which tuberosity remains attached to the head. "Four-part displacements" are characterized by detachment of both tuberosities from the head, and the articular surface of the head is displaced out of contact with the glenoid. Crushing or fragmentation of the articular surface produces the "impression fractures" and the "head-splitting fractures." (Modified from Neer, C. S., II: J. Bone Joint Surg. *52A*:1077, 1970.)

peutic implications of the four-segment classification are summarized in Table 5–1.

The term fracture-dislocation has, at times, caused confusion.[214] It is used in this classification to imply that the articular segment is out of contact with the glenoid rather than subluxated or rotated. Anterior, posterior, lateral, and inferior fracture-dislocations are associated with characteristic two-, three-, and four-part lesions. Finally, fractures of the articular surface (the "impression fracture" or "head-splitting fracture") are given separate consideration (Fig. 5–4).

One of the advantages of this system is that it describes the anatomical problem present. It demands good initial x-rays prior to considering treatment and prognosis. It is important to have at least two views of the upper humerus made at right angles to each other. The technique of accomplishing this in an acutely injured and painful shoulder requires special consideration. A "trauma series" of x-ray views (see Fig. 1–12B) made in the scapular planes should be standardized for the first examination of all shoulder fractures. Previous classifications based on the level of the fracture or on the mechanism of injury as well as the more recently proposed AO classification do not describe the pathology of displaced fractures of the proximal humerus and have led to confusion in the literature.[8]

Diagnosis of Upper Humeral Fractures

Physical Signs

Because the upper humerus is well covered by soft tissue and the displacement is often minimal, early signs are usually limited to direct and indirect tenderness. The diagnosis depends on radiographic studies, which should be made in any patient with continuing shoulder pain subsequent to an injury. Within a few days, ecchymosis, which may extend from the chest wall to the elbow, appears and strongly suggests the diagnosis.

Fracture-dislocations are more difficult to recognize clinically than simple dislocations, because although the contour of the shoulder may be flattened, the break in the continuity of the bone allows the shaft to fall into normal alignment and to be moved without the characteristic limitations of movement. This is especially true of posterior fracture-dislocations, and, statistically, over 50 per cent of these are missed on initial examination. The true Velpeau or supine axillary view (see Fig. 1–12) is the most reliable method for establishing the diagnosis of a posterior dislocation. This axillary view should always be obtained if the lesion is suspected from other views or from the physical findings. The physical signs of posterior dislocation include prominent coracoid; loss of external rotation and abduction; prominence of the head posteriorly; and altered axis of the arm, so that it is directed posteriorly (Fig. 5–32). However, in fracture-dislocations, these signs are less apparent than in posterior dislocations without fracture.

Upper humeral fractures are most frequently missed or underdiagnosed in patients with multiple injuries because the physician is distracted by other, more obvious injuries and because it is more awkward to obtain good radiographic evaluation of the shoulder. However, even in this situation it is possible to obtain views of the upper humerus in two planes by tilting the patient 35 degrees, injured side down, and to supplement as needed with supine axillary views (see Fig. 1–12B). Radiographic techniques are most important as discussed further in the next section.

Associated injuries to the axillary nerve and brachial plexus are not rare, and the axillary vessels are occasionally torn. The status of these structures should be documented before and after instituting treatment. Displacements at the surgical neck level and anterior fracture-dislocations are especially apt to cause neurovascular damage. Violent trauma to the shoulder with avulsion of the roots of the plexus can occur in the absence of a fracture.

Radiographic Diagnosis

Oblique and poorly centered films of any fracture cause confusion and make logical treatment impossible because the glenohumeral joint lies in neither the coronal or the sagittal plane. Two-plane views of this joint and the upper humerus are best made by placing the beam vertical and then parallel to the scapular plane (see Fig. 1–12), rather than in the coronal and sagittal planes. This can be done without removing the arm from the sling and without discomfort to the patient. The patient may be standing, sitting, or supine. These two initial survey views, which are called the "trauma series," should be standardized in every hospital emergency service.

Supplemental studies are made at the discretion of the surgeon, the most important of which is the axillary view.[118] In severely injured patients, this can be made with the patient supine with minimal abduction of the injured arm by placing the x-ray tube near the patient's hip and holding the film superior to the glenohumeral joint, the standard supine axillary view (see Fig. 1–12). In

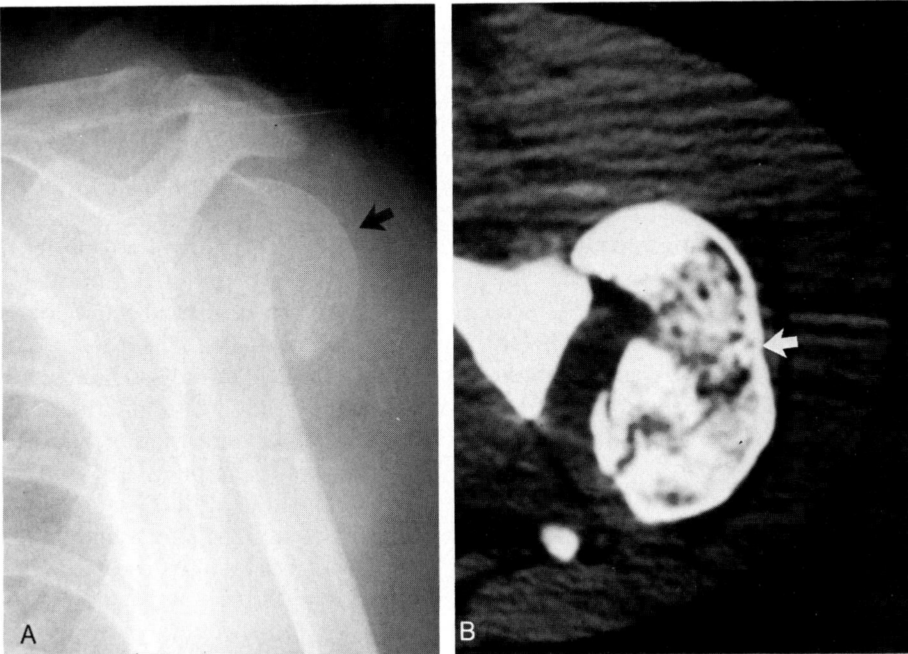

Figure 5–5. Computerized tomography is a help for seeing details in fracture-dislocations of articular surface fractures, as shown in this patient.

A, Lateral radiographic view showing the head (arrow) is posteriorly dislocated but suggesting it is in continuity with the greater tuberosity and a closed reduction might be attempted.

B, Computerized tomogram of the same fracture showing the head is broken from the greater tuberosity (arrow) and its anterior 30 percent has been crushed, making it unwise to attempt a closed reduction.

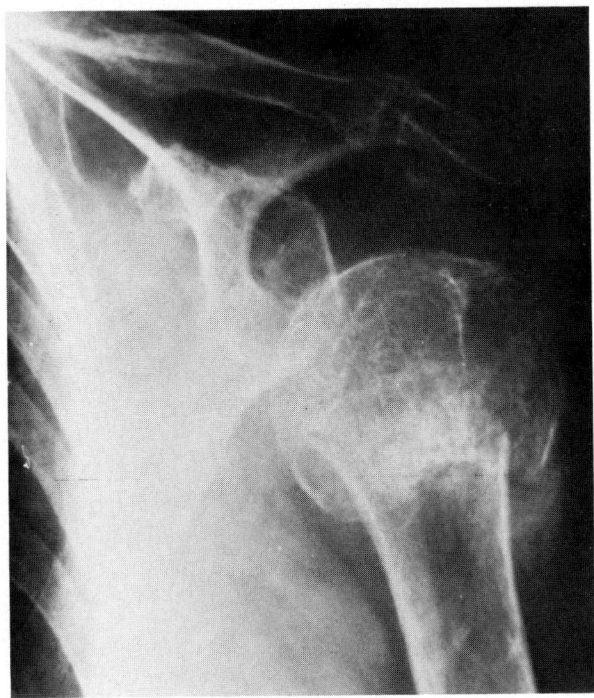

Figure 5–6. Typical "minimal displacement" seen four weeks after injury with early callus and a transitory subluxation of the head. The subluxation disappeared when the rotator cuff and deltoid muscles regained tone.

In addition to the impacted surgical neck component, there are nondisplaced fissure fractures of the greater and lesser tuberosities; nevertheless, this lesion is termed a "minimal displacement" and is not considered with the displaced fracture terminology (see Fig. 5–4). If this terminology were used, the lesion would be called a "one-part" fracture.

ambulatory patients, the axillary view can be obtained with the patient standing, supine, or prone. I prefer the Velpeau method shown in Figure 1–12. This is the most valuable method of diagnosing posterior dislocations and is also the best way to identify glenoid fractures. Other supplemental x-rays include transthoracic views, anterior-posterior views with the humerus in various positions of rotation, and laminograms. All are at times helpful in estimating the amount of displacement of specific segments. Laminograms can be especially useful in judging the size of articular surface defects. Computerized tomography (CT scan) is helpful for determining the size of the head defects, the condition of the glenoid, and whether the head is dislocated (Fig. 5–5).

Treatment

The therapeutic implications of the four-segment classification are summarized in Table 5–1.

Minimal Displacement

This important group constitutes approximately 80 percent of upper humeral fractures. No segment is displaced significantly (less than 1.0 cm. or less than 45 degrees). These lesions might well be called "one-part fractures" (Fig. 5–5). The fragments are usually held together by the intact rotator cuff and periosteum and move together as one piece when the humeral shaft is rotated. This allows early functional exercises as healing occurs and callus appears in x-ray films. At times, one of the fragments is disimpacted, so that false motion is present. This requires initial immobilization with a sling and swathe or similar appliance (see Fig. 7–2) until sufficient clinical union has occurred for the head and shaft to rotate in unison before exercises can be started.

It is important to test carefully for false motion as a guide to when the functional exercises can be begun. The examiner stands behind the patient and with one hand palpates the outlines of the acromion and then slides his or her fingers down around the head of the humerus. With the other hand at the bent elbow, the examiner gently rotates the humeral shaft.

When clinical continuity is present, the sling and swathe are removed for pendulum exercises, which progress as pain permits (see Fig. 7–8A). I believe that the patient feels more secure and makes better progress when some of the early exercises are performed lying supine. The "good" arm supplies the power. Assistive elevation is

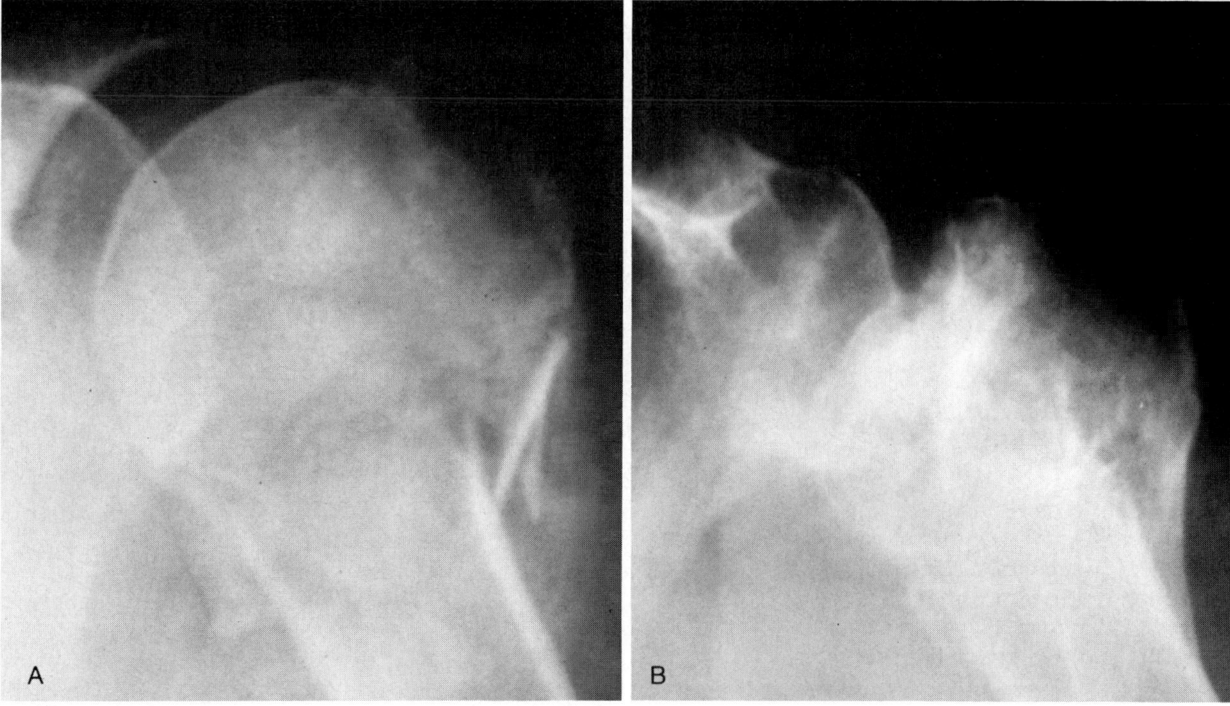

Figure 5–7. Rare complications of minimally displaced proximal humeral fractures. Occasionally, minimal displacements cause late avascular necrosis of the head. A, Original fracture (anterior-posterior view). B, Advanced avascular necrosis three years later.

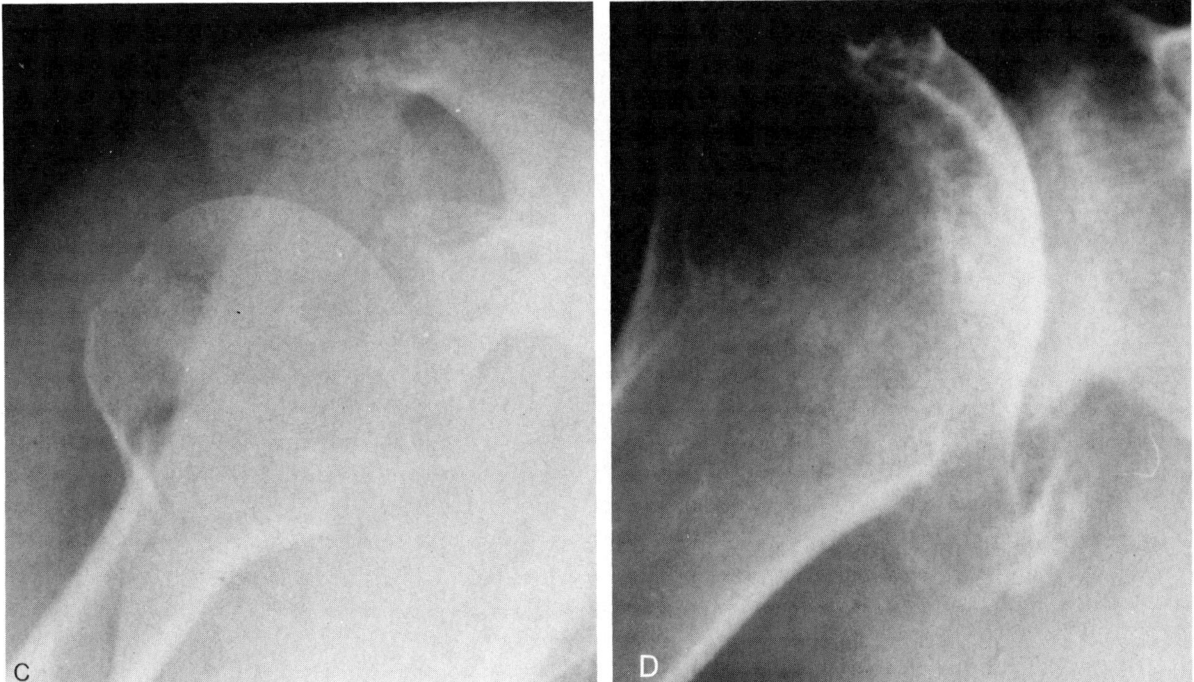

Figure 5–7 *Continued* C and D, Occasionally, a minimal displacement causes later post-traumatic arthritis. C, Original fracture (Velpeau axillary view). D, Post-traumatic arthritis five years later (anterior-posterior view).

usually added before rotation. After union, stretching exercises, as from the top of a door and sliding up the wall (see Fig. 7–9A), are very helpful. "Wall climbing" (creeping up the wall with the fingers) is not an effective exercise for regaining range of motion.

The first objective is to establish a good passive range of motion with heat and passive exercises. Active and resistive exercises to restore strength are not attempted until union is quite advanced and a good passive range has been accomplished. Fractures through cancellous bone heal with almost predictable regularity, and union can be expected at six to eight weeks. However, optimal functional recovery requires the exercises to be continued for a number of months. Occasionally, a patient with minimal displacement develops late avascular necrosis or post-traumatic arthritis (Fig. 5–7A to D).

A "transitory subluxation" of the humeral head often follows upper humeral fractures of all types and can cause considerable concern, as seen in Figure 5–6. It is best explained by two facts: (1) the deltoid and rotator cuff muscles become atonic after injuries, and (2) the ligaments and capsule of the glenohumeral joint are normally loose enough to allow the head to descend. Thus, the weight of the arm can lead to a transitory subluxation that disappears as the muscles regain tone. Treatment consists of a sling to support the arm and isometrics between regular exercise periods.

Two-Part Displacements

In two-part displacements, because only one segment is displaced, it is usually possible to accomplish and maintain reduction by closed methods. There are exceptions to this generalization, however, and each lesion merits individual discussion.

Two-Part Anatomical Neck Displacement (Fig. 5–8)

Isolated displacement of the articular segment at the anatomical neck, perhaps in association with hairline tuberosity components but without accompanying displacement of the tuberosities, is quite rare. Its presence is easily overlooked unless a good anterior-posterior x-ray of the upper humerus is obtained in the scapular plane and in the proper rotation of the humerus. There is a threat of late avascular necrosis of the head regardless of the method of treatment.

Because no surgeon has had a great deal of experience with these fractures, it is not possible to be dogmatic about treatment. Because the tuberosities are in good position, it seems logical to treat an acute lesion in the way recommended for other large displaced fragments of the articular surface in other major joints—namely, by open reduction and internal fixation. The alternative is to accept the displacement and hope for a comfortable malunion that does not go on to avascular necrosis with collapse of the head or allow the

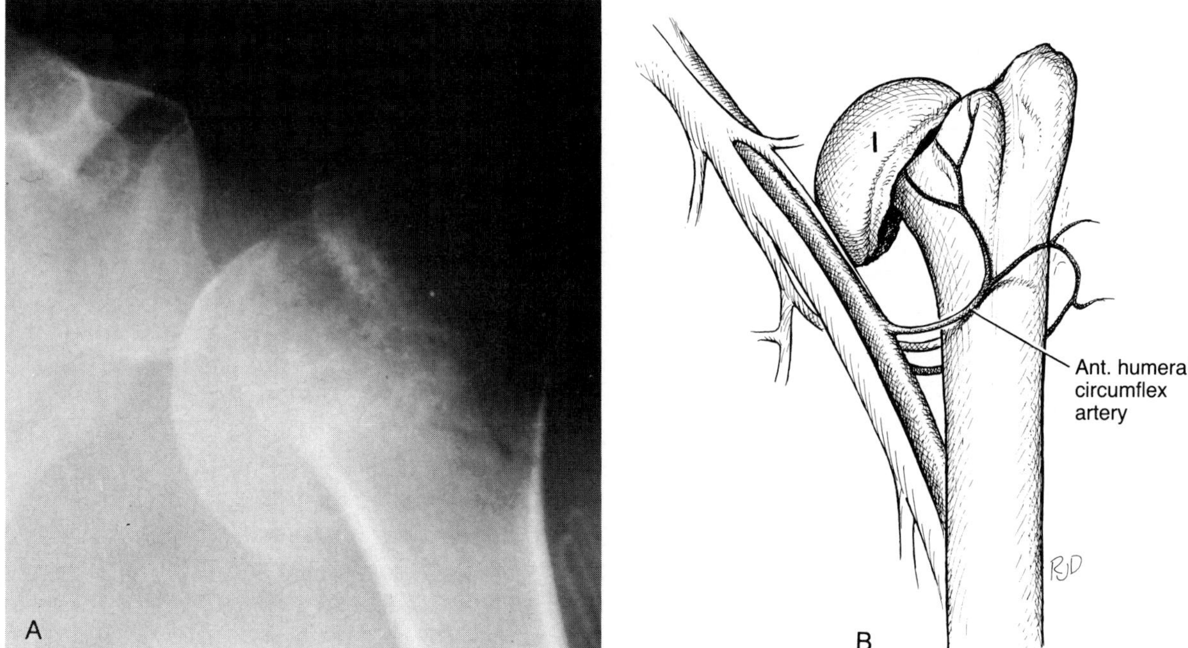

Figure 5–8. Two-part anatomical neck displacement. The author treated the recent fracture shown in the anterior-posterior roentgenogram (A) with the same exercise program as for a minimal displacement but with a more guarded prognosis for incongruity from avascular necrosis or from the malaligned head and for possible impingement from the prominent tuberosity. The two year follow-up result in this patient was satisfactory.

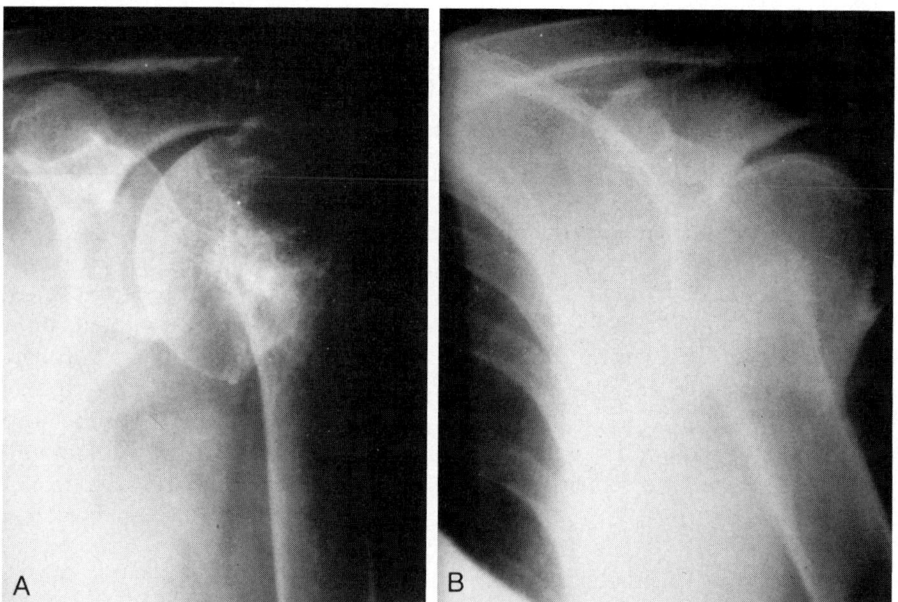

Figure 5–9. Impacted two-part surgical neck fracture with only mild displacement seen two years after injury in anterior-posterior views with the arm in external rotation (A) and internal rotation (B). This fracture has been allowed to unite in this position, and function was quite good. If there had been more angulation, closed reduction would have been considered. Epiphyseal fractures of the proximal humerus are of this type. The anterior angulation, muscle forces, and intact posterior periosteum characteristic of these lesions are illustrated in Figure 5–37.

These two films of the same fracture in different rotations show why classification of proximal humeral fractures according to the mechanism of injury caused confusion. With the shoulder externally rotated (A), the head appears to be in varus (the "adduction fracture"); with the shoulder in internal rotation (B), the head appears to be in valgus (the "abduction fracture").

patient to have pain from a prominent and impinging greater tuberosity or from an incongruous, inferiorly subluxated head. I have come to favor this latter course (Fig. 5–9). If avascular necrosis or incongruity pain occurs, it may be sufficiently disabling to require prosthetic replacement.

Two-Part Surgical Neck Displacement

Displacement of the shaft (or surgical neck displacement) is common and occurs in patients of all ages. Epiphyseal fractures are of this type (see Fig. 5–37). A displacement of at least 1.0 cm. or more than 45 degrees angulation is present at the surgical neck level just distal to the tuberosities. Although fissure fractures may exist proximally, the rotator cuff is intact and holds the head in neutral rotation. The head is only slightly abducted, unless tilted by an overriding shaft (Fig. 5–10A and B). Three variations are seen in adult patients (Fig. 5–4).

Impacted and Angulated. The apex of the angle is usually anterior, and the posterior periosteum is intact (Fig. 5–9). If the segments are allowed to unite in this position, shoulder elevation will be permanently limited in direct proportion to the amount of residual angulation. Therefore, I prefer to treat active patients by closed reduction. The periosteal sleeve posteriorly affords sufficient stability, so that the fracture may be disimpacted with traction and the angulation corrected by full-forward elevation. The reduction is performed with image intensification fluoroscopic checks to find a position of adequate stability. After the alignment is corrected, the arm is usually immobilized in the Velpeau position across the chest (see Fig. 7–2C). This position relaxes the pectoralis and is usually more effective and comfortable than an abduction cast or a hanging cast. An abduction cast puts tension on the pectoralis major that may cause the fracture to displace. A hanging cast may distract the fracture. I usually use a stockinette and swathe until clinical union is strong enough to allow gentle exercises, usually about three to four weeks. Rehabilitation is then continued as for minimally displaced fractures.

Unimpacted. The shaft is displaced forward and medially by the pull of the pectoralis major, while the head remains in neutral rotation (Fig. 5–10A and B). This fracture is often unstable after closed reduction. An abduction cast may increase the deformity by intensifying the pull of the pectoralis. However, occasionally the reduction is more stable in abduction, in which case an abduction spica cast is used. A hanging cast levers the shaft forward when the patient lies supine and can lead to nonunion (Fig. 5–10D), especially if it distracts the fracture. A tight sling increases the anterior angulation.[114] I consider three possibilities in treatment:

1. *Closed reduction can be obtained and is stable.* Closed reduction has usually been accomplished best by traction, pulling the shaft forward and adducting it to relax the pectoralis, and then displacing the upper end of the proximal humerus laterally to lock it under the tuberosities as the traction is released. The arm is then secured across the chest in the Velpeau position because in this position the pectoralis major is relaxed. I prefer a stockinette Velpeau and swathe with an axillary pad (see Fig. 7–2C). Rarely, because of the direction of the fracture surfaces and the way they interlock, the reduction is better maintained in a salute position or in abduction, in which case a plaster spica cast is applied in this position.

2. *The fracture can be reduced but is too unstable to maintain reduction.* It is percutaneously transfixed with a stiff-threaded pin inserted anteriorly into the shaft through the deltopectoral interval and then on into the head. The Velpeau dressing is then applied. The pin is removed within three weeks, prior to starting exercises. If the patient has multiple injuries requiring access to the chest, overhead olecranon traction is used.

3. *The fracture cannot be reduced closed.* Interposition of the deltoid muscle (Fig. 5–10C and D) or the long head of the biceps (Fig. 5–10E and F) must be suspected and an open reduction with internal fixation performed. An AO T-plate can be used if the proximal fragment is not too soft to hold screws, but a compression band nonmetallic suture with an intramedullary rod (Fig. 5–10H) is often necessary because of softening. As previously stated, this lesion may be associated with arterial injuries and with injuries of the infraclavicular part of the brachial plexus. Fortunately, the prognosis for spontaneous recovery of nerve function following infraclavicular injuries is generally good.

Comminuted. When the fragmentation extends distally for several centimeters, the fragments of bone undergo twist displacement if the arm is placed in internal rotation across the chest (see Fig. 5–11). This occurs because the tuberosities and the head are held in neutral rotation by the intact rotator cuff. Intermediate fragments may be retracted by the pectoralis. This fracture cannot be adequately aligned across the chest because it collapses with overriding. It is well aligned by overhead traction. However, a spica cast applied in neutral rotation to accommodate the position of the proximal segments and in adduction and forward flexion to relax the pectoralis is usually adequate and much more convenient for the pa-

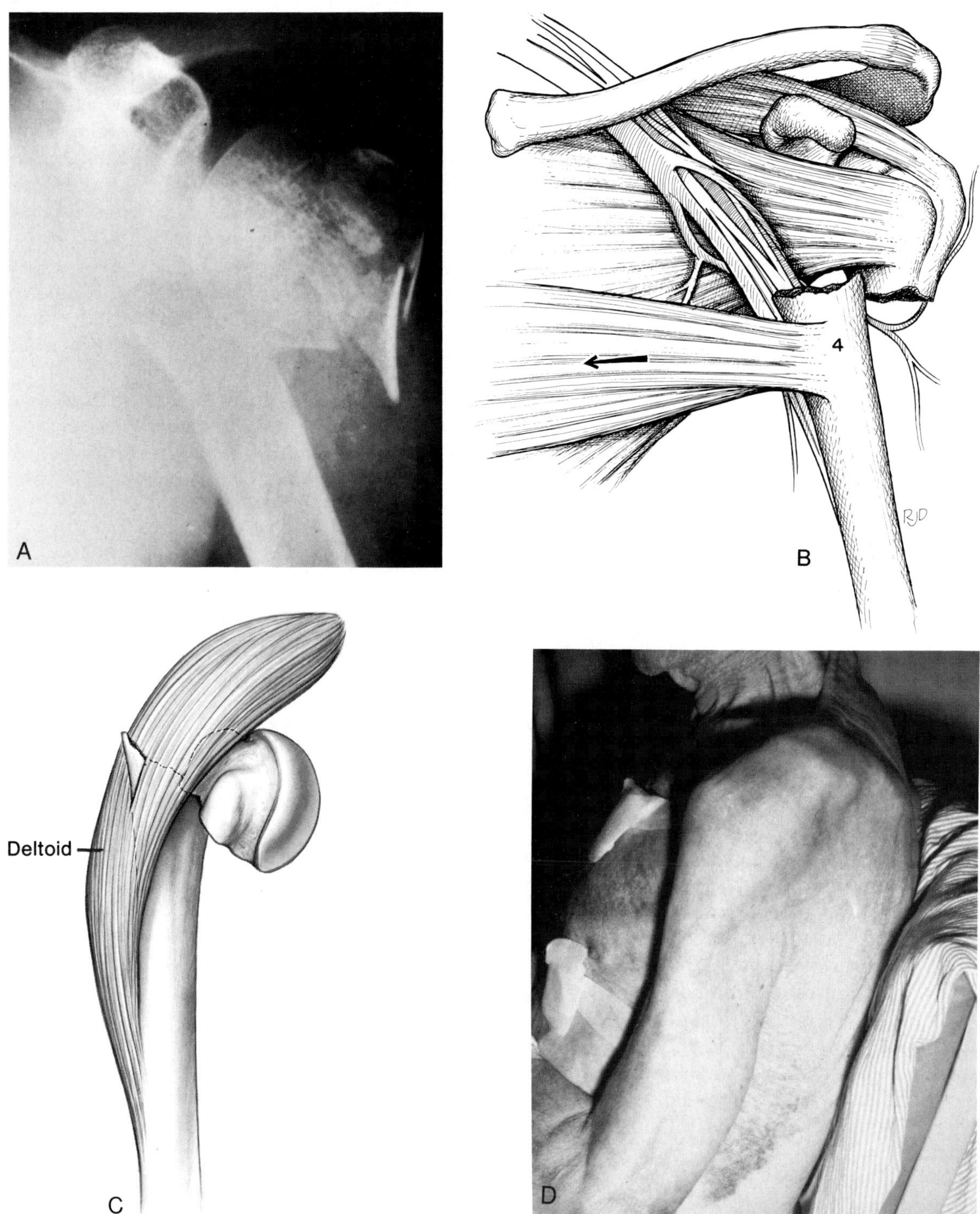

Figure 5–10. ***Two-part Unimpacted Surgical Neck Displacement.*** Three types of treatment are discussed in the text.

A and B, Example of the lesion.

C and D, Two-part unimpacted surgical neck displacement may be complicated by interposition of deltoid muscle. The shaft is usually angulated anteriorly by the pectoralis major puncturing the anterior deltoid (right).

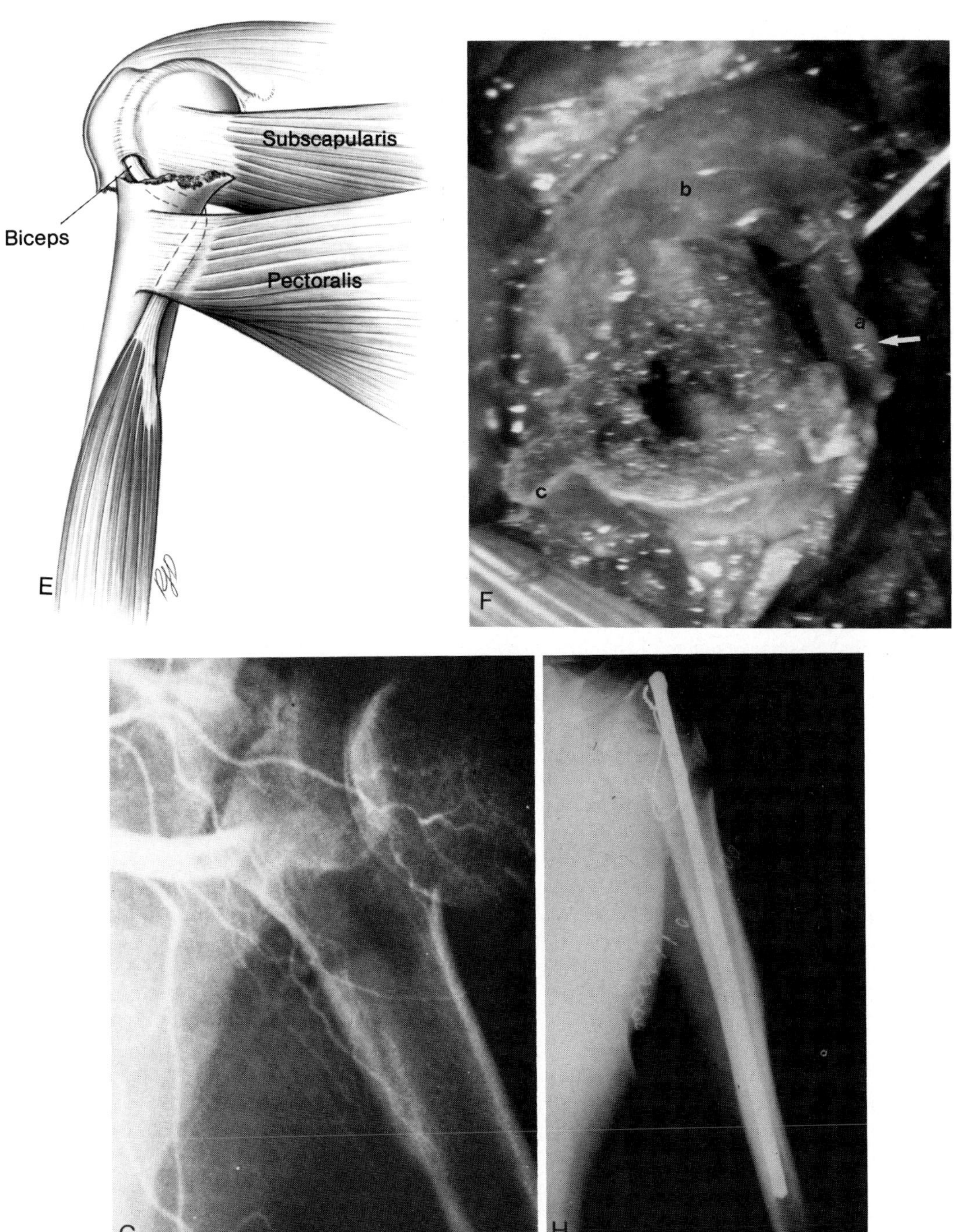

Figure 5–10 *Continued* E and F, Interposition of biceps (a) and subscapularis (b) tendons can occur preventing closed reduction of a two-part unimpacted surgical neck displacement. The stump of the shaft (c) is anterior to these tendons. The skin hook is pulling the long head of the biceps out of the way so that the shaft can be returned under the subscapularis.

G and H, Arteriogram (G) after an unimpacted two-part surgical neck displacement showing interruption of the axillary artery. The fracture was fixed quickly with the compression band technique (H) (see Fig. 3–68) and the vessel was repaired.

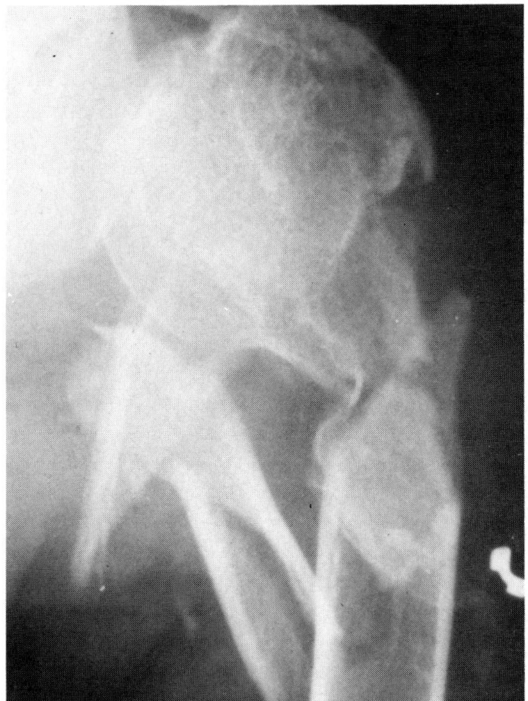

Figure 5–11. Anterior-posterior view of a comminuted two-part surgical neck displacement with the arm in a sling. The sling is causing overriding and tilts the head (rather than, as has commonly been misinterpreted, the head being tilted by the rotator cuff). The rotator cuff ordinarily holds the head in near-neutral adduction-abduction and rotation (see Fig. 5–10B). The sling is also internally rotating the arm, which twists the comminuted fragments. The pectoralis major is displacing several fragments of the shaft of the humerus medially. This lesion is usually treated with a lightweight, plastic spica cast, which holds the arm in neutral rotation (de-rotating the shaft to align it with the head), with the arm at the side (rather than in abduction). Abduction would place the pectoralis major under tension. Distraction delays union and is avoided.

tient. Internal fixation is not necessary, and attempts to accomplish this have failed to allow discontinuing external support because of the comminution.

Two-Part Lesser Tuberosity Displacement

Lesser tuberosity fractures are often seen with posterior dislocations but may be seen either as an isolated lesion (for example, following a seizure) or in association with an undisplaced fracture of the surgical neck (Fig. 5–12). Although this displacement produces spreading of the anterior fibers of the rotator cuff and results in a bony prominence, prominence of the lesser tuberosity alone has not had clinical significance. However, when a portion of the articular surface of the humeral head is broken off with the lesser tuberosity, a serious block against internal rotation occurs, as

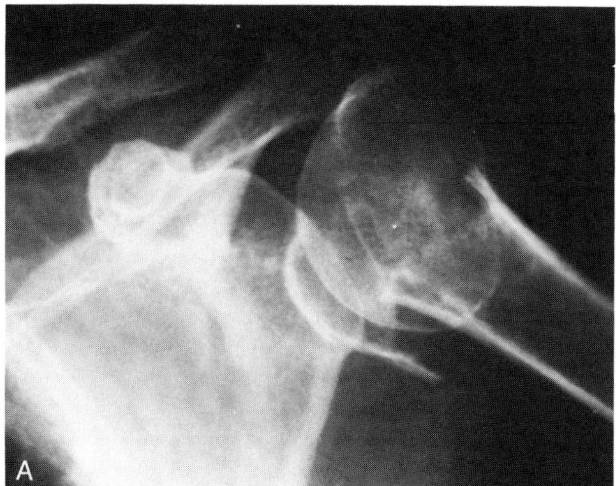

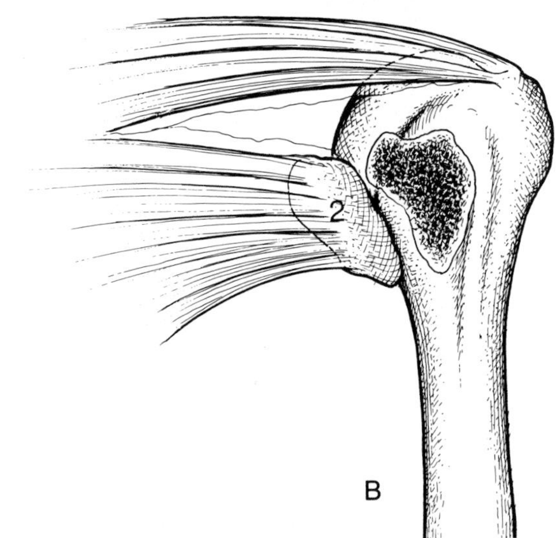

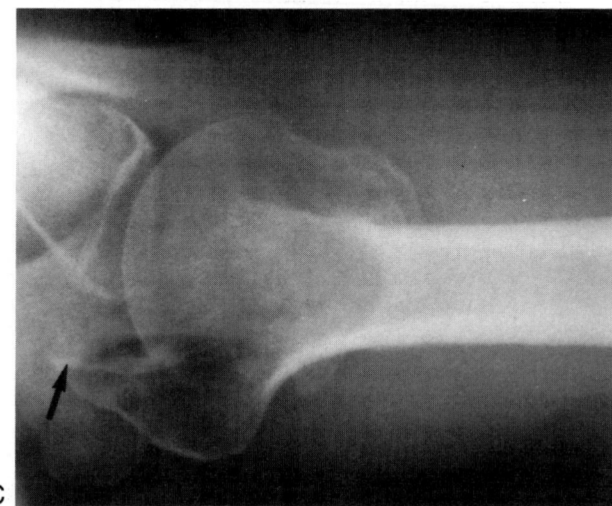

Figure 5–12. Two-part lesser tuberosity displacement (A and B) may be harmless. However, if a piece of the articular surface is displaced with the lesser tuberosity, as shown in the axillary view of the malunited fracture (C), it may block internal rotation and cause a stiff and painful shoulder. CT scan helps evaluate this lesion. Treatment of the latter is discussed in the text.

illustrated in Figure 5–12C, requiring open reduction and internal fixation.

Several malunited lesser tuberosity fractures of the type shown in Figure 5–12C have been treated by excision of the bone projecting in front of the glenoid, an extensive release of adhesions, and an intensive exercise program, with good results.

Two-Part Greater Tuberosity Displacement

The greater tuberosity has three distinct facets for the insertions of the supraspinatus, infraspinatus, and teres minor. Retraction and displacement of the entire greater tuberosity or one of its facets are pathognomonic of a longitudinal tear in the rotator cuff (see Fig. 5–13A to C). In general, the

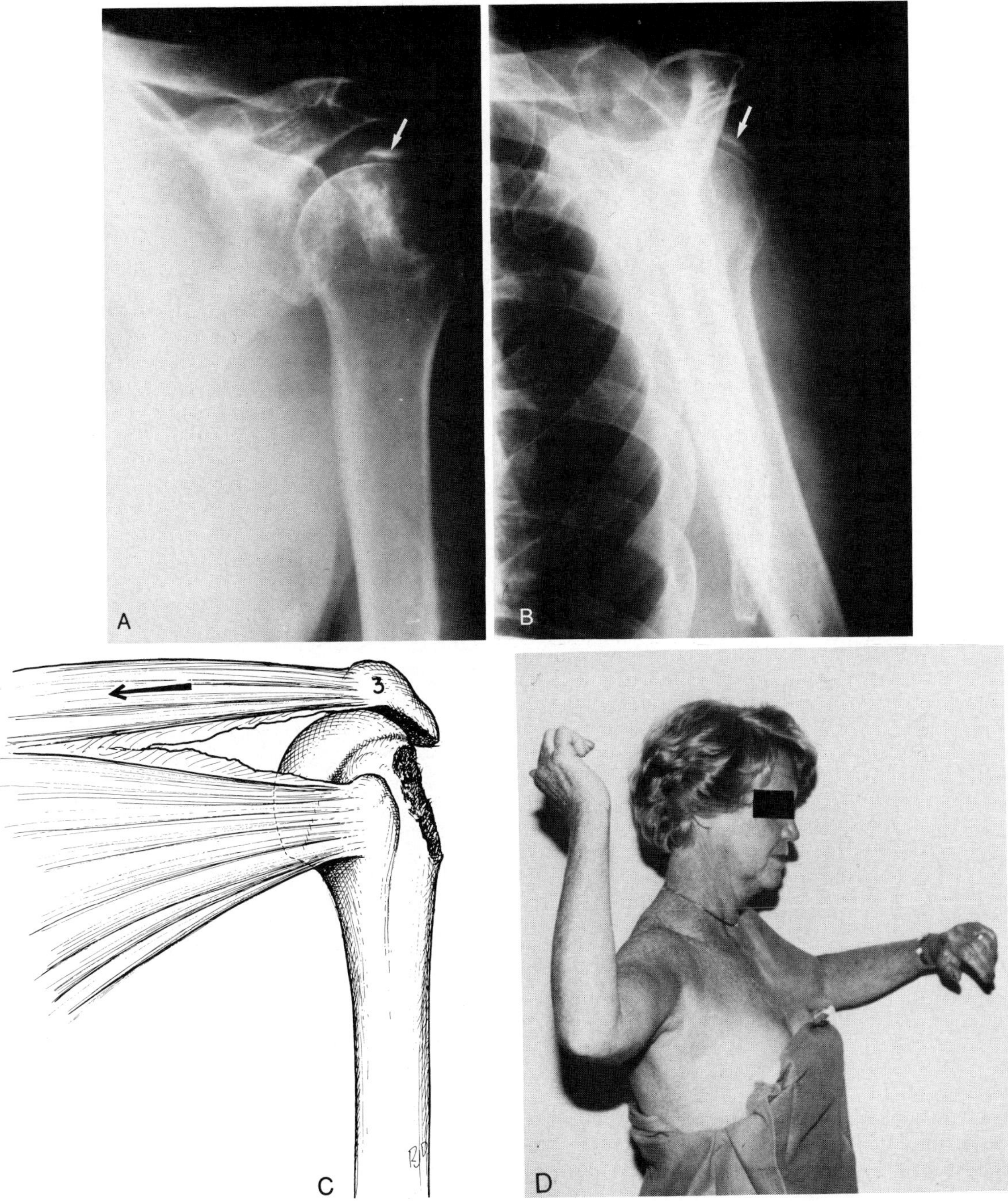

Figure 5–13. *Two-Part Greater Tuberosity Displacement.*

A, Anterior-posterior view (A) and lateral view (B). (Arrow indicates the retracted greater tuberosity.)

C, The rotator cuff is torn and retracted. Fragments block elevation and external rotation.

D, In the evaluation of two-part greater tuberosity displacements, loss of external rotation in abduction is a much more sensitive test than loss of external rotation with the arm at the side or loss of elevation.

Illustration continued on following page

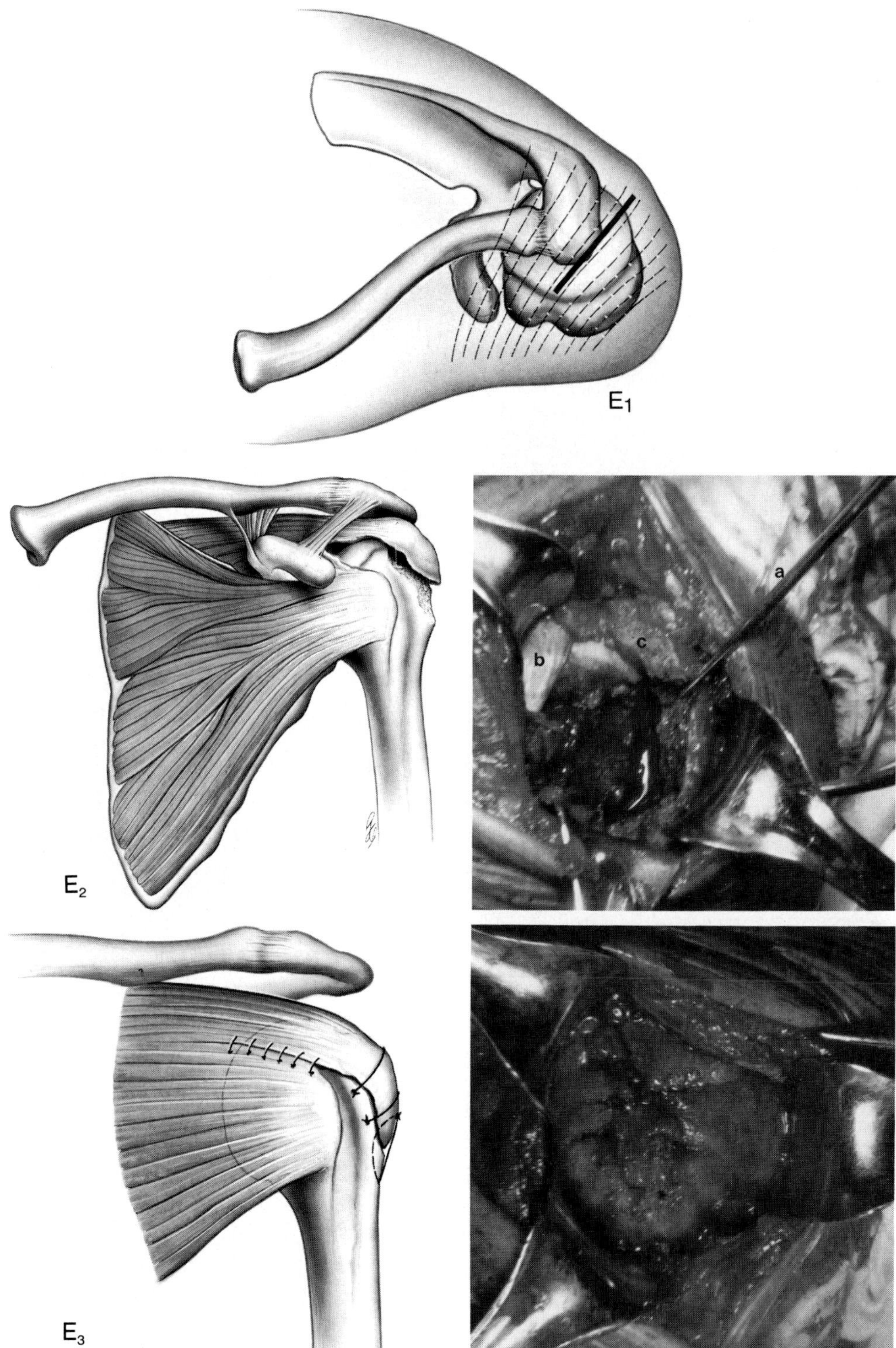

Figure 5–13 *Continued* E, Open reduction and rotator cuff repair for a two-part greater tuberosity displacement.

1, Skin incision and approach. A 6.0 cm. skin incision is made just lateral to the acromion in the skin lines. The deltoid muscle is split 5.0 cm. from above downward and is detached from the acromion for a distance of 1.0 cm. on each side of the split.

2, Hemorrhagic bursa is removed, and a skin hook (a) is used to pull the fragment of greater tuberosity (c) forward into the wound and against the raw bone from which it came (b). The biceps tendon may be exposed because the posterior side of the biceps groove is often fractured.

3, The fragment of greater tuberosity is usually reduced in size with a rongeur before suturing it in its normal anatomical location with three No. 5 or No. 2 nonabsorbable sutures as illustrated (left). The tear in the rotator cuff is sutured with 0 or 00 nonabsorbable sutures (right). The deltoid muscle is re-attached with care.

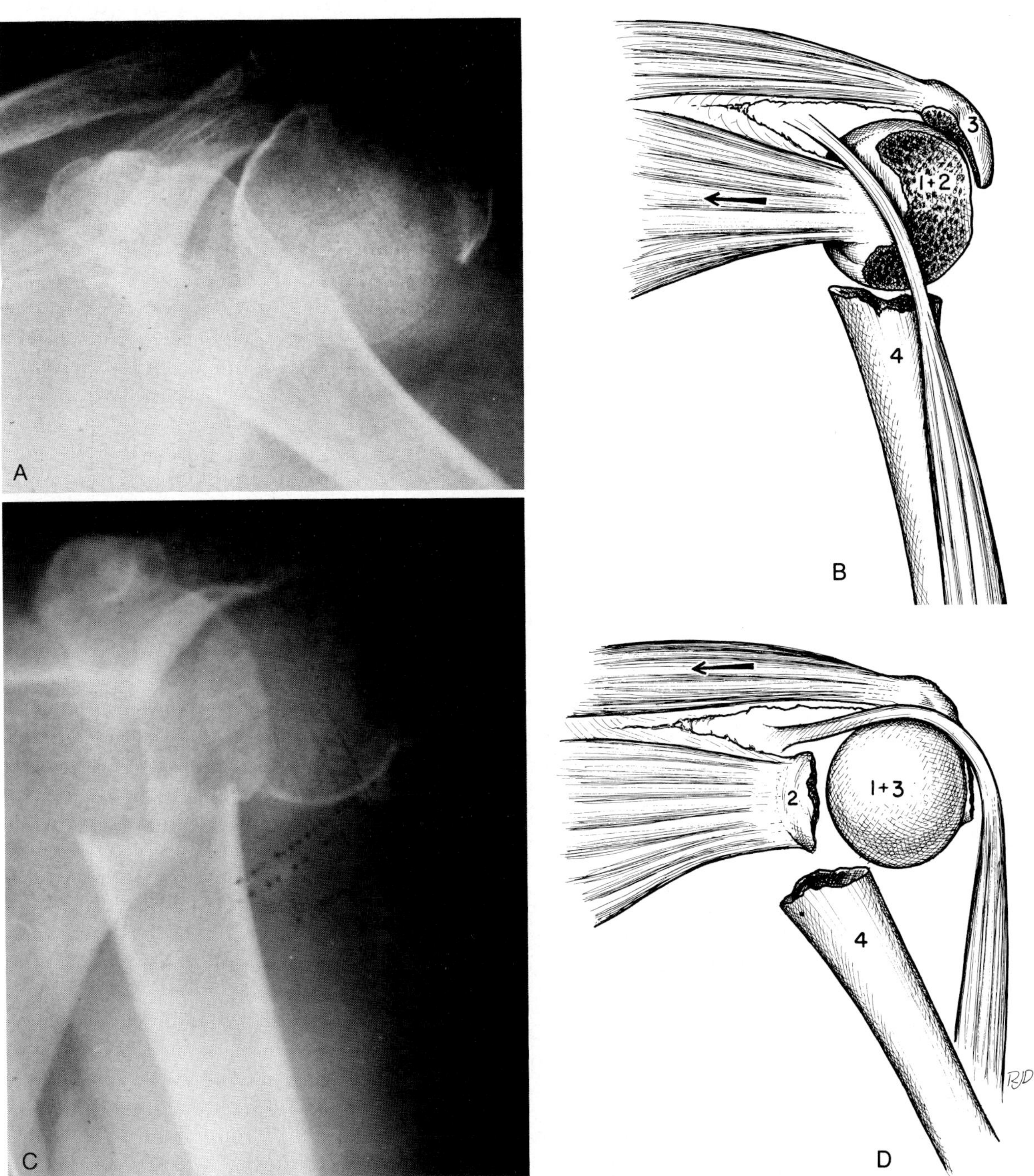

Figure 5–14. ***Three-Part Displacements. Pathology and Indications.*** A and B, Greater tuberosity three-part displacement. The articular surface of the head faces backward. The lesser tuberosity remains attached to the head, but the blood supply to the head is less abundant than in the lesion shown in C and D. C and D, Lesser tuberosity three-part displacement. The articular surface of the head faces anteriorly. The greater tuberosity remains attached with adequate blood supply for the head.

tuberosity fragment is large in younger patients and smaller in older patients. In addition to the cuff deficiency, the retracted tuberosity further impairs motion by impinging under the acromion and against the posterior glenoid, where it blocks external rotation and abduction (Fig. 5–12). It is now generally accepted that more than a 1.0 cm. displacement of this type in an active patient is best treated by open reduction and cuff repair. This can be accomplished through a two-inch, deltoid-splitting incision with minimal detachment of the deltoid muscle from the acromion, as described in Figure 5–12E. I usually excise part of the fragment and prefer to suture it in place with nonabsorbable sutures using a similar suture material for repairing the cuff (Fig. 5–12E). If a stable, minimally displaced fracture at the surgical neck level is also present, it is not disturbed.

Three-Part Displacements

Three-part displacements have been called rotary fracture-subluxation or rotary fracture-dislocations. The two types of three-part displacements are illustrated in Figure 5–14, which shows the muscle forces involved. An unimpacted surgical neck fracture is present, which is associated with detachment and retraction of one of the tuberosities. The other tuberosity remains attached to the articular segment and rotates it so as to open the defect in the rotator cuff. The anatomical distortion is much greater than that of two-part fractures because of these opposing forces on the muscle attachments. They cannot be reduced by closed methods (Fig. 5–15). However, because the articular segment retains soft-tissue attachments, it usually has sufficient blood supply to survive after carefully performed open reduction and internal fixation (Fig. 5–16).

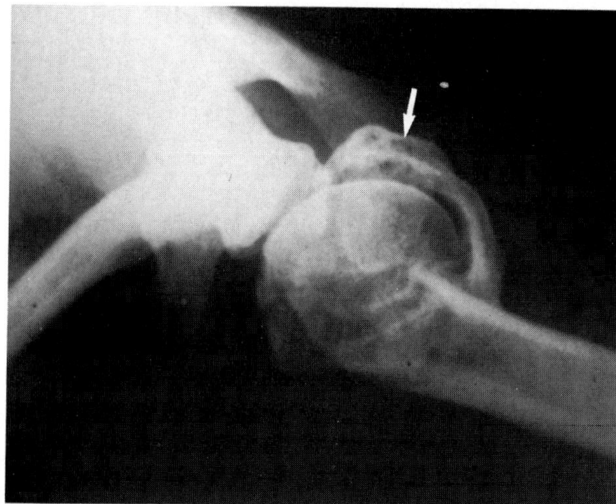

Figure 5–15. Axillary view after unsuccessful closed treatment of a three-part greater tuberosity displacement. There is marked rotary displacement of the head, causing it to face posteriorly. The retracted greater tuberosity (arrow) has malunited on the head, covering much of the articular surface and blocking external rotation.

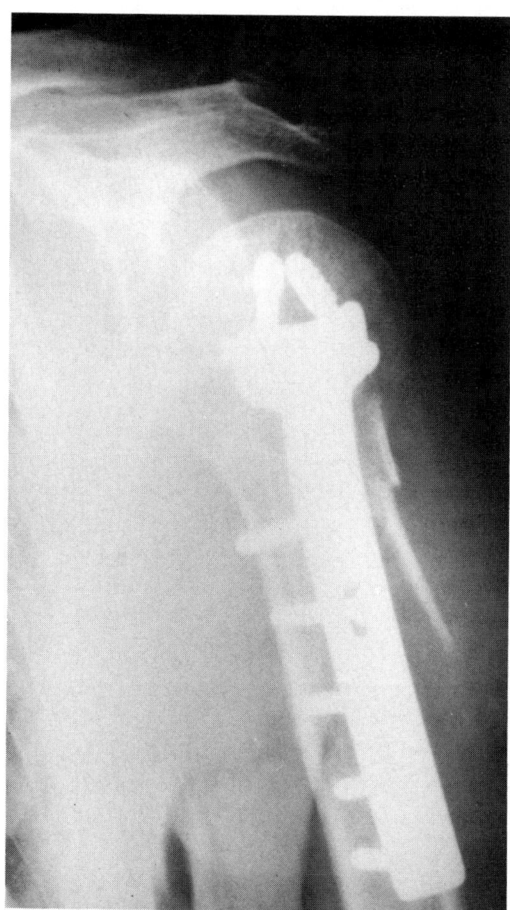

Figure 5–16. Internal fixation of a three-part displacement is often difficult because of soft bone and the short proximal fragment. Fortunately, in this case the bone was hard enough to hold a T-plate despite the comminuted surgical neck component. The patient is warned pre-operatively that removal of the internal fixation device and release of adhesions are often necessary after healing of the fracture to obtain optimal results.

Indications for Three-Part Displacement

A few surgeons have claimed adequate results following closed treatment, but on close scrutiny the majority of these authors have included some minimally displaced fractures with multiple fissure lines. A true "three-part displacement" has an unimpacted surgical neck component with rotary deformity and displacement of one of the tuberosities to block motion. Of course, in poor risk patients and those with doubtful ability to comply with a complicated post-operative exercise regimen, closed treatment (accepting considerable loss of movement and the possibility of continuing pain) is best. Other patients, when they learn of

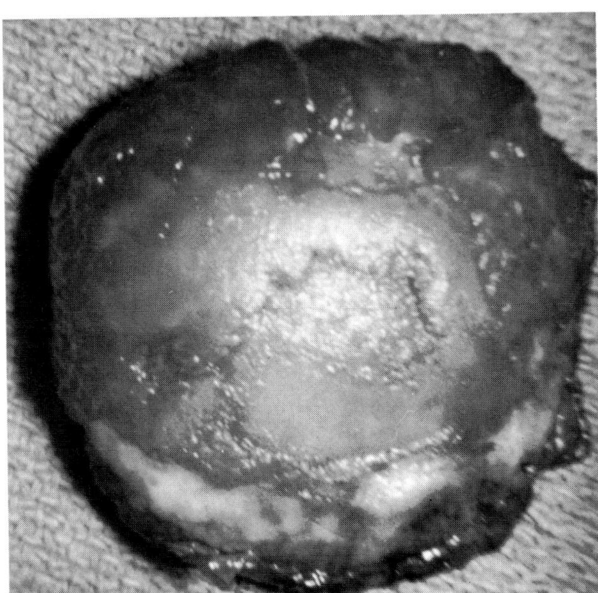

Figure 5–17. The humeral head removed at total shoulder arthroplasty for post-traumatic arthritis 11 years after an open reduction and internal fixation of a greater tuberosity three-part displacement. The shoulder had functioned satisfactorily for 9 years before it became arthritic and painful.

the limitations of closed treatment, want to strive to achieve something better and are offered surgical repair. However, the long post-operative exercise program and the possibility of further surgery to remove the internal fixation materials should be clear. Prior to open reductions for three-part fractures, I routinely explain to the patient that a further procedure will probably be necessary after the fracture has healed, to remove the fixation device and release adhesions.

Many of these lesions can be treated by open reduction; however, I now prefer prosthetic replacement with tuberosity and cuff repair (see Figs. 5–23 to 5–25) in older patients and those who have three-part greater tuberosity displacements with flimsy, tenuous soft-tissue attachments on the articular segment. I have seen a patient who had a good open reduction go on to develop traumatic arthritis requiring total shoulder arthroplasty (see Fig. 5–17), and other patients, as Cofield and Tanner observed,[148] who have had slow recoveries and less satisfactory and uncertain results.

Technique of Open Reduction of Three-Part Displacements

Open reduction is performed through a 15.0 cm incision and extended deltopectoral approach without detachment of the origin of the anterior deltoid (Fig. 5–18). After division of the clavipectoral fascia, the tendon of the biceps long head serves as a guide to the rotator interval (between the supraspinatus and subscapularis tendons and between the lesser and greater tuberosity seg-

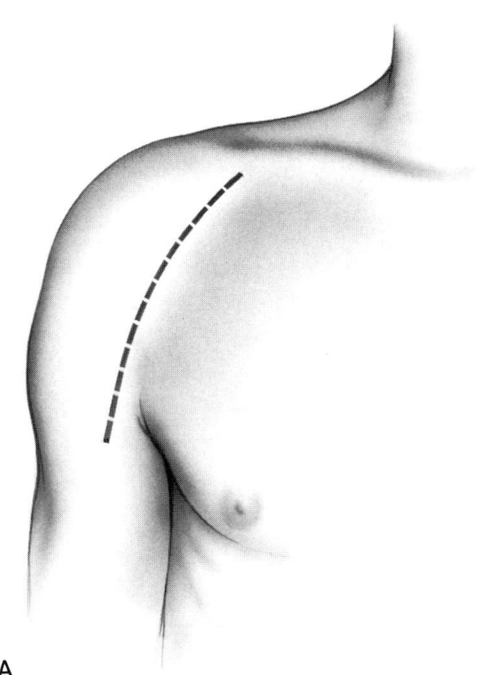

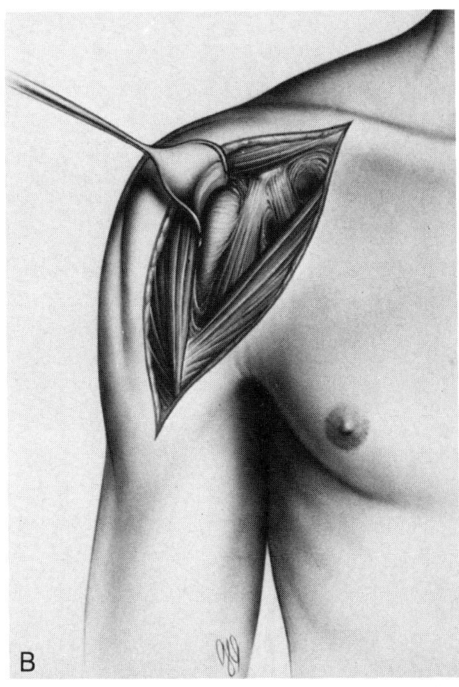

Figure 5–18. Technique of open reduction and internal fixation of three-part displacements. Position and draping as in Figure 5–23.

A, A 15.0 cm. incision is made over the deltopectoral interval.

B, Extended deltopectoral approach.

Illustration continued on following page

ments). Surgical trauma to the soft-tissue attachments of the articular segment is carefully avoided.

When the bone is hard enough to hold screws, an AO T-plate with transfixing screws is used (Figs. 5–16 and 5–18E). Otherwise, the compression band technique (Fig. 5–18E) is used. The displaced tuberosity is first reduced and fixed to the articular segment with No. 2 or No. 5 nonabsorbable sutures or screws. The displaced surgical neck component is then reduced and secured with an intramedullary rod and compression band or with the T-plate and screws. The choice depends on the quality of the bone. The tear in the rotator cuff is closed with nonabsorbable sutures.

Although I have found these methods of internal fixation to be superior to pins, staples, or intramedullary rods, the bone is rarely adequate for immediate unprotected movement of the shoulder. Pendulum and gentle passive exercises (see Fig. 7–7) are usually permissible, but a sling and swathe is usually worn between exercise sessions until early callus appears in the x-ray films (usually at four weeks). At that point, the self-assistive exercises (aimed at minimizing adhesions by maintaining adequate motion) are progressed (see Fig. 7–8), as for fractures with minimal displacement.

After six to nine months, when mature healing has occurred, the fixation devices are usually removed, at which time adhesions around the upper humerus are often released to obtain better motion because the T-plate is bulky or the intramedullary rod is usually backing out and prominent. In some

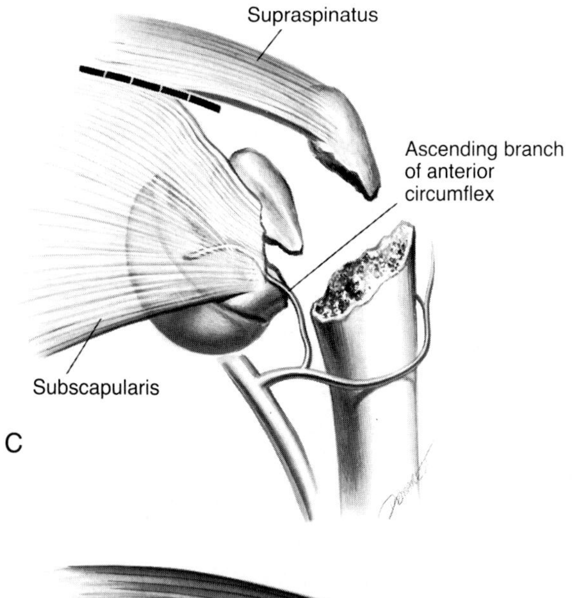

Figure 5–18 *Continued* C, Preserve the blood supply to the head.

D, Reduction forces. If the greater tuberosity is displaced (left), externally rotate the head and pull the greater tuberosity forward. If the lesser tuberosity is displaced (right), internally rotate the head and pull the lesser tuberosity laterally.

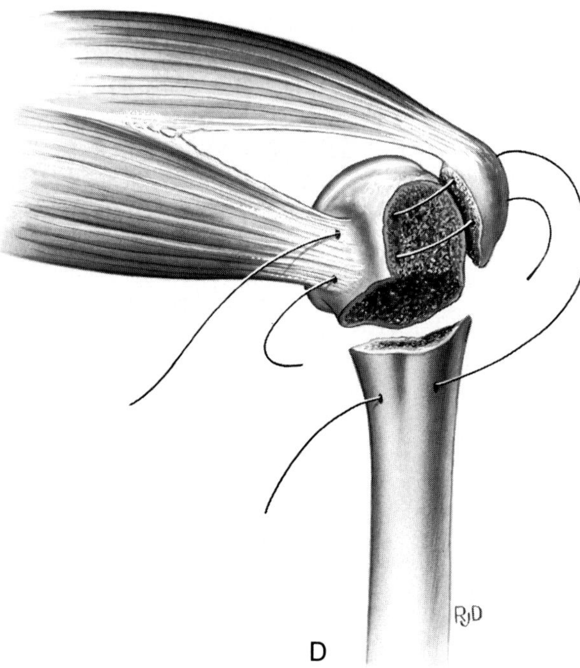

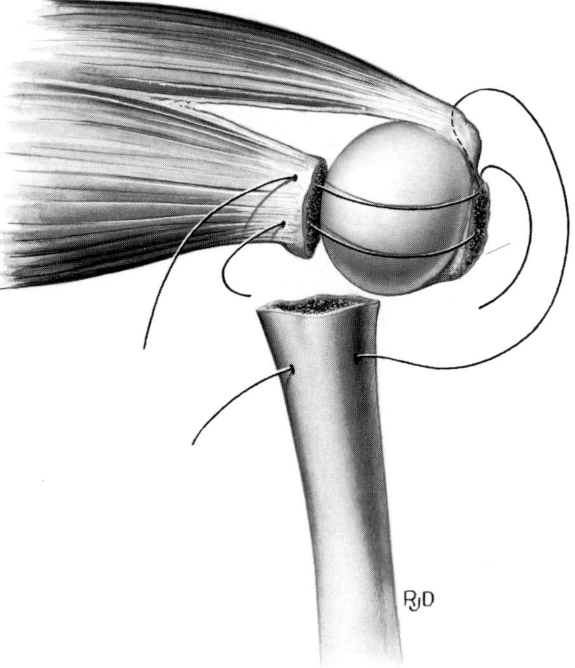

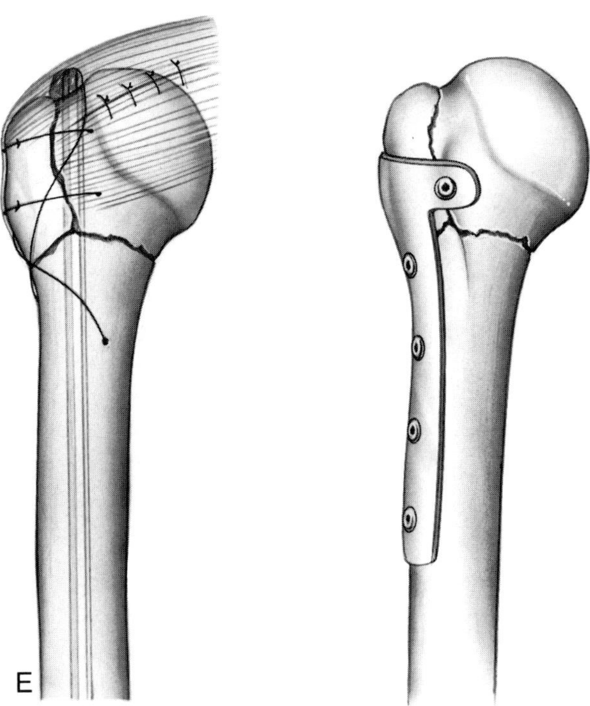

Figure 5–18 *Continued* E, Fixation requires ingenuity. The two types most often used are shown. The compression band (left) is used when the bone is soft, and the AO T-plate (right) is employed when the bone is hard.

Procedure for closure and suction drains is same as for a replacement arthroplasty (see text and Fig. 5–23).

cases with good motion, the rod can be removed earlier through a stab-wound incision made over the prominence of the rod. If a release is necessary, it is done through the upper three-quarters of the previous approach.

Because of the long rehabilitation program and less certain outcome of open reduction and internal fixation, I have, as discussed above, come to favor prosthetic replacement with tuberosity and cuff repair in older patients and those with three-part greater tuberosity displacements with frail soft-tissue attachments on the articular segment.

Four-Part Displacements

When both tuberosities are detached and retracted (see Fig. 5–19), the articular segment remains as a "shell fragment" devoid of soft-tissue attachments and without a blood supply. To distinguish four-part displacements from minimal displacements with multiple fissure lines, in the four-part displacement the head is out of contact with the glenoid. The head may be displaced (dislocated) out of contact with the glenoid laterally, anteriorly, posteriorly, or inferiorly (Fig. 5–19). When the head is displaced laterally, the term lateral fracture-dislocation aptly applies. Closed

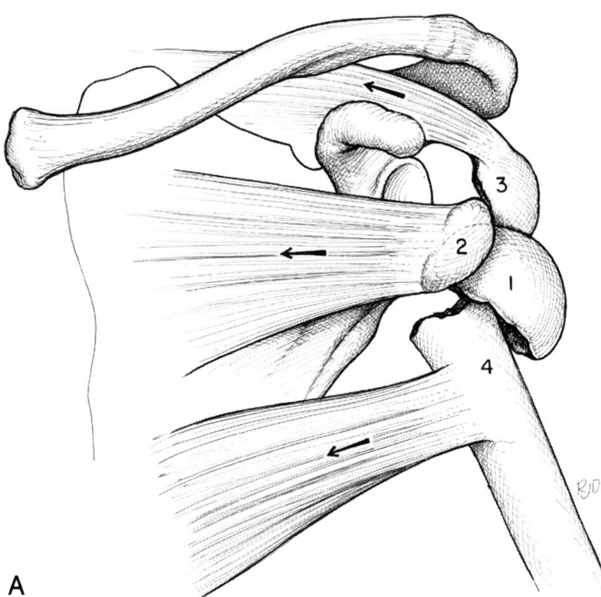

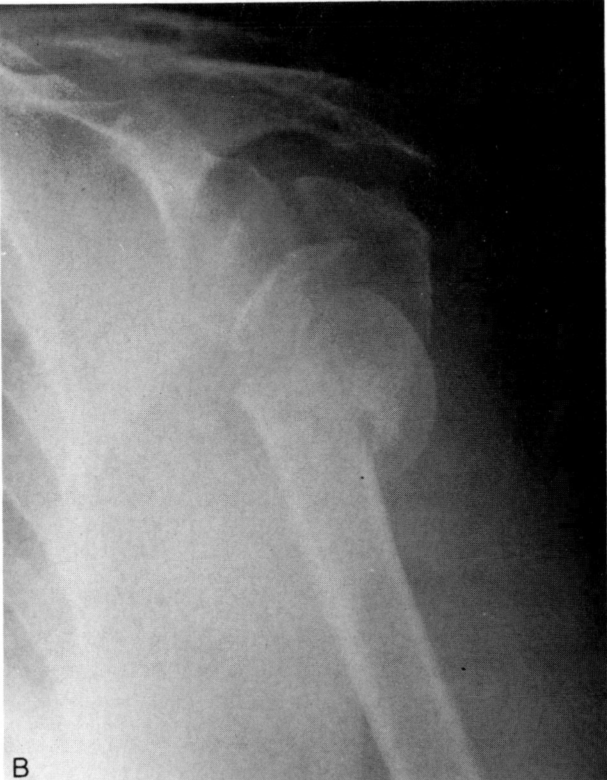

Figure 5–19. *Four-Part Displacements.* The articular surface is dislocated out of contact with the glenoid and is separated from both tuberosities. The tuberosities may be retracted or may be together.

A, Lateral four-part fracture-dislocation.

B, Lateral four-part fracture-dislocation.

Illustration continued on following page

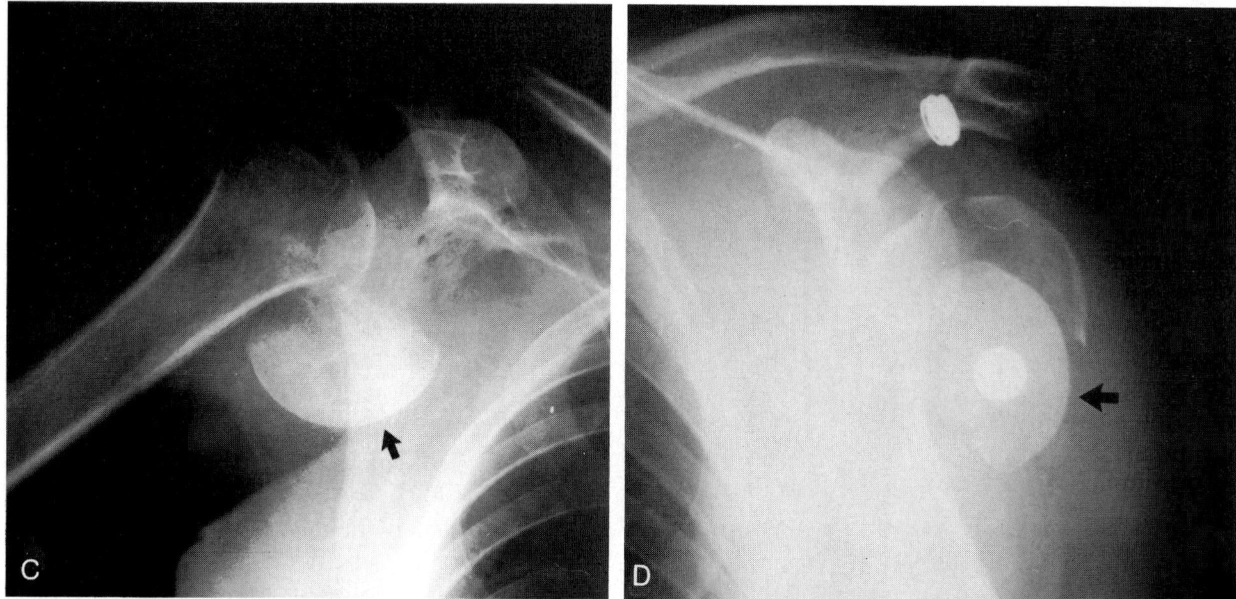

Figure 5–19. *Continued* C, Anterior four-part fracture-dislocation. D, Posterior four-part fracture dislocation.

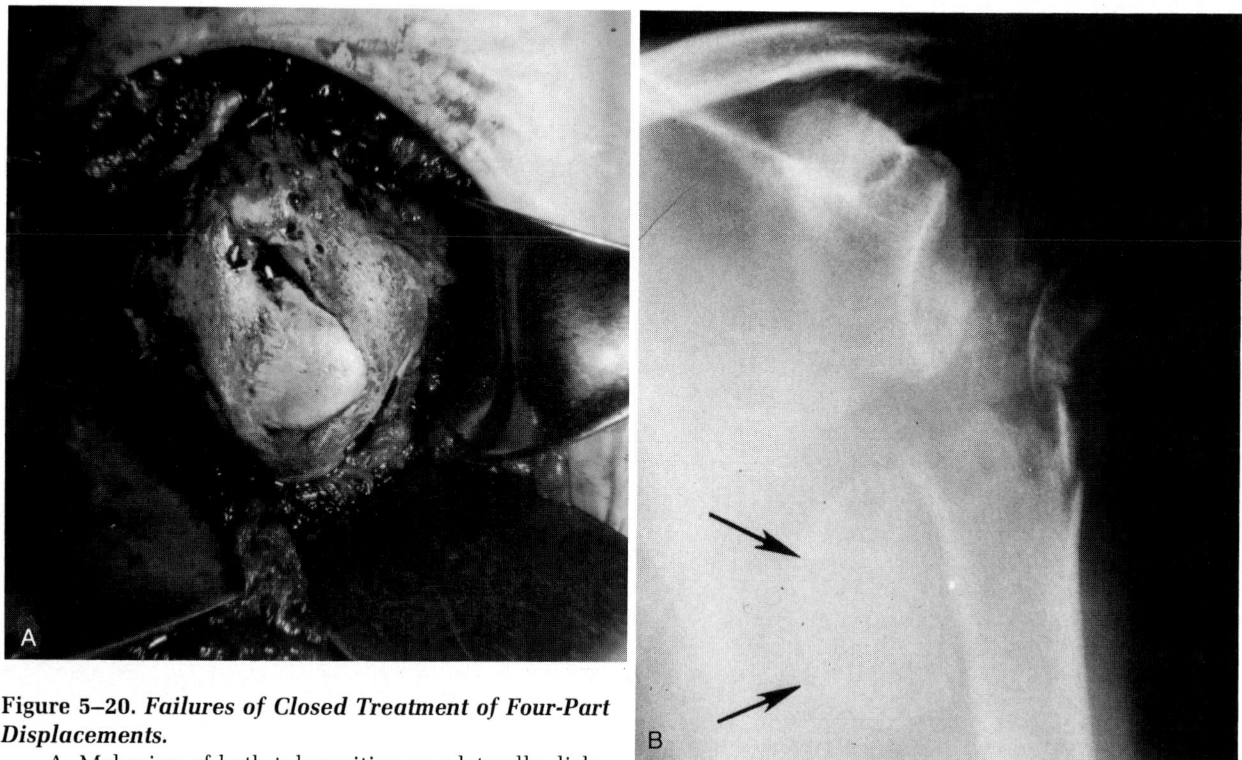

Figure 5–20. *Failures of Closed Treatment of Four-Part Displacements.*

A, Malunion of both tuberosities on a laterally dislocated head (as in Fig. 5–19B) seen two years later at the time of total shoulder arthroplasty.

B, Marked displacement of the head after two attempts at closed reduction, which resulted in injury to all three major nerve components of the arm and hand.

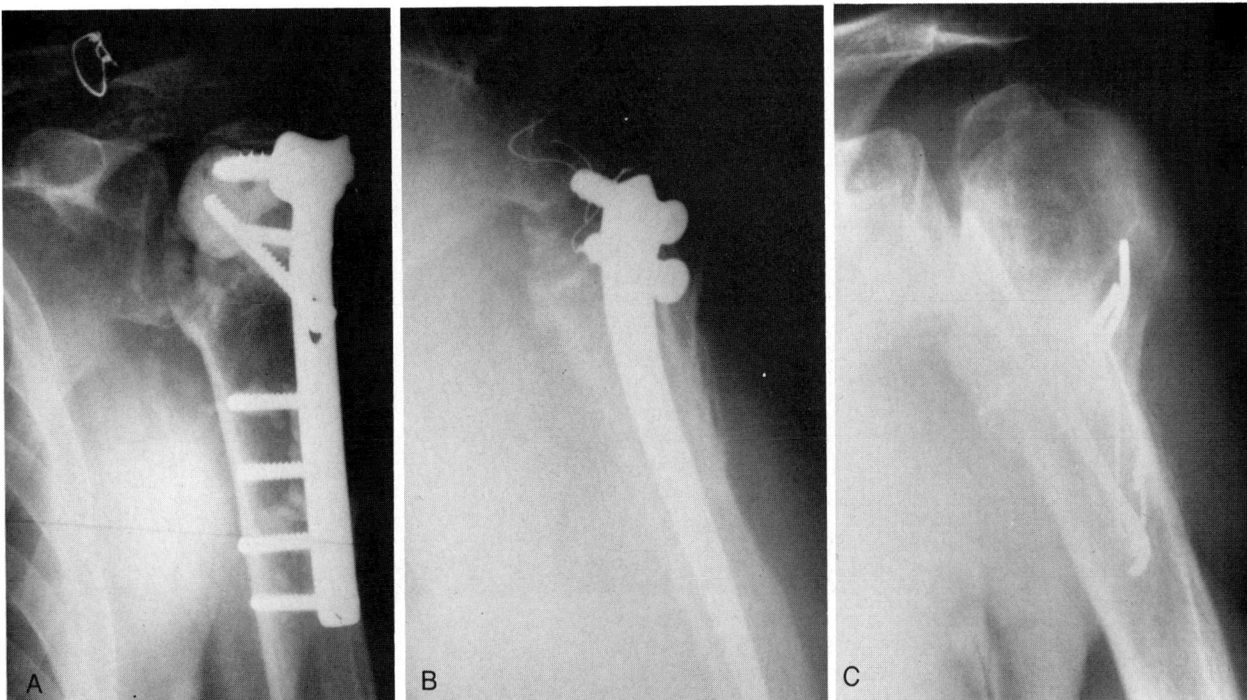

Figure 5–21. ***Failures of Open Reduction and Internal Fixation of Four-Part Displacements.***

A, Avascular necrosis and severe pain four years after the second AO T-plate fixation. Cement had been used at the screw holes because the screws of the first attempted plating had pulled out of the head shortly after their insertion. At the time of total shoulder arthroplasty, a few Staphylococcus aureus organisms were cultured, although there had never been a clinical infection.

B, Avascular necrosis three years after open reduction and internal fixation with a Mouradian intromedullary device. This was treated with a total shoulder arthroplasty.

C, Avascular necrosis two and one-half years after open reduction and multiple AO tension-band pin fixation. There was pain and little glenohumeral motion.

treatment is unsatisfactory (Fig. 5–20), and the incidence of avascular necrosis and resorption of the head following open reduction and internal fixation has been so high (Figs. 5–21 and 5–22) that I prefer to treat this lesion initially with a prosthesis (Fig. 5–23).[8, 149, 150, 241, 264] The prosthesis replaces the articular segment and provides firm anchorage for accurate nonmetallic suture fixation of the tuberosities and repair of the cuff. It is of key importance to restore the length of the humerus so that the deltoid power and glenohumeral stability are retained (Figs. 5–23 to 5–25). This allows early gentle passive exercises and minimizes adhesions. Following this procedure, it should be possible to begin EPM (early passive motion) exercises on the first or second day. Active exercises are not attempted until the tuberosities have united. The importance of a good rehabilitation program cannot be overemphasized, and exercises should be continued until near-normal motion and function are achieved, working first for passive range and later for strength.

Glenohumeral Fracture-Dislocations

In a fracture-dislocation, the articular segment is outside the joint space, anteriorly, posteriorly, laterally, or inferiorly. The associated humeral fracture is almost always displaced and can be a two-, three-, or four-part displacement (see Figs. 5–26 through 5–33). It is of clinical value in analyzing these lesions to note that the anterior dislocations are associated with displacement of the greater tuberosity, whereas posterior dislocations are associated with displacements of the lesser tuberosity. Both tuberosities are usually displaced in four-part fracture-dislocations; however, in some cases the tuberosities remain together and the head is dislocated out from under them. As stated previously, the head is out of contact with the glenoid in all four-part displacements, so all of these lesions should be considered to be fracture-dislocations.

Because fracture fragments and damaged soft tissue are present outside the joint space, these

Text continued on page 391

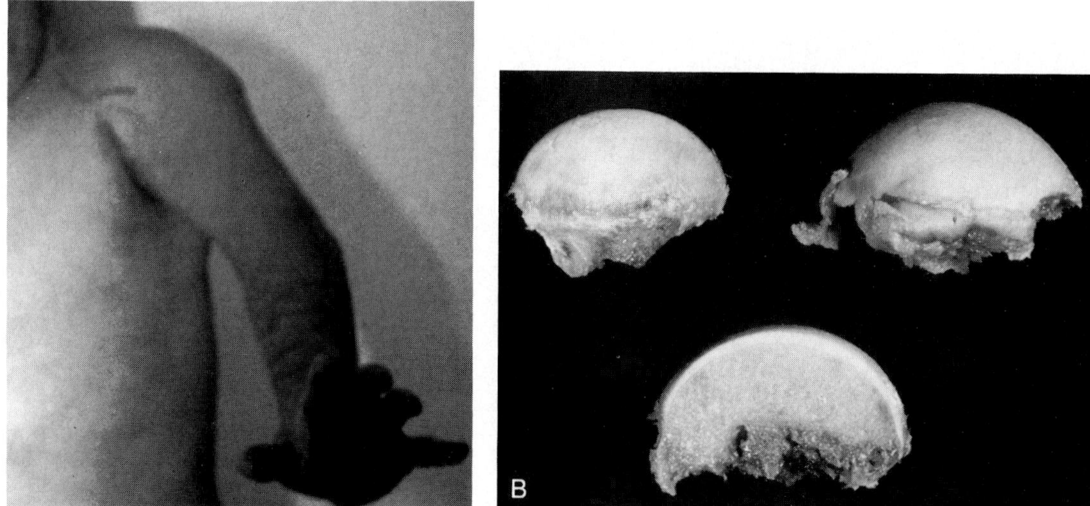

Figure 5–22. The logic of early humeral head replacement for four-part fracture-dislocations.

A, A typical disability with a failed open reduction. There was extensive scar and pain.

B, A detached head fragment removed at the time of replacement of the head for a recent four-part displacement. It is not worth the risk of losing all of the soft tissue around the shoulder in an effort to save this little piece of bone.

Unfortunately, prosthetic replacement can be a difficult procedure and demands dedication to the rehabilitation program for optimal results.

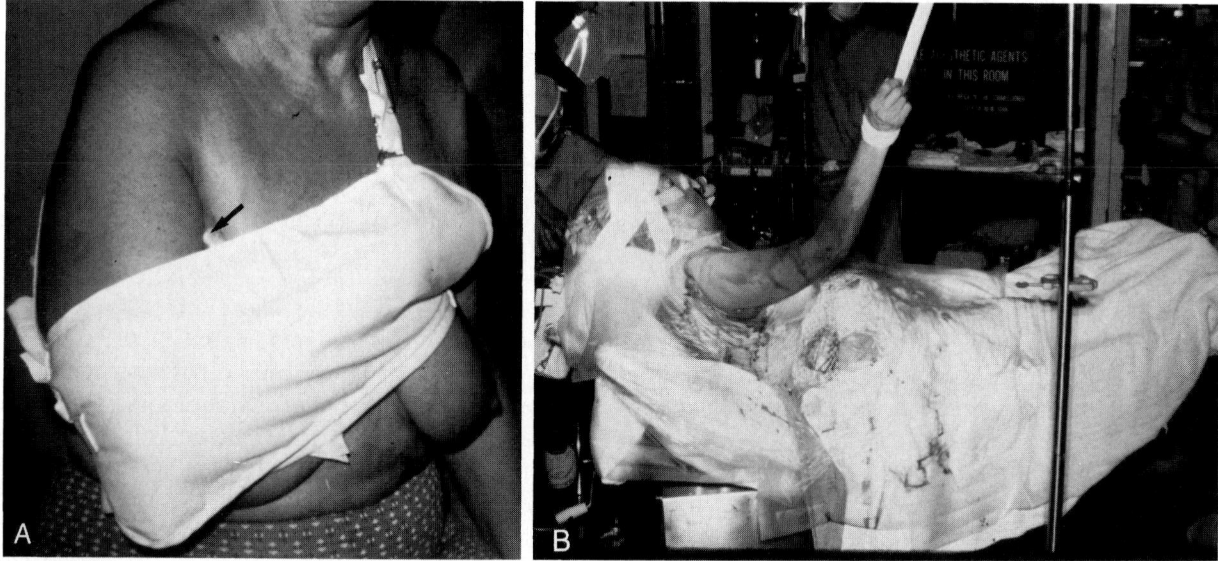

Figure 5–23. Technique of prosthetic replacement for four-part displacements. A four-part lateral fracture-dislocation is illustrated.

A, While awaiting surgery, a sling and swathe protects the arm and an axillary pad (arrow) with antiseptic solution is changed daily to prevent excoriation of the skin.

B, With the patient under intratracheal anesthesia (or scalene block anesthesia), the arm is suspended from an intravenous pole to immobilize the fracture during the skin preparation. Positioning and draping are performed with the same care as described in Figure 3–24.

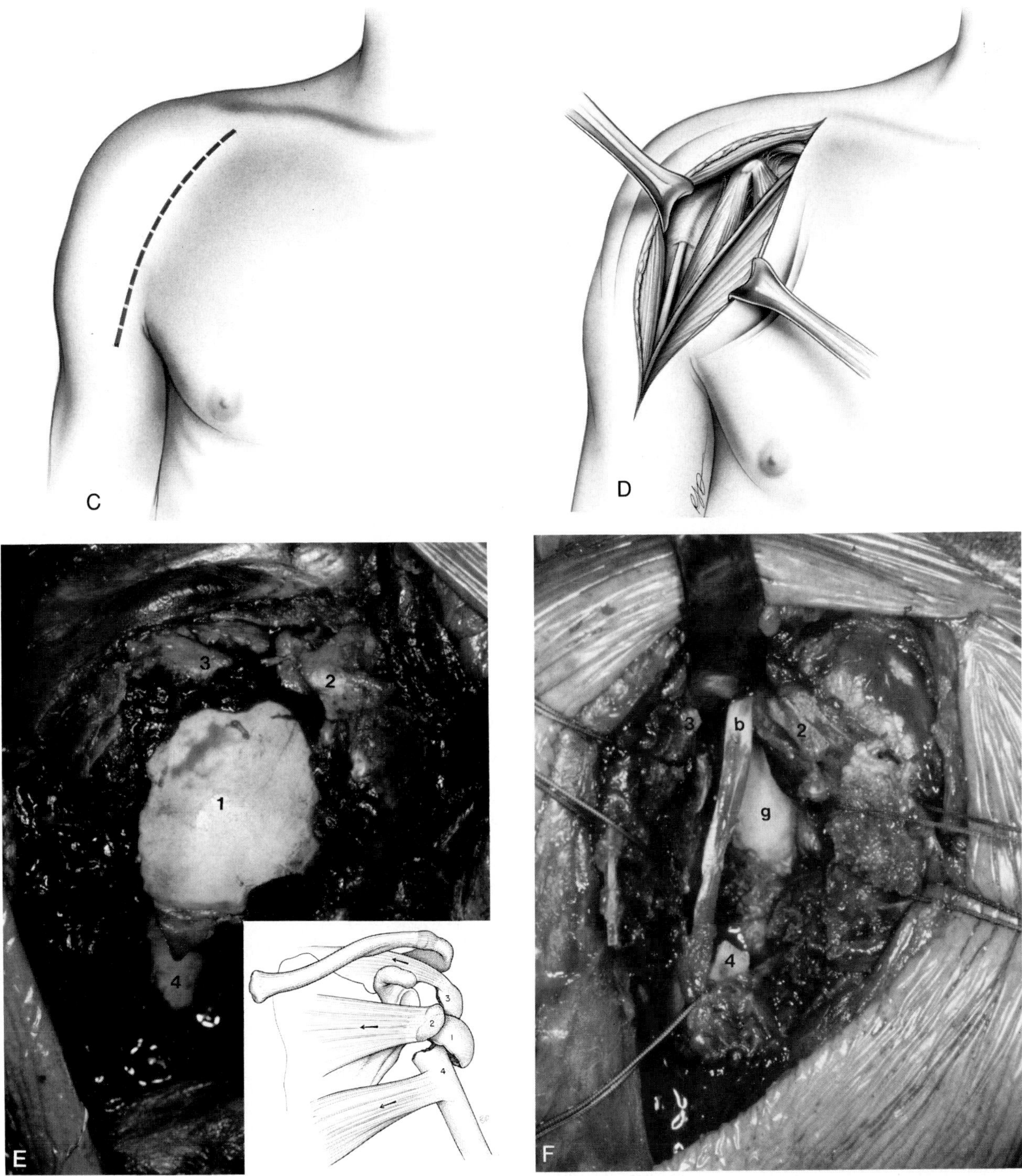

Figure 5–23 *Continued* C, The extended deltopectoral approach is used (see Fig. 3–25). A 15.0 cm. incision is made from the clavicle across the coracoid and down to the deltoid insertion.

D, The approach is developed between the deltoid and the pectoralis major, retracting the cephalic vein medially. The clavipectoral fascia is divided, exposing the long head of the biceps, which is a guide to the interval between the supraspinatus and subscapularis tendons and between the lesser and greater tuberosities.

E, The appearance of this lateral fracture-dislocation at surgery and as depicted in the inset. The interval between the greater tuberosity (3) and the lesser tuberosity (2) is developed (without dividing the long head of the biceps) so that the head and bone fragments inside the joint can be removed.

F, No. 5 or No. 3 nonabsorbable sutures are placed around the tuberosities for retraction and later for anchoring the tuberosities to the prosthesis. In this illustration, the head and bone fragments have been removed from the joint and the empty glenoid (g) can be seen. The biceps (b) is intact, and the tuberosities (2 and 3) are being retracted by the nonabsorbable sutures. The upper end of the shaft (4) can be seen.

Illustration continued on following page

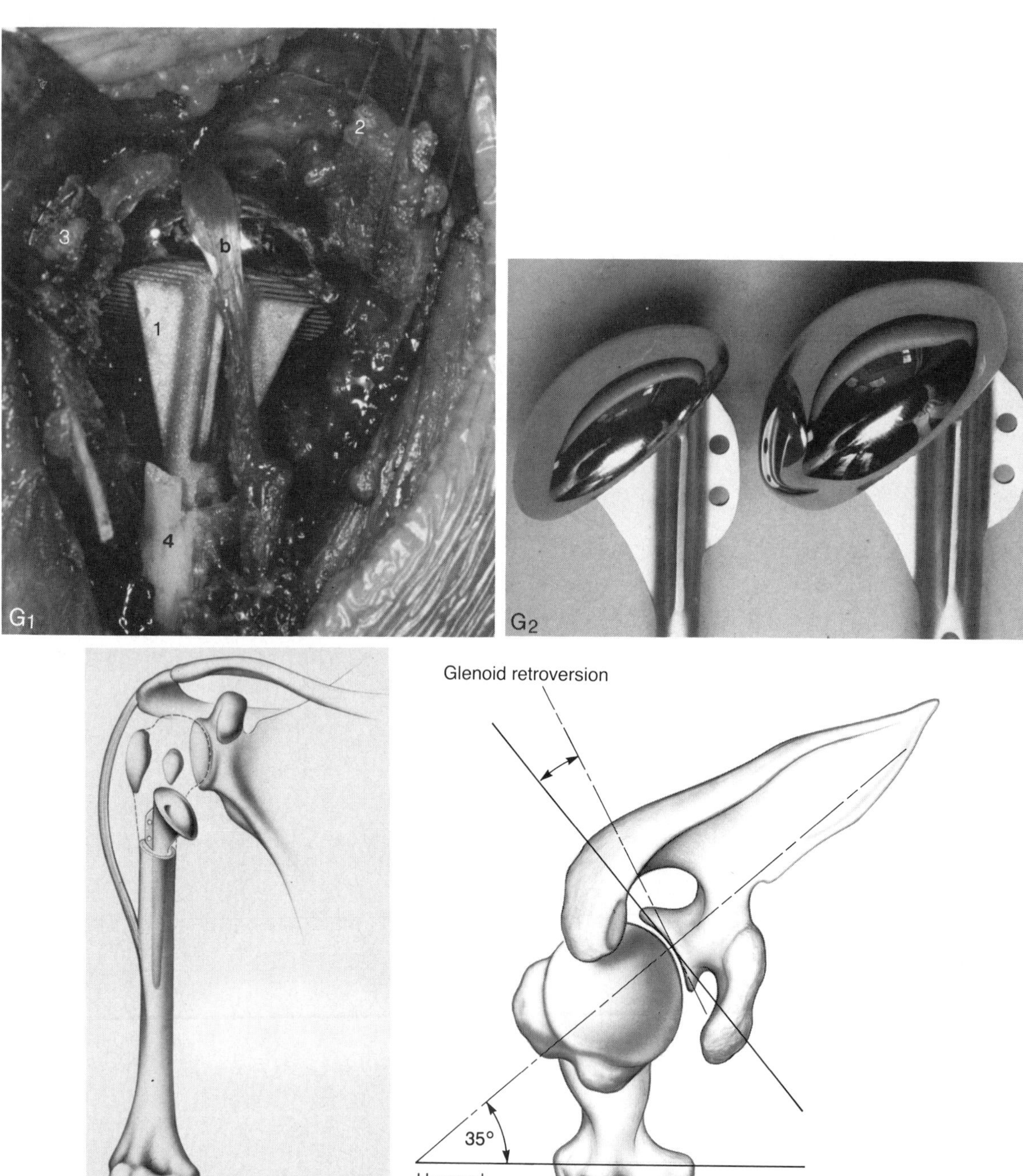

Figure 5–23 *Continued* G, After reaming the medullary canal (see Figs. 3–26 and 3–29), a trial prosthesis is inserted to determine the proper length of the head (tuberosity-glenoid space), height of the head (preserving the length of the arm), and version of the head G1. Depicted is the trial prosthesis in place in the medullary canal (4) between the tuberosities (2 and 3) and beneath the biceps (b). The head is against the glenoid. The proper prosthetic head length is determined by pulling the tuberosities together (with the stay sutures) around the prosthesis. If the length of the capsule and rotator cuff does not permit the tuberosities to be approximated, the shorter head (G2, left) is used. The longer head (G2, right) is used whenever possible because it affords better leverage for the muscles G3. The height of the head is determined by putting traction on the arm to place tension on the myofascial sleeve and by placing the head of the prosthesis opposite the glenoid while measuring the amount of the prosthesis that is protruding above the shaft of the humerus. The prosthesis will later be cemented at this level, as shown in Figure 5–52E and F. If the prosthesis is implanted too low, as illustrated, it will dislocate and the deltoid muscle will be too long to raise the arm (G4). The prosthetic head is placed at 35 degrees retroversion. The head should point directly toward the glenoid when the arm is held in neutral rotation. Neutral rotation is determined by flexing the elbow 90 degrees and by palpating the epicondyles at the elbow. The shaft of the humerus is marked by an osteotome to ensure proper rotation at the time of cementing.

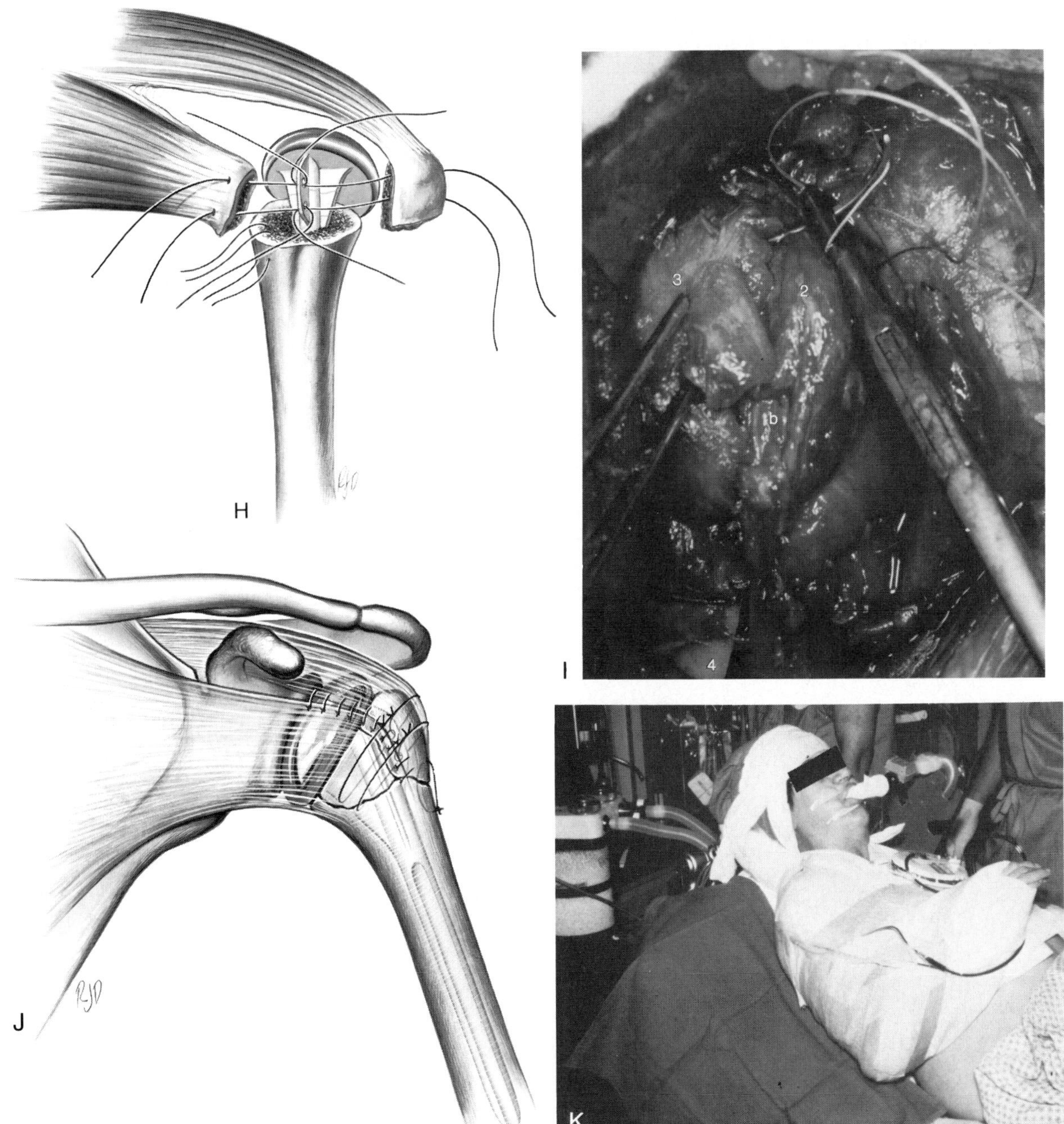

Figure 5–23 *Continued* H, After making a drill hole in the shaft and placing a No. 2 suture in it to be used in attaching the greater tuberosity, the prosthesis is cemented in the shaft using a vent tube as depicted in Figure 3–29. The tuberosities are then firmly attached to the prosthesis with No. 5 and No. 2 nonabsorbable sutures. It is important that the tuberosities be below the level of the head of the prosthesis so that they will not impinge against the acromion.

I, The biceps tendon (b) is aligned between the greater (3) and lesser (2) tuberosities and is incorporated in the rotator cuff repair with 0 and 00 nonabsorbable sutures.

J, At the conclusion of the repair, the tuberosities lie below the level of the top of the head of the prosthesis and are securely fastened to the prosthesis. The greater tuberosity is attached to the shaft, with the suture inserted prior to cementing. Fragments of bone are wedged in between the greater tuberosity and the shaft to expedite bone union.

K, Suction drains are placed between the deltoid and the rotator cuff; the deltopectoral interval is closed with interrupted 00 sutures, and the skin is approximated with a removable subcuticular suture. A sling and swathe is applied as shown in Figure 3–32.

The suction drains are removed at 24 hours, and early passive motion (EPM) (see Fig. 7–7) is begun at about 48 hours.

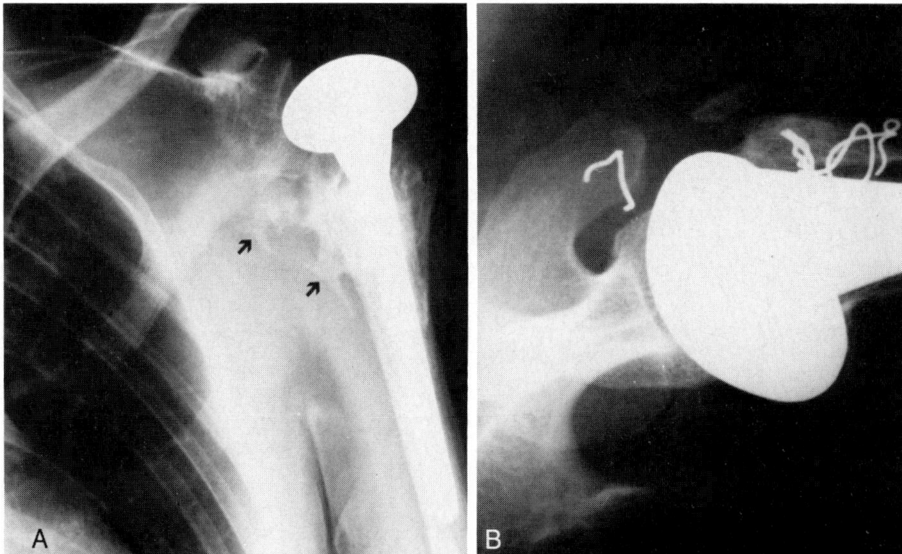

Figure 5–24. Complications of replacement of the humeral head for four-part fracture-dislocations.

A, Heterotopic bone (arrows) formed in 7 of 61 shoulders in our recent series,[149, 150] usually after delayed surgery beyond ten days. All but 5 regained adequate motion spontaneously.

B, Late breakage of wires used to fix the tuberosities can occur years after the repair and can necessitate wire removal. Therefore, wire is no longer used.

The most important complication following this procedure for fractures is stiffness of the shoulder due to inadequate supervision of post-operative exercises.

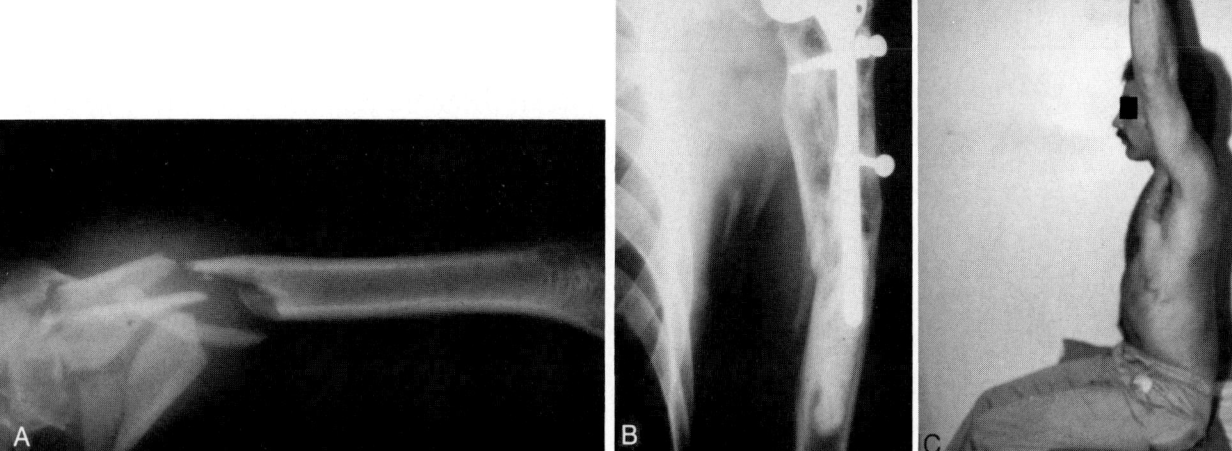

Figure 5–25. ***Results of Humeral Head Replacement for Four-Part Fracture-Dislocations.*** Because of the improvements in technique and aftercare outlined in Figure 5–23, in my more recent series of four-part fracture-dislocations, presented in 1987,[150] the typical result was "excellent," in contrast to the 1970 series,[8] in which the typical result was "satisfactory" (using the criteria for rating shown in Figures 3–101 and 3–102). Preservation of the attachment of the origin of the deltoid muscle, preservation of the normal length of the humerus, better anchorage of the stem of the component, and earlier passive motion along with the improved exercise program were considered to be responsible for the improvement.

A, Pre-operative axillary view of a comminuted, head-splitting, four-part fracture-dislocation.

B, Prosthetic reconstruction of this lesion.

C, Result of this reconstruction shown in B was rated "excellent," seen here six years after surgery.

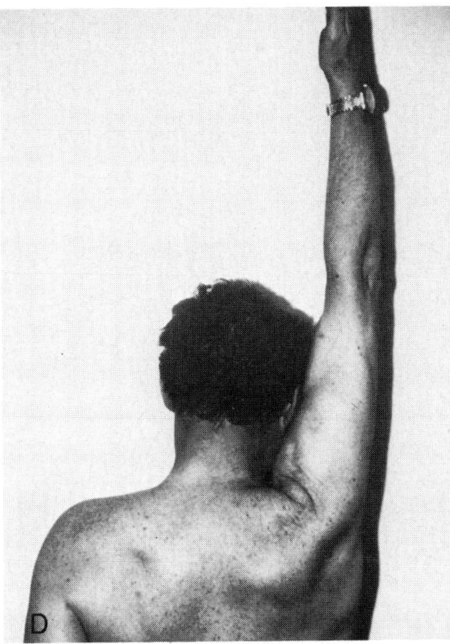

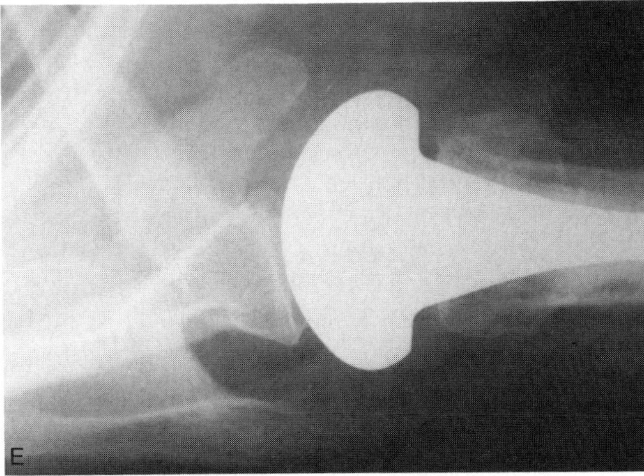

Figure 5–25 *Continued* D, An excellent result 12 years after replacement showing preservation of the muscles around the shoulder. Excellent ratings were given to 51 of the 61 shoulders in the recent series.

E, Axillary view made 11 years after humeral head replacement for a four-part fracture-dislocation showing good preservation of the contour of the glenoid. Erosion of the glenoid has not been a problem following this procedure provided that good joint motion is obtained.

lesions are prone to cause unwanted pericapsular bone formation, which restricts motion and is usually referred to as "myositis ossificans." Factors that appear to be related to the production of this complication are (1) repeated unsuccessful attempts at manipulative reduction, (2) open reduction delayed beyond ten days, and (3) possible variations in the tissue responses to repair in individual patients. This complication appears to be related to the effect of re-injury on early repair responses. In any event, it is important to reduce fracture-dislocations within the first week, avoiding repeated manipulations and unnecessary trauma.

A second feature of fracture-dislocations is the association of nerve injuries, which may require prompt decompression from either the displaced head or the shaft.

ANTERIOR FRACTURE-DISLOCATIONS

Two-Part Anterior Fracture-Dislocations

The greater tuberosity is displaced in approximately 15 per cent of anterior dislocations (Fig. 5–26). This is the most common type of fracture-dislocation. The ligaments and capsule usually cause the fragment to fall in good position after closed reduction of the dislocation. When this happens, no further surgical reduction of the fragment or suture of the rotator cuff is needed. The most atraumatic reduction possible should be used. I prefer traction with gradual abduction until the head can be gently lifted into the joint (see Fig. 4–30).

Occasionally, the greater tuberosity remains displaced and retracted more than 1.0 cm. after reduction of the dislocation. The problem is then that of a two-part greater tuberosity displacement. This is best treated by open reduction of the tuberosity and cuff repair (see Fig. 5–12E).

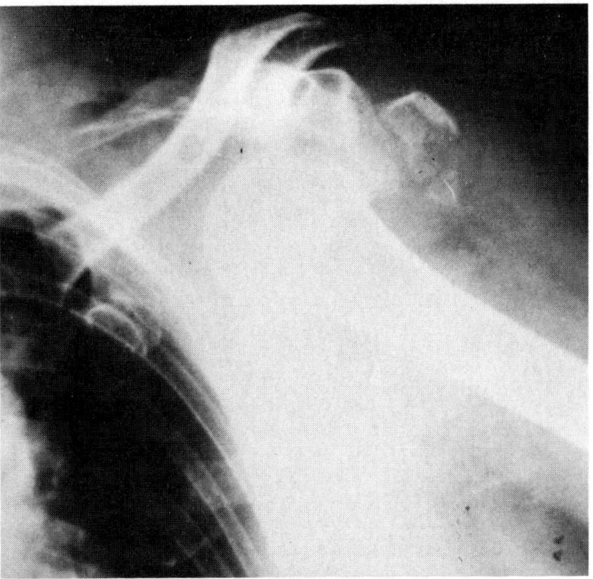

Figure 5–26. Two-part anterior fracture-dislocation almost always occurs with a displacement of the greater tuberosity, as shown.

Two common errors in assessing these lesions are failure to test for axillary nerve palsy and mistaking a facet avulsion for "calcium deposits." Prognostically, it is of interest that dislocations associated with this fracture rarely become recurrent dislocations. This is explained by the fact that the anterior ligaments have not been torn, and once fracture healing occurs the joint is stable.

Three-Part Anterior Fracture-Dislocations

The articular segment and lesser tuberosity are in continuity, so that the subscapularis and anterior capsule remain attached to provide circulation to the head (Figs. 5–14 and 5–27). I believe that a more gentle and accurate reduction can be accomplished surgically than by closed reduction. The subscapularis interferes with closed reduction and tends to rotate the head, even when it can be relocated into the joint. Residual internal rotation of the head after closed reduction may make it appear to be upside down on x-rays. Internal fixation as for other three-part lesions and cuff repair is preferred when feasible (see Fig. 5–18), and especially in younger patients; however, immediate prosthetic reconstruction is performed in selected cases (see Fig. 5–23).

Four-Part Anterior Fracture-Dislocations

Four-part anterior fracture-dislocation is not uncommon. Both tuberosities are usually retracted, but in about one-third the soft tissue holds the tuberosity fragments in contact (without retraction), so that the head is dislocated out from under them (Figs. 5–19C and 5–28). In all four-part lesions, the head is detached from all or nearly all soft-tissue attachments, and the incidence of late avascular necrosis is so high that I prefer prosthetic replacement and tuberosity repair, as described in Figures 5–23 to 5–25.

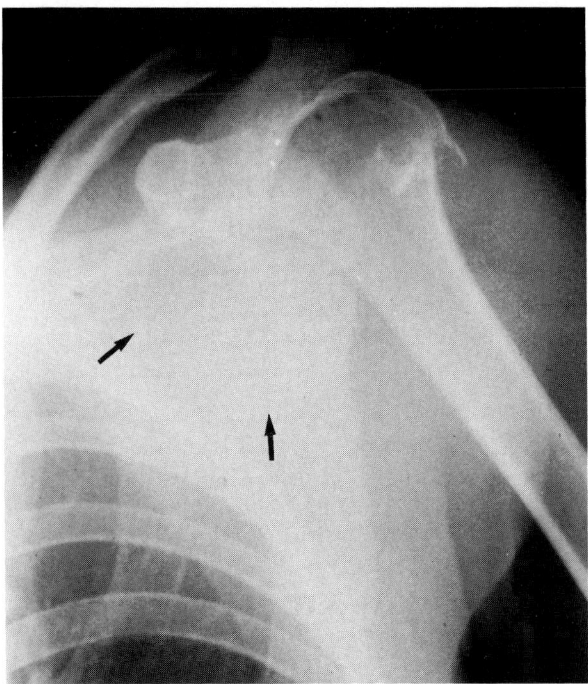

Figure 5–27. Three-part anterior fracture-dislocation. The lesser tuberosity remains attached to the head (arrows), while the greater tuberosity is usually retracted by the external rotators.

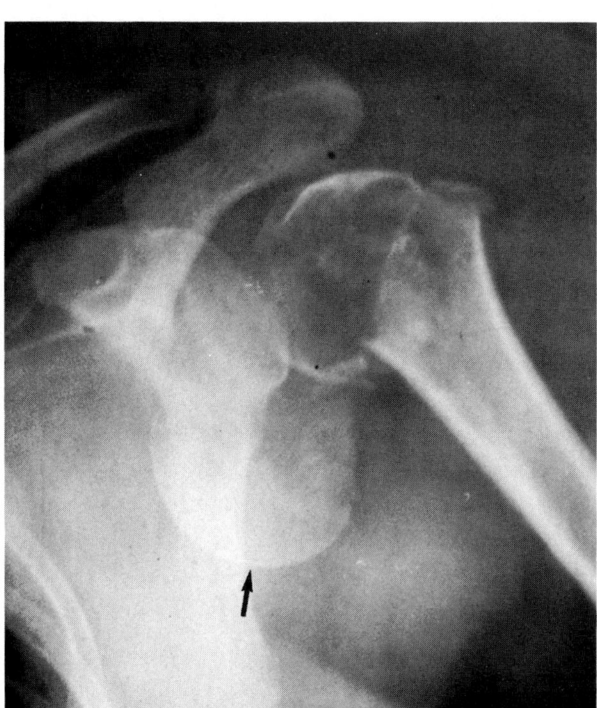

Figure 5–28. Four-part anterior fracture-dislocation. In this case, as in about 40 percent of four-part displacements, the tuberosities remain in approximation despite marked displacement of the head (arrow). In the majority, the tuberosities are retracted by the rotator cuff more than in this example.

POSTERIOR FRACTURE-DISLOCATIONS

Two-Part Posterior Fracture-Dislocations

Avulsion of the lesser tuberosity often accompanies posterior dislocation because of the tension placed on the subscapularis tendon and anterior capsule (Fig. 5–29). This fracture per se is of no importance, and closed reduction is indicated. The method I prefer for reducing a posterior dislocation is to apply traction while the arm is held in 90 degrees forward flexion and gradually adducting it across the chest (see Fig. 4–33), causing the glenoid to lever the neck of the humerus laterally. This unlocks the head from behind the glenoid, so that the head can be re-located with minimal risk of further fracture. Following reduction, the arm is immobilized at the side but in slight external rotation and extension for four weeks.

Three-Part Posterior Fracture-Dislocations

This lesion is often missed because of inadequate radiographic studies. An axillary x-ray is the best way to establish the diagnosis (Fig. 5–30). This should always be obtained if the lesion is suggested in other views. If it is recognized early, closed reduction by traction in forward flexion and gradual adduction may be successful, but I usually find it necessary to do an open reduction and internal fixation (see Fig. 5–18). Immediate prosthetic replacement is not considered for this lesion because the greater tuberosity is attached to the head and affords an abundant blood supply to the articular segment.

Four-Part Posterior Fracture-Dislocations

This lesion (Figs. 5–19D and 5–31) cannot be adequately reduced by closed means, and because the incidence of avascular necrosis is very high, I prefer early prosthetic replacement and tuberosity repair (see Figs. 5–23 to 5–25).

Fractures of the Articular Surface

Impression Fractures

Small lesions are often seen at the posterior edge of the articular surface in patients with recurrent anterior dislocation, as described by Malgaigne;[161] and the roentgen appearance was later described by Hill and Sachs.[162] Bone loss at this site may be the source of osteochondral bodies that become detached to float free in the joint. Larger impression fractures result from acute dislocations when there is severe impact of the head against the rim of the glenoid, usually with posterior dislocations (Fig. 5–32). The bone beneath the in-

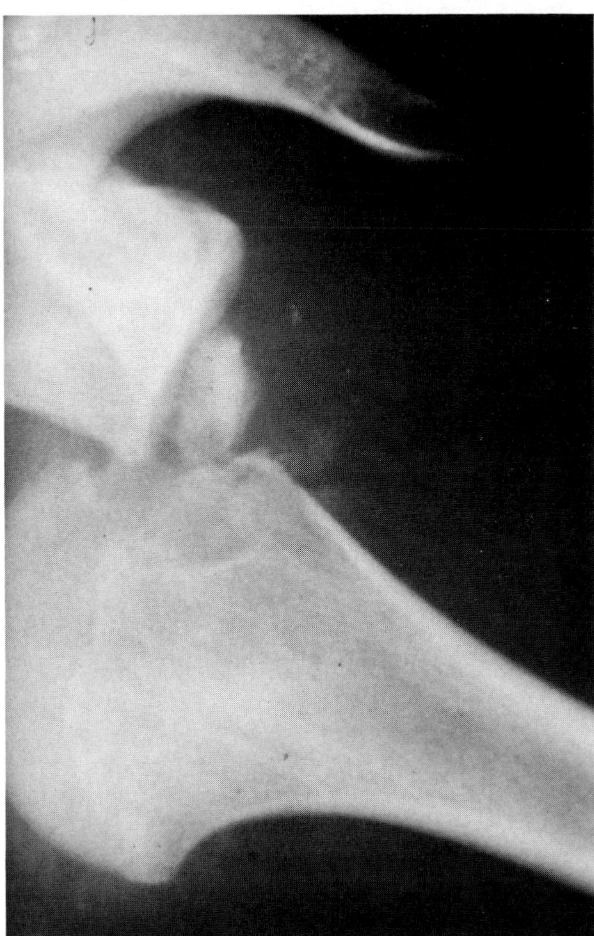

Figure 5–29. Axillary view of two-part posterior fracture-dislocation. The lesser tuberosity was avulsed.

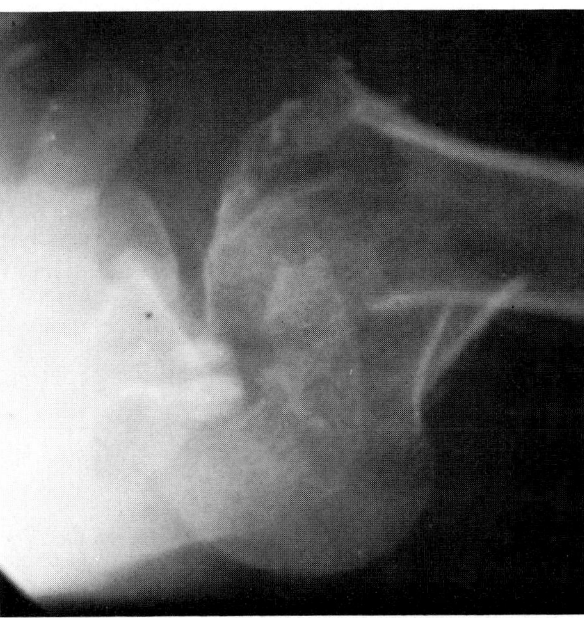

Figure 5–30. Axillary view of a three-part posterior fracture-dislocation. The greater tuberosity remains with the head.

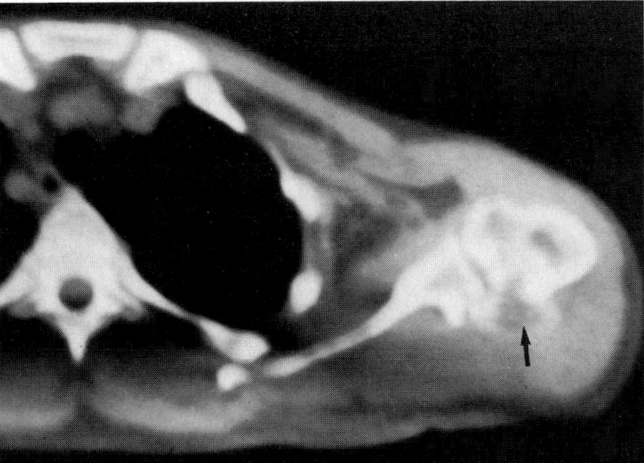

Figure 5–31. Computerized tomographic scan of a three year old, unreduced four-part posterior fracture-dislocation. Part of the head (arrow) was crushed, avascular, and collapsed. The posterior part of the head (arrow) had united to the shaft; however, it was soft from disuse atrophy.

The value of the computerized tomographic scan in recent posterior fracture-dislocation is illustrated in Figure 5–5.

dented cartilage is compressed and crushed. The indentation locks the head behind the glenoid, where it remains unless the posterior dislocation is recognized and reduced.

Treatment varies with the age of the lesion and the size of the head defect. There are three possibilities:

1. When the lesion is recognized early, if less than 20 per cent of the articular surface is involved, the joint is stable after closed reduction. Reduction is accomplished by traction forward with adduction, and the arm is immobilized in a cast in slight external rotation (Fig. 4–32E).

2. If from 20 to 40 per cent of the articular surface is indented, the joint is often unstable after closed reduction. In this situation, I prefer to transplant the lesser tuberosity with the attached subscapularis tendon into the head defect (Fig. 5–32F).

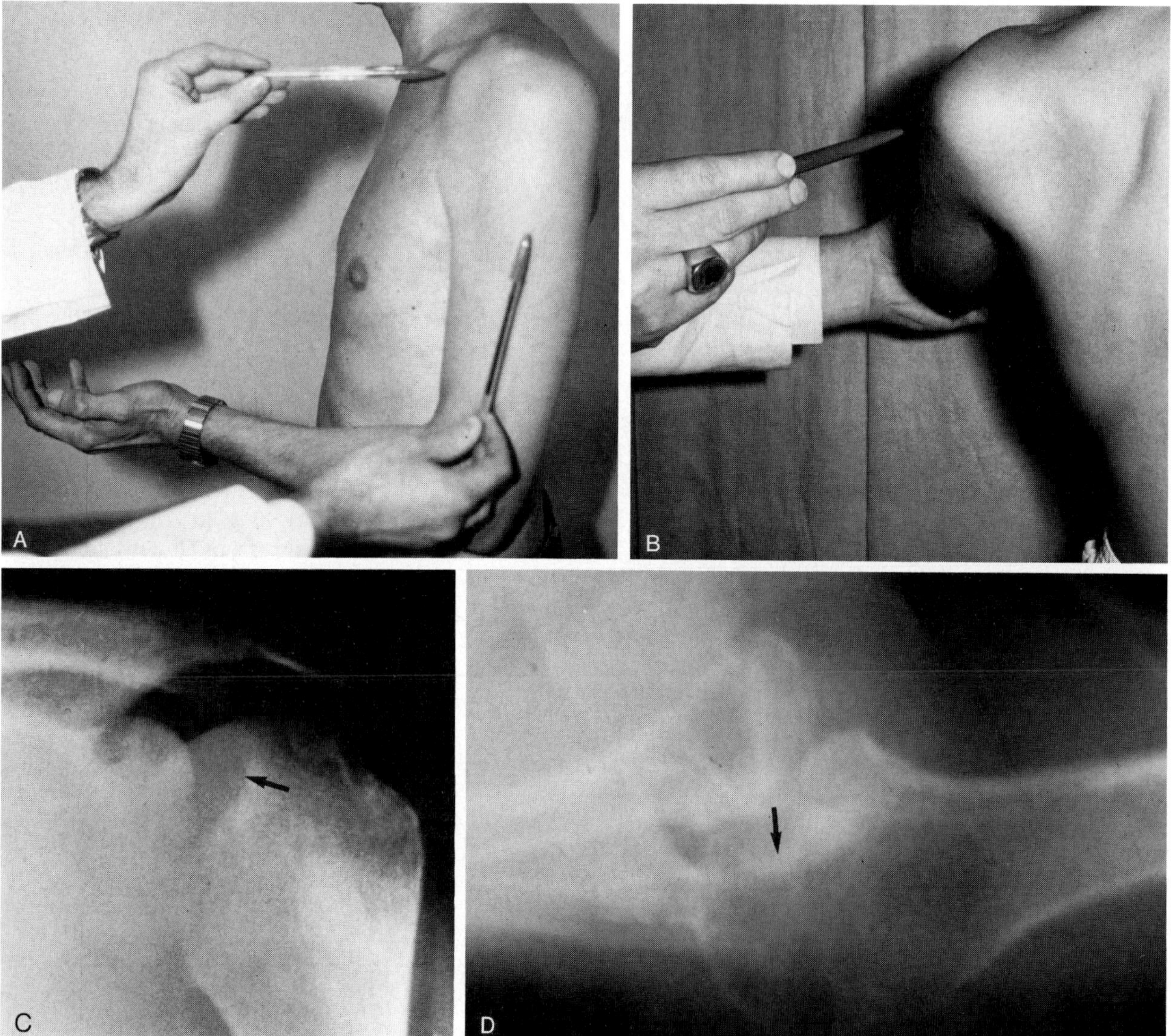

Figure 5–32. Clinical and roentgen diagnosis of an "impression fracture" with a locked posterior dislocation. Impression fractures occur more often with posterior dislocations than with anterior dislocations. The treatment of anterior fracture-dislocations with posterior head defects follows the same principles. Over 50 percent of these lesions continue to be missed by the initial examining physician.

A and B, The classic physical findings are prominence of the head posteriorly, loss of external rotation, and prominence of the coracoid. These signs are hard to see in a muscular or obese patient, especially if there is swelling. I find an unpublished sign to be more helpful and more reliable. I look for the altered axis of the arm (A). The arm points toward the posterior acromion rather than toward the anterior acromion.

C and D, Anterior-posterior and axillary x-rays of a "locked" posterior fracture-dislocation with a 15 percent impression fracture.

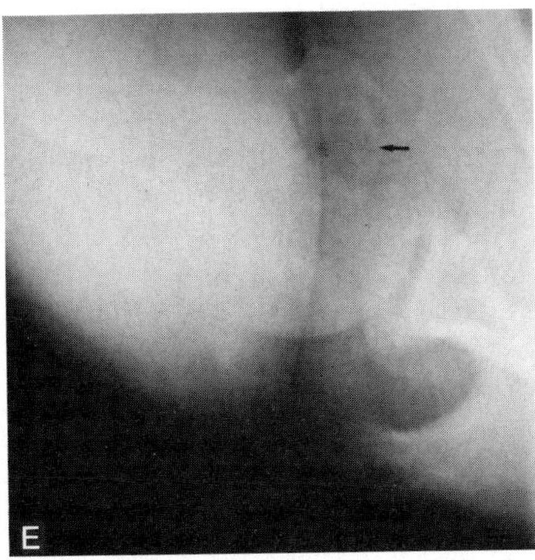

Figure 5–32 *Continued* Treatment of locked posterior fracture-dislocations with impression fractures depends on the size and duration of the head defect.

E, Twenty percent impression fracture that has had a closed reduction of the posterior dislocation (see Fig. 4–33) with good result.

This is a modification of the McLaughlin procedure.[253] This is also followed by an "external rotation" and extension lightweight cast for four to six weeks.

3. When 50 per cent or more of the head is impressed, I prefer to use a prosthesis to replace the articular surface. If the glenoid articular surface is worn or deformed by a long-standing lesion, a total shoulder replacement is preferred (see Figs. 3–57 to 3–63). CT scans of the glenohumeral joint as well as axillary view tomograms can be of great value in assessing the condition of the head and glenoid pre-operatively.

Head-Splitting Fractures

Head-splitting fracture, an uncommon injury, is produced by a violent central impact of the head against the glenoid. The articular surface is fragmented into a number of separate pieces (Fig. 5–33). The tuberosities may also be broken and retracted. This lesion is treated with a prosthesis, and the tuberosities and cuff are repaired; however, the patient often has serious multiple injuries that delay shoulder surgery.

Results to Be Expected

There has been a tendency in the literature to underestimate the disability time that follows frac-

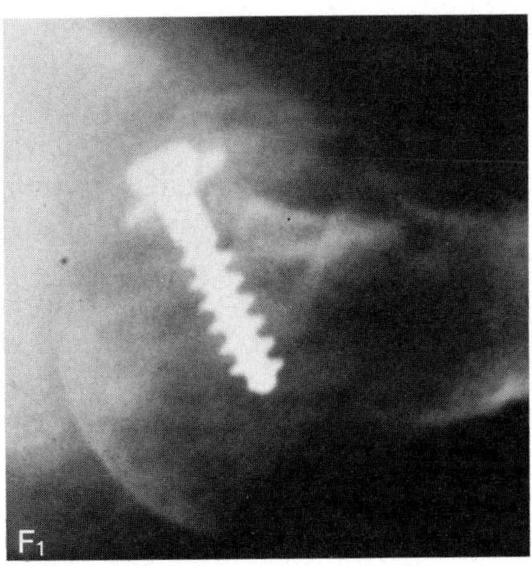

Figure 5–32 *Continued* F, (1) Thirty percent impression fracture that had been unstable after closed reduction of the posterior dislocation and was treated by transfer of the lesser tuberosity into the head defect. (2) Technique of transfer of lesser tuberosity for unstable locked posterior fracture-dislocation, as discussed in the text. An extended deltopectoral approach is used. The subscapularis tendon must be left attached to the lesser tuberosity. In order to keep the subscapularis tendon attached, inspection of the joint is made through the rotator interval to decide if the transfer of the lesser tuberosity is necessary before osteotomizing the lesser tuberosity. The head is "shoe-horned" away from the posterior glenoid as the arm is externally rotated in order to reduce the head with minimal damage (center).

Illustration continued on following page

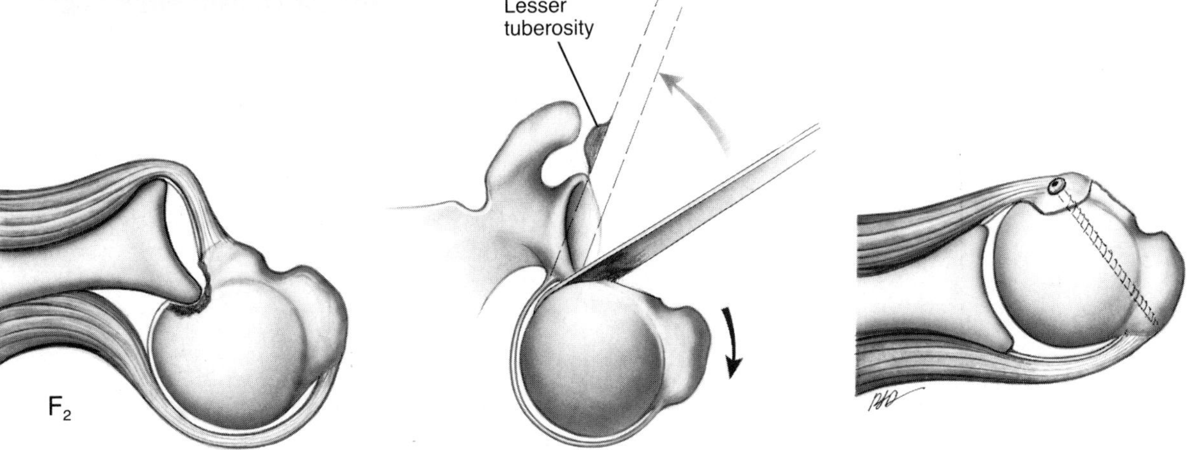

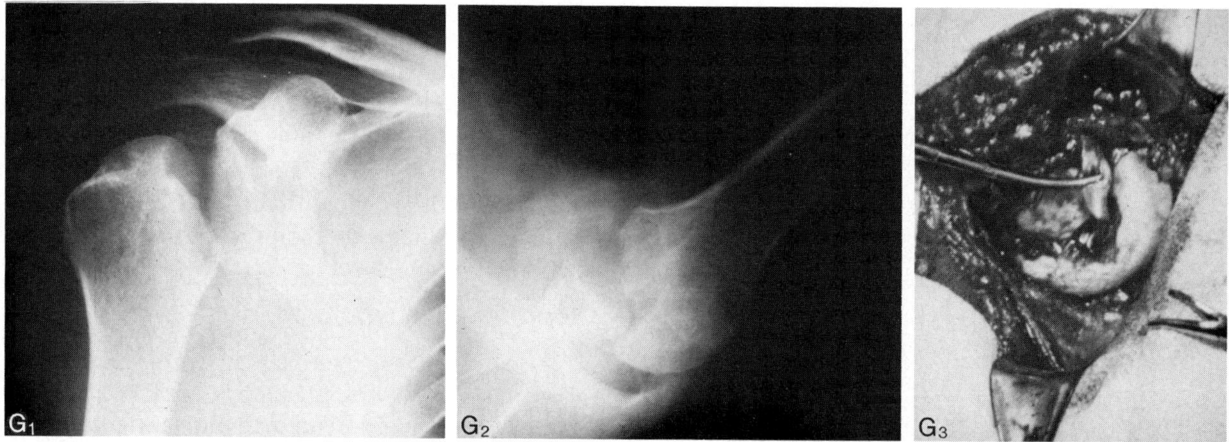

Figure 5–32 *Continued* G, (1) Anterior-posterior view of a 50 percent impression fracture with a posterior dislocation. (2) Axillary view of (1). Humeral head replacement was advised (see Fig. 5–23). (3) Appearance at surgery of a similar case in which a humeral head replacement was performed.

Long-standing, locked fracture-dislocations (over 9 months) usually have wear of the articular surface of the glenoid requiring a total arthroplasty (see Figs. 3–57 to 3–63).

tures with minimal displacement. A few patients do recover motion and function within three months, but they are exceptional. Lingering stiffness, pain at the extremes of motion, and "weather-ache" usually persist for at least six months. Strength and coordination return even more slowly. The results of treatment of fractures with minimal displacement are much better after an adequate exercise regimen.

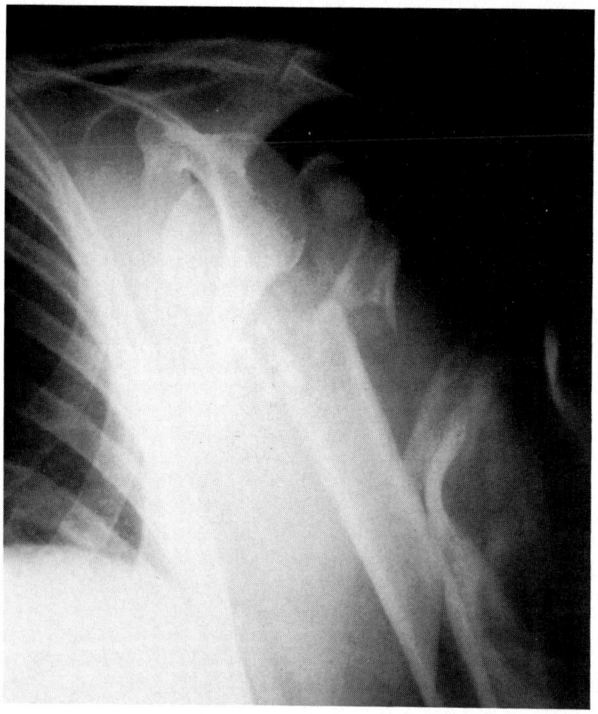

Figure 5–33. Head-splitting fracture with part of the head dislocated anteriorly and part dislocated posteriorly. An attempt at closed reduction had been made, and the patient had been referred for a prosthesis wearing an ineffective hanging cast.

Displaced lesions requiring tuberosity and cuff repair, with or without prosthetic replacement, can be expected to require longer periods of recovery. Approaches avoiding detachment of the origin of the deltoid and EPM (see Fig. 7–7) have been of great value in expediting recovery. Improvement in range, strength, and comfort can occur for a number of months, provided that patients continue with occasional stretching and strengthening exercises, which are best performed after a shower or bath. As illustrated in Figure 5–25, the results in 61 shoulders with recent four-part fracture-dislocations in my personal series[149] were rated "excellent" in 51 and "satisfactory" in 9, and "unsatisfactory" in 1. These results are much better than those reported in the 1970 series.[8]

Complications of Upper Humeral Fractures

Joint Stiffness

Bursal and capsular adhesions that restrict range and cause pain at the extremes of motion can usually be overcome by applications of warmth and stretching exercises. Forceful manipulation may fracture the weakened and osteoporotic bone and is to be avoided. In rare instances, usually in patients treated surgically with inadequate aftercare, open release of adhesions can be helpful. It is, of course, mandatory that this latter procedure be followed by an adequate exercise regimen.

Unless edema and immobilization of the hand have been avoided throughout the course of treatment, shoulder injuries may be complicated by stiffness of the finger joints. This can be overcome by range of motion exercises, but is best prevented by active and passive exercises of all finger joints during the period of shoulder rehabilitation.

Malunion or Nonunion of the Greater Tuberosity

Reconstruction after malunion or nonunion of the greater tuberosity may be required when the greater tuberosity restricts external rotation and elevation and causes pain (Figs. 5–34 and 5–36). The procedure is technically difficult because of joint and bursal adhesions, adherence of the greater tuberosity to the posterior part of the articular surface of the humeral head, and fixed retraction of the external rotators. The reconstruction is discussed in Figs. 5–12E and 3–62. Passive exercises for elevation overhead and for external rotation are especially important throughout the recovery period.

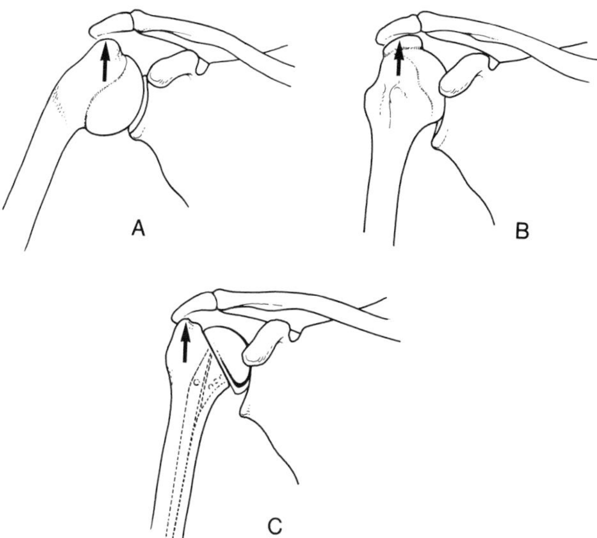

Figure 5–34. Treatment of symptomatic malunion of the greater tuberosity with impingement as is seen in three situations.

A, Varus malunion at the surgical neck level can usually be relieved by a liberal anterior acromioplasty (however, without shortening the acromion) rather than an osteotomy of the neck of the humerus.

B, Malunion of the greater tuberosity as shown here and in Figure 5–36, requires an osteotomy to remove the tuberosity from the articular surface and re-attachment of the tuberosity in its normal location. If the articular surface of the humeral head has been damaged, it may be necessary to replace the head and possibly the glenoid (see Fig. 3–62).

C, Prominence of a greater tuberosity above a prosthesis is usually treated by re-setting the humeral component higher but may be treated by osteotomizing and lowering the tuberosity, depending on the amount and type of displacement of the tuberosity.

Malunion of the Surgical Neck

Although malunion with varus and anterior angulation at the surgical neck level can permanently restrict elevation (Fig. 5–35), it has rarely been treated by an osteotomy. An adequate result can usually be obtained by releasing adhesions and obtaining clearance for the greater tuberosity with an anterior acromioplasty, and, if the cuff is torn, by removing some of the prominent greater tuberosity and re-attaching the cuff.

Malunion of Three-Part and Four-Part Fracture-Dislocations

Malunited three-part and four-part fractures and fracture-dislocations can be very disabling and are formidable lesions because of joint incongruity, fixed retraction of the tuberosities, loss of bone length, nerve deficits, and scar tissue. They are much harder to reconstruct than acute injuries, as described in Figures 3–57 to 3–71. Nevertheless, I prefer prosthetic reconstruction rather than arthrodesis unless there has been infection or permanent loss of the axillary and suprascapular nerves. Pres-

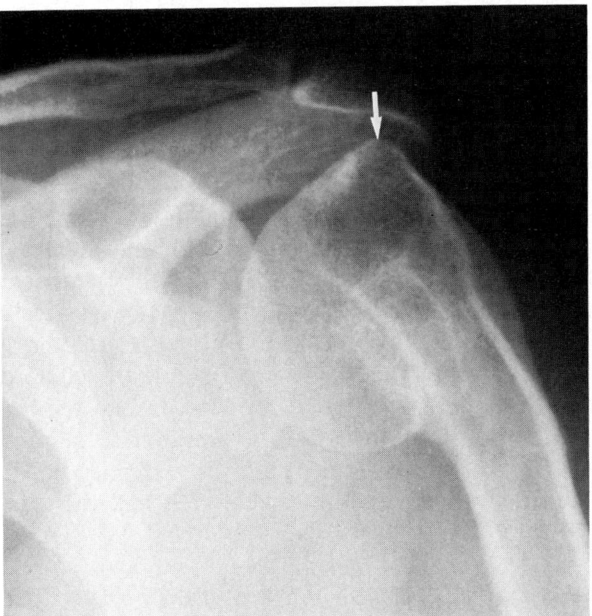

Figure 5–35. Anterior-posterior view of a varus malunion of the surgical neck successfully treated with a generous anterior acromioplasty without an osteotomy of the neck of the humerus.

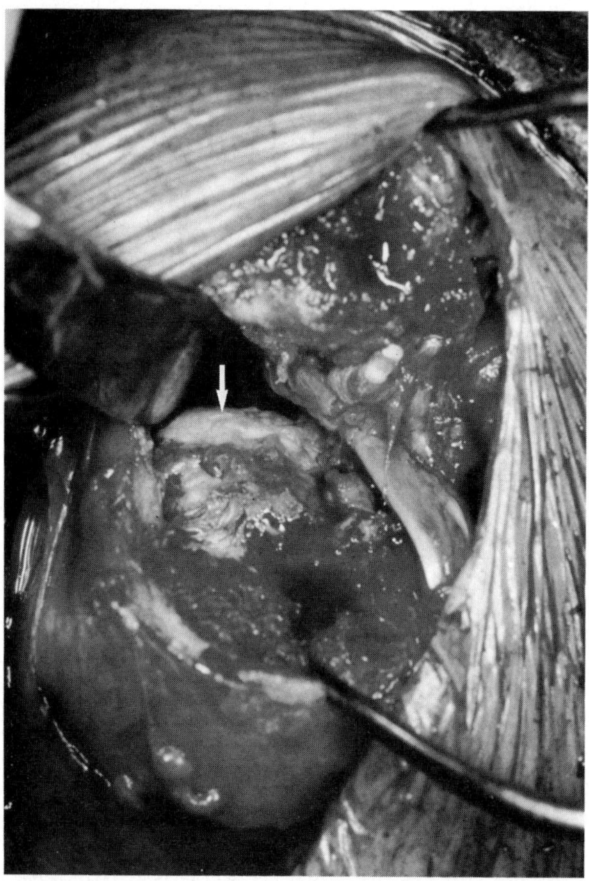

Figure 5–36. A retracted malunion of the greater tuberosity with a cuff tear and scar. The displaced greater tuberosity (under the retractor) has become attached to the articular surface of the head of the humerus, as shown in Figure 5–20A. The arrow points to the scarred articular surface. The long head of the biceps is seen on the right, as was seen in the acute two-part displacement of the greater tuberosity shown in Figure 5–12E.

ervation of the deltoid attachments, mobilization and re-attachment of the rotator cuff and tuberosities, and meticulous aftercare are all of critical importance (see Figs. 3–57 to 3–71). I generally prefer to resurface the glenoid as well as replace the head when the articular surface of the glenoid and the tuberosities are abnormal, especially if the cuff is defective, because the conforming surface of the glenoid component affords a slightly better fulcrum for the rehabilitation of the weak muscles.

Avascular Necrosis of the Humeral Head

Fractures with minimal displacement are occasionally followed by collapse of the head, but these cases are rare and are easier to treat by prosthetic replacement because the tuberosities and cuff are intact (see Fig. 5–7).[71] When the incongruity of the head has caused wear on the glenoid and painful post-traumatic arthritis has developed, I prefer total shoulder replacement rather than fusion of the glenohumeral joint.

Untreated four-part fractures often develop avascular necrosis with resorption of the articular segment. As described previously (see Figs. 3–57 to 3–71), prosthetic reconstruction is unfortunately more difficult than in an acute lesion because of fixed retraction of the rotator cuff and adhesions.

Nonunion of the Surgical Neck

As discussed with Figures 3–64 to 3–71, nonunion of the surgical neck is not rare. It may be due to interposition of the deltoid muscle or long head of the biceps but may follow treatment with traction or a hanging cast, especially when it distracts the fracture. It is occasionally due to disregard for immobilization in patients with multiple injuries and in alcoholic patients. The lesion is usually painful. Characteristically, the arm cannot be actively elevated to the horizontal. The lesion and its pathology and treatment are illustrated in Figure 3–65. Repair by an overconfident surgeon often fails. The bone is usually too soft for plate or screw fixation. If the head is adequate and the bone is hard, I use an AO T-plate. If the bone is soft, a compression band is used. In either case, iliac bone grafts and a spica cast for external fixation are used. I wait for radiographic evidences of consolidation before discarding the cast. A prosthesis is used when the head has collapsed or been resorbed.

"Heterotopic Bone"

As previously stated (see Fig. 5–24A), this complication is rarely seen except after fracture-dislocations. Callus formation occurs around the extruded head fragment and remains after relocation or removal of the head as "pericapsular bone."

The pericapsular bone usually diminishes with time and very rarely requires excision (see Fig. 5–24A). In no case should an attempt to remove the unwanted bone be made before it has reached maturity. The new bone is observed for at least one year after injury, and observation is continued as long as there are even gradual gains in motion or radioactive bone scans show the hypervascularity of active bone formation (see Fig. 3–108).

FRACTURES OF THE PROXIMAL HUMERAL EPIPHYSEAL PLATE

These lesions are not rare and compose about 3 percent of epiphyseal fractures (Fig. 5–37).[151] I became interested in them in 1963 because of some personal experiences with remarkable remodeling and recovery of function after displacements of this type treated by a policy bordering on laissez faire.

Dr. F. M. Smith[152] of our Fracture Service at the Columbia-Presbyterian Medical Center in New York made a study of 43 of these injuries treated prior to 1953.[152] He concluded that the attempts to correct displacement by reduction under anesthesia, skeletal traction, and open reduction frequently constituted overtreatment. My study[151] compared the results of 46 of these lesions subsequent to 1953 (treated with simple measures and little regard for anatomical restoration) with the results of Smith's series, which had been treated with efforts to obtain and maintain anatomical reductions. In addition, the anatomical problem

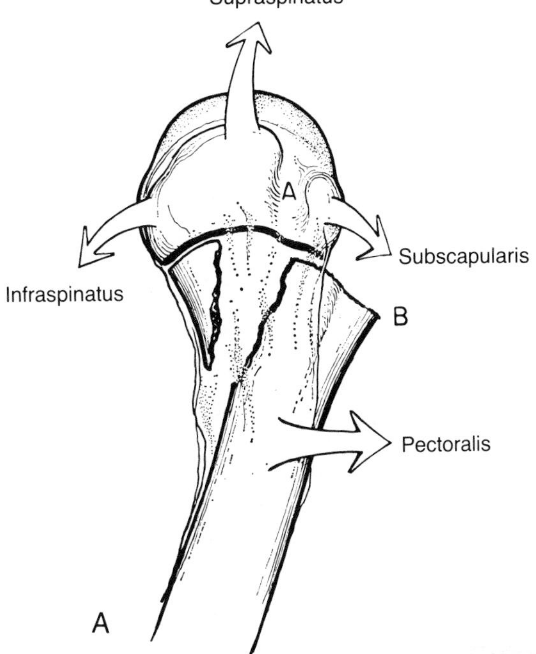

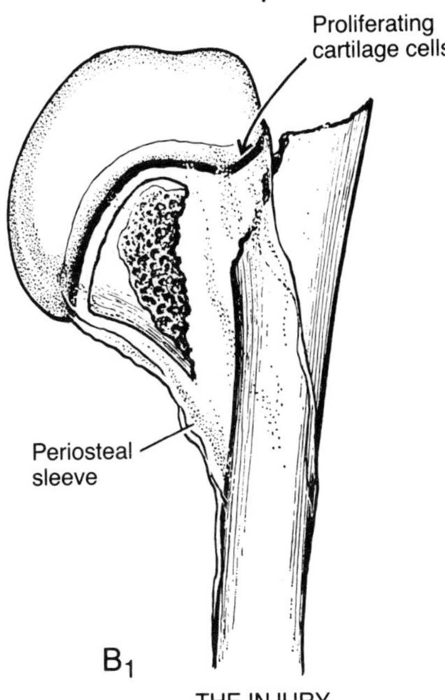

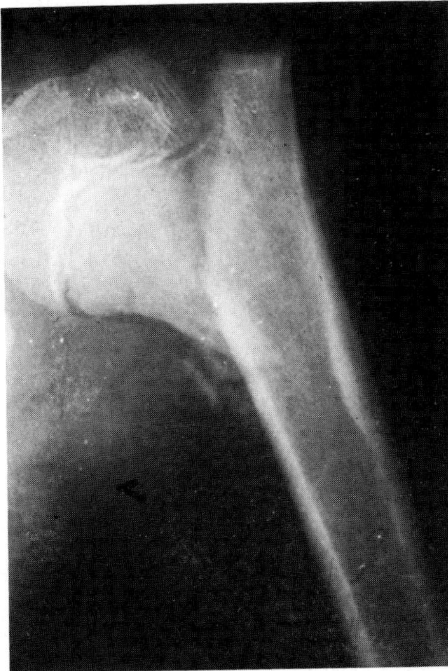

Figure 5–37. ***Fractures of the Proximal Humeral Epiphyseal Plate.***

A, The anatomical problem in fractures of the proximal epiphyseal plate. The head is held in neutral rotation by the rotator cuff, and the pectoralis major is the deforming muscle.

B, The remarkable epiphyseal growth contributes to correcting the deformity. (1) The injury in a 13 year old boy treated without reduction by 6 weeks immobility in a sling.

Illustration continued on following page

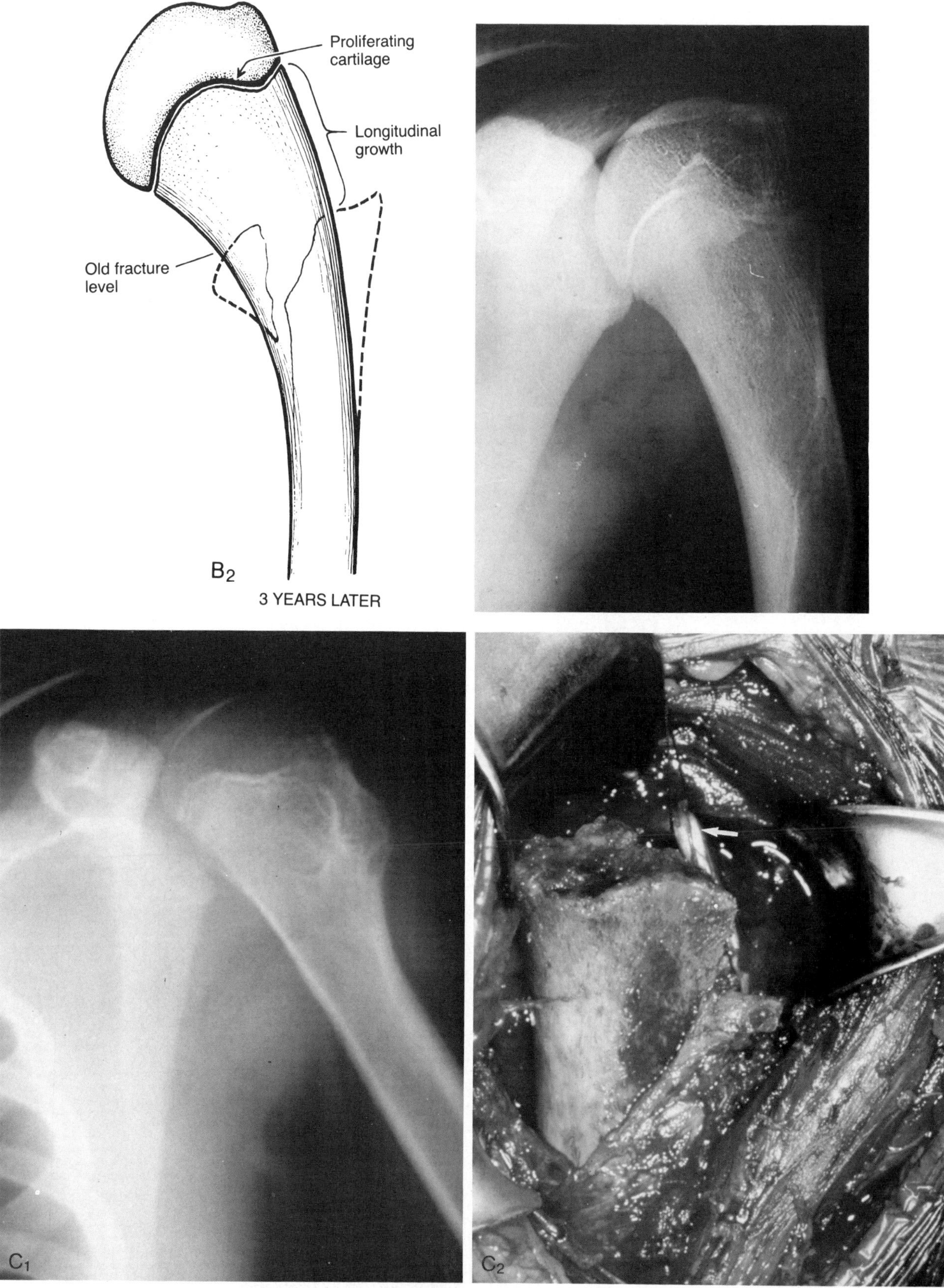

Figure 5–37 *Continued* B, (2) Three years later, at the completion of growth, there is 2.0 cm. shortening and mild anterior bowing, but function is normal. C, Very rare problems in proximal humeral epiphyseal fractures. (1) Salter IV fracture with early closure of the epiphysis. The growth plate is usually spared (Salter II fractures), as illustrated in A (see text). (2) Interposed biceps (arrow) and subscapularis, as in the adult surgical neck fracture (see Fig. 5–11E), treated by open reduction.

was analyzed, as described in this section, and the unique importance of epiphyseal growth to the remodeling process was recognized.

Personal Series

The 89 patients in our 1965 series from the Fracture Service of the Columbia-Presbyterian Medical Center in New York[151] ranged in age from 12 months to 17 years and were most often between 11 and 15 years. Male patients predominated by a ratio of 3 to 1. On our review of the literature, it was noted that this fracture has been reported at any age, while the epiphysis is open from birth to age 23 years in a patient who had pituitary gigantism.[153]

The majority (59 of 89) of these patients or their parents described the mechanism of injury as a blow on the shoulder rather than a fall on the outstretched hand.

Follow-up of from 2 to 11 years had been obtained on 62 patients, and their functional and anatomical results were recorded. These lesions were graded according to the amount of displacement in the original films as follows:

Grade I: Less than 5.0 mm. displacement
Grade II: Up to one-third the diameter of the shaft
Grade III: From one-third to two-thirds the diameter of the shaft
Grade IV: Greater than two-thirds the diameter of the shaft

Angulation of varying degrees was also present in Grade III and Grade IV lesions. Of the combined series, 64 patients had Grade I or II lesions, 7 had Grade III, and 18 had Grade IV displacements.

The results were reviewed on the basis of (1) the severity of displacement, and (2) the age of the patient at the time of injury. The results of the 62 patients with minimum follow-up of 2 years and average follow-up of 4.8 years were as follows:

1. Permanent discrepancy in length of from 1.0 cm. to 3.0 cm. occurred in 9 per cent of the patients with Grades I and II displacement and in 33 per cent of those with Grade IV displacement.
2. No instance of persistent inequality was seen in a child who was under age 11 years at the time of injury.
3. Although moderate anatomical defects in length and alignment were not infrequent in children 11 years of age and older at the time of injury because of mobility of the glenohumeral joint, the functional results were "acceptable."

We concluded that Grades I and II displacement should be treated with simple immobilization. Grade IV lesions should have closed reduction and a spica cast to correct angulation and rotation, but only partial end-on apposition was required because of the effectiveness of "epiphyseal remodeling." Open reduction was thought to be rarely justified. However, although "epiphyseal remodeling" is more complete at this location than any other and moderate anatomical discrepancies in length and alignment are better tolerated by the glenohumeral joint, parents should be warned that some permanent shortening may occur, which is more prevalent when the displacement is marked.

Anatomical Problem in Proximal Humeral Epiphyseal Fractures

We analyzed the anatomical derangement as shown in Figure 5–37A. The secondary ossification center for the humeral head is present at birth or appears soon after. A secondary center for the greater tuberosity appears at about age 3 years, and one for the lesser tuberosity at about age 5 years. These three centers coalesce at age 6 years to form one epiphysis. Therefore, when a fracture passes through the epiphyseal plate, the rotator cuff, which inserts on the tuberosities, remains attached to the proximal fragment.

In the four-segment classification, this is a "subtuberous" or "surgical neck" level fracture, which when displaced more than 1.0 cm. or angulated more than 45 degrees would be equivalent to the two-part surgical neck displacement (shaft displacement) (see Fig. 5–4). Just as in two-part surgical neck displacements in adult patients, the head is in neutral position (unless tilted by the overriding shaft) because the pull of the external rotators is neutralized by the subscapularis and because the abducting effect of the supraspinatus is neutralized to a large extent by the intact lower parts of the infraspinatus and subscapularis and by the teres minor as well as the intact posterior periosteum. Thus, the proximal segment is held near neutral position unless it is tilted by pressure on it from the distal fragment, such as can be caused by a tight sling.

The pectoralis major acts to displace the shaft anteriorly and medially. This force can be overcome by placing the arm in the Velpeau position (adduction and internal rotation position) but is intensified by placing the arm in abduction.

Another factor in the displacement that should be considered when planning a closed reduction is the possible presence of internal rotation of the shaft, which may have been caused by placing an unstable lesion in a sling.

Unique Epiphyseal Remodeling

The epiphyseal plate remains open until approximately 19 years of age in males, and a year or two earlier for females. It is very active and contributes 80 to 81 per cent of the longitudinal growth of the humerus. The weakest area is just distal to proliferating cartilage cells in the "zone of degenerating cartilage"—cells in which the cartilage is being converted to bone and calcifying on the metaphyseal side of the plate. Thus, this fracture usually spares the important zone of proliferating cartilage cells. The glenohumeral joint is the most mobile joint in the body; therefore, compressive force with crushing or splitting of the epiphyseal plate is less likely. All of the 89 epiphyseal fractures in the series cited previously were Salter[154] Type II or Type I lesions, in which the cells responsible for longitudinal growth are largely spared. Since then, as discussed below, a very few exceptions have been seen. Continuing epiphyseal growth displaces the epiphyseal plate away from the fracture site, correcting moderate angulatory deformities and assisting in the remodeling process (see Fig. 5–37B).

Anterior angulation at the fracture site and medial displacement of the shaft are the most common deformities in Grades III and IV displacements. This deformity is probably produced by the force of injury augmented by the pull of the pectoralis major. Interestingly, 59 of the 89 patients or their parents described a direct blow on the shoulder rather than a fall on the outstretched hand as the mechanism of injury. A shearing force displacing the shaft is probably more common than end-on compressive force, which would be more likely to crush the growing cells of the epiphyseal plate.

Present Treatment

The age of the patients at the time of injury has a bearing on the ability of future epiphyseal growth to correct the deformity (just as is true of any epiphyseal injury).

Open reduction, which harms an actively growing epiphyseal plate, would seem to be ill advised. After the mid-teens, however, open reduction should be safer and more logical in extreme displacements that cannot be reduced to even partial end-on contact in which interposition of the long head of the biceps and the subscapularis and periosteal sleeve are suspected. However, these problems are extremely rare (see Fig. 5–37C).

Since the 1965 series, I have seen a few epiphyseal injuries that were Salter III or IV displacements, as shown in Figure 5–37C1. These should be mentioned, but with emphasis on their rarity. In the vast majority of these cases, epiphyseal growth can be expected to correct reasonable deformities in a remarkable way, provided that the patient has a few years of growth remaining.

In patients under 16 years of age, reduction with even slight end-on contact and with correction of angulation to within 40 degrees is considered to be acceptable. This position should be achieved by closed manipulation and should be maintained with a spica cast (with the arm just below the salute position in most cases). The closed reduction should be achieved without crushing or injury to the epiphyseal plate, appreciating the fact that a partially intact periosteal sleeve along with the configuration of the fracture surface may prevent more than incomplete end-on reduction without the risk of damaging the plate. Greater angulation can be overcome and maintained, provided that the arm is positioned so that the pull of the pectoralis major is neutralized. The maneuver for closed reduction may vary but is along the lines of correcting internal rotation: The arm is brought to neutral rotation, judged with the elbow flexed 90 degrees, followed by light traction and flexion of the arm to above the horizontal. Finally, after traction has been discontinued and the major fragments have locked together, the arm is lowered to about 90 degrees flexion and neutral rotation, where it is immobilized in a spica cast for four to six weeks.

As mentioned previously, the parents should be alerted to the possibility of moderate, permanent shortening and loss of the final degrees of overhead elevation. Some athletic patients with this injury who have extremely ambitious and aggressive parents have been referred because there is some residual deformity in post-reduction x-rays that the parents are unwilling to accept. An explanation is generally indicated rather than an open reduction, emphasizing how important future growth of the epiphyseal plate is and how an open reduction may damage the growth line of the plate, causing a greater anatomical deformity. Even the most ambitious parents of Little League baseball players are usually willing to accept this advice.

I have participated in only one open reduction for this injury during the last 18 years, and that lesion was in a 16 year old boy whose epiphyseal fracture could not be brought into even slight end-on contract and in whom the long head of the biceps and the periosteum were found to be interposed, as shown in Figure 5–37C2. This type of interposition, as is seen in adults with two-part surgical neck displacement, is rare but is possible. Fluoroscopic control with the image intensifier is helpful in assessing problem reductions for the decision as to whether open reduction is indicated. I have never seen a nonunion following this injury, as one would expect to see if interposition occurred more than extremely infrequently.

FRACTURES OF THE CLAVICLE

Anatomy of Clavicular Fractures

Mechanical Forces and Design

Anchored securely to the scapula by the acromioclavicular and coracoclavicular ligaments and to the trunk by the sternoclavicular and costoclavicular ligaments, the clavicle serves as the only osseous strut to maintain the width of the shoulders.[153a] Fractures of the clavicle allow the shoulder to slump downward and forward, owing to spasm of the muscles crossing from the thorax to the arm and to the effect of gravity (Fig. 5–38). The proximal fragment tends to be displaced upward by the sternomastoid muscle. With violent trauma, the subclavian vessels may be torn and the brachial plexus contused or its roots avulsed.

Whereas the midclavicle is tubular, the outer clavicle is flattened, and either the coracoclavicular ligaments or the acromioclavicular joint capsule is attached to the entire length of the undersurface of this flattened portion. Fractures of the outer clavicle have been subdivided into three categories (Fig. 5–39). The inner end of the clavicle is rotated 40 degrees and moved in all directions as the scapula is rotated (see Chapter 1, p. 3). It is thought to be moved more often than any other joint, with the exception of the costovertebral articulations. Considering its poor support by the sternum, it is surprising that it is only infrequently deranged (see pp. 355 and 436).

Mechanism of Injury

Because the clavicle is an S-shaped bone, mechanical forces from the side cause a shearing effect on its middle third, where the majority of clavicle fractures occur.

Tell-tale skin contusions show that fractures of the distal portion of the clavicle result from a blow on the point of the shoulder from above downward, whereas acromioclavicular separations usually result from a force that strikes somewhat more posteriorly. The impact that produces displaced fractures of the outer clavicle may drive the scapula against the chest wall with such force as to produce rib fractures, and when this injury is sustained from a high fall, accompanying head and cervical spine injuries are not uncommon.

Fractures of the inner clavicle usually result from direct trauma. Articular surface fractures at either end are caused by compression of the joint surfaces.

Classification

It is customary to classify these lesions in three groups: (1) mid-third, 80 per cent; (2) distal or interligamentous, 15 per cent; and (3) inner third, 5 per cent of clavicle fractures.

Because of differences in clinical behavior, it has proved helpful to me[155, 156] to subdivide fractures of the distal clavicle, as shown in Figure 5–39: Type I, minimal displacement with intact ligaments; Type II, displaced with detachment of the ligaments from the proximal fragment; and Type III, fractures of the articular surface. Type I is a minor injury, but Types II and III can be troublesome.

Articular surface fractures are less common at the inner end than at the distal clavicle, but inner end fractures do occur and can cause permanent symptoms because of subsequent arthritic changes. As discussed with Figure 4–69, prior to age 17 years, epiphyseal fractures occasionally occur at the inner end of the clavicle.

Diagnosis of Clavicular Fractures

Signs and Symptoms

When a middle-third fracture is displaced, the shoulder slumps downward and inward and the patient holds the arm against the chest to protect against shoulder movements. Because the superior surface of the clavicle is subcutaneous, there is direct and indirect tenderness and often palpable deformity and crepitus at the fracture. However, nondisplaced clavicular fractures in children are easily missed.

Fractures of the articular surfaces do not cause deformity and can easily be overlooked unless special x-ray views are obtained.

Radiographic Assessment

Fractures of the middle and inner thirds are studied by an anterior-posterior view and a 45

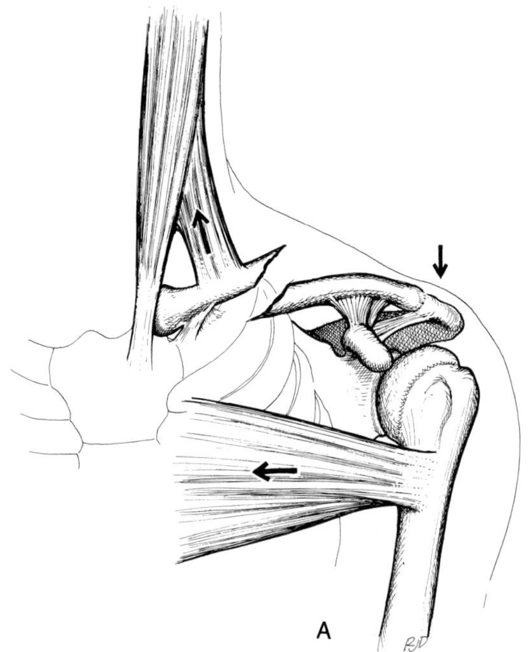

Figure 5–38. ***Midclavicular Fractures. Forces Acting on the Clavicle.***

A, The distal fragment is pulled down by the weight of the arm and medially by the pectoralis major and latissimus dorsi. The proximal fragment is pulled upward by the sternomastoid.

B, Typical x-ray appearance of a middle third fracture.

C, "Clavicular cast" for displaced fractures in adults.

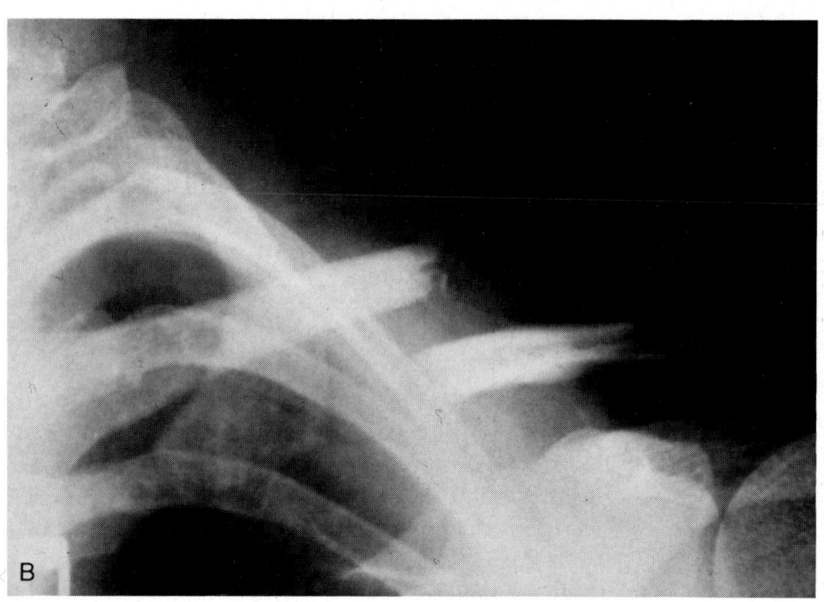

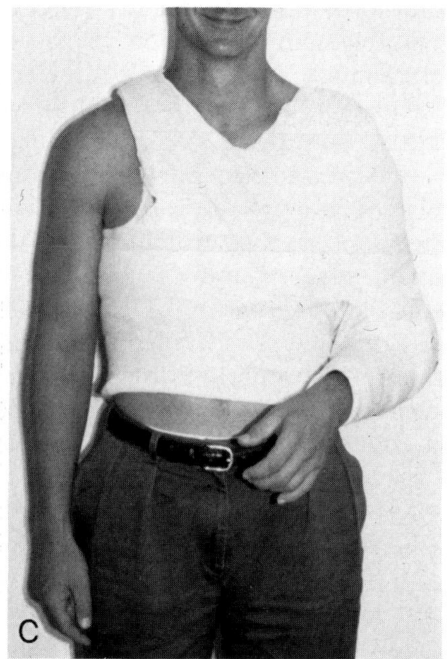

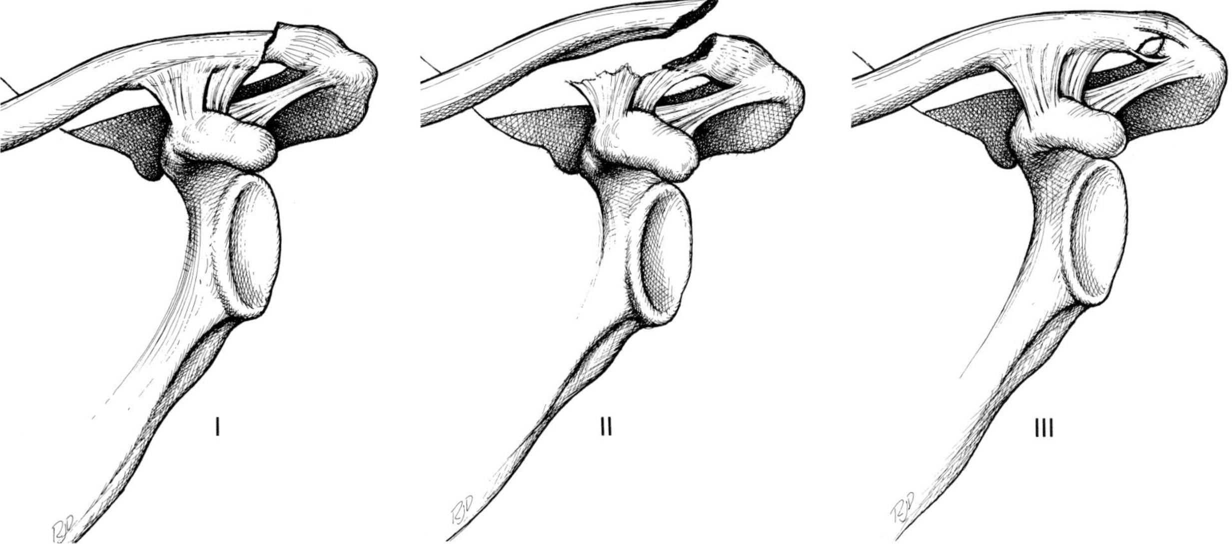

Figure 5–39. ***Classification of Distal Clavicle Fractures.***
Type I, Minimal displacement with intact ligaments.
Type II, Displaced with detachment of the ligaments from the medial fragment.
Type III, Articular surface fracture.

degree view, which is made with the tube directed from below (see Fig. 1–12F).

Fractures of the distal clavicle require special roentgen studies to determine the integrity of the coarcoclavicular ligaments. The presence of displacement can be shown by anterior-posterior and lateral views in the scapular plane (the "trauma series") (see Fig. 5–40). Disruption of the ligaments attaching on the proximal fragment can be further demonstrated by an anterior-posterior view of both shoulders on a single large film made with patient erect and with 10 pounds of weight attached to each wrist to show widening of the space between the coracoid and the medial fragment of clavicle on the injured side.[155, 156]

Fractures of the articular surfaces in the acromioclavicular and sternoclavicular joints may require laminograms or CT scans for accurate diagnosis (see Fig. 5–40).

Treatment of Clavicular Fractures

Authors from Hippocrates to the present have been dissatisfied with the anatomical results of treating unstable clavicular fractures, regardless of the method used. However, the clavicle has unusual healing powers, perhaps because it behaves like a membranous bone (like the skull), and functional results after closed treatment are usually good. Hundreds of methods of closed treatment have been described, including use of metal, leather, wood, plastic, muslin, and plaster.

Open reduction has rarely been considered to be the preferred treatment for uncomplicated fractures. Open reduction may have a place in the management of a few complicated fractures.

Fractures of the Middle Third

Reduction can usually be accomplished by drawing the shoulders upward and backward as the ends of the fragments are manipulated into alignment. This may be done with the patient sitting on a stool between two tables to support the arms or lying supine on a canvas sling. Local anesthesia—10 mg. of 1 percent lidocaine—may be used. Reduction is usually easy, but, as noted previously, maintenance of reduction is not a simple matter. For adult patients, I prefer a modified shoulder spica cast ("clavicular cast") (see Fig. 5–38), which presses backward against the anterior deltoid regions. Whereas children may heal in three or four week, union of these fractures in adults requires at least eight weeks. Use of the cast (as shown in Fig. 5–38) is followed by the patient wearing a sling. In my experience, figure-of-eight dressings have been inadequate for adult patients. The few situations in which operative treatment is considered are discussed on page 408.

Fractures of the Distal Clavicle

Type I Distal Clavicle Fractures

Type I fractures (Fig. 5–40), with minimal displacement and intact ligaments, require only a sling, and activities are extended as pain subsides.

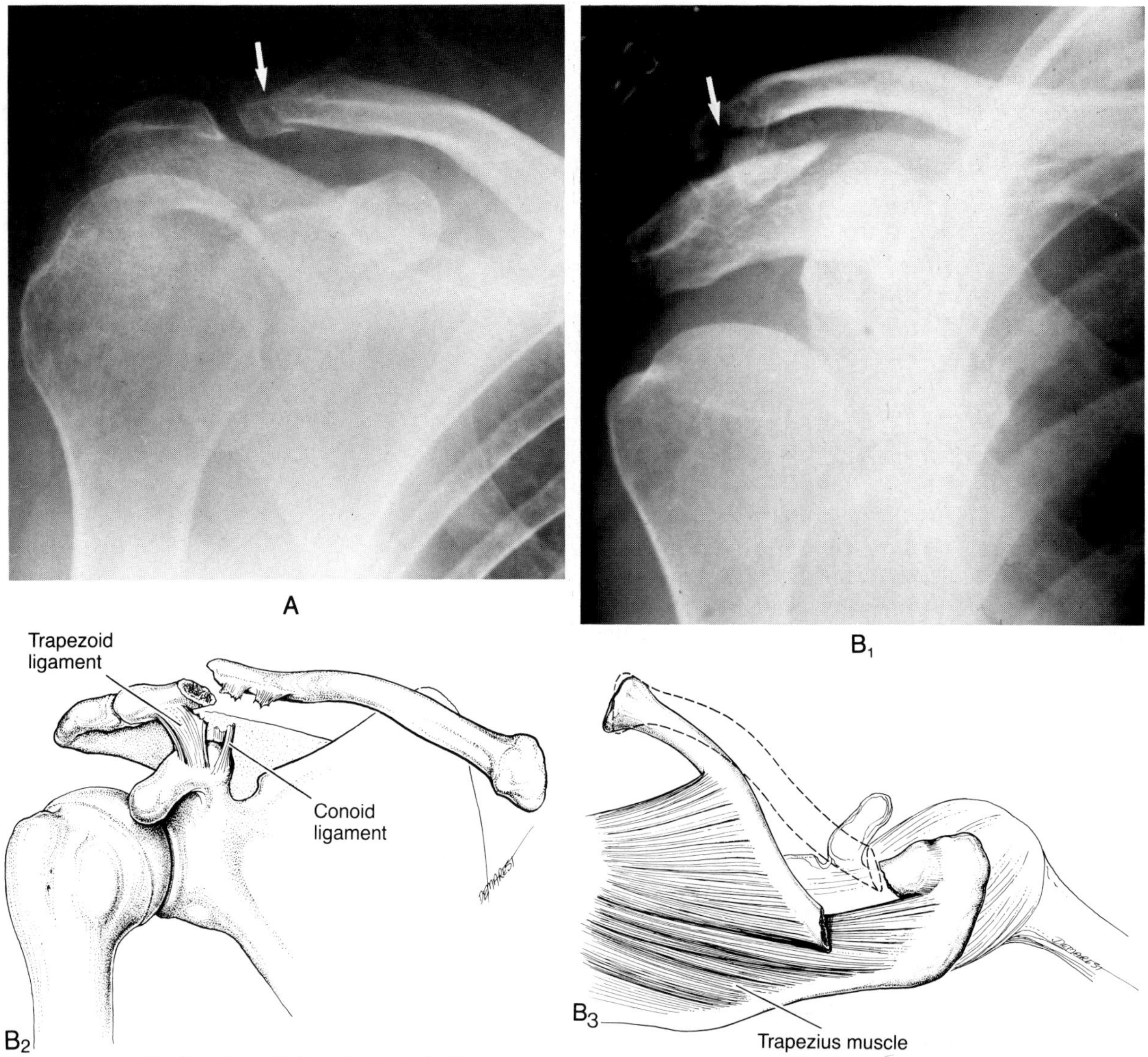

A

B1

Trapezoid ligament

Conoid ligament

B2

B3

Trapezius muscle

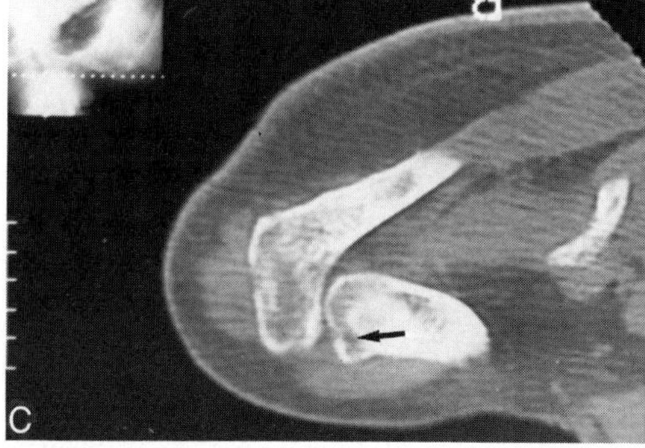

Figure 5–40. ***Evaluation of Distal Clavicle Fractures.***

A, Type I fracture (arrow) seen in the anterior-posterior view of the "trauma series" (see Fig. 1–12B). There is no significant displacement, and the coracoclavicular ligaments are intact.

B, Type II fractures (arrow) have consistent, characteristic displacement. 1. In the anterior-posterior view of the trauma series, the distal fragment retains its normal anatomical relationship with the coracoid and acromion. The proximal fragment appears high because it has been detached from the coracoclavicular ligaments while the distal fragment has dropped downward and forward with the weight of the arm. There is widening of the distance between the coracoid and the medial fragment, which can be brought out by x-rays made with the patient standing with weights on each wrist (see Fig. 1–12E). 2. In Type II lesions, the coracoclavicular ligaments and the acromioclavicular joint capsule remain attached to the distal fragment but are detached from the proximal fragment. 3. In Type II lesions, the distal fragment drops forward and downward, causing the proximal fragment to be surrounded by the trapezius muscle. This posterior displacement of the proximal fragment can be seen well in the lateral view of the trauma series (see Fig. 1–12B).

C, Type III lesions can be easily overlooked in the initial films. Computerized tomography (illustrated) can show an occult fracture of the articular surface. A tense hemarthrosis of the acromioclavicular joint occasionally occurs.

Type II Distal Clavicle Fractures

Type II, displaced, fractures are unstable, because the coracoclavicular ligaments are detached from the proximal fragment (Figs. 5–40 and 5–43). The proximal fragment is retracted upward and backward within the substance of the trapezius muscle, while the distal fragment drops downward and forward and is rotated by any movements of the scapula. The usual figure-of-eight dressing should not be used because it presses the proximal fragment backward and exaggerates this deformity. Closed treatment requires a type of strapping that draws the point of the shoulder upward and backward, and although closed treatment may succeed, it is difficult to maintain reduction, union is usually slow with some deformity, and occasionally a nonunion develops. However, exceptions can be made if one is willing to accept these disadvantages of closed treatment.

I previously used a transacromial wire that transfixed the distal clavicular fragment between

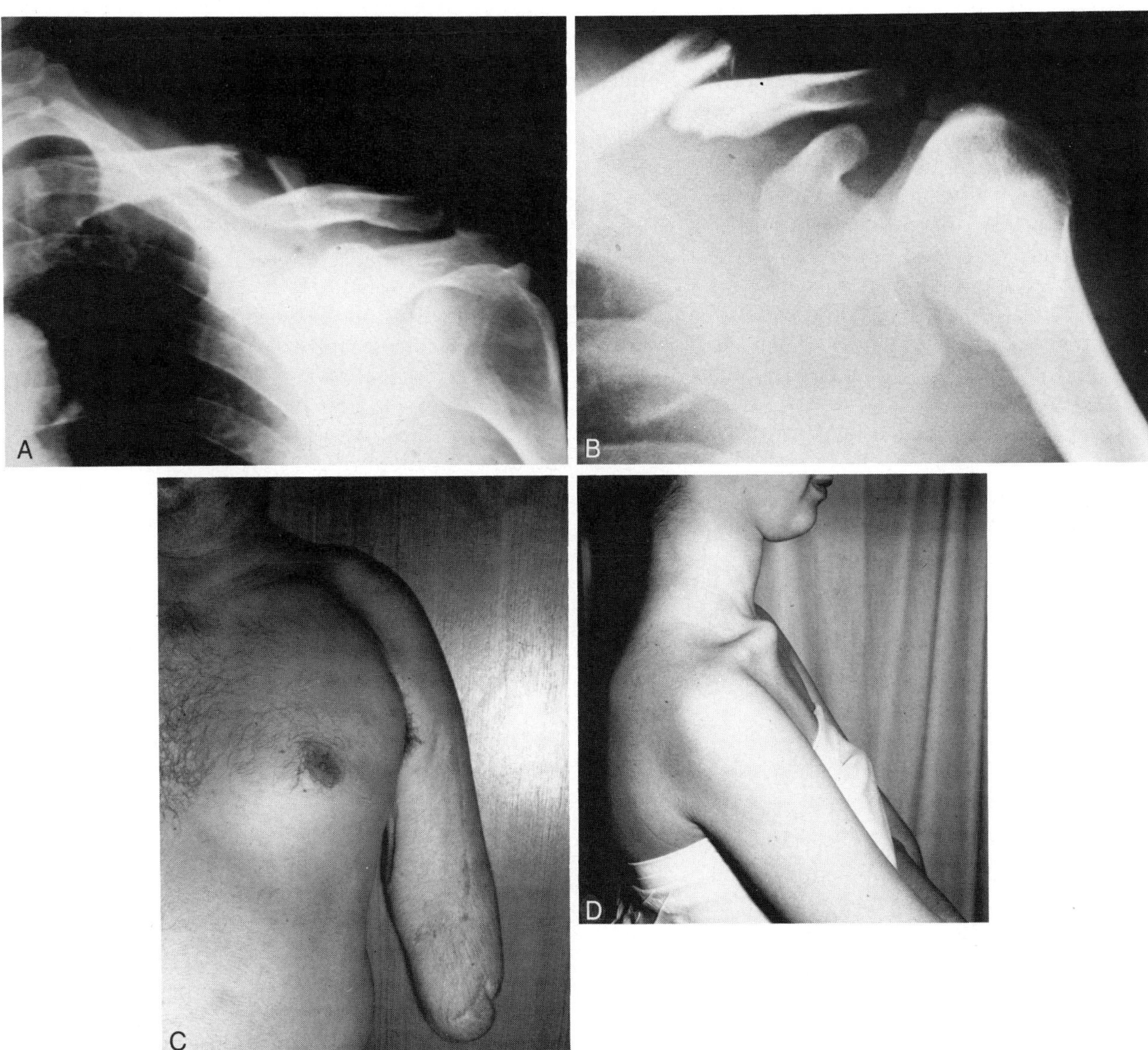

Figure 5–41. ***Complications of Midclavicular Fractures.***

A, Rotated intermediate fragment, which was caught in the cervical fascia and eventually eroded through the skin.

B, Nonunion of the middle third from inadequate immobilization in a patient who had multiple injuries.

C, Laceration of the subclavian artery and infraclavicular plexus with paralysis of the deltoid muscle and below, loss of sensation to the middle of the arm, and gangrene below the elbow.

D, An ugly malunion in a young woman.

The indications for internal fixation are considered on page 408.

the acromion and the proximal fragment. In most cases, I now prefer to use two strands of No. 5 nonabsorbable, nonmetallic suture material passed around the proximal fragment of clavicle and under the coracoid. This technique is almost the same as that described in Figure 4–62 for acute acromioclavicular dislocations, except in this case the fracture fragments are pulled into apposition. This is done through a 9.0 cm. incision that starts superiorly over the fracture site and extends down anteriorly to the coracoid.

If a transacromial pin is used, a 3.0 cm. incision is made over the fracture site and a rigid, smooth, 3/32-inch pin is passed through the distal clavicular fragment out laterally, and the blunt end of the pin is passed back retrograde into the proximal clavicular fragment, similar to the technique for internal fixation of midclavicular fractures (Fig. 5–42). This technique requries careful positioning of the patient with a sandbag under the scapula and the patient's head turned away from the operating field, or else the pin cannot be passed out laterally. A smooth pin seems less apt to break than a threaded pin, but it must be bent over subcutaneously at right angles (lateral to the acromion) to prevent migration. Following either method of fixation, a sling is worn for six weeks. If a transacromial pin is used, it is removed at this time.

In any operative repair of this lesion, it is important to appreciate that the distal fragment retains intact ligamentous attachments to the coracoid that contribute to the strength of the repair. For this reason, the distal fragment should not be excised except in very rare instances when its articular surface has been hopelessly distorted by the injury.

Type III Distal Clavicle Fractures

Type III fractures, those of the articular surface of the clavicle, frequently lead to symptomatic arthritic changes, and apparently because of the abundant blood supply, they may be followed by extensive resorption of the end of this bone. Resorption of the articular surface is also seen in "weightlifter's clavicle" and in other athletic patients who have repeated microtrauma, which I believe can produce small fractures of the articular surface of this type.

When this injury is followed by persistent symptoms, it can be treated satisfactorily by excision of the acromioclavicular joint leaving most of the coracoclavicular ligament intact. It is important in acromioclavicular arthroplasty to suture the trapezius muscle to the deltoid muscle so that it covers the stump of the clavicle and fills the dead space (see Fig. 6–8).

Fractures of the Inner Clavicle

Fractures of the inner clavicle can be treated with a supporting sling, but occasionally, when the articular surface is involved, they lead to arthritic changes with persistent pain and disability. These arthritic changes are treated by excision of the inner clavicle. In performing sternoclavicular arthroplasty, it is important to leave most of the costoclavicular ligament intact and to transfer the clavicular head of the sternomastoid into the dead space, to minimize hematoma formation and to reduce the tendency of the stump to ride upward (see Fig. 6–11).

Indications for Operative Treatment

The indications to consider for operative treatment of acute fractures of the clavicle may be summarized as follows:

1. Neurovascular involvement (Fig. 5–41C).
2. Interposition of soft tissues or rotated intermediate fragment (Fig. 5–41A).
3. Open fractures.
4. Electively for severe, uncontrolled deformity in young women (Fig. 5–41D).
5. Electively for the management of selected patients with multiple injuries (Fig. 5–41B).
6. Electively for Type II distal clavicle fractures.

Technique of Open Reduction and Internal Fixation

Unless the surgeon approaches internal fixation of clavicular fractures with the same precautions and scrupulous technique accorded any other long-bone fracture, the incidence of complications is high.

Various methods have been used for the internal fixation of fractures of the distal end of the clavicle. I usually prefer to use intramedullary fixation of midclavicular fractures, as illustrated in Figure 5–42, rather than plates and screws. The clavicle may be too small in diameter to accept a Knowles pin, which when feasible may be inserted through a drill hole in the anterior cortex of the proximal fragment across the fracture site and into the medullary canal of the distal fragment. I usually use a smooth, 3/32-inch Steinmann pin inserted

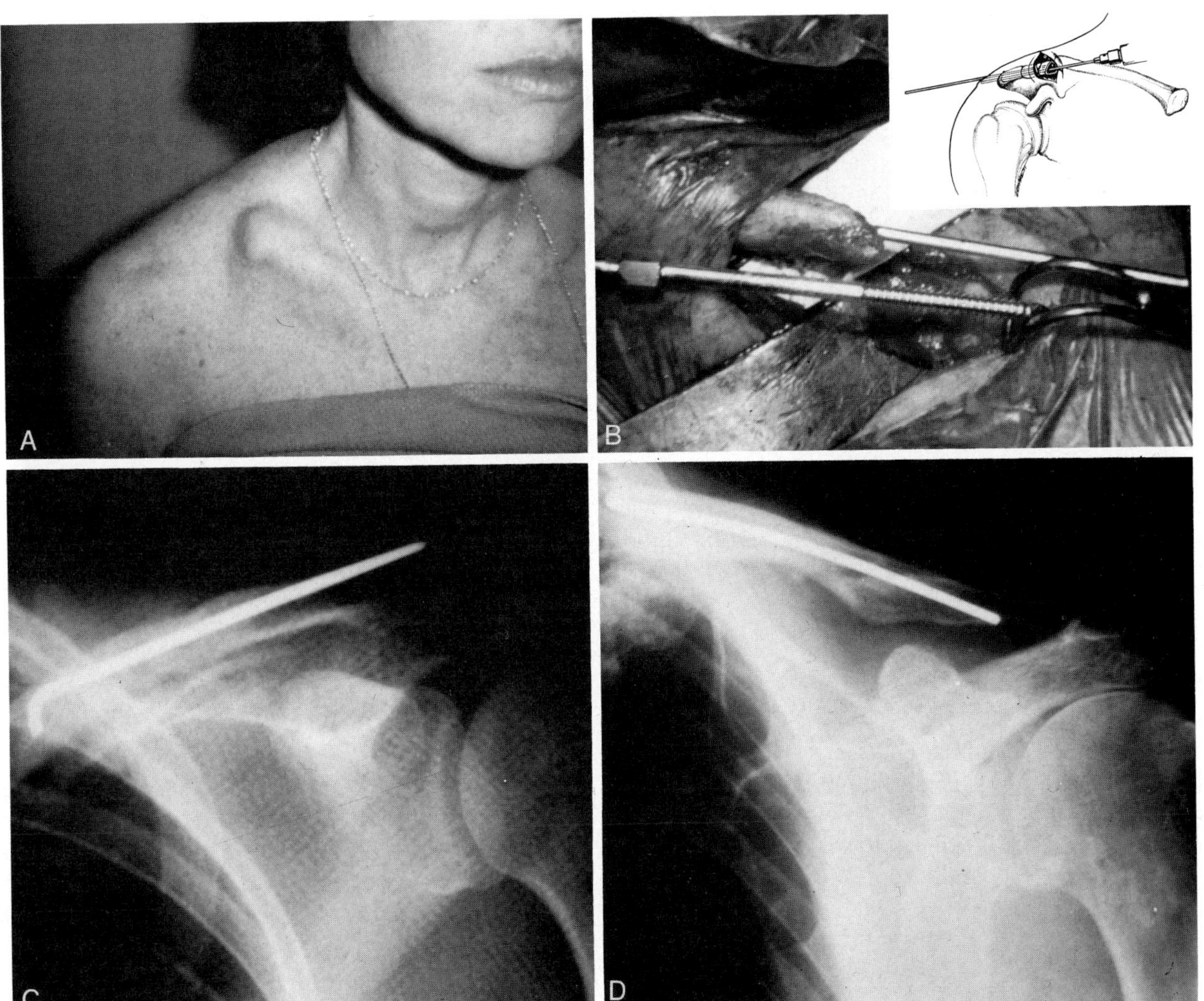

Figure 5–42. Technique of repair of nonunion of the middle third of the clavicle by the method described in the text.

A, Pre-operative appearance; patient had pain on use of the arm or on sleeping on that side.

B, Nonunion with retrograde wire as in the inset. A Knowles pin (in the field) was considered as an alternative but was too large for this clavicle. Iliac bone grafts were placed posteriorly.

C, Immediate post-operative x-ray; patient in a plastic clavicular cast. A single pin was used in this case. The bone grafts can be seen.

D, A 45 degree angle view of the clavicle nine months after repair showing good healing. The bone grafts had been placed posteriorly, avoiding a bump on the subcutaneous surface and avoiding pressure on the neurovascular bundle. The pin was removed with local anesthesia.

retrograde from the fracture site into the proximal fragment after having pre-drilled the medullary canal of the proximal fragment to make a hole in the anterior cortex, with the drill used from inside out at the point at which the drill engages the anterior cortex. The blunt end of the Steinmann pin is then inserted retrograde from the fracture site up the medullary canal and out the anterior cortex. The fracture is then reduced, and the sharp end of the pin is inserted down the medullary canal of the distal fragment and allowed to protrude a short distance outside the posterior cortex of the distal fragment. The pin is then bent over near the hole in the anterior cortex to prevent lateral migration and is cut off at this site. This is a modification of Rowe's intramedullary pin method of fixation.[272] The procedure is performed through an oblique incision in Langer's lines (which parallel the curve of a necklace) made just inferior to the fracture site below the bone prominence. For repairing a nonunion with bone grafts, a 7.0 cm. incision is used (a shorter incision is used for a fresh fracture). A sling or shoulder spica is used post-operatively, depending on the security of the fixation, until early union occurs.

Results to Be Expected

Nonunion of the clavicle is rare.[157] It is more likely to occur in poorly immobilized and neglected fractures, such as in patients with multiple injuries or in unstable Type II (displaced) fractures of the distal end. Malunion is common, and for this reason it may be justifiable occasionally to consider elective internal fixation in selected displaced fractures of the middle third in young women with unsightly, unstable fractures who require a good cosmetic result (see Fig. 5–42); however, this is unusual.

The time required for enough consolidation to permit adult patients to resume heavier activities is considerably greater than that for children—at least five months. The incidence of re-fracture is high in mature clavicles that are subjected to violent activities prior to that time.

Complications of Clavicular Fractures

Neurovascular

Exuberant callus, residual deformity, and scarring in the middle third may be associated with persistent neurological defects and circulatory changes as a result of compression of the subclavian vessels and brachial plexus against the first rib. It is important to consider the possibility that a cervical root avulsion or brachial plexus injury could have occurred at the time the fracture was sustained. The presence of anomalous cervical ribs predisposes the patient to this problem, and cervical spine radiographs should be obtained. When chronic neurovascular symptoms are severe, decompression by excision of the middle third of the clavicle may be indicated. Acute laceration to the subclavian vessels and brachial plexus is less common but can occur, demanding expert vascular surgery and neurosurgery and posing dire consequences (Fig. 5–41B).

Malunion

An ugly prominence in the middle clavicle can be extremely disturbing to a young woman (Fig. 5–41D). Shaving away the bone may be inadequate, and an osteotomy for realignment and internal fixation might have to be considered but has not been necessary in my experience.

Nonunion

Nonunion of the clavicle is rather rare but is a threat, especially in adults (see Figs. 5–41 and 5–42). Factors predisposing the patient to nonunion of the clavicle include (1) inadequate immobilization (as in patients with multiple injuries), (2) operative treatment with inadequate internal fixation, and (3) Type II (interligamentous) fractures of the distal clavicle (Fig. 5–43). The nonunion, in my experience, is usually symptomatic and is treated by internal fixation and iliac grafts, which are placed posteriorly (away from the neurovascular bundle and subcutaneous surfaces)[157] (see Fig. 5–42). In nonunions of the distal end, I prefer to save the distal fragment unless its articular surface is too incongruous, as discussed with Fig. 5–43D, in which case if it is excised the coracoacromial ligament is transposed to the proximal fragment to reinforce the coracoclavicular ligament repair, and the proximal fragment is internally fixed with No. 5 nonabsorbable sutures passed under the coracoid, as shown in Figure 4–67C.

Post-traumatic Arthritis

Post-traumatic arthritis is discussed with Type III fractures of the distal clavicle (Fig. 5–43E) and in Chapter 6, page 436. The acromioclavicular joint is much more frequently involved than the ster-

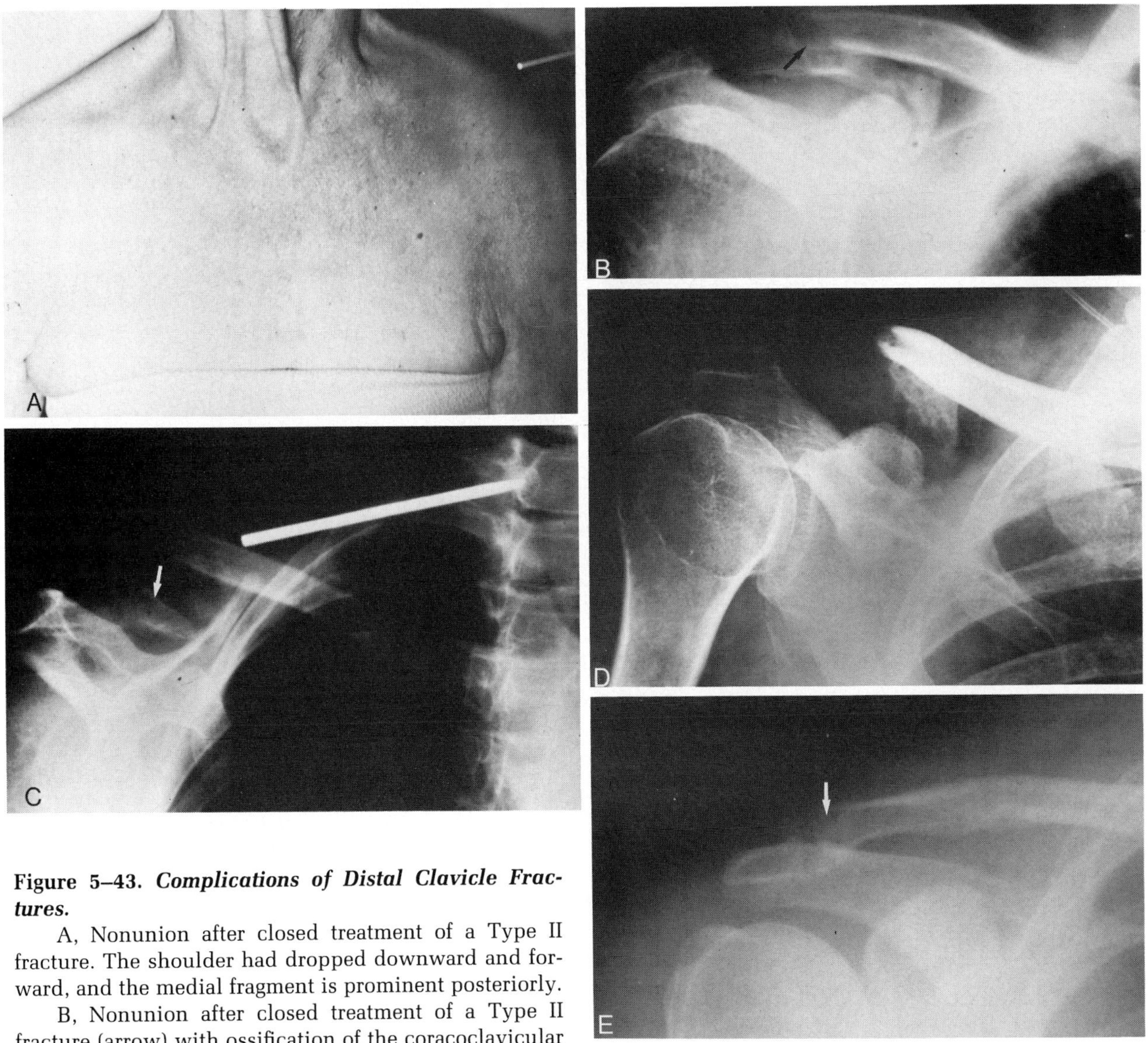

A B C D E

Figure 5–43. ***Complications of Distal Clavicle Fractures.***

A, Nonunion after closed treatment of a Type II fracture. The shoulder had dropped downward and forward, and the medial fragment is prominent posteriorly.

B, Nonunion after closed treatment of a Type II fracture (arrow) with ossification of the coracoclavicular ligaments outlining their attachment on the distal fragment and detachment from the proximal fragment (see Fig. 5–40B2).

C, Migration of a straight pin used to internally fix a Type II fracture (arrow).

D, Prominent medial stump and pain two years after excision of the distal fragment of a Type II fracture. Excision of the distal fragment should be avoided in this injury because it removes the only intact ligaments remaining attached to the clavicle. These ligaments attach the distal fragment to both the coracoid and the acromion (see Fig. 5–40B2).

E, Osteolysis of the distal clavicle and painful post-traumatic arthritis (arrow) 2 years after a Type III fracture.

noclavicular joint. The articular surface defect has often been overlooked at the time of the injury. Comparison radiographs of the normal side, laminograms, and CT scans are helpful in establishing the diagnosis (see Fig. 5–40C). A therapeutic test injection of 1 percent lidocaine into the joint should temporarily eliminate pain. This is routine before recommending surgical excision of the joint. In acromioclavicular arthroplasty, after the outer clavicle is excised, the trapezius muscle is sutured to the deltoid muscle. In sternoclavicular arthroplasty, the clavicular head of the sternomastoid is used to fill the dead space, as described in Figure 6–8, page 435.

FRACTURES OF THE SCAPULA

The scapula acts as a flat surface against the ribs for stabilization of the upper extremity against the thorax. Because it is firmly attached to the clavicle and articulates with the humerus, it is subjected to a large variety of injuries. The surgical anatomy, mechanism of injury, and therapeutic implications of each of the major patterns will be considered individually.

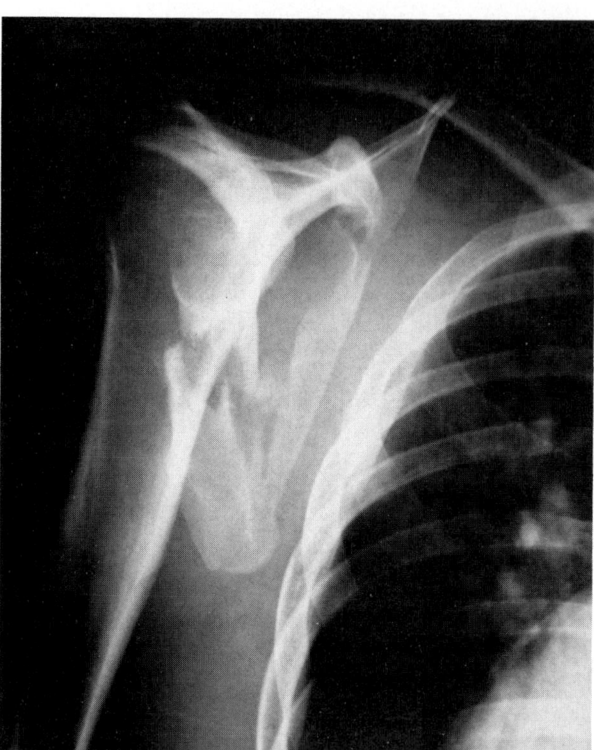

Figure 5–44. ***Scapular Fractures.*** Fractures of the body of the scapula are surrounded by muscles and heal rapidly; however, adjacent structures may have been injured, as discussed in the text.

Fracture of the Body of the Scapula

The body and spine of the scapula are surrounded by muscles and heal rapidly with little residual disability (Fig. 5–44). The scapula's muscle coverage and "give" on impact by recoil on the chest wall protect it from both direct and indirect trauma. Fractures of the scapula, therefore, usually require trauma of appreciable magnitude and should alert the surgeon to search for associated injuries (e.g., multiple rib fractures, pneumothorax, subcutaneous emphysema, vertebral compression fractures, and extremity fractures). Because of the gravity of associated injuries, fractures of the scapula may be missed initially. Scapula fractures may also occur from indirect trauma. For example, avulsion fractures of the coracoid process may result from psychiatric electroshock therapy as a result of muscle contraction or may occur with a severe blow directly on the top of the shoulder, in which case there are often associated neurological deficits (see Fig. 5–51).

Clinical and Radiographic Findings

The patient with a fractured scapula usually holds the arm adducted and protects it from all movements, especially abduction. This posture is caused by intramuscular hemorrhage into the supraspinatus, infraspinatus, and subscapularis, resulting in secondary spasm, which produces loss of arm abduction and may mimic a rotator cuff injury. Abduction power returns as the hematoma and spasm resolve. In my experience, the amount of swelling and ecchymosis present with scapular fractures is soon generally much more extensive than that seen with a tear of the rotator cuff and direct tenderness over the scapula distinguishes these lesions from cuff tears.

Radiographs should include anterior-posterior and tangential oblique views of the scapula as well as a true axillary view to evaluate the glenoid ("trauma series").

Treatment

I believe that fractures of the body and spine of the scapula can be treated in the same way that the surrounding soft-tissue injury is treated: by cold applications to minimize bleeding for the first 48 hours, followed by low heat to increase local resorption, and by continuing immobilization so long as needed to relieve pain. Considerable displacement is compatible with a good result and can be accepted. However, in patients with severe trauma, associated glenoid displacement, and rib displacements, "a locked scapula" may result in permanent limitation of scapular movement (Fig. 5–45).

Complications

Fractures with displacement may heal with sufficient bony irregularities to cause rubbing on the ribs. If chronic irritation causes pain, crepitus, and limitation of motion, this may necessitate excision of irregular areas on the scapula.

"Locked" Scapula

Intrathoracic dislocation has been reported in which the entire body of the scapula is displaced forward and outward and its lower angle is locked between the ribs. I have never seen this lesion. DePalma[17] states that the injury responds to closed

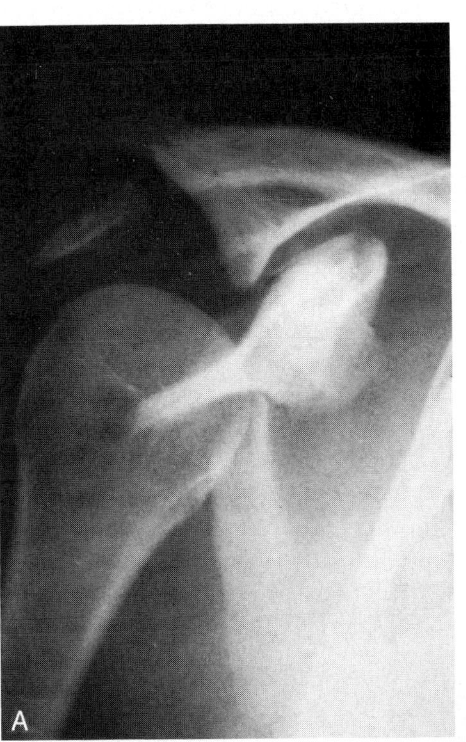

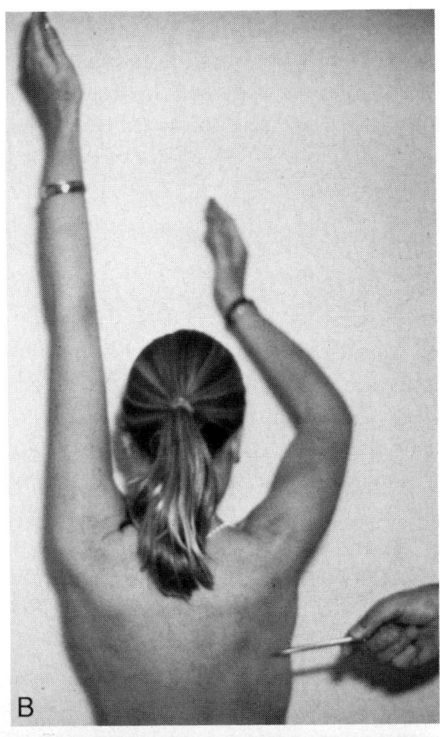

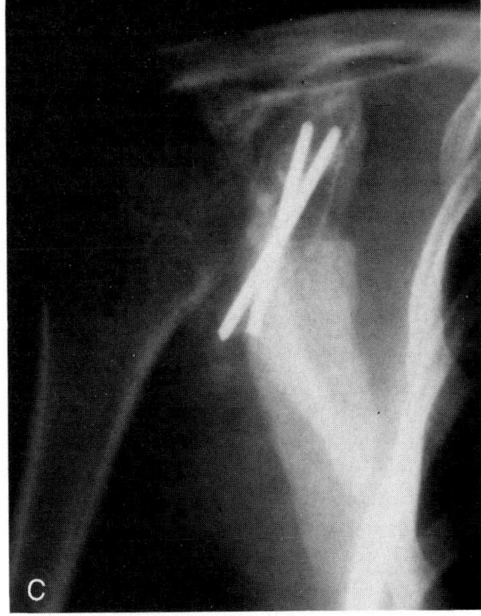

Figure 5–45. ***"Locked Scapula."*** A and B, Trauma severe enough to produce this fracture also fractured eight ribs, collapsed the lung, and ruptured the liver. One-third of the glenoid remained with the coracoid, and two-thirds with the "lateral mass." The coracoid muscles were pulling the coracoid caudalward, while the teres muscles were displacing the lateral mass laterally, producing marked distortion of the articular surface of the glenoid. An open reduction was performed with threaded pin fixation (C), with recovery of much of the glenohumeral motion; however, the scapula did not rotate because of the rib deformities.

reduction. His technique of reduction is as follows: While an assistant applies steady traction on the hyperabducted arm, the surgeon grasps the axillary border of the scapula, and in one movement, rotates it forward and pushes it directly backward. After reduction is obtained, the scapula is fixed to the chest wall, followed by use of a sling and swathe for ten days.

I have seen, as shown in Figure 5–45, several patients with limited motion following violent injuries that produced multiple depressed rib fractures that created a cavity locking the scapula and prohibiting scapulothoracic movement. I have heard of chest surgery with rib osteotomies being performed for this; however, none of my patients had enough disability to want such treatment, probably because their glenohumeral motion was normal.

Fractures of the Neck of the Scapula

When these fractures are minimally displaced and stable, I treat them by early functional exercises, as described previously for minimally displaced upper humeral fractures. There is rarely an indication for open reduction of a fracture of the neck of the scapula unless the glenoid is involved (see Figs. 5–45 to 5–48). The functional results of the fractures are much better than the disturbing radiographs might indicate.

I have seen only three isolated scapular neck fractures (without articular surface components of the glenoid) that were unstable, and they were associated with displaced midclavicular fractures, as illustrated in Figure 5–48. These patients were treated satisfactorily with internal fixation of the clavicle fracture and gentle passive exercises. However, it should be added that I have never seen an ununited scapular neck fracture and have not seen this combination of scapular neck and clavicle fracture treated without internal fixation of the clavicle.

Fracture of the Glenoid

A small fragment of the rim of the bony glenoid or reaction bone is often seen after traumatic glenohumeral dislocation (see Fig. 4–49), which is best seen in axillary view x-rays made with the film held above the shoulder and the tube near the patient's hip. It is helpful to determine the presence of these fragments, because they confirm the diag-

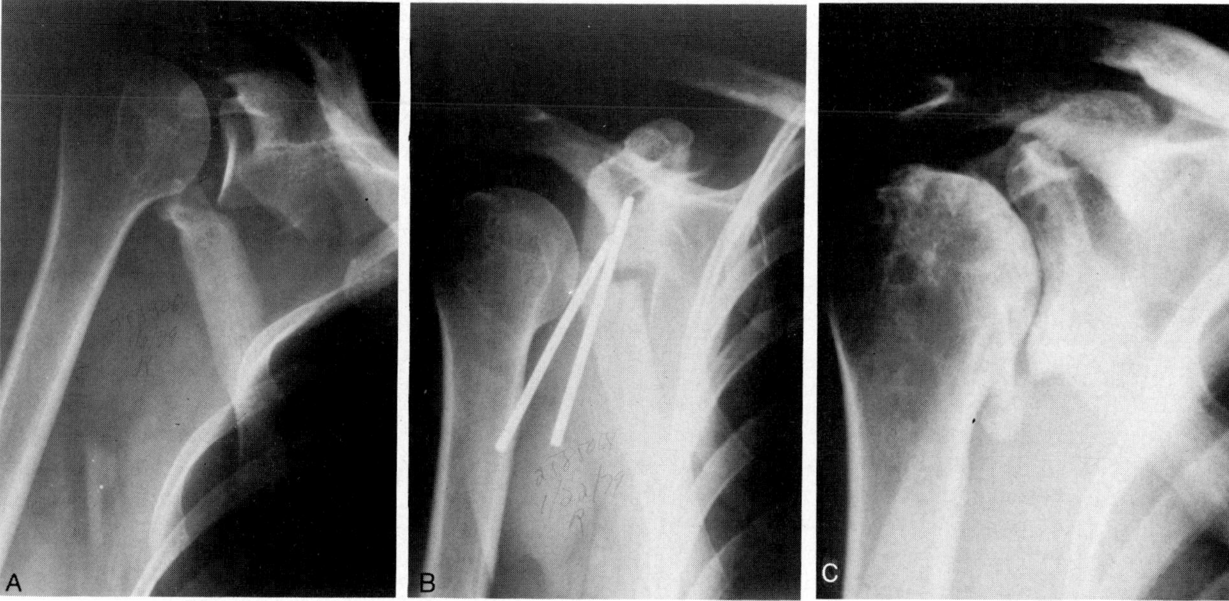

Figure 5–46. A 30 year old woman with another displacement of part of the glenoid with the "lateral mass" of the scapula by the teres muscles and caudal tilt of the coracoid and proximal fragment of the glenoid (A). Open reduction and removeable pin fixation were performed, which appeared to be satisfactory (B). Nine years later, the patient returned with painful post-traumatic glenohumeral arthritis requiring an arthroplasty (C).

nosis and may be useful in repairing recurrent dislocations. In shoulders with recurrent posterior dislocations, there may be a posterior rim fragment. The extent of larger glenoid fractures can be demonstrated by CT scan. Their treatment is shown in Figures 4–45, 4–46, and 4–49.

Large portions of the articular surface of the glenoid are occasionally seen with comminuted fractures of the scapula, as shown in Figure 5–47, or displaced with either anterior or posterior fracture-dislocations. These lesions are caused by a violent central impact on the head of the humerus, and they render the joint incongruous and unstable. They may require open operative treatment.

As shown in Figure 3–14, there is a strong mass of bone along the lateral margin of the scapula that we have come to refer to as the "lateral mass." This may fracture as a separate piece, which is usually in continuity with some of the articular surface of the glenoid. It is usually abducted by the teres major and teres minor muscles, requiring open reduction if the contour of the articular surface of the glenoid is to be restored (see Figs. 5–45 and 5–46).

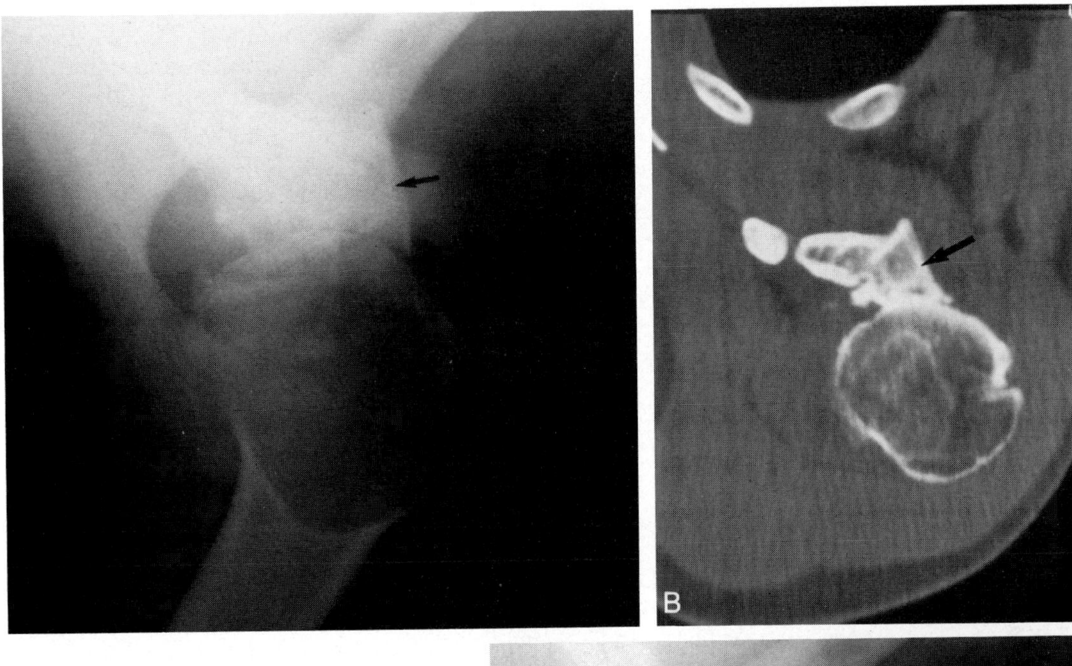

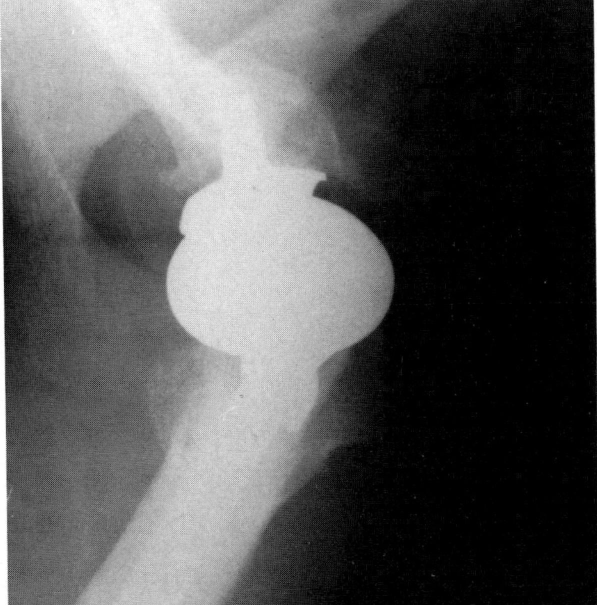

Figure 5–47. Markedly displaced fracture of the neck of the glenoid seen one year after injury in a 20 year old man requiring total shoulder arthroplasty.

A, Axillary view showing the articular surface of the glenoid pointing anteriorly (toward the arrow) and the head, which is articulating against the side of the glenoid and has become devoid of cartilage and arthritic.

B, CT scan showing the malunited glenoid (articular surface pointing toward the arrow) and the loss of joint space.

C, Total arthroplasty using a glenoid component but leaving the malunited glenoid in place gave an excellent result.

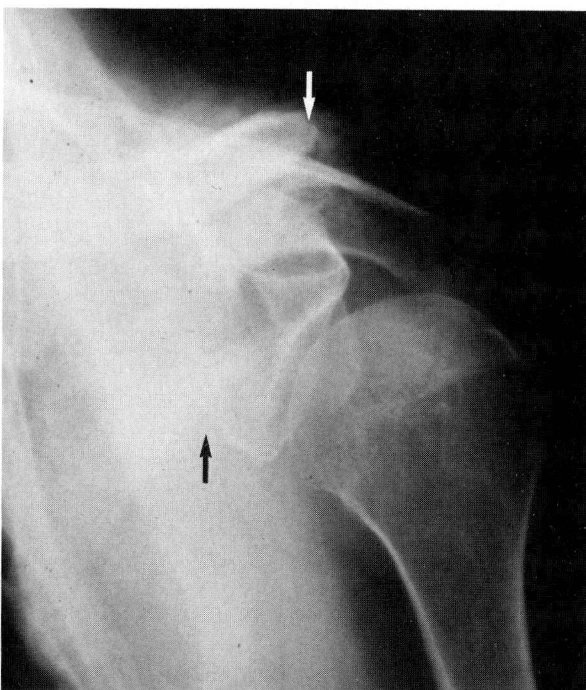

Figure 5–48. Fracture of the neck of the scapula (black arrow) and fracture of the midclavicle (white arrow). Treatment is discussed in the text (see p. 414).

Fracture of the Acromion

Fractures of the acromion usually result from a direct downward blow on the shoulder. A careful neurological examination is important, because an impact of this magnitude often produces avulsion lesions of the roots of the brachial plexus (Fig. 5–49A).

Acromial fractures may also be produced by upward displacement of the humeral head—that is, a "superior dislocation." In this case, an extensive traumatic tear of the rotator cuff should be suspected and an arthrogram performed (Fig. 5–49B).

Clinical and Radiographic Findings

Diagnosis is confirmed on anterior-posterior and lateral views ("outlet view"; see Figs. 1–12 and 2–28) of the shoulder made in the scapular plane and supplemented with an axillary view. An unfused acromial epiphysis, or os acromiale, may be confused roentgenographically with a fracture of the acromion; however, lack of tenderness and swelling differentiates it from a fracture. When one is in doubt, both shoulders should be x-rayed, the os acromiale being bilateral in about 60 per cent of the cases; a CT scan can help in some instances. In litigation cases, distinguishing between an old fracture and an os acromiale may be important. Arthrograms should be obtained to demonstrate an associated tear of the rotator cuff when a superior dislocation is suspected (see Fig. 5–49B).

Treatment of Acromial Fractures

Acromial fractures are usually without significant displacement and can be treated symptomatically. Depressed fractures, as shown in Figure 5–49A, occasionally require elevation and screw fixation to eliminate impingement on the subacromial space and to eliminate a derangement of the acromioclavicular joint.

When the acromion is fractured by the upward impact of the humeral head ("superior dislocation" of the glenohumeral joint; Fig. 5–49B), there is usually extensive tearing of the rotator cuff, which requires surgical repair. The lesion is underdiagnosed. It should be suspected if the acromial fragment is displaced upward and the subacromial space (acromiohumeral distance) is reduced. An arthrogram of the glenohumeral joint demonstrates a tear in the rotator cuff. Every effort should be made to repair the rotator tendons and the acromion. Acromionectomy should be especially avoided because it weakens the deltoid muscle, which, in the face of cuff impairment, can be disastrous (see Fig. 2–46). In symptomatic nonunion or malunion of the acromion, no more than a very small fragment of acromion should be excised (see Fig. 2–46).

Fracture of the Coracoid

The coracoid process stands out from the anterior-superior aspect of the scapula, and its attached muscles and ligaments play an important role in stabilizing the scapula as well as in contributing to flexion of the shoulder and elbow. The muscles that attach to it are the short head of the biceps, the coracobrachialis, and the pectoralis minor. Its attached ligaments are the coracohumeral, coracoacromial, and coracoclavicular. A hard blow on the point of the shoulder, such as that which produces a displaced fracture of the distal clavicle or an acromioclavicular dislocation, may avulse the coracoid by exerting traction on the coracoclavicular ligament (Fig. 5–51A). It may be avulsed by strong muscle pull, as in a seizure; fractured by the impact of a dislocating humeral head; or fractured by direct trauma.

Clinical and Radiographic Findings

Acute injuries are associated with local pain and tenderness, as well as pain on forced adduction

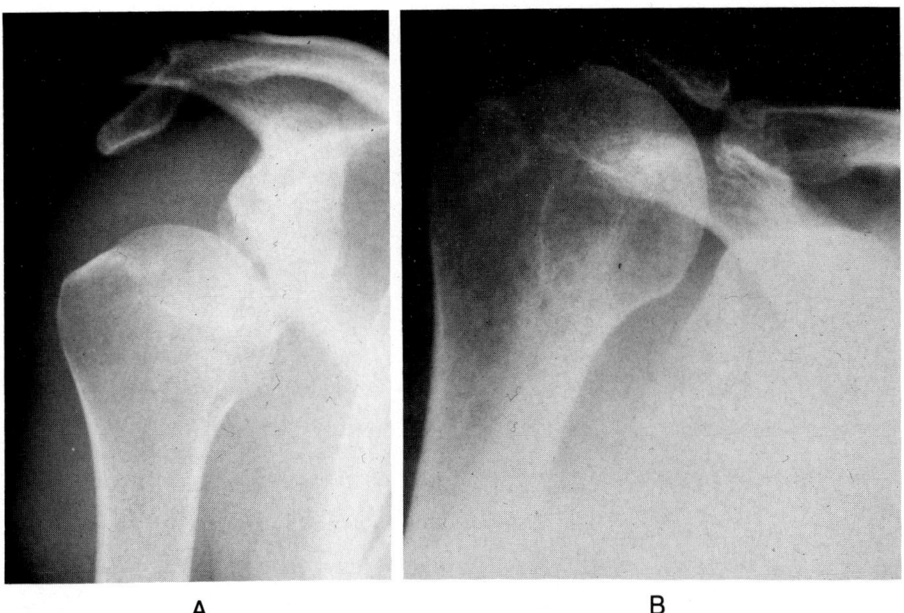

Figure 5–49. The direction of the displacement of fractures of the acromion is important.

A, If the acromion is depressed, as in this shoulder, think of root avulsions and nerve injuries.

B, If the acromion is displaced upward, think of a "superior dislocation" of the humeral head with a large rotator cuff tear, and obtain an arthrogram.

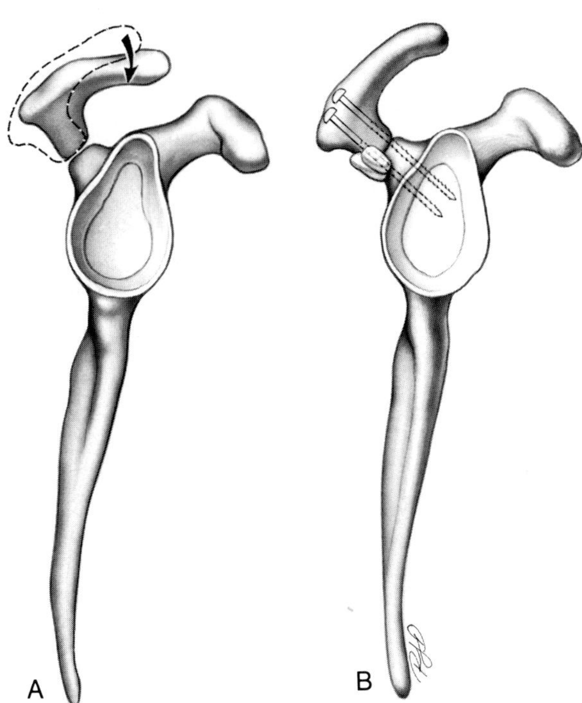

Figure 5–50. A and B, Nonunion or malunion of the acromion can cause impingement (see Chapter 2, p. 53, and Fig. 2–11B). It is possible to obtain rigid fixation of the base of the acromion with two screws as depicted in B, shown with bone grafts, either to repair a nonunion of the base of the acromion or after an osteotomy for a malunion.

of the shoulder and flexion of the elbow. Old injuries may cause impingement symptoms (see Chapter 2, p. 53) aggravated by specific motions of the shoulder.

The initial force may cause the coracoid to contuse the cords of the brachial plexus, which lie just beneath it (Fig. 5–51B). This can produce subtle and occult neurological defects, which are easily overlooked initially.

When the suprascapular nerve is caught in the notch (Fig. 5–51C), its paralysis has been mistaken for a tear of the rotator cuff. Electromyograms are important in diagnosing and prognosticating this injury. As to be discussed, exploration of the nerve is usually indicated.

Anterior-posterior radiographs may demonstrate a fractured coracoid, but a good lateral view is essential to avoid missing the lesion. The distal fragment is usually displaced downward and medially.

Fractures may be confused with accessory ossification centers, which may occur at the proximal and distal aspects of the coracoid process. These are generally shell-like and are characteristically located medial to the base, or they may be small and located at the tip to the coracoid process.

As shown in Figures 5–45 and 5–46 and discussed[161] in a following paragraph, displaced fractures of the "lateral mass" of the scapula and

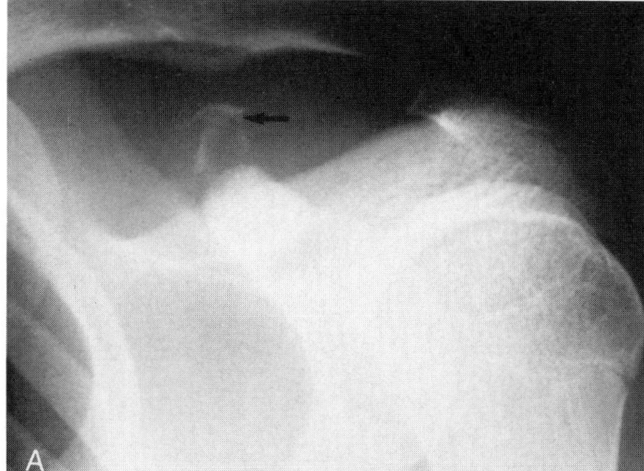

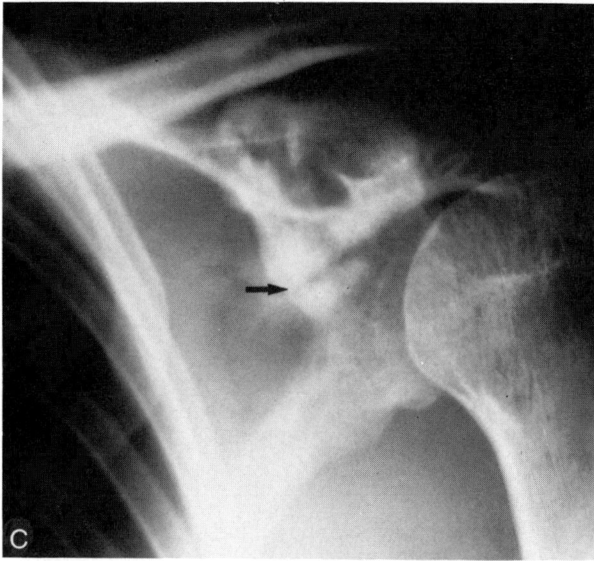

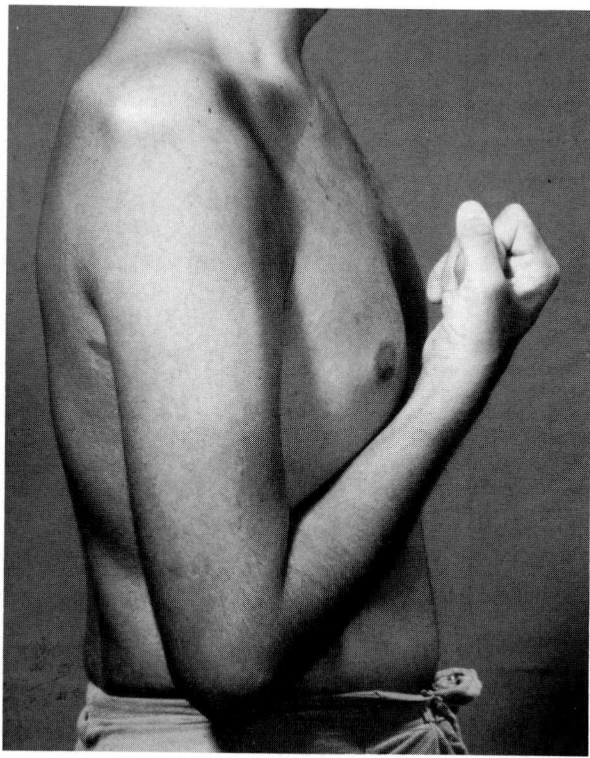

Figure 5–51. Coracoid fractures may be associated with occult, serious, and unexpected neurological deficits.

A, Avulsion of the coracoid by the coracoacromial ligaments and a dislocation of the acromioclavicular joint with extensive neurological injuries, as illustrated in B.

B, Loss of the posterior cord and peripheral motor weakness after an avulsion of the coracoid in a motorcycle accident.

C, Fracture of the base of the coracoid with suprascapular nerve paralysis due to callus and deformity in the suprascapular notch. The differential diagnosis between this lesion (with paralysis of the infraspinatus and supraspinatus muscles) and a tear of the rotator cuff was made by a negative arthrogram and electromyographical findings.

articular surface of the glenoid are often associated with a displaced fracture at the base of the coracoid, which is rotated by the coracoid muscles.

Treatment of Coracoid Fractures

In most instances, no special treatment of the coracoid fracture is needed other than to ensure decompression of the neurovascular bundle. Dislocation of the acromioclavicular joint with avulsion of the coracoid may require transacromial fixation and may be associated with a more violent injury (as shown in Fig. 5–51A) with neurological damage. A severe displacement of the coracoid that threatens persistent coracoid impingement may be best treated by operative repair. In symptomatic

Figure 5–52. A composite of several patients to illustrate the reconstruction of an old gunshot injury.

A and B, The appearance nine months after initial debridement and injury.

C, The gap between the glenoid and the humeral shaft.

D, With traction on the arm, the height for seating the prosthesis is determined to keep tension on the myofascial sleeve. The prosthesis is cemented in the shaft at this level.

E, Roentgen appearance six months after cementing the prosthesis with the arm at proper length, assembling the fragments around it, and re-attaching the muscles to the fragments of bone. Bone union has occurred.

F, The appearance of the patient in B seven years later. Good use below the horizontal was recovered.

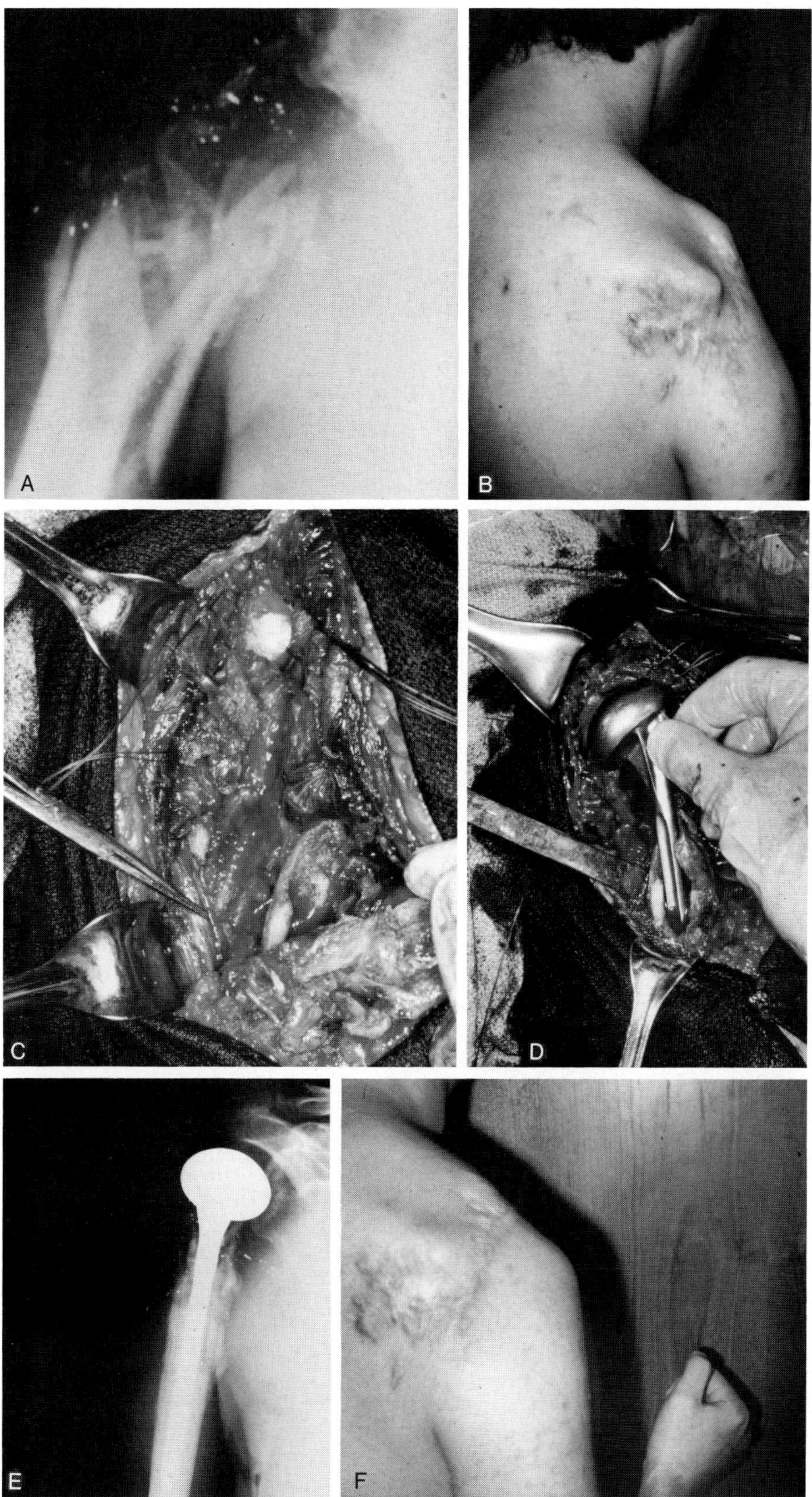

Figure 5–52 *See legend on opposite page*

old injuries, excision of the distal fragment and reattachment of the conjoined tendon are indicated.

In my experience, suprascapular nerve entrapment with fracture of the base of the coracoid (Fig. 5–51C) has a very poor prognosis for recovery once callus forms. I now favor earlier exploration of the nerve (once paralysis of the spina is definitely identified) rather than a long period of watchful waiting.

Fractures of the "Lateral Mass"

A special fracture that I described[71] is a displacement of the "lateral mass of the scapula" (the thick bone along the lateral margin of the scapula), which is usually broken in continuity with the inferior part of the glenoid and is displaced by the teres major and minor muscles, which are attached to the lateral margin of the scapula (see Figs. 5–45 and 5–46). These muscles abduct the lateral mass. In several instances, I have seen this to be associated with displacement of the superior part of the articular surface of the glenoid, which is in continuity with the coracoid. The coracoid is fractured at its base, allowing the coracoid and attached upper portion of the articular surface of the glenoid to be adducted by the short head of the biceps and coracobrachialis. This creates severe distortion of the articular surface of the glenoid and is, I believe, an indication to consider open reduction and internal fixation with pins, AO screws, or nonmetallic sutures.

GUNSHOT AND PROPELLER INJURIES

Mangled shoulders with shattering of bone and soft tissue (Fig. 5–52A) are often associated with nerve injuries and greater risk of infection.

The initial debridement should aim at removing crushed and devitalized tissue and gross contamination, yet preserving bone whenever possible (or in doubt) and of course, evaluating the nerves that present during the dissection (e.g., the axillary nerve is usually seen). The initial surgical treatment aims at preventing infection following the principles of early secondary closure when in doubt. When there is blast injury or crushing of the tissue, antibiotic coverage should be continued longer than for other wounds.

If the glenohumeral joint has been destroyed, it is, of course, a matter of judgement whether any type of reconstruction or steps in preparation for later reconstruction should be made during the initial procedure. In general, I prefer waiting to perform a prosthetic reconstruction until the wound has healed and has remained free of infection. It may be helpful to approximate the tuberosities or rotator cuff tendons with one or two absorbable sutures at the time of debridement to prevent their retraction.

Later, when the wound is healed, it is possible to better estimate the extent of the nerve and muscle damage and the degree of disability. Those patients who have had extensive nerve injuries and possible infection are better left alone. Others might be considered for replacement arthroplasty at the time of exploration of the nerves (Fig. 5–52).

In older lesions, the alternatives are replacement arthroplasty, perhaps with tendon transfers and limited goals rehabilitation (see Figs. 3–57 to 3–71); glenohumeral arthrodesis (see p. 438); or, in some patients who are free of pain, exercises to make the most of what they have rather than surgery.

6

LESS FREQUENT PROCEDURES

FROZEN SHOULDER

Although "frozen shoulder" (Fig. 6–1) is a very frequent cause of chronic shoulder pain, it is relegated to this part of the book because conservative treatment is usually successful. Manipulation under general anesthesia and open release are both rarely indicated; therefore, it is appropriate to list them with the less frequent procedures.

Etiology and Pathology of Frozen Shoulders

The more recent literature[17, 208–210] on frozen shoulder generally agrees with my belief that stiffness of the glenohumeral joint can result from many different pathological conditions. The initiating cause may be situated in the shoulder (intrinsic) or at some distance away from the shoulder (extrinsic). Confusion begins when one believes that a frozen shoulder occurs as a "primary" entity.

It has been best for me to think of frozen shoulder as a symptom (like a headache) that can be produced by any condition that causes the patient to hold the arm against the chest to protect it from painful movements (the "protected position") for a protracted period of time. The initiating pain could be due to inflammation of the bursa from an injury, overuse, a calcium deposit, a cardiac disorder, cervical radiculitis, or a Colles' fracture. The initial cause for holding the arm against the chest has often mended and disappeared by the time the patient is seen by the physician, at which time pain is due to residual stiffness.

Stiffness pain (the pain caused by the frozen shoulder) is due to the shortening and thickening of the soft tissue and to reduction in the volume of the bursal and glenohumeral joint spaces that occurs, as from the immobilization of a joint with a plaster cast. The only difference between the effect of immobilization on the shoulder and that on other joints is the unusually large excursion of motion and the normally loose capsule, ligaments, and bursae present in the shoulder.

It has been a deterrent to logical treatment to think of one single anatomical structure, such as the biceps tendon or glenohumeral joint capsule, as responsible for frozen shoulders.[67] On the rare occasion when my colleagues and I perform open release for intractable frozen shoulder, it has been apparent that indeed the glenohumeral joint capsule is tight and the joint volume is reduced. In addition, the subacromial bursa is also partially obliterated and, what I believe is an important practical point, the coracohumeral ligament is shortened. A short coracohumeral ligament restricts external rotation and always requires division during an open release (see Fig. 1–24). The shoulder stiffens with the arm at the side in internal rotation just as it has been held in the "protected position." The elbow is inactive and may stiffen in a bent position. The hand is inactive and may also stiffen, producing the "shoulder-hand syndrome." This is clear evidence that immobilization affects all of the tissue in the upper extremity and not just one anatomical structure and is not specific to one joint (the shoulder) alone.

In addition, it has been a deterrent to effective treatment to think of a specific pathological process, such as inflammation, as causing all frozen shoulders. To be sure, inflammation can be asso-

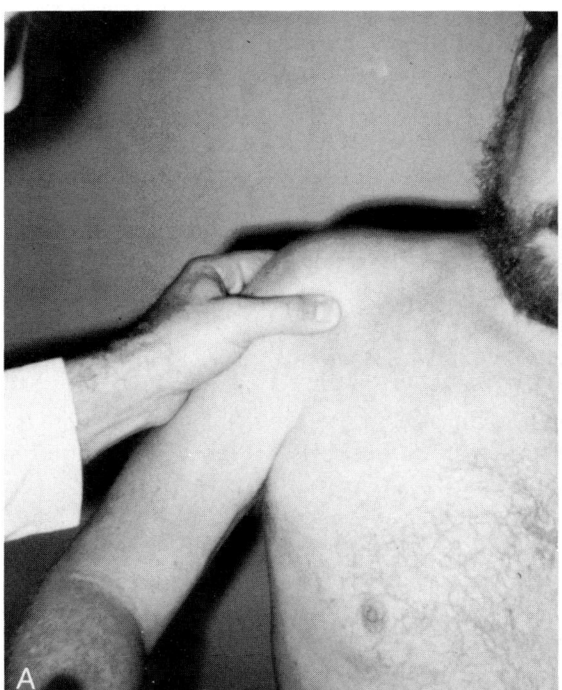

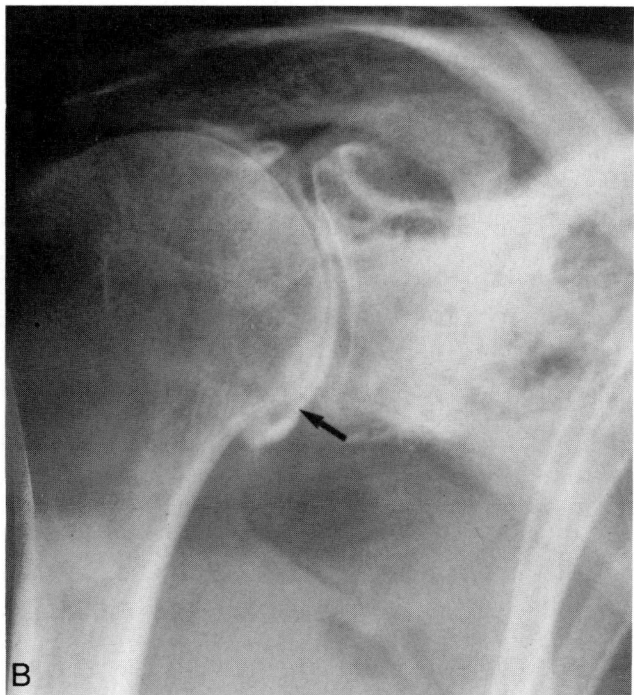

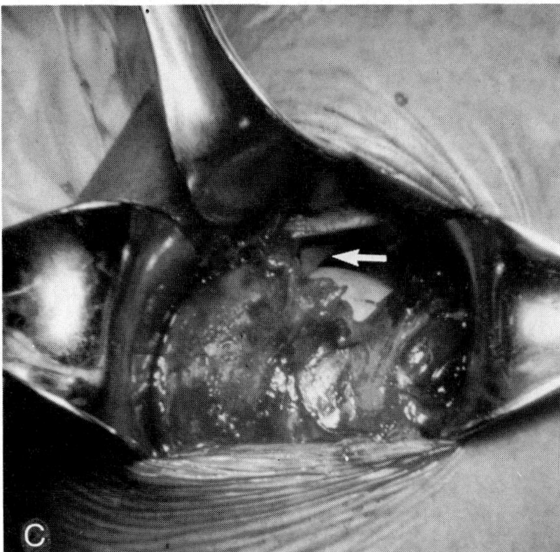

Figure 6–1. ***Frozen Shoulder.***

A, Frozen shoulder pain is elicited at the extremes of passive motion. There is no tenderness. Frozen shoulder is caused by many different conditions and, like a headache, is not considered a primary diagnosis. The safest policy until recovery is complete is to suspect that a hidden, underlying cause may surface later.

B, This arthrogram shows complete obliteration of the capsular pouch (arrow) and early break-out of dye from the subscapularis bursa, as is characteristic of arthrograms of frozen shoulders. Roentgenograms are normal except for eventual decalcification and osteopenia from disuse.

C, Photograph taken in the operating room of a tear at the rotator interval and upper part of the tendon of the subscapularis (arrow) (right shoulder, biceps tendon above arrow) produced by closed manipulation of a frozen shoulder, which had been done just prior to exploration for removal of a calcium deposit. Despite this finding in this case, in my experience closed manipulation before surgery rarely produces a tear of the rotator cuff. If the cuff is torn during closed manipulation, I believe it might heal spontaneously provided that the tear is not superimposed on an impingement lesion.

ciated with pain that leads to a frozen shoulder, but the underlying cause of the inflammation must be sought. The inflammation might have been due to early rheumatoid arthritis, gout, or an injury. Treatment of the stiffness, which is nonspecific, is apart from the treatment of the underlying initiating lesion, which may require some separate medication (anti-inflammatory medication, anti-gout medication, etc.).

The point is that it is extremely helpful and effective to think of the treatment for the residual stiffness as the same in all instances—namely, heat and progressive exercises. If some underlying condition is recognized, it is treated concomitantly. In most instances, however, the initiating condition has either cleared spontaneously and disappeared or has not yet surfaced to be diagnosed.

The fact that similar chemical changes have been found in the joint capsule in a series of frozen shoulders[209] lends further support to my belief that the alterations caused by immobilization—thickening and retraction of the joint capsule and surrounding structures—are nonspecific and occur similarly regardless of the initiating cause for immobilizing the arm. In my clinical experience, similar treatment for all patients with this syndrome (rather than cold for some and heat for others, rest for some and exercise for others, or stellate ganglion blocks for some) has been simple and effective in the vast majority.

Frozen Shoulder Is a Clinical Syndrome

"Frozen shoulder" is a symptom or syndrome rather than a diagnosis. This point emphasizes the need to continue to search for the underlying cause rather than assume that a definite diagnosis has been made.

The clinical picture of this syndrome is as follows:

1. There is a limitation of motion, both active and passive, at the glenohumeral joint. Stiffness varies in intensity from a few degrees loss of external rotation and elevation to rigid glenohumeral ankylosis. Pain is produced by moving the shoulder beyond the range of its free excursion. Pain is almost absent when the shoulder is moved within its range of free excursion (Fig. 6–1A).
2. There is no local tenderness (unlike bursitis, acute calcium deposits, or metastatic lesions).
3. Roentgenograms are normal except for possible osteopenia from disuse atrophy (Fig. 6–1B).
4. Routine laboratory data (see Chapter 1, Table 1–2) are negative.
5. The underlying or precipitating cause for the initial immobilization and inactivity of the extremity may or may not be diagnosable as discussed previously. At the time that the frozen shoulder is recognized, there is usually no evidence of the initiating cause.
6. Relief of pain occurs as glenohumeral joint motion improves.
7. Patients with this condition are most often between 40 and 60 years of age. Although emotional instability has been said to be characteristic, I believe that it is the exception rather than the rule.

Patients with frozen shoulders may be tearful and difficult when first seen because of failure of previous treatment, but given the confidence that comes with reduction of pain as motion improves, most become normal in their mental outlook and become grateful.

During recent years with better diagnosis of shoulder conditions, it is remarkable how few patients are seen in our shoulder clinic who are considered to have emotional disorders. Of course, a patient with continuing pain can become very emotional and uncooperative. If the progress is at a standstill for four months, all laboratory and diagnostic procedures are repeated and the diagnosis is re-appraised.

Treatment of Frozen Shoulder

Conservative Treatment

As discussed previously, I never found it helpful to consider this condition as a primary entity occurring in phases—e.g., "freezing phase," "frozen phase," and "thawing phase"—each with a different treatment. Those who believe in a primary frozen shoulder consider that it occurs in these three phases with more "reaction" and inflammation in earlier phases, which are treated with rest and cold or perhaps arthroscopic irrigation and steroids. They might treat the frozen phase with stellate ganglion blocks and the thawing phase with heat and cautious exercises. If inflammation is present, one should look for the cause of the inflammation (e.g., rheumatoid arthritis, gout, or infection) rather than considering this a primary condition.

My approach has been as follows. After a careful preliminary diagnostic work-up, the range of motion is recorded (see Figs. 1–5, 1–6, 1–7, and 1–9) and a careful explanation is given to the patient regarding the effect of immobilization of the arm against the side (these patients may not have been aware they were doing this) and the importance of light use and passive exercises. The aim of re-establishing external rotation and elevation to eliminate the pain caused by the "checkreign"[211] is explained.

Exercises as described in Figs. 7–7, 7–8, and 7–9 are advised three to five times daily, preceded by low heat, and are advanced according to the amount of stiffness and the amount of pain. Some nonaddicting medication for analgesia is given prior to exercise as needed. Short exercise sessions (five to ten minutes) that are repeated through the day have been most effective. Discomfort should be experienced at the extremes of motion, but the pain should not linger for more than a few minutes. Five repetitions of each exercise are advised, using the first three to warm up and the last two to stretch for a little more motion. It is considered a deterrent to recovery for the patient to worry about keeping the shoulder blade down during exercises.

Those with only minor restriction of movement usually have had pain on certain activities during the day and only in certain positions at night. They can be expected to lose most discomfort within a month, and before full recovery of motion. They are advised to continue stretching exercises at least twice daily until the passive range of motion matches that of the "good" side. Otherwise, there is a tendency to avoid using the arm at the extremes of the excursion of shoulder motion and stiffness tends to return.

At the other extreme are those patients with severe stiffness and a long history of shoulder pain, often after failed treatment. These patients may require the careful guidance of a knowledgeable and understanding physical therapist (who communicates with the physician), as discussed in Chapter 7, Rule 2, page 488. Conservative treatment is continued as long as any improvement is occurring. The therapist sees the patient two or three times a week, and the physician evaluates the patient at intervals of from one to three months, depending on the rate of progress. It is important for the physician to supervise the program, checking the range of motion at intervals and discussing goals of therapy with the therapist until the recovery of range of motion is complete and the patient is comfortable. If exercises are discontinued before recovery of motion, the patient may be disinclined to use or move the arm into the extreme positions and stiffening of the shoulder may gradually recur.

If the patient with a significant deficiency in motion reaches a plateau at which no further improvement in the range occurs for four months, closed manipulation under general anesthesia is considered, as to be discussed.

Manipulation Under General Anesthesia

Indications for Manipulation

Closed manipulation under general anesthesia is considered when, despite an adequate trial of exercises, as described previously and in Chapter 7, a plateau without improvement for four months is reached and significant restriction of movement and pain persist. All diagnostic tests and x-rays are repeated to exclude the appearance of some now diagnosable underlying condition. For example, the finding of a calcium deposit may indicate an injection of the deposit, possibly with local steroids, or an excision of the deposit at the time of manipulation. An elevated uric acid level indicates medical treatment and continuing exercises.

If there are doubts about the diagnosis, arthroscopy prior to the examination and manipulation under anesthesia is considered. An arthrogram might be obtained prior to manipulation if there is the possibility of an impingement lesion interfering with recovery. If an incomplete tear of the rotator cuff was present, it might have lead to the frozen shoulder and prevent recovery with exercises.

Arthrography has been observed to increase motion by distending the joint in some patients (see Fig. 6–1B), although I have not used it for this purpose. Arthrography has been used by some physicians for the treatment of frozen shoulders.[212]

If x-rays show severe osteopenia of the proximal humerus, it is unwise to attempt closed manipulation because of the possibility of fracturing the humerus; an open release is preferred.

Technique of Manipulation Under General Anesthesia

A short-acting general anesthetic agent is used with the patient supine. As soon as the patient is asleep, the range of elevation and external rotation is recorded, and when indicated, the joint is tested for instability. With traction on the arm with one hand and the other hand applying pressure on the humerus near the surgical neck level (to reduce leverage that might fracture the shaft), the arm is raised to as near full elevation (scapular plane) as possible with two-fingers' pressure. With the arm lowered to the side and with the elbow bent 90 degrees, the arm is externally rotated with two-fingers' pressure. More force is avoided. The arm is then abducted (coronal plane) and, with the elbow bent 90 degrees, it is rotated in internal rotation and in external rotation using two-fingers' pressure (see Fig. 2–41B).

These maneuvers are repeated in the same order until a normal range of motion is obtained. Palpable and audible breakage of adhesions is heard during the initial part of this procedure. The final passive range of motion is again recorded. An intra-articular steroid injection at the conclusion of this procedure was discontinued years ago because the ease of maintaining motion post-operatively seems as good without it.

Early passive motion (EPM) (see Fig. 7–7) is begun within 24 hours, and the full passive and self-assistive exercise program is advanced as rapidly as possible (see Chapter 7, Figs. 7–8 and 7–9). A narcotic is used for a few days to relieve pain during exercises. Low heat is applied prior to exercises to relax the muscles. These patients, who have been thoroughly indoctrinated in their role in the exercise program and are made to expect some soreness after this procedure, usually have minimal complaints of pain. Most patients recover their range of motion very rapidly, with gratifying relief.

Post-operatively, the exercise program is closely supervised by the surgeon during the first two or three weeks and at regular intervals thereafter until complete recovery has occurred.

Causes of Failure of Closed Manipulation

Some patients are referred who failed to improve after closed manipulation or who soon become stiff again. The usual cause for this is an unrecognized associated lesion that prevented recovery. The lesion may be impingement, hidden calcium, some unrecognized systemic disorder, arthritic process, or any of many intrinsic or extrinsic disorders. The first step is to repeat all diagnostic studies and x-rays in an effort to find an underlying problem, and if so, treat it.

Failure may have been due to inadequate manipulation at the time of the procedure with inadequate restoration of motion.

A frequent cause of failure is inadequate aftercare after the manipulation. Breaking adhesions creates two raw ends that form even more adhesions unless an adequate range of passive motion can be established within a week or ten days after the manipulation.

A possible cause of failure is tearing the rotator cuff during the manipulation. I have explored a few shoulders after closed manipulation and appreciate that Dr. H. L. McLaughlin,[208] for whom I have only the deepest admiration and respect, was correct in stating that tears of the rotator cuff may be produced by a closed manipulation. He abandoned this procedure for that reason. However, in my experience, more often there is no tear, and even if a tear occurs, provided that it is not superimposed on an impingement tear, it can heal spontaneously.

I have explored a shoulder after manipulation in search for calcium deposits. This patient had developed a frozen shoulder because of painful calcium. At exploration, there was a longitudinal tear at the rotator interval and upper part of the subscapularis insertion, apparently owing to a short coracohumeral ligament. I believe that this tear could have healed without suturing because there was no impingement (see Fig. 6–1C).

Results After Closed Manipulation

The overall results of closed manipulation have been quite good. I believe that significant cuff tears at the time of properly performed manipulation are rare, as discussed above.

I have seen several patients in whom disuse osteopenia had led to fracture of the shaft of the humerus during manipulation. This created a difficult problem. The fracture must be allowed to heal before exercises can be begun to alleviate the stiffness. This complication can necessitate an open release.

With respect for the pitfalls and precautions described previously, the results of closed manipulation have, in my experience, been outstanding. It is performed routinely when doing anterior acromioplasties, repairing tears of the rotator cuff, and arthroscopic procedures. It has not been required more often than once or twice a year for "frozen shoulders," but when indicated for the reasons described previously, the results have been good and lasting.

Open Release of a Frozen Shoulder

Indications

Closed manipulation under anesthesia is contraindicated if (1) there is severe osteopenia of the upper humerus, (2) there has been a previous fracture, or usually (3) if prior closed manipulation has failed. In the case of a failed prior manipulation, the shoulder is explored for evidence of impingement, calcium deposit, or other local lesion that requires correction at the time of the release.

Technique of Open Release

A 7.0 cm. superior incision is made just as for an anterior acromioplasty (see Fig. 2–41). The deltoid is split two inches from above downward. Adhesions are cleared by excising some of the subacromial bursa and using a flat elevator beneath the acromion and deltoid muscle (keeping in mind the axillary nerve in front of the subscapularis and beneath the inferior capsule), freeing all of the rotator cuff superficially with the arm positioned in flexion and external rotation for subscapularis exposure and positioned in extension and internal rotation for infraspinatus and teres minor exposure. The arm is then gently manipulated to determine the amount of residual stiffness.

The coracohumeral ligament is very important in frozen shoulder. It is divided next near the base of the coracoid. This usually improves external rotation and elevation more than would be expected and may be all that needs to be done.

If firm resistance to motion persists or it is thought desirable to explore the joint for diagnostic reasons, the rotator interval is opened. This allows freeing any tight structures inside the joint by prying with a blunt elevator.

In some cases, the subscapularis tendon requires lengthening. If so, it is divided transversely half way through near the lesser tuberosity, and after separating the superficial half of the subscapularis tendon from the deep half, the ends of the two halves are approximated with 00 nonabsorbable sutures, as depicted in Figure 3–30.

If during this procedure there is unexpected evidence of impingement, hidden calcium, or unexpected arthritis, appropriate decompression by anterior acromioplasty or calcium excision is performed. Cultures and biopsies are performed routinely.

The deltoid closure and skin closure are as for anterior acromioplasty (see Fig. 2–41). EPM is started within 24 hours, and the post-operative exercise regimen as described previously after closed manipulation is followed.

Results After Open Release for Frozen Shoulder

The results to be expected are similar to those of closed manipulation under anesthesia, as described on page 426, with the exception of somewhat more initial soreness as would be expected from the incision. However, within ten days the rate of improvement should be about the same as that of closed manipulation.

Although this procedure is rarely indicated, in the right situation, it is of value in clarifying the diagnosis and the long-term results have been lasting.

CALCIUM DEPOSITS

Pathology and Four Types of Pain

Calcium deposits occur at the shoulder more frequently than at other joints. The deposits are located in the tendons of the rotator cuff but may

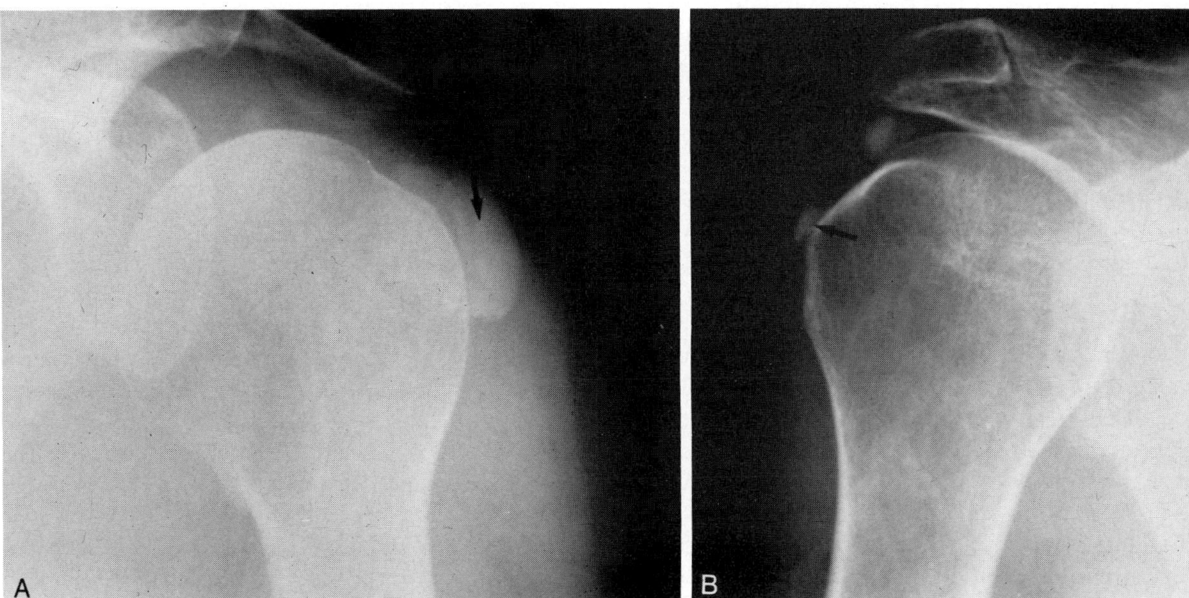

Figure 6–2. *Calcium Deposits.* The routine x-ray views (see Fig 1–12A) bring calcium deposits into profile.

A, Large deposit at the junction of the supraspinatus and infraspinatus tendons (arrow) seen in the anterior-posterior in neutral rotation view.

B, Deposits in the teres minor (arrow) and infraspinatus tendon seen in the anterior-posterior view with internal rotation.

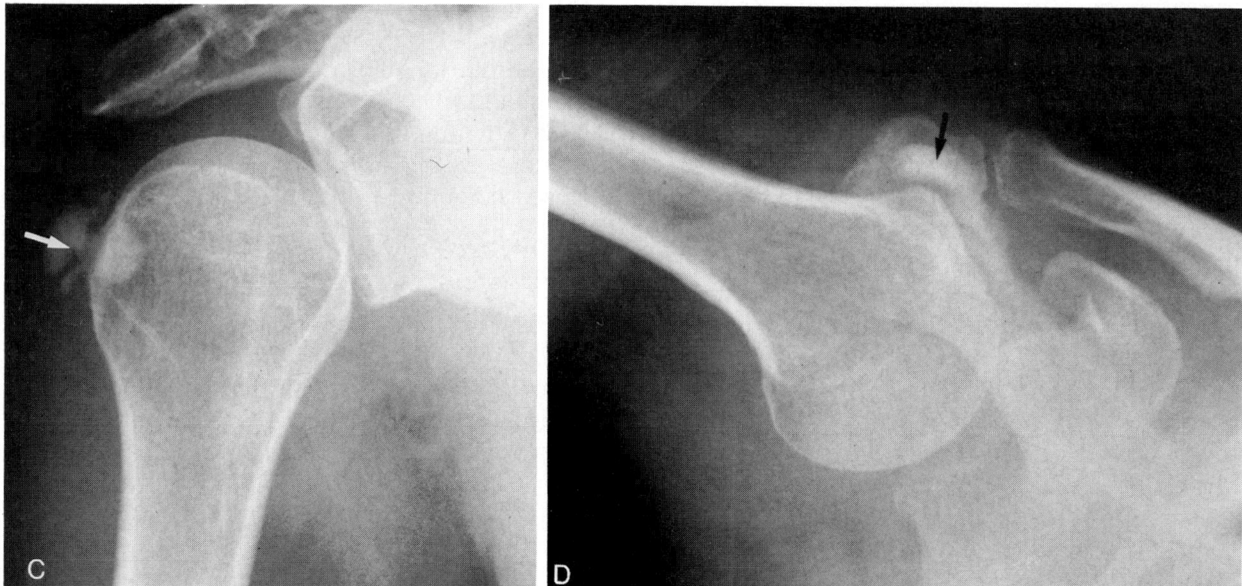

Figure 6–2 *Continued* C, Deposit in the teres minor (arrow) seen in the anterior-posterior view with more internal rotation.

D, Axillary view showing deposit in the subscapularis tendon on the lesser tuberosity (arrow).

break and extrude into the subacromial bursa. They vary in consistency from a milky fluid to chalk-like material (see Figs. 6–2 and 6–3).

In long-standing calcium deposits the subacromial bursa adheres to the area of calcification and becomes thickened. The local thickening of the bursa is thought to occur because the calcium not only acts like a foreign body, but also chemically irritates the tissue. It is this chemical inflammation that might be relieved temporarily by a corticosteroid. A calcium deposit may lie "dormant" and symptomless, or in the "acute" state cause unrelenting agony. In between these extremes is a "subacute" state in which the discomfort, like Stage II impingement, is brought out by the mechanical irritation of activity and subsides with rest. Four types of pain are seen.

First, pain may be due to the ability of the calcium to irritate the tissue chemically.

Second, calcium has the ability to imbibe water and swell under certain conditions. The swelling produces tension in the tissue and can generate enough pressure to cause the calcium to squirt up when first broken open or incised at surgery. Pressure in the tissue causes unrelenting, throbbing pain that can be almost unparalleled. Dr. McLaughlin referred to an acute calcium deposit as a "chemical furuncle" if, when the calcium was incised at surgery, it oozed out under pressure.

Third, thickening of the bursa may occur, which is due to the fibrosis caused by chemical irritation, the amount of room in the subacromial space is reduced and impingement-like pain develops. The prominence caused by a large collection of calcium may also cause impingement pain. This type of impingement pain occurs when the individual is putting on a coat or using the arm overhead.

A fourth type of pain associated with a chronic calcium deposit is that caused by the stiffening of the glenohumeral joint ("frozen shoulder") that occurs when overhead use is avoided for a protracted period of time and the arm is maintained at the side in an effort to avoid irritating the calcium deposit.

Etiology and Behavior

The etiology of a calcium deposit is obscure. I believe that it results from some local insult or injury to one of the tendons in the rotator cuff. This injury to the local blood supply within the tendon causes an alteration in the local pH and leads to "calcific degeneration" with the precipitation of calcium soaps. Whether the "local insult" to the tendon is an injury, a virus, or some other process is not clear. As discussed in Chapter 2, page 142, impingement does not appear to cause the "local insult" in most cases. Once the deposit is formed, it may persist as a potentially irritating foreign body (as described previously) or break out into the bursa to be resorbed; as this break-out occurs, a new blood supply is formed and repair takes place in the tendon where the calcium has been situated.

If the calcium is irritated by some mechanical force, such as raising a window, it may become "acute" with intense pain. It may be broken by this mechanical force, in which case it usually resorbs spontaneously after a period of acute pain caused by chemical irritation. Portions of the deposit may become dormant again, persisting in x-ray films after the period of acute pain has subsided.

Diagnosis of Calcium Deposits in the Shoulder

Because the intensity of the local inflammation and tension in the tissue at the site of the calcium deposit varies, as described previously, the presenting symptoms vary from constant, throbbing pain that prohibits sleep to mild, low-grade discomfort noted only intermittently after activity or when the arm is in certain positions (such as in abduction on the back of the sofa).

On examination, the classic findings are as follows:

1. Tenderness over the deposit, which in the acute phase is marked but is difficult to elicit in the low-grade, subacute phase. In trying to determine whether or not a deposit in a low-grade phase is symptomatic, it is helpful to stand in back of the patient, palpating the tuberosities with one hand as the other hand rotates the humerus. Tenderness is the most important test because even though a deposit is visible in x-ray films, it may not be causing pain at the time of the examination. The patient's pain at that time may be from another cause, such as a neoplasm, or from a frozen shoulder that has developed because of the deposit.

2. Shoulder motion is guarded and restricted, both active and passive motion. In the acute phase, even the slightest movement is extremely painful.

3. Roentgenograms show the characteristic calcium deposits, provided that the deposits are brought into profile. This requires anterior-posterior views with the arm in internal and external rotation and an axillary view. The external rotation view places the supraspinatus tendon in profile. The internal rotation view places the infraspinatus tendon in profile. The axillary view demonstrates deposits in the subscapularis tendon.

Small deposits can cause considerable pain. The amount of discomfort does not correspond to the size of the deposit.

Occasionally, the deposit can be seen to be extruding out from the tendon into the bursa because the calcium is breaking under the tension. This is a good prognostic sign in that the pain, although perhaps worse for a brief period because of the irritation of the tissue caused by the calcium, will soon abate. Calcium breaking into the bursa in this manner is apt to be resorbed and disappear.

4. Routine laboratory data are negative except in the extremely acute phase, in which there may be a low-grade fever and elevation of the white blood cell count, which are in part due to loss of sleep and dehydration from loss of appetite and are often augmented by nausea and vomiting from analgesia. Because of chemical inflammation at the site of an acute deposit, the appearance of the tissue can suggest an infection; however, unless the shoulder had been contaminated by an injection, the local cultures are negative.

Treatment of Calcium Deposits

When I was a resident, the most frequent shoulder operation in our hospital was excision of calcium. Since then, with better parenteral anti-inflammatory medication and corticosteroids, excision of calcium has become a relatively rare procedure in our shoulder clinic.

Conservative Treatment

Calcium Deposit Dormant with Pain from a Frozen Shoulder

The first step is to determine whether the site of the deposit is inflamed and painful or whether the symptoms are secondary to a frozen shoulder (stiffness) that may have developed because of chronic, intermittent discomfort from the deposit but without current inflammation. Limitation of glenohumeral motion without tenderness over the deposit is my indication to try low heat and exercises as for a frozen shoulder but avoiding movements in the directions that irritate the deposit. If this exercise regimen causes the deposit to become tender, a limited number of local steroid injections may be given to reduce the inflammation sufficiently to resume exercises. If this fails, removal of the calcium and thickened bursa with manipulation under anesthesia (see Fig. 6–4) may be required before the patient can tolerate exercises.

Treatment of this combination is made difficult by the fact that exercises are helpful for the frozen shoulder but irritate the deposit. Low heat locally is helpful for the frozen shoulder but irritates the calcium.

Calcium Deposit Acutely Inflamed

In this situation, the calcium deposit is so tender it can hardly be touched. The patient has constant pain, and the pain is made worse by any

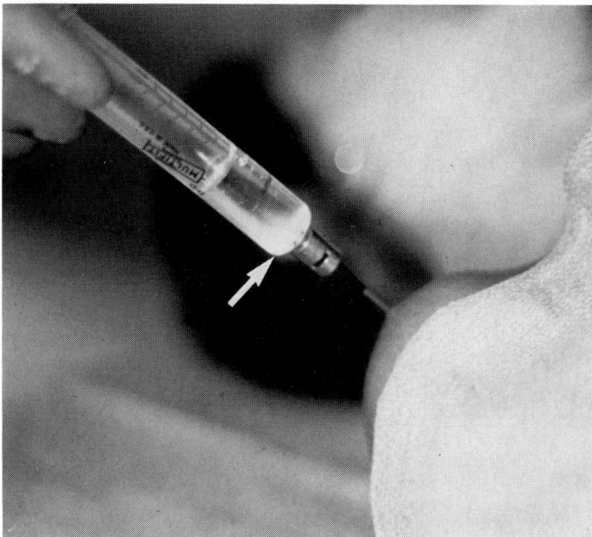

Figure 6–3. Aspiration of soft calcium (arrow) using a syringe with a clear anesthetic agent. This usually relieves pain dramatically by relieving tension in the tissue as well as removing some of the irritating calcified substance. Breaking into the deposit may introduce a blood supply and help the deposit to be resorbed.

movement of the arm. Immobilization ("rest"), applications of cold, and the trial of systemic anti-inflammatory medication may be given first, but if these are not immediately effective, an injection of lidocaine (Xylocaine) and "needling" with local steroids are given. This is the condition in which needling of the deposit is most effective. If a deposit under pressure is present and it is entered with the needle, pain relief is dramatic. The intent is to puncture the deposit to break tension in it. The needle is directed in multiple directions, starting over the point of maximum tenderness. Calcium may be aspirated into the syringe during this procedure to prove that the deposit was entered, and if so, the prognosis for recovery is good (Fig. 6–3).

Subacute Deposits

Intermittent symptoms may be treated with anti-inflammatory medication; a local inection; and, if glenohumeral motion is restricted, cautious exercises. Injections are less apt to be successful when symptoms have been present for years and there are multiple deposits. Excision of the deposit and thickened bursa may eventually be advisable.

Technique of Needling Calcium

An inquiry is made as to the possibility of sensitivity to procaine hydrochloride (Novocain) or Xylocaine. The patient is warned of a possible reaction to the steroid.

Complete surgical precautions are followed with the same skin preparations and use of sterile gloves. I use a fenestrated towel centered over the point of the shoulder for draping (Fig. 6–3).

Two syringes are needed. One syringe with a clear anesthetic agent is used first for local anesthesia and for needling the deposit. If calcium is aspirated back into this syringe, it can be seen. The second syringe has the corticosteroid, which is deposited at the end of the procedure.

The anterior and posterior acromial edges are located, and while the patient or assistant rotates the humerus, the point of maximum tenderness on the upper humerus is identified. With the arm held immobile, this point is anesthetized (with 1 percent Xylocaine) using an 18 or 22 gauge cannulated needle. Next, multiple perforations are made in the rotator cuff in this area, aspirating with each insertion of the needle and irrigating with the solution of anesthetic agent to see if flakes of calcium return. After this attempt to perforate the deposit, the steroid is deposited in the bursa just beneath the acromion.

The patient is given a prescription for pain medication and is advised to use it and an ice bag if an inflammation with pain (from the steroid) should occur.

Those with acute deposits usually have instant and gratifying relief. If the deposit has been punctured, after a few days of soreness (from the calcium in the tisue) relief is usually permanent. The results are less likely to be good in those with long-standing, chalk-like deposits.

Excision of Calcium

Indications

I advise removal of calcium and thickened bursa when conservative treatment, as outlined previously, has failed and there are multiple hard, gritty deposits with long-standing symptoms, indicating the likelihood of associated thickening of the bursa. Using these indications, this procedure has become much less frequently performed than in the past. It is now done in my practice as an isolated procedure only once or twice a year. However, there are a few patients with these criteria and they are helped a great deal.

In my experience, the recovery period for those with long-standing lesions is longer than would be expected. I warn the patients of this pre-operatively and stress the importance of the exercise program following surgery. Under anesthesia, the shoulder

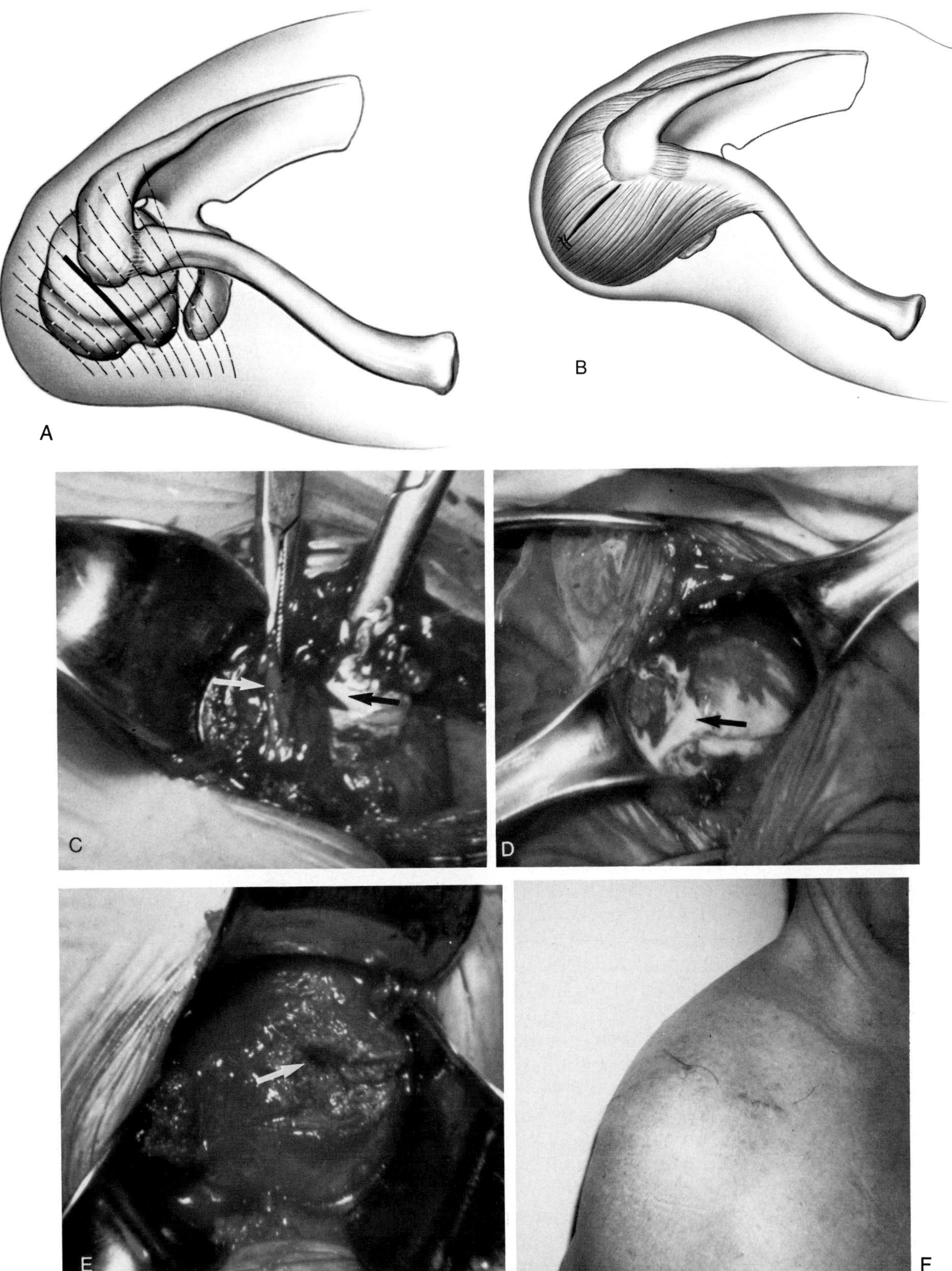

Figure 6–4. Removal of calcium. Patient is positioned in the 30 degree beachchair position. The shoulder is manipulated to eliminate "frozen shoulder" (as shown in Fig. 2–41B and discussed on p. 425) prior to the skin preparation. A, A 6.0 cm. incision is made in the skin lines. B, The deltoid muscle is split 5.0 cm. C, Bursectomy to remove thickened and inflamed bursa (white arrow). Deposits are located with a large needle or clamp (black arrow). D, Soft calcium may exude under pressure (illustrated at the arrow). Hard, gritty calcium requires sharp dissection and curettage with minimal removal of tendon, as described in the text. E, After curettage, all but unusually large cuff defects are left open. No attempt was made to suture the defect (arrow) illustrated. F, After closing the deltoid with two interrupted sutures, a meticulous skin closure is performed with a removeable subcuticular stitch.

is manipulated at the time of the procedure to make sure that associated frozen shoulder has been freed.

Technique

The technique is shown in Figure 6–4. The patient is positioned in a beachchair position with the arm draped free of the side of the table so it can be moved, as for an anterior acromioplasty (see Fig. 2–41). I prefer a general anesthesia, although a supraclavicular block or local anesthesia can be used. The arm is manipulated to obtain a full passive range of motion, as illustrated in Figure 2–41B. A 6.0 cm. skin incision is made in the skin lines. The deltoid muscle is split 5.0 cm. from the anterior acromion. Thickened subdeltoid bursa is excised. The arm is rotated by the assistant to display the subscapularis tendon (by flexion and external rotation of the humerus), the supraspinatus tendon (in neutral rotation), and the infraspinatus and teres minor tendons (when the humerus is held in internal rotation and extension). The location of areas with calcium or hyperemia ("strawberry spot," indicative of a probable site of calcium with inflammation of the tissue) is noted. The bursa is apt to be adherent over the site of the calcium, acting as another guide to help locate the deposits.

When the sites in the cuff to be explored for calcium have been determined, a large No. 15 cannulated needle is inserted into the tendon in various directions at each site. If flakes of calcium are encountered, small longitudinal incisions are made into the tendon so that the deposit can be curetted and removed as much as possible with minimal removal of tendon. Some small flakes of calcium may be left in the floor of the cavity in the tendon rather than remove excessive amounts of tendon.

No attempt is made to close the defects in the rotator cuff except for a few with large, full thickness holes in the cuff. Because there is no impingement present, these defects in the rotator cuff can heal spontaneously within a few months, provided that there has not been too much excision of the cuff during surgery (Fig. 6–4).

The wound is irrigated to remove all fragments of calcium (because calcium can irritate the tissue). An x-ray or fluoroscopic study may be made when indicated to determine how much calcium has been removed. The deltoid muscle is closed with a few interrupted nonabsorbable sutures, and the skin is closed with a pull-out subcuticular stitch.

A sling and swathe is applied for transportation back to the patient's room. This is removed within 24 hours. EPM (see Fig. 7–7) is started within 24 hours and is progressed as rapidly as possible to obtain a full range of motion. Strengthening exercises are deferred until later.

Results to Be Expected After Calcium Excision

As mentioned previously, the patients have been warned pre-operatively of the possibility of a lengthy exercise program following surgery. This can be explained as the time required "until the bursa has had a chance to form" after excision.

Small, full thickness defects in the rotator cuff are at times created during removal of the calcium (Fig. 6–5). I have seen arthrograms to prove that these can heal spontaneously within six months. There is no subacromial impingement to prevent healing of the cuff, as discussed earlier.

We performed anterior acromioplasties at the time of calcium removal in a few patients in hope of easier aftercare. Unfortunately, anterior acro-

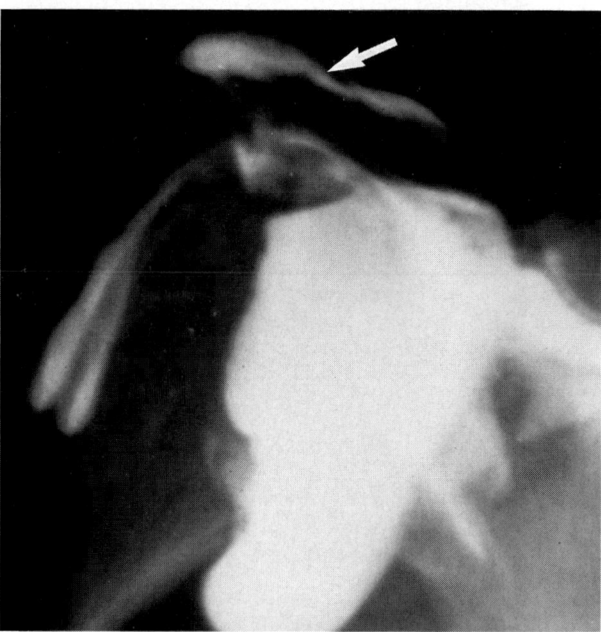

Figure 6–5. Arthrogram of a patient referred for a repair of the rotator cuff because this film showed a leak of dye (arrow) three months after surgical removal of a calcium deposit, at which time a full thickness opening was made in the rotator cuff. Surgery was deferred and exercises were carefully supervised to regain shoulder motion. The pain disappeared. A repeat arthrogram nine months later indicated that the tear in the cuff had healed. This case lends support to the belief that impingement is not a significant factor in the etiology of calcium deposits and anterior acromioplasty is unnecessary at the time of removal of calcium.

mioplasty at the time of this procedure seemed to retard recovery and has been abandoned.

Small areas of residual calcium left in the tendon after calcium removal tend to resorb spontaneously with time as a new blood supply enters. Larger isolated deposits that were not entered during surgery are, of course, unlikely to resorb very soon. It is remarkable how infrequently calcium is seen to recur at the site of excision.

The majority of our patients have been quite pleased with their eventual result following this procedure, although a few who had large deposits have had some dissatisfaction in their strength and performance.

Arthroscopic Excision of Calcium

Ellman,[212a] Zarins,[212b] and other investigators in the United States have had satisfactory results with arthroscopic excision for selected chronic calcium deposits. This has been less satisfactory when there are deep or multiloculated, multiple-foci deposits.

To me, this should be a logical procedure for selected single and accessible deposits, especially because calcium deposits are not associated with ongoing subacromial impingement and no subacromial decompression is required. Arthroscopic calcium removal is a procedure somewhere between needling and excision. It would seem to have merit for the right type of chronic deposit.

ACROMIOCLAVICULAR ARTHRITIS

Acromioclavicular separations are discussed in Chapter 4, page 341. Fractures of the distal clavicle are considered in Chapter 5, page 405. Osteolysis of the distal clavicle ("weightlifter's shoulder") and arthritis of the acromioclavicular joint can require excision of the distal clavicle. These lesions are considered in this section along with the technique of excision of the distal clavicle when the ligaments are intact.

Osteolysis of the Distal Clavicle ("Weightlifter's Shoulder")

Unique resorption of bone occurs at the distal clavicle after Type III articular surface fractures of the distal clavicle (see Chapter 5, p. 411 and Fig. 5–43E). Osteolysis or resorption is also seen after certain types of athletic activity, especially weight lifting. Minute fractures can be seen microscopically in the remains of the articular surface of the distal clavicle after the distal clavicle has been excised from weightlifters. These fractures are in various states of healing, indicating that they occurred at different times. The force of the weights upon the end of the clavicle produced these microfractures. The microfractures in time produce the hyperemia of injury that causes resorption of bone. Bone resorption in the distal clavicle is greater than in other parts of the body, probably because of the vascularity of the clavicle, as depicted in Figure 6–6.

Upon physical examination, there is direct tenderness over the acromioclavicular joint. The horizontal adduction test (see Figs. 4–58 to 4–62) brings out pain. Xylocaine injected into the acromioclavicular joint, as to be described, temporarily stops the pain. The resorption and irregularity of the distal clavicle can be made more evident with tomograms or CT scans (Fig. 6–7). Comparison

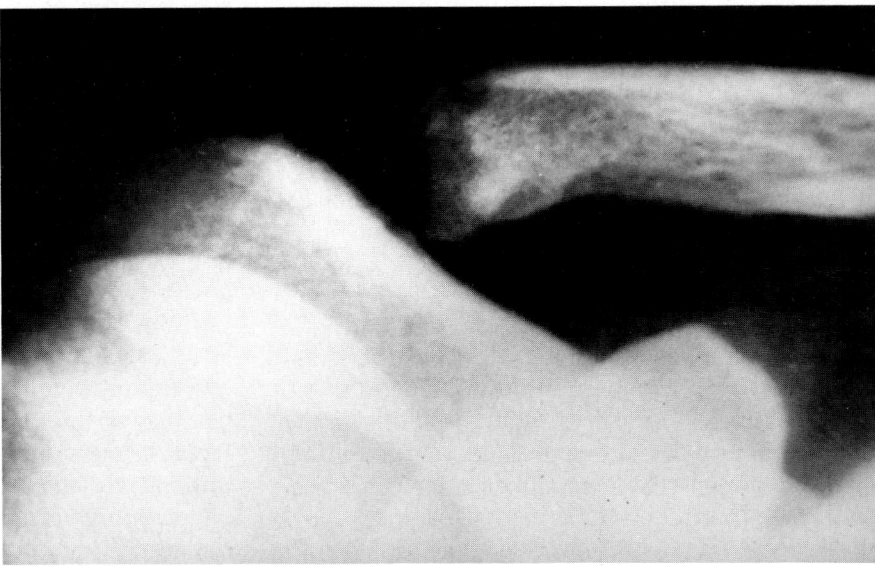

Figure 6–6. ***Acromioclavicular Arthritis.*** "Weightlifter's clavicle." Osteolysis and arthritis from minute articular fractures are seen.

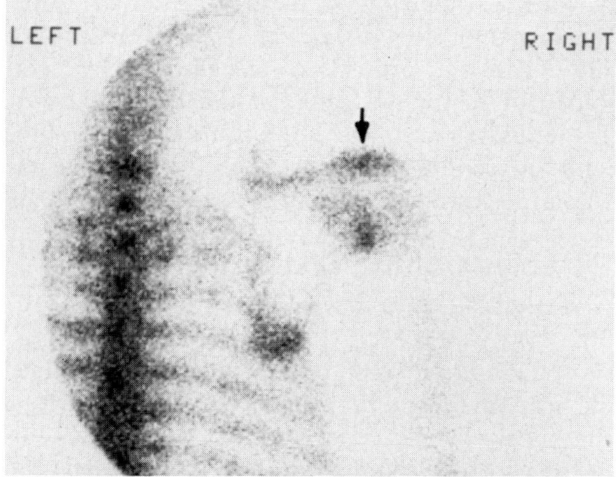

Figure 6–7. Radioactive technetium bone scan of acromioclavicular arthritis. Radioactive scans, CT scans, and tomograms can help document acromioclavicular arthritis (arrow). The most reliable clinical test is relief of pain after an anesthetic agent is injected into the acromioclavicular joint.

with the opposite shoulder is not always helpful because both shoulders may be involved. When these clinical findings are present, excision of the distal clavicle as described in Figures 6–6 to 6–8 is considered.

Other Types of Acromioclavicular Arthritis

Other types of arthritis of the acromioclavicular joint are seen that may be benefited by excision of the acromioclavicular joint. Aside from post-traumatic arthritis discussed previously, the most common are osteoarthritis and rheumatoid arthritis.

With osteoarthritis and rheumatoid arthritis, in addition to local tenderness at the acromioclavicular joint, as elicited by standing behind the patient and palpating both acromioclavicular joints (simultaneously comparing the two sides), Xylocaine injected into the joint temporarily stops pain when the horizontal adduction test is performed.

Acromioclavicular Injection Test

As mentioned in Chapter 2 in the differential diagnosis of impingement, and in Chapter 4 in the differential diagnosis of glenohumeral instability and in the analysis of the cause of pain in a long-standing acromioclavicular dislocation, an injection of Xylocaine or some equivalent local anesthetic agent into the acromioclavicular joint can be a great help in diagnosis. Of course, relief of pain is specific for acromioclavicular joint derangement. This test is most important diagnostically and is an indication of the probable result of excision of the distal clavicle.

I prefer to inject the acromioclavicular joint while standing in back of the patient, with the patient seated on the examining table. After the injection of Xylocaine, the arm is moved through a full range of motion and the horizontal adduction test is repeated to determine the amount of pain relief. If a frozen shoulder, glenohumeral instability, or impingement is present, the pain will not be relieved. If the pain is due to acromioclavicular arthritis, pain relief is usually complete.

Excision of the Distal Clavicle (Ligaments Intact)

This procedure is illustrated in Figure 6–8. A 7.0 cm. incision is made from the anterior edge of the acromioclavicular joint toward the coracoid. The skin is undermined to expose the capsule of the acromioclavicular joint and distal 2.0 cm. of clavicle. A thin elevator is placed posterior to the distal end of the clavicle (through the trapezius muscle) for retraction. The capsule is incised longitudinally and by sharp dissection is elevated off the distal clavicle. This creates a flap of deltoid muscle anteriorly and of trapezius muscle posteriorly. These two flaps are marked with stay sutures. A second thin elevator is placed under the distal clavicle and lateral to the coracoclavicular ligaments. This elevator is pressed firmly against the coracoclavicular ligaments, exposing the distal 1.5 cm. to 2.0 cm. of clavicle, which is removed with a rib cutter, as shown in Figure 6–8, removing more of the clavicle posteriorly than anteriorly. This creates a space 2.0 cm. wide between the stump of the clavicle and the acromion. The superior edge of the stump of the clavicle is beveled off with a rongeur, as shown in Figure 6–8. The trapezius flap and deltoid flap with their capsular attachments are approximated with interrupted, nonabsorbable sutures. This fills the dead space and covers the stump of the clavicle. The skin is closed with a removeable, continuous subcuticular pull-out stitch. The arm is placed in a sling and swathe, which is discarded within a few days.

Because the coracoclavicular ligaments are intact, use of the arm may be advanced as rapidly as wound healing allows. All activities can be permitted, with the exception of active forward elevation, which is prohibited for three weeks to allow the anterior deltoid to re-attach firmly.

The glenohumeral joint is normal in this situation, and motion is easily preserved without special exercises.

The results have been excellent; however, the following points should be kept in mind:

1. Loose fragments of bone can grow, causing spurs and impingement. Avoid burrs and rasping instruments that leave bone dust. This can cause re-growth of unwanted bone.

2. Failure to remove the posterior corner of the stump of the clavicle can leave a prominence that may hit against the base of the acromion when

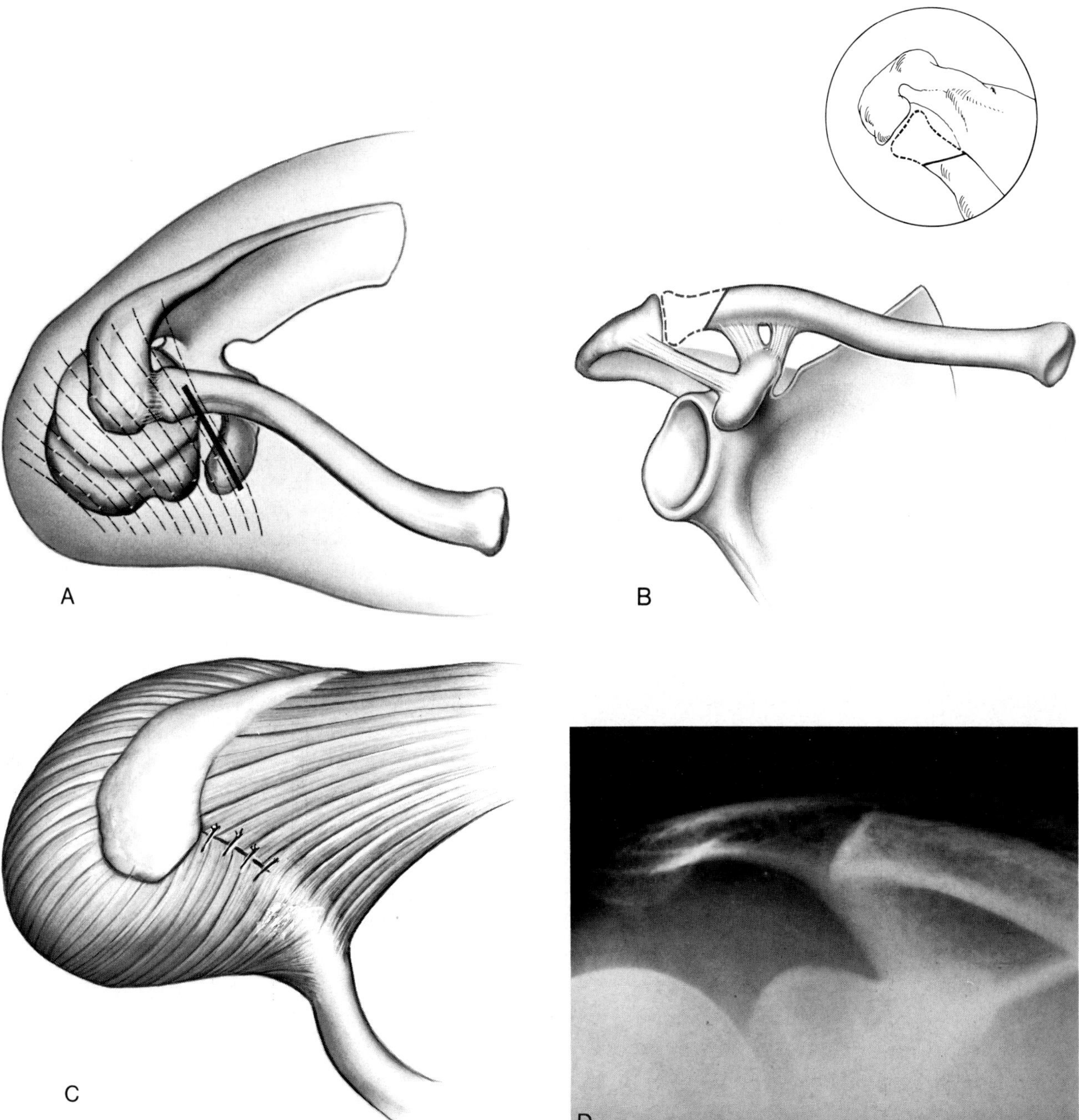

Figure 6–8. ***Acromioclavicular Arthritis.*** Excision of the distal clavicle when the ligaments are intact.
A, Incision.
B, Bone removed. More of the clavicle is removed superiorly and posteriorly.
C, Closure with trapezius and deltoid to fill the dead space. Skin closure is as shown in Figure 6–4F.
D, Post-operative appearance (x-ray).
Technique of excision of the distal clavicle when the ligaments have been torn is shown in Figure 4–67.

the arm is adducted. Create an even 2.0 cm. space all the way across between the acromion and the clavicle.

3. Leave the coracoclavicular ligaments attached to the clavicle.

Excision of the Distal Clavicle When the Coracoclavicular Ligaments Have Been Torn

This procedure for long-standing acromioclavicular dislocations is described in Chapter 4, Fig. 4–67.

STERNOCLAVICULAR ARTHRITIS

Types of Sternoclavicular Arthritis

Because there is a great deal of mechanical stress and motion at the sternoclavicular joint, degenerative arthritis of this joint is very common and is almost a normal part of aging. Many older patients have a prominence of the inner clavicle caused by excrescences (Fig. 6–9). It is not unusual to see that a biopsy has been performed at this site to exclude a neoplasm. Older patients with a swelling at this joint can be watched without treatment and without a biopsy unless there is clear roentgen evidence of bone destruction. Giving reassurance that the prominence is "nothing to worry about" is the only treatment indicated.

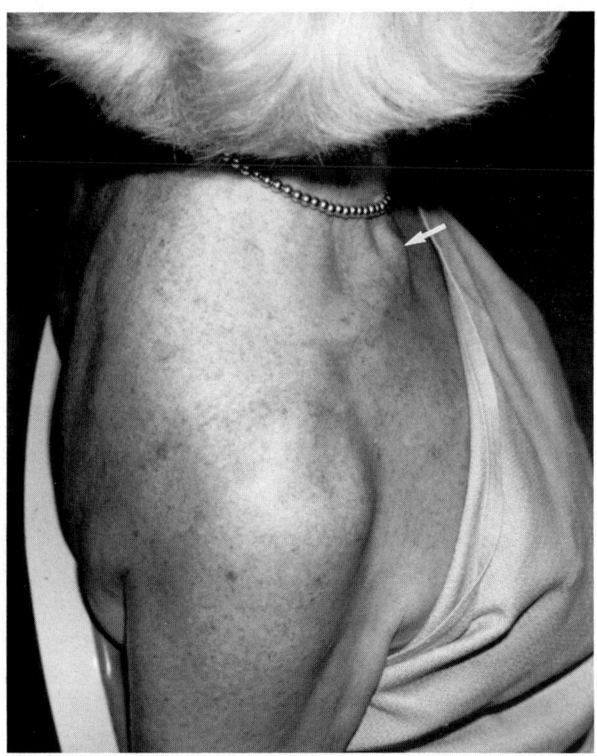

Figure 6–9. ***Sternoclavicular Arthritis.*** Prominences of the sternoclavicular joint as a result of osteoarthritis are common, are usually asymptomatic, and in the past have too often been biopsied in error with the mistaken tentative diagnosis of a neoplasm.

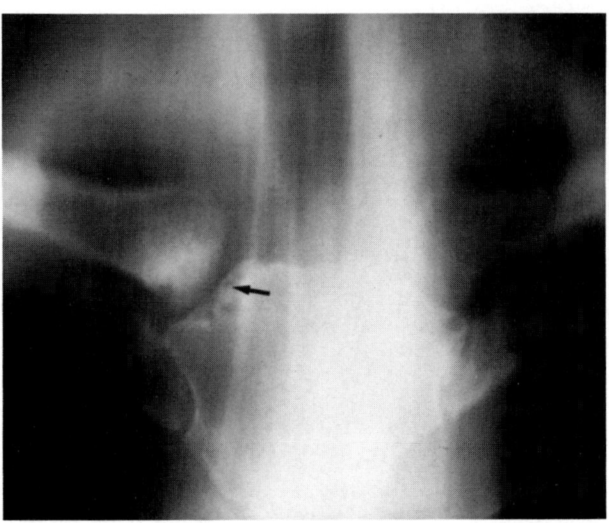

Figure 6–10. ***Sternoclavicular Arthritis.*** Tomogram showing sternoclavicular arthritis (arrow). Pain was temporarily relieved with a local injection of anesthetic agent into the sternoclavicular joint (arrow); subsequent excision of the inner clavicle (see Fig. 6–11) relieved the pain and gave an excellent functional result.

Rarely, younger patients develop degenerative changes, rheumatoid arthritis, or post-traumatic arthritis that is painful. Laminagrams and 45 degree angle views may clarify the existence of arthritis (Fig. 6–10). If a Xylocaine injection into the joint temporarily stops the pain, excision of the inner clavicle may be in order.

Dislocations of the sternoclavicular joint are discussed in Chapter 4, page 355; and fractures in Chapter 5, page 408.

Excision of the Inner Clavicle (Ligaments Intact)

With the patient in a beachchair position and the arm draped free, as shown in Figure 2–41, a 5.0 cm. incision is made in line with a necklace inferior to the bone prominence. The skin is undermined, exposing the sternoclavicular joint capsule and the tendon of the clavicular head of the sternocleidomastoid. By subperiosteal dissection and staying very close to bone, the capsule and clavicular head are elevated first off of the superior

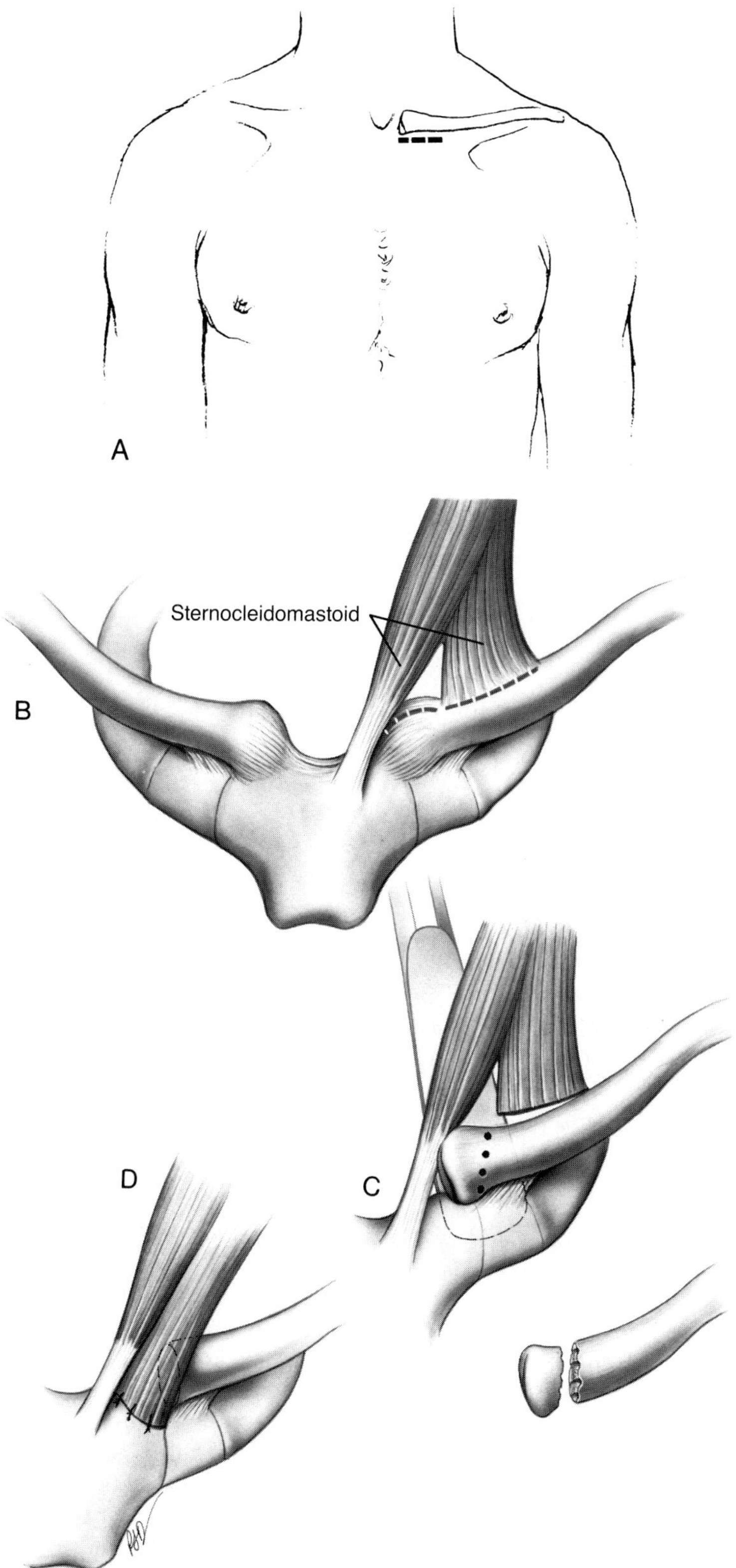

Figure 6–11. ***Sternoclavicular Arthritis.*** Excision of the inner clavicle (ligaments intact).

A, A 5.0 cm. incision is made in line with the necklace.

B, The clavicular head of the sternocleidomastoid is detached.

C, Bone is removed with a flat elevator guarding behind to prevent injury to the great vein. The costoclavicular ligament is retained intact.

D, Closure with clavicular head of sternocleidomastoid placed into the dead space.

Repair of old sternoclavicular dislocations (with the ligaments torn) is shown in Figure 4–72.

and posterior sides of the inner clavicle and then the inferior capsule is detached with care to leave the costoclavicular ligament intact (Fig. 6–11). Note that the costoclavicular ligament is very close to the capsule inferiorly and can easily be detached in error. Only 0.5 cm. of the distal clavicle is removed inferiorly, and 1.0 cm. is removed superiorly. This is done with a hand drill; small, sharp osteotome; and rongeur. The edges of the stump of the clavicle are made even with the rongeur. The clavicular head of the sternocleidomastoid is sutured into the dead space. The cervical fascia and platysma are approximated with 000 interrupted sutures, and the skin is closed with a continuous subcuticular suture. A sling and swathe is applied, which is discarded within a few days.

The glenohumeral joint is normal in these patients, and motion can easily be maintained without special exercises. Activities can be advanced as rapidly as wound healing permits. The special points to keep in mind about this procedure are as follows:

1. Know where the great vein is behind the clavicle. Spend extra time making sure it is protected. If you are unaccustomed to this procedure, alert a vascular surgeon to be available in case the vein is torn and be prepared to hold your finger on the vein until the vascular surgeon can arrive to repair it.

2. Fill the dead space with the clavicular head of the sternocleidomastoid. This accomplishes two things: it is a deterrent to hematoma formation and re-growth of bone; and it removes the pull of the sternocleidomastoid, which otherwise tends to displace the stump of the clavicle upward.

A good functional result of this procedure is seen in Figure 6–12.

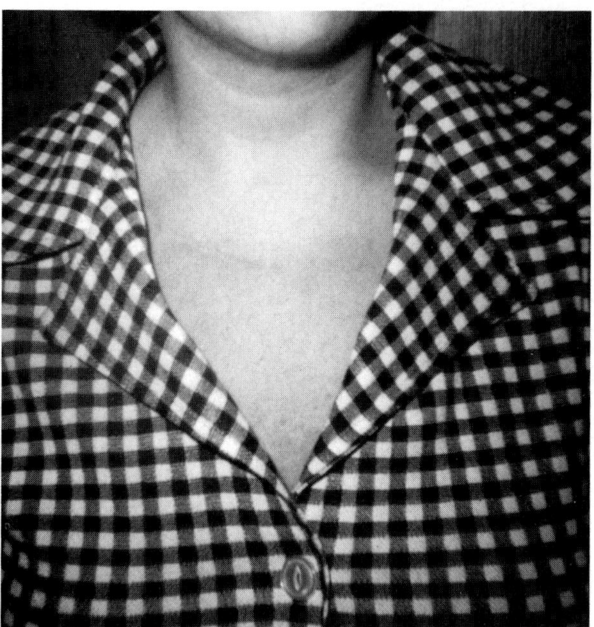

Figure 6–12. ***Sternoclavicular Arthritis.*** Acceptable scar and good functional result after excision of right inner clavicle (see Fig. 6–11).

Excision of the Inner Clavicle When the Costoclavicular Ligament Has Been Torn

This procedure for long-standing sternoclavicular dislocations is described in Chapter 4, Figure 4–72.

GLENOHUMERAL ARTHRODESIS

With the advent of glenohumeral arthroplasty for destruction of the glenohumeral joint by arthritis and injuries and with the control of poliomyelitis and tuberculosis, there are very few indications for glenohumeral fusions. This fact is welcome news for mankind because shoulder fusions, which were common in the past, severely restrict shoulder motion, as illustrated in Figures 3–19, 3–96, and 6–13B, and are frequently associated with discomfort[213] and dissatisfaction[78] because of limitation of daily activities.

Glenohumeral arthrodesis eliminates all rotation and 120 degrees of the 180 degrees of elevation of the shoulder.[3] The most important function of the shoulder is to rotate the humerus so that the elbow in flexion and extension positions the hand where it is needed. The glenohumeral joint supplies virtually all of this rotation. It supplies nearly 180 degrees of rotation. After a shoulder fusion, the only motion remaining is 60 degrees of scapulothoracic elevation, and rotation is impossible.

A fusion in the best possible position allows the hand to reach from just below the hip pocket to the eyebrows. The most critical position to consider in a fusion is the position of rotation. If the fusion is in more external rotation, the hand may reach to the top of the head but cannot reach the opposite axilla to clean it and cannot reach the belt buckle or zipper on the front of pants. With a fusion in more internal rotation, the hand can reach the anal region but has difficulty in reaching the mouth. The position of elevation of the arm is less critical, but a fusion in excessive forward elevation or abduction causes a prominence of the scapula and extra fatigue of the scapular muscles. A fusion in too much abduction also causes inability to lower the arm to the side of the body. This is a conspicuous deformity both during ambulation and in recumbency.

Personal Series

Hawkins and I reviewed 17 glenohumeral fusions that I had performed between 1966 and 1976. This study was presented to the Canadian Orthopaedic Association in 1977 and has since been published.[78, 78a] The results are summarized in Table 6–1. To show how rarely fusions are performed today, during the ten years since that study, I have performed only three glenohumeral fusions—two on patients from outside the United States who had poliomyelitis paralysis of the deltoid, rotator cuff, and biceps muscles; and one in a patient referred with a prior failed attempt at glenohumeral fusion for an infected prosthesis.

Table 6–1. FUNCTIONAL ANALYSIS AFTER GLENOHUMERAL ARTHRODESIS

Optimum position from medial border of scapula.	Abduction: 20 to 40 degrees Flexion: 20 to 30 degrees Internal rotation: 25 to 30 degrees
Optimal position at surgery.	The hand touches the eyebrows when the elbow is flexed.
Reaching	
Overhead	No
Mouth	Yes
Opposite axilla	Yes
Belt buckle	Yes
Side pocket	Yes
Back pocket	No
Brassiere strap	No
Sleep on fused side	Rarely
Work as carpenter (hammer overhead)	No
Work as housepainter (from ladder)	No

Data compiled from Hawkins, R. S., and Neer, C. S. II: A functional analysis of shoulder fusions. Clin. Orthop. *223*:65, 1987.

Indications for Glenohumeral Arthrodesis

Arthrodesis is now considered in only two situations:

1. *Paralysis or destruction from trauma of both the rotator cuff muscles and the deltoid muscle (with functioning scapulothoracic muscles).* Deltoid palsy alone with intact rotator cuff muscles, which was once considered an indication for fusion,[216] is almost never treated with a fusion today because it is preferable for most patients to retain active glenohumeral rotation. Massive destruction of the rotator cuff, such as by excision for tumor, is rarely an indication for fusion because soft-tissue operations for stability and muscle transfers for the rotator cuff (see Fig. 3–31) retaining the function of the deltoid muscle are preferred by patients who do light work. A fusion may be better for a patient who has pain and does heavy work below the horizontal. A fusion will not allow work above shoulder level (Table 6–1). I no longer attempt a fusion of a neurotrophic (Charcot's) shoulder (see p. 455).

2. *Inactive infection of the glenohumeral joint with painful incongruity that has not been relieved by "resection," immobilization and antibiotics, when bone involvement precludes a prosthesis,* as discussed in the next section and illustrated in Figure 3–92.

The most satisfied patients in our series of shoulder fusions were males who had severe pain prior to the fusion and who did heavy work below the horizontal, such as a farmer or a machine worker. House painters and carpenters did not return to this work because they could not use their hands above shoulder level.

Another extremely happy category of patients following fusions were those with old poliomyelitis paralysis with loss of deltoid, rotator cuff, and biceps (but with adequate hand and scapular musculature). In these patients, a transfer of the pectoralis major for elbow flexion was performed at the time of stabilization of the shoulder to restore elbow flexion (see Fig. 6–13C). However, when there are good rotator cuff muscles to rotate the humerus, fusion for paralysis of the deltoid muscle alone impedes positioning the hand by making rotation impossible and is less desirable for most patients.

The most dissatisfied patients following fusions were young females, most of whom objected to the appearance of the shoulder as well as to the restriction of motion and inability to sleep on that side. I have seen several young women with shoulder fusions who wanted to have their shoulder replaced with a prosthesis to put it back to previous condition (see p. 253 and Fig. 3–96).

No patient should be advised to have a glenohumeral arthrodesis who has not been schooled in the functional limitations and who does not accept these limitations, as outlined in Table 6–1. When fusion has occurred in optimum position, the best possible excursion of the hand is from the eyebrows to just below the back pocket as illustrated in Figure 6–13B1 and 6–13B2.

The impaired function imposed by bilateral shoulder fusions, in our experience, has been un-

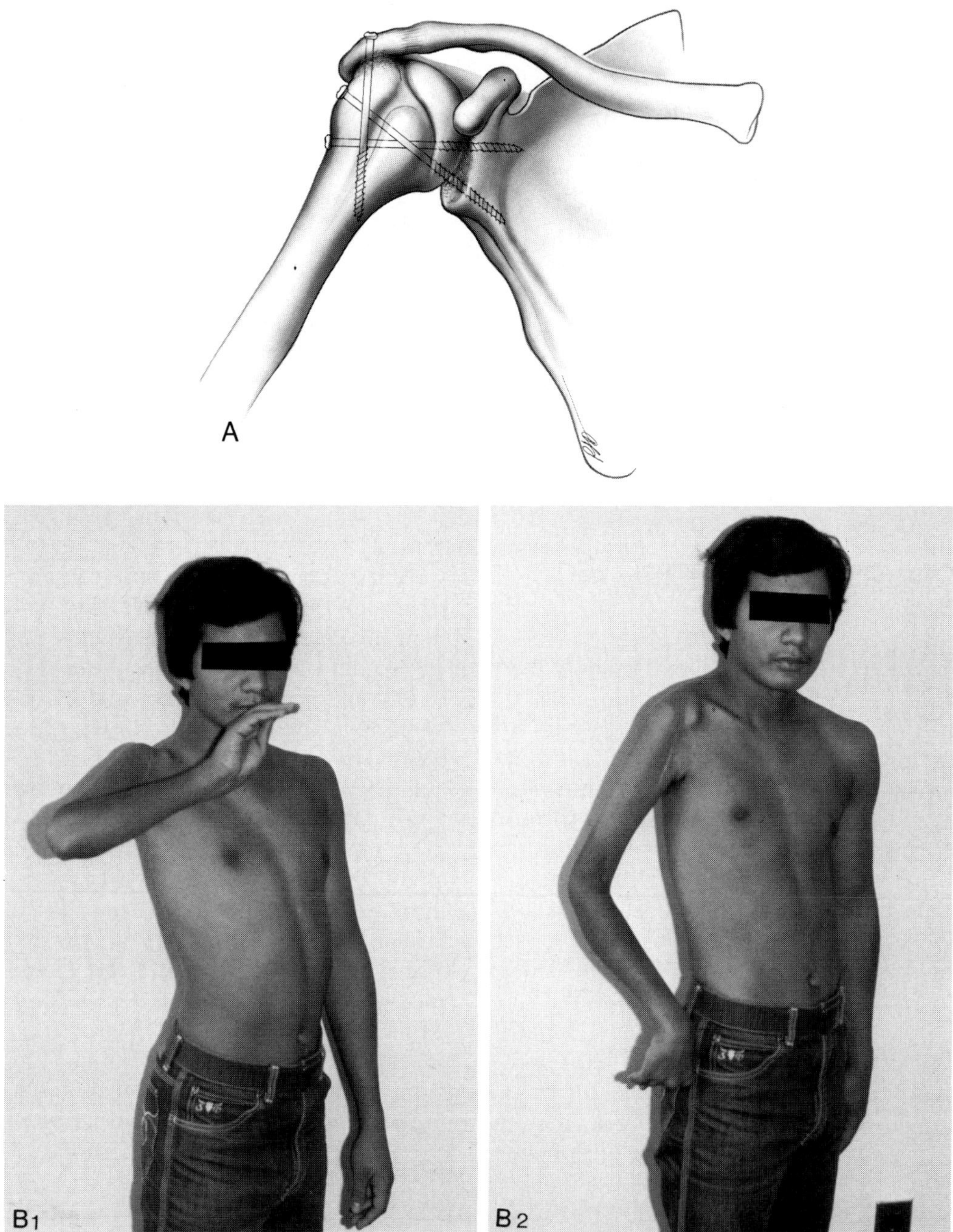

Figure 6–13. ***Glenohumeral Arthrodesis.*** A, Better appearance results are achieved if the acromion and acromioclavicular joints are left intact and the humerus is displaced upward against the acromion. Regardless of technique, with the fusion in optimal position the best obtainable excursion of the hand is from the eyebrow to just below the back pocket (see B1 and B2 and Fig. 3–19).

B1 and B2, Shoulder fusion with transfer of the pectoralis major for biceps is especially rewarding, as in this 18 year old man, when there is post-poliomyelitis paralysis of the deltoid, rotator cuff, and biceps muscles. This man had a useless arm pre-operatively and now uses it in eating and all light activities below shoulder level.

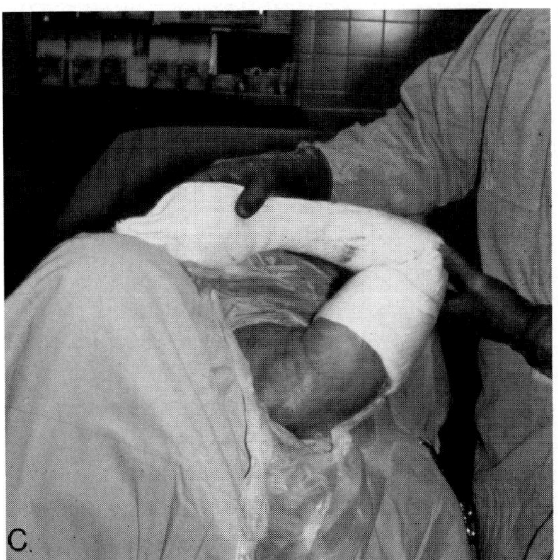

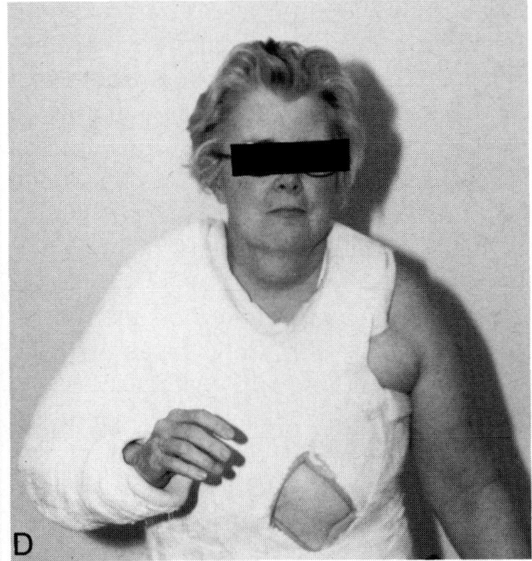

Figure 6–13 *Continued* C, Practical method for obtaining the optimal position for a glenohumeral fusion at surgery. The arm is abducted about 20 to 30 degrees, and, with the elbow flexed 90 degrees, the arm is internally rotated until the hand reaches the eyebrows when the elbow is flexed further. This position of rotation is the most important factor to consider. With a fusion in too much internal rotation, the patient cannot reach the mouth. With a fusion in too much external rotation, the patient cannot clean the opposite axilla or buckle the belt.

D, Optimal functional position in the post-operative spica cast after glenohumeral arthrodesis. Lightweight plastic material is used for the spica.

acceptable. An arthrodesis is avoided in rheumatoid shoulders because both shoulders are often involved.

Regarding the youngest age of the patient at the time of fusion, the Research Committee of the American Orthopaedic Association concluded that a fusion could be performed for a paralytic shoulder at any age after 6 years. It should be remembered, however, that over 80 percent of the length of the humerus comes from the proximal humeral epiphysis and if this is destroyed, the arm will be severely shortened. The oldest patient in my series was 74 years, and the youngest was 15 years of age at the time of fusion.

Contraindications to fusion include active infection, paralysis of both trapezius and serratus anterior muscles, and contralateral fusion.

Technique of Glenohumeral Arthrodesis

A routine can be developed for arthrodesis of paralytic shoulders with normal bones; however, old fractures and failed arthroplasties usually lack bone stock, require supplemental bone grafts, and require individualization of internal fixation rather than a routine. Furthermore, previously infected fractures and arthroplasties are required to have been inactive for least one year and to receive appropriate antibiotics for six weeks following fusion. Nevertheless, as illustrated in Figure 3–93, even when there has been past infection and severe bone loss, fusion can be obtained if distraction at the fusion site can be prevented with internal fixation, iliac grafts are used, and spica cast external fixation is continued until bony union occurs (at least six months).

Despite these differences posed by the condition of the bone, several technical points are worthy of emphasis:

1. *No patient should be advised to have a fusion who has not been schooled in the functional limitations inherent in fusions as outlined in Table 6–1.* The patient must accept these limitations.
2. *Preserve the contour of the shoulder.* Avoid an osteotomy of the acromion to flatten it against the humerus, but rather displace the humerus upward to contact the acromion. This is important in the appearance of the shoulder.
3. *Preserve the acromioclavicular joint intact unless it is painful.* Resection of the distal clavicle does not increase shoulder motion after an arthrodesis. Actually, I have found it to be a mistake to resect the distal clavicle to increase motion in a fused shoulder because an unusually deep and ugly indentation often occurs between the acromion and the clavicle, which upsets the patient without gaining motion.
4. *Individualize internal fixation.* When there

is loss of bone and the bone is soft, a wire loop through the glenoid and humerus[217] to maintain contact is helpful. Under most circumstances, I prefer three AO cancellous screws, as depicted in Figure 6–13A. Plate fixation on the spinous process and shaft of the humerus to avoid a cast has been advocated and may be all right for paralytic shoulders, but it has the disadvantages of a long scar, lack of adjustability if the position is incorrect, and causes flattening of the contour of the shoulder.

5. *Use iliac bone grafts* (from the inner table of the iliac crest) when the bone is deficient.

6. *Regarding the ideal position for glenohumeral arthrodesis, consider the position of the hand foremost in positioning the fusion.* In the past, the accepted position for fusion was 45 to 55 degrees abduction, 15 to 25 degrees flexion, and 15 to 25 degrees *internal* rotation, using the medial border of the scapula for reference, as recommended in 1942 by the Research Committee of the American Orthopaedic Association[216] for poliomyelitis paralysis. Rowe[215] in 1974 correctly emphasized that the position of abduction should be lower for the modern-day fusions in adult patients. He advised 20 degrees abduction, 30 degrees flexion, and 40 to 50 degrees internal rotation, using a "clinical measurement" from the side of the body rather than from the medial border of the scapula. Cofield[213] concluded that a "broader range" of abduction was acceptable for function. I have found it of great interest to ask residents, fellows, and visitors in my examining room to measure independently and secretly record the position of the arm in patients with shoulder fusions. It is remarkable how different these recorded measurements are, even with the patient awake and sitting on the examining table. It is obviously impossible to be precise about the exact degrees of flexion or abduction or rotation of the arm when the patient is in the operating room covered with drapes. For practical purposes in the operating room, we have found it best to position the arm in about 20 to 30 degrees of abduction and 20 degrees of flexion, and then rotate the forearm (with the elbow flexed 90 degrees) to the position at which the hand touches the eyebrows when the elbow is flexed further (Fig. 6–13D and Table 6–1). The arm is internally fixed in that position and is held until the cast has been applied.

7. *Continue external immobilization* until there is roentgen proof of bone consolidation, which is usually at four to five months for adult patients and longer for those with loss of bone. Tomograms through the cast are helpful in determining when the cast can be removed.

GLENOHUMERAL RESECTION

Excision of the Proximal Humerus

As discussed in Chapter 3, Figure 3–1, a study showed the results of removal of the humeral head to be unacceptable and stimulated the design of the original shoulder prosthesis. Resection of the proximal humerus, as was once frequently performed for serious fractures and arthritis, has since been abandoned and prosthetic replacement is now used instead. The disappointing results of debridement and resection for osteoarthritis and rheumatoid arthritis have been discussed. There is no place for excision of the proximal humerus except for control of osteomyelitis or removal of neoplasms. Superficial infections without bone involvement may, if quiescent for a year, be amenable to prosthetic replacement (see Figs. 3–90 and 3–91). En bloc resections for neoplasms of the proximal humerus are reconstructed with a prosthesis and bone grafts unless the muscles have been too extensively involved (Figs. 3–94 and 3–95).

TREATMENT OF GLENOHUMERAL INFECTION WITH BONE INVOLVEMENT

A clean-out to control infection is of great importance and may have to be repeated. Following removal of all involved tissue, bone prominences that are noted to catch and hang up are excised. After thorough irrigation with antibiotics and with systemic antibiotic coverage for at least six weeks, the arm is immobilized in a sling and swathe for three months. The aim is a fibrous ankylosis with elimination of dead space. Following this, gradual resumption of function and later strengthening exercises (with the arm at the side and not above the horizontal) are begun. The result can be extremely satisfying (Fig. 6–14B and C). Usually the patient is disinterested in further surgery. If pain and disability persist after one year, a fusion is considered, as in Figs. 3–93B and 6–14A.

GLENOIDECTOMY

Glenoidectomy has been advocated for rheumatoid shoulders. This, of course, removes the fulcrum. A possible advantage I have considered is that it displaces the head more medially where the rotator cuff is more easily re-attached. However, as discussed in Chapter 3, the rotator cuff is

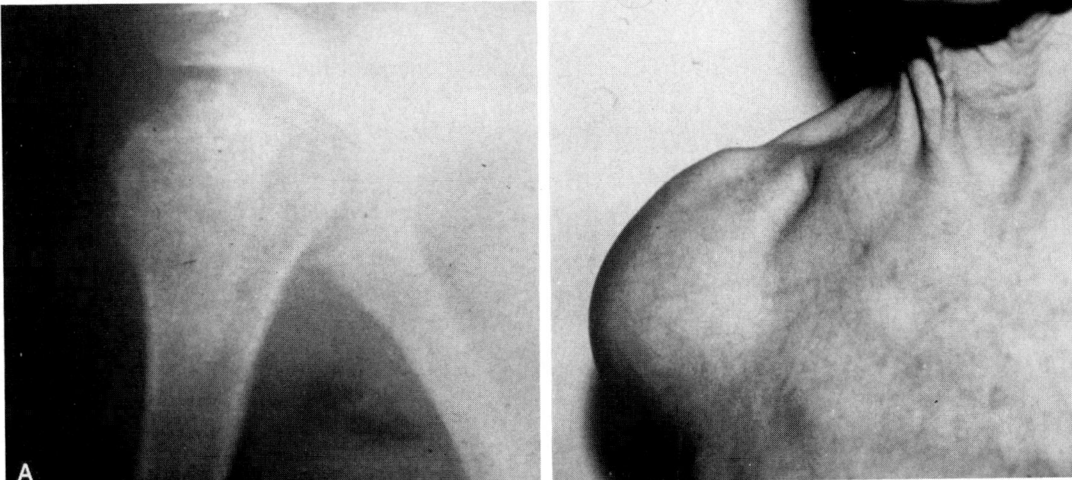

Figure 6–14A. Glenohumeral "resection" ("clean-out" of devitalized bone and irrigation) may be necessary to control infection. Pre-operative appearance and roentgenogram of a shoulder one year after an infected injection of the glenohumeral joint with destruction of the humeral head. This was treated with a "clean-out," antibiotics, and immobilized as described in the text. Pain persisted, and after one year an arthrodesis was performed.

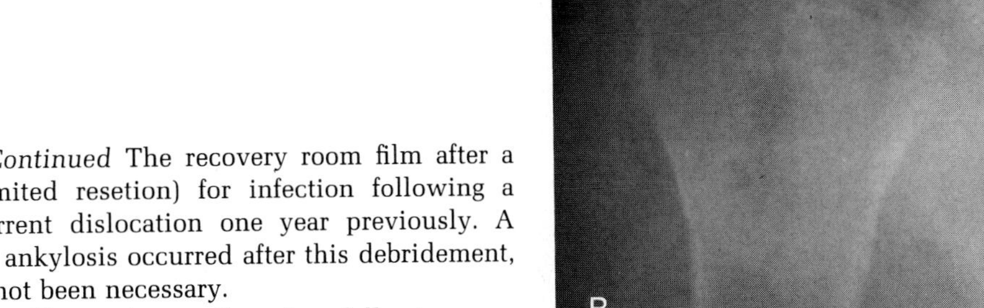

Figure 6–14B *Continued* The recovery room film after a "clean-out" (limited resetion) for infection following a repair for recurrent dislocation one year previously. A painless fibrous ankylosis occurred after this debridement, and fusion has not been necessary.

Illustration continued on following page

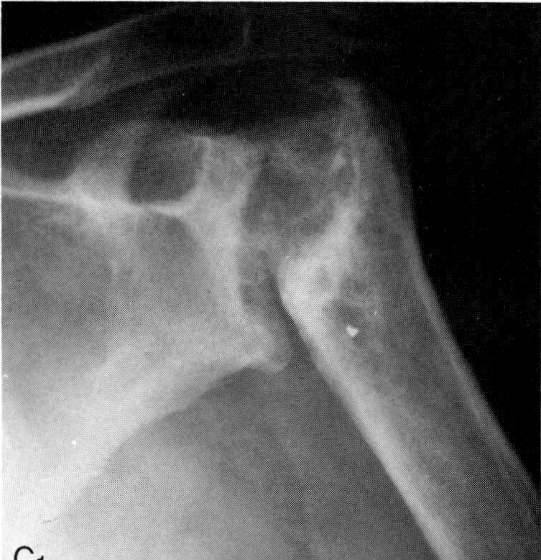

Figure 6–14C1 to C3 *Continued* Unusually good result six years after removing an infected, uncemented humeral head prosthesis; debridement; and immobilization as described in the text. Irregular prominences on the humerus that tended to catch on the glenoid were removed with a rongeur at this last procedure.

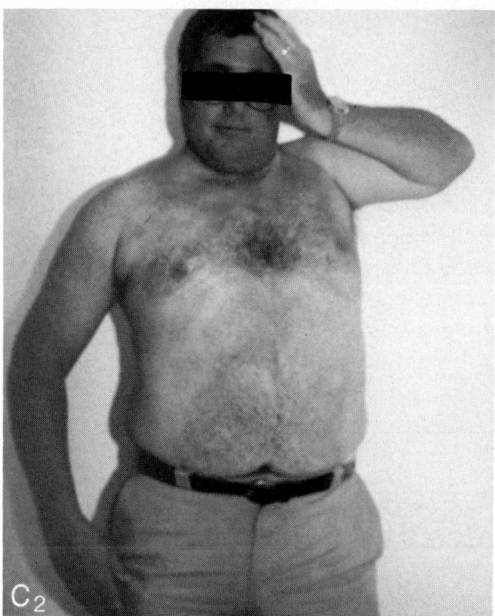

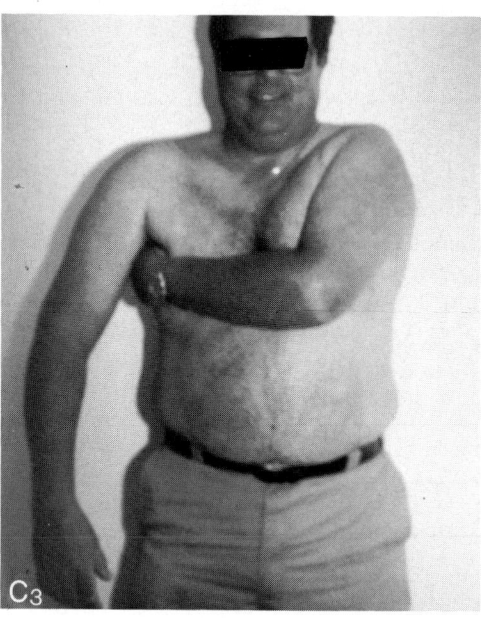

usually intact or repairable in rheumatoids and the results of replacement arthroplasty have been far superior to those of glenoidectomy.

ROTATIONAL OSTEOTOMY OF THE HUMERUS

There are very few indications for a rotational osteotomy of the humeral shaft. As previously discussed (see Chapter 4, p. 333), rotational osteotomies for glenohumeral instability are of no value when the bones are normal and the instability is due to lack of soft-tissue support. Derotational osteotomy may be considered in the rare situation when a rotational deformity is interfering with function; glenohumeral motion is painless, making an arthrodesis unnecessary; and there are extensive muscle deficits at the shoulder precluding an arthroplasty. Such muscle deficits at the shoulder may be seen after multiple trauma, head injuries, and in severe Erb's paralysis (see Chapter 3).

I have performed proximal humeral osteotomy on only two patients, both of whom had been in serious accidents with head injuries and coma that interfered with the treatment of displaced proximal humeral fracture-dislocations. Months later, after recovery from coma, their shoulders had ankylosed in malposition with so much fixed internal rotation they were unable to use a walker or reach their face. The shoulder muscles were spastic and too

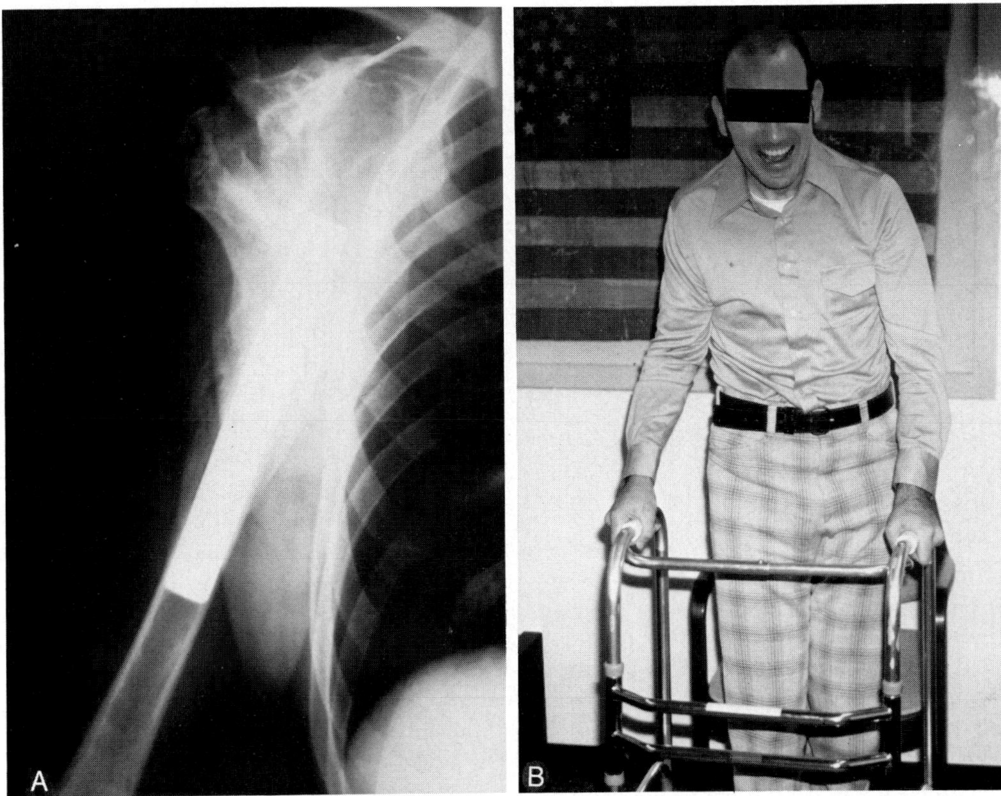

Figure 6–15. ***Rotational Osteotomy of the Humerus.*** A and B, Derotational osteotomy (externally rotating the shaft) and plate fixation of the humeral shaft for an old unreduced fracture-dislocation (with the arm fixed in internal rotation) and spastic shoulder muscles two years after head injury. Following the osteotomy, the patient could reach a walker and ambulate as shown.

uncoordinated for an arthroplasty to be considered. There was no pain at the old fracture-dislocation of the shoulder. A derotational osteotomy without disturbing the old fracture was of great functional value to both of these patients, one of whom is shown in Figure 6–15.

The technique of this procedure consisted of an extended deltopectoral approach and an osteotomy near the surgical neck level where there is better osteogenesis than in pure cortical bone, but low enough to permit firm internal fixation. The arm was derotated at the osteotomy site, with the elbow bent 90 degrees, until the forearm pointed straight ahead (neutral rotation). T-plates or plates and screws were used for internal fixation. The position obtained was protected with a lightweight spica cast in 20 degrees of abduction.

RECONSTRUCTION FOR LOSS OF THE DELTOID MUSCLE (DELTOIDPLASTY)

Reconstruction of the Deltoid Muscle After Injuries

Paralysis or destruction of the deltoid muscle usually results from an injury or surgery. Usually the anterior or anterior and middle parts of the deltoid muscle have been damaged. Because the most frequent indication to reconstruct a damaged deltoid muscle is in conjunction with an arthroplasty, the technique of deltoidplasty is described with arthroplasty (see Fig. 3–33).

Reconstruction for Paralysis of the Deltoid Muscle

The treatment of axillary nerve injuries is discussed in the next section (p. 446).

Muscle transfers for permanent paralysis of the deltoid muscle have been disappointing. Transfers of the trapezius muscle have been inadequate for several reasons. Not only is the available part of the trapezius muscle obviously too small to compensate for all three parts of the massive deltoid muscle, but also the transferred part of the trapezius muscle re-attaches to the acromion or humerus and loses its pull.

As depicted in Figure 6–16, transfer of all or part of the pectoralis major, with biceps and triceps transfer to the acromion with an inferior capsular shift, can stabilize the humeral head against dislocation but is inadequate to raise the arm.

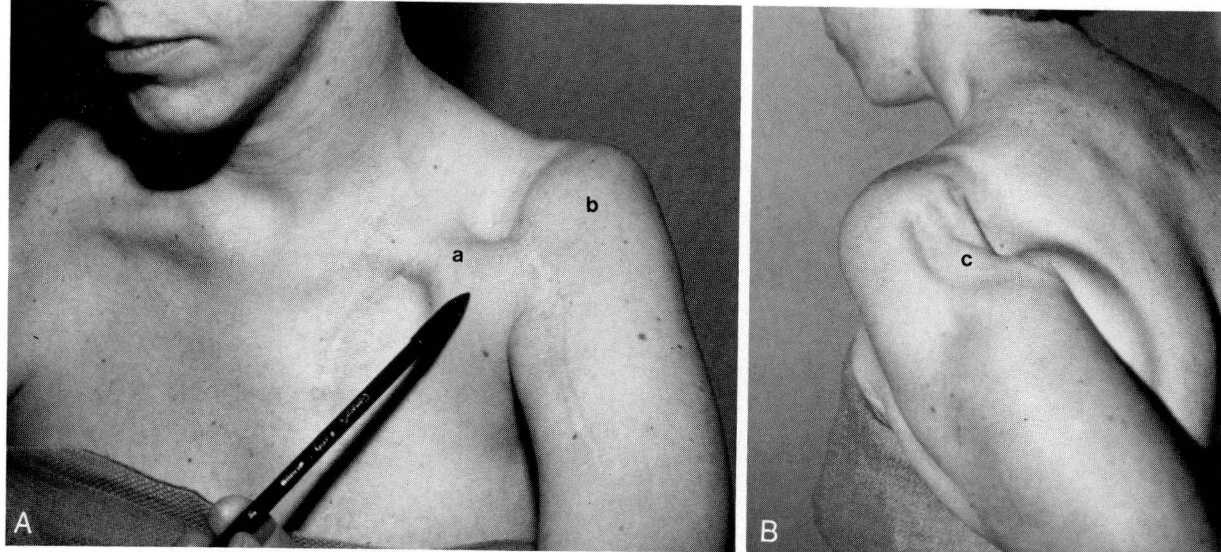

Figure 6–16. ***Deltoidplasty.*** A and B, Typical imperfect result after a deltoidplasty. This reconstruction was for post-poliomyelitis palsy of the left deltoid muscle. The opposite shoulder had been fused, and therefore a fusion of this shoulder was unacceptable. The shoulder dislocated inferiorly, anteriorly, and posteriorly with pain. Inferior capsular shift (see Fig. 4–40) was performed, followed by transfer of the biceps and both heads of the pectoralis major to the clavicle and acromion (a) and transfer of the posterior deltoid anteriorly (b) to substitute for the anterior deltoid. This was followed by transfer of the triceps (c) to substitute for the posterior deltoid. These procedures eliminated her pain and stabilized the shoulder, but provided inadequate strength to raise the arm.

The various types of deltoidplasties are illustrated in Figure 3–32 and p. 123.

Transfer of the latissimus dorsi with its neurovascular bundle, as described in Fig. 3–32D and on p. 192, is the most hopeful type of reconstruction, but the functional results in the limited numbers of patients I have seen with severe deltoid muscle loss were not encouraging. The inadequate results in those cases were at least in part due to concomitant weakness of other parts of the upper extremity.

Arthrodesis is considered when there is paralysis or destruction of both the deltoid muscle and the rotator cuff muscles. However, when the rotator cuff muscles are intact and functioning, it is better for most patients to accept the loss of elevation caused by the paralyzed deltoid muscle and, for the sake of retaining rotation of the humerus by the rotator cuff, leave the shoulder unfused. The disadvantages and advantages of arthrodesis are discussed on page 438.

NEUROLOGICAL CONDITIONS

Axillary Nerve Palsy

This discussion considers isolated lesions of the axillary nerve. Complex brachial plexus conditions are excluded.

Treatment of Acute Injuries

Injuries to the axillary nerve with surgical neck fractures, dislocations, or traction injuries usually cause only temporary paralysis of the deltoid muscle (Fig. 6–17). The prognosis for recovery, as in all blunt infraclavicular nerve injuries, is good. (Stab wounds and penetrating wounds are excluded.)

In the series of four-part fracture-dislocations described in Chapter 4,[150] 14 patients had axillary nerve palsies, of which 12 recovered spontaneously.

The condition of the deltoid muscle is followed with electromyograms at intervals of about every six weeks, and exploration of the axillary nerve is deferred. If there has been concomitant detachment of the rotator cuff or if the glenohumeral joint has been destroyed or is unstable, these structures are repaired without waiting for return of the axillary nerve function, because improving the cuff and fulcrum action of the glenohumeral joint seems to augment the recovery of the axillary nerve. Although spontaneous recovery of the axillary nerve usually occurs within six to nine months, in the patient depicted in Figure 2–24, axillary nerve function did not return until 22 months after injury.

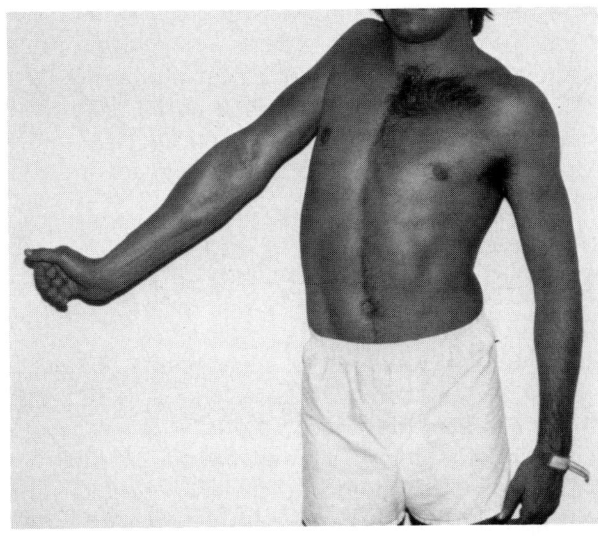

Figure 6–17. Axillary nerve palsy after an anterior dislocation.

Exploration, Neurolysis, and Repair of the Axillary Nerve

If there are displaced fragments of bone, foreign bodies, or penetrating wounds in the vicinity of the paralyzed axillary nerve, it is explored without unnecessary delay to make sure that the nerve is free of compression by these objects. In recent injuries, this is usually in conjunction with repair of the fracture using an anterior, extended deltopectoral approach.

In older, healed fractures or when the humerus is intact, the exploration is usually, not always, made first from a posterior approach along the posterior border of the deltoid muscle with visualization of both the branch to the teres minor muscle (which may be divided before entering the quadrilateral space) and the branches to the deltoid muscle and skin. However, the shoulder is prepared so that an additional anterior approach can be made if desired during this same procedure. This nerve can be exposed first beneath the glenohumeral joint capsule and in front of the subscapularis muscle from the anterior approach depending on the clinical problem. In special cases, wide exposure of the nerve from the posterior cord and radial nerve to the quadrilateral space can be obtained by detaching the clavicular head of the pectoralis major and the coracoid muscles.

There are several points to keep in mind:

1. Accurate pre-operative assessment of the patient's neurological status is essential. Associated involvement of the suprascapular nerve or other nerves suggests a more proximal brachial plexus or cervical root lesion than in the axillary nerve itself, and may contraindicate exploration of the axillary nerve.

2. Electromyographic testing and repeated clinical testing of deltoid contraction (by palpation) are both important. Exploration of the nerve is deferred as long as any suggestion of recovery is occurring (so long as there is no roentgen evidence of skeletal or foreign body encroachment on the nerve). Clinical testing of contraction of the deltoid muscle can be developed with practice by the examiner until it becomes actually more accurate in some cases than electromyography.

3. It is my impression that electrical stimulation of the deltoid muscle is of definite value in preserving muscle tone until stimulation by the axillary nerve itself returns.

4. The patient should be advised pre-operatively (and positioned at surgery accordingly) that if the nerve is seen to be intact on one side of the quadrilateral space from either a posterior or an anterior approach, it may be necessary to make a second approach on the opposite side to explore the nerve from that side.

5. If the nerve is involved in scar tissue but its neurons are intact, neurolysis is performed. If the nerve is divided or its neurons are interrupted by a traction injury, repair may be difficult or impossible; therefore, neuromicrosurgical assistance should be available and the patient must be draped so that the full length of the nerve can be exposed from the front and back. Encouraging reports[218] have been made of sural nerve grafts effectively filling the gap using microsurgical technique when the axillary nerve has been severed and retracted or when a segment of the nerve has to be removed because the nerve fibers have been interrupted and the nerve has been fibrosed because of a stretch injury. I know of one patient in whom a sural nerve graft worked well. Other neurosurgical techniques are said to hold promise.

6. Following exploration of the nerve, deltoid

muscle tone is maintained with electrical stimulation. If a nerve repair is performed, an appropriate period and position in a spica cast (to take tension off of the repair) is indicated. If only a neurolysis has been performed, shoulder motion may be begun early and shoulder rehabilitation advanced as tolerated.

Suprascapular Nerve Entrapment

Suprascapular nerve entrapment where the nerve passes under the transverse scapular ligament has been described as one of the causes of chronic shoulder pain by a number of surgeons, some of whom I hold in the highest respect. This entrapment probably does occur; however, I have never seen a definite example except with fractures of the coracoid process and with traction injuries, although I have looked for it for many years.

The case I've recognized as closest to suprascapular nerve entrapment was in a middle-aged professor whom the neurologists assured me was a classic example; this individual had the electromyographic evidence of supraspinatus, infraspinatus, and teres minor paralysis with weakness and atrophy (Fig. 6–18). He also had a negative arthrogram for a tear of the rotator cuff. After noting failure of disappearance of the symptoms for several months, I explored the suprascapular nerve at the suprascapular notch in the prescribed fashion (by a 10 cm. incision parallel to and cephalic to the spine of the scapula, elevating the trapezius muscle to expose the supraspinatus muscle and gently retracting the supraspinatus muscle to expose the nerve where it passes through the suprascapular notch under the ligament). The transverse scapular ligament was carefully excised, retracting the suprascapular artery (which is superficial to the ligament) out of harm's way. The suprascapular nerve appeared to be normal. After enlarging the notch very liberally with a rongeur, I explored the suprascapular nerve further at the suprascapular notch without positive findings. This patient never regained strength in his external rotators. About six months later, he began to show other neurological symptoms in his arm and eventually proved to have a degenerative disc lesion at the C5–C6 level of his cervical spine rather than suprascapular nerve entrapment.

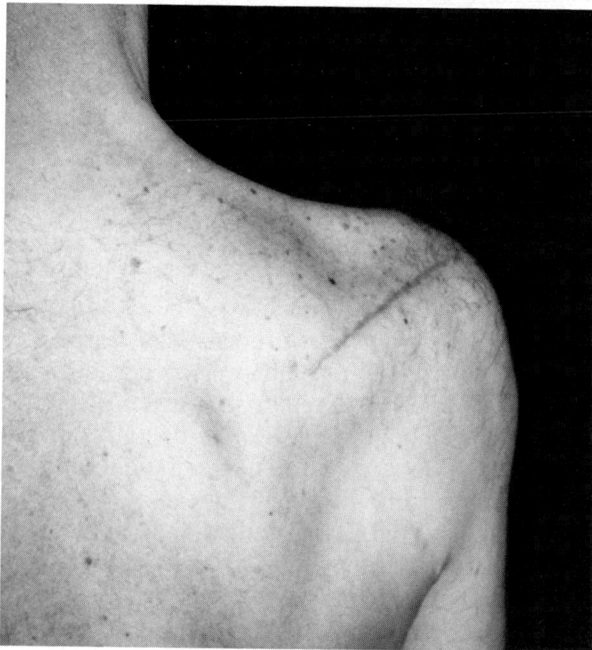

Figure 6–18. Unsuccessful neurolysis for what was diagnosed as suprascapular nerve entrapment. Rotator cuff tears or C5–C6 root lesions are far more likely diagnostic possibilities when a patient presents with weakness of external rotation.

I have seen a large number of patients who have had similar surgery elsewhere without relief of symptoms. Most of these patients had undiagnosed tears of the rotator cuff. Some, as shown in Figures 4–63 to 4–68 and Figures 6–17 to 6–23, had other causes of scapular pain. The causes of scapular pain are described on pages 482 to 485. The typical clinical picture of a patient with suprascapular nerve entrapment is shoulder discomfort, especially scapular discomfort, and weakness of external rotation. However, any cause of pain may cause apparent weakness because the patient does not resist as hard on the painful side. Thus, it is easy to be misled, as is true of most entrapment syndromes anywhere in the body.

A traumatic dislocation of the glenohumeral joint or traction injury can cause transitory changes in the electromyogram of the spinati muscles; however, these neurological findings tend to disappear spontaneously and no treatment is required. I believe that this type of traction injury of the suprascapular nerve causes edema at Erb's point (where C5 and C6 join), which is like a transitory "birth palsy" in an adult.

Surgeons who explore the suprascapular nerve regularly for entrapment say that the nerve often appears to be normal, but, nevertheless, the patient's symptoms often disappear following surgery. Perhaps the symptoms would have disappeared in time without surgery.

The suprascapular nerve is occasionally but rarely injured by penetrating trauma and by fractures at the coracoid and suprascapular notch (see Chapter 5, Fig. 5–51C, p. 418). Compression of this nerve by ganglion-like lesions and neoplasms has been described. The suprascapular nerve does require neurolysis for these conditions, using the approach described previously, and the results are rewarding. However, I caution my students against the impression that suprascapular nerve entrapment is a frequently seen and important cause of shoulder pain and weakness. I advise them, when shoulder discomfort and external rotation weakness are present, to think of a tear of the rotator cuff or a C5–C6 spinal lesion as being far more likely.

Long Thoracic Nerve Palsy

Isolated serratus anterior paralysis may result from injury or after carrying objects on the shoulder without injury. Injuries include both sharp and blunt trauma and traction on the neck or shoulder, which cause the shoulder to be depressed. Unexplained paralysis of the long thoracic nerve also occurs after viral infections and without clear cause. The paralysis usually disappears spontaneously but may persist.

The patient usually has scapular pain and inability to raise the arm above the horizontal. Examination of the shoulder must include observation of the scapular region from in back of the patient; otherwise, this lesion will be missed. Furthermore, winging of the scapula (Fig. 6–19A) will be overlooked unless especially tested for by asking the patient to elevate the arms actively. The winging can be brought out by having the patient push against a wall with both hands (Fig. 6–19B). Electromyographic studies assist in confirming the isolated paralysis.

Treatment initially is conservative. Passive exercises are given daily to avoid contractures, and muscle-setting exercises are begun when recovery starts. Progress is followed at intervals. If the paralysis persists over one year and the patient has sufficient disability and symptoms to desire surgery, the repair I have used is substitution for the serratus anterior by transfer of the sternal head of the pectoralis major using a fascial extension into a hole through the inferior angle of the scapula (Fig. 6–19C and D), essentially as described by Marmor and Bechtol (Fig. 6–19B).[219]

Pectoralis Transfer for Serratus Anterior Palsy

The patient is positioned on the "good" side (with care to place a rolled blanket under the chest to relieve pressure on the arm underneath). The arm on the involved side is draped free so that it can be fully elevated overhead. A 17.0 cm. incision is made along the inferior margin of the pectoralis major insertion, across the chest to the anterior axillary line, and down the lateral margin of the scapula to the inferior angle of the scapula (Fig. 6–19D). The sternal insertion of the pectoralis major is detached from the humerus and is dissected free from the clavicular head of the pectoralis major. The pectoralis major is split about 6.5 cm., the surgeon keeping its nerve supply in mind and avoiding injury to this nerve. The inferior one-third of the lateral margin of the scapula is exposed, and a hole is made through the scapula about 2.0 cm. from its inferior angle and about 1.5 cm. medial to its lateral border. A piece of fascia lata about 10.0 cm. long and 3.5 cm. wide is rolled on itself and is sutured to the stump of the pectoralis; it is passed through the hole in the scapula and is sutured upon itself at only slight tension. The skin is closed with a subcuticular pull-out stitch, and the arm is immobilized with a Velpeau sling (with the shoulder in internal rotation and flexion) for eight weeks. After removal of the sling, progressive passive and later strengthening exercises are begun.

My results using this procedure in three patients have been good. All of these individuals lost their fatigue pain and could elevate the arm to within 25 degrees of the opposite side. One returned to heavy work as a roofer (Fig. 6–19D). I have seen one patient who had a similar procedure performed elsewhere and who had persistent discomfort because a bone prominence had developed near the site where the hole had been made near the inferior angle of the scapula. The discomfort was relieved by removing this bone prominence.

Spinal Accessory Nerve Paralysis

The spinal accessory nerve is very exposed to injury in the posterior triangle of the neck where it emerges at the midpoint of the posterior margin of the sternocleidomastoid muscle and crosses very superficially to enter the trapezius muscle. It is usually injured during surgery in this area, by necessity in radical neck dissections for tumors and accidentally during lymph node biopsies. I have also seen severe weakness of the trapezius muscle with injuries at the C2–C3 level. It is well to remember that some of the motor supply to the trapezius is obtained from the C2–C3 (or C3–C4) roots, although this is less important than the accessory nerve.

Paralysis of the trapezius muscle, as illustrated in Figures 1–16 and 6–20A, causes the scapula to

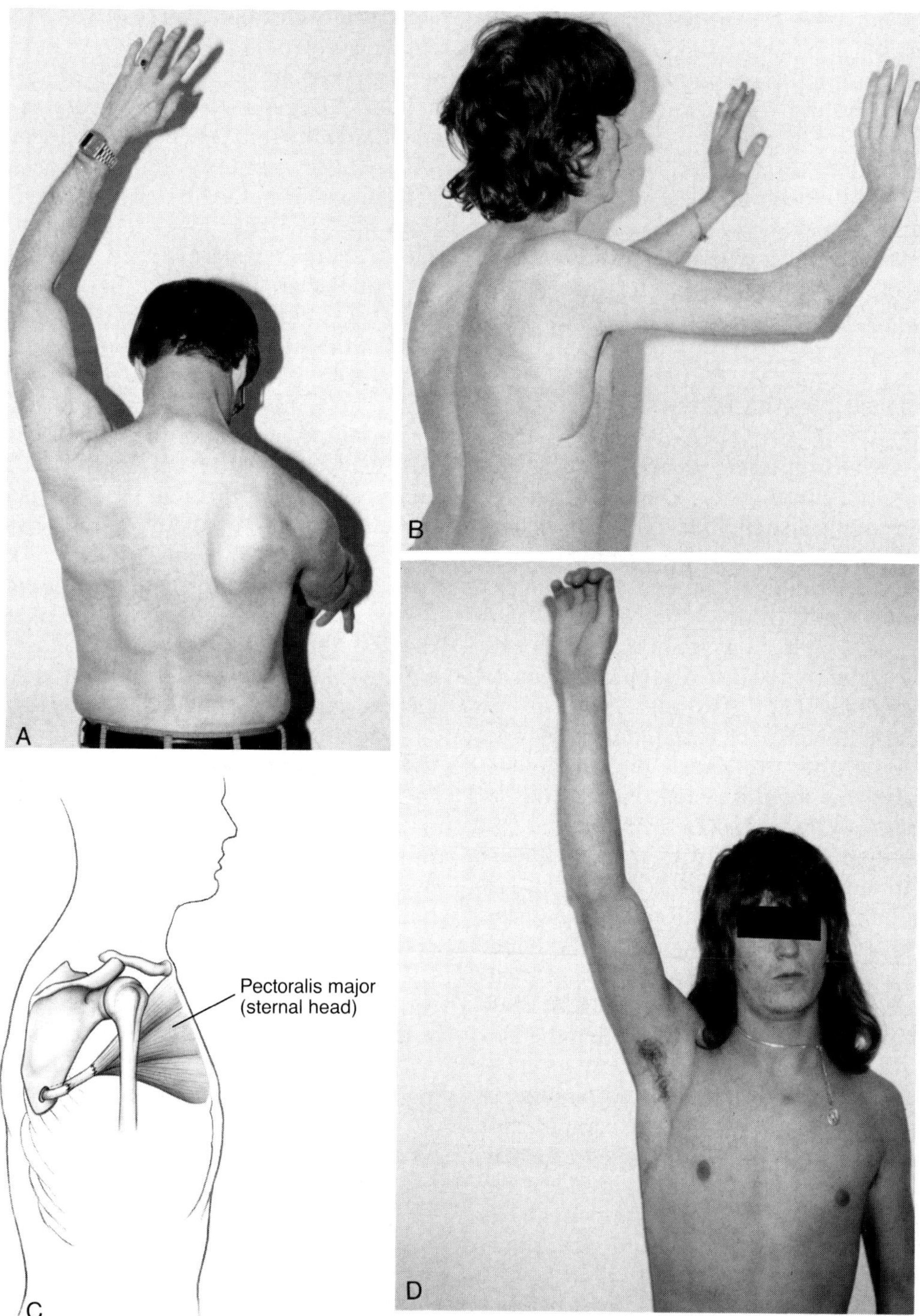

Figure 6–19. ***Serratus Anterior Paralysis.***

A, Serratus anterior paralysis with winging of the scapula and inability to raise the arm.

B, Winging of the scapula can be demonstrated by having the patient push against a wall with both hands.

C, Drawing of the transfer of the pectoralis major for serratus anterior using a fascial extension as described in the text.

D, Depicting scar and a good result after pectoralis major transfer for serratus anterior paralysis in a 28 year old roofer.

drop and fail to rotate properly. Trapezius palsy may cause two types of pain, similar to some old acromioclavicular dislocations (see p. 349 and Fig. 4–63):

1. Fatigue pain from loss of the major suspensory muscle (see Fig. 1–16, p. 349, Fig. 4–63, and Table 4–3, p. 343).

2. Impingement from failure to rotate the acromion out of the way of the greater tuberosity. This original clinical observation is discussed in Chapter 2, Figure 2–10A and page 139.

The presence of fatigue pain can be diagnosed with the "weight duration test" (see Fig. 4–63)—lifting a chair with the involved arm and holding it off of the floor until pain begins. Impingement pain can be identified by eliminating pain with an injection of Xylocaine beneath the acromion—the impingement injection test (see Fig. 2–30). Long-standing impingement of this type can lead to an impingement tear of the rotator cuff, which can be seen in an arthrogram and, as we have observed on several occasions, in the operating room.

It is important during the early period after an injury to determine whether the spinal accessory nerve should be explored.

The damage to the nerve may be complete, partial, or neuropraxia. Electromyograms are indicated to follow the recovery of the nerve and to help in the decision regarding exploration of the nerve with possible microsurgery for neurolysis or to repair the nerve.

Later, in long-standing lesions, the indications for treatment are less easily determined. Most articles on this subject by orthopaedic surgeons fail to consider that the majority of spinal accessory nerve injuries are produced by necessity during radical neck dissections for tumors. Orthopaedic surgeons usually see only lesions that result from accidental injury to the spinal accessory nerve during a lymph node biopsy. The contrast in motivation of these two groups of patients is striking. The group with tumors would prefer to have no shoulder disability, whereas the second group usually has a personal injury attorney. Such motivational factors are of great practical importance in evaluating these patients.

The indications for stabilization of the scapula (Dewar-Harris)[61] are not entirely clear. Head and neck surgeons have more experience with this problem than orthopaedic surgeons, and many of

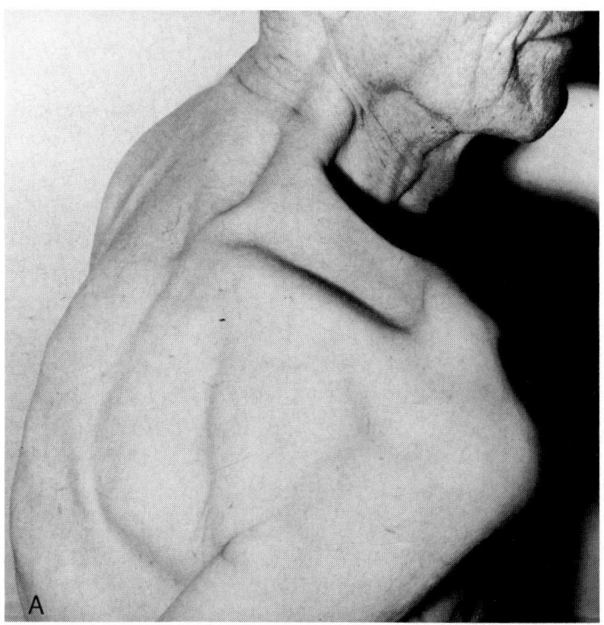

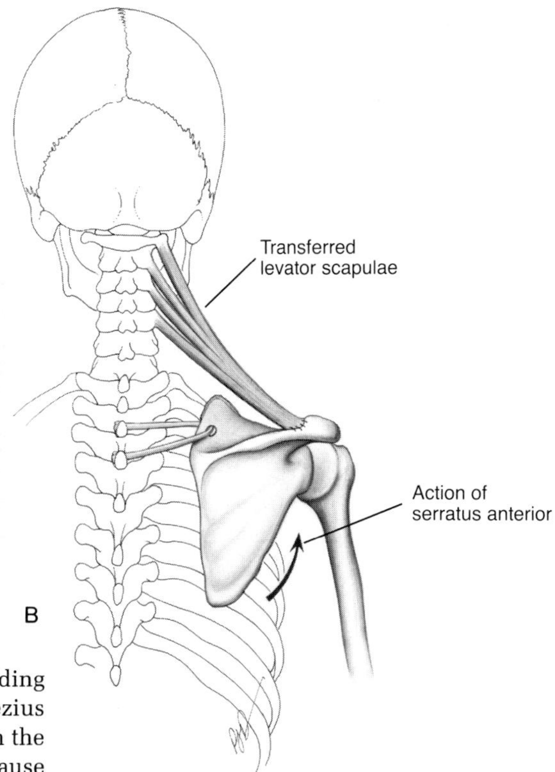

Figure 6–20. *Trapezius Paralysis.*

A, Photograph of a 65 year old man with a long-standing trapezius paralysis. The levator scapula stands out. Trapezius palsy interferes with normal scapular rotation and, when the arm is raised, may be associated with impingement because the acromion is not properly rotated out of the way of the greater tuberosity. A cuff tear caused by this type of impingement was demonstrated in this patient by a positive arthrogram.

B, Dewar-Harris scapular suspension for trapezius palsy uses a fascial sling from the second and third dorsal vertebrae to stabilize the mid-scapula, allowing the serratus anterior to rotate the scapula, as described in the text. Some surgeons prefer to transfer the rhomboids laterally in place of or in addition to the fascia.

them[101] have found the disability insufficient to justify extensive surgical procedures to stabilize the scapula; however, the activities and life expectancy of their patients are usually more limited. Patients with accidental, iatrogenic injuries are usually younger, are more active, and have a normal life expectancy.

Scapular suspension (Fig. 6–20B) is limited to those who have truly disabling scapular fatigue symptoms and have a good life expectancy. This precludes most of those who have had radical neck dissections for malignant tumors.

I have found that the primary cause of pain in some of these patients is subacromial impingement. Patients with this type of pain can be satisfactorily relieved of symptoms by anterior acromioplasty alone (see Figs. 2–41 and 4–63 to 4–68), with a repair of the rotator cuff if it is torn. If the impingement injection test (see Fig. 2–30) completely relieves the pain, anterior acromioplasty is considered rather than the Dewar-Harris procedure. An arthrogram may show a tear, as was one case in the patient illustrated in Fig 6–20A.

Technique of Scapular Stabilization

The technique is essentially that of Dewar and Harris.[61] The levator scapulae are transferred to the acromion, and a sling of fascia is implanted (as shown in Fig. 6–20C) from the vertebral border of the scapula to the spinus processes of the second and third thoracic vertebrae. Of course, the small levator scapulae alone are nowhere near strong enough to substitute for the trapezius muscle. The fascial sling is intended to stabilize the middle scapula so that the strong serratus anterior can cause the lower angle of the scapula to rotate forward, assisting the levator in tilting the acromion out of the way as the arm is raised. Bigliani[113] prefers transferring the rhomboid insertions laterally, in place of the fascial sling. Other surgeons advise using both procedures.

I have performed scapular suspensions for trapezius palsy too infrequently to have a meaningful personal experience or knowledge of late results.

Erb's Palsy (Upper Arm Birth Paralysis)

In Patterson's study,[254] injury to the upper part of the brachial plexus (C5–C6), partial or complete, occurred about every 3000 births, even in the best obstetrical units. I have seen a number of adult patients with partial birth palsies who have gone undiagnosed throughout their lives. However, today detection is perhaps more efficient in our obstetrical units and by our pediatricians than it was 20 years ago.

In a complete lesion, the arm hangs at the side, as shown in Figure 6–21A, adducted and internally rotated. Abduction is lost because of paralysis of the deltoid and supraspintatus muscles. External rotation is lost because of paralysis of the infraspinatus and teres minor muscles. Biceps and brachioradialis paralysis causes inability to flex the elbow and weakness of supination. In my experience, the distribution of motor weakness is not always the same. Segmental motor deficits may occur of any of the muscles supplied by the C5–C6 roots medial to the branching off of the long thoracic and dorsal scapula nerves. The serratus anterior, levator scapulae, and rhomboids may be partially affected. Electromyographic studies are of practical assistance in older patients.

Initial Treatment of Erb's Palsy

The aim of treatment in infants and prior to age four years is the prevention of contractures and bone deformities by passive motion performed by the parents each time the diapers are changed and by the therapist. The humeral head tends to dislocate posteriorly because of the internal rotation contracture and the retroversion of the glenoid and humerus. Spontaneous neurological recovery may continue for two years.

In untreated older children and adult patients, the glenoid faces backward and the proximal humerus is in retrotorsion (see Figs. 3–87 to 3–89). The acromion becomes elongated and hangs down over the humeral head (Fig. 6–21C). The coracoid becomes prominent (as with all posterior dislocations) but tends to develop laterally, impinging against the front of the humeral head. The objective of passive exercises in infants is to prevent fixed contractures and minimize these bone changes until spontaneous neurological recovery occurs or until releases can be performed. Older patients with fixed contractures may require releases; tendon transfers; and, eventually, bone surgery.

Releases, Tendon Lengthening, and Transfers for Erb's Palsy

After age four years, release or lengthening of the subscapularis and the pectoralis major with or without transfer of the latissimus dorsi and teres major to the posterior humerus can be considered.

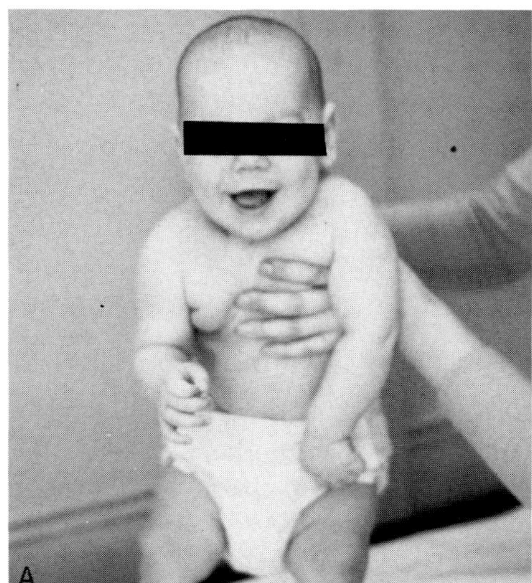

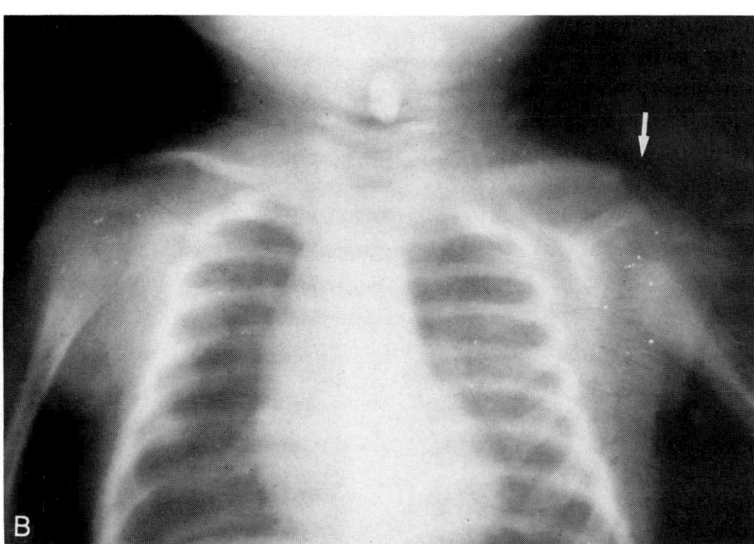

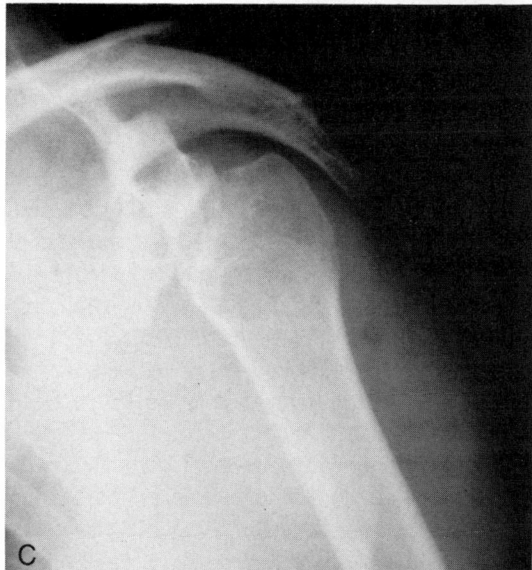

Figure 6–21. ***Birth Paralysis.***

A, The arm hangs at the side in a complete lesion, internally rotated and elbow straight.

B, Roentgen evidence of the Erb's paralysis in infants is easily overlooked; however, on close inspection in severe cases the retroversion and posterior displacement of the upper humerus can be seen (arrow) even before ossification of the epiphysis for the head.

C, Roentgen findings in those with residual paralysis after skeletal maturity include a retroverted and posteriorly subluxated humeral head; a retroverted glenoid; a long, overhanging acromion; and a protruding coracoid. Some patients with partial paralysis go on to develop painful glenohumeral arthritis in later life (see Chapter 3, Figs. 3–87 and 3–88).

I have done this through a deltopectoral approach with and without a posterior approach. Great care is necessary to avoid injury to the axillary nerve.

Fairbanks (1913)[256] is credited with the first releases for these internal rotation contractures. He divided the upper part of the pectoralis major tendon, the subscapularis tendon, and anterior joint capsule. When necessary, he also divided the coracohumeral ligament, supraspinatus tendon, and coracoid process. A few years later, Sever[257] modified this procedure by dividing the entire pectoralis major tendon, the subscapularis tendon, and when necessary the short head of the biceps and coracobrachialis from the coracoid and divided the coracoid and acromion. Steindler[258] pointed out that contractures of the latissimus dorsi and teres major may also limit external rotation and should be released if present. L'Episcopo[255] was the first to suggest balancing the muscle power by transferring the latissimus dorsi and teres major to the posterior humerus. Zachery[259] suggested the addition of a posterior incision for this transfer.

The severity of the contracture and residual muscle imbalance is, in my experience, inconsistent. I have seen patients whose parents had been dedicated to passive exercises of the shoulder who had incomplete residual paralysis of the external rotators and deltoid muscles but without a contracture of the subscapularis or pectoralis major. In this situation, lengthening of the subscapularis tendon was unnecessary and after detachment of the pectoralis major tendon, the latissimus dorsi and teres major tendons could be transferred to the back of the humerus through the anterior (deltopectoral) approach without a second (posterior) approach. This is done by making two drill holes from the front through the back of the upper humerus just below the epiphyseal line and with the arm in extreme external rotation passing the nonabsorbable sutures through these holes from back to front to hold the latissimus dorsi and teres major against the posterior humerus. Alternatively, with the arm in external rotation, teres major and latissimus dorsi may be sutured to the posterior musculotendinous cuff. During this step, great care is taken to avoid injury to the axillary nerve. The arm is held in an abducted and externally rotated position until a spica cast can be applied. The cast is worn for six to eight weeks, following which the parents continue passive exercises and the therapist instructs in active external rotation and deltoid strengthening exercises. In more severe cases, more extensive releases or lengthenings of the tendons may be required, and a second incision posteriorly is always an option if needed.

Because an internal rotation contracture limits function of the shoulder (see Fig. 1–20), eliminating this contracture alone improves function. However, active motion is dependent on the strength of the muscles and although the strength of the deltoid and infraspinatus muscles may improve with exercises after the contracture has been eliminated, it should be clear to the parents that the operation per se does not increase the number of muscle fibers. The latissimus dorsi and teres major transfer is of less importance than the release of the internal rotation contracture in most cases.

In those with more severe motor involvement of the upper extremity, arthrodesis or derotation osteotomies (when there is no pain) may eventually be alternatives to consider. Some patients with missed Erb's palsy are not recognized until later life, at which time painful glenohumeral arthritis may complicate the picture.

Arthritis of Erb's Palsy Deformity in Adults

As I indicated in Chapter 3, Figures 3–87 to 3–89, and reported to the American Shoulder and Elbow Surgeons,[260] I have encountered several adult patients with old deformities of the shoulder secondary to incomplete C5–C6 birth paralysis who in later life had painful arthritis with spurs and excrescences at the glenohumeral joint. Several of these patients knew they had something wrong with their shoulder all of their life, but the underlying cause had never been diagnosed. Neurological consultations and electrical studies confirmed the diagnosis. I treated them with the arthroplasty as described in detail in Figures 3–88 and 3–89, with relief of pain and improved function.

If these patients had less muscle power, they might not have the arthritis or the pain because they would have subjected the joint to less use. For extensive paralysis of the shoulder without pain, arthrodesis (see Chapter 6, p. 438) may be preferable. If there is fairly good stability and the glenohumeral joint is free of pain, an osteotomy (see p. 454) to eliminate the internal rotation deformity might be considered. For a long-standing Erb's deformity with fairly good muscles and painful arthritis with incongruity of the glenohumeral joint, the arthroplasty as described (see Figs. 3–87 to 3–89) has been a very rewarding procedure. This type of arthroplasty leaves the shoulder stable, restores passive external motion, and relieves impingement on the coracoid and acromion. The exercise program can be advanced rapidly.

In this total shoulder arthroplasty, the pectoralis major is detached early and later is transferred to substitute for the short subscapularis. The subscapularis and anterior glenohumeral joint capsule are released. The subscapularis tendon is lengthened if possible; however, it is usually too deficient to be lengthened. The posterior capsule and infraspinatus and teres minor tendons are maintained intact to stabilize the prosthesis. The glenoid component is implanted on the deformed glenoid in whatever retroversion is present (usually about 80 degrees retroversion). The humeral component is implanted in anteversion (usually about 40 degrees anteversion) to make a combined retroversion of 30 to 40 degrees. The coracoid process and undersurface of the acromion are beveled to eliminate impingement, with care to avoid detachment of the deltoid muscle. The pectoralis major is transferred upward to augment the subscapularis.

Charcot Neuropathy; Neurotrophic Shoulders

Charcot shoulders are not rare. They are usually caused by syringomyelia rather than, as in the recent past, by syphilis. Neurotrophic shoulders are said to occur with diabetes; however, I have not seen such a case. I have seen a juvenile diabetic who had daily seizures and daily shoulder dislocations who developed a Charcot-like shoulder after hundreds of painful dislocations. This patient was treated successfully with control of the seizure (by medication) and surgical stabilization of the shoulder, and was not a true neurotrophic joint with loss of protective reflexes.

It is a common misconception to think that Charcot shoulders are always free of pain. Shoulder pain and instability may be the first sign of syringomyelia. I average seeing and making the initial diagnosis of syringomyelia in one or two new patients each year. These patients have usually been referred for an arthroplasty because of pain and "degenerative changes" in the x-ray films of the glenohumeral joint, as illustrated in Figure 6–22A and B. One recent patient was referred to me with the diagnosis of idiopathic avascular necrosis of the humeral head.

The age of the patients with undiagnosed Charcot shoulders when first seen has ranged from 40 to 60 years. In the earlier stages, roentgenograms show a head defect like that in recurrent dislocations but larger. The head defect is usually anterior, as is associated with posterior dislocations; however, it may be posterior, eventually is present on both sides, and ultimately the entire articular surface is destroyed, as shown in Figure 6–22C to E. On examination, there is instability of the shoulder. Instability without trauma and more alterations in the bones than in ordinary recurrent dislocations should alert the examiner to the possibility of syringomyelia. It is a simple matter to test sensation in the hands with a pin and cotton and temperature sensation with one test tube filled with hot water and a second filled with cold water. The diagnosis can thus be made in the surgeon's office before sending the patient to the neurologist. Electromyography, CT scans of the cervical spine, and other tests confirm the diagnosis.

Patients with undiagnosed early neurotrophic changes at proximal humeral fractures may be seen. The diagnosis becomes obvious in the late stages (Fig. 6–22E), but initially the neuropathy must be recognized to avoid unsuccessful treatment of the nonunion.

Patients with an established diagnosis of Char-

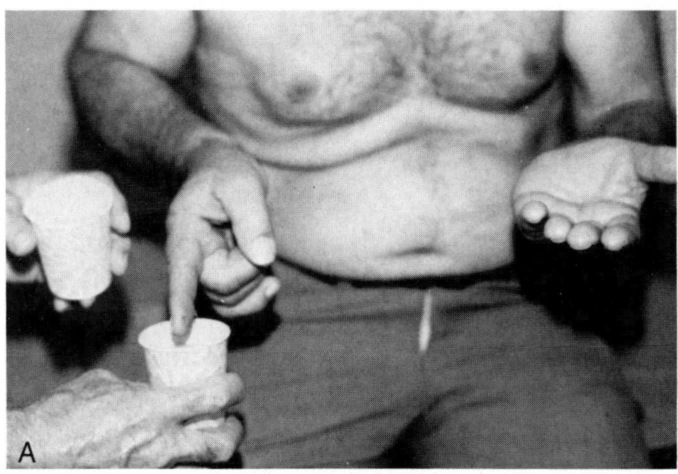

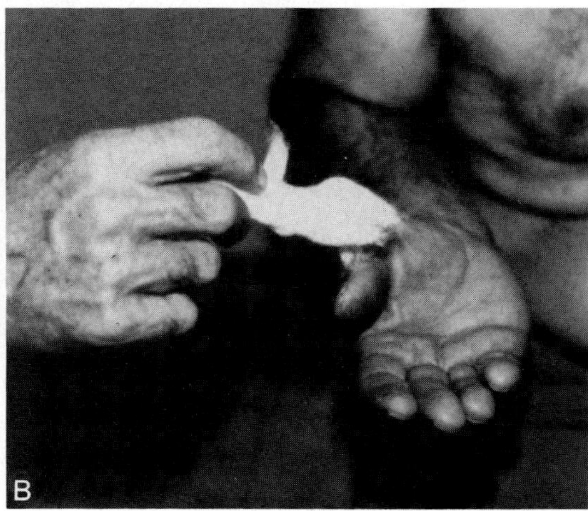

Figure 6–22. *Neurotrophic Shoulders.*

A and B, The shoulder surgeon is often the first to diagnose syringomyelia with cups of hot and cold water, a wisp of cotton, and a pin.

Illustration continued on following page

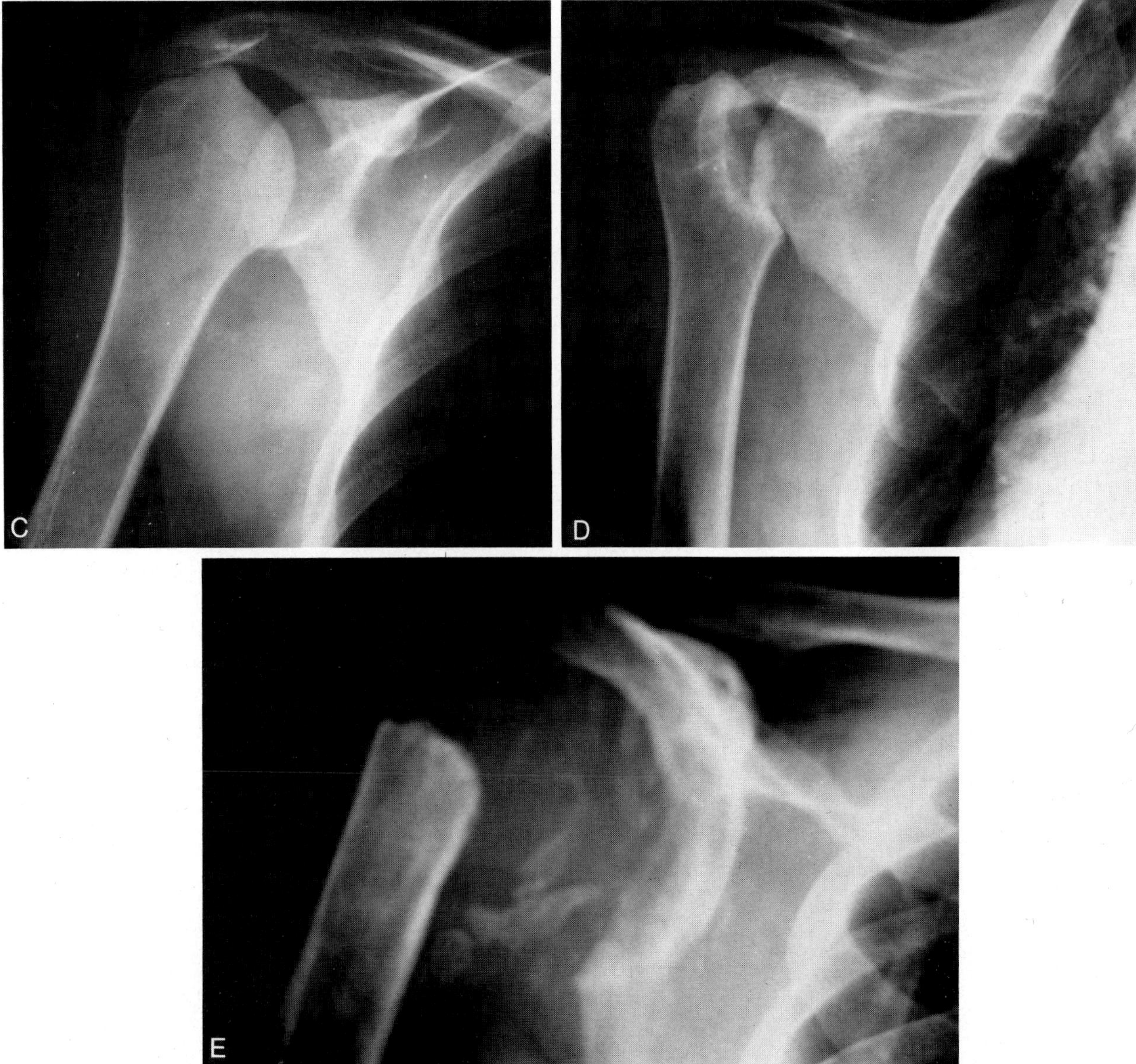

Figure 6–22 *Continued* C to E, Progressive roentgen changes in a Charcot shoulder. C, Peculiar change in density and shape of the unstable head.

D, Same patient a few months later. There was gross instability.

E, Advanced neurotrophic changes after a fracture with the typical osteochondrol fragments outside of the huge joint cavity.

cot shoulders may also be referred to the surgeon for treatment of the shoulder. Because the disintegration of the joint is due to the loss of protective reflexes allowing repeated injuries, the patient can be advised about the nature of the problem, given a strap or sling to wear selectively, and told to avoid pushing up and leaning on the involved arm. It is also important to have the patient receive the appropriate treatment for the underlying disease.

Surgical treatment of the shoulder has little to offer. After several unsuccessful attempts to fuse Charcot shoulders, I no longer desire to attempt this again. In the 1960s, I performed two replacement arthroplasties on painful Charcot shoulders with the following modifications of the usual technique described in Chapter 3. In both cases, the capsular space was greatly enlarged and was filled with bone fragments and fluid. The joints were very unstable. My procedure consisted of removing the bone debris and fluid, inserting a prosthesis to replace the humeral head, closing the redundant capsule as tightly as possible, overlapping the capsular flaps for reinforcement against becoming lax again, and immobilizing the joint for four months to allow healing of the soft tissue. It was hoped that sufficient fibrosis would occur to prevent a recurrence of the instability. One of these patients was a 56 year old male subway conductor who returned to his previous occupation about nine months after the arthroplasty but unfortunately never returned to me again for follow-up. I was unable to obtain a further report from his local orthopaedic surgeon. The second patient was a 59 year old woman who also had syringomyelia. Her prosthesis dislocated within six months after the arthroplasty, and she continued to have shoulder discomfort with traction symptoms in her arm. I removed the humeral prosthesis and used fascia to anchor the humerus to the scapula. This failed to relieve her symptoms.

Thoracoscapular Fusion for Muscular Dystrophy

Thoracoscapular fusion is occasionally indicated for fascioscapulohumeral dystrophy (Fig. 6–23). Copeland and Howard[220] consider the indication to be symptomatic winging of the scapula caused by thoracoscapular muscle paralysis with intact function in the deltoid muscle. This situation occurs almost exclusively in fascioscapulohumeral dystrophy. In this condition, the deltoid muscle is nearly always spared. Although the course of this type of muscular dystrophy is variable, there is fairly good life expectancy. The benefits of the operation are said to be slow to deteriorate with the progression of the disease.

When the thoracoscapular muscles are paralyzed, the deltoid muscle loses its stable origin. When the deltoid muscle contracts, it tilts the

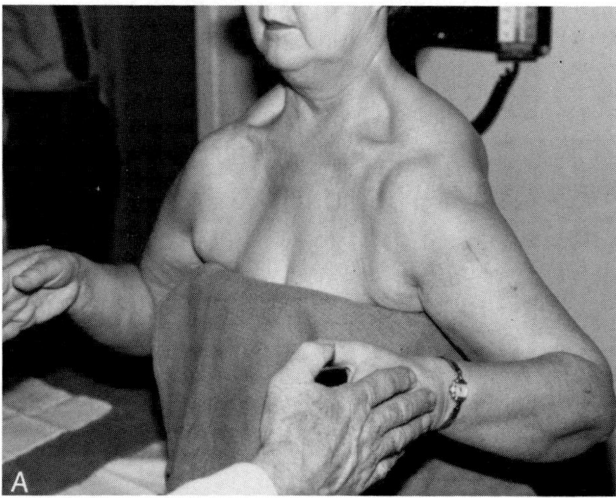

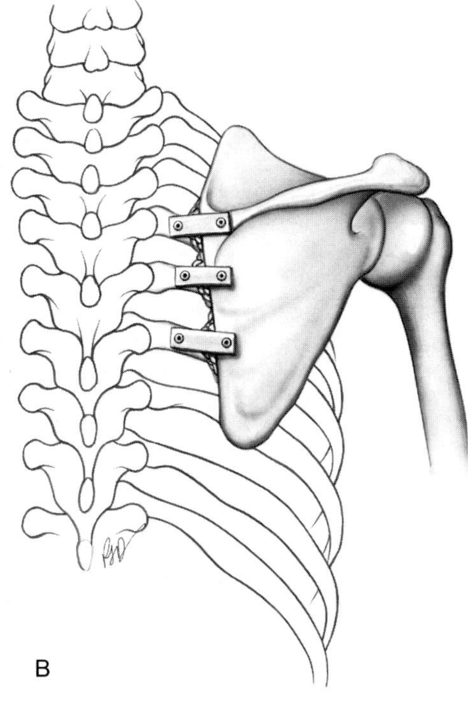

Figure 6–23. ***Copeland-Howard Thoracoscapular Fusion 220 for Muscular Dystrophy.***

A, In fascioscapulohumeral muscular dystrophy, the scapular muscles cannot stabilize the scapula and contraction of the deltoid muscles rotates inferior angles of the scapula medially rather than raises the arms.

B, Thoracoscapular fusion stabilizes the scapula so that the deltoid can raise the arm. Cancellous-cortical iliac crest grafts are now used rather than tibial grafts.

scapula rather than raises the humerus. The patient is unable to raise the arm. The objective of the procedure is to transmit this force to the humerus by anchoring the scapula to the fourth, fifth, and sixth ribs with bone grafts.

In the technique of Copeland and Howard,[220] with the patient supine to obtain the tibial grafts and prone with the arm off the side of the table for the procedure, an incision is made along the medial border of the scapula. The muscles on the undersurface and superficial surface of the scapula are detached (they are atrophied), and the undersurface, superficial surface, and vertebral border of the scapula are denuded 2.0 cm. laterally. The presenting ribs (usually the fourth, fifth, and sixth ribs) are exposed by subperiosteal dissection, placing retractors under them to protect the pleura from damage by the screws. In the original technique, tibial grafts were used. Cancellous-cortical iliac crest grafts are now preferred. The grafts are attached to each of the three ribs and to the scapula with screws, taking care that the tips of the screws do not protrude on the deep surface of the ribs. Cancellous chips of bone from the posterior iliac crest are packed between the grafts. After the patient is carefully turned, a shoulder spica cast is applied with the arm at 80 degrees abduction and 30 degrees flexion with the hand in front of the mouth. The patient is nursed after this operation in the sitting position. At three months, the top of that part of the cast on the involved arm is removed so that the arm may be moved. The cast is discarded when motion allows; a triangular pillow is used to allow gradual adduction; and after one week, physical therapy is begun to strengthen the deltoid muscle.

The purpose of this procedure is to regain elevation and flexion of the arm for reaching forward and upward and to relieve fatigue ache. The average range of motion recovered by the 11 shoulders in the series of Copeland and Howard was 90 degrees flexion and 100 degrees abduction. All patients had relief of pain. Rapid progression of disease occurred in two of the six patients.

This is a very rare condition, and I have had little personal experience with it except for seeing several patients in consultation who appeared to be good candidates for thoracoscapular fusion. Fascia to anchor the scapula is an alternative, but it tends to stretch and lose fixation and is less satisfactory.

TUMORS OF THE SHOULDER

The shoulder is the site of predilection for certain tumors and tumor-like conditions that will be considered briefly along with the special procedures of the shoulder for these lesions. The general principles of diagnosis and treatment of neoplasms of the shoulder do not differ from those for other parts of the body, and for more details, the reader is referred to the excellent existing literature.[222–229]

Tumors have always been of special interest to me.[116, 142, 230, 231] I was very fortunate to study in Dr. H. L. Jaffe's first course on orthopaedic tumors. I served as the orthopaedic surgeon for the Delafield Cancer Hospital in New York City at one time. I participated in the International Workshop on the Design and Application of Tumor Prostheses for Bone and Joint Reconstruction in 1983 and 1984.

Indications for Surgery on Shoulder Tumors

"Staging" of Tumors

It is essential that all surgeons use terms with the same connotation when discussing these lesions. The system for describing malignant tumors and their size, extensions, activity, and operability ("staging") generally used in the United States is that of Enneking.[228, 229] This staging system depends on the definition of three critical factors: grade (G_0 is benign, G_1 low-grade [well differentiated], G_2 is high-grade [undifferentiated]), whether the tumor is localized or spreading (T_1 is intracompartmental, T_2 is extracompartmental), and whether there is metastasis to the lungs as lymph nodes (M_0 is no metastasis, M_1 is metastasis). Disagreements on cell type are avoided by this system, the surgical implications can be agreed upon, and meaningful comparisons of the results of treatment can be made. Examples of surgical procedures requiring evaluation regarding the adequacy of the margin and the role of radiotherapy and chemotherapy are the following:

Benign: Unicameral bone cyst, chondroblastoma, or osteochondroma = curettage or marginal resection.

IA: Low-grade (G_1), intracompartmental (T_1), without metastases (M_0) = marginal or wide resection.

IB: Low-grade (G_1), extracompartmental (T_2), without metastasis (M_0) = wide or radical excision

IIA: High-grade (G_2), intracompartmental (T_1), without metastasis (M_0) = wide or radical excision.

IIB: High-grade (G_2), extracompartmental (T_2), without metastasis (M_0) = radical excision

III: Low-grade or high-grade, either intracompartmental or extracompartmental with regional or distant metastasis (M_1) = resection of pulmonary lesions, palliative resections, radiotherapy, and/or chemotherapy.

The two problems with this system requiring special definition in the shoulder are (1) an accurate definition of a compartment, and (2) an accurate definition of what is an adequate margin. To clarify these points, tumors confined to one muscle or bone are designated as confined to one compartment. Those extending beyond fascial planes or from the soft tissue extending into a bone or into the neurovascular bundle are extracompartmental. A malignant tumor breaking into the subdeltoid bursa from a tumor in the humerus raises a point for judgment. It is probably extracompartmental, but whether the deltoid muscle must be sacrificed should be decided upon depending on the nature of the tumor and whether the axillary nerve is involved. A malignant tumor breaking out from the proximal humerus into the glenohumeral joint or involving the glenohumeral joint capsule and axillary nerve requires en bloc excision of the glenohumeral joint, including the articular surface of the scapula and humeral head, as well as the axillary nerve (see Fig. 6–34). This sacrifices the deltoid muscle, which may as well be excised if it would add safety to the margin. Radical excision for a tumor of the upper humerus (or a tumor of the adjacent soft tissue) with extracompartmental invasion or for high-grade undifferentiated tumors without metastasis may be either by massive resection of all tissue in the area except the neurovascular bundle (Tikhoff-Linberg procedure)[232, 234] (see Fig. 6–38) if the neurovascular bundle is spared, or by amputation (see Fig. 6–39) if the neurovascular bundle is involved. Radical excision of a tumor of the scapula may be by scapulectomy, Tikhoff-Linberg procedure, or interscapulothoracic amputation and chest wall resection, depending on the lesion.

There must be some room for individual decision as to what is a safe margin. As mentioned on page 468, Fig. 6–31, a frozen section biopsy at the margin or stump of the bone is made during surgery. "Skip areas" of tumor in another part of the humerus or scapula must be excluded preoperatively as far as possible by appropriate imaging studies.

Most Frequent Shoulder Tumors

Metastatic tumors and myelomas occur more often than primary tumors in the shoulder, as they do elsewhere in the body. Excluding these lesions, the primary tumors and tumor-like lesions most frequently encountered in the shoulder are the following:

Scapula. The most frequent primary benign lesion in the scapula is an osteochondroma. The most frequent primary malignant lesion is a chondrosarcoma.

Proximal Humerus. Frequent primary benign conditions in the proximal humerus are unicameral bone cysts and osteochondromas. This is also a site of predilection for the less common chondroblastoma. Frequent low-grade malignancies, which are seen in patients over age 40 years, are chondrosarcoma, fibrosarcoma (desmoplastic fibroma), and giant cell tumor. Frequent high-grade malignancies, which are usually seen in patients under age 25 years, are osteogenic sarcoma and Ewing's sarcoma.

Soft Tissue. By far, the most common soft-tissue tumor of the shoulder region is a lipoma. The more frequent malignant soft tissue tumors are liposarcoma and malignant fibrous histiocytomas (undifferentiated fibrosarcomas).

Of course, the metaphyseal area of the proximal humerus is one of the most actively growing areas of the body and almost any tumor or tumor-like condition can occur here or in the shoulder region. However, the lesions just cited are especially prevalent and are worth keeping in mind.

Pre-operative Tests

Staging of tumors requires a meticulous physical examination and work-up and, in addition to the routine laboratory data (see Table 1–2), may be supplemented as indicated with other tests such as serum acid phosphatase and protein electrophoresis. Roentgen studies of the shoulder often include, in addition to the routine views (see Fig. 1–12A), tomograms, CT scans, arteriograms, venograms, and magnetic resonance imaging (MRI). Technetium bone scans can help show the extent of the bone tumor and metastases that are at a distance. CT scans and tomograms of the chest may be required to augment plain films.

Biopsy

A biopsy is the most definitive test and must be carefully planned. If at all possible, it should be done by the surgeon who will be performing the definitive treatment of the tumor. The surgeon consults with the pathologist and radiologist pre-operatively. The pathologist makes the judgement as to whether a needle biopsy will be adequate and the amount of tissue required. The surgeon performs the biopsy as follows:

1. Subsequent procedures are kept in mind, and involvement of vital tissue is avoided.
2. The biopsy tract is placed so that the sample can be excised with minimal loss of deltoid muscle.
3. The surgeon avoids spreading tumor cells outside of the bone or to another compartment.

The pathologist is in the operating room to perform a frozen section and to decide if an adequate specimen has been obtained. The pathologist also decides what special stains or special studies of the tissue will be performed. For more technical details, the reader is referred to Chapter 3, pages 250 and 253.

Treatment of Common Shoulder Tumors

Unicameral Bone Cyst

Unicameral bone cysts consist of cavities containing varying amounts of serous fluid and are lined by a thin connective tissue membrane that has usually been modified by fractures (Fig. 6–24A to C). Juxta-articular (subchondral) cysts and those in the small bones of the hands and feet were not considered in our study of 250 of these lesions,[230, 231] of which 133 (53 percent) occurred in the proximal humerus and none occurred in the scapula.

Etiology of Bone Cysts

I believe that a shoulder with a bone cyst should be considered a failure of repair following an injury, either trauma or infection, rather than a neoplasm. Injuries with bleeding and hematoma formation in soft tissue heal without a cavity because the soft tissue allows a potential space to collapse. However, bone is rigid, preventing collapse of the space. A fibrous lining forms in the cavity, probably in an effort to repair the injury. Some fluid remains in the cavity. The fibrous lining does not act as a semi-permeable membrane. Trauma, major fractures, or microfractures often modify the shell of bone surrounding the cyst. We studied the nature of the fluid. The level of electrolytes, proteins, and alkaline phosphatase in cyst fluid differs from that in interstitial fluid and plasma.[231, 238] Chemical analysis of the fluid compared with simultaneous analysis of venous blood showed the protein content to be elevated above that of venous blood. In some cases, the alkaline phosphatase value was as much as ten times greater than that of venous blood. We measured the hydrostatic pressure in the cysts. A pulse was transmitted to the cyst fluid with values between 200 mm. and 250 mm. of saline, as compared with 180 mm. for intact bone.

It was hoped that this study, which continued for several years, might not only shed light on the etiology of cysts but also be of prognostic value in predicting which cysts would be more likely to recur after curettage and bone grafting. The facts

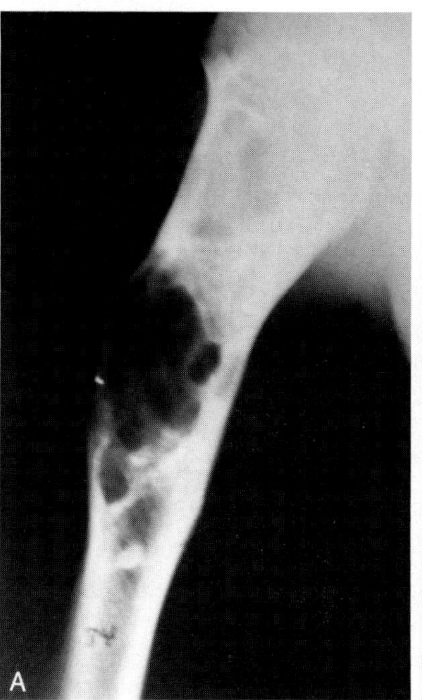

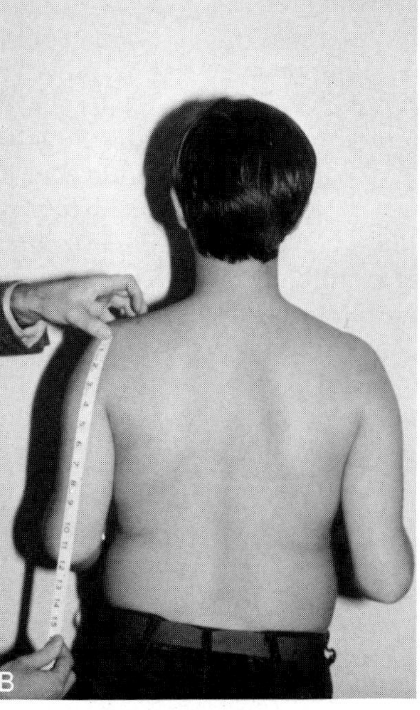

Figure 6–24A and B. ***Unicameral Bone Cyst of the Proximal Humerus*** A true recurrence of a unicameral bone cyst in a 16 year old boy who had three previous operations. This lesion was associated with 6.2 cm. of shortening.

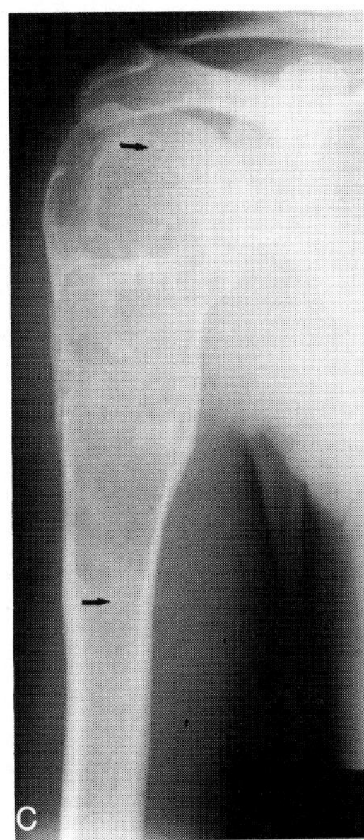

Figure 6–24C *Continued* An unusual unicameral bone cyst in a 19 year old man that persisted after closure of the epiphysis, crossed the epiphyseal line, and was associated with shortening of the arm. The arrows indicate the highest and lowest margins of the cystic cavity.

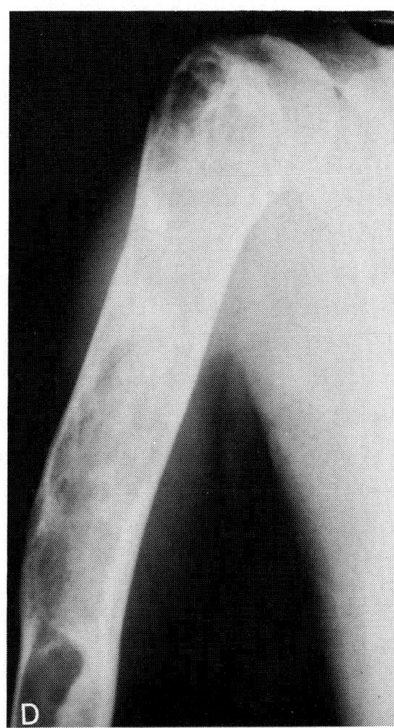

Figure 6–24D *Continued* Fibrous dysplasia. This can resemble a bone cyst and, if it fractures, may develop a nonunion.

just described may have some significance to anyone studying the effects of methylprednisolone acetate on cysts, as introduced by Scaglietti in 1979.[236, 237]

Diagnosis of Unicameral Bone Cysts

Bone cysts in the proximal humerus are extremely rare after closure of the proximal humeral epiphysis, whereas in other bones, which are less frequent locations for cysts, these lesions are commonly seen in adult life. They occur twice as frequently in male patients as in females. The diagnosis can be strongly suspected in plain x-ray films. The diagnosis can be confirmed by CT scans; the aspiration of fluid; or by filling the cavity with a radiopaque dye, as is done at the time of methylprednisolone injections.

The differential diagnosis includes fibrous dysplasia (Fig. 6–24D), cartilage lesions, and aneurysmal bone cysts (dilated sinus filled with blood with

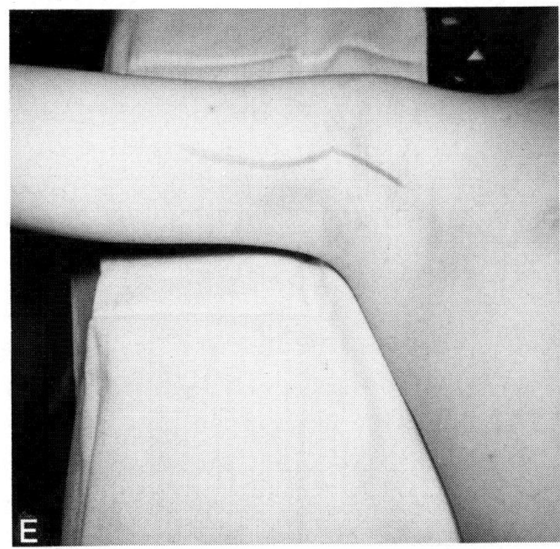

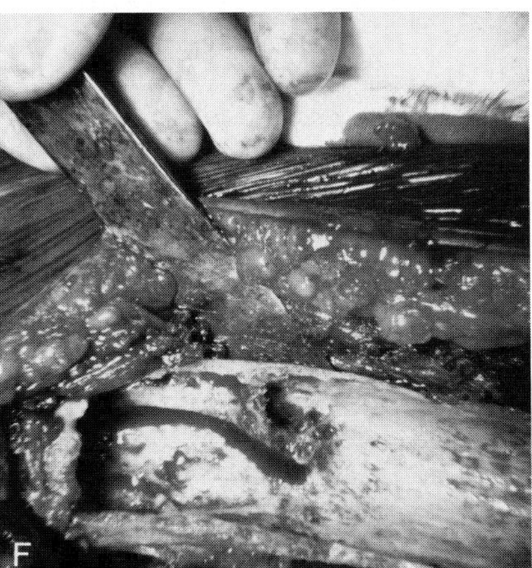

Figure 6–24 *Continued* Technique of surgical obliteration of a unicameral bone cyst.

E, The "concealed incision." The skin is undermined and retracted upward to permit a deltopectoral approach.

F, A window two-thirds the circumference of the humerus allows complete obliteration of the cavity and preserves length. The periosteal sleeve is used to enclose the bone grafts. Care is taken to fill the full length of the cavity with grafts.

a thickened fibrous lining). I have seen a patient with fibrous dysplasia who had been treated as having a unicameral cyst by watchful waiting for years. The diagnosis was made only after a nonunion occurred in one of her fractures. As is true of fibrous dysplasia, cartilage rests cannot be expected to heal and disappear (as occurs in bone cysts in the upper humerus by adulthood). Of course, the treatment and prognosis for recurrence of aneurysmal bone cysts are quite different from those for unicameral cysts. It was of interest that during our study, areas of the lining of some unicameral cysts were noted to contain foci of aneurysmal nature and it was thought that this might be an explanation for why some unicameral cysts are more prone to recur.

Treatment of Unicameral Bone Cysts in the Proximal Humerus

Bone cysts in the upper humerus, where 80 percent of the growth of that bone occurs, behave differently than cysts in the less frequent locations, and they tend to disappear after puberty. Only 4 percent of the patients in our study[231] with upper humeral cysts were over 17 years of age, whereas 50 percent of the patients with upper femoral cysts, the next most frequent location, were over 17 years of age and their ages ranged as high as 54 years. Some of the rare locations, such as the ilium, were characteristically found in adults.

Not only do cysts in the upper humerus tend to heal spontaneously before adulthood, but also fractures through the cyst in the upper humerus, which often occur with minimal trauma, tend to heal without serious deformity, in contrast to fractures through cysts in the lower extremity. Thus, a policy of watchful waiting after the diagnosis of a cyst in the upper humerus is safer than in the case of cysts in the femur.

Three forms of treatment are considered:

1. If the diagnosis is certain and the cyst in the upper humerus has adequate walls without fractures, the cyst can be observed. The epiphyseal plate tends to grow away from the cyst, and as maturity approaches, the cyst may disappear. Unfortunately, the majority of patients in our experience eventually have some procedure to obliterate the cyst. The epiphyseal plate did not grow away from the cyst in 70 percent, and in some cases, it remained near the epiphyseal line until the humerus was mature. In two of our patients, the cyst eventually crossed the epiphyseal line, undoubtedly contributing to the shortening of the humerus beyond that which occurred from repeated fractures.

2. If the cyst has a thin wall and repeated fractures, something should be considered to accelerate obliteration of the cyst so that the patient can get on with a more normal life. If the diagnosis is still certain, the injection of methylprednisolone acetate is the treatment of choice. The diagnosis can usually be substantiated, as discussed previously, by CT scan and by aspirating fluid and the "cystogram" performed with radiopaque dye just prior to the injection of methylprednisolone acetate.

3. If the diagnosis is in doubt, a biopsy is indicated and open surgical obliteration of the lesion may be performed at that time. If treatment with methylprednisolone acetate injection fails, surgical obliteration of the cyst is considered. It is important to define a failure of treatment.[230] Surgical intervention with bone grafts is unnecessary for residual defects in the bone surrounded by strong cortical bone that do not pose a threat of fracture nor present uncertainty as to the diagnosis. A "true recurrence" requiring surgical repair is an expanding lesion with a thin cortex and the threat of fracture rather than a residual hole in the bone surrounded by sclerotic bone.

Technique of Methylprednisolone Acetate Injection. A "cystogram" is made by aspirating (and culturing) any fluid obtainable and injecting radiopaque dye into the cystic cavity. An x-ray is made to determine if there are separate loculations in the cyst, which require separate injections of methylprednisolone. With two needles placed in the cystic cavity (with radiographic control), 80 to 200 mg. of methylprednisolone acetate (Depo-Medrol) is injected into each loculation. The injection of this steroid is repeated with radiographic control in two or three months if necessary. This is done in the majority of cases.

Most reports indicate about a 75 percent chance of satisfactorily obliterating the cyst in this way. The exact mechanism is unclear. Our findings in the study of the nature of the fluid within the cyst, the hydrostatic pressure in the cyst, and the nature of the cyst lining were discussed previously. One of the factors might one day prove to have bearing on the prognosis after this form of treatment.

Technique of Surgical Obliteration of the Cyst. The following points are emphasized:

1. Use a "concealed" incision along the anterior axillary line and medial side of the arm to avoid an unsightly scar (Fig. 6–24E). The skin flap is mobilized to permit a conventional deltopectoral approach or, if necessary, extended down the medial side of the arm to permit a conventional approach laterally between the biceps and brachialis anteriorly and the triceps posteriorly.

2. Elevate the periosteum and create a window two-thirds the circumference of the humerus but retain the periosteal sleeve. This allows complete obliteration of the cavity and yet leaves a strut of bone one-third the diameter of the shaft to maintain the length of the humerus. The periosteal sleeve is later used to keep the bone grafts in place. A liberal "window"[231, 235] or diaphysectomy[240] has been shown to reduce the recurrence rate.

3. Curette away the fibrous lining so that it will not interfere with filling the space with bone grafts. During this step, avoid injury to the proximal humeral epiphysis. The fragments of cortex removed for the large window may be used for grafts after the fibrous lining has been removed.

4. Supplement the pieces of local cortical bone removed (cleaned of soft tissue) with grafts as required with the objective of filling the space, taking care to fill the remote corners of the cavity.

5. Immobilize the arm to avoid fractures until some healing of the bone has occurred.

6. Follow with roentgenograms at yearly intervals to check for recurrence until the humerus has reached maturity.

"True recurrence rate" after this type of obliteration of the cyst is lower than when a smaller, narrow window is used. However, in the series of Fahey and O'Brien,[235] 5 of their 20 (25 percent) proximal humeral cysts recurred. In our study of 179 humeral cysts, of which 129 were followed more than one year, 30 of the 129 (23 percent) recurred. In patients under ten years of age and those referred with large lesions, the recurrence rate is higher than in adolescent patients with smaller lesions.

Enchondroma

The term enchondroma implies a chondroma in the central part of the bone (rather than on the surface of the bone, or "ecchondroma"). Whereas 50 percent of solitary chondromas occur in the small bones of the hands and feet, a large percentage of central chondromas in the large bones occur in the proximal humerus (Fig. 6–25). These lesions are considered by most pathologists to be cartilage "rests" (from embryonic development); however, later in life (usually after age 40), these lesions may "degenerate" to become "secondary chondrosarcomas."

As mentioned previously, the most common primary malignant tumor in the scapula is a chondrosarcoma.[221, 234] It is usually treated with scapulectomy. Proximal humeral chondrosarcomas, along with the less frequent fibrosarcomas and giant cell tumors, are the most frequent indications for en bloc resection of the proximal humerus, as described on page 249 in Chapter 3 and Figures 6–30 and 6–31.

The most important question with cartilage

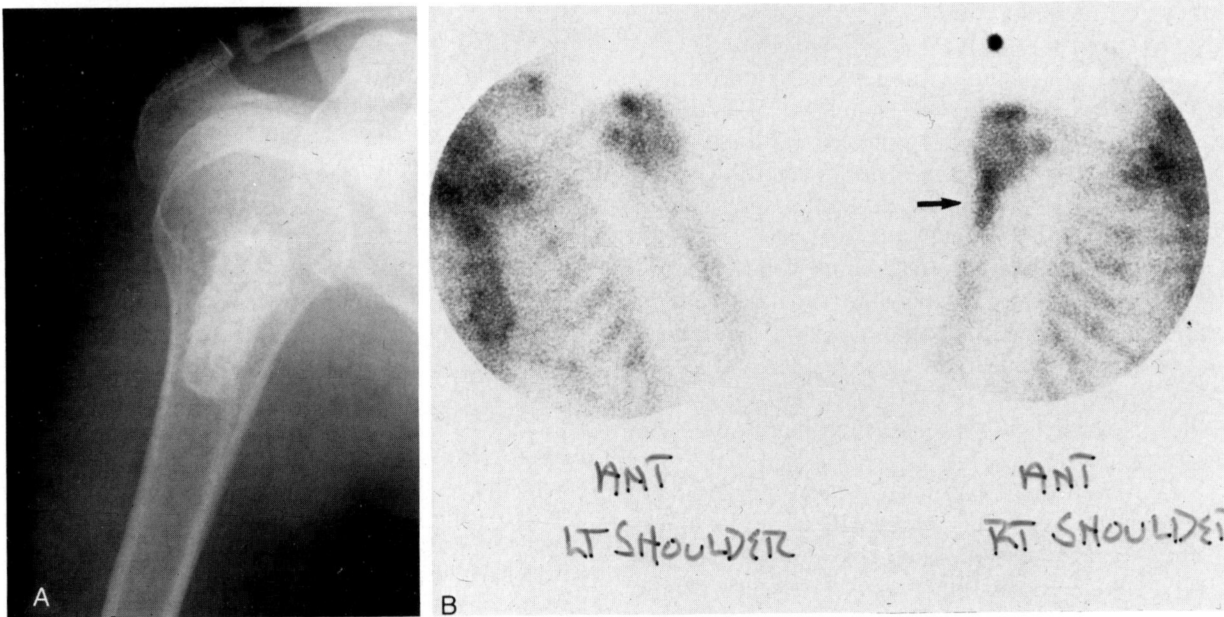

Figure 6–25. Example of an enchondroma of the humerus with enough uptake in the technetium bone scan that a biopsy is indicated. In this case, after the biopsy the pathologist advised local excision, as a prophylactic measure. This was done through a large window so that the tumor could be lifted out with a large gouge in one piece. The cavity was partially filled with iliac bone grafts. A, Original x-ray. B, Technetium radioactive scan.

Illustration continued on following page

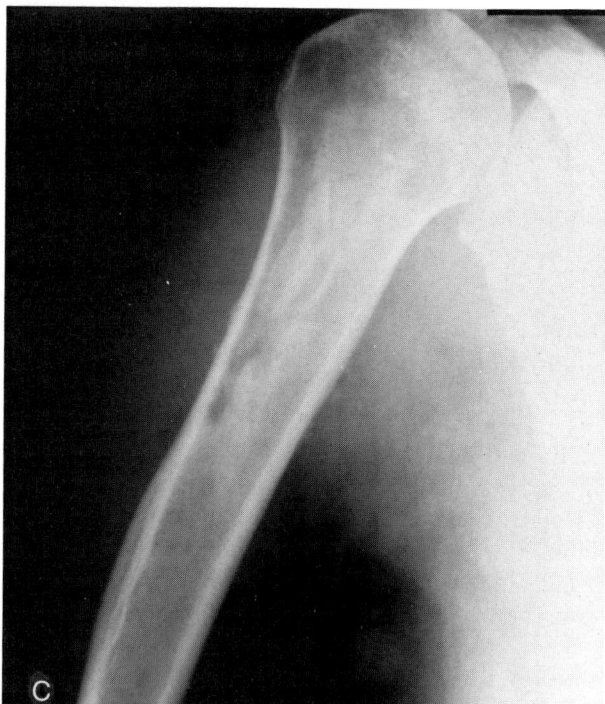

Figure 6–25 *Continued* C, Postoperative appearance, after local removal and grafts.

tumors in the proximal humerus, scapula, or clavicle is whether they are aggressive, low-grade malignancies with the potential for local invasion, local recurrence, and eventual metastasis to the lungs, or are benign "rests." As is the case of low-grade secondary chondrosarcomas in other large bones of the body, this can be a very difficult distinction (see Figs. 6–25 and 6–26).

The histological appearance can be disarming, especially if an inadequate sampling of different parts of the tumor has been obtained. Biopsy samples of several parts of the tumor should be obtained with a trochar or an angulated curette through a small window (see Chapter 3, p. 253). The "seeding" of chondrosarcoma cells into the soft tissue outside of the bone is especially easy to do during a biopsy or en bloc resection. Therefore, biopsies of enchondroma must be performed extremely carefully and placed where the biopsy tract can be resected if there is subsequent en bloc resection or local excision.

Enchondromas are usually seen for the first time in a middle-aged patient with shoulder pain. In many cases, another cause of shoulder pain is present, such as calcium deposits, impingement, and acromioclavicular arthritis. One of my patients with a proven chondrosarcoma of the proximal humerus was noted during en bloc resection to have a small impingement tear of the rotator cuff (Fig. 6–26). The question then arises as to whether the "enchondroma" should be observed or biopsied.

Factors favoring possible malignancy and the need for biopsy are as follows:

1. Uptake in the tumor during a technetium scan is evidence for the possibility of activity, whereas no uptake is reassurance for further observation.

2. Cortical erosion—this can be brought out with computerized tomography. A soft-tissue mass outside the bone is, of course, surely indicative of advanced malignancy.

3. As in other parts of the body, large cartilage tumors should be treated as if they were low-grade malignancies. Biopsies of several parts of the tumor are mandatory.

4. "Tumor pain" or constant, low-grade pain that is present at rest should be a strong point in favor of biopsy. However, as mentioned previously,

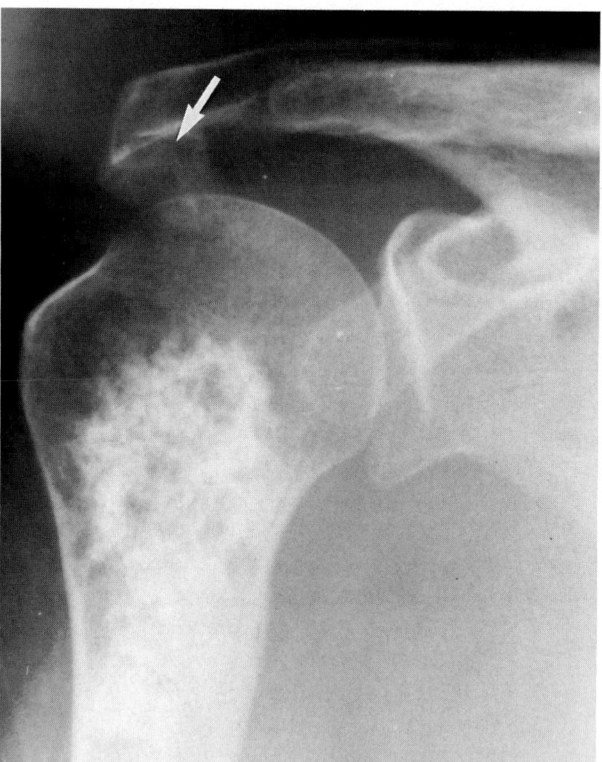

Figure 6–26. It can be difficult to distinguish between enchondroma and chondrosarcoma. This lesion was graded by the pathologist as a chondrosarcoma of the upper humerus. There was an incidental finding of an anterior acromial spur (arrow). Also, there was an impingement tear of the rotator cuff noted during the en bloc resection of the upper humerus. Pain from the cuff tear was undoubtedly a factor in drawing attention to this tumor, although the chondrosarcoma was threatening to break out of the cortex and may well have been contributing to the pain.

some concomitant lesion may be present to cause the pain. Almost every type of shoulder pain is worse at night. The absence of pain is a point strongly in favor of observation without biopsy.

Treatment often consists of further observation. Intralesional excision with bone grafting to reinforce against future fractures is performed if the pathologist believes this is indicated as a prophylactic measure against the insidious transition to a chondrosarcoma (see Figs. 6–25 and 6–26). En bloc resection is indicated if the lesion is proved to be a chondrosarcoma.

Chondroblastoma of the Proximal Humerus

Chondroblastoma of the proximal humerus is a rare tumor, but a large proportion of chondroblastomas occur in the shoulder. The nine examples Codman[6] collected were all in the upper humeral epiphysis. However, Jaffee[223] showed that these lesions also occur at other sites and are somewhat more common in the bones at the hip and knee. I have treated only two chondroblastomas of the proximal humerus primarily and four others referred from other orthopaedic surgeons after attempts at excision had failed.

The term "benign chondroblastoma" is used by pathologists to suggest that in these often calcifying tumors of mixed chondroid cells and giant cells that occur in ossification centers just beneath articular surfaces, the histological appearance may be more frightening than the benign clinical behavior. Although more than 75 per cent of these lesions occur in patients between 12 years and 20 years of age, they are occasionally reported in younger patients and after age 50 years.

The diagnosis is strongly suggested by the calcifications; the epiphyseal location; and, in most cases, by the age of the patient. If a good bone pathologist is available for interpretation of a frozen section biopsy or needle biopsy sample, under ideal circumstances one may proceed with intralesional excision of the tumor and bone grafts if needed. If there is any doubt, we wait for formal sections, especially at re-operation on recurrences.

In my experience, all of the patients with "recurrences" after previous surgery had incomplete removal of the lesion and the lesion continued to grow—rather than a recurrence. In one case (see Figs. 3–94 and 3–95), after two attempts at excision by other surgeons, the lesion had re-grown to involve a large area around the proximal humerus and into the glenohumeral joint. Because of this unusual behavior, the pathologists advised an en bloc excision, as was done, including removal of the glenohumeral joint. A prosthesis and autogenous fibular bone graft were used, and recurrence was not seen after nine years follow-up.

Technique of Local Excision and Bone Graft for Proximal Humeral Chondroblastoma

A deltopectoral approach is made to the anterior surface of the lesser tuberosity, where a window 1.5 cm. by 1.5 cm. is made, without injury to the long head of the biceps or articular surface. This entails detaching some of the subscapularis tendon, which provides exposure of the articular surface of the humeral head as needed to prevent perforations into the glenohumeral joint. The joint can be opened further by developing the interval between the supraspinatus and subscapularis tendons. Through the window in the lesser tuberosity, the tumor is excised with osteotomies and gouges. An effort is made to excise it rather than curette it out. After all of the lesion has seemingly been excised, a curette is used to check all of the crevices, making sure that no pieces of tumor have been left behind.

These lesions tend to encroach immediately beneath the articular surface, and only a thin layer of cartilage and subchondral bone may remain in the central area. This can be reinforced by taking a plug of cancellous bone from the iliac crest, which has been shaped to fill the hole and implanted through the window (Fig. 6–27). Other fragments of donor site bone are used to plug the crevices. No internal fixation is needed.

Shoulder exercises to preserve motion are begun in about seven days, but strengthening exercises are deferred several months until it is thought that the graft has revascularized and re-attached sufficiently to lend some support to the articular surface.

I have followed two patients with this procedure for over ten years, and neither has symptoms or degenerative changes yet.

Recurrent Chondroblastoma in the Proximal Humerus

All four of the patients referred to me for this problem were thought to have had incomplete removal of the tumor rather than a recurrence. In two patients, it was possible to make a window in the lesser tuberosity, through which the residual tumor was excised and bone grafted as described previously. One patient had so much damage as a result of collapse and scarring of the humeral head that a humeral head prosthesis was used with iliac grafts to fill the defects in the proximal humerus

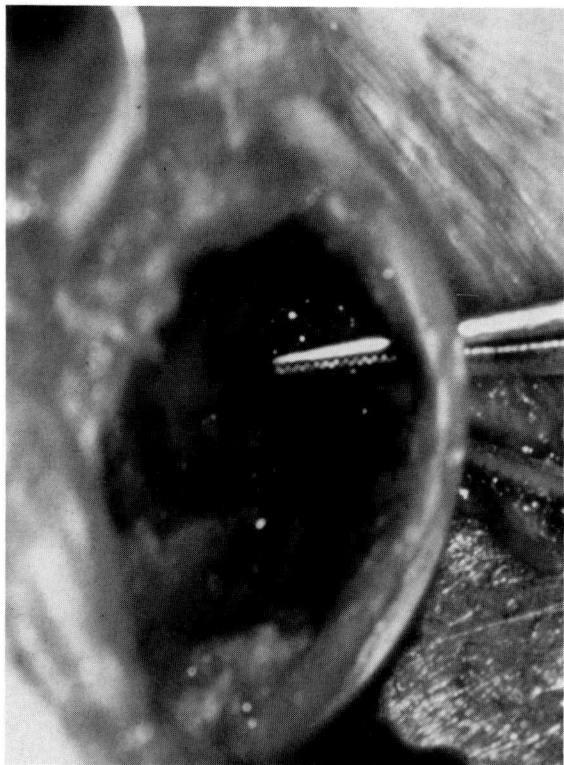

Figure 6–27. Chondroblastoma in the humeral head requiring an iliac bone graft to support the articular surface after removal of the tumor.

created when the tumor was excised and to support the stem of the prosthesis. The fourth patient had the en bloc resection described in detail in Chapter 3, page 251, Fig. 3–95. None of these patients had further recurrence of the tumor.

Osteochondroma of the Scapula

Osteochondromas occur as solitary lesions or in patients with multiple cartilaginous exostoses. As is true of osteochondromas at other sites, osteochondromas of the scapula grow throughout the second decade of life and even a few years later.

On the undersurface of the scapula, these lesions come to cause pain as a result of pressure. A bursa develops between the ribs and the exostosis. The scapula is elevated from the chest wall, giving the appearance of "winging." I have seen patients who have been treated for several years as having neurological problems without the true underlying lesion recognized because an x-ray showing the full length of the scapula had never been obtained.

The diagnosis depends upon the x-ray films including the *entire scapula,* and although the lesion may be suspected in the anterior-posterior view, a true lateral view of the scapula is the critical film to establish the diagnosis (Fig. 6–28). Imaging is usually unnecessary although a CT scan shows the lesion quite well. The benign nature of the lesion can be assumed from the characteristic shape of its stalk and cartilage cap seen in patients in the second or third decade of life. Broad-based, sessile lesions with atypical cartilage that begin to grow in older patients, especially those with multiple osteochondromas, must be suspected of possible secondary malignant transformation to chondrosarcomas; however, the typical solitary lesions in adolescents and young adults are assuredly benign.

Technique of Excision of Osteochondroma of the Scapula

The patient is positioned on the uninvolved side in a 45 degree face-down tilt position with a pad under the chest to relieve pressure on the shoulder of the uninvolved side. A longitudinal incision is made over the medial border of the scapula 15.0 cm. long and centered over the site of the tumor. The lateral margin of the trapezius muscle is identified, and this muscle is retracted cephalically. The rhomboids are temporarily detached. The lateral margin of the trapezius muscle is identified, and this muscle with the terminal branches of the accessory nerve is retracted upward, exposing the medial border of the scapula. It may be necessary to free the medial angle of the scapula from a little of the attachment of the trapezius muscle. The rhomboids and serratus anterior are temporarily detached from the medial border sufficiently to expose the tumor (which can easily be palpated deep to the subscapularis). The tumor is exposed by elevating the subscapularis and is cut off smoothly at its base. It is removed with its entire cartilage cap. Elevated ridges near the base of the lesion often remain, which are removed with a rongeur. The bursal sac is left intact if it serves to fill dead space. After reattachment of the muscles on the medial border of the scapula, the skin is closed with subcuticular 000 nonabsorbable suture. A sling is used for a few days for comfort.

Low-Grade Malignancies of the Shoulder Region

The staging of these lesions has been discussed (see p. 458), including the pre-operative assessment, biopsy, and surgical implications. Biopsies must be performed with the same caution for all of these lesions (see pp. 253 and 464; Fig. 6–29). Treatment is by complete excision with a tumor-free margin in each case, usually by en bloc resec-

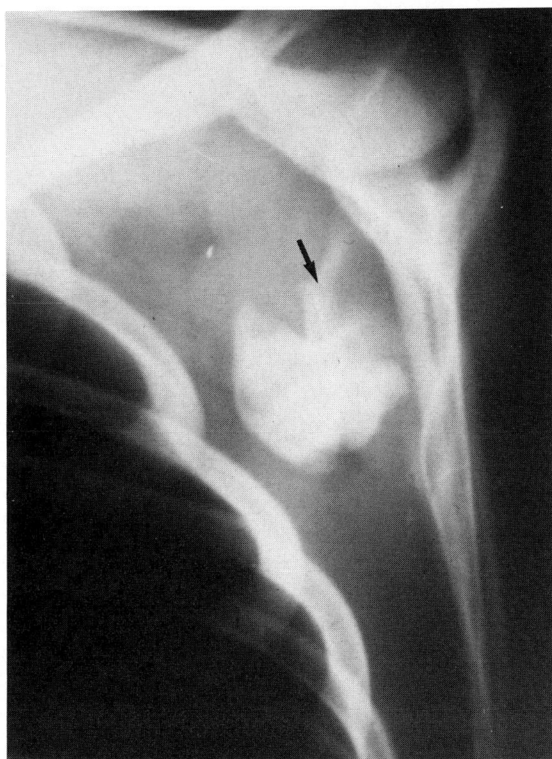

Figure 6–28. Osteochondromas of the scapula are best seen in a lateral view of the scapula, as in the "trauma series" (see Fig. 1–12B), but with the arm raised (as illustrated) or in CT scans of the scapula. These lesions can be missed unless the full length of the scapula is known.

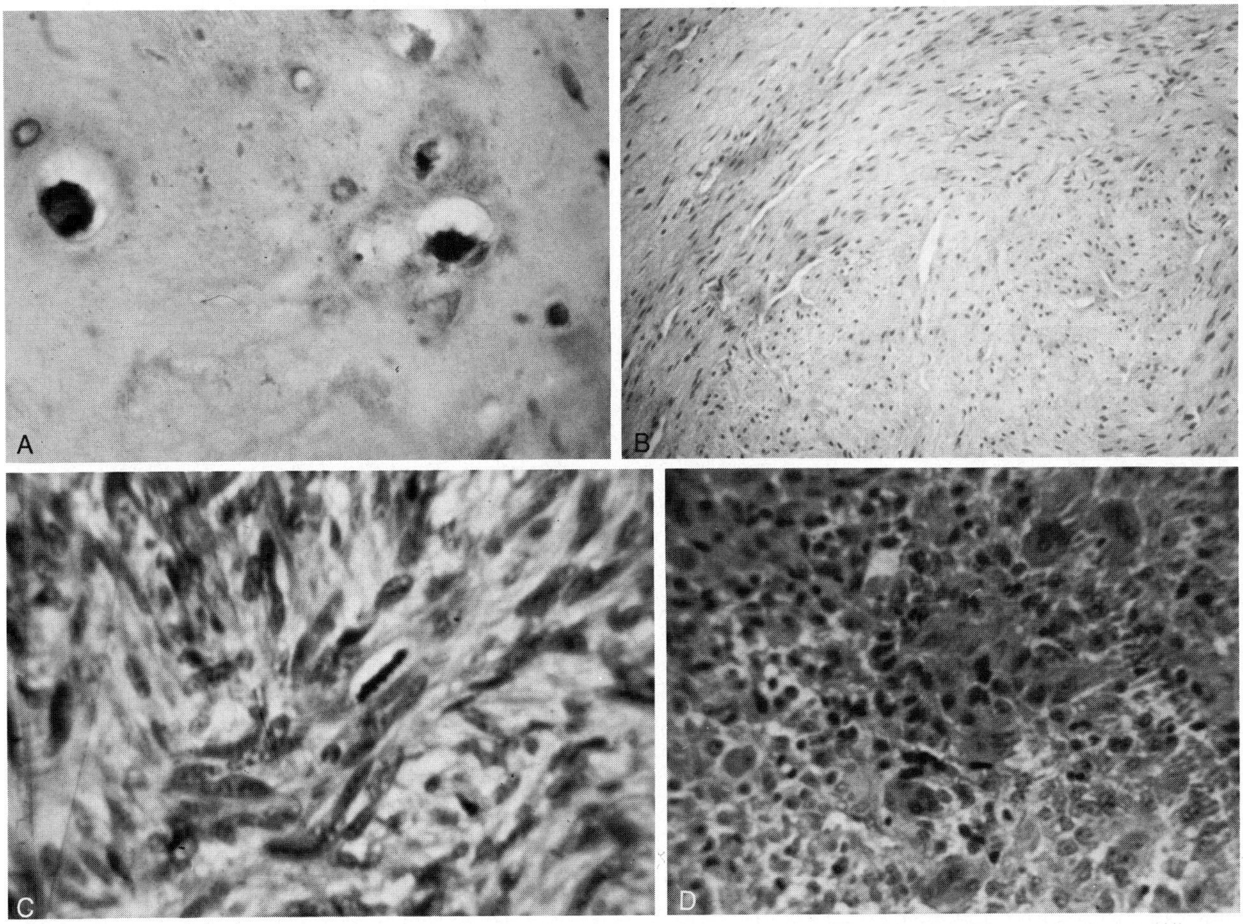

Figure 6–29. Microscopic picture of the low-grade malignancies most likely to occur in the shoulder. A, Chondrosarcoma. B, Fibrosarcoma of bone (desmoplastic fibroma). C, Extraosseous fibrosarcoma. D, Giant cell tumor.

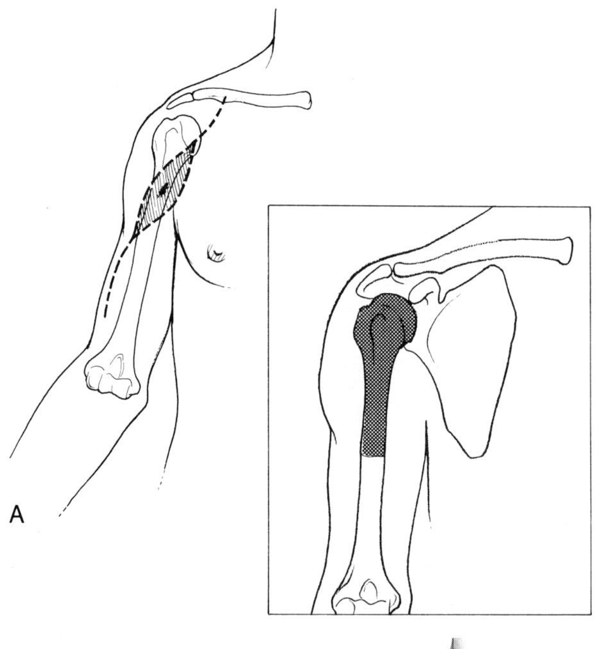

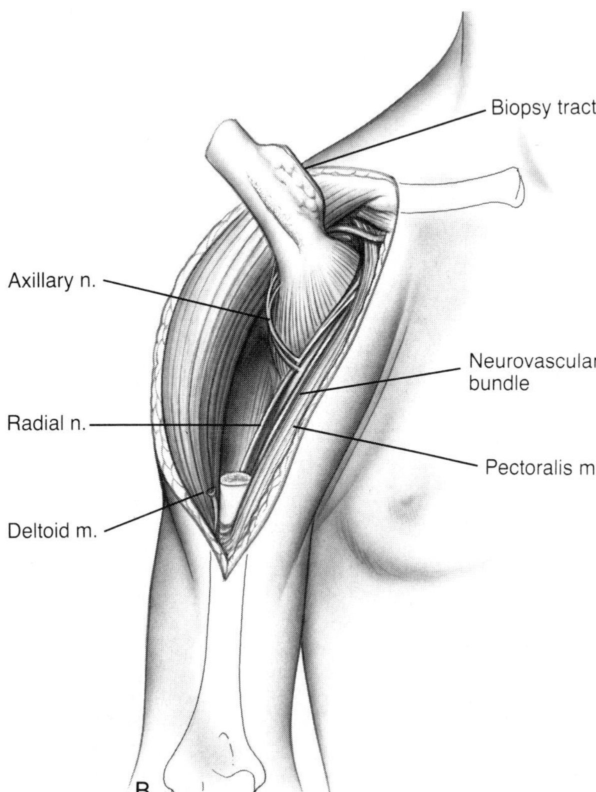

Figure 6–30. Technique of en bloc resection of the proximal humerus when the glenohumeral joint and deltoid muscle have been spared.

A, Skin incision and approach remove the biopsy tract with the specimen.

B, Depicting the biopsy tract remaining intact with the specimen. Major anatomical structures are shown.

Details of the technique for prosthetic replacement and fibular bone grafting after removal of the tumor are shown in Figure 3–95, and alternatives are discussed in the text.

tion of the proximal humerus (see pp. 249 to 253, Figs. 3–94, 3–95, and 6–30) or scapulectomy (see Figs. 6–36 and 6–37).

Chondrosarcoma

Chondrosarcoma is the low-grade malignancy most likely to occur in the proximal humerus or scapula. The diagnosis and its differentiation from enchondroma are discussed on page 463. These lesions are diagnosed after the second decade of life, and usually treatment by en bloc resection is considered (see Fig. 3–95; Figs. 6–30 and 6–31) after age 40.

Fibrosarcoma (Desmoplastic Fibroma)

Of the musculoskeletal system, the shoulder is the third most frequent site for fibrosarcomas. These lesions may be intraosseous or extraosseous.

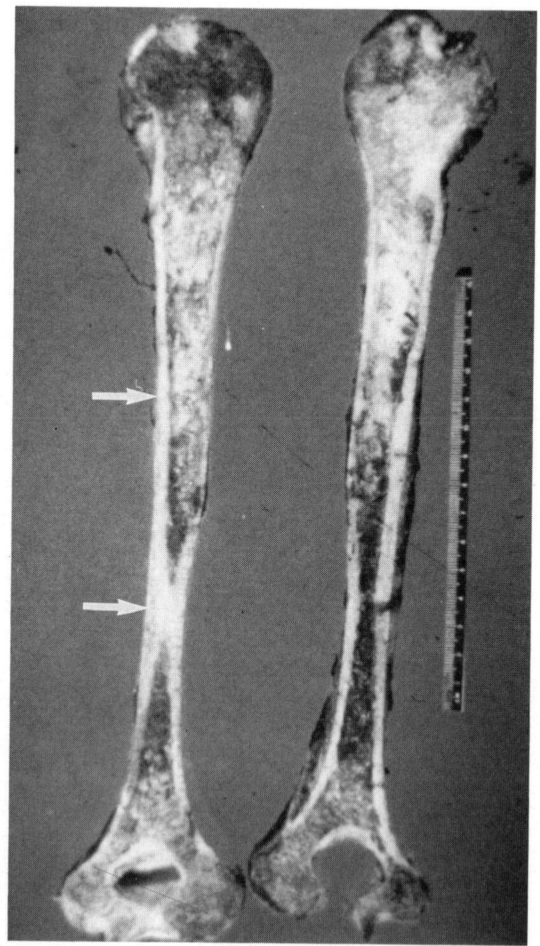

Figure 6–31. Chondrosarcoma with "skip" areas (arrows), as must always be feared in en bloc resection of the proximal humerus for this lesion. A frozen section biopsy of the contents of the distal stump of the humerus is obtained during this procedure when there is any doubt.

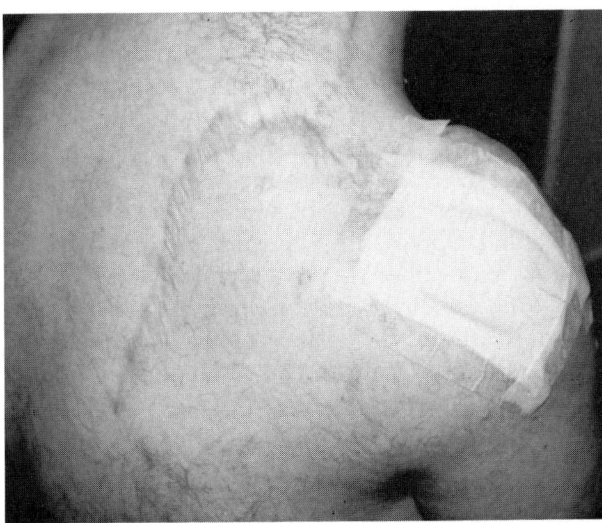

Figure 6–32. Extraosseous fibrosarcoma with five failed attempts at excision treated with a Tikhoff-Linberg radical resection. This tumor has an awesome tendency to recur locally unless completely excised.

They occur in adult life. Fibrosarcomas should be remembered for their awesome tendency to recur locally despite their often rather disarming histological appearance. They must be completely removed.

Extraosseous Fibrosarcoma. I have seen a soft-tissue fibrosarcoma in the scapula region of a 55 year old man who had eight local recurrences after incomplete removal, similar to the lesion illustrated in Figure 6–32. A Tikhoff-Linberg radical en bloc resection of the scapula and upper humerus with excision of some of the ribs and chest wall was used to rid him of the tumor. These lesions usually do not metastasize to distant sites until very late.

Extraosseous lesions may erode bone from outside.

Fibrosarcoma of the Proximal Humerus. Low-grade fibrosarcoma of the proximal humerus eventually metastasizes to the lungs by the hematogenous route, but it is slow to do so. Like the other low-grade malignancies in the upper humerus, it slowly destroys bone, breaking through the cortex, as can be seen in computerized tomography or plain films. It may involve the former epiphyseal center of the head of the humerus (as well as the metaphysis) like a giant cell tumor. It may involve the glenohumeral joint, requiring excision of the joint (Fig. 6–33).

Giant Cell Tumor

Giant cell tumors are rare, but the proximal humerus is next to the distal radius and knee region

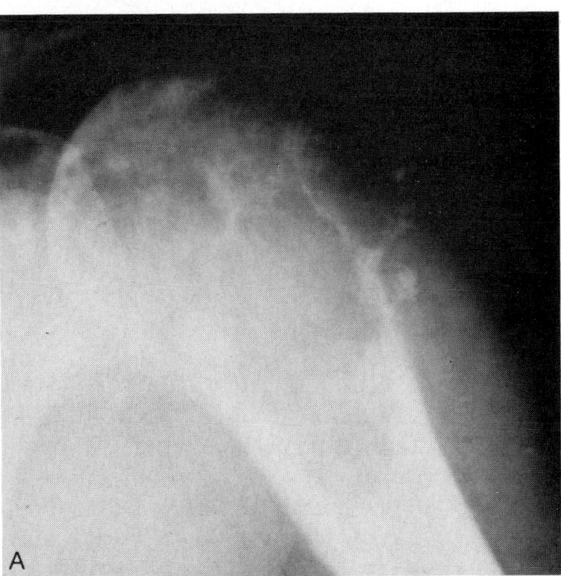

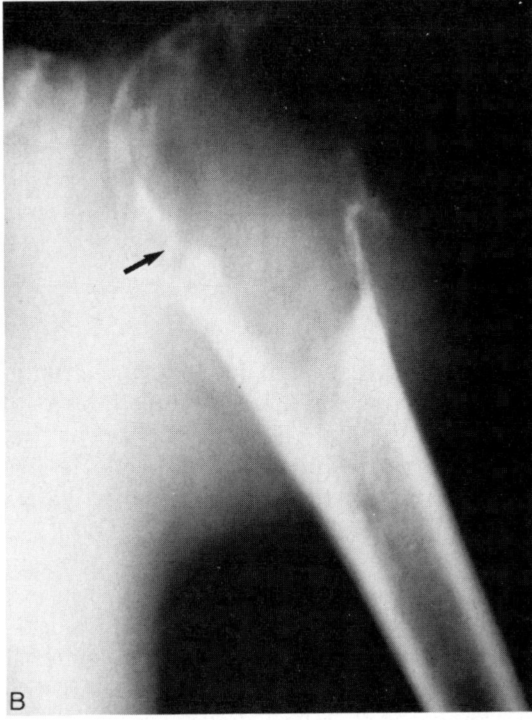

Figure 6–33. Fibrosarcoma with glenohumeral joint extensions requiring excision of the joint at en bloc resection. A, Anterior-posterior view. B, Tomogram shows break into the joint (arrow). CT scan and MRI can assist in the preoperative evaluation.

Illustration continued on following page

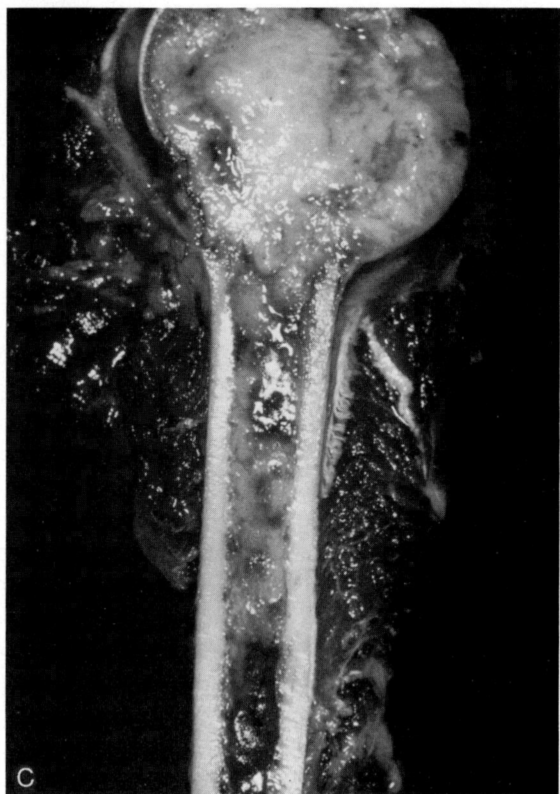

Figure 6–33 *Continued* C, Specimen with joint excised intact.

as the site of most frequent occurrence (see Fig. 6–29D). As is true of all giant cell tumors elsewhere, it involves the epiphysis; is seen in adult life; and although its histological appearance may be benign, it may metastasize and is more apt to recur after a second operation if not completely excised the first time. Therefore, it is treated with respect and a good margin.

Technique of En Bloc Resection of the Proximal Humerus

This procedure is used for low-grade malignancies of the upper humerus. Complete removal of the tumor is the first objective, and reconstruction of the proximal humerus with available surrounding muscles is the secondary objective, as described in Chapter 3, Figures 3–94 and 3–95.

A posterior approach with the patient lying on the uninvolved side can be considered because it is important to retain the anterior deltoid muscle for function and because the important external rotators (infraspinatus and teres minor) are detached during this operation anyway to remove the tumor. If a posterior approach is used, the patient is positioned on the uninvolved side and an incision is made along the posterior margin of the deltoid muscle and extended downward over the lateral intermuscular septum; superiorly, this incision swings laterally sufficiently to allow detachment of the origin of the posterior deltoid. Distally, the approach reaches the humerus along the lateral intermuscular septum (with care to avoid injury to the radial nerve). In a posterior approach, the axillary and radial nerves are in the center of the field and the slope of the acromion causes it to be a little in the way. Neither of these findings is an overriding objection to this approach. However, because the biopsy or previous surgery has usually been performed anteriorly and since the biopsy tract and previous scars must be excised, the anterior deltopectoral approach is usually used.

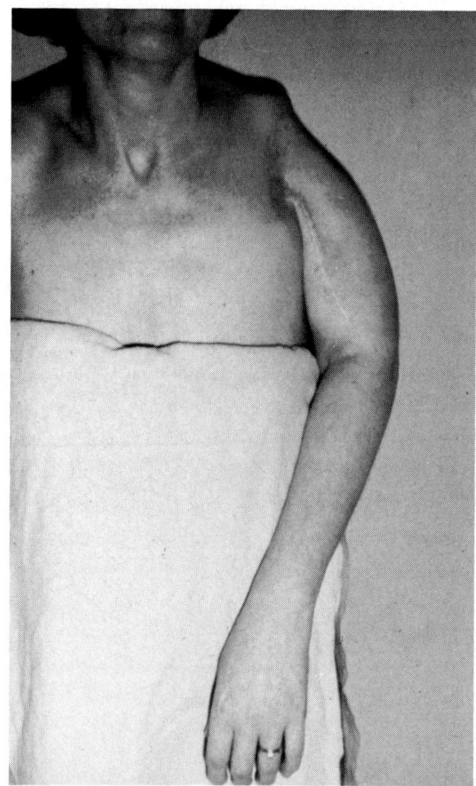

Figure 6–34. Arthrodesis after en bloc resection of the upper humerus can be difficult because it requires long grafts that often fracture and develop nonunion. In this patient, fibrosarcoma involved the axillary nerve and deltoid muscle, requiring removal of these structures during en bloc resection of the proximal humerus. Because of both the loss of the deltoid muscle and detachment of the rotator cuff, arthrodesis was attempted using autogenous fibular grafts. Even though two long metal plates were used to protect the grafts, the grafts fractured a few minutes after their insertion. Nonunion at these fractures in the grafts followed, which persisted despite two further attempts to repair them.

For the anterior approach, the patient is positioned supine with the head of the table raised 35 degrees and the knees bent to prevent the patient from sliding down. Folded towels are placed under the scapula, and the arm is draped free so it can be moved. With the extended deltopectoral approach (see Figs. 3–94 and 6–30), the biopsy tract and previous scars and any tissue involved in previous procedures are taken with the specimen. The objective is to maintain a tumor-free margin without entering tumor cells at any time during the procedure. If the subdeltoid bursa laterally and posteriorly is free of tumor and the axillary nerve is tumor free, the deltoid muscle can be saved except for that part of the anterior deltoid involved with previous surgery.

Tomograms and imaging prior to surgery are depended upon for the decision as to whether the glenohumeral joint is involved and whether the joint capsule intact with the articular surface of the glenoid must be taken with the specimen (Fig. 6–33).

The humerus is divided at least 3.0 cm. below the lower extent of the tumor. The content of the medullary canal of the distal stump of the humerus is sent for frozen section studies to be sure that it is free of tumor.

After removal of the tumor from the field, the prosthetic replacement with autogenous fibular grafts is performed, as described in Figure 3–95. If the glenoid is intact and normal, no glenoid component is used. If it has been necessary to excise the glenohumeral joint, there may be enough bone in the neck of the scapula and coracoid to support a glenoid component. If not, the humeral component is used alone. In either case, the humeral component is stabilized against the stump of the scapula by securing the rotator cuff muscles to the bone grafts.

Alternative methods for reconstruction after en bloc resection of the proximal humerus have serious disadvantages. Allograft replacement of the upper humerus is complicated by avascular necrosis of the head and slow incorporation of the bulk of the graft. Autogenous grafts for arthrodesis also require a very long time for incorporation of the grafts, during which time the grafts break unless supported by metal rods or plates (Fig. 6–34).

Disarticulation at the Shoulder

Amputation through the glenohumeral may be required for a few lesions distal to the shoulder. The procedure is performed through incisions as shown, the axillary vessels are doubly ligated and divided early, and the remaining structures severed through the joint (Fig. 6–35).

Technique of Scapulectomy

Coley[234] credits Syme with the first successful complete excision of the scapula (1855!). This procedure is indicated when a low-grade malignancy is confined to the scapula. The entire scapula should be removed when the margin is in doubt (Figs. 6–36 and 6–37).

If imaging and tomograms show the lesion is confined to the body of the scapula, the glenoid (with the attached glenohumeral joint capsule) and the coracoid process (with the coracoclavicular ligament) may be preserved to suspend the arm. This simplifies the procedure and aftercare.

If the tumor invades the glenohumeral joint, the head of the humerus and glenohumeral joint capsule are taken with the scapula. It is then important to attach the long and short head of the biceps and the triceps to the clavicle to support the weight of the arm.

In any case, that part of the trapezius muscle that was attached to the scapula should be attached to the clavicle, where it can continue to act as the main suspensory muscle. Detached deltoid muscle is also re-attached to the clavicle.

With the patient positioned on the uninvolved side, the skin incision starts at the inferior angle of the scapula and goes along the medial border of the scapula and along the spine of the scapula until opposite the acromioclavicular joint, where it swings forward to the coracoid process. The skin flap is elevated to expose the trapezius muscle so that it can be detached from the spine of the scapula. The deltoid is detached from the spine of the scapula and from the acromion. The rhomboids and serratus anterior are detached next, taking care to ligate the descending branch of the transverse cervical artery if encountered. The scapula can now be retracted away from the ribs. The subscapularis, infraspinatus, teres minor, and supraspinatus are usually left with the specimen to cover the scapula for a safe margin. The tendons of the infraspinatus, teres minor, and supraspinatus are divided, taking care to preserve the full length of the long head of the biceps, which will be used later to tenodese the humeral head to the clavicle. The long head of the biceps is tagged with a stay suture and is divided at the glenoid. The coracoid process is exposed from in front, and the structures attached to it are divided after tagging them with stay sutures. The suprascapular nerve and artery are severed. The acromioclavicular joint capsule and subscapularis tendon are divided. After dis-

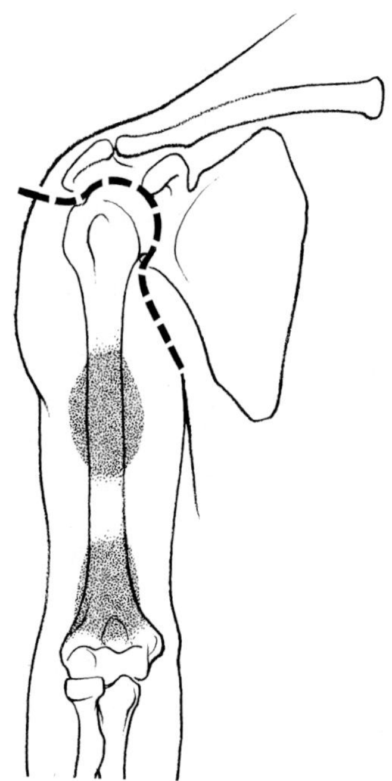

Figure 6–35. Disarticulation at the shoulder is occasionally indicated for trauma or tumors in the upper arm distal to the shoulder.

secting the inferior capsule free of the axillary nerve, it is detached from the scapula. The origin of the triceps is tagged with a stay suture and is detached close to bone. The specimen is removed from the table.

The long head of the biceps is passed through a hole in the humeral head and through a hole in the distal clavicle to anchor these structures together. This is reinforced by attaching the short head of biceps, coracobrachialis, and triceps to the clavicle. The trapezius muscle and deltoid muscle are attached to the clavicle and to each other. Suction drains are placed, and the skin flaps are trimmed and approximated with a few subcutaneous fascial sutures to eliminate dead space and subcuticular stitches. A pressure dressing and sling and swathe are applied.

Post-operatively, the sling is worn for 12 weeks, and heavy lifting is deferred for at least 6 months.

Scapulectomy with Resection of the Glenohumeral Joint. If it has been necessary to resect the glenohumeral joint (including the humeral head), the stump of the humerus is tenodesed to the clavicle using the long head of the biceps through holes in the bones and reinforcing with the other long muscles and deltoid on the clavicle, essentially as described previously.

Partial Scapulectomy. The procedure is simplified if only a partial scapulectomy is required and the glenoid, coracoid, coracoclavicular ligaments and glenohumeral joint capsule remain as attachments for the humerus to the clavicle. The long head of the biceps and the triceps and coracoid muscles also remain intact (Fig. 6–37).

Results of Scapulectomy. Although the proximal humerus has lost its fulcrum, so the arm cannot be raised and the humeral rotators are lost, the patient retains good strength for carrying objects at the side and, of course, has normal function of the elbow and hand. One of my patients continued to play golf with a low handicap after a complete right scapulectomy with resection of the glenohumeral joint and humeral head. His long head of biceps and surrrounding muscles had been used to secure the stump of the humerus to the clavicle (see Fig. 6–36).

Radical Resection; Tikhoff-Linberg Procedure

Low-grade fibrosarcomas of the soft tissue, chondrosarcomas of the coracoid process with soft-tissue extensions, and other lesions that have spread locally and are locally recurrent but have not involved the neurovascular bundle are treated with removal of all structures necessary to get

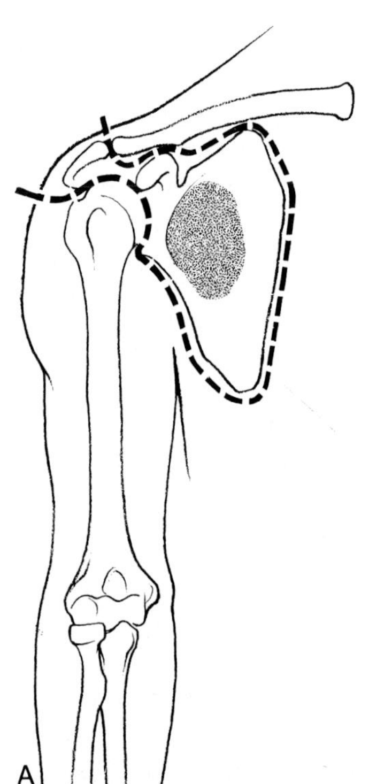

Figure 6–36. ***Complete Scapulectomy.***

A, This procedure is used for selected malignancies involving the body, neck, and coracoid process as determined by tomograms, CT scans, radioactive scans, and MRI as indicated.

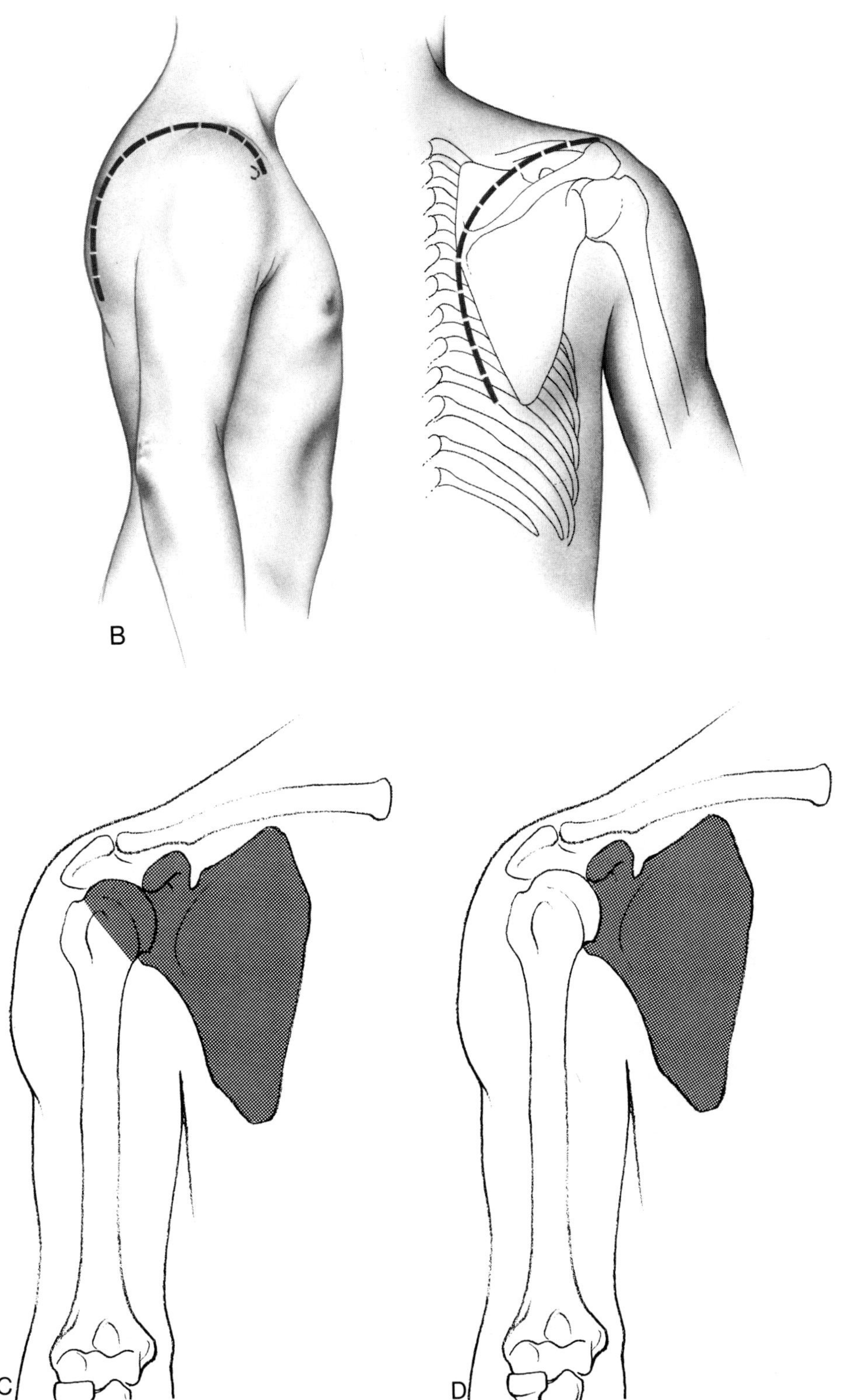

Figure 6–36 *Continued* B, *Left and right,* The skin incision.

C, If the glenohumeral joint is involved it is removed with the specimen.

D, Usually the glenohumeral joint is spared and the scapula is removed by dividing the glenohumeral joint capsule. In either case, the rotator cuff muscles, serratus anterior, and teres major muscles are left intact to cover the scapula to prevent spilling tumor cells in the field and are removed with the specimen to give a safer margin. The humerus is attached to the clavicle with the long tendon of the biceps. The posterior deltoid muscle is attached to the clavicle.

Illustration continued on following page

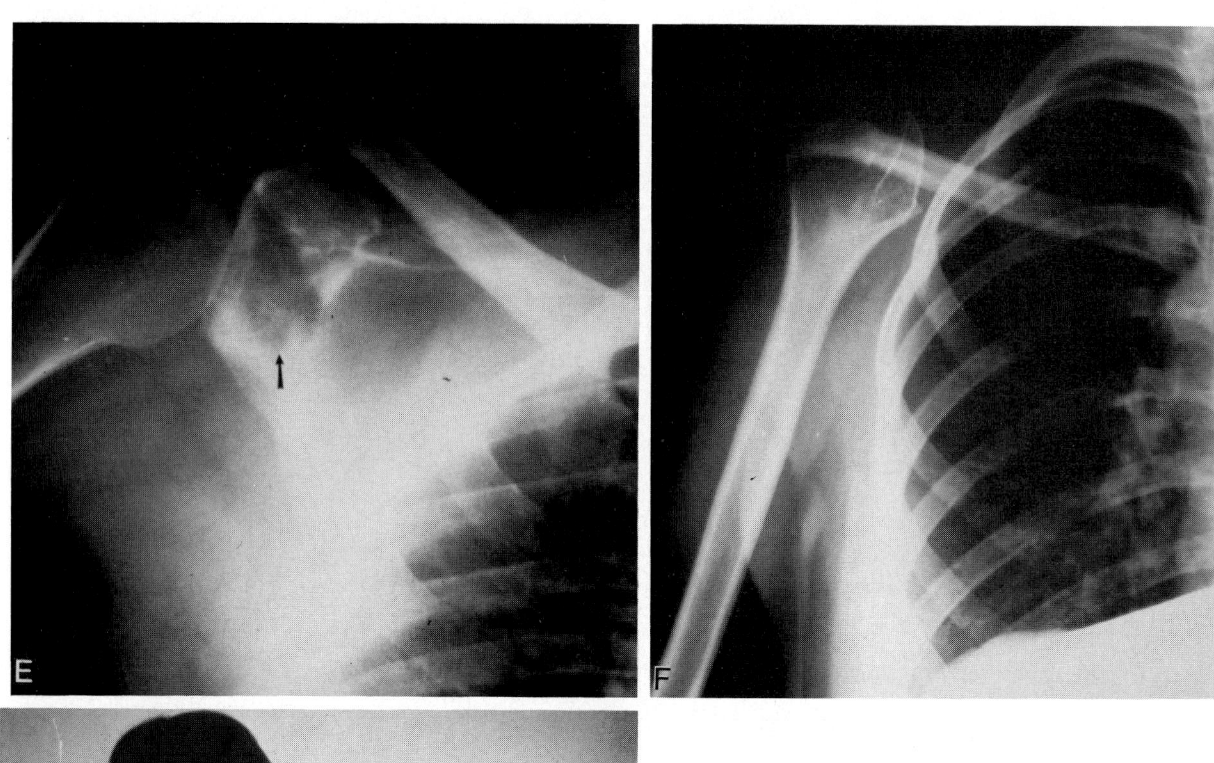

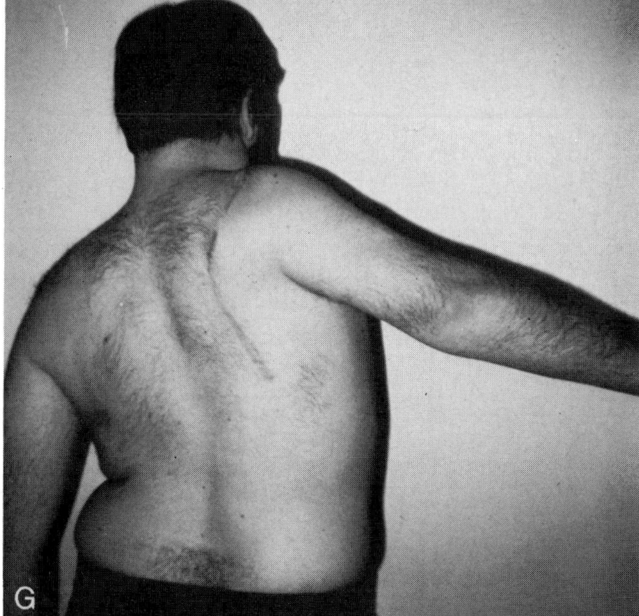

Figure 6–36 *Continued* E, Pre-operative tomogram of a chondrosarcoma in the neck of the scapula (arrow) to illustrate complete scapulectomy.

F, Post-operative view. The humerus was suspended from the clavicle with the long tendon of the biceps and the deltoid muscle.

G, Result six years later. Patient was unable to raise the arm but was playing golf; he had no pain and no recurrence of the tumor.

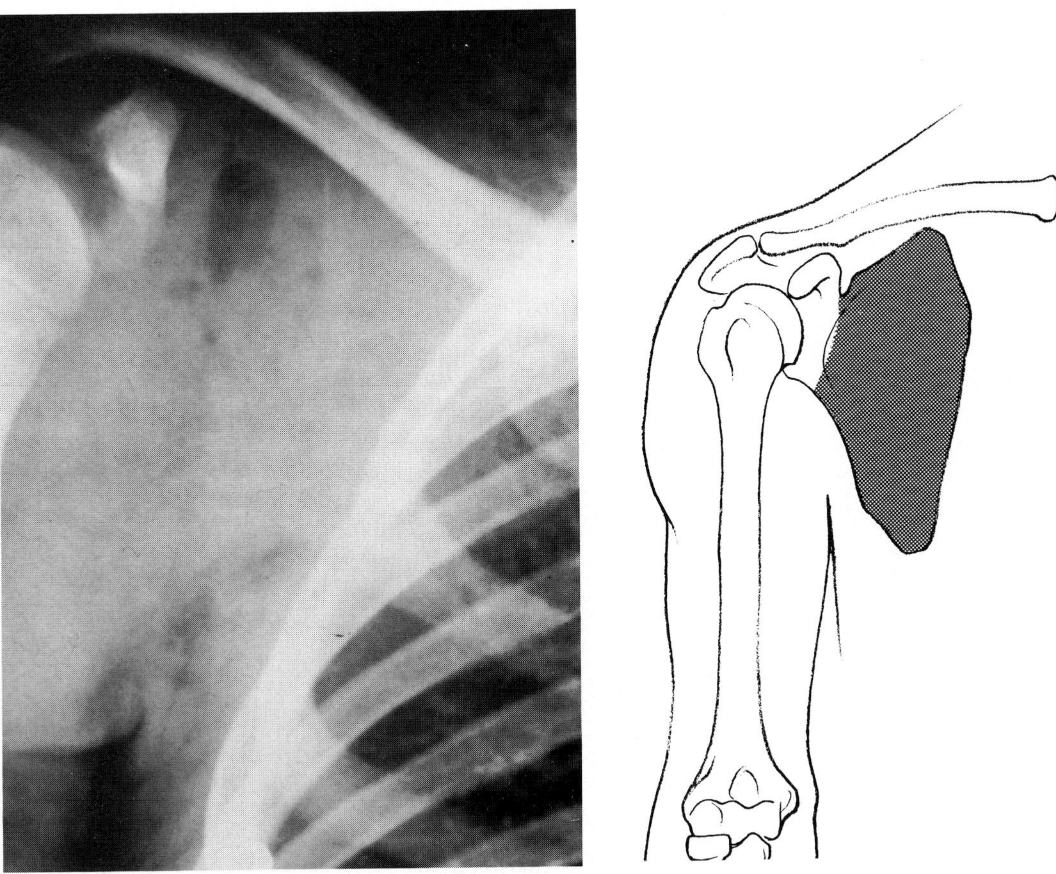

Figure 6–37. Partial scapulectomy. If the glenoid and coracoid process can be retained safely, it simplifies scapulectomy because the glenohumeral joint capsule and coracoclavicular ligaments are preserved to stabilize the humerus.

around the tumor. This may entail removal of not only the scapula and humeral head as described previously, but also the clavicle and upper shaft of the humerus.[232] Only the neurovascular bundle and skin remain, but the procedure leaves a useful hand and elbow (Fig. 6–38).

High-Grade Malignancies of the Shoulder

Almost any type of undifferentiated tumor can occur in the shoulder. Osteogenic sarcoma is the most frequent example of the type of bone tumor under discussion. Undifferentiated chondrosarcoma is another. A malignant fibrous histiocytoma (from fibroblastic tissue—e.g., high-grade fibrosarcoma) is an example of a high-grade soft tissue malignancy.

The role of chemotherapy and radiotherapy and the timing and extent of surgical procedures for the lesions are beyond the scope of this book. This is an active and changing field. However, occasionally, when the neurovascular bundle is involved or the shoulder girdle is extensively infiltrated with tumor, an interscapular amputation is indicated. I will review some points about this procedure.

Interscapulothoracic Amputation (Forequarter Amputation)

The technique I have used and found to be satisfactory is that of Berger (1887).[242] It considers the operation to be divided into two parts: the "anterior part," for early ligation of the subclavian vessels to minimize bleeding followed by division of all the anterior structures connecting the scapula or humerus to the thorax or neck; followed by the "posterior part," for divison of the structures connecting the scapula to the trunk or neck.

The patient is positioned on the uninvolved side with access to both the front and back of the shoulder. The incision may have to be varied from that shown in Figure 6–39, if there are local soft-tissue recurrences in the way or for some other reason. About 7.0 cm. of the clavicle is resected with a rib cutter, and after division of the pectoralis major and minor, the subclavian artery and veins are triple ligated and divided with two ligatures

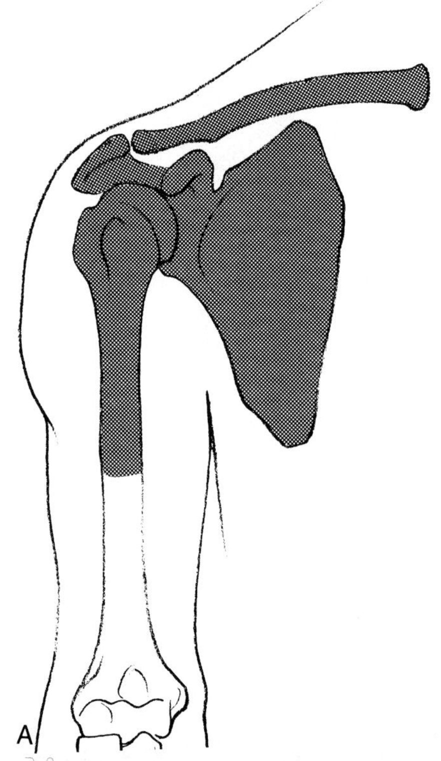

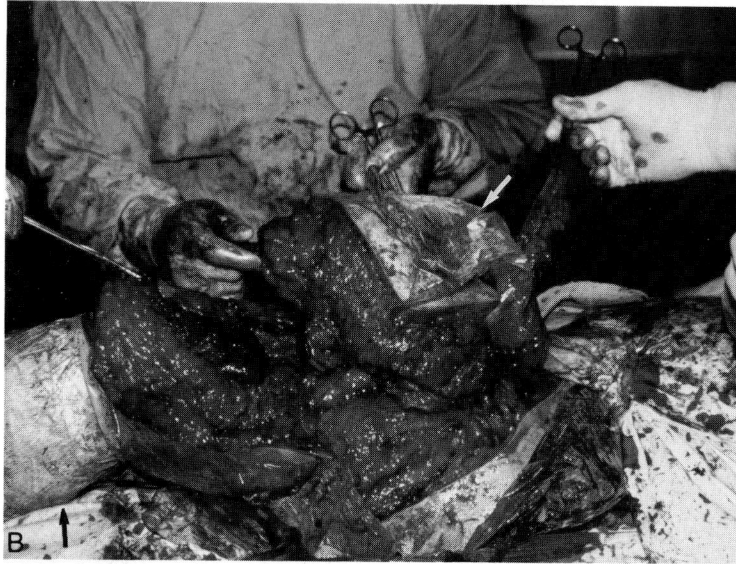

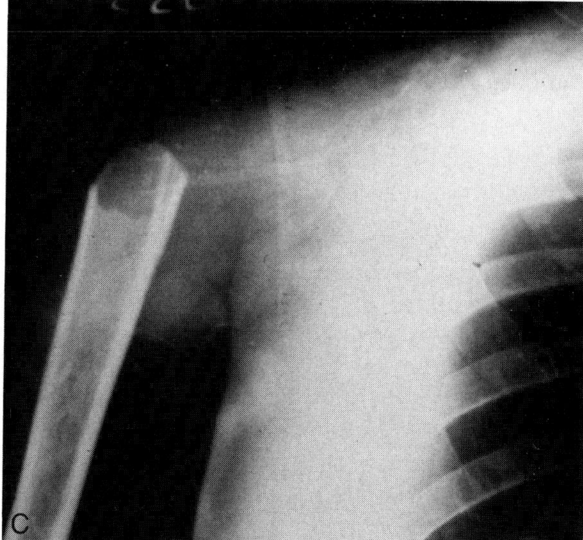

Figure 6–38. Tikhoff-Linberg procedure after multiple failed operations for fibrosarcoma.

A, The inner clavicle may be spared or removed, depending on the nature and extent of involvement.

B, In the operating room just prior to removal of the specimen, which includes all previous operative and biopsy scars (white arrow). The arm (black arrow) and neurovascular bundle remain.

C, Post-operative roentgen appearance. The patient was pleased at late follow-up because he had a useful hand, and could flex and extend the elbow and carry 25 pounds of weight with his arm at the side.

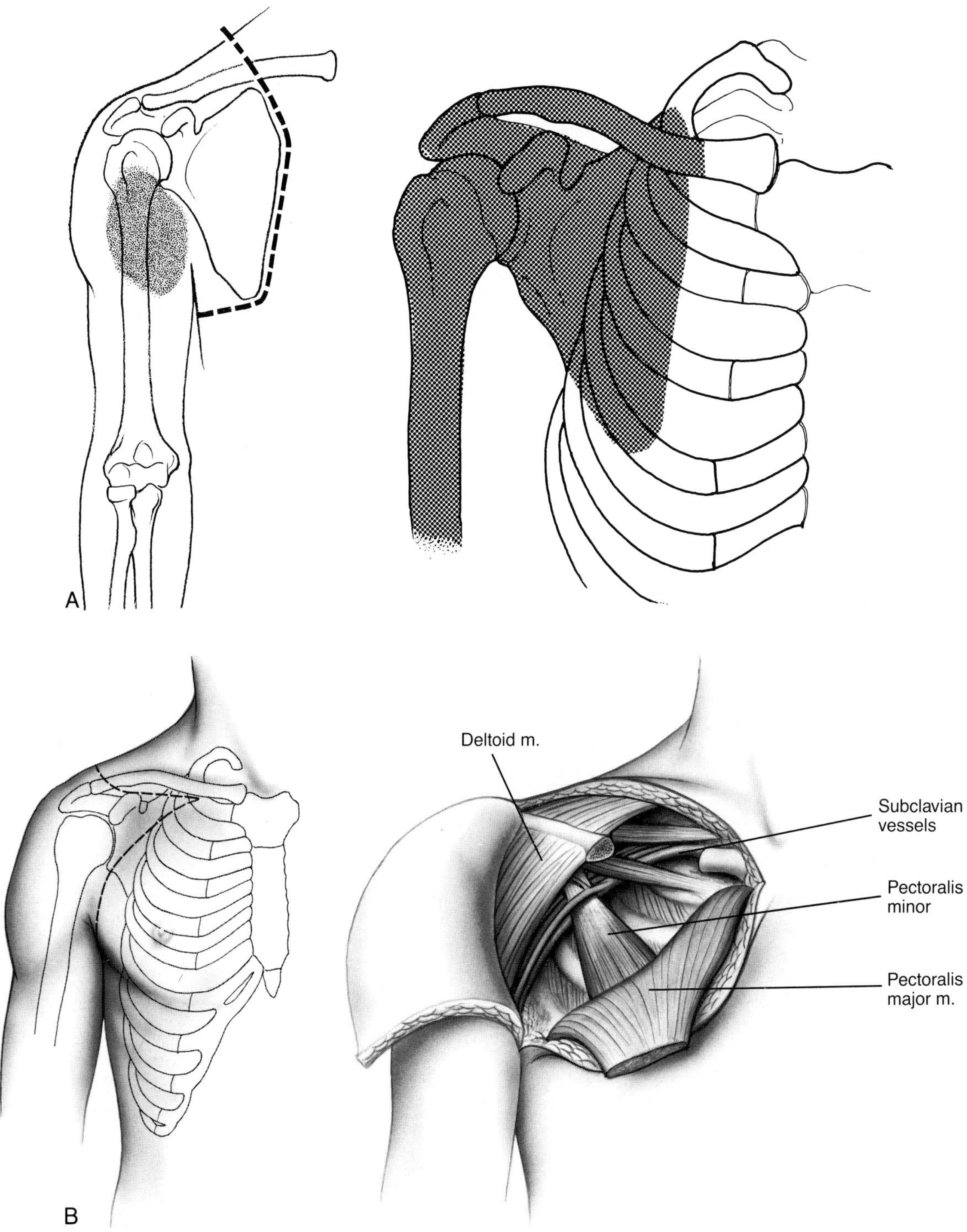

Figure 6–39. ***Interscapulothoracic Amputation.***

A, *Left and right,* When the neurovascular bundle is involved and the shoulder girdle infiltrated with a high-grade malignancy, this procedure must be considered.

B, Anterior part is started first with ligation of the subclavian vessels early.

The skin incision is shown on the left and division of the clavicle to expose the neurovascular bundle on the right.

Illustration continued on following page

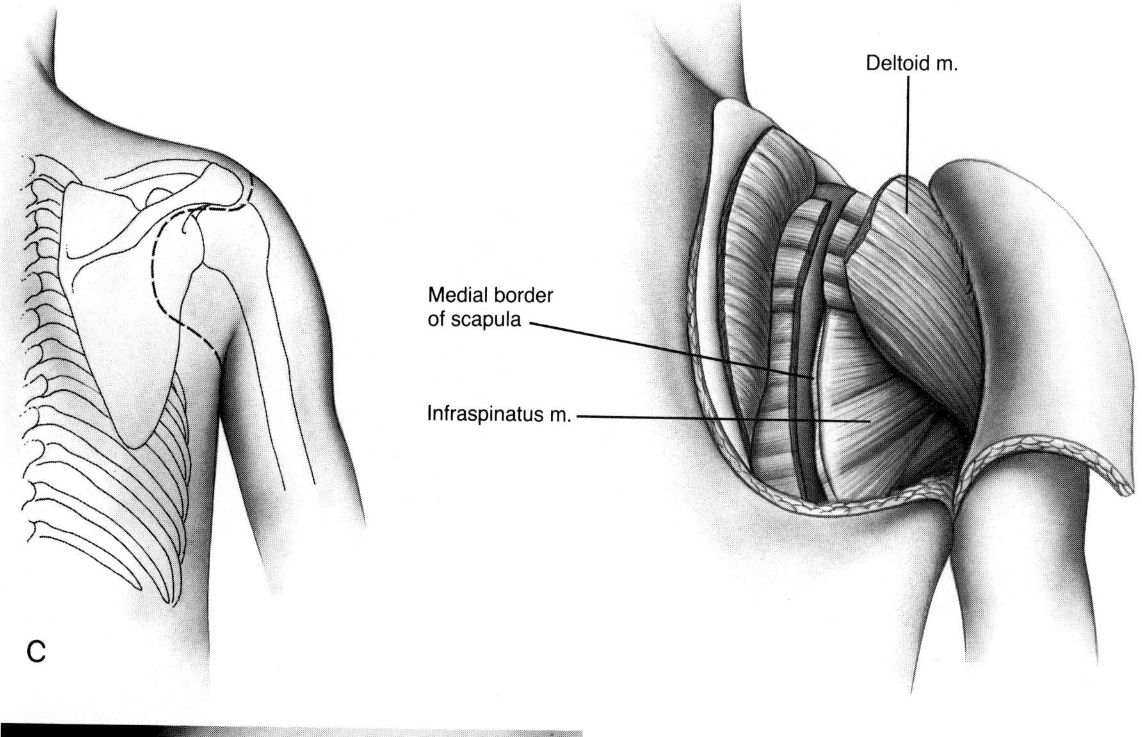

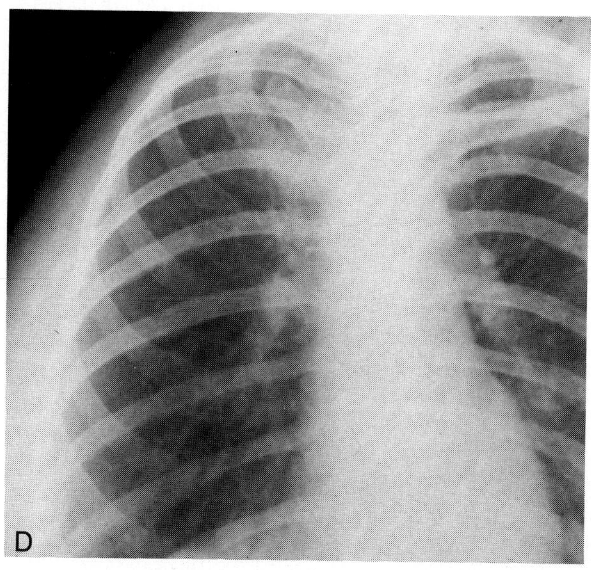

Figure 6–39 *Continued* C, Posterior part of the procedure is with the incision shown on the left, and removal of the scapula and its attached muscles is as depicted on the right, as described in the text.

D, Post-operative roentgen appearance of a 23 year old man who had this procedure for a high-grade, undifferentiated fibrous histiocytoma. He died two years later of lung involvement.

remaining on the side of the thorax and one ligature remaining on the side of the arm. All other anterior structures connecting the arm to the trunk or neck are divided—e.g., trapezius, omohyoid, and levator scapulae. The posterior part of the operation detaches the lower part of the trapezius, rhomboids, and serratus anterior (Fig. 6–39). At times, the stumps of the pectoralis major and trapezius may be sutured together to close dead space to minimize hematoma. The skin flaps are trimmed and approximated with suction drains; a few subcutaneous, interrupted sutures are used to close dead space; and subcuticular sutures are placed. Dry pressure dressing is applied.

RARE SHOULDER LESIONS

Glenohumeral Osteochondromatosis ("Primary" vs. "Secondary")

"Primary" glenohumeral osteochondromatosis, without associated instability or arthritis, is extremely rare. I have performed synovectomies on only two such lesions. Total synovectomy in the glenohumeral joint is not difficult, but it involves temporarily detaching the subscapularis tendon and humeral attachments of the anterior glenohu-

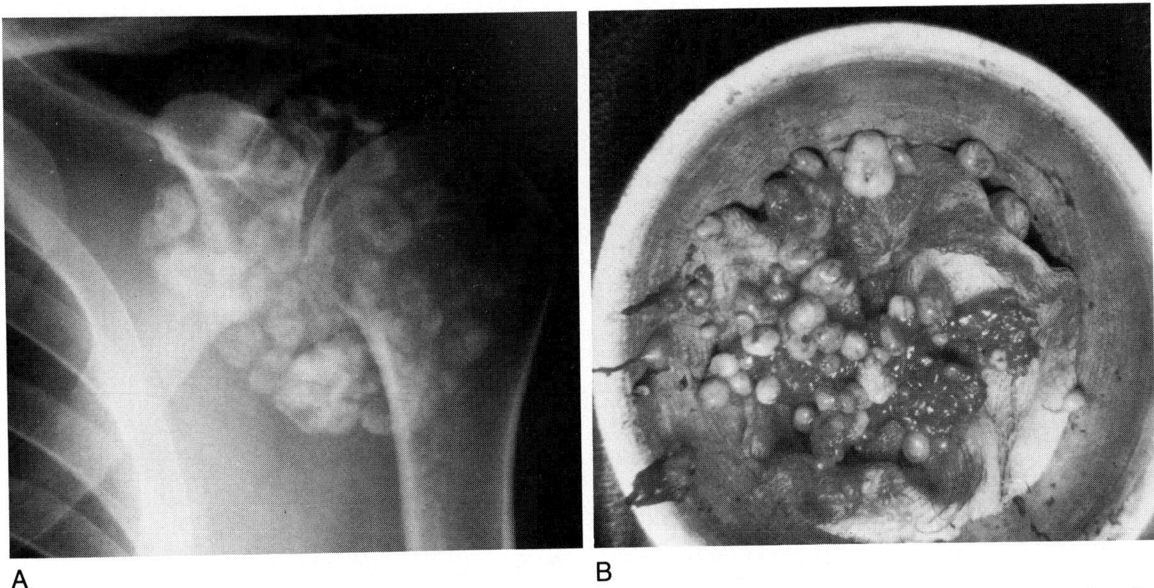

Figure 6–40. Glenohumeral osteochondromatosis. A, Pre-operative appearance of the rare primary osteochondromatosis with subsynovial osteochondral bodies and minimal damage to the articular surfaces. B, Specimen removed at synovectomy.

meral ligaments sufficiently to subluxate the humeral head (Fig. 6–40).

"Secondary" subsynovial and intra-articular osteochondral bodies are commonly present in a very unstable shoulder with frequent dislocations. Repair of the instability and removal of the loose bodies and presenting abnormal synovium are indicated. For example, Charcot-like charges of osteochondral subsynovial bodies are frequent in an unstable shoulder with a large cuff tear or cuff-tear arthropathy. "Secondary" subsynovial osteochondral bodies are also commonly present in glenohumeral osteoarthritis. In this case, it can be difficult at times to know whether the loose synovial bodies lead to the degenerative changes or whether they resulted from the spurs and incongruity of degenerative arthritis. In any case, prosthetic replacement is performed with removal of loose bodies and removal of synovium containing osteochondral bodies.

Posterior Glenoid Spur (Bennett[243])

This exostosis of the posterior glenoid rim has been attributed to pull of the triceps tendon on the glenoid rim in baseball pitchers. I believe the exostosis occurs too far superiorly to have this as its cause (Fig. 6–41). I have seen several patients with undiagnosed pain who had this lesion. One was an archer whose shoulder was explored only to find an early degenerative osteophyte at the rim, as is seen in degenerative arthritis. He had a loose shoulder, apparently acquired from archery.[243a] A posterior capsular repair was performed. Years later, his arthritis had progressed, requiring a total shoulder arthroplasty (see p. 314).

Exploration of this ridge of bone in two other patients seemed unrewarding. Only a smooth mound of bone was found. Pre-operatively, one patient had acromioclavicular joint symptoms, and the other had impingement symptoms. At the time of exploring the posterior glenoid lesion, an acromioclavicular joint excision (see Fig. 6–8A and B) was performed on one individual and an anterior acromioplasty (see Fig. 2–41) was done on the other. Both patients were permanently relieved of pain. Apparently, the pain was relieved because of these other procedures and not because of exploring the posterior rim prominence. Now when I see this lesion in roentgenograms, I look for another cause of shoulder pain and do not explore the posterior glenoid rim.

Bands in the Deltoid Muscle (Congenital)

Bands of dense fibrous tissue in the deltoid muscle occasionally occur congenitally[244] or result from injections.[252]

These bands cause an abduction contracture and abnormal forces on the humeral head, which in children with immature bones can in time de-

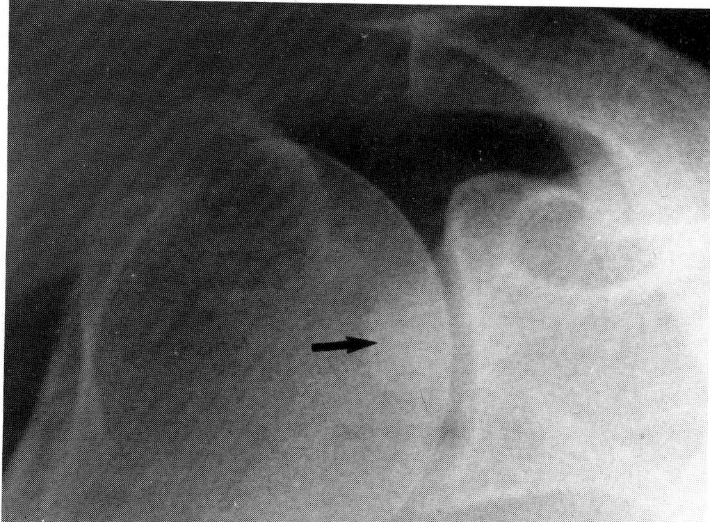

Figure 6–41. Anterior-posterior view of a "posterior glenoid spur."

form the shape of the humeral head. The bands cause winging of the scapula when the arm is at the side (Fig. 6–42).

The presence of fibrous bands in the deltoid muscle is determined by palpation of the deltoid muscle itself. No complicated test gives a lead, and I have seen patients who have gone for years with some incorrect neurological diagnosis.

The treatment is to excise the bands through a transverse incision made just lateral to the acromion prior to the development of a humeral head deformity. All bands should be divided and a section of each band removed to avoid recurrence. The operation is performed by splitting the deltoid longitudinally directly over the bands, rather than by detaching the origin of the deltoid muscle. It is important to have the axillary nerve in mind and to section the fibers near the acromion cephalically to the level of this nerve. The incision usually becomes keloid in children, as it true of almost all shoulder incisions in youngsters.

Osteitis Condensens Clavicle

This rare clinical entity was first described by Brower and colleagues in 1974.[245, 246] It usually

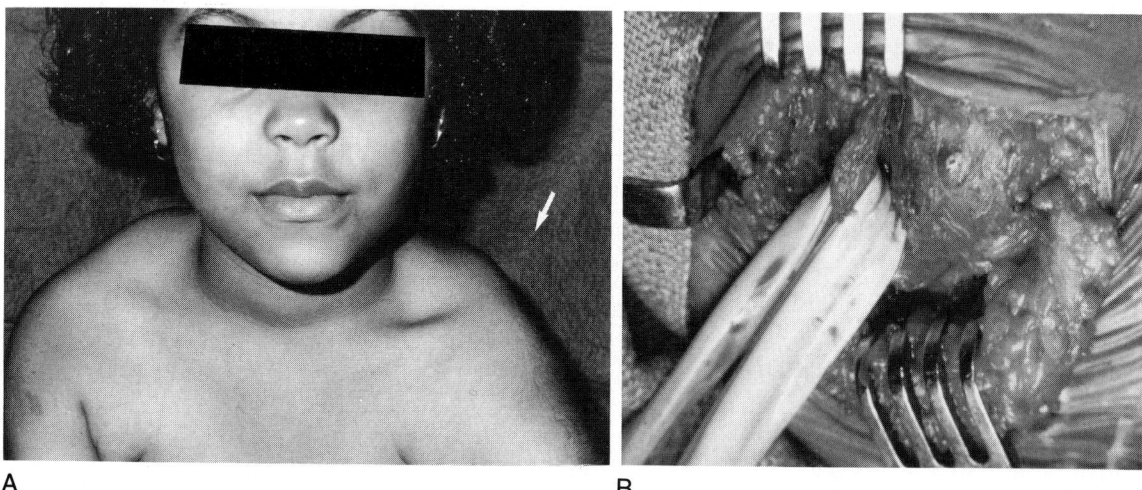

Figure 6–42. Congenital bands in the deltoid muscle may cause an abduction contracture with winging of the scapula requiring excision of the bands.

A, A three year old child with the typical deformity (arrow) who had been misdiagnosed as having a neurological defect because of winging of the scapula.

B, At surgery, the band was excised with the least detachment of deltoid muscle possible. A rubber drain is being used to pull the band away from the deltoid muscle during the dissection.

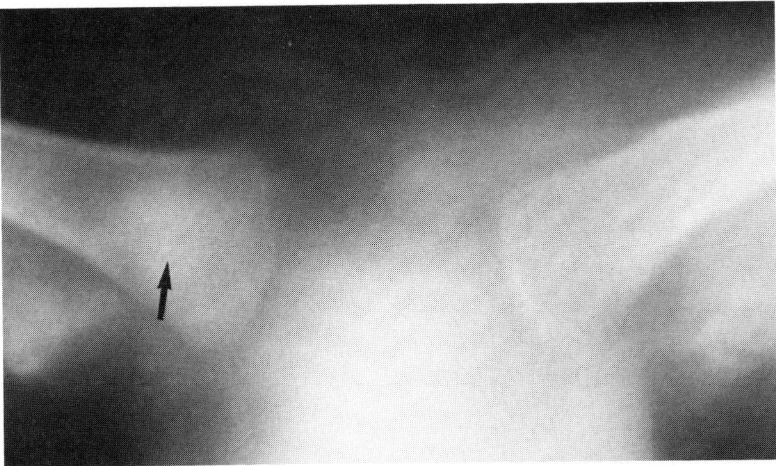

Figure 6–43. Osteitis condensans clavicle seen in a tomogram (arrow) in a 29 year old woman who had pain for 2 years. The pain stopped following the biopsy and has not returned.

occurs in women between 25 and 50 years of age. Chronic pain and swelling of varying degrees of intensity appear at the medial third of the clavicle with density of the clavicle seen in good quality x-rays (comparing the two clavicles and sternoclavicular joints), but is better seen with tomograms of both inner clavicles (Fig. 6–43). There is increased uptake in a technetium radioactive bone scan. Cultures of the bone are negative, and a biopsy shows only normal bone in excessive amounts. The differential diagnosis includes osteomyelitis and neoplasms (lymphomas, histiocytosis X, Ewing's tumor, metastatic disease, etc.). The benign nature is confirmed by the finding of only normal bone in the biopsy sample.

The patients I have seen have been relieved of their pain after the biopsy and reassurance as to the benign nature of the condition. Some are said to have no pain, and the temporary use of nonsteroidal anti-inflammatory medication is said to control the discomfort in others until the pain spontaneously disappears. I believe that continuing clinical and roentgen follow-up at yearly intervals is important to make sure nothing further develops, since the etiology of this condition is unknown.

Cleidocranial Dysostosis

The clavicle is unusual. It is the first bone to ossify in the embryo (at five weeks). Its central portion is developed by intermembranous bone formation, and its ends are developed by cartilaginous bone formation. Occasionally, the middle clavicle and frontal area of the skull fail to ossify (Fig. 6–44). These patients have no symptoms, and no treatment is required.

I believe that some of the unilateral failures of union of the midclavicle seen in children that have been classified as unilateral congenital dysostosis may be nonunions of mid-third clavicular fractures from unrecognized injuries sustained in early life.[253] I have treated two of these unilateral pseudarthroses, which were symptomatic after age six years, with bone grafting and intramedullary fixation similar to treatment of nonunion of the clavicle

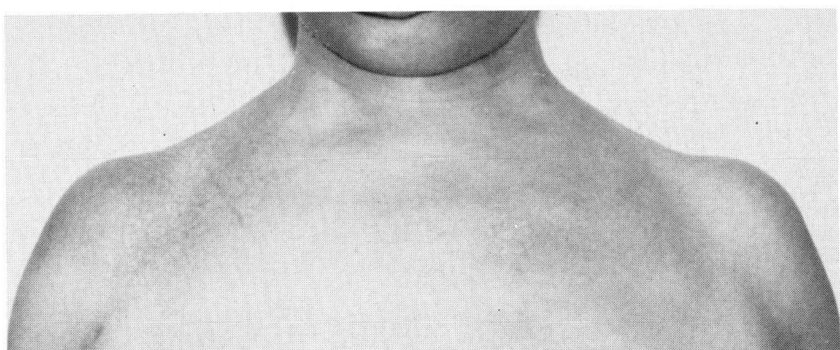

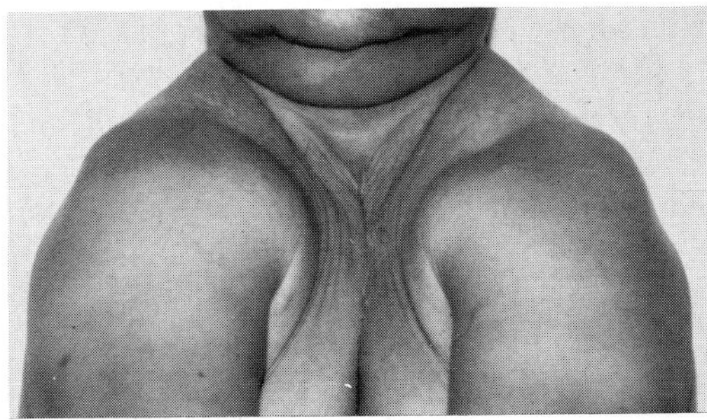

Figure 6–44. Cleidocranial dysostosis in a 60 year old man who has an indentation in the front of his skull. The shoulder lesions are not very obvious when he stands erect (A), but he can approximate the shoulders in an amazing way (B). He has no shoulder pain.

in adults. Traumatic nonunion of the clavicle can be disabling and symptomatic; however, I have never seen cleidocranial dysostosis with pain in an adult.

SCAPULAR PAIN

In the recent past, a number of vague syndromes were described to account for scapular pain. In my experience, it has usually been possible to find some real anatomical basis for the pain rather than falling back on some unexplained "syndrome" to account for the pain. There are a number of real anatomical conditions that usually cause scapular pain. A good physical examination and laboratory and roentgen work-up are of critical importance to the determination of the true basis for the pain. In the initial examination, not only should the scapula be examined for masses and tender points, but also its movements must be observed and it must be tested for winging (see Fig. 6–19). Anterior-posterior and lateral x-rays of the whole scapula, with the arm raised out of the way for the lateral view, are routine (see Fig. 1–12B). These are supplemented by imaging studies of the scapula and cervical spine, electromyograms, and other neurological tests as indicated.

We will consider some of the scapulothoracic syndromes of the recent past to emphasize that they are not the usual causes of scapular pain. We will then discuss briefly the common causes of scapular pain.

Scapulothoracic Syndromes of the Past

Although these syndromes are not the usual cause of scapular pain, terms frequently used in the past[247–249] are listed for historic interest and completion.

"Fibrositis"[247] or "Myositis." "Toxic" or "metabolic" products are blamed for tenderness or soreness in the trapezius muscle or scapular muscles.

"Tension." Psychogenic stress causing tension pain of the scapular and neck muscles.

"Atmospheric." Dampness, drafts, and changes in barometric pressure.

"Postural." Bad posture, asthenic habitus, poor muscle conditioning, etc., causing scapular pain.[249]

"Intercostal Neuralgia." Nerve root irritation causing scapular pain.

"Scapulocostal Tendinitis." Poorly understood inflammation at the point of attachment of the muscles along the medial border of the scapula causing scapular pain.

"Grating Scapula" or "Snapping Scapula." Crepitus and noises when the scapula is moved on the chest.[248] When I was a resident, this was often treated by excision of the medial border or superior angle of the scapula as in the patient in Figure 6–46C. I have not performed this procedure for many years. Partial scapulectomy has been performed occasionally for a deformed scapula after a fracture. Grating scapula, as is usually seen in teenage girls, is treated with reassurance and observation (Fig. 6–45).

"Suprascapular Nerve Syndrome." The entrapment of this nerve in the notch is discussed on page 448. It is at best very rare. Other than with fractures involving the base of the coracoid and suprascapular notch, I have never seen a clear example.

Common Causes of Scapular Pain

The important causes of scapular pain in approximately the order of frequency are the following (see Fig. 6–39).

Internal Derangements of the Glenohumeral Joint

The most frequent cause of scapular pain is a lesion that causes pain or restriction of motion at the glenohumeral joint. Examples include "frozen shoulders," calcium deposits in the rotator cuff tendons, cuff tears, and glenohumeral arthritis (Fig. 6–46A and B). Impaired glenohumeral motion throws extra load on the scapular muscles because scapular movements are increased. This can result in fatigue aching. Rotator cuff tears and osteoarthritis of the glenohumeral joint can also be associated with this same type of scapular pain.

The treatment of this type of scapular discomfort is the correction or elimination of the underlying glenohumeral problem and then exercises to recover coordinated scapulohumeral rhythm and strength.

Cervical Radiculitis

Inflammation of the cervical nerve roots as a result of degenerative changes or other lesions of the cervical spine is a common cause of scapular pain. This has been the source of many diagnostic errors, as illustrated in Figure 6–46C.

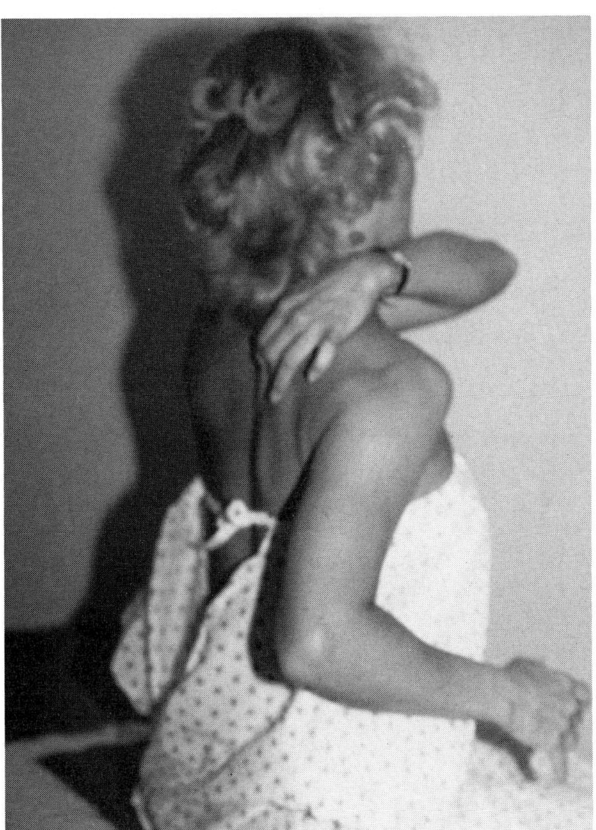

Figure 6–45. "Grating scapula" in young patients who have had no trauma and have normal laboratory findings is treated with reassurance and light exercises rather than by surgery, as discussed in the text.

The pain in the scapular region is usually intensified by hyperextension of the neck as the head is tilted toward the involved side. There may be biceps, deltoid, or other muscle weakness, and electromyographic changes (see Fig. 2–37). Alterations can usually be demonstrated in the plain films and computerized tomograms of the cervical spine.

This type of scapular pain regresses with the correction of the problem of the cervical spine, which, in the case of degenerative lesions of the cervical spine, is treated conservatively with a large pillow, "rest," and avoidance of activities that entail hyperextension or stress on the cervical spine.

Scapulothoracic Bursitis (Darrach, Jobe)

Darrach[250] has shown how a scapulothoracic bursa, between the scapula and the chest wall, can become acutely inflamed and painful. The proof that this bursa is responsible is the relief of the pain when 5.0 to 10.0 cc. of 1 percent lidocaine (Xylocaine) is injected into the bursa. Excision of the bursa for this type of bursitis is rarely indicated because it is usually self-terminating.

Jobe[251] has described how a hypertrophied scapulothoracic bursa can cause disability in baseball pitchers requiring surgical excision (Fig. 6–46E and F). In this condition, there is a palpable lump under the lower angle of the scapula and the pain is localized to that area. The pain is intensified by throwing and is temporarily relieved by Xylocaine injected locally.

Tumors of the Scapula Region

Scapular pain may be due to a neoplasm, as has been discussed in this part of the book. The most frequent benign lesion is an osteochondroma of the scapula (see Fig. 6–28 and p. 466). The most frequent primary malignancies are chondrosarcoma of the scapula or fibrosarcoma of the soft tissue overlying the scapula.

These lesions can be easily overlooked unless a careful examination of this region is made during the initial physical examination and repeated as indicated until the correct diagnosis has been established. Good x-ray films of the *entire scapula* in the anterior-posterior and lateral view, computerized tomograms, and MRI scans are indicated when the diagnosis is in doubt.

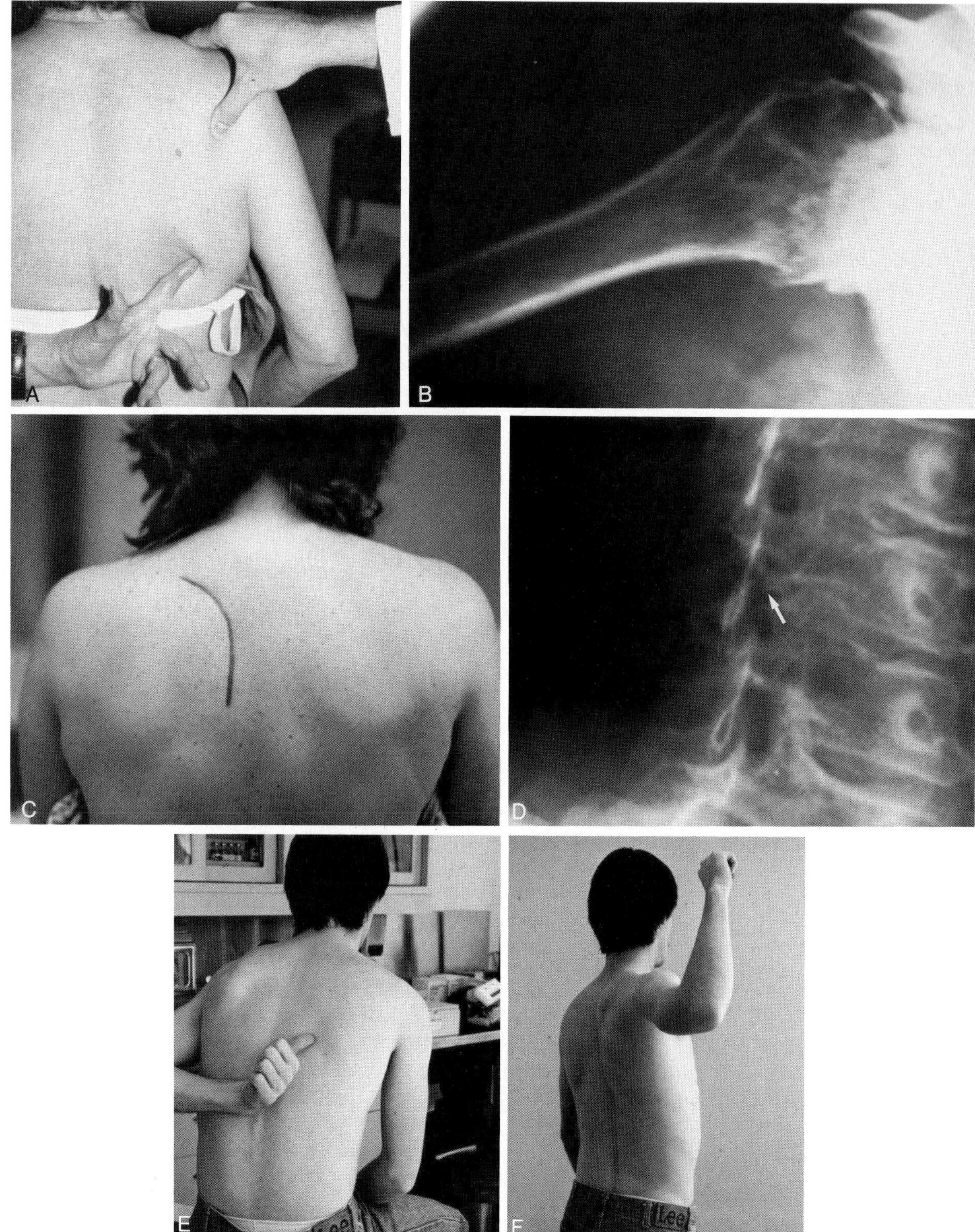

Figure 6–46. ***Common Causes of Scapular Pain.***

A and B, Derangement of the glenohumeral joint is the most frequent cause of scapular pain, as in this patient with glenohumeral arthritis.

C and D, Cervical radiculitis frequently causes scapular pain, as in this man who had the medial border of his scapula erroneously excised (scar is outlined), when the trouble was due to a spur in the neural foramen of the cervical spine (arrow).

E and F, Scapulothoracic bursitis, tumors, malunion of fractures, and neurological conditions are other causes of scapular pain, as discussed in the text.

Malunion of the Scapula or Ribs

Old fractures of the scapula or ribs can cause chronic pain requiring partial scapulectomy. The diagnosis is made by the deformity as is seen in roentgen and imaging studies; and by the injection test, in which pain is temporarily relieved by a local Xylocaine injection.

Most scapular and rib fractures heal well without symptoms. It is unusual to see them cause chronic pain. More often, scapular fractures are usually well tolerated because of the padding provided by the muscles surrounding the scapula (see Fig. 5–44).

Winging of the Scapula

Neurological or muscle disorders that cause weakness of the scapular muscles are often associated with fatigue pain in the scapular region. Long thoracic nerve paralysis with weakness of the serratus anterior is a good example (see p. 449).

Winging should be especially looked for in any patient complaining of pain in the scapular region. During the examination, with both scapulae exposed, observe the patient actively raise the arms overhead and push against a wall supported by the outstretched arms (see Fig. 6–19A and B).

Sprengel's Deformity

In this congenital deformity, the scapula fails to descend completely and is small and misshapened, and other congenital anomalies are usually associated, including malformed ribs, anomalies of the cervical and thoracic vertebrae (often with scoliosis), and, in the more severe cases, a cartilaginous bone, the omovertebral bone, connecting the scapula to one or two lower cervical vertebrae. The degree of deformity varies from so mild that shoulder motion is good and no treatment is indicated to moderate or severe with restricted elevation, in which case surgery may be considered.

I believe surgery can be helpful in those with a fixed scapula without rotation and loss of shoulder elevation above 110 degrees provided that associated deformities are not so severe as to prevent a functional scapula. The family must have a realistic discussion on the limitations of surgery and the fact that it has little effect on the appearance of the associated deformities.

I prefer a modification of the Woodward[287] procedure with more emphasis on re-establishing rotation of the scapula by freeing the muscles on the medial border and superior angle of the scapula and working early stretching exercises (see Fig. 7–7, 7–8, and 7–9) (depending on the age of the child). The operation is performed through a straight midline incision from C3 to T9 without curving the incision even if scoliosis is present. The trapezius and rhomboid muscles are released from the spines of the vertebrae and from the chest wall, all fibrous bands are divided, and if an omovertebral bone is present, it is excised. The superior angle of the scapula usually projects forward and is excised. When indicated (not routinely), the trapezius muscle is divided transversely at the level of C4, taking care to avoid injury to the spinal accessory nerve or nerve to the rhomboids. A few deep sutures are used at the upper and lower ends of the release to maintain the proper level of the scapula, but the medial border of the scapula is left untethered so that the scapula can rotate. A sling and swathe with the arm in the Velpeau position is used for 5 days, at which time passive stretching exercises for elevation are begun and progressed as rapidly as possible.

Usually the glenohumeral joint is essentially normal in this condition; and if active scapular rotation is re-established, glenohumeral elevation can be enhanced, since the acromion is then rotated out of the way of the humerus when it is raised.

7

SHOULDER REHABILITATION

Because of the unique anatomical arrangement and function of the rotator cuff, rehabilitation of the shoulder after surgery is more difficult than that of any other joint. The shoulder has more motion than other joints. There is little bony stability. The muscles that stabilize the humeral head also move it. In most patients all of the muscles involved in the complex muscle couplings used in synchronous movements of the scapula and humerus have been atrophied by months of disuse.

Nevertheless, because a good rehabilitation program is critical and is of special importance in restoring optimum function in this complex joint, the shoulder surgeon must not only understand this type of rehabilitation but also remain actively involved with the patient and therapist to make it work. It is not enough to perform a technically perfect, clean shoulder reconstruction. The shoulder surgeon must have an equal fervor for preventing adhesions and strengthening muscles while preserving the integrity of his or her repair.

The real pleasure for the shoulder surgeon occurs some time following the operation when patients have recovered enough function and comfort to know, often with tremendous relief at being free of their dreadful pain, that there is a new life ahead for them. The other members of the shoulder team—the therapist, assistants, and office personnel—share in the pleasure of this reward.

Methodical planning and cooperation between the patient, surgeon, and therapist are often required to achieve this goal. Patients cannot perform exercises with confidence if they do not know the current objectives and exactly what they are supposed to do. A therapist cannot work with confidence unless the specific anatomical problem is clearly in mind, and current objectives and limitations are understood. Only the surgeon knows the stability and strength of the repair, the capabilities of the muscles, and whether the goal is stability (as after a repair for recurrent dislocations) or mobility (as after most repairs for cuff tears and fractures and most arthroplasties). Only he or she can direct the post-operative program and explain new and changing objectives of the exercise program as they develop. A confident therapist is of great assistance to the patient. An informed, confident patient is a happy patient who is proud of his or her accomplishments and progress rather than worried and disappointed at the slow speed or incompleteness of recovery.

In this discussion, I will include only information that has seemed helpful for my patients, with no attempt to describe or disagree with other systems of shoulder rehabilitation used by others. I will outline some of the general rules I follow, describe the specific shoulder exercises I use and their purpose, and finally, discuss special precautions that apply to the various diagnostic categories.

RULES OF SHOULDER REHABILITATION AFTER SURGERY

The following generalizations are helpful to me in the pre-operative assessment, in discussions with the patient and therapist, and in planning the post-operative exercise program. Some points in the pre-operative assessment are illustrated in Figure 7–1.

Rule 1. "The Results of Surgery Are Made Before Surgery"*

Beyond an accurate diagnosis and complete understanding of the anatomical problem, the surgeon must understand the motivation and character of the patient. Not all patients are suited for surgery, and the time to find out is before surgery rather than after.

*Professor Mario Randelli, Milan, Italy.

Rule 2. A Joint Effort Is Made (Patient, Therapist, and Surgeon) with All Participants Informed

Details of the expected exercise program are outlined to the patient before surgery. This is done by means of diagrams (see Figs. 7–8 to 7–12) prior to the patient's admission to the hospital. Following surgery, it is the surgeon's responsibility to initiate the exercise program and later to continue to explain the aims and objectives to the patient and to the therapist as the program advances. The therapist instructs and assists the patient, makes a progress report, and discusses an updated treatment plan with the surgeon at appropriate intervals. The patient must know the details of the self-assistive exercise program and what it is accomplishing. Doubts or confusion must be promptly eliminated.

Rule 3. Specify Warm or Cold Applications or Neither

In my experience, cold applications are helpful when there is acute inflammation (as in an acute calcium deposit, see p. 427) or after overuse of the shoulder in athletics. Cold applications are also helpful after recent injuries in which there is a threat of internal bleeding and hematoma formation. I know that many advocate cold applications prior to exercises for a frozen shoulder; however, I prefer warm applications for the preparation of the shoulder for exercises aimed at regaining motion. I believe that low, dry heat applied for five minutes before passive, assistive, and later gentle stretching exercises makes the tissue more supple and relaxes the muscles in preparation for these exercises. However, I do not start heat applications until at least five days after surgery because of fear of dilating the blood vessels and the greater likelihood of internal bleeding with hematoma formation. During the first five days following surgery and indefinitely after procedures that do not call for range of motion exercises, neither heat nor cold is used.

Rule 4. Exercises to Regain Motion Generally Are Given Priority Over Exercises to Build Strength

Exercises to regain motion are indicated following most surgery to repair rotator cuff defects and glenohumeral arthroplasties. These exercises should be started before strengthening exercises for

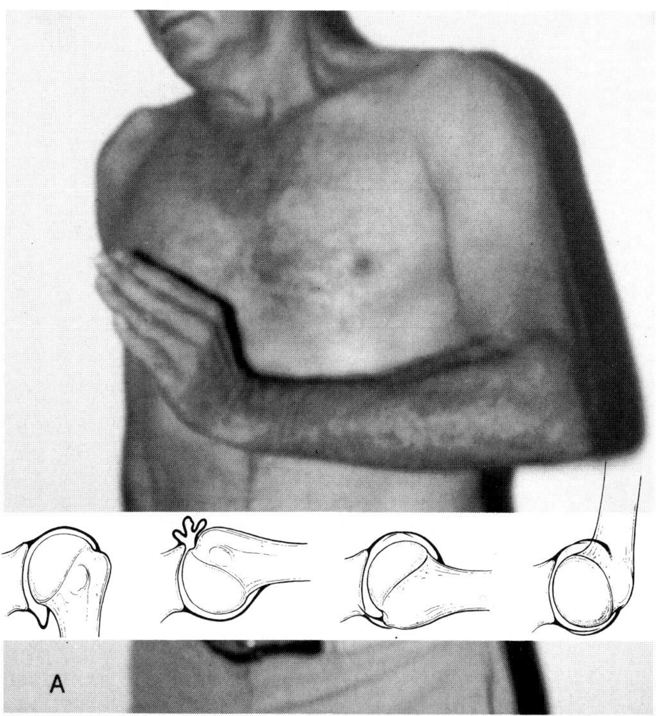
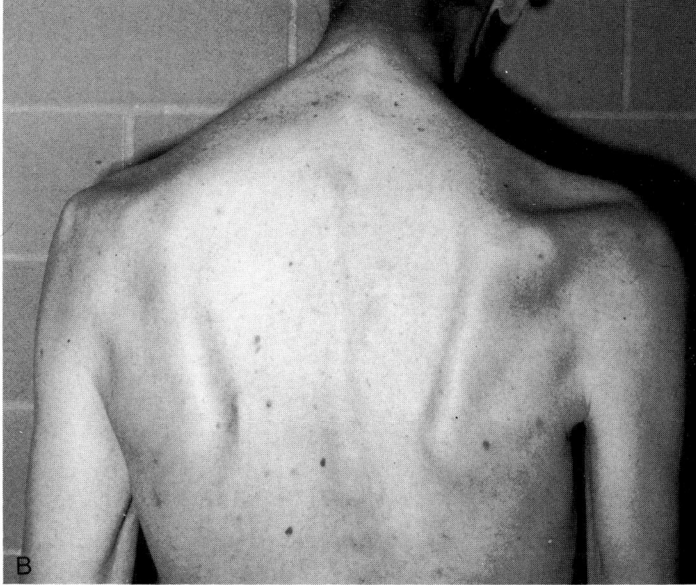
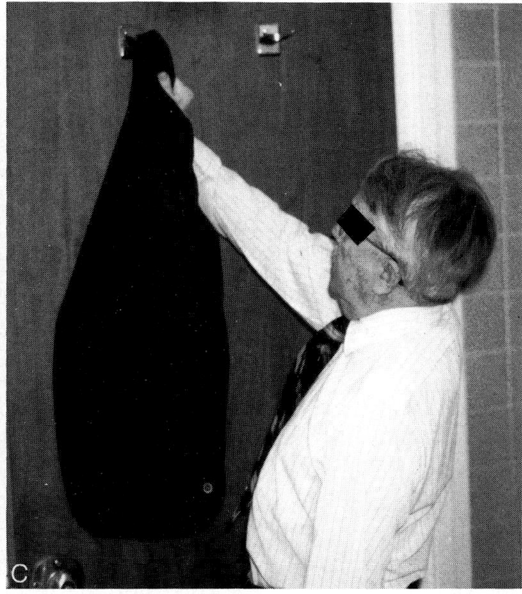

Figure 7–1. ***Pre-operative Assessment for Rehabilitation.*** A, Loss of motion characteristically occurs with the arm clasped against the side in internal rotation. Exercises to recover motion emphasize external rotation as well as elevation. As shown in Figure 1–20 and in the inset, external rotation is essential for overhead elevation because at 90 degrees abduction it provides an articular surface for further elevation and rotates the greater tuberosity so that it does not impinge on the acromion.

B, All of the muscles, including the scapular muscles as well as the rotator cuff muscles and deltoid muscle, atrophy and lose strength when there has been long-standing arthritis or injuries. Exercises to recover strength consider all of these muscles.

C, In the late aftercare following shoulder reconstruction, the patient may need to be taught to use the arm. The man shown, seen one year after a total shoulder arthroplasty for long-standing rheumatoid arthritis of the shoulder, had not hung his coat on a hook for over 15 years and had to break his old patterns of use.

three reasons. First, motion must be re-established prior to the maturation of adhesions to prevent failure of the procedure with a need for further surgery to release the adhesions. There is a specific time limit within which exercises for motion are maximally effective, whereas strengthening exercises are equally effective if started months later. Second, the too early initiation of active exercises aggravates muscle soreness. Painful muscles interfere with the recovery of motion. Third, strengthening exercises are more effective if begun after a good passive range of motion has been obtained and the initial muscle soreness that follows surgery has subsided.

Rule 5. Exercises to Regain Motion (Passive, Assisted, and Later Stretching Exercises) Are Done Repeatedly for Short Periods with Muscles Relaxed

It is more effective to perform exercises for motion for five minutes four or five times a day than to exercise for thirty minutes once a day. The muscles become fatigued and tighten with long exercise periods, making it impossible to obtain the excursion of movement that is possible when the muscles are relaxed. Rule 3 indicates that warm applications also help to relax the muscles. Slight, fleeting pain is to be expected because of undesired tightening of the muscles, but the pain should not cause tightening of the muscles and should not persist after exercising. Unless contraindicated, recovery of external rotation is emphasized (see Figs. 1–20, 1–21, and exercises illustrated in this Chapter) as well as elevation.

Rule 6. During Exercises to Regain Glenohumeral Motion, Allow the Scapula to Rise First

It is necessary to rotate the acromion out of the way, as in normal shoulder motion; otherwise, the greater tuberosity impinges on elevation. Do not tell the patient to "keep the shoulder blade down as the arm is raised."

Rule 7. Exercises to Regain Strength (Isometric, Active Assisted, Active, and Resisted Exercises) Are Followed by a Rest Period for Recovery

A period of rest is important for recovery of the muscles after strengthening exercises. Isometric, active assisted, active, and resisted exercises are performed progressively when muscle soreness subsides. These exercises are done no more frequently than once a day. Some temorary ache due to muscle fatigue may occur, but if persistent soreness develops, exercises causing soreness should be discontinued.

Rule 8. Record Motion and Function at Each Session Using a Simple, Reproducible System

Making a record (as in Figs. 1–6, 1–7, and 1–9) of the amount of motion, comfort, and function achieved helps to define deficiencies and objectives and has a good motivating effect on the patient.

Rule 9. Compliment the Patient on Achievements

An attitude of cheer and optimism is important. The patient can be made aware of deficiencies by pointing out the good features of his or her efforts and improvements made since the last session. This is followed by instruction in the exercises needed to eliminate weaker areas. Patients are easily discouraged and frightened, especially about three months after surgery when progress may seem slow and the newness of the effort has worn off. A gloomy physician or therapist is a huge deterrent to recovery.

Rule 10. Establish a Realistic Final Goal According to the Capability of the Muscles and the Excursion and Stability of the Glenohumeral Joint

Prior to surgery the surgeon should establish with the patient a realistic picture of the function and comfort level to be expected after the procedure and the time expected to achieve this goal. It is better to overestimate the length of time so that the patient can feel ahead of schedule in the exercise program after surgery rather than behind. The therapist must know whether the patient is on the "full exercise program" (see below), has specific "restrictions," or is on the "limited goals" program (see p. 530). For example, a patient with a cuff-tear arthropathy can accept and appreciate being on the limited goals program (see p. 530) provided that he or she knows from the beginning, even before surgery, that overhead use of the arm is beyond his or her expected capability. It is equally important for the therapist to know the range of motion that is to be restricted and for the patient to be taught how to avoid stress on the cuff repair.

FULL EXERCISE PROGRAM

Indications for Full Exercise Program

The exercises in the full exercise program are used when the surgeon believes that the quality of the rotator cuff and the stability of the glenohumeral joint are good enough that near-normal range of active motion and function might be obtained eventually. The full exercise program is used in 95 percent of patients with repairs for tears of the rotator cuff and over 80 percent of those with glenohumeral arthroplasties. The exceptions are patients with such severe loss of deltoid muscle, rotator cuff, or bone that they require the limited goals program, which aims at a lesser range of motion and greater stability (see p. 530).

The full exercise program usually begins with earlier passive motion exercises (see Fig. 7–7) and then progresses to the self-assisted exercises for recovering range of motion (see Fig. 7–8). Later, when the strength of the repair and comfort allow, the patient progresses to the stretching exercises (see Fig. 7–9) and strengthening exercises (see Fig. 7–10). In the late rehabilitation program, stretching exercises are continued and resistive exercises (see Fig. 7–11) are added to work against residual deficiencies in motion or strength.

The speed with which the exercises are added in the full exercise program varies according to the condition of the specific shoulder being treated. The surgeon makes this determination and instructs the therapist and patient about timing. The sequence and timing of the exercises I usually follow are outlined below according to diagnostic category. In practice, however, the surgeon who performed the procedure should make this judgment, and the exercise schedule may not follow the one to be outlined.

Precautions According to Diagnosis

I repeat, the surgeon who did the procedure should plan the schedule of exercises because only he or she knows the true pathology and strength of the repair. The surgeon instructs the therapist and patient when changes in the program are to be made. The schedules described below are guides for the average patient in each category.

Precautions Following Anterior Acromioplasty with Intact Cuff or Small Incomplete Tears

Aftercare following anterior acromioplasty when the rotator cuff is intact is described on pages 106 and 118, Chapter 2. The program starts with early passive motion (EPM) (see Fig. 7–7) on the first day after surgery, and the patient is discharged from the hospital when he or she can do the self-assisted exercises (see Figs. 7–8 to 7–12) and is allowed active use of the arm in all directions except forward elevation. Active forward elevation is deferred for two weeks to allow the deltoid muscle to heal. The full exercise program can be advanced rapidly without precautions. Patients are advised pre-operatively of the need to do stretching exercises at least twice a day for the first five months after surgery until the subacromial bursa has had time to re-form.

The exceptions are those who require manipulation at the time of anterior acromioplasty for a frozen shoulder. They are retained in the hospital or followed daily until a full range of motion is re-established just as in other patients with frozen shoulders who require manipulation.

The aftercare program for anterior acromioplasty in those with incomplete cuff tears is discussed on page 118, Chapter 2. Those with small incomplete tears are treated in the same way as if the cuff were intact, as briefly described above. Those with larger incomplete tears requiring suture repairs are usually treated the same as patients with complete supraspinatus tears (Chapter 2 and below), except that they can usually return to activities such as tennis and golf somewhat sooner.

Precautions Following Complete Cuff Tear Repairs

The exercise program for patients with repairs of complete supraspinatus tears is outlined in detail on page 118, Chapter 2. To summarize, EPM (see Fig. 7–7) is started within two or three days after surgery, but the excursion of motion is restricted to 160 degrees of elevation and 60 degrees of external rotation to avoid stressing the repair. The first four self-assisted exercises for motion are performed four or five times daily for the first six weeks (see Fig. 7–8A through D). During the next six weeks, the other exercises to regain motion are added (see Figs. 7–8E through 7–9). Strengthening exercises are delayed until at least three months, at which time isometric exercises are prescribed (see Fig. 7–10), and advanced so that at four months the patient is able to hold the arm overhead, lower it, and eventually raise it using a stick, as shown in Figure 7–12. Heavy use of the shoulder (lifting more than 15 pounds) is avoided for at least one year. Other details are discussed in Chapter 2.

The exercise program for patients with repairs of massive tears and re-operations with tenuous repairs or deltoid muscle damage is discussed on page 119, Chapter 2. A brace is used for four to eight weeks, during which time the arm is passively raised to at least 160 degrees elevation each day (see Fig. 7–3). The brace is discarded, as depicted in Figure 7–15, following which self-assisted exercises are begun and slowly advanced at the discretion of the surgeon in the sequence described above for repairs for complete supraspinatus tears. In difficult cases, active use of the arm is guarded, often for more than one year and as long as any chance of further recovery remains.

Precautions After Arthroplasties

Special problems that are frequently seen after humeral head replacement arthroplasty and total glenohumeral arthroplasty are discussed in Chapter 3 according to diagnostic category. The characteristic pathology requiring precautions can be summarized for each as follows.

Precautions After Arthroplasties for Avascular Necrosis (see Chapter 3, pp. 198 and 199). Muscles and bone are ideal. As in all arthroplasties, avoid crutches for at least six months to allow the rotator interval and subscapularis to heal.

Precautions After Arthroplasties for Osteoarthritis (see Chapter 3, p. 206). Muscles are ideal, but patient may have posterior glenoid wear with a loose posterior capsule, posing the threat of posterior subluxation. Avoid early supine elevation (see Fig. 7–8E). Avoid overhead exercises (pulley, etc.) with the arm in forward flexion and adduction.

Precautions After Arthroplasties for Arthritis of Recurrent Dislocations (see Chapter 3, pp. 211 and 212). Instability is common, owing to uneven glenoid wear and a capsule that is short on one side and long on the other. Deltoid muscle is usually weakened by prior surgery.

Precautions After Arthroplasties for Rheumatoid Arthritis (see Chapter 3, p. 221). Often arthritis of the neck, opposite shoulder, elbows, wrists, and hands is present, requiring improvisation. Twenty percent of patients have rotator cuff defects that may delay the strengthening program. The muscles are involved in rheumatoid disease and require longer to respond to exercises. Expect everything to be slow, and encourage the patient. When the patient is not ambulatory, transfers must be avoided until the rotator cuff has healed (i.e., at least six months), during which time the type of rehabilitation illustrated in Figure 7–16 is required (see p. 167 and Table 3–2a, p. 168).

Precautions After Arthroplasties for Old Trauma (see Chapter 3, p. 228). The shoulder may be unstable because of inadequate height or length of the head of the humeral component or because of a capsular pouch from a longstanding dislocation. Nerve injuries, bone loss, cuff defects, deltoid muscle defects, and dense scar make rehabilitation especially challenging, requiring individualization.

Precautions After Arthroplasties for Cuff-Tear Arthropathy (see Chapter 3, p. 238). Limited goals rehabilitation is advised (p. 530).

Precautions After Arthroplasties for Congenital Defects (see Chapter 3, p. 238), Erb's Palsy Deformity (see Chapter 3, p. 243), Neoplasms (see Chapter 3, p. 249), and so on. Often these conditions require limited goals rehabilitation and individualized exercises.

Precautions After Repairs for Recurrent Dislocations

Precautions After Anterior Repairs (see Chapter 4, p. 307). The repair must be given time to heal before it is subjected to stress. The position of greatest stability is holding the arm at the side in internal rotation and flexion (as in a Velpeau sling). I use a stockinette Velpeau sling during the first 24 hours after surgery (see Fig. 7–2C) and then use a removable sling (see Fig. 7–2A). Conversely, exercises used to regain motion in a shoulder that becomes too stiff after a repair for anterior instability emphasize recovery of external rotation, elevation, and extension. I believe it is unwise to set a routine because of the great variability in type of patients involved. A young, hypermobile female patient may well require a sling most of the time for six weeks, whereas a male patient over 60 years may be stiff and better off without immobilization.

Almost all patients are allowed to use the arm for light activities out of the sling when awake during the first week following surgery, except for overhead use and more than 25 degrees external rotation. All patients are re-evaluated at three weeks after surgery; if the shoulder is overprotected and stiff, pendulum and pulley exercises are started. After six weeks patients are allowed full light activities, but they are advised against carrying more than 20 pounds of weight and impact loads for 10 to 12 months. Other self-assisted exercises to improve the range of motion are added after three months if indicated, but most patients are allowed to limber up at their own speed during a nine month to one year period. I believe it is wrong to prescribe exercises to recover motion in most patients (throwing athletes are an exception) unless the patient has less than 140 degrees of passive elevation and less than 40 degrees of external rotation. At one year after surgery the patient is expected to have within 10 degrees full elevation and within 20 degrees full external rotation compared with the opposite side. Motion should not always equal that of the opposite side because the opposite side is often hypermobile.

Beginning at three months after repair, strengthening exercises for the subscapularis (see Fig. 7–13A and B) are begun starting with isometric exercises and advancing to resistance with the rubber. I avoid overhead strengthening exercises because of the fear that they will make the shoulder too loose. I advise patients against future overhead weightlifting or use of bench presses of more than 50 pounds. Activities are discussed further in Chapter 4, page 314.

Precautions After Posterior Repairs (see Chapter 4, p. 314). The position of greatest stability for protection of a posterior repair is external rotation and slight flexion with the elbow held at the side. A cast is used for six to eight weeks in some patients with bone blocks (see Fig. 4–34). Following this, pendulum exercises are begun, and the patient is allowed to limber up at his or her own speed. Starting at three months, strengthening exercises for the infraspinatus (see Fig. 7–13A and C) are begun. However, carrying more than 20 pounds of weight and heavy use of the shoulder are avoided for ten months to a year. Other details of aftercare are discussed in Chapter 4, page 314.

Precautions After Repairs for Multidirectional Instability (see Chapter 4, p. 326). Aftercare following an inferior capsular shift entails holding the arm in near-neutral rotation (without tension on either the front or the back of the glenohumeral capsule) to allow healing of the soft tissue to bone. These patients usually require little in the way of exercises to recover motion; however, the surgeon should check their range of motion carefully at three months and make a decision then and at subsequent interval examinations whether some exercises for range of motion are indicated. Strengthening exercises are given with great caution, usually starting with gentle isometrics at three months and mild resistance after six months (see Fig. 7–13). Activities are often restricted for 18 months (see discussion on page 326 for details).

Precautions After Acromioclavicular Joint Repairs (see Chapter 4, p. 336)

Since the glenohumeral joint is normal, little rehabilitation is needed; however, the repair of the coracoclavicular ligaments must be protected until mature healing occurs. Light use of the shoulder is allowed soon after surgery, but heavy activities should be avoided for nine months.

Precautions After Fracture Repairs (see Chapter 5)

The speed with which exercises are allowed must be individualized and directed by the surgeon, as discussed in Chapter 5. One exception is the patient in whom prosthesis is used to replace the humeral head in a four-part or head-crushing displacement. An early aggressive exercise regimen to recover range of motion is routine when a prosthesis has been used unless some rare technical problem had been encountered.

Precautions After Prosthesis for Fracture (see Chapter 5)

After secure implanting of the prosthesis and tuberosity repair, EPM (see Fig. 7–7) is started within two days after surgery. The patient continues with self-assisted exercises for motion (see Fig. 7–8A through D and H) four or five times a day until the tuberosities unite to the shaft with early callus. After the tuberosity has healed, the full exercise program is advanced as rapidly as possible, stressing exercises to recover motion initially and strength later. Finally, stretching exercises to eliminate any residual defects can continue daily for as long as necessary to achieve near-normal motion.

Equipment for Exercises

Stretching Material For Resistive Exercises

Initially, we used surgical tubing in various thicknesses. Later, we used the type of rubber sheeting dentists were using at the time ("dental dam"). This has since been manufactured in colors to signify various strengths of elasticity. All of these materials are satisfactory.

Slings

Some of the slings used after shoulder surgery are illustrated in Figure 7–2. A sling with hooks or Velcro connectors that is easily removed for exercises (Fig. 7–2A) or no sling is used once exercises are begun. A sling and swathe (Fig. 7–2B) is usually applied immediately after surgery to protect the shoulder during transportation back to the patient's hospital room. I prefer a stockinette Velpeau (Fig.

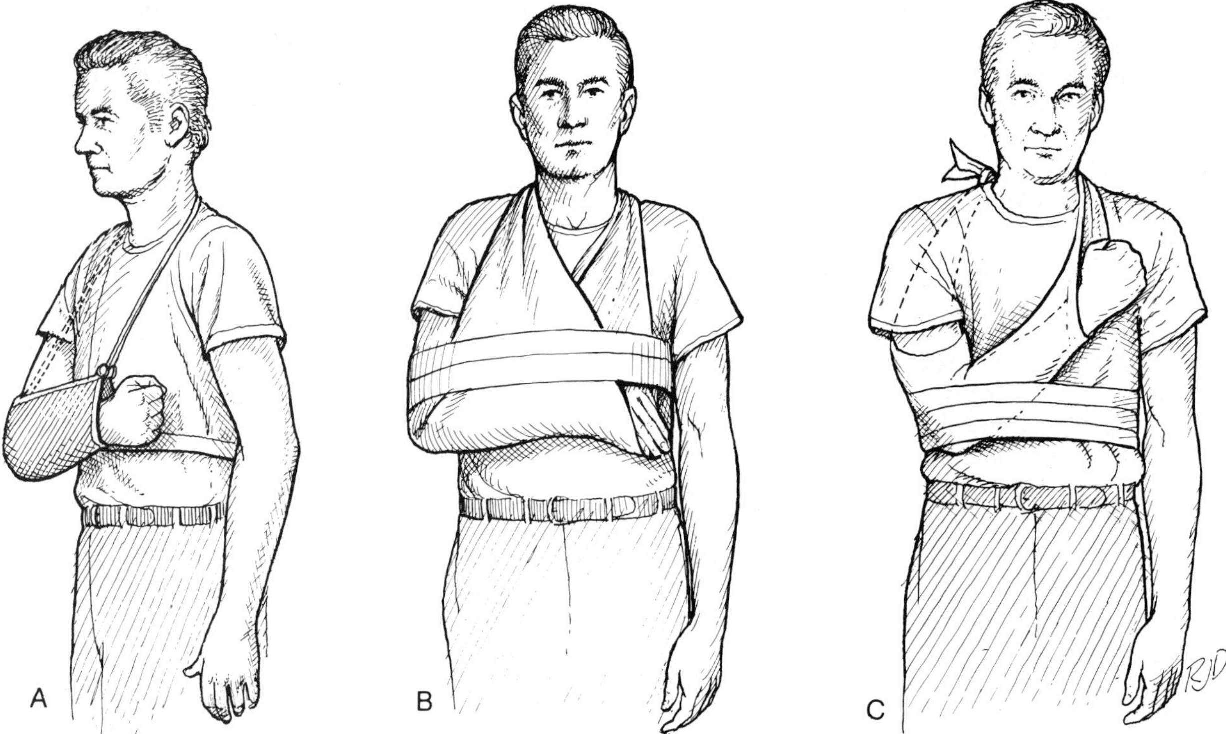

Figure 7–2. ***Equipment for Exercises.*** A, Removable sling with hooks (shown) or Velcro connections or no sling is used once the exercise program begins.

B, Sling and swathe, as is often applied immediately after surgery for temporary protection of the shoulder.

C, Stockinette Velpeau sling I prefer during the immediate period after a repair for recurrent anterior dislocations to prevent excursive movement of the shoulder even when the patient reacts violently after the anesthesia (see Chapter 4, p. 306) and for two-part surgical neck fractures (see Chapter 5, p. 375).

(From Neer, C.S. II: Fractures about the shoulder, Chapter 11. *In* Rockwood, C.A., and Green, D.P. (eds): Fractures in Adults, 2nd ed. Philadelphia, J.B. Lippincott, 1984.)

7–2C) after a repair for recurrent anterior dislocations to protect the shoulder against violent movements of the arm in the immediate post-operative period.

Braces or Pillows

A lightweight brace, well padded to prevent nerve injuries, is used occasionally to protect a tenuous repair of the rotator cuff or to protect the deltoid muscle (Fig. 7–3).The brace holds the arm at about 90 degrees elevation and neutral rotation. This position relieves tension from all of the tendons at the rotator cuff. The arm can be passively elevated once or twice daily from the brace to maintain motion (see Fig. 7–15). A small pillow is placed under the elbow when the patient is recumbent to prevent extension of the shoulder. The exercises in a brace and the method of discarding the brace are illustrated in Figure 7–15.

A wedge of foam or pellets may be used in place of the brace. In either case, straps across the uninvolved shoulder and around the body support

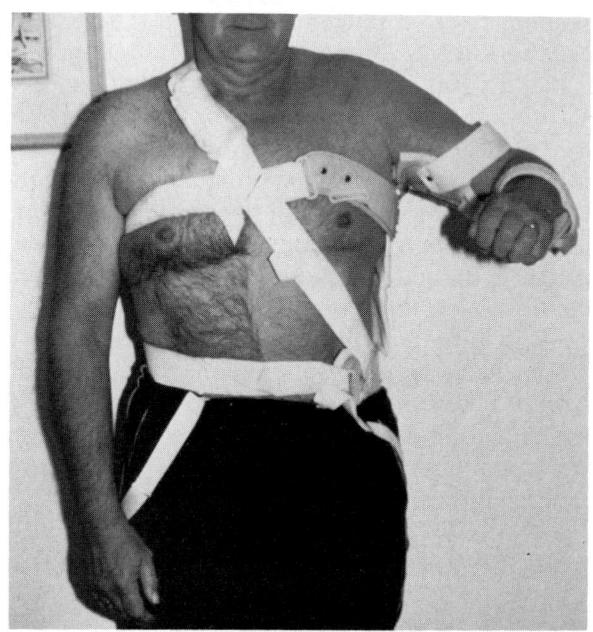

Figure 7–3. ***Equipment for Exercises.*** A brace is occasionally used to protect a tenous rotator cuff repair or deltoidplasty. The care of the shoulder in a brace is illustrated in Figure 7–15.

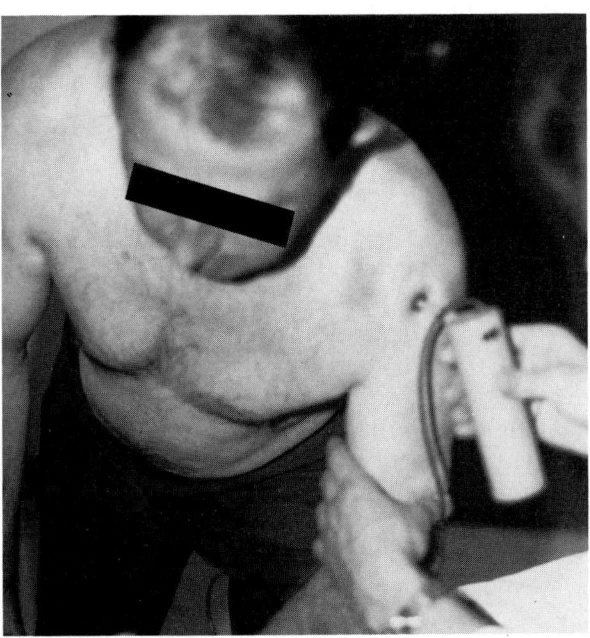

Figure 7–4. ***Equipment for Exercises.*** Electrical stimulation (portable unit) being applied to a paralyzed deltoid six months after a displaced proximal humeral fracture, as discussed in the text.

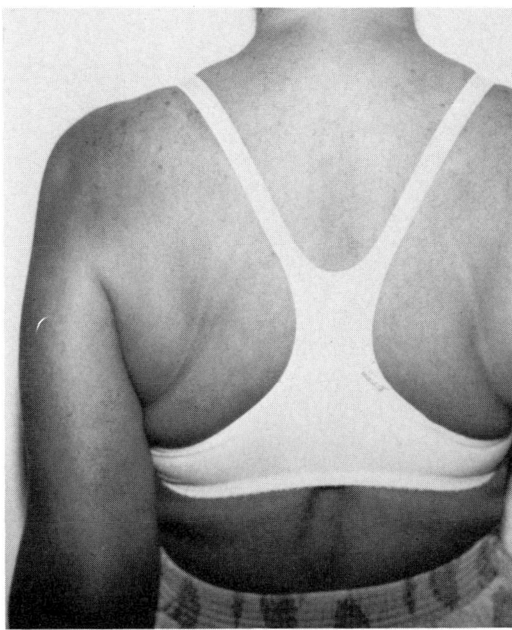

Figure 7–5. ***Equipment for Exercises.*** Loose clothing and a brassiere that snaps in front and with straps crossed in the back or no straps are worn during the period of shoulder rehabilitation.

the weight of the arm to prevent downward drag on the repair.

Electrical Stimulation

I believe that electrical stimulation to maintain muscle tone is beneficial when the deltoid muscle is paralyzed. A portable unit is illustrated in Figure 7–4.

Loose Clothing

Clothing should not restrict the scapula or humerus. Brassieres without shoulder straps or, as illustrated in Figure 7–5, with straps that cross in back with the hooks in the front are used.

EXERCISES TO REGAIN MOTION

Earlier Passive Motion (EPM)

In the past, when the repair permitted, emphasis has been on self-assisted exercises to restore motion, usually starting with pendulum exercises about the fourth or fifth day and adding one or two exercises daily.[74] Continuous passive motion (CPM) has been used in the shoulder in our clinic since its inception, but mainly in patients who have both shoulders involved precluding the self-assistive exercise program. I discussed the use of CPM in the shoulder with Doctor Salter[263] early in its development, and used one of the initial shoulder CPM machines especially in patients with bilateral shoulder disorders.

Craig[265] reported the beneficial effects of early CPM on the earlier recovery of motion after shoulder surgery. This stimulated my interest.[7] Because of the limited supply of CPM machines (as illustrated in Fig. 7–6), the questionable safety of these devices after a major cuff repair and shoulder arthroplasty, the limited excursion of CPM machines, and, since articular cartilage and ligamentous defects were not of concern in these patients (making continuous motion seem unnecessary), a manual technique for earlier passive motion (EPM) was developed, which dramatically improved our exercise program.

In a consecutive series of my patients with rotator cuff repairs and shoulder arthroplasties, a prospective study has been completed as presented to the American Shoulder and Elbow Surgeons in 1987.[89]

It is critical that the length of the tendons and freedom of adhesions necessary for free passive motion be obtained at surgery. Otherwise, no amount of exercise can overcome fixed contractures. It is especially easy and disastrous to fail to release the internal rotation contracture and short subscapularis so frequently present in long-standing disorders of the shoulder.

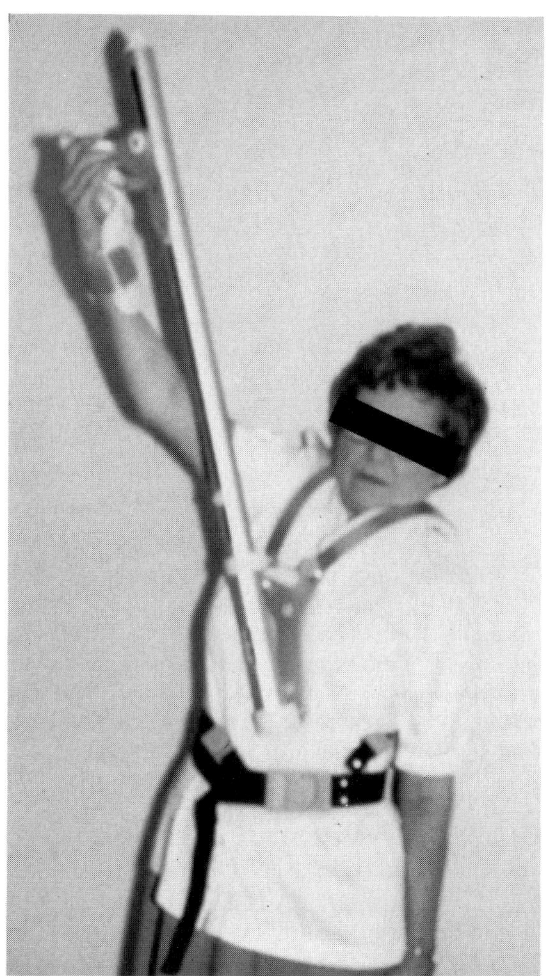

Figure 7–6. Photograph of the continuous passive motion (CPM) machine once used by the author. It has been replaced by earlier passive motion (EPM) (see Fig. 7–7A) because of the limited supply and limited excursion of motion of CPM machines, as discussed in the text.

The importance of the prerequisites for this method should be emphasized, especially a knowledgeable and able person to move the arm. The necessary relaxation of the patient's muscles depends upon the skill and communication of this person. Gloom, lack of knowledge, lack of confidence, and rough handling are sure to cause a failure.

It is easier to perform EPM on patients with repairs of the rotator cuff and arthroplasties for conditions with good muscles. Old trauma with previous failed surgery, revision arthroplasty, and long-standing and stiff rheumatoids are much more difficult and require patience. However, the most valuable contribution of EPM has probably been in improving the motion in many of these difficult problems. Many of the 15 percent of this series who did not achieve the designated range of passive motion by the sixth day after surgery had a friend or relative instructed in the EPM maneuver so it could be continued after discharge from the hospital for gradual improvement in motion.

Early Passive Motion Study[89]

A prospective study was made of 160 shoulders, 49 cuff repairs and 111 glenohumeral arthroplasties,[261] performed by the author at the Columbia-Presbyterian Medical Center in New York between March 1986 and June 1987. Ten men and 1 woman had bilateral shoulder arthroplasties and 1 woman had bilateral rotator cuff repairs during the course of this study. Thus, the 160 shoulder operations were performed in 149 patients. Fourteen shoulders with extreme loss of bone and soft tissue were excluded from the study because they required "limited goals rehabilitation" aimed at less motion and more stability. Their diagnoses were: four cuff-tear arthropathies, three long-standing rheumatoids, one arthritis of dislocations, two old fracture-dislocations, three revisions of prostheses implanted elsewhere, and one massive cuff tear. Seven of the limited goals shoulders were in women and seven were in men. Thus, there were 146 shoulders, 48 with cuff repairs and 98 with arthroplasties, in 135 patients who had the full normal rehabilitation program who were suitable for this analysis.

The ages of the 135 patients ranged from 20 to 91 years and averaged 60 years. The right shoulder was involved in 74, the left in 71. Of those with tears of the rotator cuff, the tear was complete in 45 and incomplete in 3. Nine with massive tears were given an abduction brace for six weeks following surgery, but EPM was performed in the usual way from the brace.

Of the 98 arthroplasties evaluated, the diagnosis was osteoarthritis in 41, rheumatoid arthritis in 16, arthritis of dislocations in 7, acute proximal humeral fracture in 10, inactive infection followed by degenerative arthritis in 1, avascular necrosis in 4, old fractures in 14, and revision prosthesis in 5.

There were no early complications precluding EPM. The ranges of passive elevation and passive external rotation were recorded by the surgeon and therapist. Special attention was given to the motion achieved by the sixth day following surgery compared with that observed in similar patients with the same procedures[22, 28, 107, 108] prior to March 1986.

Prerequisites for EPM

The requirements for use of this technique were considered to be:

1. Adhesions and short tendons must be freed at surgery to allow a full passive range of elevation and external rotation.

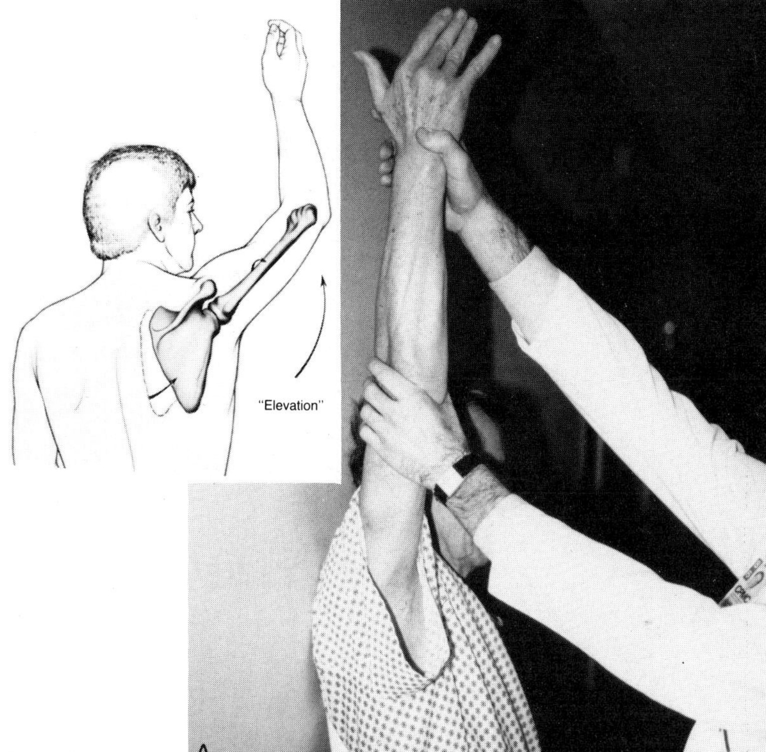

Figure 7–7. ***Technique of Earlier Passive Motion (EPM).*** As described in detail in the text, after 24 to 48 hours following surgery, pendulum exercises (see Fig. 7–8A) are begun and the patient is taught to relax the shoulder muscles as the arm is moved by the surgeon or therapist. Premedication (analgesia) may be helpful.

A, Elevation in the scapular plane (as shown in the inset) is accomplished by supporting the full weight of the arm by the surgeon or therapist and, after 90 degrees elevation, traction is applied at the wrist and steady pressure at the elbow to move the arm upward. The same forces are maintained when the arm is lowered.

Illustration continued on following page

2. In the case of glenohumeral arthroplasties, the implant must be stable.

3. In the case of massive tears of the rotator cuff, the repair must be sufficiently strong to permit this amount of passive motion without disrupting the repair.

4. A knowledgeable person raising the arm is essential. Scapular plane movement (Fig. 7–7A) must be maintained, avoiding force that would damage the repair. This must be done with the type of assurance that breeds confidence.

5. The patient must relax the muscles in the shoulder ("like a rag doll"); otherwise, the patient will experience pain.

Technique of EPM

Starting on the second day after surgery, EPM was performed twice daily, once by the surgeon and once by the therapist. Between these sessions, the patient did pendulum exercises every two hours and discarded the sling as rapidly as possible.

A moderate oral pain medication given 45 minutes before EPM; and low, dry heat to relax the muscles were quite helpful in some patients but were unnecessary in many.

EPM was begun with instructions to the patient in deltoid muscle relaxation and pendulum exercises. Pendulum exercise was done with the patient bent well forward, in circles and backward and forward with the palm of the hand turned in and also with it turned out, always striving for complete muscle relaxation. Following this, the surgeon or therapist raised the relaxed arm in the scapular plane with traction at the wrist while the other hand pushed above the elbow (Fig. 7–7A). The excursion of the arm was maintained at about 35 degrees lateral to forward flexion, and the arm was raised slowly. The patient's facial expression was watched, stopping whenever apprehension was noted. It was considered important to talk to the patient almost constantly during this maneuver to remind him or her to relax the muscles ("like a rag doll") to avoid pain. The arm was held overhead for five seconds at the highest point. The patient was warned before starting its descent that lowering the arm is often more uncomfortable than raising it unless the patient makes a special effort to relax. After brief rest periods to relax, this maneuver was repeated three to five times, attempting to gain a little more height with each movement.

On the fourth day after surgery, passive external rotation was added (Fig. 7–7B). The elbow was bent 90 degrees and held close to the side as the hand was gently assisted away from the midline to externally rotate the humerus as far as possible, holding five seconds and resting between each movement. These were also repeated three to five times.

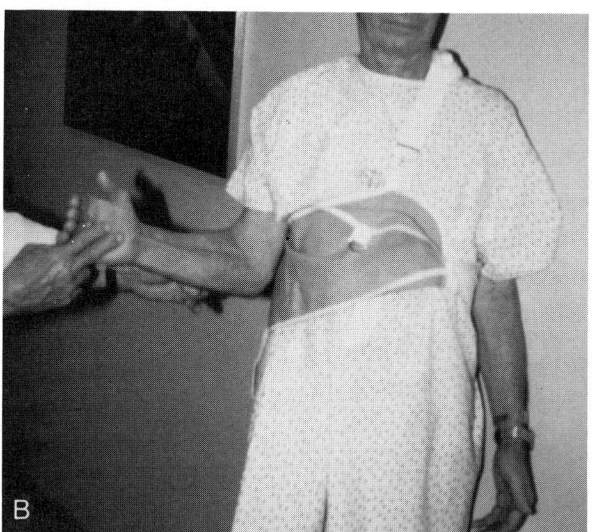

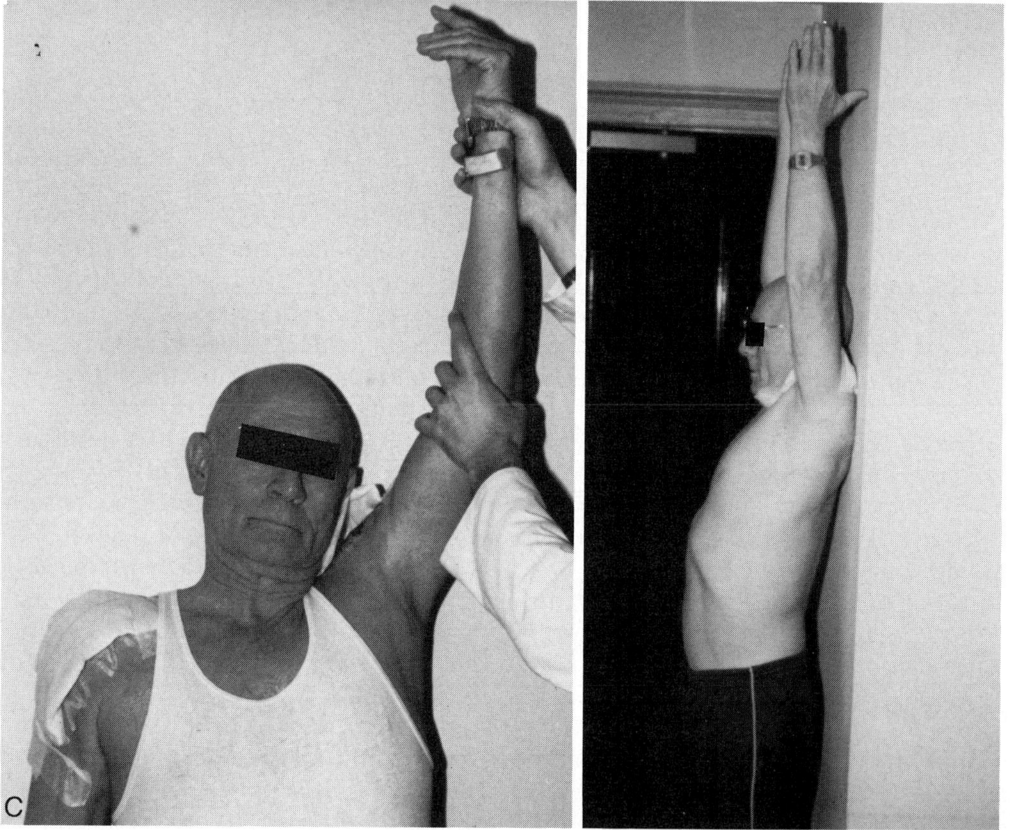

Figure 7–7. ***Technique of Earlier Passive Motion (EPM)*** *Continued* B, Passive external rotation with the arm at the side is begun as muscle soreness subsides, usually starting on the fourth day after surgery.

C, An unusually strong patient seen 12 days after total shoulder arthroplasty on the right and 4 days after total shoulder arthroplasty on the left for osteoarthritis receiving EPM (left). At that time, he was able to hold the arms overhead (right) after the arms had been placed in that position by the therapist, demonstrating the excellent motion already obtained.

The self-assisted exercises to regain motion (see Fig. 7–8A through D) are usually begun on the fifth day after surgery, and other assistive exercises for motion are added as tolerated. Active motion is deferred until muscle soreness has disappeared.

On the fifth or sixth day, the regular self-assisted program of exercises was advanced (i.e., pulley, external rotation with a stick, extension, internal rotation, etc. was begun) and advanced as rapidly as tolerated (see Fig. 7–8).

Active exercises were deferred until all muscle soreness had disappeared, which was often after discharge from the hospital.

Results

In patients who were good relaxers, it was usually possible to elevate the arm over 140 degrees the first time. Apprehensive patients required three or four days to achieve this.

Those with anterior acromioplasties and cuff repairs had little trouble in gaining motion. It was thought best to stop at 160 degrees early passive elevation and 60 degrees early passive external rotation in this group. All but 1 of the 48 shoulders achieved over 140 degrees elevation and 40 degrees external rotation by the sixth day following surgery. The one patient in this group with less motion had an unfused anterior acromial epiphysis requiring closure at the time of cuff repair.

All but 14 of 98 shoulders (85 percent) with arthroplasties achieved over 140 degrees passive elevation by the sixth post-operative day. The exceptions were as follows: 0 of 48 osteoarthritis, 3 of 16 rheumatoid, 2 of 7 arthritis of dislocations, 2 of 10 acute four-part fractures, 0 of 1 inactive infection, 0 of 4 avascular necrosis, 4 of 14 old fracture-dislocations, and 3 of 5 revisions.

Characteristically, these patients were discharged from the hospital several days sooner than those with similar arthroplasties and cuff repairs prior to EPM. After leaving the hospital, they maintained and usually improved their motion with the self-assisted exercises, as illustrated in Figures 7–8 and 7–9. Strengthening exercises (Figs. 7–10 through 7–12) were advanced over several months, depending on the capabilities of the muscles.

Clinical follow-up examinations have continued for over two years in 50 percent of these patients and for over one year in the majority of the rest without observing complications or detrimental effects of EPM.

Self-Assisted Exercises to Regain Motion

These exercises (Fig. 7–8A to J) are designed to increase motion. In these exercises, the stiff shoulder is assisted by the "good" arm, by gravity, or by a pulley. Whenever possible, apply heat (hot water bottle, heating pad, and so on) for two minutes before starting the exercises. Five exercise sessions are done daily, and each exercise is done five times during each session.

Pendulum Exercise

Emphasize muscle relaxation. More passive motion can be obtained if the sensitive muscles can be relaxed (Fig. 7–8A).

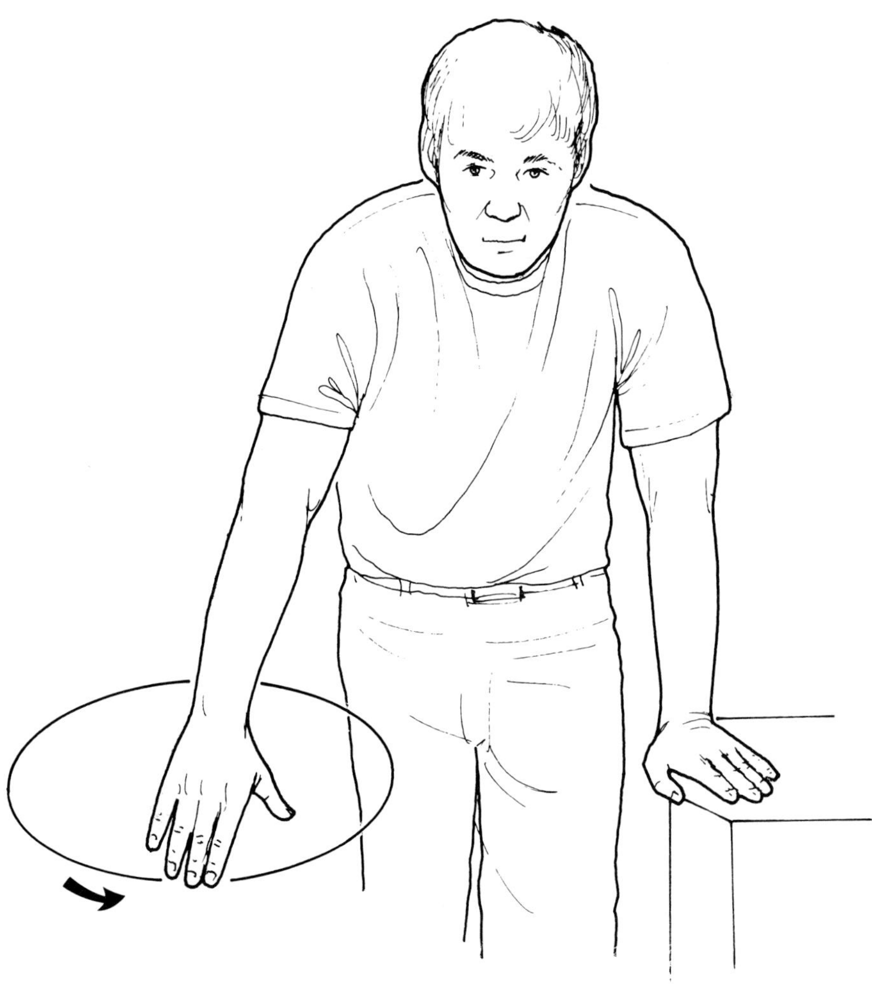

Figure 7–8A. Pendulum Exercise

While bending over at the waist and balancing with the good arm, let the stiff side relax and swing with gravity:

1. Circle with the hand turned inward.

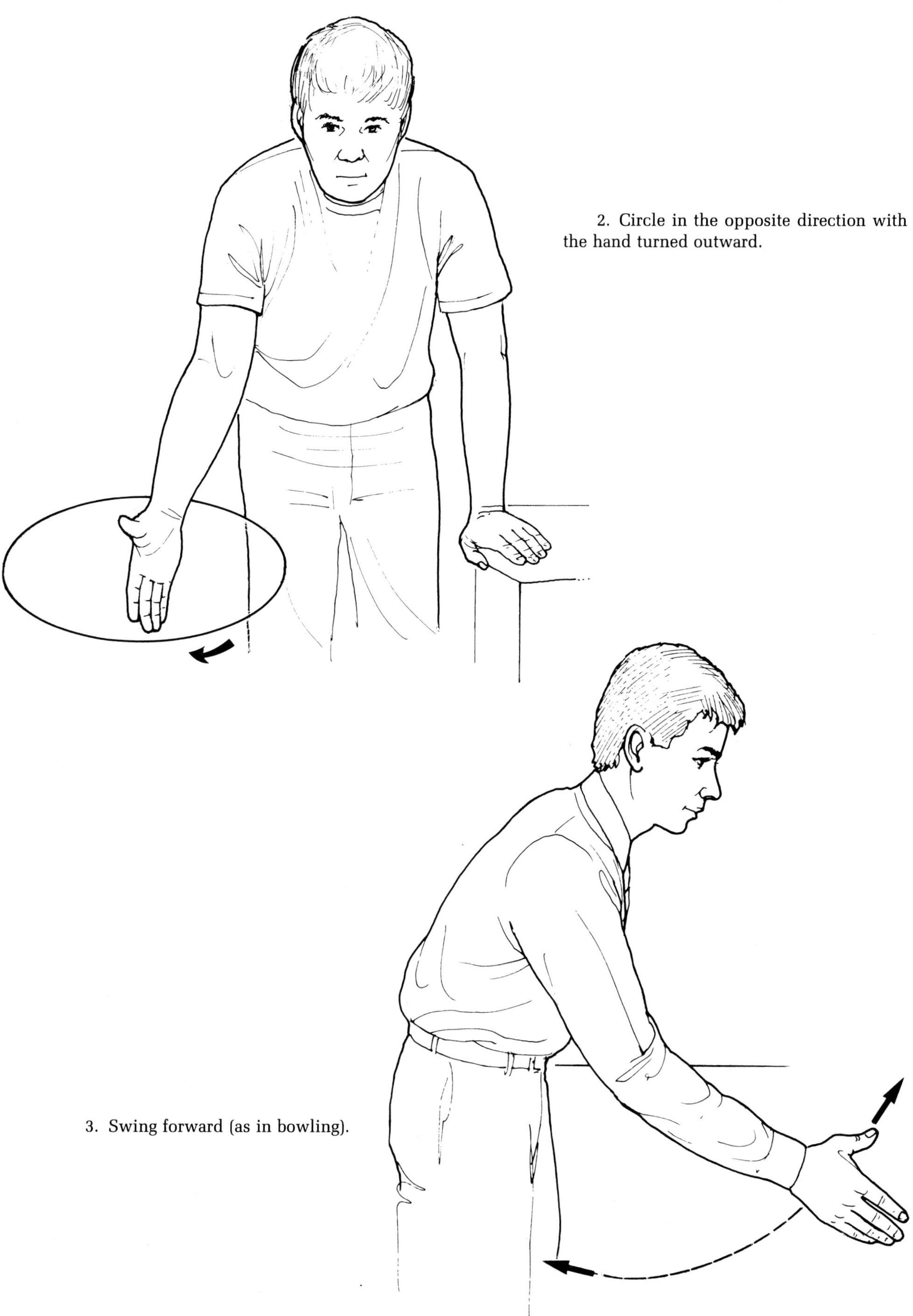

2. Circle in the opposite direction with the hand turned outward.

3. Swing forward (as in bowling).

Assisted External Rotation Supine

A towel is placed under the elbow to relax the anterior deltoid. Keep the elbow bent (Fig. 7–8B).

The therapist may gently assist more effectively while the patient does this exercise because the stick gives the patient control of the arm and the patient relaxes better while holding it than without it.

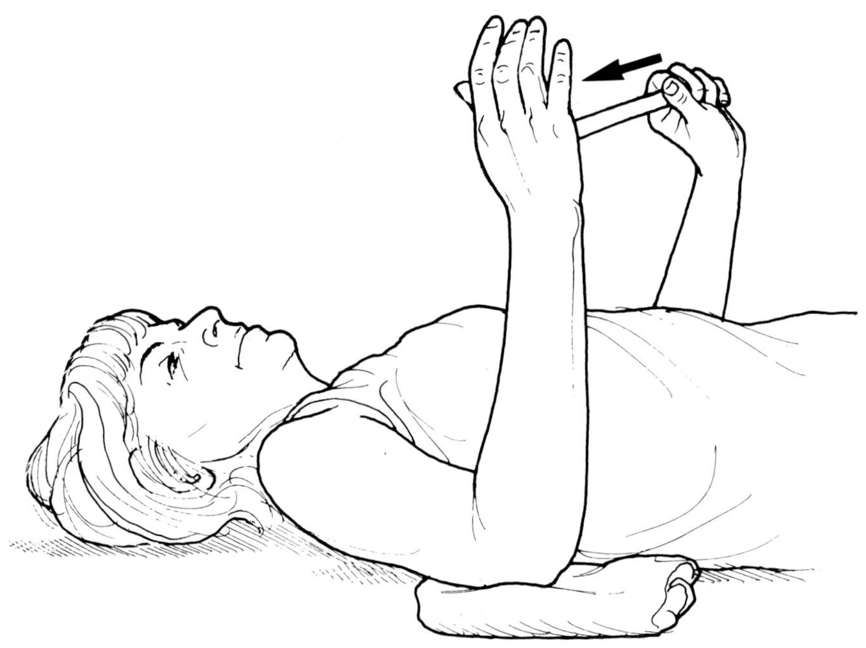

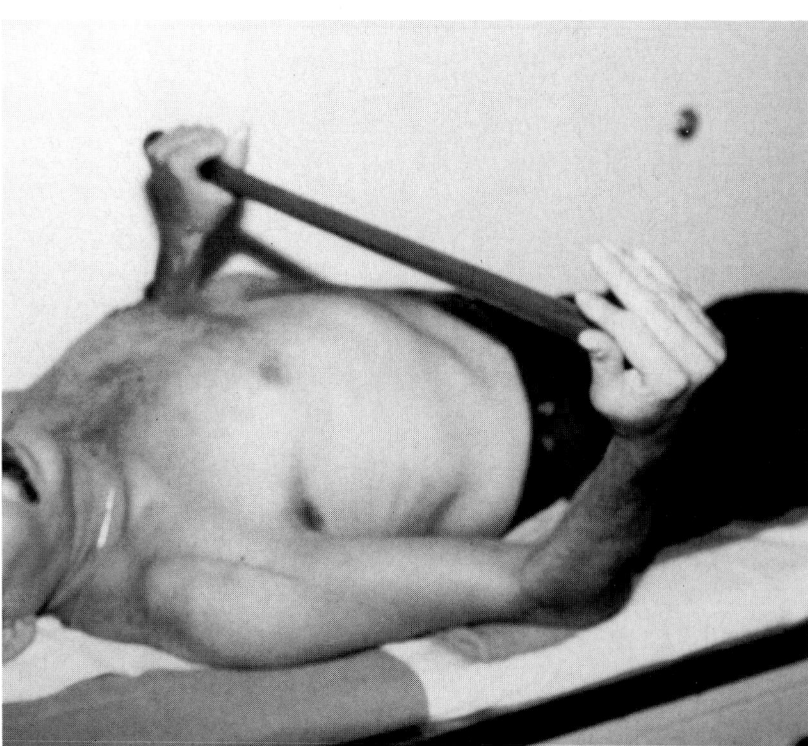

Figure 7–8B. Assisted External Rotation Supine

Lying on the back with the elbow of the stiff side supported on a folded towel and both elbows bent 90 degrees and held closely to the body, push the hand of the stiff side outward away from the chest with the stick, using the good arm to supply the power.

Assisted Extension

This exercise (Fig. 7–8C) is done in preparation for the exercise shown in Figure 7–8F, which is done when the hands can be brought together in back. This exercise also helps to condition the anterior deltoid.

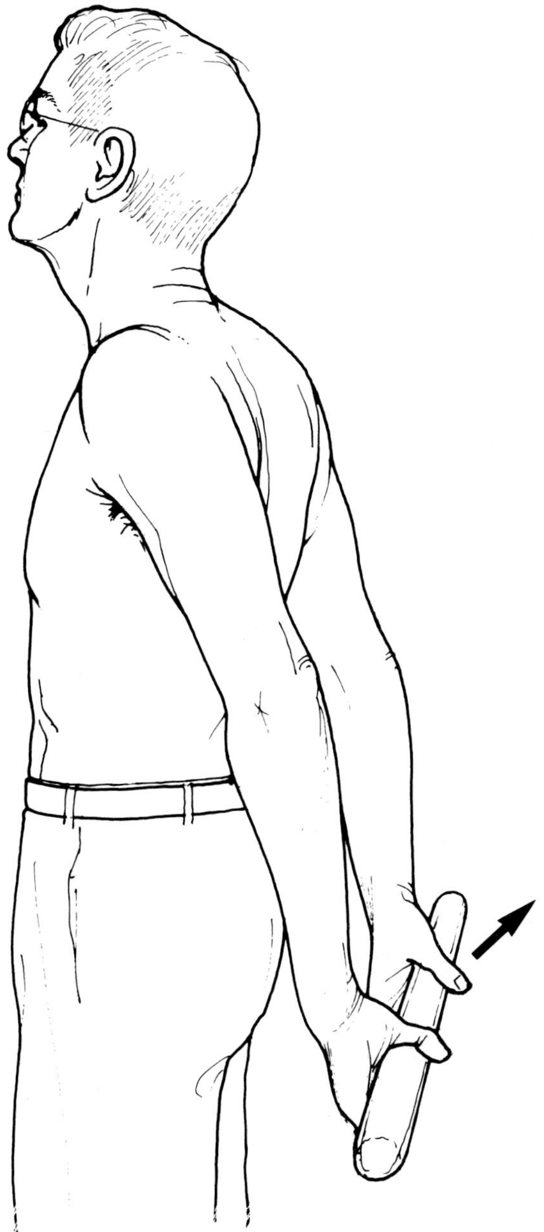

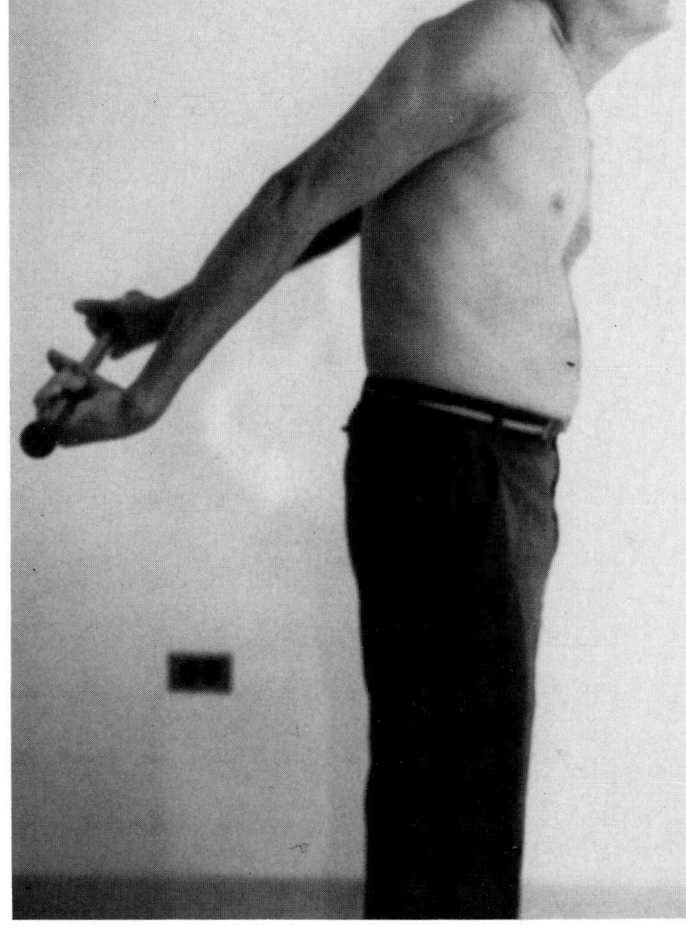

Figure 7–8C. Assisted Extension

While standing, grasp the stick with both hands and push backward using the good arm to supply the power.

Pulley-Assisted Elevation

This exercise (Fig. 7–8D) involves stress using the uninvolved arm for power while the muscles of the shoulder that was operated on relax. It cannot be used as early as early passive motion (EPM) because it is harder to relax the involved side.

Avoid stressing either the anterior or posterior capsule by raising the arm in the scapular plane (unless special circumstances require it).

Have the pulley high enough to give good traction—in front at first and later more overhead.

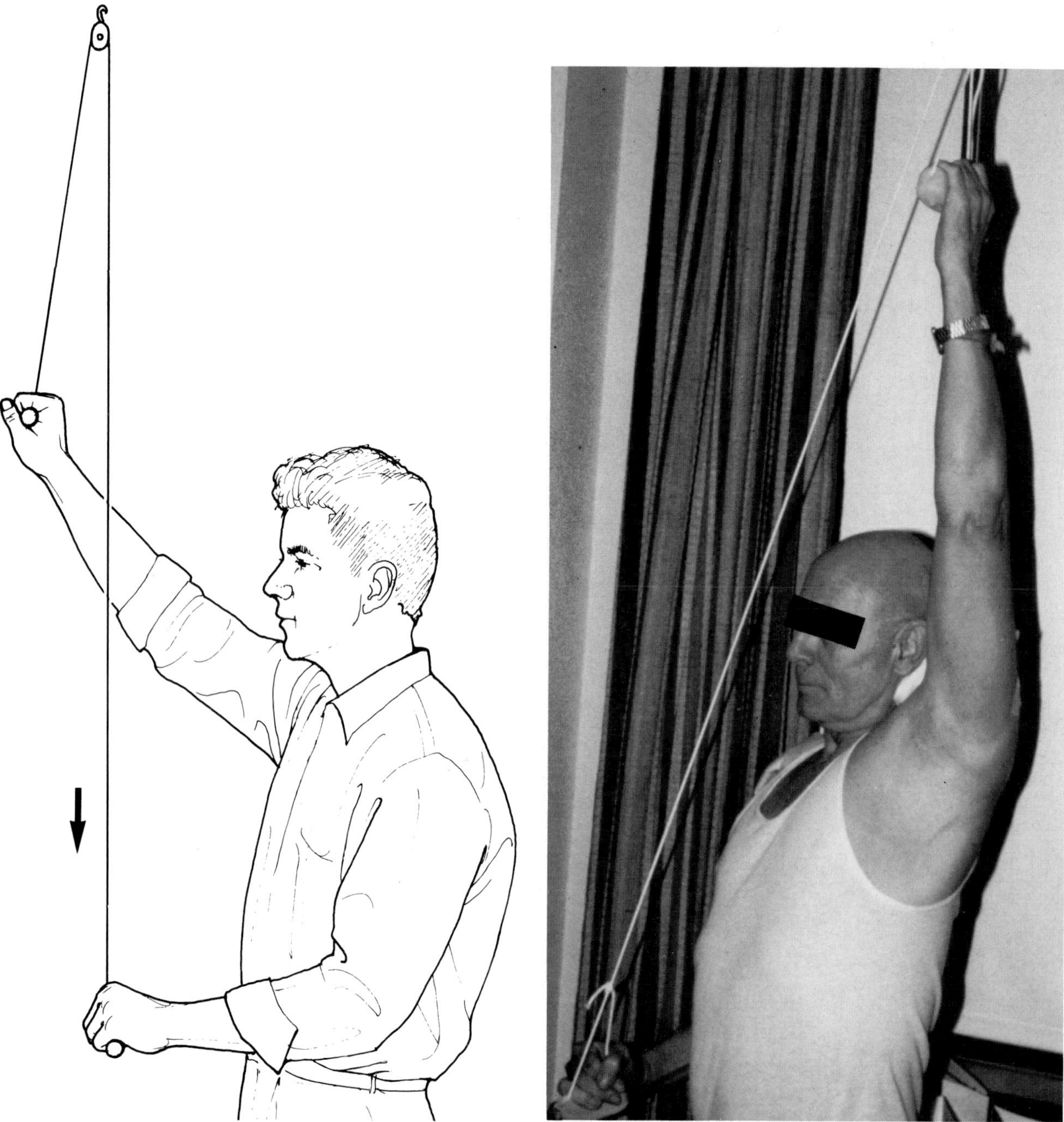

Figure 7–8D. Pulley-Assisted Elevation

While standing, with the pulley two feet higher than the good arm can reach overhead, the good arm supplies the power to bring the hand as near the pulley as possible. If the pulley is lower, the patient sits with his or her back to the pulley.

Assisted Elevation Supine

The uninvolved arm takes the weight of the arm off the posterior capsule by pulling it forward and then overhead (Fig. 7–8E). Let the shoulder muscles relax.

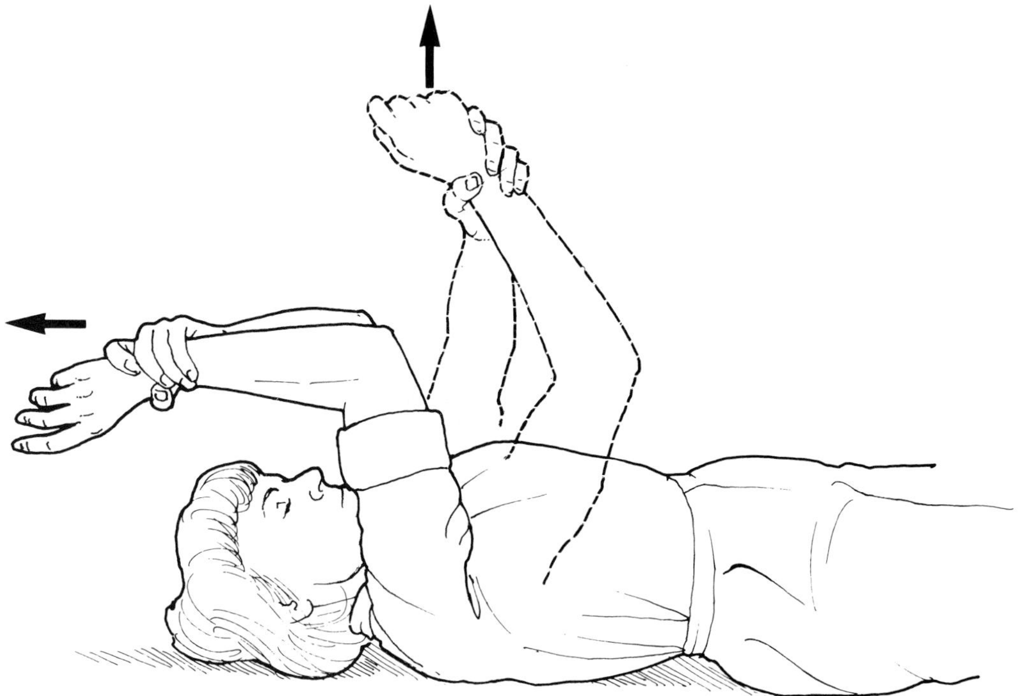

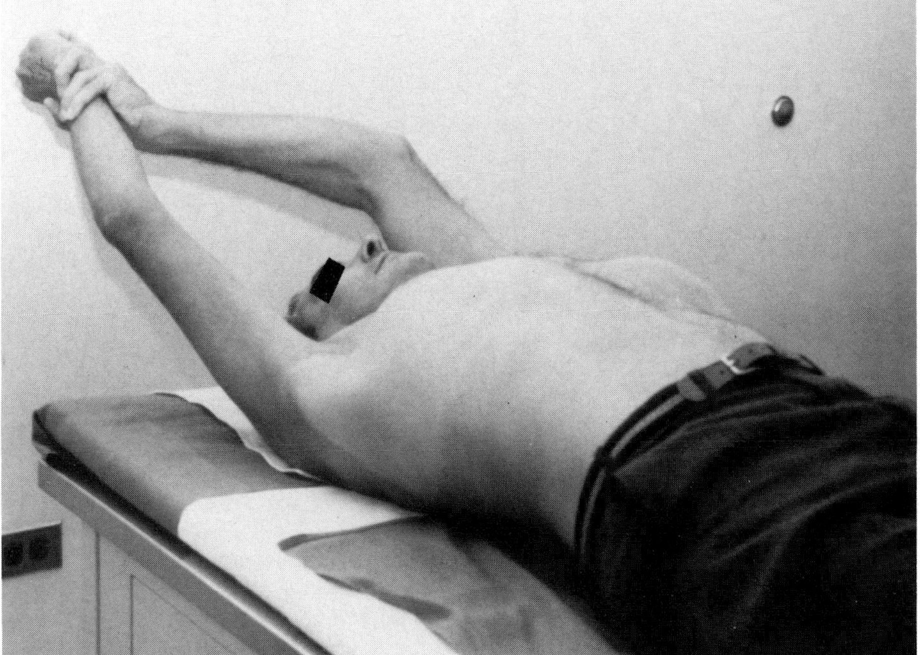

Figure 7–8E. Assisted Elevation Supine

Lying on the back, grasp the wrist of the stiff side with the good hand and pull the stiff arm:

A. Toward the ceiling and then,
B. Overhead.

Assisted Internal Rotation

Push the hands away from the body first and then bend the elbows (Fig. 7–8F).

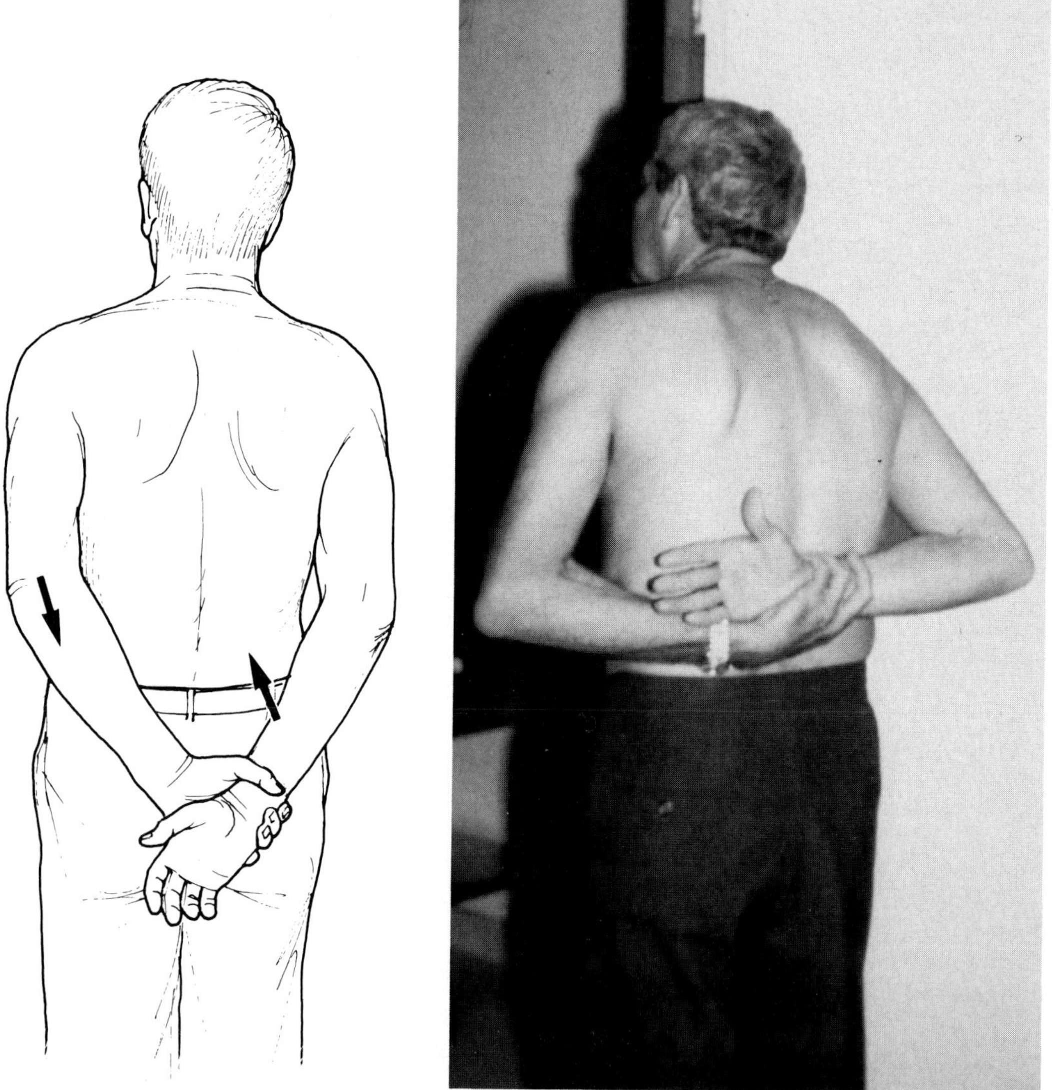

Figure 7–8F. Assisted Internal Rotation

While standing, grasp the wrist of the stiff arm with the good hand.

A. Push the arm backward as far as possible (as in Fig. 7–8C), and then,

B. Bend the elbows as far as possible, bringing the hand up between the shoulder blades.

Assisted Abduction

This exercise (Fig. 7–8G) introduces movement in the coronal plane (abduction) without the strain of raising the arm from the side (which is more difficult and can be discouraging for the patient).

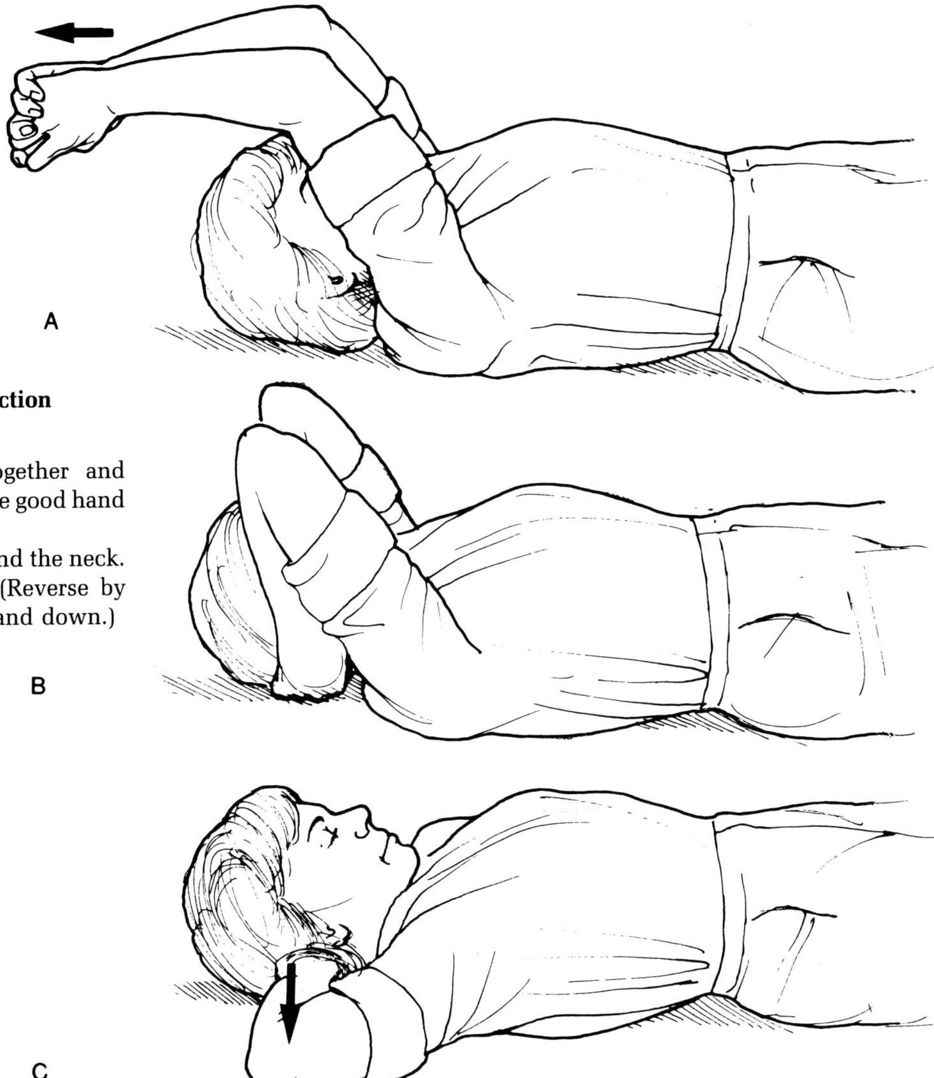

Figure 7–8G. Assisted Abduction

Lying on the back

A. Lock the fingers together and stretch the arms overhead (the good hand supplies the power).

B. Bring the hands behind the neck.

C. Flatten the elbows. (Reverse by sliding the hands overhead and down.)

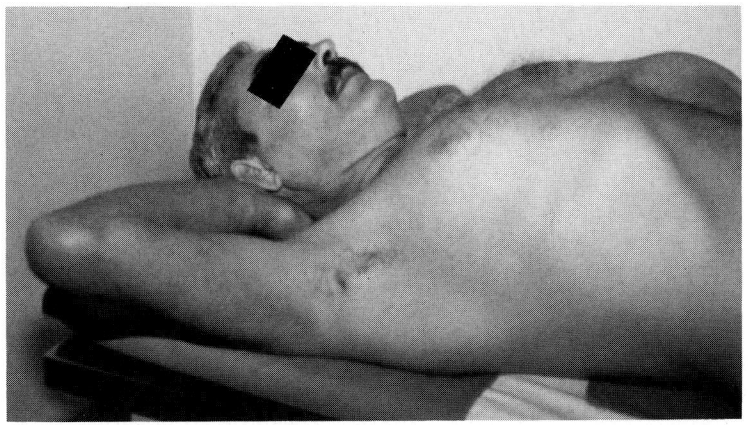

Assisted Elevation at Top of the Door

Patient faces the side of a door (Fig. 7–8H). Emphasize leaning forward to press the armpits on the door. An overhead bar in an open doorway is not as effective because the patient tends to lean over backward without a point of reference.

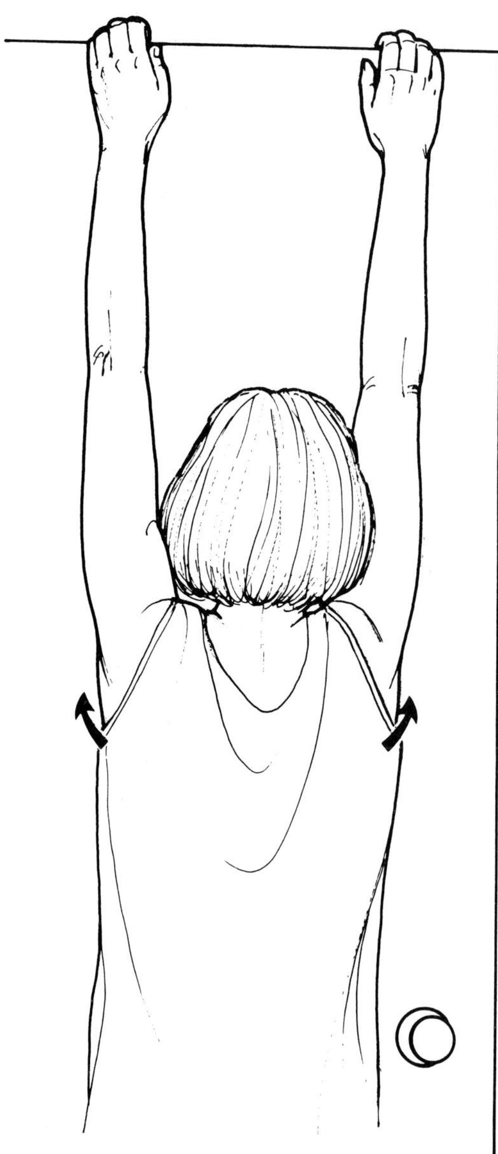

Figure 7–8H. Assisted Elevation on Top of the Door

Facing a door, help the stiff arm up with the good arm, hook the fingertips of both hands over the top of the door, bend knees to stretch, and lean forward, pressing the armpits forward against the door. *Do not* lean backward.

Assisted External Rotation in a Doorway

Emphasize keeping the elbow bent and walking in place (Fig. 7–8I).

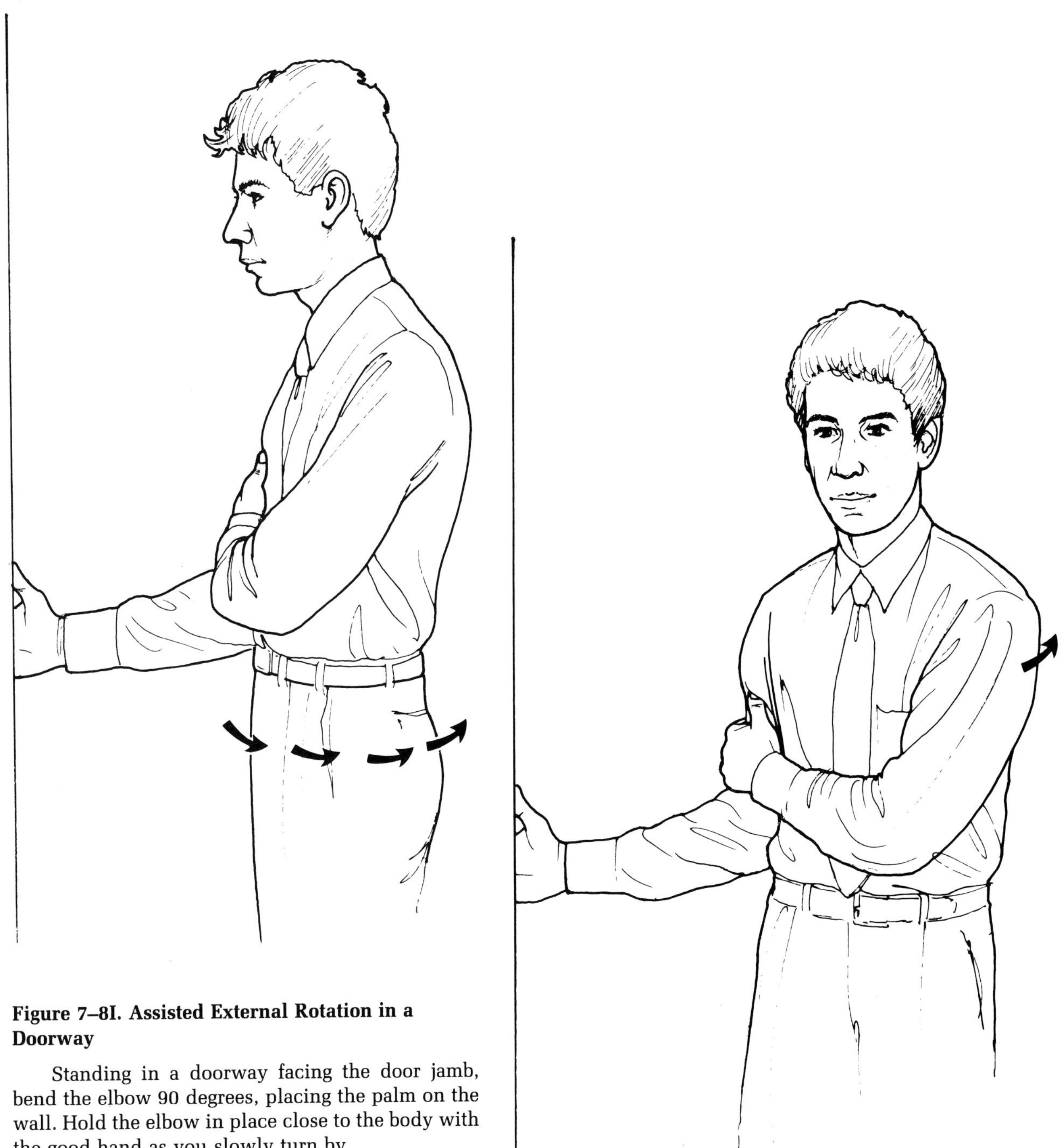

Figure 7–8I. Assisted External Rotation in a Doorway

Standing in a doorway facing the door jamb, bend the elbow 90 degrees, placing the palm on the wall. Hold the elbow in place close to the body with the good hand as you slowly turn by

A. Moving your feet in place, and

B. Dropping your good shoulder back until you face into the room.

Assisted Internal Rotation

This exercise (Fig. 7–8J) is used when the opposite shoulder, elbow, or wrist is too involved to assist the operated arm. This has been more effective than a towel or pulley in back because the arm is forced back away from the body.

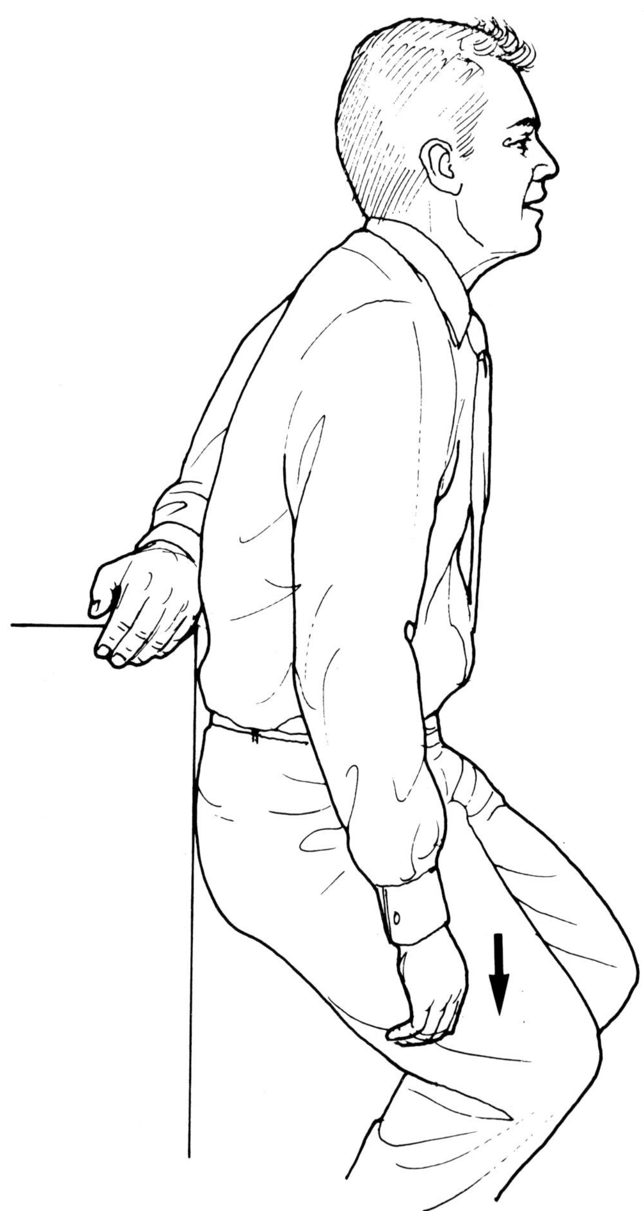

Figure 7–8J. Assisted Internal Rotation

Place the stiff arm behind you on a cabinet top and bend the knees to force the hand to move upward between the shoulder blades.

Self-Stretching Exercises for Motion

These exercises (Fig. 7–9A to E) are designed to eliminate any remaining stiffness after muscle sensitivity has subsided. The goal is to equal range of motion on the normal side. The exercises are done for five minutes at a time, two to four times a day as directed. When possible, precede each session with a brief warm-up period of pendulum exercises and heat (heating pad, hot water bottle, hot shower, and so on). Although existing shoulder motion may seem adequate, residual stiffness may cause pain at the extremes of motion, preventing the shoulder from "feeling right." Therefore, these exercises are often continued once daily for many months after an arthroplasty or fracture to achieve optimal results.

Sliding Up the Wall (Elevation)

The elbow is held rigid and straight. The feet are away from the wall to permit leaning forward, which causes the hand to slide up the wall. In the early stages the uninvolved arm is used to place the hand on the wall to start and to help it down when finished (Fig. 7–9A).

This is my favorite exercise in both the early and late stages. It is less strenuous than wall climbing with the fingers. It is superior to a pulley.

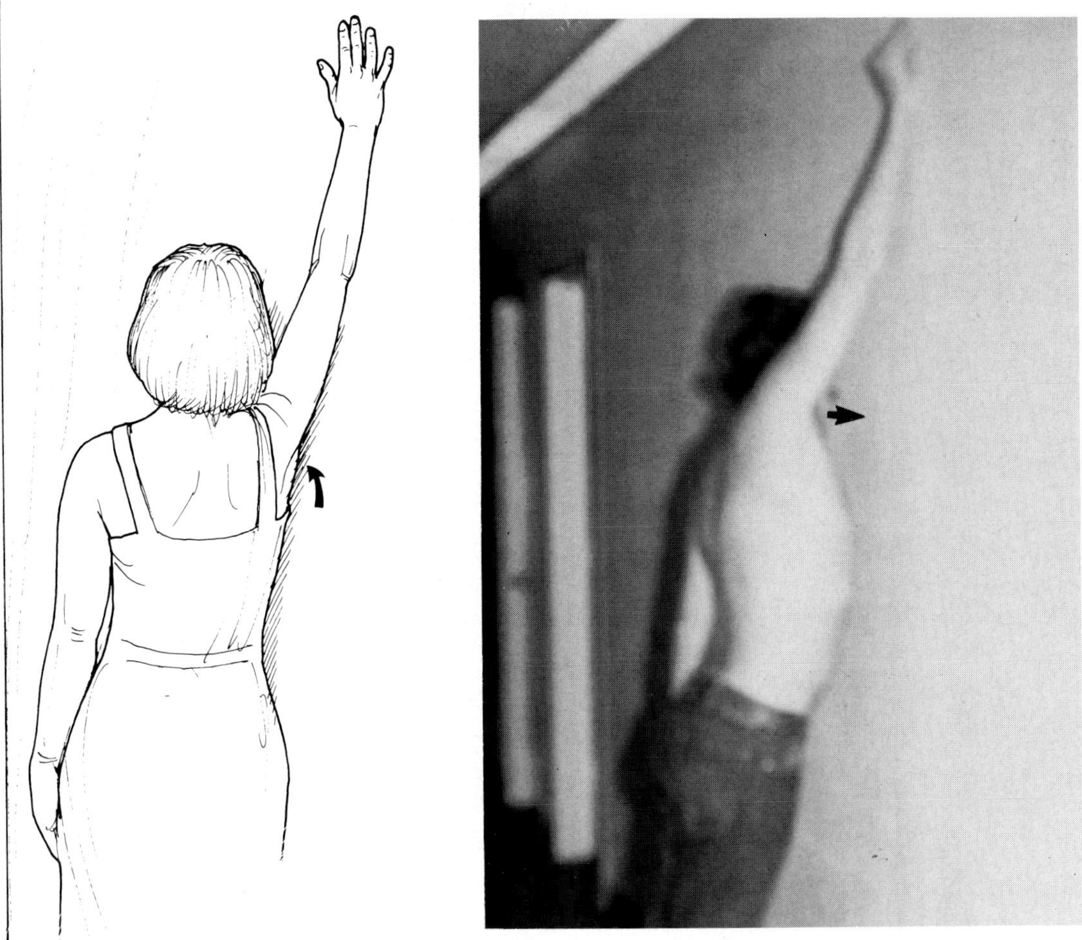

Figure 7–9A. Sliding Up the Wall (Elevation)

With the elbow straight, lean forward, sliding the hand up the wall as high as possible, then push the armpit forward against the wall. *Do not* lean backward.

End of Door (Elevation)

Patient faces the end of the door, standing to one side so the body does not collide with the door. The knee bend gives a gentle stretch as the armpit is pressed forward against the door (Fig. 7–9B).

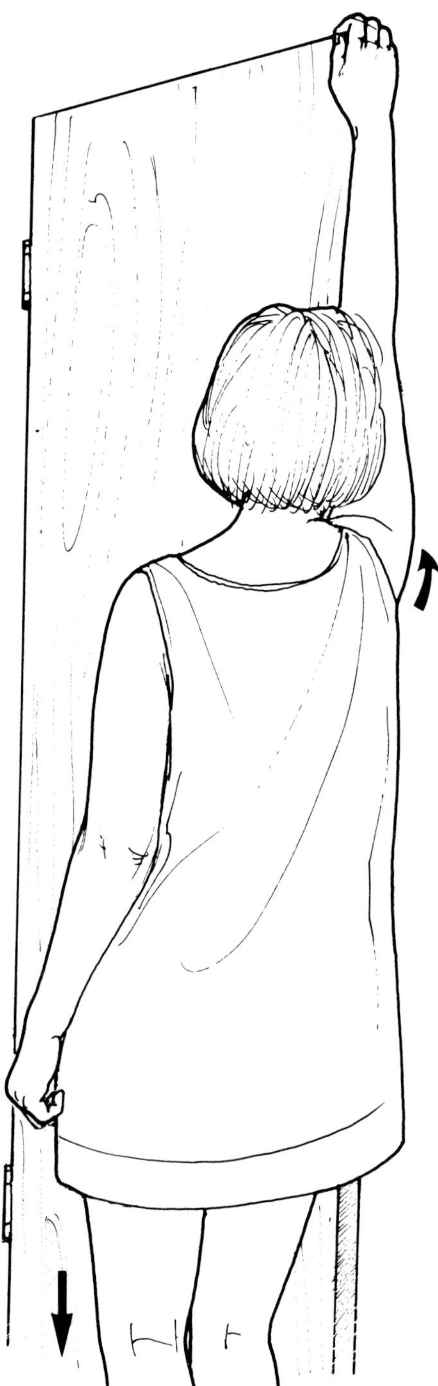

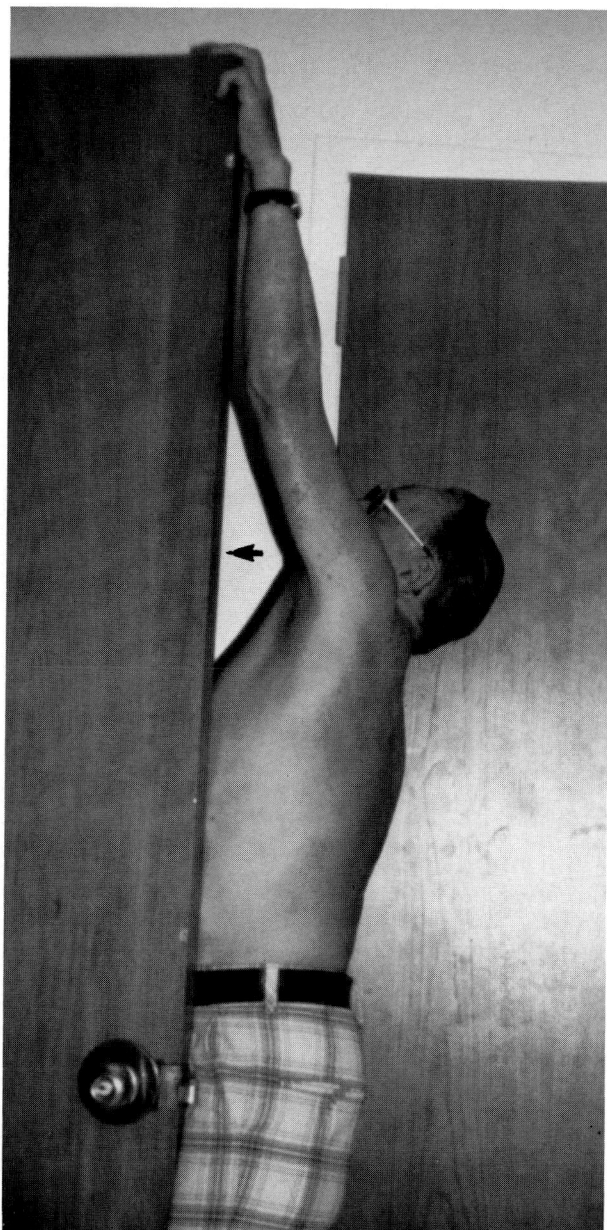

Figure 7–9B. End of Door (Elevation)

Hook the fingertips over the end of a door; then (a) bend the knees to stretch the arm upward, and (b) lean forward to flatten the armpit against the edge of the door. *Do not* lean backward.

Abduction in the Doorway

This exercise is important for reaching the back of the head, throwing, executing a serve in tennis, and reaching overhead (Fig. 7–9C). Think of the head moving in front of the hands.

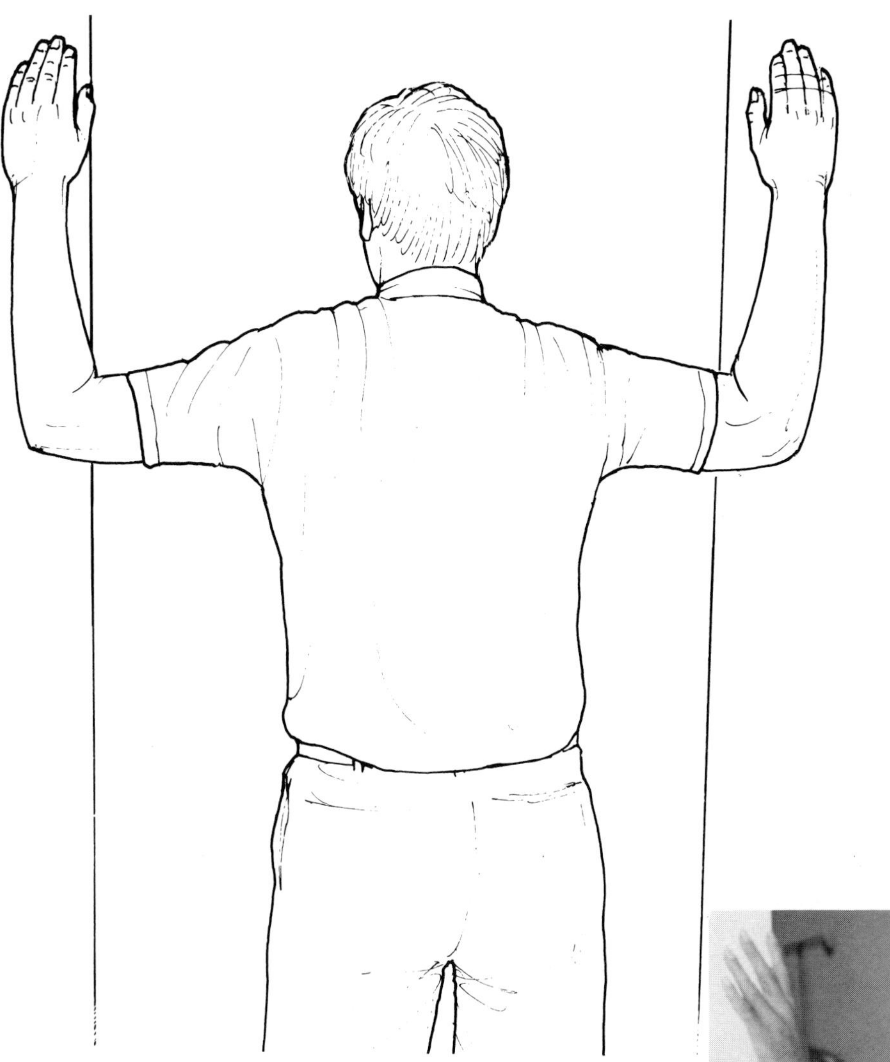

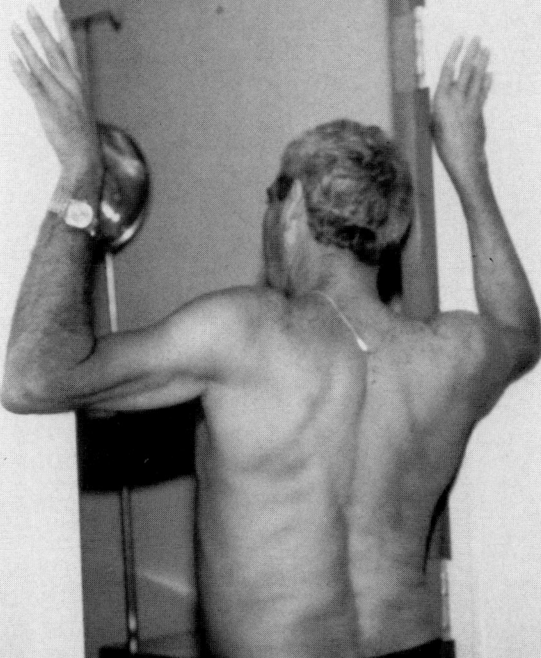

Figure 7–9C. Abduction in the Doorway

Stand in a doorway with the elbows bent 90 degrees and the arms held parallel to the floor. Hold the elbows against the door jamb and lean forward, stretching the arms backward as the body pushes forward.

Horizontal Adduction

This "diagonal" exercise helps to eliminate discomfort when sleeping on the involved side (Fig. 7–9D).

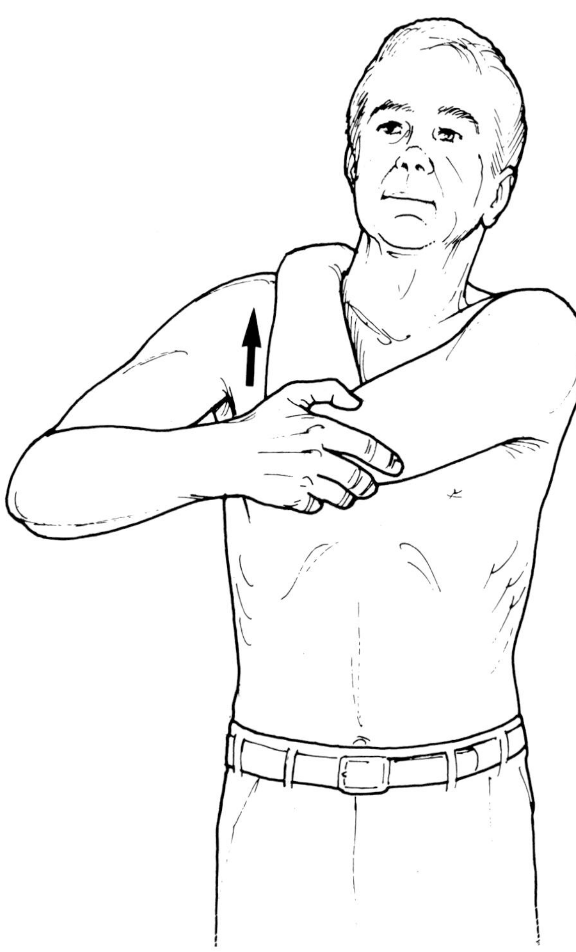

Figure 7–9D. Horizontal Adduction

Reach across the chest toward the back of the neck as far as possible, then grasp the elbow with the good hand and hug the elbow further across the body and flat against the chest.

Elevation Prone

This exercise (Fig. 7–9E) can be helpful when both shoulders are involved.

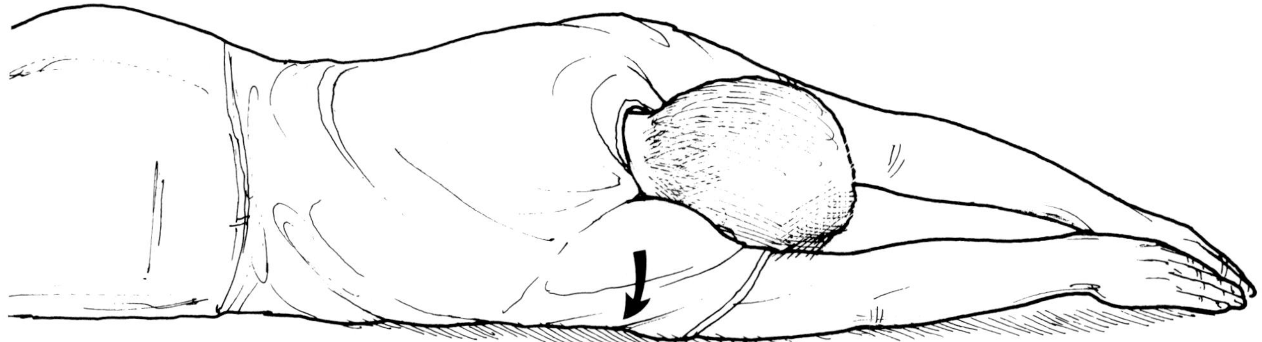

Figure 7–9E. Elevation Prone

Lying face down with the arms straight overhead, roll from side to side, flattening the armpits against the bed.

EXERCISES TO RESTORE STRENGTH

Isometric Exercises

These exercises (Fig. 7–10A through D) are designed to gain strength without moving a sensitive joint. Note that in isometric exercises no motion is allowed (i.e., motion is resisted and prevented by either the good arm or an immovable object such as the arm of a chair or a wall). These exercises can be done lying, sitting, or standing and can be repeated as often as desired throughout the day. Use only about two pounds of force. Set the muscles for five seconds and relax for five seconds with each movement, doing five movements during each exercise session.

Internal and External Rotators

Lying on the back, sitting, or standing, with the elbows bent 90 degrees and held close to the body, grasp the wrist of the weak side with the good hand and attempt to rotate the weak arm inward and outward, pushing against the good hand to prevent it from moving (Fig. 7–10A).

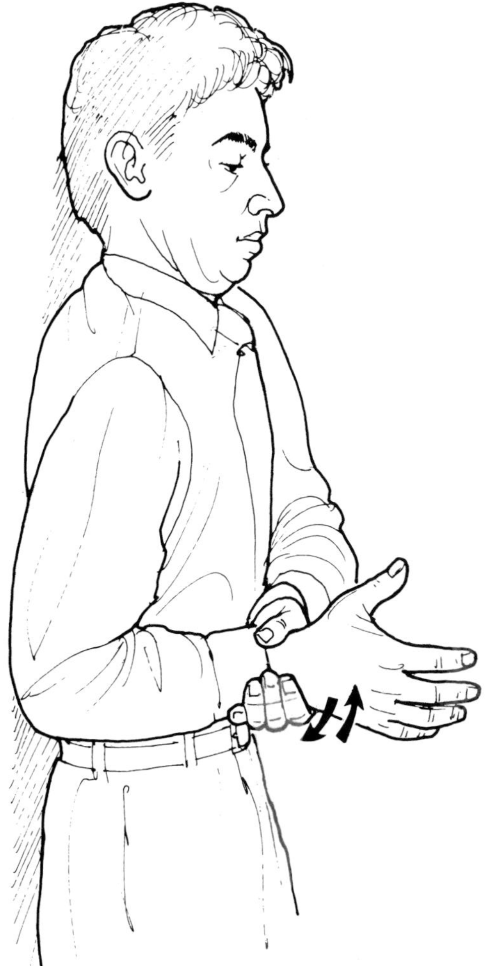

Figure 7–10A. Internal and External Rotators

Lying on the back, sitting, or standing, with the elbows bent 90 degrees and held close to the body, grasp the wrist of the weak side with the good hand and attempt to rotate the weak arm inward toward the chest and outward, pushing against the good hand. The good hand prevents the weak arm from moving. If sitting, the arm of a chair or, if standing, a wall may be used for resistance.

Extensors

This exercise (Fig. 7–10B) primarily strengthens the posterior deltoid muscle and latissimus dorsi muscle.

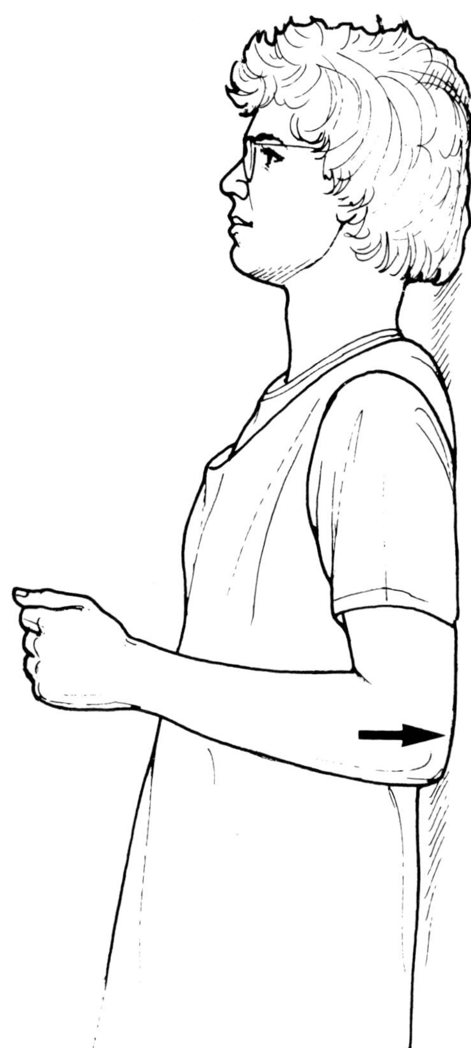

Figure 7–10B. Extensors

With the elbow flexed 90 degrees and held close to the body, press the body backward against a wall (standing), back of a chair (sitting), or bed (lying).

Middle Deltoid

This exercise (Fig. 7–10C) primarily gives tone to the middle deltoid muscle and supraspinatus muscle.

Anterior Deltoid

This exercise (Fig. 7–10D) begins to give tone to the anterior deltoid muscle, which is usually sensitive after surgery.

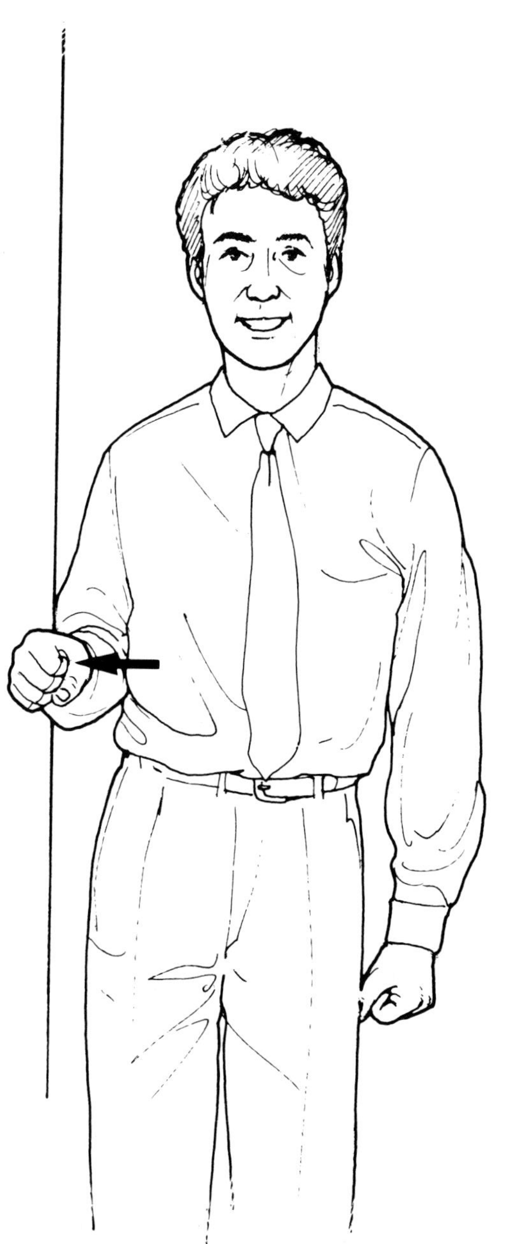

Figure 7–10C. Middle Deltoid

With the elbow flexed 90 degrees, attempt to push the arm out and away from the side against a wall (if standing) or arm of a chair (if sitting).

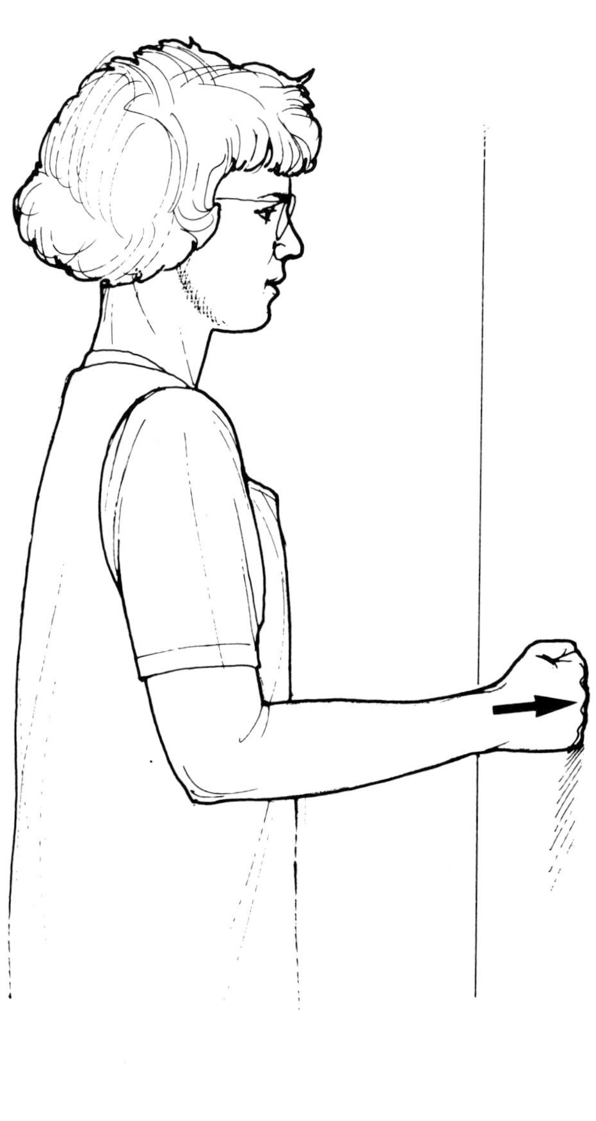

Figure 7–10D. Anterior Deltoid

While standing with the elbow bent 90 degrees, push the fist against a wall. (The good hand can provide resistance when sitting or lying.)

Active-Resisted Exercises for Strength

These exercises (Fig. 7–11A through E) are designed to build strength by progressive resistance. Hold each movement five seconds and rest five seconds between movements. Repeat each exercise five to ten times, once (or at most twice) a day. It is important to use the arm in daily activities. It is also important to do strengthening exercises infrequently enough to allow the muscles to recover between sessions.

Extensors

This exercise (Fig. 7–11A) is usually easy for the patient because the latissimus dorsi and posterior deltoid are rarely involved in the surgery.

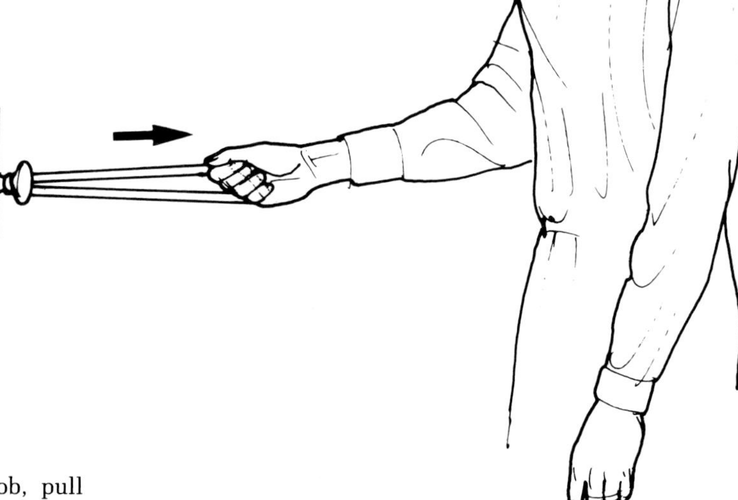

Figure 7–11A. Extensors

Holding a rubber around the door knob, pull backward and hold five seconds. Relax five seconds. Repeat.

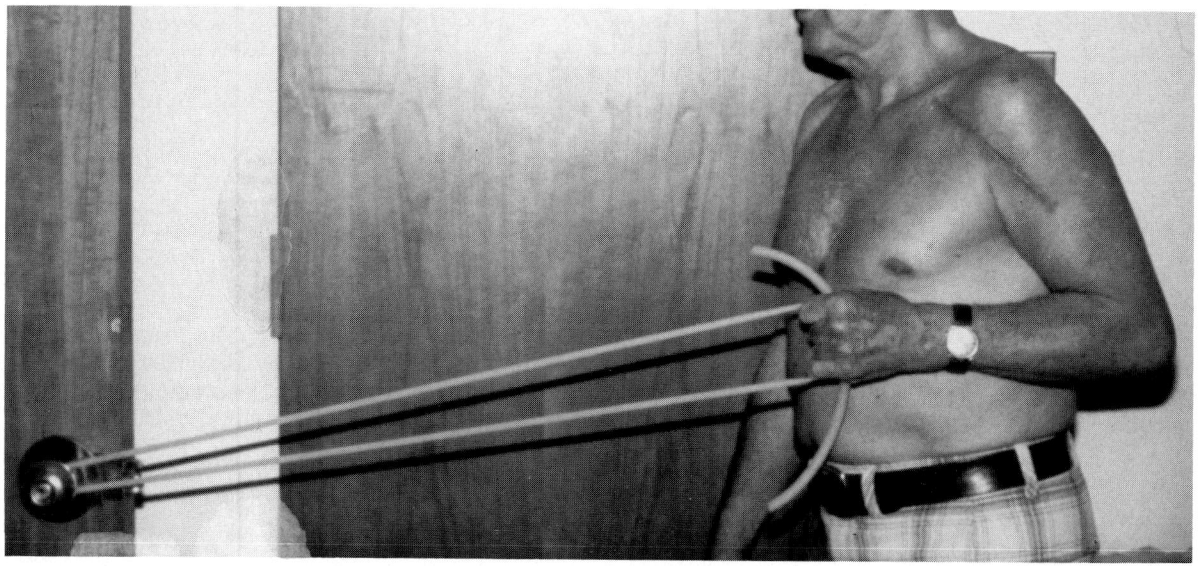

External Rotators and Middle Deltoid

When the deltoid is too weak, this exercise (Fig. 7–11B) can be done with the elbows held against the sides to strengthen the external rotators.

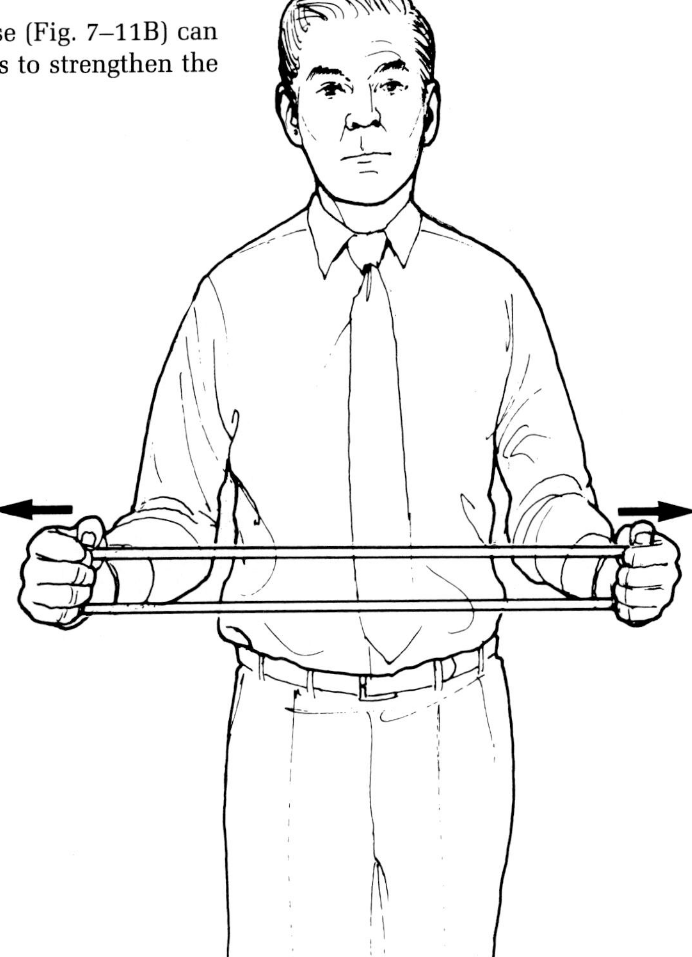

Figure 7–11B. External Rotators and Middle Deltoid

With both elbows bent 90 degrees and a rubber placed over the wrists, stretch the rubber by pulling the arms apart so that the elbows and hands leave the side of the body equally. Look in a mirror to be sure both arms are held in the same position. Hold five seconds. Relax five seconds. Repeat.

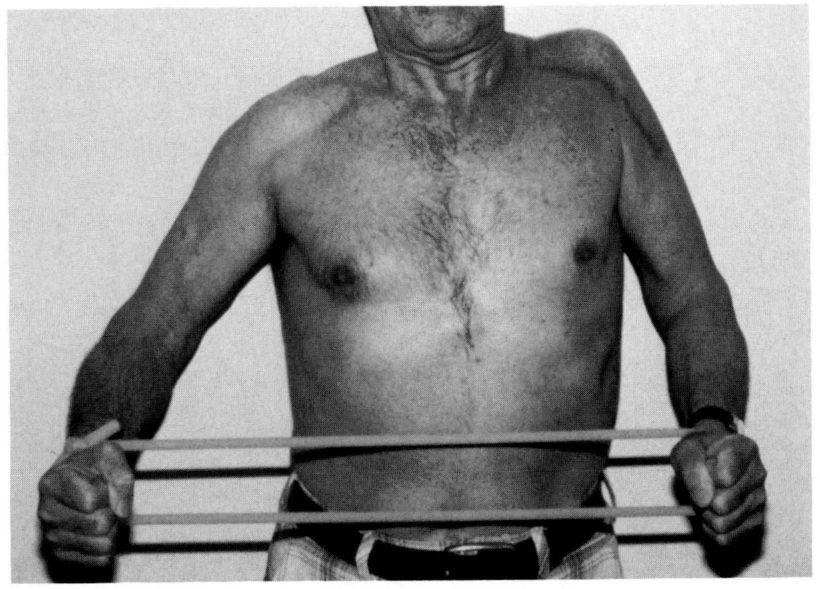

Anterior Deltoid

This exercise (Fig. 7–11C) usually starts with lighter strengths of rubber because the anterior deltoid is often sensitive from surgery.

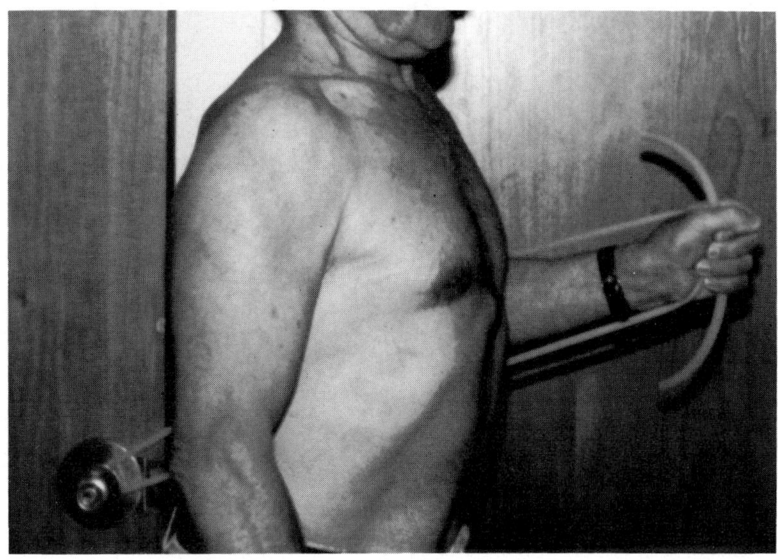

Figure 7–11C. Anterior Deltoid

With a rubber around the door knob and the elbow bent 90 degrees, push forward. Hold five seconds. Relax five seconds. Repeat.

Elevation ("Upper Cut")

This exercise (Fig. 7–11D) is especially useful if glenohumeral impingement or instability is present because it avoids the overhead position. (This exercise is used in the conservative regimen for instability and impingement [see Fig. 7–13].)

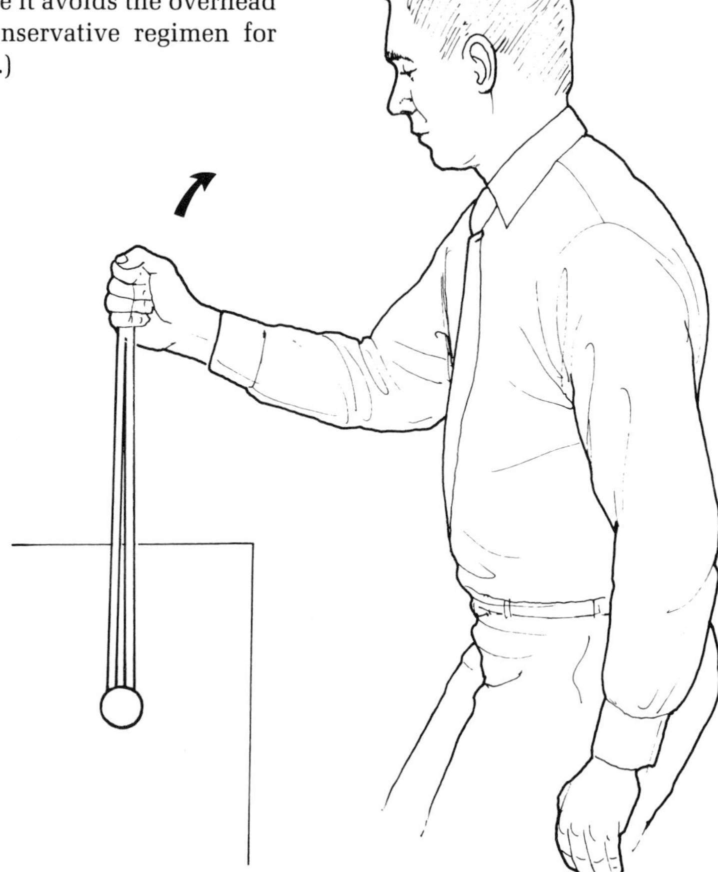

Figure 7–11D. Elevation ("Upper Cut")

With a rubber placed around the low knob of a cabinet and the elbow bent 90 degrees, lift forward and upward ("upper cut"). Hold five seconds. Relax five seconds. Repeat.

Weightlifting

This exercise (Fig. 7–11E) is used in selected patients who have good muscles and good stability. Heavy overhead exercises ("flies," etc.) and overhead weights should be avoided after most repairs for instability (see Chapter 4).

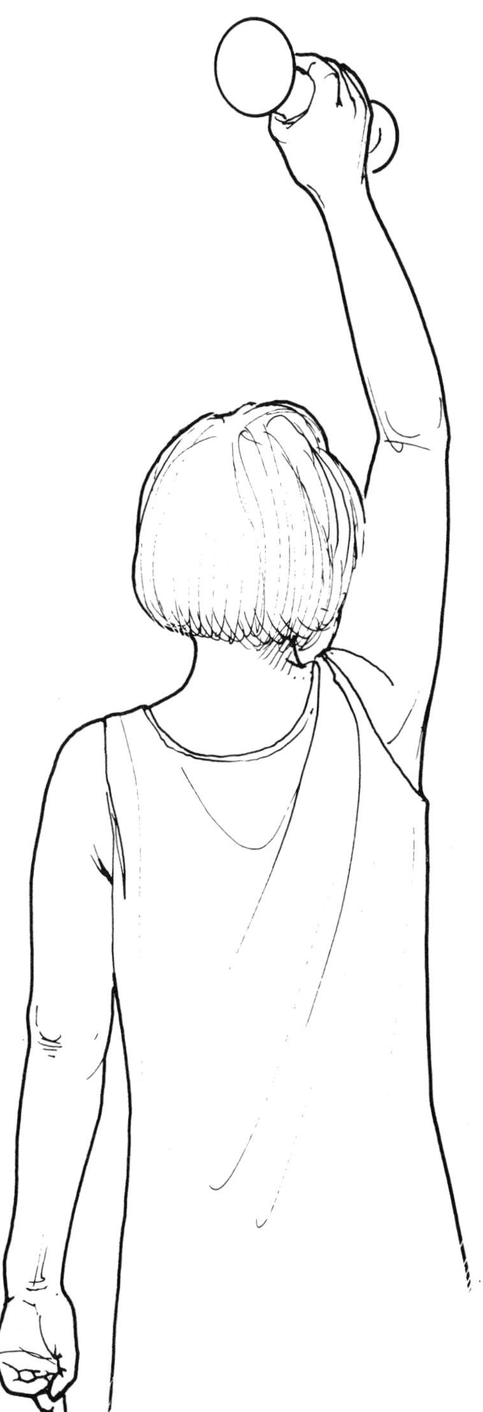

Figure 7–11E. Weightlifting

When one can easily raise the empty hand straight overhead, weights of from one to five pounds may be added progressively as directed. Heavier weights are rarely indicated in a post-operative program.

LEARNING HOW TO RAISE THE ARM OVERHEAD

These active-assistive exercises are shown in Figure 7–12A through E. Explain to the patient that just as in training for athletics, the muscles must be gradually strengthened. I teach my patients to hold the hand overhead and lower it slowly in a controlled manner before they attempt to raise it. Of course, adequate passive elevation is a prerequisite for these exercises.

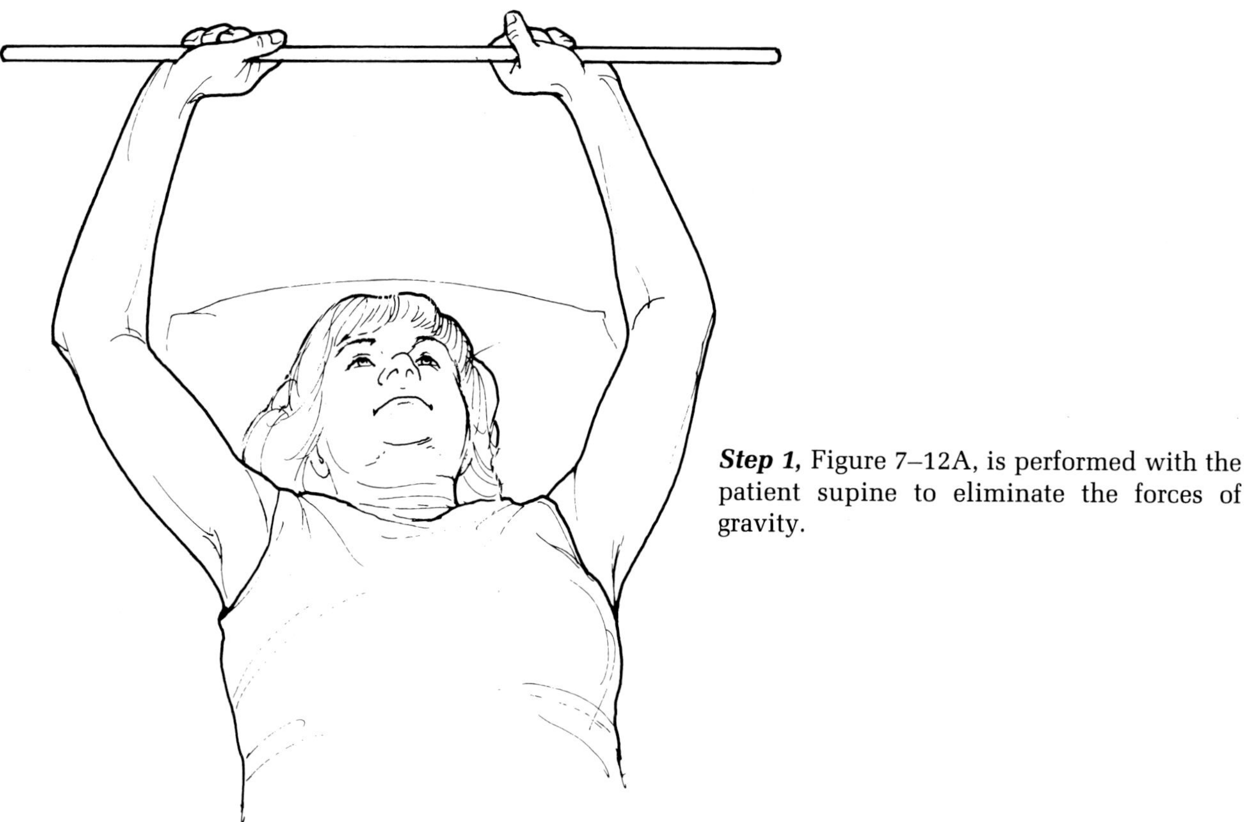

Step 1, Figure 7–12A, is performed with the patient supine to eliminate the forces of gravity.

Figure 7–12A. When Other Arm Is Strong, Supine Elevation with a Stick

In the *supine* position, grasp a stick in both hands and push straight upward and down as the elbows are bent and straightened. Later, let go of the stick when the hand is overhead and finally use less and less help as the arm is raised until the arm can be raised without the stick.

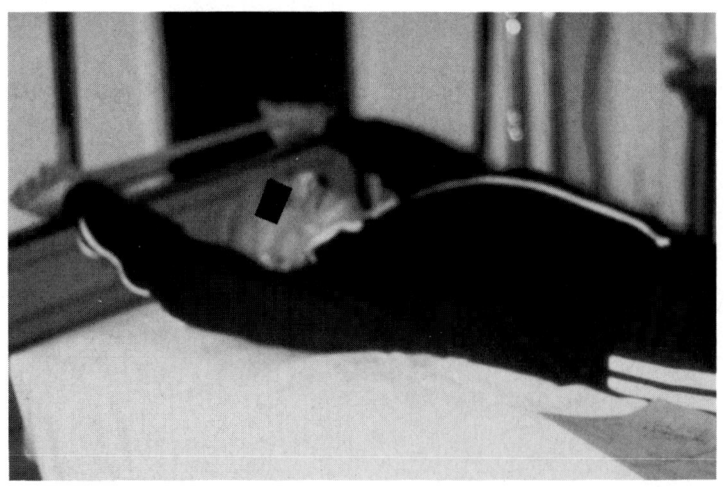

Step 2, Figure 7–12B, is performed without the stick and later with light weights for resistance.

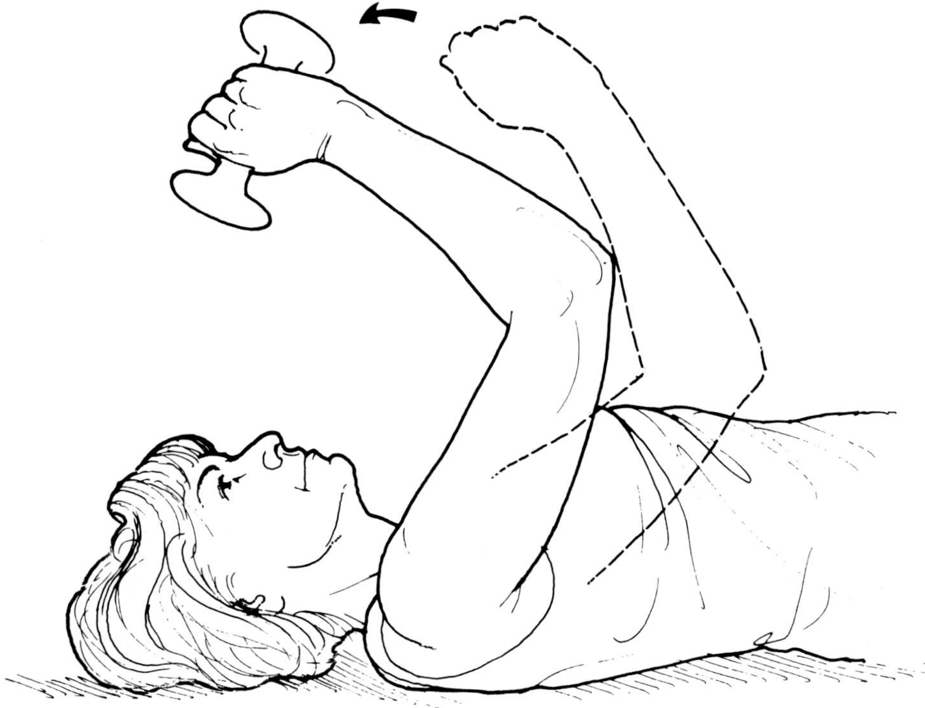

Figure 7–12B. Supine Elevation

While lying on the back, bend the elbow and stretch the arm overhead, then gradually lower it. Later the arm can be raised with the elbow straight and lifting graduated amounts of weight (from one to five pounds). (In special cases a similar exercise may be done while lying on the good side, with and without weights, to strengthen the external rotators and middle deltoid.)

Step 3, Figure 7–12C and D, teaches the patient to hold the arm overhead first, then to lower the arm, and finally to raise the arm with less and less help from the stick or pulley.

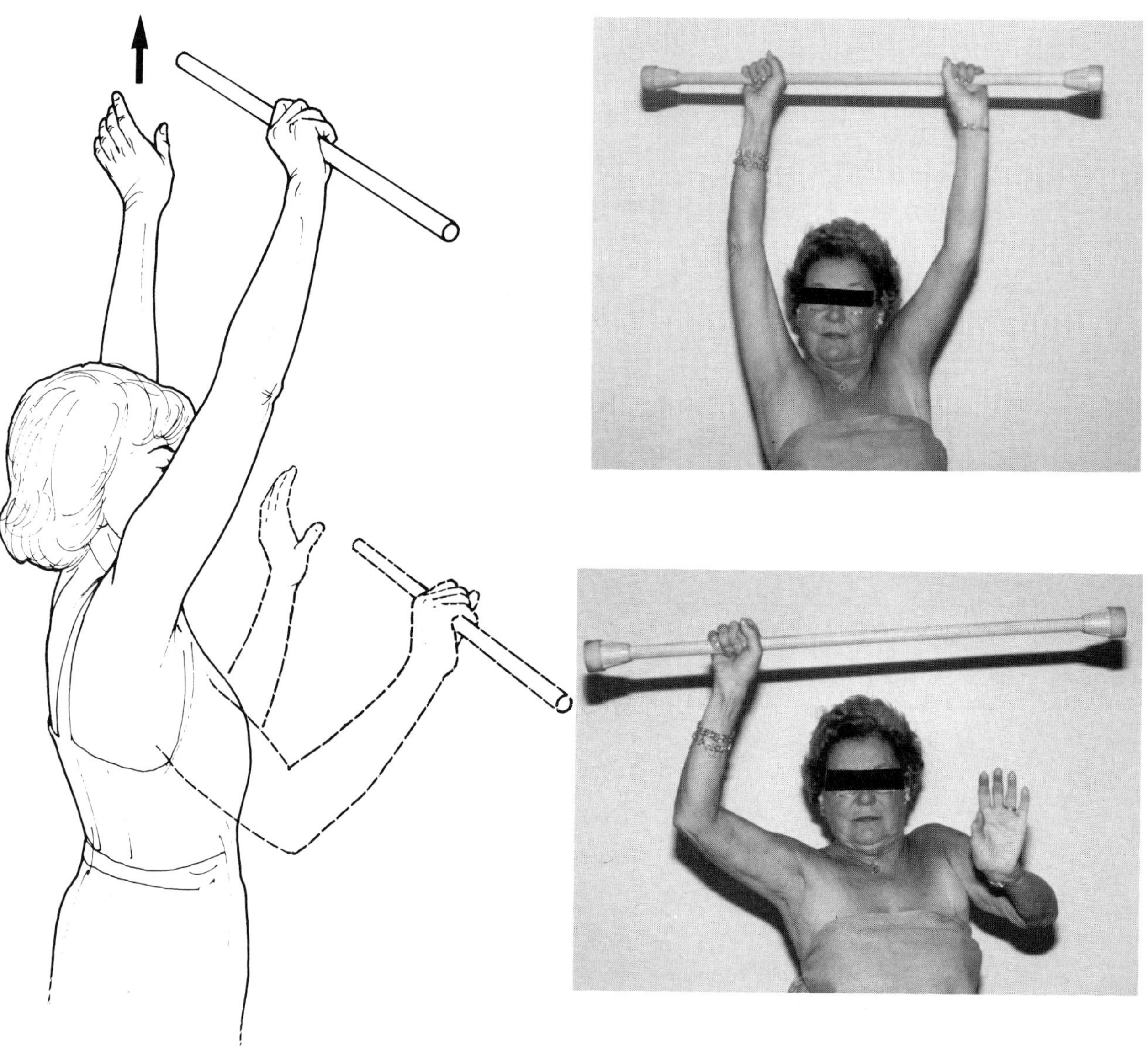

Figure 7–12C. Standing Elevation with a Stick

Standing, raise the arm as in Step 1 with as little assistance from the good hand as possible. When the hand is overhead, hold it toward the ceiling and attempt to let go of the stick. Lower the arms together with the least possible assistance from the good hand. No attempt is made to raise the arm without assistance until good control of holding the hand overhead and lowering the arm has been obtained.

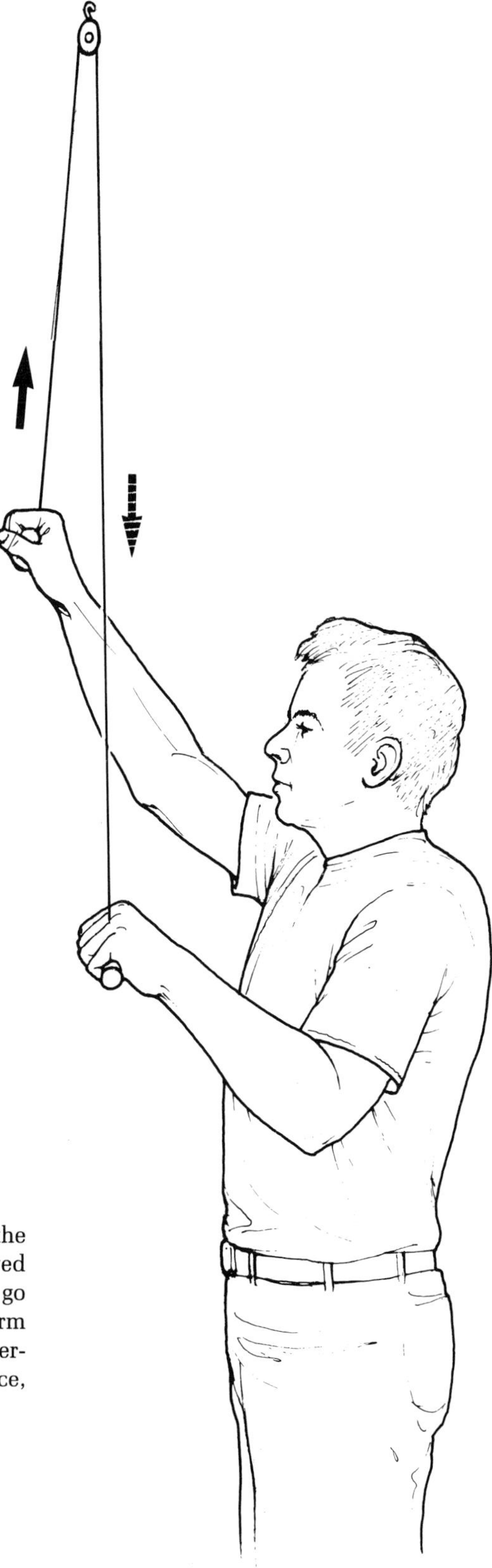

Figure 7–12D. When Other Arm Is Weak

When the other arm is weak, a pulley replaces the stick for standing elevation. *Standing*, pull the involved arm straight up overhead with the pulley and let go (progressively) with the good hand as the involved arm is lowered. When the involved arm can be held overhead and lowered in a smooth arc without assistance, begin serious work on trying to raise it by itself.

Step 4, Figure 7–12E, consists of standing elevation in front of a mirror assisted with the opposite hand (on the wrist or elbow).

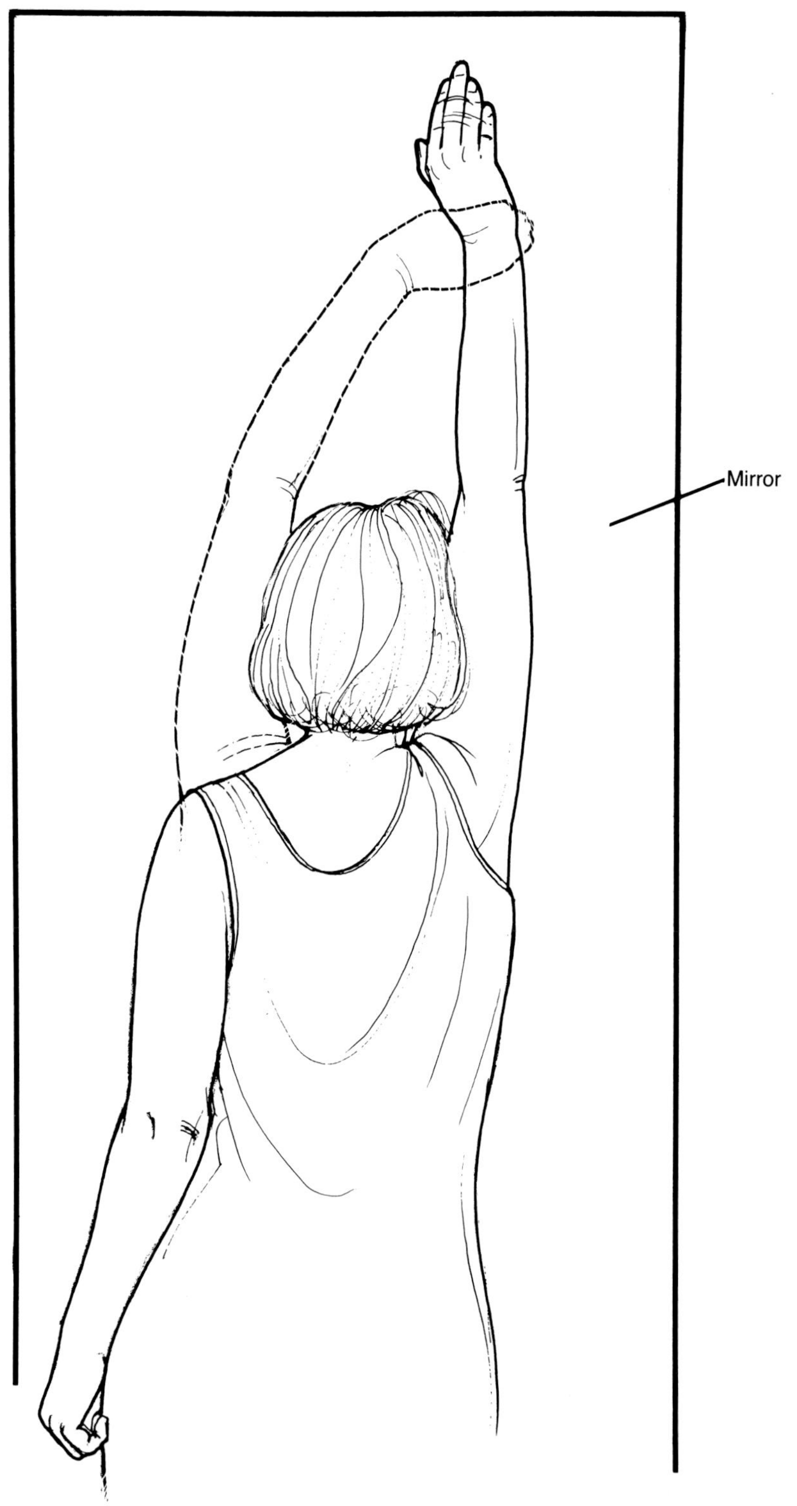

Figure 7–12E. Standing Elevation

Standing in front of a mirror, help raise the hand straight overhead with the good arm. Stretch the fingers toward the ceiling (raising the shoulder blade) and take the good arm away. Hold this position five seconds. Lower slowly. When this exercise can be done easily, try to raise the arm with less and less assistance.

STRENGTHENING EXERCISES AGAINST INSTABILITY AND IMPINGEMENT

These exercises (Fig. 7–13A to D) are used in the conservative treatment of instability and impingement as well as after surgery and are designed to strengthen the internal rotators (against anterior dislocations), external rotators (against posterior dislocation), and deltoid (against inferior dislocation) but without causing the irritation of the glenohumeral joint that results from too strenuous exercises that sublux the joint. Since the lower portions of the internal and extenal rotators are also depressors of the humeral head, these same exercises may be used to relieve subacromial impingement (for muscle tone to guard against ascent of the head). Also, these are the exercises used in the limited goals program (see p. 530). *No* exercise should be done with enough force to cause pain, and overhead exercises should be avoided. With each movement the muscles should be set five seconds and relaxed five seconds. Repeat each exercise five to ten times. One exercise session is advised daily, except for the first two exercises, which are done as often as desired.

Isometrics for Internal and External Rotators

Keep the elbow forward in line with the body to avoid stressing the anterior or posterior capsule of the glenohumeral joint (Fig. 7–13A). This exercise is repeated whenever the patient thinks about it throughout the day.

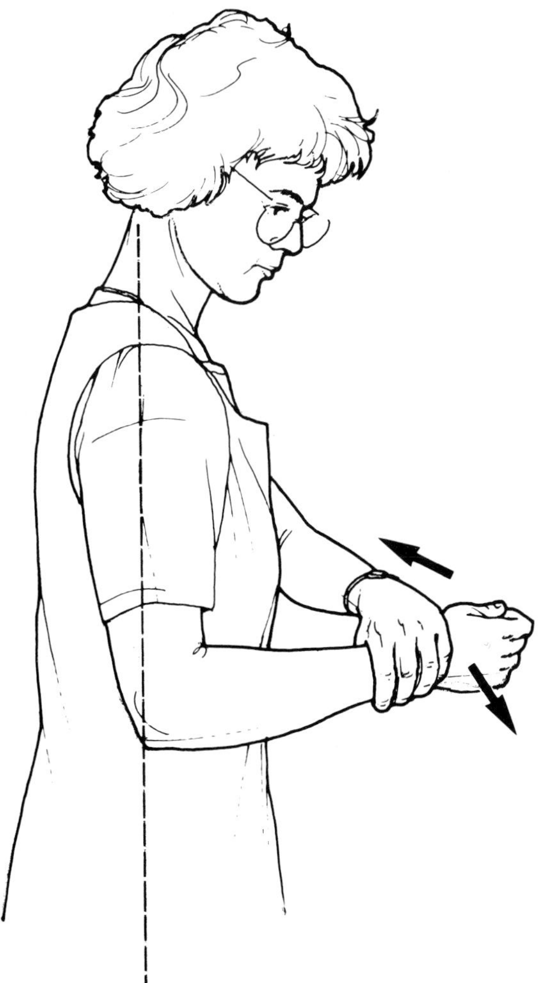

Figure 7–13A. Isometrics for Internal and External Rotators

Hold the elbow straight down at the side and bent 90 degrees. Grasp the wrist with the good hand and attempt to rotate the weak arm outward against the good hand. *Do not allow the elbow to drift backward or forward* of the dotted line.

Internal Rotators and Extensors

Keep the elbow of the involved arm forward. This exercise (Fig. 7–13B) is designed to strengthen the subscapularis without irritating the glenohumeral joint.

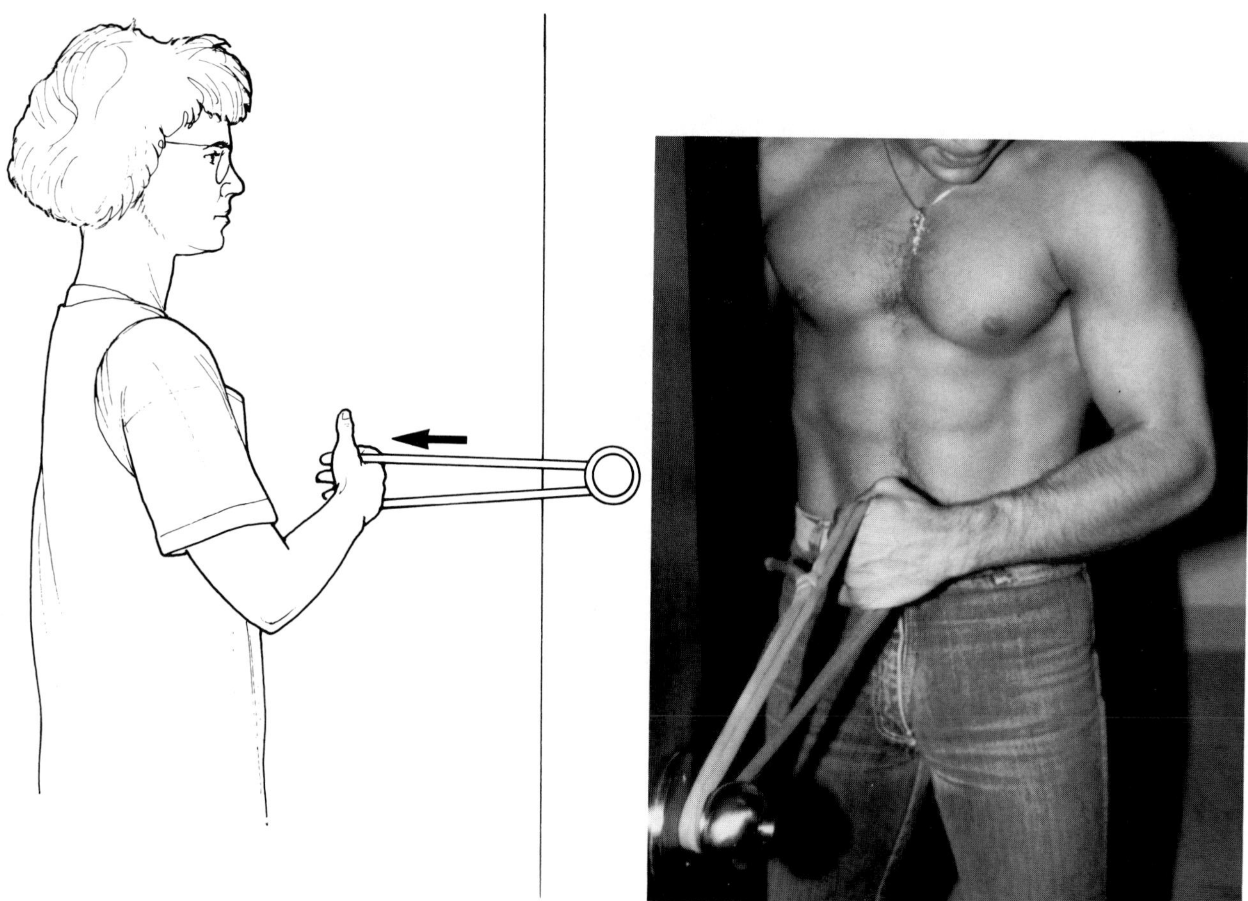

Figure 7–13B. Internal Rotators and Extensors

Hold the elbow forward well in front of the shoulder and bent 90 degrees. A rubber is placed around the door knob and hand, and the hand is held on the front of the chest. Lean back to generate resistance and hold this position for five seconds. Relax for five seconds. Repeat. It is usually helpful to use the opposite hand to help position the arm until proper resistance is obtained.

External Rotators and Middle Deltoid

Keep the elbows off the side of the body with the forearms pointing straight ahead (without external rotation, which will irritate the glenohumeral joint) (Fig. 7–13C). This exercise is especially important against posterior subluxations.

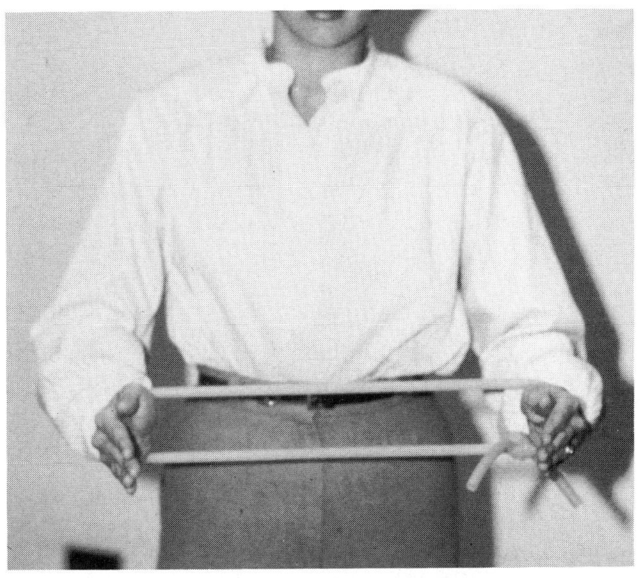

Figure 7–13C. External Rotators and Middle Deltoid

Hold the elbows off the sides and bent 90 degrees, with a rubber around each wrist. Move the arms apart equally while looking in a mirror. Hold this position for five seconds. Relax for five seconds. Repeat. *Do not* allow the elbows to drift backward of the dotted line shown in Figure 7–13A.

Anterior and Middle Deltoid and Supraspinatus ("Upper Cut")

Without irritating the subacromial space because of impingement or the glenohumeral joint because of instability by overhead activity, this exercise strengthens the muscles against inferior subluxation and also strengthens the supraspinatus against impingement (Fig. 7–13D).

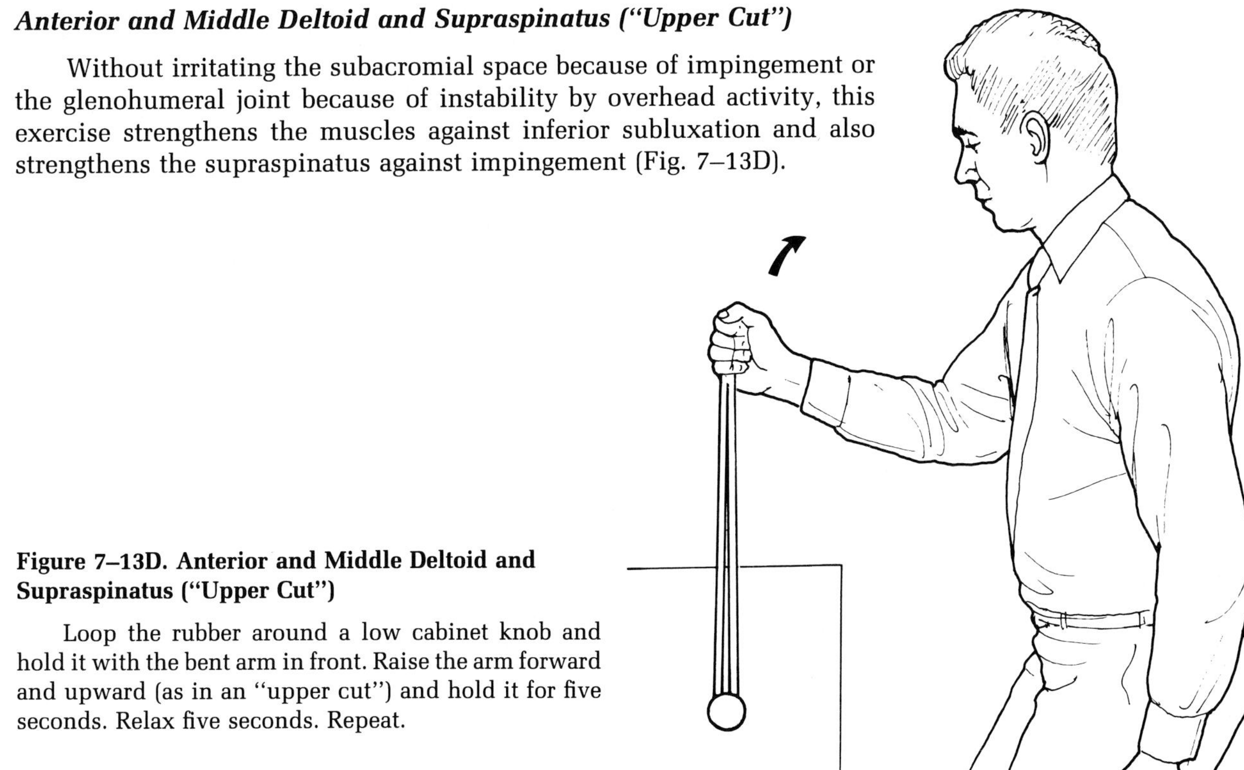

Figure 7–13D. Anterior and Middle Deltoid and Supraspinatus ("Upper Cut")

Loop the rubber around a low cabinet knob and hold it with the bent arm in front. Raise the arm forward and upward (as in an "upper cut") and hold it for five seconds. Relax five seconds. Repeat.

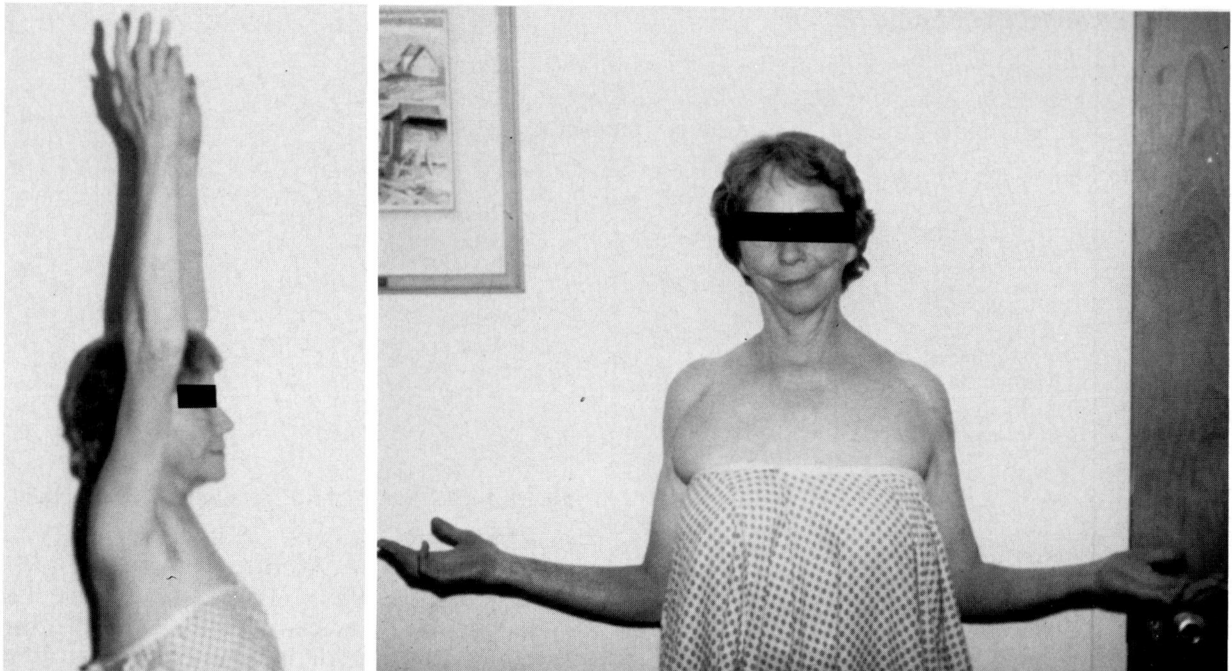

Figure 7–14. ***Late Aftercare.*** Better results after fractures, arthroplasties, and many shoulder reconstructions can be obtained by those patients who persist in occasional home self-stretching and strengthening exercises against residual defects, as illustrated by this patient, who had bilateral total glenohumeral arthroplasties for osteoarthritis (see Figs. 3–40 to 3–43). Her result as seen at 2 years is much better than it was at 6 months following surgery.

LATE AFTERCARE

Because of the large excursion of motion and many muscles supporting the normal glenohumeral joint, following fractures of the upper humerus and glenohumeral arthroplasties, improvement in range of motion and strength can continue for many months if the patient does home self-stretching and strengthening exercises against residual defects daily after a warm shower, as illustrated in Figure 7–14.

Many patients lose interest in exercises once their pain has been relieved and a functional range of motion achieved. However, those who persist in occasional brief exercise sessions and "warm-up" before activities can obtain the better results.

LIMITED GOALS EXERCISE PROGRAM

Indications for Limited Goals Rehabilitation

Some patients with extensive loss of the deltoid muscle, rotator cuff, and bone can be made comfortable and retain glenohumeral rotation without the restriction of glenohumeral arthrodesis (see Figs. 3–19 and 6–13), provided the rehabilitation program after surgery stresses use of the arm at the side and stability rather than a full exercise program. A glenohumeral arthroplasty for a resectable proximal tumor, cuff-tear arthropathy, or long-standing rheumatoid arthritis followed by this type of exercise program may provide quicker and more satisfactory results for the type of patient with these problems than an arthrodesis. A patient undergoing re-operation for a failed rotator cuff repair with a radical acromionectomy may also be suitable for this type of exercise program, which avoids overhead exercises and exercises extending into the extremes of rotation that make the glenohumeral joint unstable for no good reason because the muscles are inadequate to move the shoulder into those positions. Furthermore, because the contralateral shoulder is involved in some of these situations, glenohumeral arthrodesis is unwise.

Technique of Limited Goals Rehabilitation

The surgeon attempts to retain at least some musculature or transfer in front and in back of the humeral head to stabilize it against dislocation.

During the first three months following surgery, passive elevation to 100 degrees and external

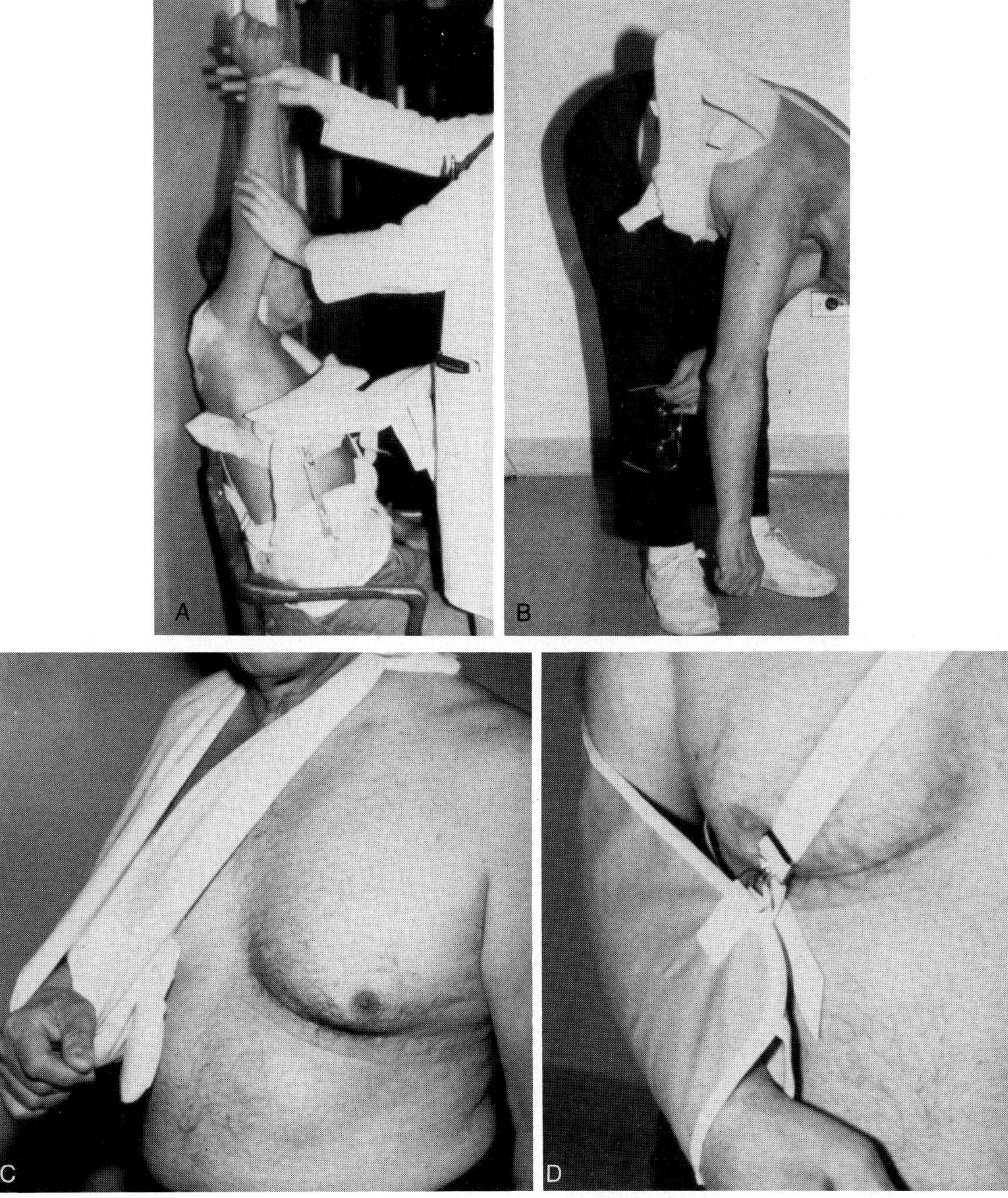

Figure 7–15. ***Rehabilitation of the Shoulder in a Brace.*** Adhesions around the rotator cuff and beneath the deltoid are prevented by the following regimen.

A, Earlier passive motion is begun about 24 hours after surgery and continued once or twice daily after discharge from the hospital by a friend or member of the family until the brace is removed.

B, About one week before the brace is to be discarded, pendulum exercises and practice lowering the arm to the side are begun.

C, On the first day after removal of the brace, a pad is worn with the sling to relieve the strain of lowering the arm. Pendulum exercises are continued.

D, On the following day, a removeable sling or no sling, depending on the nature of the repair, is used and the exercises are advanced as conditions permit.

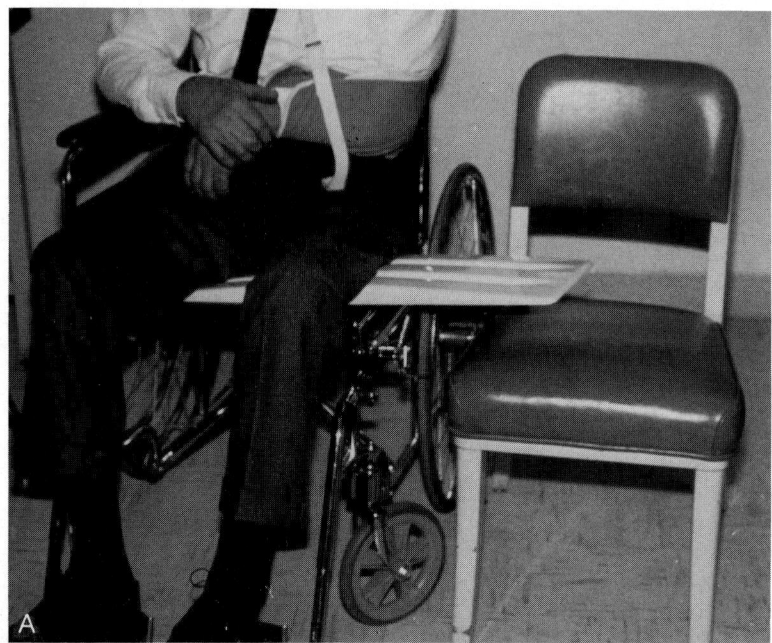

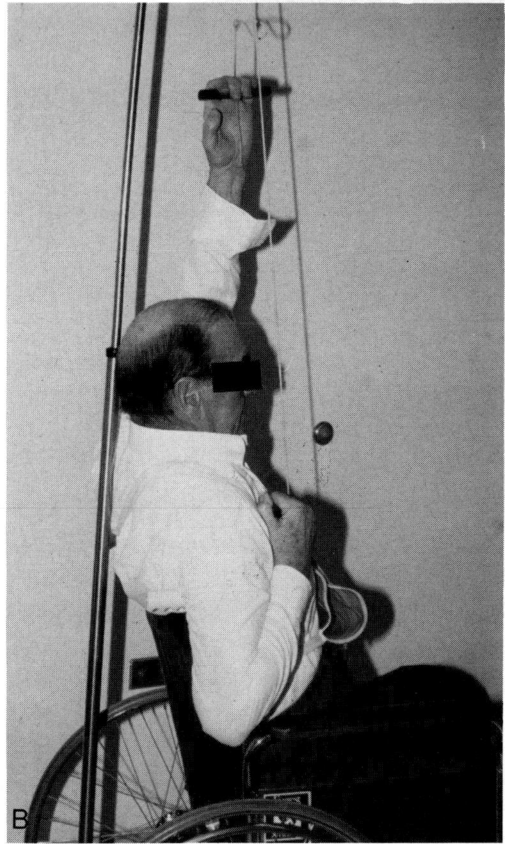

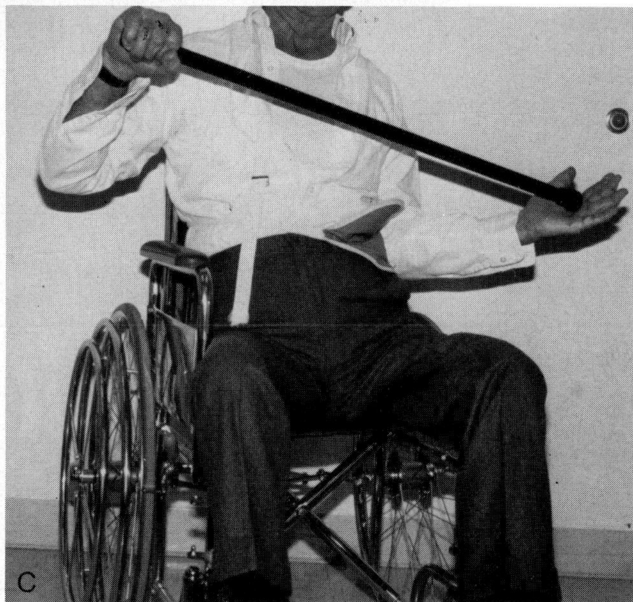

Figure 7–16. ***Shoulder Rehabilitation When There Are Nonfunctioning Lower Extremities.*** As discussed in the text, a wheelchair with a removeable arm rest and a sliding board (A) are essential. From this chair and from the bed, an almost normal shoulder exercise program can be performed, as illustrated in B and C.

A motorized tricycle with a seat that raises and lowers allows these patients to lead a good life without injuring the shoulder repair.

rotation to 20 degrees with the arm at the side are maintained easily with pendulum exercises. A sling is worn between these exercises. At three months after surgery the soft tissue is usually healed enough to discard the sling. By the fourth month the "instability exercises" (Fig. 7–13A to D) are started, beginning with isometric exercises (Fig. 7–13A). At the fifth month the patient progresses to using the rubber (Fig. 7–13B through D). After six months the patient progresses to activities as tolerated. Some patients later become strong and eventually can be advanced to some parts of the full exercise program.

The results of this procedure are discussed according to diagnosis throughout the book (e.g., acromionectomy in Chapter 2, arthroplasties for rheumatoid arthritis, old trauma, cuff-tear arthropathy, Erb's palsy deformity, neoplasms, and revisions in Chapter 3, and gunshot wounds in Chapter 5).

REHABILITATION OF THE SHOULDER IN A BRACE

Following some repairs of massive tears of the rotator cuff, re-repairs after failed cuff repairs, and re-attachment of the deltoid muscle to the acromion after prior surgery, a brace or pillow may be used to protect the repair (see Fig. 7–3; see also Chapters 2 and 3).

It is important to avoid the maturation of adhesions around the repair that can occur when the arm is in a brace. The care of the shoulder in a brace is depicted in Figure 7–15.

REHABILITATION OF THE SHOULDER WHEN THE LOWER EXTREMITIES ARE NONFUNCTIONING

Patients with paraplegia, severe lower extremity arthritis, injuries, and amputations present difficult problems in rehabilitation after shoulder reconstruction (see Chapter 2, p. 120; and Chapter 3, p. 167). The force of transfer of body weight with the arm is not tolerated by a repaired rotator cuff until healing is advanced. Unless the patient is willing to accept a full year without using the involved arm in transfers, the shoulder reconstruction should not be attempted.

For efficient movement and ambulation the first year after shoulder surgery without excessive use of the involved shoulder, it is important that the patient have proper equipment and training, preferably before the shoulder operation. An essential is a wheelchair with a removeable arm rest and sliding board (Fig. 7–16A) for transferring the body from bed to chair in the home. An almost normal post-operative shoulder exercise program can be done in this chair and in bed, as illustrated in Figure 7–16B and C. Home care is limited to one floor unless there is an elevator. Motorized tricycles with seats that raise and lower allow the patient to conduct a nearly normal life. Specially equipped automobiles may be helpful.

SHOULDER EXERCISES IN SPORTS

The exercise programs I have described above are used after shoulder surgery, to loosen frozen shoulders, and to help stabilize unstable shoulders[13, 262] and shoulders with impingement problems.[27, 262] The exercises used to restore range of motion and those aimed to stabilize the joint against instability or impingement (Fig. 7–13) have been extremely effective in the conservative treatment of athletes at all levels as well as in the conservative treatment of others. These exercises, which are for sensitive shoulders after surgery or injury (including shoulders of athletes), should be distinguished from the conditioning of normal shoulders for sports. The small traumatic cuff tears that are occasionally seen in athletes should be distinguished from the common impingement tears in the after-40-year age group (Chapter 2, pp. 62 to 70). Instability in athletes is discussed in Chapter 4, pages 277 to 327.

There has been no attempt here to consider the exercises needed for conditioning the shoulder in athletes who perform unusually strenuous tasks with their shoulders. For this the reader is referred to the existing literature.[261, 262, 282]

References

1. Kessel, L.: Clinical Disorders of the Shoulder. Ed. 1, p. 45. Churchill Livingstone, Edinburgh, London, Melbourne, and New York, 1982.
2. Neer, C. S. II: Replacement arthroplasty for glenohumeral osteoarthritis. J. Bone and Joint Surg. 56-A:1, 1974.
3. Inman, V. T., Saunders, J. B. de C. M., and Abbott, L. C.: Observations on the function of the shoulder joint. J. Bone and Joint Surg. 26:1, 1944.
4. Poppen, N. K. and Walker, P. S.: Normal and abnormal motion of the shoulder. J. Bone and Joint Surg. 58-A:195, 1976.
5. Poppen, N. K. and Walker, P. S.: Forces at the glenohumeral joint in abduction. Clin. Orthop. 135:165, 1978.
6. Codman, E. A.: The Shoulder. Ruptures of the Supraspinatus Tendon and Other Lesions In or About the Subacromial Bursa. Privately printed by Thomas Todd, Boston, 1934.
7. Brems, J. J.: Digital muscle strength measurement in rotator cuff tears. Orthop. Trans. 11:235, 1987.
8. Neer, C. S. II: Displaced proximal humeral fractures. Part I. Classification and evaluation. Part II. Treatment of three-part and four-part displacement. J. Bone and Joint Surg. 52-A:1077–1103, 1970.
9. Fukuda, K., Craig, E. V., An, K., Cofield, R. H., and Chao, E. Y. S.: Biomechanical study of the ligamentous system of the acromioclavicular joint. J. Bone and Joint Surg. 68-A:434, 1986.
10. Weaver, J. K. and Dunn, H. K.: Treatment of acromioclavicular injuries, especially complete acromioclavicular separation. J Bone and Joint Surg. 54-A:1187, 1972.
11. Vargas, L.: Repair of complete acromioclavicular dislocation utilizing the short head of the biceps. J. Bone and Joint Surg. 24:772, 1942.
12. Neer, C. S. II, Brown, T. H. Jr., and McLaughlin, H. L.: Fracture of the neck of the humerus with dislocation of the head fragment. Am. J. Surg. 85:252, 1953.
13. Neer, C. S. II and Foster, C. R.: Inferior capsular shift for involuntary inferior and multidirectional instability of the shoulder. A preliminary report. J. Bone and Joint Surg. 62-A:897, 1980.
14. Grant, J. C. B.: An Atlas of Anatomy. Ed. 3. Williams and Wilkins, Baltimore, 1951.
15. Bloom, M. H. and Obata, W. G.: Diagnosis of posterior dislocations of the shoulder with use of Velpeau axillary and angle-up roentgen views. J. Bone and Joint Surg. 49-A:943, 1967.
16. Bankart, A. S. B.: Recurrent or habitual dislocation of the shoulder joint. Brit. Med. J. 2:1132, 1923.
17. DePalma, A. F.: Surgery of the Shoulder. Ed. 2. J. B. Lippincott, Philadelphia and Toronto, 1973.
18. Ferrari, D. A.: Anterior superior anatomy of the shoulder. (Presented to the American Shoulder and Elbow Surgeons, 1984.) Orthop. Trans. 9:42, 1985.
19. Neer, C. S. II, Fithian, T. E., Hansen, P. E., Ogawa, K., and Brems, J. J.: Reinforced cruciate repair for anterior dislocation of the shoulder. Orthop. Trans. 9:44, 1985.
20. Neer, C. S. II, Cruess, R. L., Sledge, C. B., and Wilde, A. H.: Total glenohumeral replacement. A preliminary report. Orthop. Trans. 1:244, 1977.
21. Neer, C. S. II: Reconstructive surgery and rehabilitation of the shoulder. In Textbook of Rheumatology, edited by W. N. Kelley, E. D. Harris, Jr., S. Ruddy, and C. B. Sledge. Ed. 1, Vol 11: p. 1944. W. B. Saunders Company, Philadelphia, 1981.
22. Neer, C. S. II, Watson, K. C., and Stanton, F. J.: Recent experience in total shoulder replacement. J. Bone and Joint Surg. 64-A:319, 1982.
23. Neer, C. S. II, Craig, E. V., and Fukuda, H.: Cuff-tear arthropathy. (Presented to the American Orthopaedic Association, June 1981.) Orthop. Trans. 5:447, 1981.
24. Neer, C. S. II, Craig, E. V., and Fukuda, H.: Cuff-tear arthropathy. J. Bone and Joint Surg. 65-A:1232, 1983.
25. McCarty, D. J., Halverson, P. B., Carriera, C. F., Brewer, B. J., and Kozin, F.: Milwaukee shoulder. Association of microspheroids containing hydroxyapatite crystals, active collagens and neutral protease with rotator cuff defects. J. Clinical Aspects Arthrit. and Rheumat. 24:464, 1981.
26. Neer, C. S. II, Bigliani, L. U., and Hawkins, R. J.: Rupture of the long head of the biceps related to subacromial impingement. Orthop. Trans. 1:111, 1977.
27. Neer, C. S. II: Impingement lesions. Clin. Orthop. 173:70, 1983.
28. Neer, C. S. II: Anterior acromioplasty for the chronic impingement syndrome in the shoulder. J. Bone and Joint Surg. 54-A:41, 1972.
29. Neer, C. S. II and Marberry, T. A.: On the disadvantages of radical acromionectomy. J. Bone and Joint Surg. 63-A:416, 1981.
30. Saha, A. K.: Theory of Shoulder Mechanism. Charles C. Thomas, Springfield, Illinois, 1961.
31. Leslie, J. T. and Ryan, T. J.: An anterior axillary incision to approach the shoulder joint. J. Bone and Joint Surg. 44-A:1193, 1962.
32. Neer, C. S. II and Poppen, N. K.: Supraspinatus outlet. Orthop. Trans. 11:234, 1987.
33. MacNab, I. and Rathbun, J. B.: The microvascular pattern of the rotator cuff. J. Bone and Joint Surg. 52-B:540, 1970.
34. Debeyre, J., Patte, D., and Elmelik, E.: Repair of ruptures of the rotator cuff of the shoulder. J. Bone and Joint Surg. 47-B:36, 1965.

35. Armstrong, J. R.: Excision of the acromion in treatment of the supraspinatus syndrome. Report of 95 excisions. J. Bone and Joint Surg. 31-B:436, 1949.
36. Watson-Jones, R.: Fractures and Joint Injuries. Ed. 4, Vol. II, p. 449. Williams and Wilkins, Baltimore, 1960.
37. Hammond, G.: Complete acromionectomy in the treatment of chronic tendinitis of the shoulder. J. Bone and Joint Surg. 44-A:494, 1962.
38. McLaughlin, H. L.: Lesions of the musculotendinous cuff of the shoulder. The exposure and treatment of tears with retraction. J. Bone and Joint Surg. 26:31, 1944.
39. Neer, C. S. II: Chapter 111, The Shoulder, pp. 2013–2026. In Textbook of Rheumatology, edited by W. N. Kelley, E. D. Harris, Jr., S. Ruddy, and C. B. Sledge. Ed. 3. W. B. Saunders Company, Philadelphia, 1989.
40. Smith-Petersen, M. N., Aufranc, O. E., and Larson, C. B.: Useful surgical procedures for rheumatoid arthritis involving joints of the upper extremity. Arch. Surg. 46:764, 1943.
41. Skinner, H.: Anatomical considerations relative to rupture of the supraspinatus tendon. J. Bone and Joint Surg. 19:137, 1937.
42. Neer, C. S. II: Articular replacement of the humeral head. J. Bone and Joint Surg. 37-A:215, 1955.
43. Codman, E. A.: Rupture of the supraspinatus tendon. Surg. Gyn. Obst. 52:579, 1931.
44. Meyer, A. W.: The minuter anatomy of attrition lesions. J. Bone and Joint Surg. 13:341, 1931.
45. Meyer, A. W.: Further observations upon use-destruction in joints. J. Bone and Joint Surg. 4:491, 1922.
46. Grantham, A. and Neer, C. S. II: Alkaptonuric ochronosis. N. Y. Ortho. Hosp. Bull. 4:11, 1960.
47. Neer, C. S. II: Prosthetic replacement of the humeral head. Indications and operative technique. Surg. Clin. No. Am. 43:1581, 1963.
48. Neer, C. S. II: Follow-up notes on articles previously published in the journal. Articular replacement for the humeral head. J. Bone and Joint Surg. 46-A:1607, 1964.
49. Moseley, H. F. and Goldie, I.: The arterial pattern of the rotator cuff. J. Bone and Joint Surg. 45-B:780, 1963.
50. Moseley, H. F.: Shoulder Lesions. Ed. 3. E. and S. Livingstone, Edinburgh and London, 1969.
51. Neer, C. S. II and Welsh, R. P.: The shoulder in sports. Ortho. Clin. No. Am. 8:583, 1977.
52. Fukuda, H.: Study of rotator cuff in cadavers. Partial thickness tears of the rotator cuff (personal communication).
52a. Yamanaka, K. and Fukuda, H.: Pathologic studies of the supraspinatus tendon with reference to incomplete tears. In The Shoulder, p. 220, edited by N. Takagishi. Professional Postgraduate Services, Tokyo, 1987.
53. Petersson, C. J. and Gentz, C. F.: Ruptures of the supraspinatus tendon. The significance of distally pointing acromioclavicular osteophytes. Clin. Orthop. 174:143, 1983.
54. Neer, C. S. II: Chapter 17, The rheumatoid shoulder. In Surgery of Rheumatoid Arthritis, edited by R. L. Cruess and N. Mitchell. J. B. Lippincott, Philadelphia, 1971.
55. Tibone, J. E., Elrod, B., Jobe, F. W., Kerlan, R. K., Carter, V. S., Shields, C. L., Lombardo, S. J., and Yocum, L.: Surgical treatment of tears of the rotator cuff in athletes. J. Bone and Joint Surg. 68-A:887, 1986.
56. Smith, J. G.: Injury of the shoulder-joint. London Med. Gazette 14:280, 1834.
57. Keyes, E. L.: Anatomical observations on senile changes in the shoulder. J. Bone and Joint Surg. 17:953, 1935.
58. Olsson, O.: Degenerative changes of the shoulder joint and their connection with shoulder pain. Acta Chir. Scand. Suppl. 181, 1953.
59. Satterlee, C. C. and Dalsey, R. M.: Study of the incidence of complete tears of the rotator cuff in the anatomy laboratory at Columbia University (unpublished), 1988.
59a. Grant, J. C. B. and Smith, C. G.: Age incidence of rupture of the supraspinatus tendon. Anatomical Record 100:666, 1948.
60. Ellman, H.: Arthroscopic subacromial decompression. A preliminary report. Orthop. Trans. 9:49, 1985.
61. Dewar, R. P. and Harris, M.D.: Restoration of function of the shoulder following paralysis of the trapezius by fascial sling fixation and transplantation of the levator scapulae. Ann. Surg. 132:1111, 1950.
62. Neer, C. S. II: Unfused Acromial Epiphysis in Impingement and Cuff Tears. Instructional Course, American Academy of Orthopaedic Surgeons, 1978.
63. Neer, C. S. II, Bigliani, L. U., Norris, T. R., and Fischer, J.: The relationship between the unfused acromial epiphysis and subacromial impingement lesions. Orthop. Trans. 7:138, 1983.
64. Neer, C. S. II, Bigliani, L. U., Norris, T. R., and Fischer, J.: Relationship Between the Unfused Acromial Epiphysis and Subacromial Impingement Lesions. Scientific Exhibit, 50th Annual Meeting, American Academy of Orthopaedic Surgeons, Los Angeles, 1983.
65. Hitchcock, H. H. and Bechtol, C.O.: Painful shoulder: Observations on the role of the tendon of the long head of the biceps brachii in its causation. J. Bone and Joint Surg. 30-A:263, 1948.
66. Gilcrist, E. L.: The common syndrome of rupture, dislocation, and elongation of the long head of the biceps brachii. Surg. Gyn. Obst. 58:322, 1934.
67. Lippman, R. K.: Frozen shoulder, periarthritis, bicipital tenosynovitis. Arch. Surg. 47:283, 1943.
68. Neer, C. S. II: Degenerative lesions of the proximal humeral articular surface. Clin. Orthop. 20:116, 1961.
69. Cofield, R. H.: Arthroscopy of the shoulder. Mayo Clin. Proc. 58:501, 1983; Orthop. Trans. 7:141, 1983.
70. Tibone, J. E., Elrod, B., Jobe, F. W., et al: Surgical Treatment of Tears of the Rotator Cuff in Athletes. Presented at the Second Open Meeting, American Shoulder and Elbow Surgeons, New Orleans, 1986. Orthop. Trans. 10:230, 1986.
71. Neer, C. S. II: Chapter 11, Part I: Fractures About the Shoulder, p. 675. In Fractures in Adults, edited by C. A. Rockwood, Jr. and D. P. Green. Ed. 2. J. B. Lippincott, Philadelphia, 1984.
72. Yergason, R. M.: Supination sign. J. Bone and Joint Surg. 13:160, 1931.
73. Neer, C. S. II: Chapter 11, Part I: Fractures About the Shoulder. In Fractures in Adults, edited by C. A. Rockwood, Jr. and D. P. Green. Ed. 1. J. B. Lippincott, Philadelphia, 1975.
74. Neer, C. S. II and Hughes, M.: Glenohumeral joint replacement and postoperative rehabilitation. Physical Therapy 55:850, 1975.
75. Bateman, J. E.: Shoulder and Neck. Ed. 2. W. B. Saunders Company, Philadelphia, 1978.
76. Ellman, H.: Arthroscopic Subacromial Decompression: Analysis of One to Three Year Results. Symposium on "The Controversy of Arthroscopy versus Open Approaches to Shoulder Instability and Rotator Cuff Disease." Fourth Open Meeting, American Shoulder and Elbow Surgeons, Atlanta, 1988.
77. Neer, C. S. II: Four Segment Classification of Displaced

Proximal Humeral Fractures. Chapter 9, Instructional Course Lectures of the American Academy of Orthopaedic Surgeons. Vol. XXIV, p. 160, C. V. Mosby, St. Louis, 1975.
78. Neer, C. S. II and Hawkins, R. J.: A functional analysis of shoulder fusions (abstract). J. Bone and Joint Surg. 59-B:508, 1977.
78a. Hawkins, R. S. and Neer, C. S. II: A functional analysis of shoulder fusions. Clin. Orthop. 223:65, 1987.
79. Johnson, L.: Current Status of Shoulder Arthroscopy. Presidential Guest Lecture, Sixth Closed Meeting, American Shoulder and Elbow Surgeons. Orlando, 1987.
80. Rockwood, C. A. Jr.: Treatment of Large Tears of the Rotator Cuff by Anterior Acromioplasty and Debridement of the Cuff. Presented A.A.O.S. Instructional Course, 1986; and 8th Combined Meeting of the Orthopaedic Associations of the English-Speaking World, Washington, D. C., 1987.
81. Bush, L. F.: The torn shoulder capsule. J. Bone and Joint Surg. 43-A:1041, 1961.
82. Aoki, M., Ishii, S., and Usui, M.: The slope of the acromion and rotator cuff impingement. Orthop. Trans. 10:228, 1986.
83. Bigliani, L. U., Morrison, D. S., and April, E. W.: The morphology of the acromion and its relationship to rotator cuff tears. Orthop. Trans. 10:228, 1986.
84. Morrison, D. S. and Bigliani, L. U.: The clinical significance of variations in acromial morphology. Orthop. Trans. 11:234, 1987.
84a. Morrison, D. S. and Burger, P.: The use of magnetic resonance imaging in the diagnosis of rotator cuff tears. Orthop. Trans. 12:736, 1988.
85. Fukuda, H., Craig, E. V. and Yamanaka, K.: Surgical treatment of incomplete thickness tears of the rotator cuff: Long term follow-up. Orthop. Trans. 11:237, 1987.
86. Matsen, F. A. III and Kilcoyne, R. F.: Sonographic evaluation of the rotator cuff. Orthop. Trans. 8:42, 1984. Farrar, E. L., Matsen, F. A. III, et al.: Dynamic Sonographic Study of Lesions of the Rotator Cuff. Presented at 50th Annual Meeting. American Academy of Orthopaedic Surgeons, 1983.
87. Craig, E. V. and Crass, J. R.: Ultrasonography of the rotator cuff: Normal anatomy and pathologic variations. Orthop. Trans. 9:42, 1985.
88. Collins, R. A., Gristina, A. G., et al: Ultrasonography of the shoulder. Orthop. Clin. No. Am. 18:351, 1987.
88a. Conway, J. E. and Watson, K. C.: Ultrasonographic detection of incomplete rotator cuff tears. Orthop. Trans. 11:585, 1987.
89. Neer, C. S. II, McCann, P. D., Macfarlane, E. A., and Padilla, N.: Earlier passive motion following shoulder arthroplasty and rotator cuff repair. A prospective study. Orthop. Trans. 11:231, 1987.
90. Apoil, A., Dautry, P., Moinet, Ph., Koechlin, Ph.: Le syndrome dit de rupture de la coiffe des rotateurs de al l'epaule. Apropos de 70 interventions. Rev. Chir. Orthop. Suppl. II, Vol. 63, 1977.
90a. Apoil, A., Dautry, P. et al: Chirurgie de syndrome de la coiffe des rotators de l'epaule. Documenta Geigy, Paris, 1978.
91. Mansat, M. and Bonnevialle, P.: Impingement Syndrome. Surgical Treatment of Stage III. Presented at 2nd Open Meeting, American Shoulder and Elbow Surgeons, New Orleans, 1986. Orthop. Trans. 10:229, 1986.
92. Stamm, T. T. and Crabbe, W. A.: Paraglenoid Osteotomy of the Scapula. Clin. Orthop. 88:39–45, 1972.
93. Imbriglia, J. E., Neer, C. S. II, and Dick, H. M.: Resection of the proximal one-half of the humerus in a child for chondrosarcoma. Preservation of function using a fibular graft and Neer prosthesis. J. Bone and Joint Surg. 60-A:262, 1978.
94. Bigliani, L. U., Neer, C. S. II, Parisien, M., and Johnston, A. D.: Dysplasia epiphysealis hemimelica of the scapula. A case report. J. Bone and Joint Surg. 62-A:292, 1980.
95. Neer, C. S. II and Takagishi, K.: Bilateral replacement for avascular necrosis of the humeral heads after paraplegia. Strategies in Ortho. Surg. Learning Technology, Inc. (Medical), Albany, Vol. 1, No. 5, 1981.
96. Ha'eri, G. B. and Wiley, A. M.: Advancement of the supraspinatus muscle in repair of ruptures of the rotator cuff. J. Bone and Joint Surg. 63-A:232, 1981.
97. DeOrio, J. K. and Cofield, R. H.: Surgical repair of failed rotator cuff repairs. Orthop. Trans. 6:362, 1982; Results of a second attempt at surgical repair of a failed initial rotator cuff repair. J. Bone Joint Surg. 66-A:563, 1984.
98. Clayton, M. L. and Ferlic, D. C.: Surgery of the shoulder in rheumatoid arthritis. Clin. Orthop. 106:166, 1974.
99. Allman, F.: Fractures and ligamentous injuries of the clavicle and its articulations. J. Bone and Joint Surg. 49-A:774, 1967.
100. Post, M.: Constrained total shoulder arthroplasty. Long term results. Orthop. Trans. 11:238, 1987.
101. Connley, J.: Personal communication. (Head and Neck Surgical Service, Columbia-Presbyterian Medical Center, New York, 1988.)
102. Ferlic, D. C., discussed by Neer, C. S. II: Subacromial Spacer. Ortho. Consultation, H. P. Publishing Company, New York. Vol 3, October, 1981.
103. Cofield, R. H.: Glenohumeral Arthroplasty for Rheumatoid Arthritis (incidence of rotator cuff tears). Instructional Course, 54th Annual Meeting, American Academy of Orthopaedic Surgeons, 1987.
104. Barrett, W.P., Tornhill, T. S., Thomas, W. H., Gebhardt, E. M., and Sledge, C. B: Nonconstrained total shoulder arthroplasty for patients with polyarticular rheumatoid arthritis. Orthop. Trans. 11:238, 1987.
105. Gerber, C., et al: Latissimus Dorsi Transfer for the Treatment of Massive Tears of the Rotator Cuff. Presented at 4th Open Meeting, American Shoulder and Elbow Surgeons, Atlanta, 1988. Clin. Orthop. 232:51, 1988.
106. Takagishi, N., Okabe, Y., Matsuzaki, A., et al: Treatment of the rotator cuff tear. J. Jpn. Orthop. Ass. 49:698, 1975.
107. Neer, C. S. II, Flatow, E. L., and Lech, O.: Tears of the Rotator Cuff. Long Term Results of Anterior Acromioplasty and Repair. Presented at 55th Annual Meeting, American Academy of Orthopaedic Surgeons, and 4th Open Meeting, American Shoulder and Elbow Surgeons, Atlanta, 1988; Orthop. Trans. 12:735, 1988.
108. Neer, C. S. II and Satterlee, C. C.: Re-operation for Failed Cuff Repairs. Presented at 6th Closed Meeting, American Shoulder and Elbow Surgeons, Orlando, 1987.
109. Dennis, D. A., Ferlic, D. C., and Clayton, M. L.: Acromial stress fractures associated with cuff-tear arthropathy. A report of three cases. J. Bone and Joint Surg. 68-A:937, 1986.
110. Neer, C. S. II and Kirby, R. M.: Revision of humeral head and total shoulder arthroplasties. Clin. Orthop. 170:189, 1982.
111. Darrach, W.: Surgical approaches for surgery of the extremities. Am. J. Surg. LXVII:237, 1945.
112. Berquist, T. H., McCough, P. F., Hattrup, S. J., and Cofield, R. H.: Arthrographic Analysis of Rotator Cuff Tears. Presented at Fourth Open Meeting, American Shoulder and Elbow Surgeons, Atlanta, 1988.
113. Bigliani, L. U., Perez-Sanz, J. R., and Wolfe, I. N.: Treat-

ment of trapezius palsy. J. Bone and Joint Surg. 67-A:871, 1985.

114. Neer, C. S. II: Nonunion of the surgical neck of the humerus. Orthop. Trans. 7:389, 1983.

115. Mansat, M.: Acromial obstructions and rupture of the rotator cuff. Ann. Chir. 35:835, 1981.

116. Neer, C. S. II: Importance of the Technique of Biopsy to Successful Replacement for Proximal Humerus Tumors. In the Proceedings, 2nd International Workshop on the Design and Application of Tumor Prostheses for Bone and Joint Reconstruction, p. 69, Vienna, 1983.

117. Neer, C. S. II: Unconstrained shoulder arthroplasty. In Surgery of the Shoulder, edited by J. E. Bateman and R. P. Welsh. Decker and Mosby, Toronto, p. 240, 1984.

118. Hawkins, R. J. and Neer, C. S. II: Missed posterior dislocations of the shoulder. In Surgery of the Shoulder, edited by J. E. Bateman and R. P. Welsh. Decker and Mosby, Toronto, p. 117, 1984.

118a. Hawkins, R. J., Neer, C. S. II, Pianta, R. M., and Mendoza, F. X.: Missed posterior dislocations of the shoulder. J. Bone and Joint Surg. 69-A:9, 1987.

119. Neer, C. S. II and Brems, J. J.: Shoulder replacement in the athletic and active patient. In Shoulder Surgery in the Athlete, edited by D. W. Jackson. Aspen Press, Rockville, Maryland, 4:93, 1985.

120. Neer, C. S. II: Unconstrained Shoulder Arthroplasty. Instructional Course Lectures of the American Academy of Orthopaedic Surgery. C. V. Mosby, St. Louis, 34:278, 1985.

121. Fukuda, H.: A Ceramic Glenohumeral Prosthesis. Presented to Annual Meeting of the Japanese Shoulder Society, 1984.

122. Bigliani, L. U. and Neer, C. S. II: Normal humeral head sizes in very large adults (unpublished).

123. Kenmore, P. I.: A Simple Shoulder Replacement. Read at Clemson University Biomaterials Symposium, 1973.

124. Zippel, J.: Vollstandiger Schullergelenkersatz ans Kunstoff und Metall. Biomed. Techink. 17:87, 1972.

125. Neer, C. S. II: Nonconstrained Shoulder Arthroplasty. Indications and Special Steps in Technique. (Invited Lecture: 100th Birthday of Sir Harry Platt, Manchester, England.) Current Trends in Orthopaedic Surgery, edited by C.S.B. Galasko and J. Noble. Manchester University Press, Manchester, England, 1988.

126. Neer, C. S. II and Morrison, D.: Glenoid bone grafting in total shoulder arthroplasty. J. Bone and Joint Surg. 70-A:1154, 1988.

127. Fukuda, H., Mikasa, M., and Ogawa, K.: Ring retractor. J. Bone and Joint Surg. 64-A:289, 1982.

128. Petersson, C. J. and Redlund-Johnell, I.: Joint space in normal glenohumeral radiographs. Acta Orthop. Scand. 54:274, 1983.

128a. Petersson, C. J.: Degeneration of the glenohumeral joint. Acta Orthop. Scand. 55:277, 1983.

129. Parrish, F. F.: Partial and total half joint transplantation of tumors involving ends of major long bones. J. Bone and Joint Surg. 53-A:1653, 1971.

130. Parrish, F. F.: Neer prosthesis with allograft and Silastic cuff repair (personal communication).

131. Cofield, R. H.: Status of total shoulder arthroplasty. Arch. Surg. 112:1088, 1977.

132. Lugli, T.: Artificial shoulder joint by Pean (1893). Clin. Orthop. 133:215, 1978.

133. Clayton, M. L., Ferlic, D. C., and Jeffers, P. D.: Prosthetic arthroplasties of the shoulder. Clin. Orthop. 164:184, 1982.

134. Cruess, R. L.: Steroid induced avascular necrosis of the head of the humerus. J. Bone and Joint Surg. 58-B:313, 1976.

135. Takagishi, K. and Neer, C. S. II: Avascular Necrosis of the Humeral Head. Presented to the Alumni Association, New York Orthopaedic Hospital, 1980; and at the Annual Meeting, Japanese Shoulder Society, 1982.

136. Springfield, D. S. and Enneking, W. J.: Surgery of aseptic necrosis of the femoral head. Clin. Orthop. 130:175, 1978.

137. Ficat, R. P. and Arlet, J.: Ischemia and Necrosis of Bone. Chapter IV, Necrosis of the Femoral Head. Williams and Wilkins, Baltimore, p. 53, 1980.

138. d'Aubigne, Merle R., et al: Avascular necrosis of the femoral head in adults. J. Bone and Joint Surg. 47-B:612, 1965.

139. Mankin, H. J., Doppel, S. H., et al: Osteoarticular and intercalary allograft transplantation in the management of malignant tumors of bone. Cancer 50:613, 1982.

140. Olivier, H., Duparc, J., and Romain, F.: Fractures of the greater tuberosity of the humerus. Orthop. Trans. 10:223, 1986.

141. Lech, O.: (re: latissimus dorsi transfer) Personal communication, 1987.

142. Neer, C. S. II: The design and technical considerations for proximal humerus and shoulder prostheses. In the Design and Application of Tumor Prostheses for Bone and Joint Reconstruction, edited by E. C. Chao and J. C. Ivins. Theime-Stratton, New York, 1983.

143. Withington, E. T.: Hippocrates. Hinemann, London, 1922.

144. Moseley, H. F.: Recurrent Dislocation of the Shoulder. McGill University Press, Montreal, 1961.

145. Rowe, C. R.: The Shoulder. Churchill Livingstone, New York, 1988.

146. Rockwood, C. A. Jr.: Chapter 11, Part II: Subluxations and Dislocations About the Shoulder, p. 722. In Fractures in Adults, edited by C. A. Rockwood, Jr. and P. Green. Ed. 2. J. B. Lippincott, Philadelphia, 1984.

147. Laing, P. G.: The arterial blood supply of the adult humerus. J. Bone and Joint Surg. 38-A:1105, 1956.

148. Tanner, M. W. and Cofield, R. H.: Prosthetic arthroplasty for fractures and fracture-dislocations of the proximal humerus. Clin. Orthop. 179:116, 1983.

149. Neer, C. S. II and McIlveen, S. J.: Recent Results and Technique of Prosthetic Replacement for 4-Part Proximal Humeral Fractures. Presented at 53rd Annual Meeting, American Academy of Orthopaedic Surgeons. Orthop. Trans. 10:475, 1986.

150. Neer, C. S. II and McIlveen, S. J.: Remplacement de la tete humerale avec reconstruction des tuberosities et de la coiffe dan les fractures deplacees. Resultats actuels et techniques. Rev. Chir. Orthop. Suppl. II, 74:31, 1988.

151. Neer, C. S. II and Horwitz, B. S.: Fractures of the proximal humeral epiphyseal plate. Clin. Orthop. 41:24, 1965.

152. Smith, F. M.: Fracture-separation of the proximal humeral epiphysis. Am. J. Surg. 91:627, 1956.

153a. Robin, G. C. and Kedar, S. S.: Separation of the upper humeral epiphysis in pituitary gigantism. J. Bone Joint Surg. 44-A:189, 1962.

153b. Neer, C. S. II: The clavicle. Editorial comment. Clin. Orthop. 58:3, 1968.

154. Salter, R. B. and Harris, W. R.: Injuries involving the epiphyseal plate. J. Bone and Joint Surg. 45-A:587, 1963.

155. Neer, C. S. II: Fractures of the distal third of the clavicle. Clin. Orthop. 58:43, 1968.

156. Neer, C. S. II: Fractures of the distal clavicle with detachment of the coracoclavicular ligaments in adults. J. Trauma 3:99, 1963.

157. Neer, C. S. II: Nonunion of the clavicle. J. Am. Med. Assn. 172:1006, 1960.

158. Neer, C. S. II: Involuntary Inferior and Multidirectional

Instability of the Shoulder. Etiology, Recognition, and Treatment. Instructional Course Lectures, American Academy of Orthopaedic Surgeons. C. V. Mosby, St. Louis, Vol. XXXIV, p. 232, 1985.

159. Neer, C. S. II: Recent Concepts in Glenohumeral Dislocations. Inaugural Presidental Lecture, 1st Annual Meeting of the European Shoulder Society, Paris, 1987.
160. Neer, C. S. II: Concepts in Dislocations and Subluxations. Chairman's Special Lecture of the 3rd International Conference on Surgery of the Shoulder, Fukuoka, Japan, 1986; and published in The Shoulder, p. 7, edited N. Takagishi, Professional Postgraduate Services, Tokyo, 1987.
161. Malgaigne, P. J-F.: Traite des Fractures et des Luxations. Atlas de XXX Planches. J-B. Bailliere, Paris, 1855.
162. Hill, S. A. and Sachs, M. D.: The groove defect in the humeral head. A frequent unrecognized complication of dislocations of the shoulder joint. Radiology 35:600, 1940.
163. Broca, A. and Hartman, H.: Contribution á l'étude des luxations de l'épaule. Bull. Soc. Anat. Paris, 5me Serie:4:312 and 416, 1890.
164. Perthes, G: Über Operationen bei habitueller Schulterluxation. Dtsch. Zeitschr. Chir. 85:199–227, 1906.
165. Joessel, D.: Ueber die Recidive der Humerus-luxationen. Dtsch. Z. Chir. 13:167, 1880.
166. Eden, Rudolf: Zur Operation der habituellen Schulterluxation unter Mitteilung eines neuen Verfahrens beim Abriss am inneren Pfannenrande. Dtsch. Zeitschr. Chir. 144:269–280, 1918.
167. Hybbinnette, S.: De la transplantation d'un fragment osseux pour remédier aux luxations récidivantes de l'épaule. Constatations et resultats opératoires. Acta. Chir. Scandinavica 71:411–445, 1932.
168. Bankart, A. S. B.: Recurrent dislocation of the shoulder (discussion). J. Bone and Joint Surg. 30-B:46, 1948.
169. Osmond-Clarke, H.: Habitual dislocation of the shoulder. The Putti-Platt operation. J. Bone and Joint Surg. 30-B:19–25,1948.
170. Gallie, W. E. and LeMesurier, A. B.: Recurring dislocation of the shoulder. J. Bone and Joint Surg. 30-B:9–18, 1948.
171. Rowe, C. R., Patel, D., and Southmayd, W. W.: The Bankart procedure—a long term end result study. J. Bone Joint Surg. 60-A:1, 1978.
172. Rowe, C. R., Pierce, D. S., and Clark, J. G.: Voluntary dislocation of the shoulder. A preliminary report on a clinical, electromyographic and psychiatric study of twenty-six patients. J. Bone Joint Surg. 55-A:445–460 (April), 1973.
172a. Rowe, C. R. and Yee, B. K.: A posterior approach to the shoulder joint. J. Bone Joint Surg. 26:580, 1944.
173. Rowe, C. R. and Zarins, B.: Recurrent transient subluxation of the shoulder. J. Bone and Joint Surg. 63-A:863, 1981.
174. Webber, B. G., Simpson, A., and Hardegger, F.: Rotational osteotomy for recurrent anterior dislocation of the shoulder associated with large Hill-Sachs lesions. J. Bone and Joint Surg. 66-A:1443, 1929.
175. Masnuson, P. B. and Stack, J. K.: Recurrent dislocation of the shoulder. J. Am. Med. Assoc. 123:889, 1943.
176. Nicola, T.: Recurrent dislocation of the shoulder. J. Bone and Joint Surg. 16:663, 1934.
177. May, V. R.: A modified Bristow operation for anterior recurrent dislocation of the shoulder. J. Bone and Joint Surg. 52-A:1010, 1970.
177a. Helfet, A. J.: Coracoid transplantation for recurring dislocation of the shoulder. J. Bone Joint Surg. 40-B:198, 1958.
178. Tullos. H.: Acute Shoulder Dislocations: Factors Influencing Diagnosis and Treatment. In American Academy of Orthopaedic Surgeons Instructional Course Lectures, p. 382. C. V. Mosby, St. Louis, Vol. XXXIII, 1984.
179. Jobe, F. W.: Shoulder Instability. American Academy of Orthopaedic Surgeons Continuing Education Course, Beverly Hills, September, 1987.
179a. Rokous, J. R., Feagin, J. A., and Abbott, H. G.: Modified axillary roentgenogram. A useful adjunct in the diagnosis of recurrent instability of the shoulder. Clin. Orthop. 82:84, 1972.
180. Randelli, M. and Gambrioli, P. L.: Glenohumeral osteometry by computed tomography in normal and unstable shoulder. Clin. Orthop. 208:151, 1986.
181. Hovelius, L.: Anterior Dislocation of the Shoulder. Linköping University Medical Dissertations, No. 139, Linköping, Sweden, 1982.
182. Trillat, A. and Leclerc-Chalvet, F.: Luxations Recidivante de l'épaule. Masson, Paris, 1973.
183. Mansat, M.: La Pathologie de L'épaule. University Toulouse (de Hotel Dieu), Toulouse, France, 1985.
184. Latarjet, M.: A propos du traitment des luxations recidivantes de l'épaule. Lyon Chir. 49:994, 1976.
185. Neer, C. S. II and Welsh, R. P.: The shoulder in sports. Ortho. Clin. No. Am. 8:583, 1977.
186. Rockwood, C. A. Jr. and Gerber, C.: Analysis of failed surgical procedures for anterior instability. Orthop. Trans. 9:48, 1985.
187. McIntosh, D.: On the value of immobilization after initial traumatic glenohumeral dislocations in the University of Toronto athletes. Personal communication to R. P. Welsh and author, 1976 (see ref. 185).
188. Welsh, R. P. and de'Demeter, D.: Recurrent dislocation of the shoulder. Problems encountered in the surgically treated. Ortho. Trans. 8:91, 1984.
189. Simonet, W. T. and Cofield, R. H.: Prognosis in anterior shoulder dislocation. Am. J. Sports Med. 12:19, 1984.
190. Mendoza, F. X., Nicholas, J. A., and Reilly, J. P.: Neer inferior capsular shift repair for anterior glenohumeral instability. Ortho. Trans. 10:221, 1986.
191. Leslie, J. T., Jr. and Ryan, T. J.: The anterior axillary incision to approach the shoulder joint. J. Bone and Joint Surg. 44-A:1193–1196, 1962.
192. Hawkins, R. J., Neer, C. S. II, Pianta, R. M., and Mendoza, F. X.: Locked posterior dislocation of the shoulder. J. Bone and Joint Surg. 69-A:9, 1987.
193. Hawkins, R. J., Koppert, G., and Johnston, G.: Recurrent posterior instability (subluxation) of the shoulder. J. Bone and Joint Surg. 66-A:169, 1984.
194. Owen, R.: Bilateral glenoid hypoplasia. J. Bone and Joint Surg. 35-B:262, 1955.
195. Fairbank, H. A. T.: Dysplasia epiphysealis multiplex. Brit. J. Surg. 34:225, 1947.
196. Neer, C. S. II and Hansen, P.: Multidirectional Shoulder Instability Following Proximal Humeral Epiphyseal Fractures. Unpublished study (at New York Orthopaedic Columbia-Presbyterian Medical Center), 1984.
197. Neer, C. S. II, Perez-Sanz, J. R., and Ogawa, K.: Causes of Failure in Repairs for Recurrent Anterior Dislocations. Presented at New York Orthopaedic Hospital Alumni Annual Meeting (unpublished), 1983.
198. Campbell, C. J., Kettelkamp, D. B., and Bonfiglio, M.: Dysplasia epiphysealis hemimelica. J. Bone Joint Surg. 48-A:746, 1966.
199. Rockwood, C. A. Jr.: Injuries to the acromioclavicular joint. Chapter 11, pp. 860–910. In Fractures in Adults, edited by C. A. Rockwood, Jr. and D. Green. Ed. 2. J. B. Lippincott, Philadelphia, 1984.
200. Rockwood, C. A. Jr.: Injuries to the sternoclavicular joint.

Chapter 11, pp. 910–948. In Fractures in Adults, edited by C. A. Rockwood, Jr. and D. Green. Ed. 2. J. B. Lippincott, Philadelphia, 1984.

201. Patterson, W. R.: Inferior dislocation of the distal end of the clavicle. J. Bone and Joint Surg. 49-A:1184, 1967.

202. Neer, C. S. II: Treatment of Old Acromioclavicular Dislocations. Symposium on Acromioclavicular Dislocations, 54th Annual Meeting, American Academy of Orthopaedic Surgeons, San Francisco, 1987.

203. Wilson, F. C. Jr.: Results of operative treatment of acute dislocations of the acromioclavicular joint. J. Trauma 7:202, 1967.

204. Bosworth, B. M.: Acromioclavicular separation. A new method of repair. Surg. Gyn. Obst. 73:866, 1941.

205. Alldredge, R. H.: Surgical treatment of acromioclavicular dislocations. J. Bone and Joint Surg. 47-A:1278, 1965.

206. Simmons, E. H. and Martin, R. F.: Acute dislocations of the acromioclavicular joint. Canad. J. Surg. 11:479, 1968.

207. Salvatore, J. E. Sternoclavicular joint dislocations. Clin. Orthop. 58:51, 1968.

208. McLaughlin, H. L.: On the "frozen" shoulder. Bull. Hosp. Joint Disease, Vol. XII, No. 2, pp. 383–393, October 1951.

209. Lundberg, B. J.: Glycosaminoglycans of the normal and frozen shoulder-joint capsule. Clin. Orthop. 69:279–284, 1970.

210. Neviaser, R. J. and Neviaser, T. J.: The frozen shoulder. Diagnosis and management. Clin. Orthop. 223:59–64 (October), 1987.

211. Quigley, T. B.: Indications for manipulation and corticosteroids in the treatment of stiff shoulders. Surg. Clin. No. Am. 43:1715, 1963.

212. Andren, L. and Lundberg, B. J.: Treatment of rigid shoulders by joint distention during arthrography. Acta Orthop. Scand. 36:45, 1965.

212a. Ellman, H.: Arthroscopic Treatment of Calcium Deposits in the Shoulder. Presented at the 4th Open Meeting, American Shoulder and Elbow Surgeons, Atlanta, 1988.

212b. Zarins, B.: Arthroscopic Treatment of Calcium Deposits. Abstract, 4th International Conference on Surgery of the Shoulder, New York, 1989.

213. Cofield, R. H. and Briggs, B. J.: Glenohumeral arthrodesis. J. Bone and Joint Surg. 61-A:668, 1978.

214. Duparc, J. and Largier, A.: Les luxation-fractures de l'extremite superieur de l'humerus. Rev. Chir. Orthop. 62:91–110, 1976.

215. Rowe, C. R.: Re-evaluation of the position of the arm in arthrodesis of the shoulder in the adult. J. Bone and Joint Surg. 56-A:913, 1974.

216. Research Committee of the American Orthopaedic Association: The survey of end results on stabilization of the paralytic shoulder. J. Bone and Joint Surg. 24:699, 1942.

217. Carroll, R. E.: Wire-loop arthrodesis of the shoulder. Clin. Orthop. 9:185, 1957.

218. Petrucci, F. S., Morelli, A., and Rumondi, P. L.: Axillary nerve injuries—21 cases treated by nerve graft and neurolysis. J. Hand Surg. 7:271, 1982.

219. Marmor, L. and Bechtol, C. O.: Paralysis of the serratus anterior due to electric shock relieved by transplantation of the pectoralis major muscle. A case report. J. Bone and Joint Surg. 45-A:156, 1963.

220. Copeland, S. A. and Howard, R. C.: Thoracoscapular fusion for fascioscapulohumeral dystrophy. J. Bone and Joint Surg. 60-B:547, 1978.

221. Dahlin, D. C.: Bone Tumors. General Aspects and Data in 6,221 Cases. Charles C Thomas, Springfield, Illinois, 1978.

222. Enneking, W. F.: Muscoloskeletal Tumor Surgery. Churchill-Livingstone, New York, 1983.

223. Jaffe, H.: Tumors and Tumorous Conditions of the Bones and Joints. Lea & Febiger, Philadelphia, 1958.

224. Lichtenstein, L.: Bone Tumors. C. V. Mosby, St. Louis, 1977.

225. Tooms, R. E.: Amputations of the upper extremity. Chapter 25, Campbell's Operative Orthopaedics. Ed. 7. C. V. Mosby, St. Louis, 1987.

226. Carnesale, P. G.: Tumors. Chapters 30 to 34, Campbell's Operative Orthopaedics. Ed. 7, C. V. Mosby, St. Louis, 1987.

227. Stout, A. P. and Lattes, R.: Atlas of Tumor Pathology. Tumors of the Soft Tissue. Armed Forces Institute of Pathology, Washington, D. C., 1967.

228. Enneking, W. F.: Staging of Musculoskeletal Neoplasms. Current Concepts of Diagnosis and Treatment of Bone and Soft Tissue Tumors. Springer-Verlag, Berlin–Heidelberg, 1984.

229. Enneking, W. F., Spanner, S. S., and Goodman, M. A.: A system for the surgical staging of musculoskeletal sarcoma. Clin. Orthop. 153:106, 1980.

230. Neer, C. S. II, Francis, K. C., Marcover, R. C., Terz, J., and Carbonara, P. N.: Treatment of unicameral bone cysts. Follow-up study of one-hundred and seventy-five cases. J. Bone and Joint Surg. 48-A:731, 1966.

231. Neer, C. S. II, Francis, K. C., Johnston, A. D., and Kiernan, H. A.: Current concepts on the treatment of solitary unicameral bone cysts. Clin. Orthop. 97:40, 1973.

232. Francis, K. C. and Dick, H. M.: Radical resection for tumors of the upper extremity with preservation of a functional extremity. J. Bone and Joint Surg. 52-A:823, 1970.

233. Gill, A. B.: Shoulder arthrodesis. Technique. J. Bone Joint Surg. 13:287, 1931.

234. Coley, B. L.: Neoplasms of Bone and Related Conditions. Hoeber, New York, 1949.

235. Fahey, J. J. and O'Brien, E. T.: Solitary unicameral bone cyst. J. Bone and Joint Surg. 55-A:59, 1973.

236. Scaglietti, O., Marchetti, P. G., and Bartolozzi, P.: The effects of methylprednisolone acetate in the treatment of bone cysts: Results of three years follow-up. J. Bone and Joint Surg. 61-B:200, 1979.

237. Scaglietti, O., Marchetti, P. G., and Bartolozzi, P.: Final results obtained in the treatment of bone cysts with methylprednisolone acetate (Depo-Medrol) and a discussion of the results achieved in other bone lesions. Clin. Orthop. 165:33, 1982.

238. Cohen, J.: Simple bone cysts. Studies of the cyst fluid in 6 cases with a theory of pathogenesis. J. Bone and Joint Surg. 42-A:609, 1960.

239. Mansat, M.: L'épaule douloureuse chirurgicale. Expansion Scientific Française, Paris, 1988.

240. Agerholm, J. C. and Goodfellow, J. W.: Simple cysts of the humerus treated by radical excision. J. Bone and Joint Surg. 47-B:714, 1965.

241. Stableforth, P. G.: Four-part fractures of the neck of the humerus. J. Bone and Joint Surg. 66-B:104–108, 1984.

242. Berger, P.: Ĺ'Amputation du membre superieur dans la contiguite du tróne (amputation interscapulothoracique). G. Masson, Paris, 1887.

243. Bennett, G. E.: Shoulder and elbow lesions of professional baseball pitchers. J. Am. Med. Assoc. 117:510, 1941.

243a. Fukuda, H. and Neer, C. S. II: Archer's shoulder. Recurrent posterior subluxation and dislocation of the shoulder in two archers. Orthopaedics II:171, 1988.

244. Bianco, A. J., Jr., Wolbrink, A. J., and Hsu, Z.: Abduction contracture of the shoulders and hips secondary to fibrous bands. J. Bone and Joint Surg. 55-A:844, 1973.

245. Brower, A. C., Sweet D. E., and Keats, T. E.: Condensing

osteitis of the clavicle. A new entity. Am. J. Roentgenol. 121:17, 1974.
246. Kruger, G. D., Rock, M. G., and Munro, M. D.: Condensing osteitis of the clavicle. Review of the literature and report of three cases. J. Bone and Joint Surg. 69-A:550, 1987.
247. Copeman, W. S. C.: Aetiology of fibrositic nodule: Clinical contribution. Br. Med. J. 2:263, 1943.
248. Milch, H.: Snapping scapula. Clin. Orthop. 20:139, 1961.
249. Michele, A., Davies, J. J., Krueger, F. J., and Lichtor, J. M.: Scapulocostal syndrome (fatigue postural paradox). New York J. Med. 50:1353, 1950.
250. Darrach, W.: Scapulothoracic Bursa. (Unpublished lecture, 1942.)
251. Jobe, F. W.: Enlargement of the Scapular Bursa in the Throwing Arm. American Academy of Orthopaedic Surgeons Instructional Course, 1987.
252. Kutsuma, T. and Terayama, K.: Results of surgical treatment of deltoid contracture, p. 259. In Surgery of the Shoulder, edited by J. E. Bateman and R. P. Welsh. C. V. Mosby, Toronto, 1984.
253a. Neer, C. S. II: Nonunion of the clavicle. J. Am. Med. Assoc. 172:1006, 1960.
253b. McLaughlin, H. L.: Posterior dislocation of the shoulder. J. Bone Joint Surg. 34-A:584, 1952.
254. Adler, J. B. and Patterson, R. L.: Erb's palsy. Long term results of treatment in 88 cases. J. Bone and Joint Surg. 49-A:1052, 1967.
255. L'Episcopo, J. B.: Restoration of muscle balance in the treatment of obstetrical paralysis. New York J. of Med. 39:357, 1939.
256. Fairbank, H. A. T.: Birth Palsy: Subluxation of the shoulder joint in infants and young children. Lancet 1:1217, 1913.
257. Sever, J. W.: The results of a new operation for obstetrical paralysis. Am. J. Orthop. Surg. 16:248, 1918.
258. Steindler, A.: Orthopaedic Operations. Charles C Thomas, Springfield, Illinois, 1940.
259. Zachary, R. B.: Transplant of teres major and latissimus dorsi for loss of external rotation at the shoulder. Lancet 2:757, 1947.
260. Neer, C. S. II: Arthroplasty for the Arthritis of Erb's Palsy Deformity. Presented at 7th Annual Meeting, American Shoulder and Elbow Surgeons, Santa Fe, New Mexico, 1988.
261. Jackson, D. W.: Shoulder Surgery in the Athlete. Aspen Press, Rockville, MD, 1988.
262. Jobe, F. W. and Moynes, D. R.: Delineation of diagnostic criteria and a rehabilitation program for rotator cuff injuries. Am. J. Sports Med. 10:336, 1982.
263. Salter, R. B., Hamilton, H. W., Wedge, J. H., Tile, M., Torode, I. P., O'Driscoll, S. W., Murnaghan, J. P., and Saringer, J. H.: Clinical application of basic research on continuous passive motion for disorders of synovial joints: A preliminary report of a feasibility study. J. of Ortho. Research 1:325, 1984.
264. DesMarchais, J. E. and Benazet, J. P.: Evaluation de l'hemiarthroplastie de Neer dans le traitmente des fractures de l'humerus. Canadian J. Med. 26:269–471, 1983.
265. Craig, E. V.: Continuous passive motion (CPM) after shoulder reconstruction. Orth. Trans. 19:219, 1986.
266. Charnley, J.: The bonding of prosthesis to bone by cement. J. Bone and Joint Surg. 46-B:518, 1964.
267. Charnley, J., Follacci, F. M., and Hammond, B. T.: The long term reaction of bone to self-curing acrylic cement. J. Bone and Joint Surg. 50-B:822, 1968.
268. Charnley, J.: Total hip replacement by low friction arthroplasty. Clin. Orthop. 72:7, 1970.
269. Neer, C. S. II and Satterlee, C. C.: Prospective Study of Nonconstrained Total Shoulder Arthroplasty (unpublished), June 1988.
270. Neer, C. S. II and Perez-Sanz, J. R.: Unpublished study, 1984.
271. Stimson, L. A.: A Practical Treatise on Fractures and Dislocations. Lea Brothers, New York, 1907.
272. Rowe, C. R.: An atlas of anatomy and treatment of midclavicular fractures. Clin. Orthop. 58:29, 1968.
273. Adams, M. A., Weiland, A. J., and Moore, J. R.: Nonconstrained total shoulder arthroplasty. Orth. Trans. 10:232, 1986.
274. Bade, H. A., Warren, R. F., Ranawat, C. S., and Inglis, A. E.: Long term results of Neer total shoulder arthroplasty. In Surgery of the Shoulder, p. 294. Edited by J. E. Bateman and R. P. Welsh. C. V. Mosby, Toronto, 1984.
275. Clayton, M. L. and Ferlic, D. C.: Regarding 51, minimum 2 year follow-up total shoulder arthroplasties. Personal communication, 1989.
276. Cofield, R. H.: Total shoulder arthroplasty with the Neer prosthesis. J. Bone and Joint Surg. 66-A:899–906, 1984.
277. Hawkins, R. J., Bell, R. H., and Jallay, B.: Experience with the Neer total shoulder arthroplasty. A review of 70 cases. Orth. Trans. 10:232, 1986.
278. Thornhill, T. S., Karr, M. J., Averill, R. M., Batte, N. J., Thomas, W. H., and Sledge, C. B.: Total shoulder arthroplasty. The Brigham experience. Orth. Trans. 7:479, 1983.
279. Brems, J. J., Wilde, A. H., Borden, L. S., and Boumphrey, F. R. S.: Glenoid lucent lines. Orth. Trans. 10:231, 1986.
280. Neer, C. S. II: Roentgen follow-up studies of Watson (1982) and Satterlee (1988). Presented at 5th Open Meeting, American Shoulder and Elbow Surgeons Symposium: Evolution and Current Status of Shoulder Arthroplasty, Las Vegas, Nevada, 1989 (see refs. 22 and 269).
281. Barrett, W. P., Franklin, J. F., Jackins, S. E., Wyss, C. R., and Matsen, F. A. III: Total shoulder arthroplasty. J. Bone and Joint Surg. 69-A:865, 1987.
282. Mansat, M.: L'épaule du sportif. Masson, Paris, 1985.
283. Johnson, L. L.: Arthroscopy of the shoulder. Orthop. Clin. No. Am. 11:197, 1980.
284. Andrews, J. R., Carson, W. G., and Ortega, K.: Arthroscopy of the shoulder. Technique and normal anatomy. Am. J. Sports Med. 12:1, 1984.
285. Caspari, R. B.: Shoulder arthroscopy: A review of the present state of the art. Contemp. Orthop. 4:523, 1982.
286. Lombardi, S. J.: Arthroscopy of the shoulder. Clin. Sports Med. 2:309, 1983.
287. Woodward, J. W.: Congenital elevation of the scapula: Correction by release and transplantation of the muscle origins. A preliminary report. J. Bone Joint Surg. 43-A: 219, 1961.

Index

Note: Numbers in *italics* refer to illustrations; numbers followed by t indicate tables.